INTERVENTIONAL CARDIOLOGY

INTERVENTIONAL CARDIOLOGY

EDITORS

Spencer B. King III, MD

J. B. and Dottie Fuqua Chair of Cardiology
The Fuqua Heart Center at Piedmont Hospital
Professor of Medicine, Emeritus
Emory University School of Medicine
Atlanta, Georgia

Alan C. Yeung, MD

Head, Division of Cardiovascular Medicine
Director, Interventional Cardiology
Stanford University Medical Center
Stanford, California

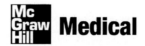

New York   Chicago   San Francisco   Lisbon   London   Madrid
Mexico City   Milan   New Delhi   San Juan   Seoul   Singapore   Sydney   Toronto

Interventional Cardiology

1 2 3 4 5 6 7 8 9 0   CTPS/CTPS   0 9 8 7 6

ISBN-13: 978-0-07-141527-9
ISBN-10: 0-07-141527-0

This book was set in Adobe Garamond by TechBooks.
The editors were Hilarie Surrena, Joe Rusko, Robert Pancotti, and Karen Davis.
The production supervisor was Phil Galea.
The cover designer was Liz Cosgrove.
The interior designer was Alan Barnett.
The indexer was Alexandra Nickerson.
China Translation & Printing Services, Ltd., was printer and binder.

This book is printed on acid-free paper.

Photo Credits:
Background photo: Branches of right coronary artery—3D Clinic/GettyImages, Inc.
Inset photo: Defective heart valve being replaced with a prosthetic implant—AJPhoto / Photo Researchers, Inc.

Library of Congress Cataloging-in-Publication Data

Interventional cardiology / [edited by] Spencer B. King III, Alan C.
    Yeung.
        p. ; cm.
    Includes bibliographical references and index.
    ISBN-13: 978-0-07-141527-9 (alk. paper)
    ISBN-10: 0-07-141527-0 (alk. paper)
    1. Coronary heart disease—Surgery. 2. Heart—Diseases—Treatment.
  I. King, Spencer B., 1937-   . II. Yeung, Alan C.
    [DNLM: 1. Cardiovascular Surgical Procedures—methods.
  2. Cardiovascular Diseases—surgery. 3. Cardiovascular Diseases—
    therapy.
  WG 168 I615 2007]
  RD598.I583 2007
  617.4'12—dc22   2006043825

To Gail, Spencer, Susan, Robert, Marie, and Liza.
— *Spencer B. King III*

To Elene, Chloe, Kara, and Tristan.
— *Alan C. Yeung*

CONTENTS

SECTION EDITORS

Nicolas Chronos, MD, FRCP, FACC, FESC, FAHA
Chief Medical and Scientific Officer
American Cardiovascular Research Institute
Adjunct Professor of Cardiology and Medicine
Duke University
Durham, North Carolina

David Cohen, MD
Associate Professor of Medicine
Harvard Medical School
Director of Interventional Cardiology Research
Beth Israel Deaconess Medical Center
Boston, Massachusetts

John S. Douglas, Jr., MD
Professor of Medicine
Director, Interventional Cardiology
Emory University School of Medicine
Director, Cardiac Catheterization Laboratory
Emory University Hospital
Atlanta, Georgia

Bernard J. Gersh, MB ChB, DPhil
Departments of Cardiovascular Diseases and Internal Medicine
Mayo Clinic
Rochester, Minnesota

John W. Hirshfeld, Jr., MD
Professor of Medicine
University of Pennsylvania School of Medicine
Philadelphia, Pennsylvania

David R. Holmes, MD
Department of Cardiology
Mayo Clinic
Rochester, Minnesota

Morton J. Kern, MD, FACC, FAHA, FSCAI
Director, Clinical Research
Pacific Cardiovascular Associates
Costa Mesa, California

Campbell Rogers, MD
Cardiovascular Division
Brigham and Women's Hospital
Boston, Massachusetts

James E. Tcheng, MD, FACC, FSCAI
Division of Cardiology
Duke University Medical Center and
Duke Clinical Research Institute
Durham, North Carolina

Paul G. Yock, MD
Martha Meier Weiland Professor
Co-Chair, Department of Bioengineering
Director, Program in Biodesign
Stanford University
Stanford, California

CONTRIBUTORS

J. Dawn Abbott, MD *(Chapter 28)*
Assistant Professor of Medicine
Brown Medical School
Rhode Island Hospital
Providence, Rhode Island

Yasushi Asakura, MD *(Chapter 35)*
Cardiopulmonary Division
Internal Medicine
Keio University
Tokyo
Japan

Donald S. Baim, MD *(Chapter 36)*
Professor of Medicine
Cardiovascular Division
Harvard Medical School
Director, Center for Integration of Medicine and Innovative
    Technology
Brigham and Women's Hospital
Boston, Massachusetts

Clifford J. Berger, MD *(Chapter 41)*
Clinical Associate Professor of Medicine
Boston University School of Medicine
Interventional Cardiologist
Boston Medical Center
Boston, Massachusetts

Robert M. Bersin, MD *(Chapter 60)*
Director, Endovascular Interventions and Clinical Research
Seattle Cardiology and the Cardiovascular Consultants of
    Washington
Seattle, Washington

Peter Bloch, PhD *(Chapter 14)*
Professor
Department of Radiation Oncology
University of Pennsylvania School of Medicine
Hospital of the University of Pennsylvania
Philadelphia, Pennsylvania

Todd J. Brinton, MD *(Chapter 47)*
Division of Cardiovascular Medicine
Stanford University Medical Center
Stanford, California

Bruce R. Brodie, MD, FACC, FACP *(Chapter 38)*
Clinical Professor of Medicine
University of North Carolina Teaching Service
The Moses H. Cone Memorial Hospital
Director, LeBauer Cardiovascular Research Foundation
Greensboro, North Carolina

Georgann Bruski, RT(R) *(Chapter 24)*
Cardiovascular Laboratories
Beth Israel Deaconess Medical Center
Boston, Massachusetts

Samuel M. Butman, MD *(Chapter 55)*
Sarver Heart Center
University of Arizona Medical Center
Tucson, Arizona

Blasé A. Carabello, MD, FACC *(Chapter 6)*
Professor of Medicine
Vice Chairman, Department of Medicine
Baylor College of Medicine
Medical Care Line Executive
Michael E. DeBakey Houston Veterans Affairs Medical Center
Houston, Texas

Ivan P. Casserly, MD *(Chapter 53)*
Director, Interventional Cardiology
Cardiology Department
Denver Veterans Affairs Medical Center
Denver, Colorado

Nicolas A. E. Chronos, MD, FRCP, FACC, FESC, FAHA
(Chapter 65)
Chief Medical and Scientific Officer
American Cardiovascular Research Institute
Adjunct Professor of Cardiology and Medicine
Duke University
Durham, North Carolina

Ricardo A. Costa, MD *(Chapter 66)*
Assistant Director
Angiographic Core Laboratory
Cardiovascular Research Foundation
New York, New York

Alain Cribier, MD *(Chapter 43)*
Department of Cardiology
Charles Nicolle University Hospital
Rouen
France

Jack T. Cusma, PhD *(Chapter 12)*
Cardiac Laboratory
Mayo Clinic
Rochester, Minnesota

Robert S. Dieter, MD, RVT, FACC, FCCP, FSVMB *(Chapter 52)*
Vascular and Endovascular Medicine
Interventional Cardiology
Loyola University Medical Center
Maywood, Illinois

John S. Douglas, Jr., MD *(Chapters 34 and 37)*
Professor of Medicine
Director, Interventional Cardiology
Emory University School of Medicine
Director, Cardiac Catheterization Laboratory
Emory University Hospital
Atlanta, Georgia

Jonathan L. Elion, MD, FACC *(Chapter 18)*
Associate Professor of Medicine
Brown University
c/o Heartlab, Inc.
Westerly, Rhode Island

Helene Eltchaninoff, MD *(Chapter 43)*
Professor of Medicine
Department of Cardiology
Charles Nicolle University Hospital
Rouen
France

William F. Fearon, MD *(Chapters 1, 2, and 27)*
Assistant Professor, Cardiovascular Medicine
Center for Research in Cardiovascular Interventions
Stanford University Medical Center
Stanford, California

Jeffrey A. Feinstein, MD, MPH *(Chapter 44)*
Assistant Professor of Pediatrics
Stanford University School of Medicine
Palo Alto, California;
Associate Director, Pediatric and Congenital
    Cardiac Catheterization Lab
Director, Vera Mouton Wall Center
    for Pulmonary Vascular Disease
Stanford University Medical Center
Palo Alto, California

Ted Feldman, MD, FACC, FSCAI *(Chapter 58)*
Cardiology Division
Evanston Northwestern Healthcare
Evanston, Illinois

Victor A. Ferrari, MD *(Chapter 15)*
Associate Professor of Medicine and Radiology
University of Pennsylvania School of Medicine
Associate Director, Noninvasive Imaging Laboratory
Cardiovascular Medicine Division
Hospital of the University of Pennsylvania
Philadelphia, Pennsylvania

Peter J. Fitzgerald, MD, PhD *(Chapter 27)*
Center for Research in Cardiovascular Interventions
Stanford University Medical Center
Stanford, California

Jon E. Gardner, CCVT, CCPT, RCIS, MBA *(Chapter 24)*
TRG Cardiovascular
Premier Heart and Vascular Consulting
East Coast Office
Research Triangle Region
Raleigh, North Carolina

Saul M. Genuth, MD *(Chapter 63)*
Division of Endocrinology
Case Western Reserve University
Cleveland, Ohio

Ziyad Ghazzal, MD *(Chapter 29)*
Associate Professor of Medicine
Director, Interventional Cardiology Fellowship Program
Emory University School of Medicine
Atlanta, Georgia

Abdul R. Halabi, MD *(Chapter 21)*
Division of Cardiology
Duke University Medical Center
Duke Clinical Research Institute
Durham, North Carolina

Robert A. Harrington, MD *(Chapter 67)*
Professor of Medicine
Division of Cardiology
Duke Clinical Research Institute
Durham, North Carolina

J. Kevin Harrison, MD *(Chapter 22)*
Associate Professor of Medicine
Division of Cardiology
Duke University Medical Center
Durham, North Carolina

Ali Hassan, MD *(Chapter 47)*
Division of Cardiovascular Medicine
Stanford University Medical Center
Stanford, California

James B. Hermiller, MD, FACC, FASCI *(Chapter 40)*
The Care Group, LLC
St. Vincent Hospital
Indianapolis, Indiana

Tomoaki Hinohara, MD *(Chapter 35)*
Pacific Foundation
Redwood City, California

John W. Hirshfeld, Jr., MD *(Chapter 17)*
Professor of Medicine
University of Pennsylvania School of Medicine
Philadelphia, Pennsylvania

Jui-Sung Hung, MD, FACC, FAHA *(Chapter 42)*
Professor of Medicine
China Medical University
Chung Shan Medical University
Taichung
Taiwan

Fumiaki Ikeno, MD *(Chapter 9)*
Research Associate
Division of Cardiovascular Medicine
Stanford University School of Medicine
Stanford, California

Alice K. Jacobs, MD *(Chapter 41)*
Professor of Medicine
Boston University School of Medicine
Director, Cardiac Catheterization Laboratory
    and Interventional Cardiology
Boston Medical Center
Boston, Massachusetts

Anna Kalynych, MD, FACC *(Chapter 19)*
Fugua Heart Center
Piedmont Hospital
Cardiology of Georgia
Atlanta, Georgia

David E. Kandzari, MD *(Chapters 20 and 67)*
Assistant Professor of Medicine
Division of Cardiology
Duke Clinical Research Institute
Duke University Medical Center
Durham, North Carolina

Osamu Katoh, MD *(Chapter 33)*
Director of Toyohashi Research Center
Toyohashi Heart Center
Toyohashi, Aichi
Japan

Young-Hak Kim, MD *(Chapter 39)*
Department of Medicine
University of Ulsan College of Medicine
Asan Medical Center
Seoul
Korea

Spencer B. King III MD *(Chapters 25 and 30)*
J. B. and Dottie Fuqua Chair of Cardiology
The Fuqua Heart Center at Piedmont Hospital
Professor of Medicine, Emeritus
Emory University School of Medicine
Atlanta, Georgia

Scott Kinlay, MB BS, PhD *(Chapter 11)*
Assistant Professor in Medicine
Harvard Medical School
Associate Physician
Brigham and Women's Hospital and
Veterans Affairs Medical Center West Roxbury
Boston, Massachusetts

Pramod Kuchulakanti, MD *(Chapter 32)*
Interventional Cardiologist
Wockhardt Heart Center
LB Nagar, Kamineni Hospital
Hyderabad
India

Iftikhar J. Kullo, MD *(Chapter 64)*
Associate Professor of Medicine
Division of Cardiovascular Diseases
Mayo Clinic College of Medicine
Gonda Vascular Center
Mayo Clinic
Rochester, Minnesota

Michael A. Kutcher, MD, FACC *(Chapter 59)*
Director, Interventional Cardiology
Associate Professor of Internal Medicine
Wake Forest University School of Medicine
Winston-Salem, North Carolina

John R. Laird, MD *(Chapter 52)*
Cardiovascular Research Institute
Washington Hospital Center
Washington, DC

Alexandra J. Lansky, MD *(Chapter 66)*
Cardiovascular Research Foundation
New York, New York

Kean-Wah Lau, MB BS, M Med, FRCP, FACC *(Chapter 42)*
Consultant Cardiologist
Associate Professor of Medicine
National University of Singapore
Singapore

David P. Lee, MD *(Chapter 45)*
Assistant Professor of Medicine
Associate Director, Coronary Intervention
    and Cardiac Catheterization Laboratory
Stanford University Medical Center
Stanford, California

Michael J. Lim, MD *(Chapter 8)*
Assistant Professor of Internal Medicine
Director, Interventional Cardiovascular
    Diseases Fellowship Program
Division of Cardiology
Department of Internal Medicine
St. Louis University School of Medicine
St. Louis, Missouri

Harold I. Litt, MD, PhD *(Chapter 15)*
Assistant Professor of Radiology
University of Pennsylvania School of Medicine
Director, Cardiac Imaging
Department of Radiology
Hospital of the University of Pennsylvania
Philadelphia, Pennsylvania

Joshua Makower, MD *(Chapter 71)*
Consulting Associate Professor
Stanford University Medical School
Stanford, California
Chairman and Chief Executive Officer
ExploraMed, Inc.
Mountain View, California

James R. Margolis, MD *(Chapter 57)*
Miami International Cardiology Consultants
Miami Beach, Florida

Laura Mauri, MD, MSc *(Chapter 11)*
Instructor in Medicine
Harvard Medical School
Associate Physician
Department of Medicine
Brigham and Women's Hospital
Boston, Massachusetts

Peter A. McCullough, MD, MPH, FACC, FACP, FCCP, FAHA
(Chapter 23)
Department of Medicine
Divisions of Cardiology, Nutrition and Preventive Medicine
William Beaumont Hospital
Royal Oak, Michigan

Annette A. Moore, RN, BSN, RCIS (Chapter 24)
Duke University Hospital
Duke Heart Center
Adult Cardiovascular Laboratories
Durham, North Carolina

Mauro Moscucci, MD (Chapter 69)
Associate Professor of Medicine
Associate Chief of Cardiology for New Program Development
Director of Interventional Cardiology Services,
    Cardiovascular Medicine
Taubman Center
University of Michigan Health System
Ann Arbor, Michigan

Joseph G. Murphy, MD, FESC, FACC (Chapter 61)
Associate Professor of Medicine
Mayo Clinic College of Medicine
Consultant, Division of Cardiology, the Coronary Care Unit,
    and the Mayo Catheterization Laboratory
Mayo Clinic
Rochester, Minnesota

Mamoo Nakamura, MD (Chapter 27)
Center for Research in Cardiovascular Interventions
Stanford University Medical Center
Stanford, California

Asha Nayak, MD, PhD (Chapter 71)
Senior Principal Advisor
Medtronic Vascular
Physician and Lecturer
Stanford University Medical Center
Stanford, California

Zoran S. Nedeljkovic, MD (Chapter 41)
Instructor in Medicine
Boston University School of Medicine
Interventional Cardiologist
Boston Medical Center
Boston, Massachusetts

Christopher D. Nielsen, MD (Chapter 46)
Assistant Professor of Medicine
Division of Cardiology
Medical University of South Carolina
Charleston, South Carolina

William O'Neill, MD, FACC, FACP (Chapter 38)
Director, Division of Cardiology
Beaumont Heart Center
William Beaumont Hospital
Royal Oak, Michigan

James L. Orford, MB ChB, MPH, FESC, FACC (Chapter 56)
Consultant Cardiologist
Mayday University Hospital
Croydon
Honorary Consultant Cardiologist
King's College Hospital
London
United Kingdom

William R. Overall, PhD (Chapter 70)
James H. Clark Centers
Stanford University Medical Center
Stanford, California

Seung-Jung Park, MD, PhD, FACC (Chapter 39)
Department of Medicine
Asan Medical Center
University of Ulsan
College of Medicine
Seoul
Korea

Manesh R. Patel, MD (Chapter 67)
Fellow, Division of Cardiology
Duke Clinical Research Institute
Durham, North Carolina

Stanton B. Perry, MD (Chapter 45)
Director, Pediatric Cardiac Catheterization Laboratory
Stanford University Medical Center
Stanford, California

Robert A. Phillips, MD, PhD, FACC, FAHA (Chapter 62)
Director, Heart and Vascular Center of Excellence
Professor and Interim Chief, Division of Cardiology
University of Massachusetts Memorial Medical
    Center and Medical School
Worcester, Massachusetts

Jan J. Piek, MD, PhD, FESC, FACC (Chapter 4)
Department of Cardiology
Academic Medical Center
University of Amsterdam
Amsterdam
The Netherlands

Sunil V. Rao, MD (Chapter 51)
Assistant Professor of Medicine
Duke University Medical Center
Director, Cardiac Catheterization Laboratories
Durham Veterans Affairs Medical Center
Durham, North Carolina

Mahmood K. Razavi, MD (Chapter 49)
St. Joseph Vascular Institute
Orange, California

Abdallah G. Rebeiz, MD (Chapter 22)
Division of Cardiology
Duke Clinical Research Institute
Durham, North Carolina

Bhagat K. Reddy, MD *(Chapter 50)*
Director of Vascular Medicine and Endovascular Interventions
Fugua Heart Center
Piedmont Hospital
Atlanta, Georgia

Johan H. C. Reiber, PhD *(Chapter 66)*
Professor of Medical Imaging
Division of Image Processing
Department of Radiology
Leiden University Medical Center
Leiden
The Netherlands

Mark Reisman, MD *(Chapter 31)*
Director, Cardiac Catheterization Laboratory
Director, Cardiovascular Research and Education
Seattle, Washington

Keith A. Robinson, PhD *(Chapter 65)*
Principal Scientist, Preclinical Division
American Cardiovascular Research Institute
Norcross, Georgia

Campbell Rogers, MD *(Chapters 7 and 10)*
Cardiovascular Division
Brigham and Women's Hospital
Boston, Massachusetts

Ramin Saket, MD *(Chapter 49)*
Interventional Radiology
University of California, San Diego School of Medicine
San Diego, California

Timothy A. Sanborn, MD, FACC, FSCAI *(Chapter 58)*
Cardiology Division
Evanston Northwestern Healthcare
Evanston, Illinois

Robert S. Schwartz, MD *(Chapter 65)*
Medical Director
Minnesota Cardiovascular Research Institute
Minneapolis, Minnesota

Norman Shaia, MD *(Chapter 55)*
Sarver Heart Center
University of Arizona Medical Center
Tucson, Arizona

Uwe Siebert, MD, MSc, MPH, ScD *(Chapter 68)*
Institute for Technology Assessment
    and Department of Radiology
Massachusetts General Hospital
Harvard Medical School
Boston, Massachusetts;
Harvard Center for Risk Analysis
Department of Health Policy and Management
Harvard School of Public Health
Boston, Massachusetts

Maria Siebes, PhD *(Chapter 4)*
Department of Medical Physics
Academic Medical Center
University of Amsterdam
Amsterdam
The Netherlands

Jose A. Silva, MD *(Chapter 26)*
Department of Cardiology
Ochsner Heart and Vascular Institute
Ochsner Clinic Foundation
New Orleans, Louisiana

Frank E. Silvestry, MD *(Chapter 16)*
Assistant Professor of Medicine
Cardiovascular Division
Director, Penn Cardiac Care at Radnor
Radnor, Pennsylvania

Daniel I. Simon, MD *(Chapter 7)*
Cardiovascular Division
Brigham and Women's Hospital
Boston, Massachusetts

Mandeep Singh, MD *(Chapter 54)*
Division of Cardiovascular Diseases and Internal Medicine and
Division of Biostatistics
Mayo Clinic College of Medicine
Rochester, Minnesota

Jos A. E. Spaan, PhD, FAHA *(Chapter 4)*
Department of Medical Physics
Academic Medical Center
University of Amsterdam
Amsterdam
The Netherlands

William H. Spencer III, MD *(Chapter 46)*
Professor of Medicine
Division of Cardiology
Medical University of South Carolina
Charleston, South Carolina

Richard E. Stewart, MD *(Chapters 1 and 3)*
Associate Professor of Medicine
Director, Vascular Interventions
Division of Cardiology
St. Louis University Health Sciences Center
Division of Cardiology
St. Louis University Hospital
St. Louis, Missouri

Rajesh Subramanian, MB BS *(Chapter 5)*
Department of Cardiology
Ochsner Heart and Vascular Institute
Ochsner Clinic Foundation
New Orleans, Louisiana

Daniel Y. Sze, MD, PhD *(Chapter 48)*
Associate Professor
Cardiovascular and Interventional Radiology
Stanford University
Stanford, California

James E. Tcheng, MD, FACC, FSCAI (Chapter 21)
Division of Cardiology
Duke University Medical Center and
Duke Clinical Research Institute
Durham, North Carolina

Daniel K. H. Thomas, MD (Chapter 15)
Fellow in Radiology
University of Cologne
Cologne
Germany

Susan P. Tourner, MD (Chapter 44)
Department of Pediatric Cardiology
Lucile Packard Children's Hospital at Stanford
Palo Alto, California

Christophe Tron, MD (Chapter 43)
Department of Cardiology
Charles Nicolle University Hospital
Rouen
France

Lou Vadlamani, MD (Chapter 31)
The Cardiovascular Group, PC
Fairfax, Virginia

Laurie A. Vancamp, RN, BSN, RCIS (Chapter 24)
Duke University Health System
Duke Heart Network
Durham, North Carolina

Bart-Jan Verhoeff, MD (Chapter 4)
Department of Cardiology
Academic Medical Center
University of Amsterdam
Amsterdam
The Netherlands

Louis K. Wagner, PhD, FACR, FAAPM (Chapter 13)
Department of Diagnostic and Interventional Imaging
The University of Texas Medical School at Houston
Houston, Texas

Ron Waksman, MD (Chapter 32)
Washington Hospital Center
Washington, DC

Paul. E. Wallner, DO, FACR, FAOCR (Chapter 14)
Senior Vice President
21st Century Oncology, Inc.
Fort Myers, Florida

Joy M. Weinberg, MD (Chapter 62)
Fellow, Division of Nephrology
Department of Medicine
Lenox Hill Hospital
New York, New York

Frederick G. P. Welt, MS, MD (Chapter 7)
Director, Cardiac Catheterization Laboratory
St. Elizabeth's Medical Center
Lecturer, Department of Cardiology
Tufts University School of Medicine
Boston, Massachusetts

Christopher J. White, MD (Chapters 5 and 26)
Department of Cardiology
Ochsner Heart and Vascular Institute
Ochsner Clinic Foundation
New Orleans, Louisiana

Tammey M. Wilkerson, RN, RCIS (Chapter 24)
Duke University Health System
Duke Heart Center
Mobile Cardiovascular Laboratories
Durham, North Carolina

David O. Williams, MD (Chapter 28)
Professor of Medicine
Brown Medical School
Rhode Island Hospital
Providence, Rhode Island

Michael S. Williams (Chapter 10)
Chief Technology Officer
Synecor, LLC
Windsor, California

R. Scott Wright, MD, FACC, FAHA, FESC (Chapter 61)
Associate Professor of Medicine
Mayo Clinic College of Medicine
Consultant, Division of Cardiology and the Coronary Care Unit
Mayo Clinic
Rochester, Minnesota

Jay S. Yadav, MD (Chapter 53)
Department of Cardiovascular Medicine
The Cleveland Clinic Foundation
Cleveland, Ohio

Alan C. Yeung, MD (Chapters 9, 30 and 47)
Head, Division of Cardiovascular Medicine
Director, Interventional Cardiology
Stanford University Medical Center
Stanford, California

Paul G. Yock, MD (Chapter 70)
Martha Meier Weiland Professor
Co-Chair, Department of Bioengineering
Director, Program in Biodesign
Stanford University
Stanford, California

Frank J. Zidar, MD (Chapter 51)
Duke Cardiology of Raleigh and
Duke University Medical Center
Durham, North Carolina

James P. Zidar, MD, FACC, FSCAI (Chapter 51)
Duke Cardiology of Raleigh and
Duke University Medical Center
Durham, North Carolina

PREFACE

Interventional cardiology was born on a kitchen table in Zurich, Switzerland. It was the child of coronary arteriography, bypass surgery, and catheter reaming of the femoral and iliac arteries. The contributions of Sones, Favalaro, and Dotter made possible the turning point of cardiology, but it took Andreas Gruentzig to bring life to this specialty. From humble beginnings, interventional cardiology has grown into a mature discipline. Cardiac training and certification have become standardized and the aspects of peripheral interventions are becoming organized as well.

This book became necessary because interventional cardiologists are expected to master a wide fund of knowledge, including radiation safety, current approaches to chronic total occlusion, and non-inferiority trial design. The knowledge base is so diverse that, until now, no single textbook was able to include all of the areas that encompass the discipline.

In this textbook, we address the anatomic, physiologic, and pathophysiologic knowledge foundation necessary for the discipline. We also explore the principles involved in the use of the catheterization laboratory to perform procedures such as x-ray and ultrasound imaging and physiologic measurements.

Several of our contributors examine the growing array of pharmacological agents used in interventional procedures and the complications related to these agents. Part Five, the largest part of the book, is devoted to the performance of specific procedures and the use of therapeutic equipment in specific anatomical conditions in the coronary, extracoronary, and peripheral domains.

Gruentzig said that complications of interventional cardiology were unusual, but such complications were his greatest concern and they should be our greatest concern today. Therefore, several chapters in this book discuss, in great detail, methods for avoiding and treating complications. The activities of the interventionalist outside the catheterization laboratory rival the importance of the activities inside the laboratory. The long-term management of patients with atherosclerosis after an intervention procedure must not be left to chance. More adverse events are caused by progression of disease than by complications related to stenting; therefore, effective medical therapies must be maintained.

Finally, the interventional cardiologist must understand experimental and clinical trials and how to critically evaluate them, the cost-effectiveness of interventional therapies, and the principles of innovation that spawned the specialty and that remain its life blood as it continues to evolve.

This book is intended for cardiology fellows in training as well as for practicing interventional cardiologists. We believe that it provides what these practitioners "must know" although there is much more to learn. The need for the subspecialty is also the reason for this book.

PART 1   Knowledge Foundation

CHAPTER 1

Coronary Artery Anatomy for the Interventionalist

William F. Fearon and Richard E. Stewart

A thorough knowledge of normal and abnormal coronary anatomy is essential for the interventional cardiologist. The direct application of this knowledge base helps in the selection of the appropriate catheter for coronary engagement in both diagnostic and intervention procedures. Knowledge of anatomy also facilitates the selection and interpretation of angiographic views during cardiac catheterization. Finally, because interventional therapy may be needed in several unusual circumstances, a working knowledge of coronary artery anomalies is also essential. This chapter addresses coronary artery anatomy and related technical issues pertinent to the interventional cardiologist.

NORMAL CORONARY ANATOMY

The coronary arterial system can be divided into the large vessels, or the epicardial coronary arteries, and the small vessels, or the microvasculature. The microvasculature consists of arterioles, which measure less than 200 μm and are poorly visualized with routine coronary angiography. These arterioles feed a broad capillary network that delivers oxygenated blood to the myocardium. They also regulate coronary pressure and flow through their ability to vasodilate and constrict in response to a variety of stimuli. The importance of the microvasculature in determining patient outcomes in both the acute setting, such as myocardial infarction, as well as the chronic setting has been highlighted.[1] Techniques for assessing the status of the microvasculature and treatment strategies for abnormal microvascular function are discussed in Chapter 4.

【 】 THE LEFT CORONARY ARTERY

Both the right and left coronary artery ostia arise from their respective aortic sinuses. Both ostia are located more than half the distance between the sinotubular junction and aortic valve annulus (Figure 1-1). The left main coronary artery originates with an elliptic ostia measuring approximately 3.2 ± 1.1 mm × 4.7 ± 1.2 mm.[2] This coronary artery continues at an acute angle and travels parallel to the aortic sinus wall, coursing between the pulmonary artery and the left atrium in the region of the left atrial appendage. The length of the left main artery ranges from 0 mm ("double-barrel ostium") to 20 mm. However, in most cases the length of the left main coronary artery is between 6 mm and 15 mm, with an average diameter ranging from 3 mm to 6 mm.[3] In two thirds of cases, the left main coronary artery bifurcates into the left anterior descending (LAD) and circumflex arteries (Figure 1-2); in one third of cases, it trifurcates into the LAD artery, the circumflex artery, and a ramus intermedius artery, which follows a course similar to either the first diagonal artery from the LAD artery or first obtuse marginal artery from the circumflex.[4]

The LAD artery follows the anterior interventricular sulcus and may pass around the cardiac apex (Figure 1-3). When it passes around the apex, the LAD travels along the posterior interventricular sulcus and can anastomose with branches from the posterior descending branch of the right coronary artery. The LAD artery has characteristic septal perforating branches that serve the anterior two thirds and the infra-apical portions of the ventricular septum. A common anatomic variant occurs when the LAD artery terminates before reaching the cardiac apex. In these cases, a large diagonal artery or an unusually large posterior descending artery

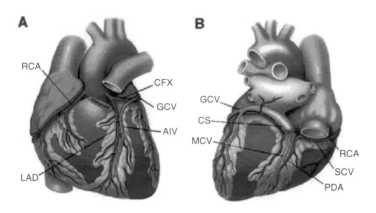

A

RCA
CFX
GCV
AIV
LAD

B

GCV
CS
MCV
RCA
SCV
PDA

FIGURE 1-1. A Diagram of coronary anatomy. The coronary arteries are located distal to the sinotubular junction at the ridge of the coronary sinuses. **B** View of the heart from the level of the mitral and aortic annulus.

from the right coronary artery should be anticipated to be present and provide the necessary left ventricular perfusion.[5]

In addition to septal perforators, the next major branches of the LAD artery are the diagonal arteries, which course along the anterolateral free wall of the left ventricle in a diagonal fashion, hence the name. On average, two major diagonal arteries are present, although smaller diagonal vessels can be identified.[6] In addition, small ventricular branches from the LAD can form an anastomotic network with similar branches from the proximal right coronary artery.

The circumflex coronary artery arises at an acute angle from the left main coronary artery and travels in the epicardial fatpad beneath the left atrial appendage, coursing through the left atrioventricular (AV) sulcus.[7] When a posterior descending artery (PDA) arises from the distal circumflex artery, the coronary circulation is defined as either left dominant or codominant. A "codominant" coronary artery system is one in which a PDA arises from both the right and circumflex coronary arteries. Codominant coronary artery systems, seen in less than 10% of patients,[8] are usually characterized by smallish PDA branches, which perfuse the posterior interventricular sulcus toward the apex of the heart. The circumflex artery gives rise to as many as three obtuse marginal arteries that supply the left ventricular lateral wall. In more than 80% of patients, the left circumflex artery transitions to a smaller AV groove artery, which is considered the distal continuation of the true circumflex artery. Usually, this artery does not pass the crux cordis, but in the 10% of cases with a left-dominant coronary circulation, the AV groove branch is large and of similar diameter to the main circumflex artery, giving rise to both posterolateral branches and a left posterior descending branch.[8]

FIGURE 1-2. Angiographic projection of the coronary artery in the RAO projection demonstrating the left main, left anterior descending, and circumflex coronary artery. *(Reproduced from Kern MJ et al. Cardiac catheterization, cardiac angiography, and coronary blood flow and pressure measurements. In Fuster V, Alexander RW, O'Rourke RA, eds. Hurst's The Heart, 11th ed. McGraw-Hill, New York, 2004:481–544.)*

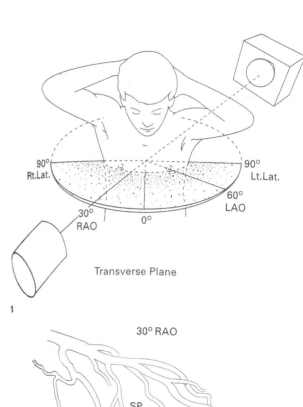

Transverse Plane

1

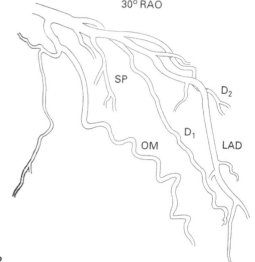

30° RAO

SP
D₂
OM
D₁
LAD

2

3

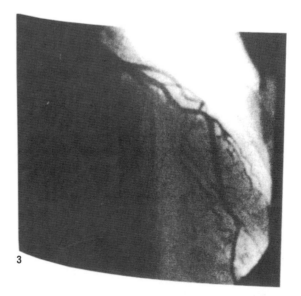

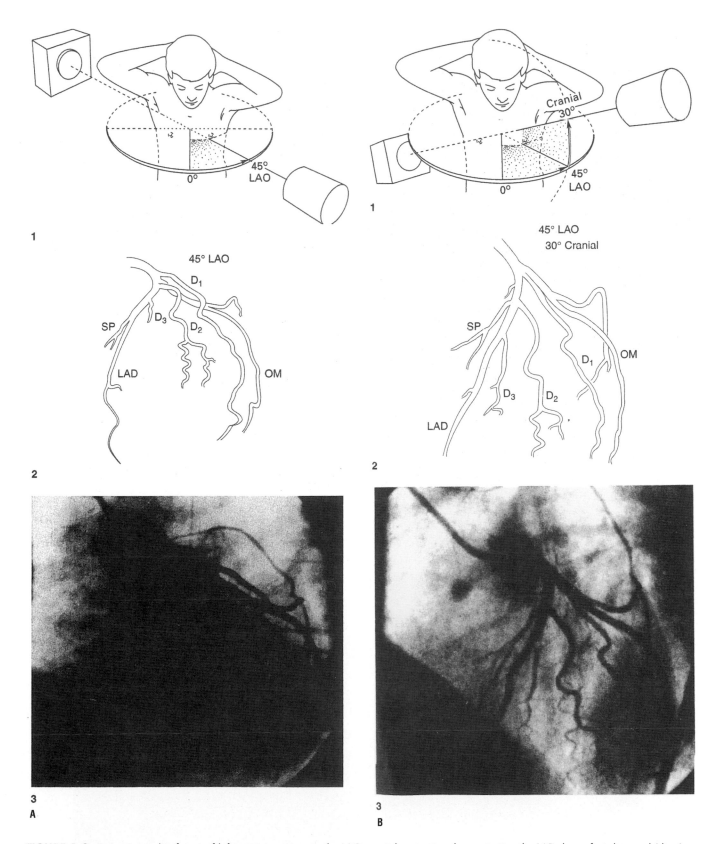

FIGURE 1-3. A Angiographic frame of left coronary artery in the LAO cranial projection demonstrating the LAD, large first diagonal (diag), and circumflex (CFX). **B** Angio frame of the left coronary artery demonstrating the LAO cranial projection A and the RAO caudal projection B. *(Reproduced from Kern MJ et al. Cardiac catheterization, cardiac angiography, and coronary blood flow and pressure measurements. In Fuster V, Alexander RW, O'Rourke RA, eds. Hurst's The Heart, 11th ed. McGraw-Hill, New York, 2004:481–544.)*

【 】 THE RIGHT CORONARY ARTERY

The right coronary artery originates from the right sinus of Valsalva and follows the right atrioventricular sulcus around the acute margin of the heart, giving off several major branches (Figure 1-4). The conus artery is the first major branch, with a separate ostium from the aorta in 50% of cases. The sinoatrial nodal artery is the second major branch, arising from the right coronary artery in 60% of cases and from the left circumflex artery in 40% of cases.[5]

The acute marginal branches of the right coronary artery arise from the proximal to midportion of the vessel, supply the free wall of the right ventricle and quite often anastomose to smaller branches of the LAD artery. The distal right coronary artery follows the posterior interventricular sulcus where it bifurcates

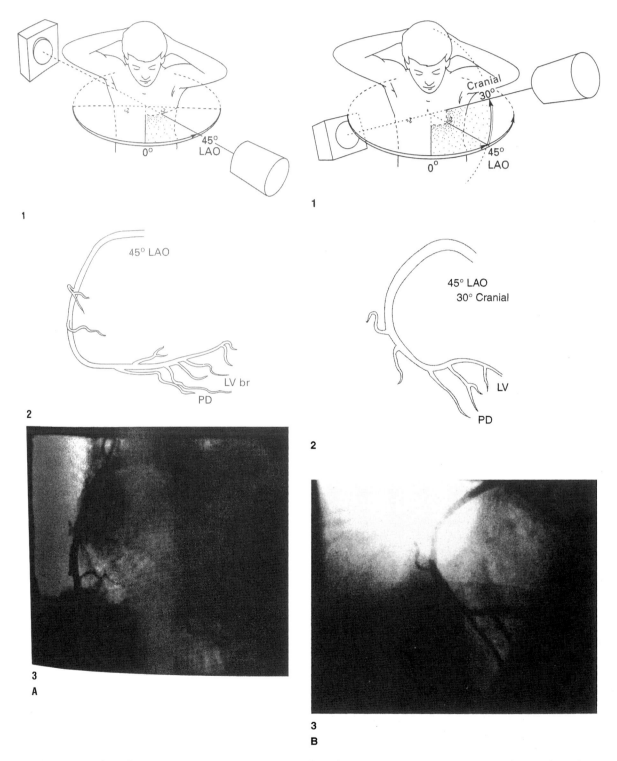

FIGURE 1-4. A The right coronary artery LAO projection. **B** The right coronary artery RAO projection. The vessel supplying the AV nodal branch is usually termed the dominant vessel. *(Reproduced from Kern MJ et al. Cardiac catheterization, cardiac angiography, and coronary blood flow and pressure measurements. In Fuster V, Alexander RW, O'Rourke RA, eds. Hurst's The Heart, 11th ed. McGraw-Hill, New York, 2004:481–544.)*

into the PDA (in 90% of patients), and major posterolateral branches.[5,6] The PDA continues in the posterior interventricular sulcus and usually terminates in the region of the cardiac apex. The posterolateral artery, a continuation of the right coronary artery, continues in the atrioventricular sulcus to the crux of the heart, frequently giving rise to the AV nodal artery. Finally, the postero-lateral artery terminates in two or three branches which course towards the cardiac apex. When the right coronary artery is non-dominant, it may terminate in the region of the acute margin of the heart.[5,6] In situations of total LAD artery occlusions, many of the branches of the right coronary artery may give rise to LAD artery collateral vessels.[1,8] The right coronary conus branch artery may become clinically significant when the LAD artery is occluded proximally. In addition, the acute marginal branches of the right coronary artery anastomose with marginal branches from the cir-cumflex artery as well as the septal perforating branches from the LAD artery. The PDA gives rise to branches that anastomose with the distal branches of the LAD artery. This angiographic visualiza-tion of the distal LAD artery by collateral arteries is especially important when performing interventions on chronic total occlu-sions of that artery. Likewise, the distal segments of the right coro-nary artery can often be visualized by left coronary angiography via collateral filling.

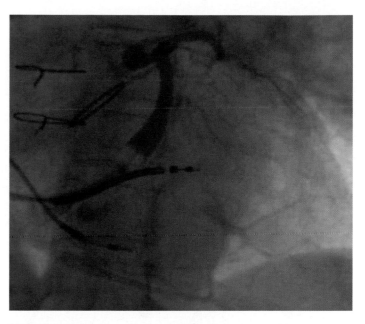

FIGURE 1-5. Coronary venous anatomy. The coronary sinus is cannu-lated with a balloon catheter, wherein contrast injection of the coronary sinus did visualize both the anterior ventricular cardiac vein as well as late phase filling of the lateral and inferior cardiac veins.

【 】 THE CORONARY VENOUS SYSTEM

Knowledge of the coronary venous system is becoming increasingly important to the interventionalist to facilitate various noncoronary and electrophysiologic cardiac interventions (Figure 1-5). The venous circulation of the heart is divided into three systems: the anterior cardiac veins, the coronary sinus and its tributaries, and the thebesian veins. The anterior cardiac veins, which originate from the right ventricular free wall surface of the heart,[3,8] drain the right ventricle and empty into the right atrium. The coronary sinus and its tributaries, which course on the surface of the left ventricle, run in parallel to the coronary arterial branches. The major tributary of the coronary sinus is the anterior interventricular branch, which

parallels the LAD artery and turns into the great cardiac vein as it enters the atrioventricular groove. The coronary sinus enters the right atrium adjacent to the tricuspid valve. Finally, the thebesian veins drain directly into the underlying right-side chambers. Flow is very minimal in these vessels, but these veins could give rise to very small and usually insignificant right-to-left shunts.[3,8]

【 】 CORONARY ARTERY ANOMALIES

Benign Anomalies

Most coronary artery anomalies are clinically benign incidental findings (Table 1-1). Separate and adjacent ostia of the LAD and left circumflex arteries is the most common anomaly, occurring in 0.41% of cases according to a large series reported from the Mayo Clinic.[9] Separate coronary ostia constitute approximately 30% of all benign coronary anomalies. Of interest, there is an association with a bicuspid aortic valve in these patients. From a practical standpoint, catheter engagement may opacify one vessel and not the other. Quite often, two separate diagnostic catheters are needed to complete the angiographic study of this anomalous left coronary artery system.

The second most common coronary artery anomaly is the anomalous origin of the circumflex artery from either the right coronary artery or the right sinus of Valsalva.[9,10] This anomaly, seen in 0.38% of diagnostic angiograms and making up 28% of benign coronary artery anomalies, is char-acterized by a retroaortic course of the cir-cumflex, with the vessel running posterior to

TABLE 1-1

Benign Coronary Anomalies (80% of total cases)

TYPE OF ANOMALY	INCIDENCE (%)	ANOMALY (%)
Separate adjacent LAD and LCX ostia	0.41	30.4
LCX origin from RCA or RSV	0.37	27.7
Anomalous LCX from PSV	0.004	0.3
Anomalous origin from aorta		
LMCA	0.01	1.0
RCA	0.15	11.2
Absent LCX	0.003	0.2
Small fistula	0.12	9.7

LAD = left anterior descending (artery); LCX = left coronary artery; RSV = right subclavian vein; PSV = peak systolic velocity; LMCA = left main coronary artery; RCA = right coronary artery.
Reproduced with permission from Yamanaka, O., and Hobbs, R.E. Coronary artery anomalies in 126, 595 patients undergoing coronary arteriography. Cathet Cardiovasc Diagnosis. 1990;21:28.

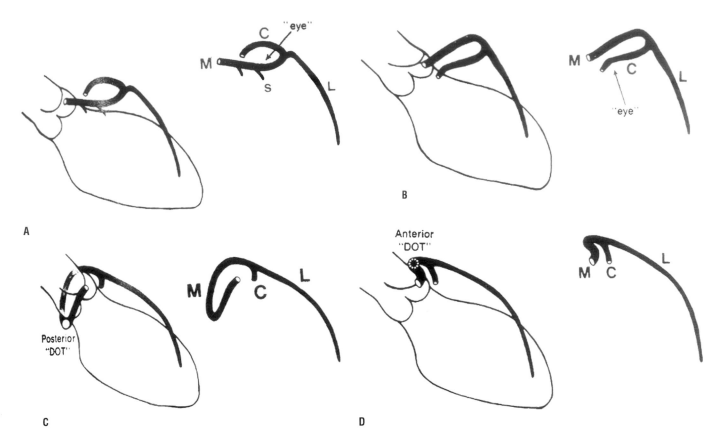

FIGURE 1-6. Diagrams of possible courses of the anomalous left coronary artery with the left main originating in the right coronary sinus. **A** The intraseptal course of the left main with an inferior loop forming an eye. **B** The anterior pathway of the left main forming the upper eye loop with the circumflex forming the lower eye loop. **C** The retroaortic course of the left main with the posterior angiographic dot of the vessel seen on end as it traverses behind the aorta. **D** The intraarterial course of the left main between the aorta and pulmonary artery with the anterior angiographic dot formed on end as the vessel turns between the two great vessels and then traverses anterior over the left ventricle. Abbreviations: M = main, C = circumflex, S = septal, and L = LAD. *(Reproduced from Kern MJ et al. Cardiac catheterization, cardiac angiography, and coronary blood flow and pressure measurements. In Fuster V, Alexander RW, O'Rourke RA, eds. Hurst's The Heart, 11th ed. McGraw-Hill, New York, 2004:481–544.)*

the aortic root. The clinical importance of identifying this anomaly is high for several reasons. First, unless the catheterizing physician has an adequate level of suspicion, this vessel may remain unvisualized. Second, for patients undergoing aortic valve replacement or mitral valve repair or replacement, this artery may be at risk for damage during surgery unless the surgeon is aware of its presence and retroaortic course. Angiographically, one imaging hallmark is a long left main coronary artery segment, often longer than 15 mm. Also, the retroaortic course of the circumflex around the aorta produces an angiographic "dot" (the end-on view of the vessel as it courses around the aorta) seen on aortography or ventriculography in the right anterior oblique (RAO) projection.[11] This coronary anomaly is best engaged with an Amplatz or Multipurpose catheter in a steep left anterior oblique (LAO) view.

The third most common benign coronary anomaly is the anomalous origin of the right coronary artery from the left sinus of Valsalva, occurring in 0.15% of cases and constituting 12% of benign coronary anomalies. The remaining benign coronary anomalies include an anomalous origin of the left main coronary artery from the aorta, constituting 1% of anomalies in the benign group, and an absent circumflex artery (seen in approximately

0.03% of all cases), constituting less than 1% of benign coronary anomalies.[9]

Coronary artery fistulas constitute a separate group of benign anomalies and occur when a coronary artery branch communicates directly with another chamber or structure, usually the right ventricle or pulmonary artery. Most fistulas, usually incidental findings during angiography, are small and clinically unimportant, and very rarely demonstrate the high flow and drainage into a right-side chamber that would produce a significant left-to-right shunt. Small fistulas have been noted to occur in 0.12%–0.14% of catheterization cases, constituting approximately 10% of all benign coronary anomalies.[9]

【 】 CLINICALLY SERIOUS ANOMALIES

Twenty percent of coronary artery anomalies are associated with potentially serious clinical consequences (Table 1-2).[9] The most common anomaly in this group is the origin of the right coronary artery from the left sinus of Valsalva, which occurs in approximately 0.12% of all cases and constitutes 8% of all coronary anomalies. In this case, the right coronary artery has an interarterial course between the aorta and pulmonary artery. This anomaly may be

TABLE 1-2

Potentially Serious Coronary Anomalies (20% of total cases)

TYPE OF ANOMALY	INCIDENCE (%)	ANOMALY (%)
Origin of coronary artery from opposite coronary sinus		
LMCA from RSV	0.02	1.3
LAD from RSV	0.03	2.3
RCA from LSV	0.11	8.1
Anomalous origin from PA		
LMCA	0.008	0.6
LAD or RCA	0.03	0.2
Single coronary artery	0.05	3.3
Multiple or large coronary fistula	0.05	3.7

LMCA = left main coronary artery; RSV = right subclavian vein; LAD = left anterior descending (artery); RCA = right coronary artery.

Reproduced with permission from Yamanaka, O., and Hobbs, R.E. Coronary artery anomalies in 126, 595 patients undergoing coronary arteriography. Cathet Cardiovasc Diagnosis. 1990;21:28.

associated with ischemic symptoms and requires surgical revascularization. The course of the vessel produces a bend point anterior to the aorta resulting in an angiographic dot sign seen on ventriculography or aortography.[12]

[ ] ANOMALOUS PATHWAYS OF THE LEFT CORONARY ARTERY ARISING FROM THE RIGHT AORTIC SINUS

Another group of coronary anomalies considered to be potentially serious involve the origin of the left main coronary artery (LMCA) from the right sinus of Valsalva (Figure 1-6).[9–12] Overall, these constitute 1.5% of all coronary anomalies and are seen in 0.2% of all catheterization cases. The LMCA from the right sinus of Valsalva has four potential pathways, with one being strongly associated with angina, syncope, or sudden death. The first pathway is a retroaortic course that takes the left main artery posterior to the aortic root. This pathway is characterized by a posterior angiographic dot sign and is considered benign (Figures 1-6C and 1-7).

In the second pathway, the LMCA may cross low and anterior through a "septal" course (Figures 1-6A and 1-8). This anomaly is usually benign, and characterized by septal perforators coming off of the LMCA, with an intramuscular course passing near the right ventricular outflow tract. As the LMCA curls downward at the bifurcation point to give rise to the circumflex artery, it creates a downward loop, or angiographic "eye" sign.

The third pathway in this group involving the LMCA coursing anteriorly over the pulmonary artery and right ventricle demonstrates an upward loop and an upgoing eye sign created by the alignment of the left main and circumflex arteries. This anomaly is also considered benign (Figure 1-6B).[9–12]

The fourth anomalous left main pathway from the right sinus of Valsalva is considered to be serious. Originating in the right sinus, the left coronary artery following an intramural path between the pulmonary artery and aorta creates an anterior dot sign as it bends and exits its intraarterial segment (Figures 1-6D and 1-9). This anomaly has been associated with angina, syncope, and sudden cardiac death. When found, surgery is usually required.[12] The slitlike ostial orifice stretching or narrowing during activity is thought to be the mechanism producing ischemia in these patients.

The anomalous origin of the LMCA, LAD, or right coronary artery from the pulmonary artery is another potentially serious coronary anomaly.[13,14] In these situations, coronary flow is antegrade in the normal coronary artery and retrograde in the anomalous vessel, allowing left-to-right shunting from the coronary artery bed to the pulmonary circulation. When the right coronary artery is involved, the situation is relatively benign. However, an anomalous origin of the LMCA or LAD from the pulmonary artery is often associated with angina and ischemic left ventricular dysfunction. Combined, anomalous origins of coronary arteries from the pulmonary artery constitute 0.8% of all coronary anomalies, and are seen in 0.04% of cases. Ligation or grafting of the aberrant vessel is the treatment of choice.

Other potentially serious coronary anomalies are rare and include a single coronary artery supplying the entire ventricle. These occur in 0.05% of catheterization cases, constitute 3.3% of all coronary anomalies, and should be considered potentially serious. There are many variations of single coronary arteries, which have been classified by Lipton et al.[15]

CORONARY ARTERY COLLATERAL CIRCULATION

The coronary collateral circulation is a potential source of blood to the myocardium that develops when blood flow via the normal route is impaired. It is believed that small anastomoses between the branches of the major epicardial coronary arteries exist in a dormant fashion. With the appropriate stimuli, these anastomoses can enlarge and allow adequate blood flow to otherwise ischemic myocardium.

Myocardial ischemia and/or development of a pressure gradient appear to be the most important stimuli to the development or maturation of coronary collateral circulation. The exact mechanism by which this is achieved remains an intense area of investigation. It appears that the increased production of growth factors induced by ischemia results in angiogenesis and/or vasculogenesis.[16] Others have proposed that the physical forces as a result of a pressure gradient might induce endothelial cells to proliferate.[16]

The presence of collateral circulation has been shown to have important clinical sequelae in both the acute and chronic settings. For example, in patients with acute myocardial infarction treated with fibrinolytic therapy, the presence of collateral circulation was associated with improved ventricular function, less aneurysm formation,

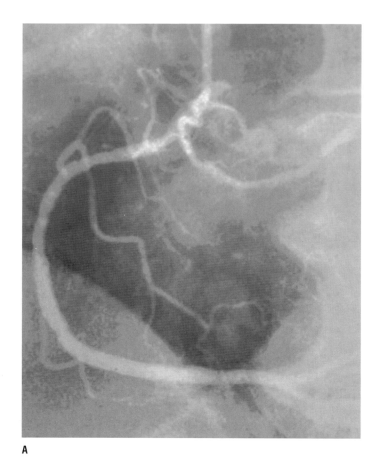

A

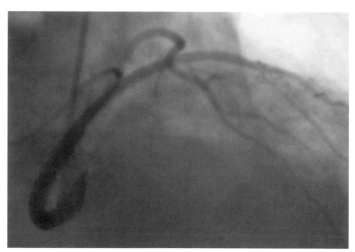

B1

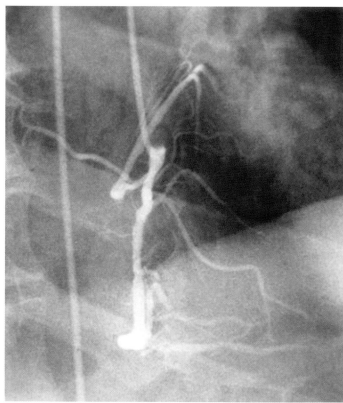

B2

FIGURE 1-7. A Anomalous circumflex coronary artery originating from the right sinus of Valsalva. This vessel forms a posterior dot similar to that of the retroaortic course of the left main. **B** Retroaortic course of the left main.

and smaller infarcts.[17–19] Long-term survival in patients with stable angina and coronary artery disease has been shown to be improved in those with good collateral circulation in comparison to patients with poor collateral circulation.[20]

Rentrop and colleagues[21] popularized a standard angiographic technique for assessing collateral circulation. The degree of contrast filling of a diseased vessel after injection of the contralateral vessel was graded on a scale of 0 to 3, where 0 equals no filling; 1 equals filling of side branches of the diseased vessel via collateral channels without visualization of the epicardial segment; 2 equals partial filling of the epicardial segment via collateral channels; and 3 equals complete filling of the epicardial segment of the diseased vessel via collateral channels. This

qualitative (and rather insensitive) method for determining the degree of collateral circulation has been replaced by coronary wire-based techniques for measuring pressure- or velocity-derived collateral flow indices.[22–24] These methods are discussed in further detail in a Chapter 4.

A number of common collateral connections between the major epicardial arteries have been described,[7] including intracoronary collaterals or connections from the proximal portion of an occluded artery to the distal portion of the same vessel. These can exist as "bridging" collaterals, which are small channels that develop around an occlusion and allow filling of the distal vessel. Alternatively, larger channels can form from a branch proximal to an occlusion, such as an acute marginal off the right coronary

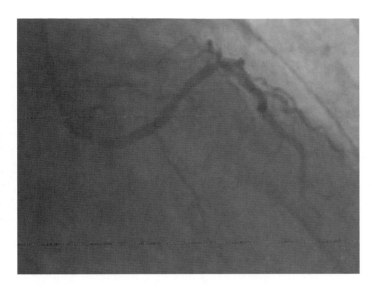

FIGURE 1-8. Anterior course of the left main originating from right coronary sinus.

artery, and anastomose to a branch distal to the occlusion, such as another acute marginal or the posterior descending artery. Another example is Kugel's artery, a branch off the proximal right coronary artery that anastomoses to the atrioventricular nodal artery, distal to a right coronary artery occlusion, and thereby fills the vessel beyond the blockage.[25]

Intercoronary collaterals are connections between branches of two of the three major epicardial coronary arteries. Common examples include septal-to-septal collaterals emanating from the posterior descending coronary artery going to the LAD artery, or vice versa; the distal LAD and posterior descending arteries often collateralize each other, as do the obtuse marginal branches of the circumflex and either the posterior left ventricular branches of the right coronary or the diagonal branches of the LAD artery. An important source of collateral flow to the LAD artery that can easily be missed at the time of angiography if not selectively injected with contrast is the conus branch of the right coronary artery.[26]

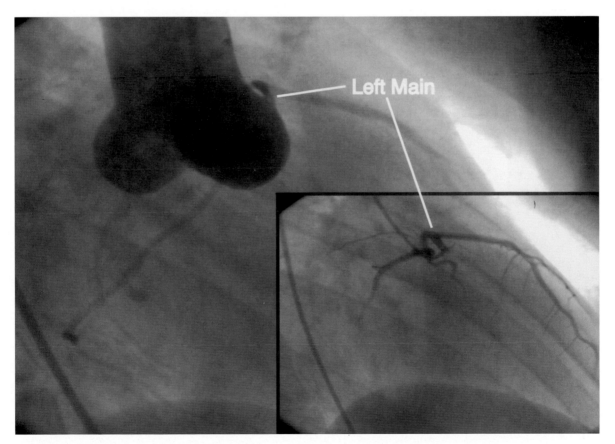

FIGURE 1-9. A Aortogram demonstrating intraarterial course of the anomalous left main from the right coronary sinus. The anterior dot is well visualized. **B** Selective coronary angiography of the same patient demonstrating the upgoing left main turning intraarterial with the left anterior descending advancing over the left ventricle, giving off septals. The dot is well visualized in this projection.

REFERENCES

1. Seiler C. The human coronary collateral circulation. *Heart.* 2003; 89: 1352–1357.
2. McAlpine WA. *Heart and Coronary Arteries: An Anatomical Atlas for Clinical Diagnosis, Radiologic Investigation, and Surgical Treatment.* Springer-Verlag, 1975:10.
3. James TM. *Anatomy of the Coronary Arteries.* Paul B. Hober, 1961:25.
4. Brandenburg RO, Fuster V, Giuliani ER, McGoon DC. Coronary arteriography. In *Cardiology: Fundamentals and Practice.* Mayo Clinic Foundation, 1987:451
5. Angelini P, Villason S, Chan AV. Normal and Anomalous Coronary Arteries in Humans. In *Coronary Artery Anomalies: A Comprehensive Approach.* Lippincott Williams & Wilkins, 1999:27.
6. Aldridge HE. Decade or more cranial and caudal angulated projections in coronary arteriography: another look. *Cathet Cardiovasc Diagn.* 1984;10:539.
7. Levin DC. Pathways and functional significance of the coronary collateral circulation. *Circulation.* 1974;50:831–837.
8. Baroldi G, Scomazzoni G. *Coronary Circulation in the Normal Heart and the Pathologic Heart.* US Government Printing Office, 1967:22.
9. Ishikawa T, Brandt PT. Anomalous origin of the left main coronary artery from the right aortic sinus: angiographic definition of anomalous course. *Am J Cardiol.* 1985;55:770.
10. Serota H et al. Rapid identification of the course of anomalous coronary arteries in adults: the "dot and eye" method. *Am J Cardiol.* 1990;65:891.
11. Levin DC, Fellows KE, Abrams HL. Hemodynamically significant primary anomalies of the coronary arteries: angiographic aspects. *Circulation.* 1978;58:25.
12. Click RL. Anomalous coronary arteries: location, degree of atherosclerosis, and effects on survival. A report from the coronary artery surgery study. *J Am Coll Cardiol.* 1989;13:531.
13. Donaldson RM, Raphael MJ. Missing coronary artery. Review of technical problems in coronary arteriography resulting from anatomical variants. *Br Heart J.* 1982;47:62.
14. Wald S, Stonecipher K, Baldwin BJ. Anomalous origin of the right coronary artery from the pulmonary artery. *Am J Cardiol.* 1971;27:677.
15. Lipton MJ, Barry WH, Obrez I, Silverman JF, Wexler L. Isolated single coronary artery: diagnosis, angiographic classification, and clinical significance. *Radiology.* 1979;130:39–47.
16. D'Amore PA, Thompson RW. Mechanisms of angiogenesis. *Annu Rev Physiol.* 1987;49:453–464.
17. Rogers WJ, Hood WP Jr, Mantle JA, Baxley WA, Kirklin JK, Zorn GL, Nath HP. Return of left ventricular function after reperfusion in patients with myocardial infarction: importance of subtotal stenoses or intact collaterals. *Circulation.* 1984;69:338–349.
18. Hirai T, Fujita M, Nakajima H, Asanoi H, Yamanishi K, Ohno A, Sasayama S. Importance of collateral circulation for prevention of left ventricular aneurysm formation in acute myocardial infarction. *Circulation.* 1989; 79:791–796.
19. Habib GB, Heibig J, Forman SA, Brown BG, Roberts R, Terrin ML, Bolli R. Influence of coronary collateral vessels on myocardial infarct size in humans. Results of phase I Thrombolysis In Myocardial Infarction (TIMI) trial. The TIMI Investigators. *Circulation.* 1991;83:739–746.
20. Hanse JF. Coronary collateral circulation: clinical significance and influence on survival in patients with coronary artery occlusion. *Am Heart J.* 1989; 117:290–295.
21. Rentrop KP, Cohen M, Blanke H, Phillips RA. Changes in collateral channel filling immediately after controlled coronary artery occlusion by an angioplasty balloon in human subjects. *J Am Coll Cardiol.* 1985;5:587–592.
22. Pijls NH, Bech GJ, el Gamal MI, Bonnier HJ, DeBruyne B, Van Gelder B, Michels HR, Koolen JJ. Quantification of recruitable coronary collateral blood flow in conscious humans and its potential to predict future ischemic events. *J Am Coll Cardiol.* 1995;25:1522–1528.
23. Matsuo H, Watanabe S, Kadosaki T, Yamaki T, Tanaka S, Miyata S, Segawa T, Matsuno Y, Tomita M, Fujiwara H. Validation of collateral fractional flow reserve by myocardial perfusion imaging. *Circulation.* 2002;105: 1060–1065.
24. Van Liebergen RA, Piek JJ, Kock KT, de Winter RJ, Schotborgh CE, Lie KI. Quantification of collateral flow in humans: a comparison of angiographic, electrocardiographic and hemodynamic variables. *J Am Coll Cardiol.* 1999;33:670–677.
25. Thompson AJ, Froelicher VF. Kugel's artery as a major collateral channel in severe coronary disease. *Aerosp Med.* 1974;45:1276–1280.
26. Levin DC, Beckman CF, Garnic JD, Carey P, Bettmann MA. Frequency and clinical significance of failure to visualize the conus artery during coronary arteriography. *Circulation.* 1981;63:833–837.

CHAPTER (2)

Cardiac Chamber Anatomy

William F. Fearon, MD

As the realm of the interventional cardiologist continues to expand beyond the coronary arteries, and as percutaneous treatments for extracoronary, but intracardiac, abnormalities continue to develop, knowledge of the relationship between the cardiac chambers and valves is of increasing importance. This chapter is a brief review of cardiac anatomy for the interventional cardiologist.

CARDIAC CHAMBERS

The orientation of the heart in the chest places the right atrium and ventricle as the most anterior structures (Figure 2-1). The posterior of the heart is comprised of the left atrium and posterior–inferior aspects of the left ventricle (Figure 2-2).

【 】 RIGHT ATRIUM

The right atrium is a cuboid structure with the capacity of approximately 60 mL. It receives blood from the superior vena cava, the inferior vena cava, and the coronary sinus. The superior vena cava drains blood from the cranial half of the body and enters the atrium at its upper and posterior portion. The inferior vena cava drains blood from the lower half of the body and enters the atrium at its lower and posterior portion. The coronary sinus returns blood from the heart itself to the right atrium, as described in the coronary venous anatomy section. The atrial septum is the result of the fusion of two embryonic septae, the primum and secundum, which mold to form the fossa ovale and ultimately seal into the common atrial septum.

【 】 RIGHT VENTRICLE

The right ventricle is triangular in shape and has the capacity of approximately 85 mL. It is an anterior structure that extends from the right atrium to the apex of the heart and rests on top of the left ventricle. The right ventricle can be divided into three components: a smooth inlet segment that extends from the tricuspid valve annulus to the insertions of the papillary muscles; a thicker trabeculated segment that extends from the papillary muscles to the apex; and an outflow segment that is also smooth and extends to the pulmonary valve. Anterior and posterior papillary muscles protrude from the anteroseptal and posterior aspects of the right ventricle and connect to chordae tendinae, which are attached to the cusps of the tricuspid valve. The right ventricle is joined to the left ventricle by the interventricular septum at its medial and posterior portion. The septum is the thickest part of the right ventricle and is the intended site for right ventricular endomyocardial biopsies. The right ventricle receives blood from the right atrium via the tricuspid valve and pumps blood to the lungs via the pulmonary valve and artery.

【 】 LEFT ATRIUM

The left atrium is a posterior structure joined to the right atrium by an interatrial septum. It receives blood from the four pulmonary veins and empties into the left ventricle. Attached to both the right and left atria are small, conical pouches termed *auricles* or *appendages*. The left atrial appendage is noteworthy because it can be a common source of thromboembolism in patients with atrial fibrillation. Percutaneous devices for excluding the left atrial appendage have been tested as a means for decreasing stroke risk

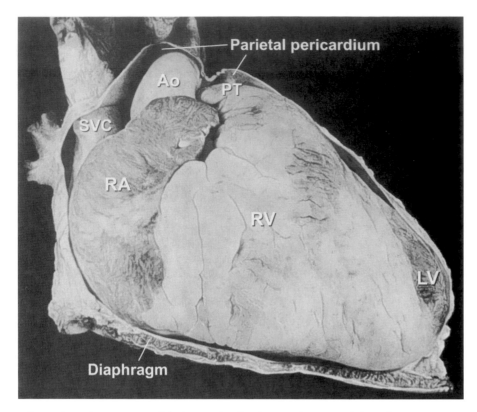

FIGURE 2-1. The orientation of the heart within the chest can be seen with the right atrium (RA) and right ventricle (RV), the most anterior structures. The great cardiac vessels arise at the top of the heart with the pulmonary trunk (PT) initially anterior to the aorta (AO) which then courses cranially up around the pulmonary artery. SVC = superior vena cava, LV = left ventricle. (Reproduced from Malouf JF, Edwards WD, Tajik AJ, Seward JB. Functional anatomy of the heart. In: Fuster V, Alexander RW, O'Rourke RA, eds. Hurst's The Heart, 11th edition. New York: McGraw-Hill, 2004; p 59.)

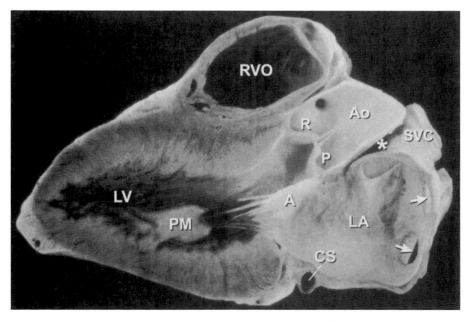

FIGURE 2-2. Left ventricular long-axis method of tomographic cardiac dissection (looking from left flank toward the midsternum). Continuity between mitral and aortic valves is clearly seen. The oblique sinus (*) abuts the wall of the left atrium. A, anterior mitral leaflet; Ao, ascending aorta; CS, coronary sinus; LA, left atrium; LV, left ventricle; P, posterior aortic cusp; PM, posteromedial mitral papillary muscle; R, right aortic cusp, RVO, right ventricular outflow; SVC, superior vena cava; arrows point to the right upper and lower pulmonary veins. (Reproduced from Malouf JF, Edwards WD, Tajik AJ, Seward JB. Functional anatomy of the heart. In: Fuster V, Alexander RW, O'Rourke RA, eds. Hurst's The Heart, 11th edition. New York: McGraw-Hill, 2004; p 56.)

and/or potentially avoiding anticoagulation in patients with atrial fibrillation.[1]

【 】 LEFT VENTRICLE

The left ventricle is a conical structure that receives blood from the left atrium and pumps blood into the aorta and to the rest of the body via the aortic valve and aorta. Its walls are much thicker and its apex is less trabeculated than those of the right ventricle. Anterior and posterior papillary muscles protrude from the anterior and posterior aspects the left ventricle and connect to chordae tendinae, which are attached to the cusps of the mitral valve.

【 】 INTERATRIAL SEPTUM

A thorough understanding of the anatomy of the interatrial septum is necessary for the safe and efficient performance of septal punctures. From the right atrium, the majority of the septum is interatrial; however, because the tricuspid annulus is more apical than the mitral annulus, a small lower portion of the septum is atrioventricular. From the left atrial side, the septum is entirely interatrial. The fossa ovalis is found in the triangular area between the two vena cavae and the coronary sinus (Figure 2-3); it is an oval depression that was the foramen ovale in the fetal heart and is the target for atrial septal punctures. In about one third of adults the foramen ovale remains patent and can be a source of paradoxical emboli.

After the bicuspid aortic valve, the atrial septal defect is the most common congenital abnormality found in adults. There are three major types of atrial septal defects found. The most common is the secundum type, which results from incomplete coverage of the fossa ovalis by either the secundum septum or primum septum and makes up approximately 70% of atrial septal defects. The next most common type is a primum atrial septal defect, which results from failure of the primum septum to fuse with the endocardial cushions and leads to a shunt at the caudal-most aspect of the atrial septum. The third type is the sinus venosus defect, which results from abnormal insertion of the superior vena cava into the right atrium and results in a shunt in the cranial aspect of the atrial septum.

【 】 INTERVENTRICULAR SEPTUM

The interventricular septum is usually divided into two parts, a much smaller thin and fibrous upper section, termed the *mem-*

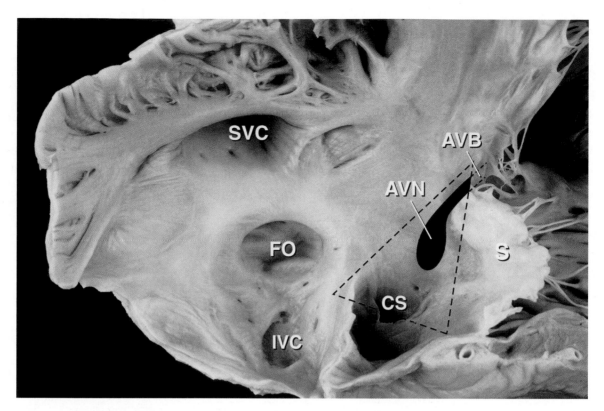

FIGURE 2-3. The fossa ovalis (FO) is found in the triangular area between the two vena cavae (Inferior vena cava, IVC and superior vena cava, SVC) and the coronary sinus (CS). *(Reproduced from Malouf JF, Edwards WD, Tajik AJ, Seward JB. Functional anatomy of the heart. In: Fuster V, Alexander RW, O'Rourke RA, eds. Hurst's The Heart, 11th edition. New York: McGraw-Hill, 2004; Figure 3–68.)*

branous septum, and a thicker and significantly more muscular segment, termed the *muscular septum.* The membranous septum is divided into the atrioventricular and interventricular components by the septal tricuspid valve leaflet. Approximately 80% of congenital ventricular septal defects occur in the membranous septum. Percutaneous closure of ventricular septal defects has been an area of investigation and device development for a number of years.[2,3]

CARDIAC VALVES

The atrioventricular valves (mitral and tricuspid) originate from the cardiac fibrous ring dividing atria from the ventricles. The semilumar valves (aortic and pulmonic) originate from the base of each great vessel, exiting the respective ventricle (Figure 2-4).

TRICUSPID VALVE

The tricuspid valve divides the right atrium from the right ventricle, allowing transmission of blood from the atrium to the ventricle during ventricular diastole and preventing reflux of blood during ventricular systole. It consists of three leaflets—anterior, posterior, and septal—that attach at their bases to a fibrous ring

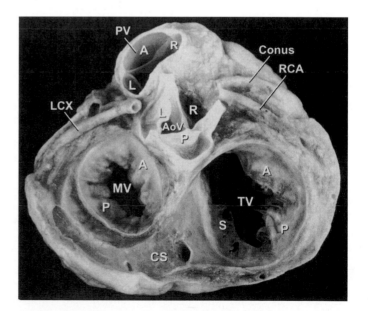

FIGURE 2-4. Base of heart. Section through the base of the heart, looking from base toward apex, with the atria and great arteries removed, shows all four cardiac valves. A, anterior; AoV, aortic valve; AV, atrioventricular; CS coronary sinus; IV, interventricular; L, left; LCX, left circumflex coronary artery; MV, mitral valve; P, posterior; PV, pulmonary valve; R, right; RCA, right coronary artery; S, septal; TV tricuspid valve. *(Reproduced from Malouf JF, Edwards WD, Tajik AJ, Seward JB. Functional anatomy of the heart. In: Fuster V, Alexander RW, O'Rourke RA, eds. Hurst's The Heart, 11th edition. New York: McGraw-Hill, 2004; p 60.)*

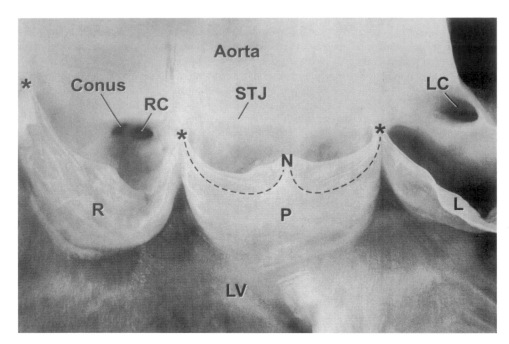

FIGURE 2-5. An opened aortic valve shows the right (R), left (L), and posterior (P) cusps. The dashed line marks the closing edge. Between the free and closing edges of each cusp are two lunular areas, representing the surfaces of apposition between adjacent cusps during valve closure. The commissures (*) attain the level of the aortic sinotubular junction (STJ). Conus, conus coronary ostium; LC, left coronary ostium; LV, left ventricle; N, nodule of Arantius; RC, right coronary ostium. *(Reproduced from Malouf JF, Edwards WD, Tajik AJ, Seward JB. Functional anatomy of the heart. In: Fuster V, Alexander RW, O'Rourke RA, eds. Hurst's The Heart, 11th edition. New York: McGraw-Hill, 2004; p 63.)*

surrounding the atrioventricular orifice and more apically to papillary muscles on the right ventricular wall via chordae tendinae. Because the bases of the valve leaflets are attached to a fibrous ring that is part of the right ventricle, right heart failure and subsequent right ventricular dilatation can result in stretching of the ring or annulus and development of tricuspid regurgitation.

[ ] PULMONIC VALVE

The pulmonic valve also consists of three leaflets—right, left, and anterior—that allow blood to flow from the right ventricle to the pulmonary artery during ventricular systole and prevent reflux of blood during ventricular diastole. The bases of the leaflets attach to a fibrous annulus surrounding the pulmonary trunk, while a fibrocartilagenous nodule at the tip of each leaflet is attached to the commissures, or junctions between the leaflet bases, by tendinous fibers. Congenital pulmonic stenosis is rarely seen in the adult population; however, it can be treated effectively by percutaneous balloon valvuloplasty.

[ ] MITRAL VALVE

The mitral valve divides the left atrium from the left ventricle, allowing blood to flow from the atrium to the ventricle during ventricular diastole and preventing reflux during ventricular systole. The valve consists of a larger anterior and a smaller posterior leaflet that attach at their bases to a fibrous ring in the atrioventricular orifice and at their tips to two papillary muscles in the left ventricular wall via chordae tendinae. The larger anterior leaflet forms part of the aortic outflow tract; in patients with hypertrophic cardiomyopathy, the anterior leaflet can appose the hypertrophied

basal septum during systole, contributing to an aortic outflow gradient, as well as to mitral regurgitation. The posterior leaflet is usually divided in to three scallops, the largest being the middle scallop, which is prone to prolapse.

Rheumatic mitral stenosis occurs uncommonly in the United States; however, it may still present in immigrants from developing countries. Percutaneous mitral valvuloplasty is a safe and effective procedure in selected populations. There has been growing interest in treating significant mitral regurgitation percutaneously.[4]

[ ] AORTIC VALVE

The aortic valve is a trileaflet structure about 2.5 cm in diameter that allows blood to flow from the left ventricle into the aorta during ventricular systole and prevents reflux during ventricular diastole (Figure 2-5). The three leaflets (right, left, and posterior) attach to the aortic outflow tract at their bases and sides, forming three distinct pockets, or *aortic sinuses*. The free edges of the leaflets are bound by fibrous tissue, termed *lunules*, each with a thick, prominent nodule at its tip. The left coronary orifice is normally found in the left aortic sinus and the right coronary orifice in the right aortic sinus. A bicuspid aortic valve is a common congenital abnormality that is associated with aortic stenosis in younger people; a left dominant coronary circulation occurs more frequently in patients with bicuspid aortic valves (Figure 2-6).[5]

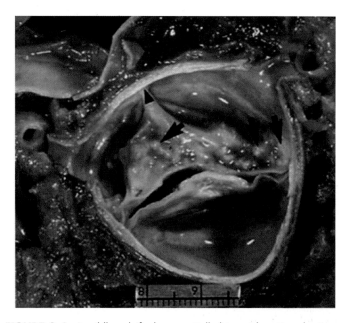

FIGURE 2-6. A mildly calcified congenitally bicuspid aortic valve in a 69 year old man. Note a nonstenotic functionally normally bicuspid valve with mild calcification (arrows) and a raphe (arrowhead) in the anterior leaflet. *(Reproduced from King SB, Douglas JS, eds. Atlas of the Heart. New York: McGraw-Hill, 1997; p 1.3.)*

REFERENCES

1. Sievert H, Lesh MD, Trepels T, et al. Percutaneous left atrial appendage transcatheter occlusion to prevent stroke in high-risk patients with atrial fibrillation: early clinical experience. *Circulation.* 2002;105:1887–1889.

2. Lock JE, Block PC, McKay RG, Baim DS, Keane JF. Transcatheter closure of ventricular septal defects. *Circulation.* 1988;78:361–368.

3. Holzer R, Balzer D, Cao QL, Lock K, Hijazi ZM Amplatzer Muscular Ventricular Septal Defect Investigators. Device closure of muscular ventricular septal defects using the Amplatzer muscular ventricular septal defect occluder: immediate and mid-term results of a U.S. registry. *J Am Coll Cardiol.* 2004;43: 1257–1263.

4. Kaye DM, Byrne M, Alferness C, Power J. Feasibility and short-term efficacy of percutaneous mitral annular reduction for the therapy of heart failure-induced mitral regurgitation. *Circulation.* 2003;108:1795–1797.

5. Hutchins GM, Nazarian IH, Bulkley BH. Association of left dominant coronary arterial system with congenital bicuspid aortic valve. *Am J Cardiol.* 1978,42: 57–59.

CHAPTER (3)

Peripheral Anatomy for the Interventionalist

Richard E. Stewart, MD

Cardiovascular catheter–based therapeutics now include peripheral arterial and venous interventions involving the great vessels, the aorta below the diaphragm, and the head and neck vessels as well as those of the lower extremities and limbs. This chapter describes the arterial and venous anatomy above and below the diaphragm, with emphasis on the radiographic examinations in the catheterization laboratory.

AORTIC ARCH AND UPPER EXTREMITIES

The vascular anatomy of the aortic arch and upper extremities begins at the level of the sinus of Valsalva. From the sinotubular ridge, the ascending aorta travels anteriorly and superiorly, passing over the main pulmonary artery and left mainstem bronchus. At this level, the mean diameter of the ascending thoracic aorta in the normal adult human is 3.5 cm.

The brachiocephalic or right innominate artery is the first major branch off the aortic arch. The next major vessel that arises from the aortic arch is the left carotid artery. The left subclavian artery is the last great artery that arises directly off the aortic arch. After the left subclavian artery arises, the aortic arch ends. This anatomic region, called the *isthmus,* is found between the last great vessel and the attachment of the ductus arteriosus, after which the descending aorta begins and continues down to the level of the iliac bifurcation.

Nine pairs of intercostal arteries arise from the descending aorta, from the level of the third through the eleventh intercostal spaces. In some cases, the bronchial arteries may arise directly off the aorta or have a common origin with an intercostal artery.

The right innominate or brachiocephalic artery gives rise to the right subclavian artery and right common carotid artery. After the bifurcation of the subclavian and carotid arteries on the right, the next vessels that arise off the right subclavian include the right vertebral artery and the right internal mammary artery. The right subclavian artery then gives rise to the thyrocervical trunk and the costocervical trunk. At this location, the subclavian artery becomes the axillary artery after it crosses the lateral margin of the first rib. On the left, the subclavian artery gives rise to the left vertebral artery and the left internal mammary artery. Anatomically, its course is similar to the right subclavian artery, giving rise to similar branches (Figure 3-1).

The axillary artery on both the left and the right gives rise to several small branches around the shoulder, including the superior thoracic, thoracoacromial, lateral thoracic, subscapular, and circumflex humeral artery. It then becomes the brachial artery at the lateral margin of the teres major muscle. The brachial artery divides into the radial and ulnar arteries in the antecubital fossa. In relationship to surface markers, the brachial artery bifurcates a few centimeters below the elbow joint. The ulnar artery then undergoes anastomosis with the median artery and forms the superficial palmar arch in the hand. The radial artery forms the deep palmar arch. The remaining axial artery at the level of the radial–ulnar bifurcation is known as the *interosseus artery* (Figure 3-2).

For the interventionalist, knowledge of common anatomic variants of the aortic arch is of great importance. Normal arch anatomy is noted in 70% of cases. The most common variant observed is the common origin of the brachiocephalic and left common carotid arteries. This occurs in 22% of patients and has been described as the "bovine arch." The next most common variant is the left vertebral artery arising directly off the aorta. Finally,

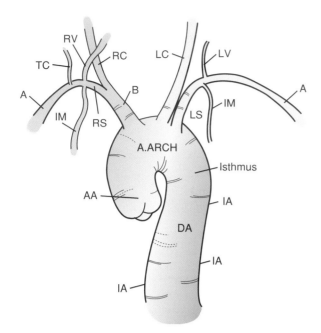

FIGURE 3-1. AA = ascending aorta; DA = descending aorta; B = brachiocephalic artery; RC = right carotid artery; LC = left carotid artery; RV = right vertebral artery; LV = left vertebral artery; IM = internal mammary artery; IA = intercostal artery; A = axillary artery; TC = cervical trunk; RS = right subclavian; LS = left subclavian; Isthmus = aortic isthmus.

the variant of the right and left common carotid arteries having a common origin is seen in less than 1% of cases.[2]

Arteriography of the aortic arch is carried out for diagnostic purposes and to plan interventions. Anteroposterior (AP) and 60° left anterior oblique (LAO) projections are initially used to image the arch and great vessels. Imaging the right brachiocephalic territory is best accomplished in a right anterior oblique (RAO) projection with caudal angulation. For selective shots of the left subclavian artery, an AP projection or steep LAO views are sought (Table 3-1).

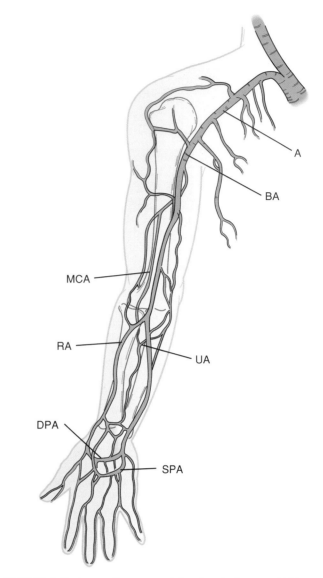

FIGURE 3-2. A = axillary artery; BA = brachial artery; MCA = medial collateral artery; RA = radial artery; UA = ulnar artery; DPA = deep palmar arch; SPA = superficial palmar arch.

VENOUS CIRCULATION OF THE UPPER EXTREMITIES

Because arteriovenous fistulas are prone to degeneration and may be suitable for percutaneous intervention, knowledge of the venous anatomy is useful. The venous system of the upper extremity is predominantly superficial. The dorsal venous network of the hand empties into the basilic vein, the cephalic vein, and the antecubital veins. The cephalic vein originates dorsally and laterally, crossing the elbow joint and entering the superior aspect of the axillary vein just above the clavicle. The basilic vein, which originates on the ulnar side of the arm, continues medially to the brachial artery. It joins the brachial vein to become the axillary vein at the border of the teres major muscle. The medial cubital veins are the veins that connect the basilic and cephalic veins in the antecubital fossa.

The deep veins in the upper arms and chest follow their respective arteries. The axillary and cephalic veins become the subclavian veins, which are continuations of the axillary veins. As the subclavian veins cross the sternum, they join with the internal jugular veins to form the brachiocephalic veins. The left brachiocephalic vein is longer than the right. The right and left brachiocephalic veins join behind the first anterior rib to form the superior vena cava. The azygous vein forms at the level of the second lumbar vertebra. It travels in the anterior aspect of the posterior mediastinum to the right of the midline, and arches anteriorly to join the superior vena cava just above the entry into the pericardium.

CAROTID AND VERTEBRAL ARTERIES

The carotid and vertebral arteries are becoming increasingly important to the interventional cardiologist. The right common carotid artery travels superiorly after bifurcating from the right

TABLE 3-1

Angiographic Views of the Aortic Arch and Upper Extremities

VASCULAR TERRITORY	ANGIOGRAPHIC VIEW	SET UP[a]
Right innominate artery	30°–60° RAO caudal	Ipsilateral
Left subclavian artery	AP	Ipsilateral
Entire aortic arch with great vessels	60° LAO	—
Carotid arteries	Lateral	Ipsilateral
	45° LAO, RAO	Ipsilateral
	AP cranial	—
Vertebral arteries	AP	Ipsilateral

RAO = right anterior oblique; LAO = left anterior oblique; AP = anterioposterior.

[a]*Ipsilateral or Contralateral indicates the angulation for a left femoral artery is best obtained with the same-side (ipsilateral) angulation (ie, LAO projection) or, if contralateral, the opposite angulation (ie, RAO projection).*

innominate artery. It then bifurcates into the right internal and external carotid arteries. Anatomically, the left common carotid artery arises directly from the aortic arch and travels cephalad to bifurcate into the left internal and external carotids. The common carotid arteries are paired vessels, located anteriorly within the neck. The bifurcation of the common carotid arteries into the internal and external arteries on both sides is generally at the level of cervical vertebra, C3 to C4.[3]

Both internal carotid arteries supply the anterior circulation of the brain as well as a portion of the skull base. The first segment of the internal carotid artery is the cervical segment, which has no branches. This is the only segment of the internal carotid artery that is extracranial. The remaining three segments of the internal carotid artery are named in relation to their location in the skull: the petrous and cavernous portions, which lie within the petrous bone and cavernous sinus, respectively; and the supraclinoid segment, which runs above the level of the anterior clinoid process. The internal carotid artery runs posterolateral to the external carotid artery and then courses medially to enter the skull base through the carotid canal (Figure 3-3).

The external carotid artery is a smaller artery in relation to the internal carotid artery. The distinguishing feature of the external carotid artery is its branches: the superior thyroid, ascending pharyngeal, lingual, facial, occipital, and posterior auricular arteries. The external carotid artery then bifurcates into the internal maxillary and superficial temporal arteries.

Arteriography of the carotid arteries is carried out primarily in two views: a lateral projection and an AP view with cranial angulation. The lateral view serves to separate the internal from external carotids and to image the bifurcation and common carotid. Many times, oblique views could also accomplish this. The AP view best characterizes the common carotid and the distal internal carotid arteries.

The vertebral arteries arise as the primary branches of the subclavian arteries, supplying the posterior circulation of the brain, spinal cord, and muscles of the neck. Vertebral arteries enter the foramina of the C6 vertebra and then run within the bony canals, exiting at the C2 foramina. These arteries then turn laterally to course around the C1 vertebra before returning medially to ascend through the foramen magnum to join and form the basilar artery. The most common views of the vertebral arteries are anterioposterior.

VENOUS ANATOMY OF THE HEAD AND NECK

The head is drained by the internal jugular veins and external jugular veins. The internal jugular vein is formed by the sigmoid and petrosal sinuses. These veins course inferiorly on both sides, running lateral to the carotid arteries and deep to the sternocleidomastoid muscle of the neck. They then join the subclavian vein on their respective sides. The external jugular vein drains portions of the face and the neck, and runs superficial to the sternocleidomastoid muscle before joining the subclavian veins. Finally, the vertebral veins drain the occipital region of the brain and adjacent to the vertebral arteries, emptying into the innominate veins.

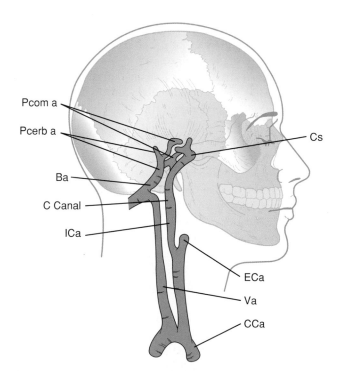

FIGURE 3-3. CCa = common carotid artery; ICa = internal carotid artery; ECa = external carotid artery; Va = vertebral artery; C canal = internal carotid artery in carotid canal; Pcerba = posterior cerebral artery; Ba = basilar artery; Pcoma = posterior communicating artery; CS = internal carotid artery in cavernous sinus.

ANATOMY OF THE ABDOMINAL AORTA

The major arteries of interest to the interventionalist that arise from the abdominal aorta are the celiac artery, the superior mesenteric artery, the inferior mesenteric artery, and the renal arteries. The celiac artery arises ventrally from the abdominal aorta at the vertebral level T12–L1. This artery is commonly called the *celiac trunk,* giving rise to the left gastric artery, common hepatic artery, and the splenic arteries. The left gastric artery branches off to the distal esophagus and stomach. The hepatic artery resides in the hepatoduodenal ligament and typically divides into the right, middle, and left branches. The cystic artery is most frequently a branch of the right hepatic artery. Further branches arising from the common hepatic artery are the gastroduodenal artery, the anterior and posterior superior pancreaticoduodenal arteries, and the right gastroepiploic artery. The splenic artery is particularly long, supplying the spleen and pancreas. The main branches are the pancreatic, short gastric, and left gastroepiploic arteries. The splenic artery then supplies the splenic parenchyma through numerous branches.

The renal arteries arise from the aorta slightly inferior to the origin of the superior mesenteric artery, at the L1–L2 level. Seventy percent of the population has a single renal artery to each kidney, with the remaining 30% having multiple renal arteries, usually separate vessels to the upper and lower poles of the kidney. This could also be seen as an early bifurcation of a single renal artery, giving the appearance of two arteries. Usually, this variant consists of a primary renal artery and an accessory artery that can supply either the upper or the lower pole of the kidney.

It should be noted that the origins of the left and right renal arteries are in different locations as they arise from the aorta. The left renal artery orifice is typically lateral, whereas the right renal artery is positioned anterolaterally. The renal arteries then divide into anterior and posterior segments at the renal hilus, continuing to divide into lobar arteries. The terminal branches are the arcuate arteries that supply the corticomedullary junction.

The superior mesenteric artery arises at the level of the L1 vertebral body. This artery supplies the midgut from the ligament of Treitz to the midtransverse colon. Its origin is caudal to the celiac artery but cephalad to the origin of the renal arteries. The major branches of the superior mesenteric artery include the inferior pancreaticoduodenal artery, jejunal and ileo branches, and the middle colic artery, which supplies the transverse colon. The colic artery portion of the superior mesenteric artery is divided into the ileocolic, right colic, and middle colic arteries. The ileocolic artery provides the blood supply to the cecum and anastomotic branches to the right colic artery. The right colic artery arises between the middle and ileocolic arteries and supplies the right colon and proximal transverse colons.

The inferior mesenteric artery is the last major artery arising from the abdominal aorta. This artery typically arises at the level of the L3 vertebra and supplies the distal transverse colon, left colon, and rectum. Its origin is from the left anterolateral surface of the aorta, which gives it a very typically arteriographic appearance. The main branches of the inferior mesenteric artery include the left colic artery, sigmoid arteries, superior rectal artery, and the marginal artery of Drummond (Figure 3-4).

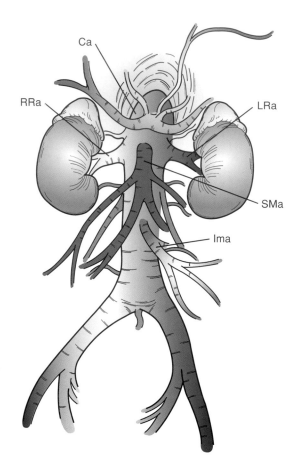

FIGURE 3-4. Ca = celiac artery; RRa = right renal artery; LRa = left renal artery; SMa = superior mesenteric artery; IMa = inferior mesenteric artery.

Arteriography of the major abdominal aortic arteries can be challenging at times. For the celiac trunk and superior mesenteric arteries, one should include both AP and lateral view projections that help engage as well as image these vessels. The renal arteries can easily be engaged and imaged in an AP projection. However, as a result of the slightly different takeoffs of these arteries, a shallow left anterior oblique projection, typically 10°–20° LAO, is the best view for both engagement and selective and nonselective imaging. The inferior mesenteric artery is typically engaged and imaged in the AP projection (Table 3-2).

THE ILIAC ARTERIES AND LOWER EXTREMITIES

The aorta bifurcates into the common iliac arteries between the level of the L4–L5 vertebrae. The common iliac arteries divide into the internal and external iliac arteries. The internal iliac artery is commonly referred to as the *hypogastric artery.* The external iliac arteries then continue, giving off the inferior epigastric and deep circumflex iliac arteries. The inferior epigastric artery anastomoses with the superior epigastric artery. The external iliac artery turns into the common femoral artery when the deep circumflex iliac artery arises from the external. It is important to recognize that there are three structures that mark the boundary between the

TABLE 3-2

Angiographic Views of the Abdominal Aorta and Lower Extremities

VASCULAR TERRITORY	ANGIOGRAPHIC VIEW	SET UP[a]
Celiac trunk	Lateral, AP	–
Superior mesenteric artery	Lateral, AP	–
Inferior mesenteric artery	Lateral, AP	–
Renal arteries (nonselective)	10° LAO	–
Right renal artery	AP, 10°–20° LAO	Contralateral
Left renal artery	AP, 10°–20° LAO	Ipsilateral
Distal aorta	AP	–
Common iliac arteries	AP	–
Right external and internal iliac arteries	10°–30° RAO	Contralateral
Left external and internal iliac arteries	10°–30° RAO	Contralateral
Right common femoral and profunda femoral arteries	20°–30° RAO	Ipsilateral
Left common and profunda femoral arteries	20°–30° LAO	Ipsilateral
Superficial femoral arteries	AP	Ipsilateral
Popliteal artery	AP	Ipsilateral
Anterior tibial artery	AP or steep oblique	Ipsilateral
Peroneal artery	AP or steep oblique	Ipsilateral
Posterior tibial artery	AP or steep oblique	Ipsilateral

RAO = right anterior oblique; LAO = left anterior oblique; AP = anterioposterior.

[a]*Ipsilateral or Contralateral indicates the angulation for a left femoral artery is best obtained with the same-side (ipsilateral) angulation (ie, LAO projection) or, if contralateral, the opposite angulation (ie, RAO projection).*

external iliac artery and the common femoral artery: the deep circumflex iliac artery, the interior epigastric artery, and the inguinal ligament.

The internal iliac artery divides into posterior internal iliac and anterior internal iliac arteries, with the posterior internal iliac giving off the superior gluteal, iliolumbar, and lateral sacral branches. The anterior internal iliac gives rise to the obturator, inferior gluteal, and internal pudendal branches. The inferior gluteal artery supplies the gluteus muscle and branches off to the sacral nerve. The internal pudendal artery then branches off the inferior hemorrhoidal branch before giving rise to the penile arteries, the dorsal artery of the penis, and the cavernosal artery. Distal branches of the internal iliac artery include the hemorrhoidal branches to the bladder as well as the genital branches (Figure 3-5).

The common femoral artery divides into the superficial femoral artery and profunda femoris artery. The profunda femoris artery courses laterally and posteriorly to the superficial femoral artery, and is also known as the *deep femoral artery*. Major branches off the profunda femoris artery include the medial and lateral femoral circumflex arteries (Figure 3-6).

The superficial femoral artery courses within the medial thigh until it divides posteriorly at the level of the adductor canal. Anatomically, this region is also known as *Hunter's canal*. This

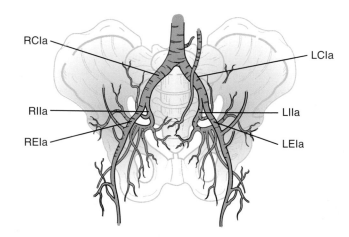

FIGURE 3-5. RCIa = right common iliac artery; LCIa = left common iliac artery; RIIa = right internal iliac artery; LIIa = left internal iliac artery; REIa = right external iliac artery; LEIa = left external iliac artery.

area is also the anatomic boundary of the superficial femoral artery and the popliteal artery. At its origin, the popliteal artery gives off the descending genicular, superior genicular, and supreme geniculate arteries, which are a rich source of collaterals in occlusive arterial disease, as is the profunda femoris artery. The popliteal arteries then divide into the anterior tibial artery and

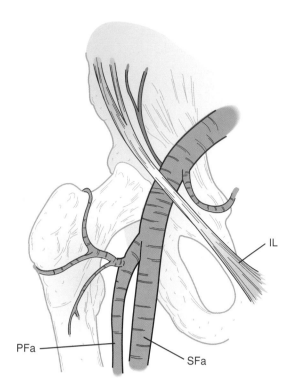

FIGURE 3-6. SFa = supperficial femoral artery; PFa = profunda femoral artery; IL = inguinal ligament.

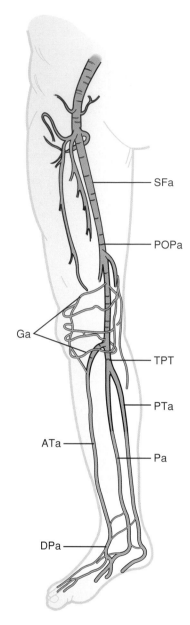

FIGURE 3-7. SFa = superficial femoral artery; POPa = popliteal artery; Ga = geniculate arteries (superior, inferior); TPT = tibioperitoneal trunk; ATa = anterior tibial artery; PTa = posterior tibial artery; Pa = peritoneal artery; DPa = dorsal pedal artery.

the tibioperoneal trunk below the level of the knee. The anterior tibial artery courses anteriorly to supply the interosseus muscles, continuing inferiorly to terminate as the dorsalis pedis artery in the foot. The tibioperoneal trunk consists of the peroneal artery, which has a medial course posterior to the interosseus membrane of the tibia and fibula. The peroneal artery terminates with the posterior communicating branch and an anterior perforating branch. The posterior tibial artery continues medially to pass posterior to the medial malleolus. Together with the branches of the dorsalis pedis branch, this artery forms the pedal arch of the foot (Figure 3-7).

Arteriography of the iliac arteries and the lower extremities involves both ipsilateral and contralateral imaging. For the aortoiliac bifurcation and common iliac arteries, an AP view is required. To image the bifurcation of the internal and external iliac arteries, a contralateral angulated view is best. For example, a left anterior oblique view would optimize imaging for the right internal and external iliac arteries. The external iliac and common femoral arteries usually require an ipsilateral angulated view, which separates out the profunda femoris artery from the superficial femoral artery. The angulation is generally between 20° and 30°. Usually, AP projections suffice for the superficial femoral arteries and the vessels of the lower extremities (Table 3-2).[4,5]

REFERENCES

1. Khan S, Haust, MD. Variations in the aortic origin of intercostal arteries in man. *Anat Rec.* 1979;195:545–552.
2. Shuford WH, Sybers RG. *The Aortic Arch and Its Malformations.* Charles C. Thomas, 1974.
3. Henry M, Ohki T, Polydorou A, Strigaris K, Kiskinis D. *Angioplasty and Stenting of the Carotid and Supra-Aortic Trunks.* Martin Donitz, 2004.4. Abrams HL, Baum S, Pentecost MJ. *Abrams' Angiography: Vascular and Interventional Radiology,* 4th ed. Little, Brown, 1997.5. Bakal CW, Filberzweig JE, Cynamon J, Sprayragen S. *Vascular and Interventional Radiology: Principles and Practices.* Thieme Medical, 2002.

CHAPTER (4)

The Coronary Circulation

Jos A.E. Spaan, PhD, Maria Siebes, PhD,
Bart-Jan Verhoeff, and Jan J. Piek, MD, PhD

The coronary circulation assumes a predominant role in the cardiovascular system because it supplies the heart muscle with blood, which in turn generates perfusion pressure for the entire circulation. Coronary blood flow amounts to 5%–10% of cardiac output, and is rapidly regulated in response to changes in myocardial metabolic demands.

This chapter relates present observations on coronary hemodynamics in the catheterization laboratory to coronary physiology as it has evolved from animal studies and theoretical models. We begin with some fundamental fluid dynamic principles, then describe basic coronary physiology and stenosis hemodynamics, and consequently apply these insights to the coronary pressure and velocity measurements as performed currently in the catheterization room. We do not strive for a full review of coronary physiology and biophysics, but restrict ourselves to those phenomena relevant for the interpretation of clinical measurements.

GENERAL FLUID DYNAMICS

The general physical laws of fluid dynamics are based on the conservation of mass, energy, and momentum. The mathematical formulations of these laws are already old, but solving these equations analytically is still feasible only for simplified geometric condition. Currently, numeric packages (computational fluid dynamics, CFD) are used to solve these equations for more realistic geometries such as curved and branching vessels with fluid–wall interactions.[9-11] It is beyond the scope of this chapter to review this literature. We present some fluid-dynamic principles for simplified geometries so that the basic phenomena in flow dynamics can be understood. Obviously, fluid velocity and shear stress are vectors.

However, in this section on fluid dynamics, we restrict ourselves in our mathematical formulations to the two-dimensional case, which can be either a flat layer, for which we use the Cartesian coordinate system, or a straight tube, for which we use cylindrical coordinates. The reader is referred to standard works on fluid dynamics for a more detailed mathematical treatment of the principles explained in this chapter.

【 】 STEADY LAMINAR FLOW

In steady-state and at low Reynolds numbers (see later), fluids flow in a laminar fashion. Such a flow type obeys Newton's law for fluid flow, which states that shear stress, τ, is proportional to shear rate, γ, with the proportionality constant equal to viscosity, μ, as

$$\tau = \mu\gamma \qquad \text{Eq. 1}$$

Shear rate is the spatial velocity gradient across the vessel lumen, and in cylindrical coordinates it equals $dv(r)/dr$, where $v(r)$ is the axial velocity in the tube as a function of radius, assuming one-dimensional flow.

In principle, blood is a non-Newtonian fluid because it is a suspension of particles. Its viscosity increases at low shear rates (< 50–100 s^{-1}) and decreases in tubes of small diameters (< 0.5 mm). However, for larger vessels such as the coronary arteries, one may assume that its behavior is Newtonian and apply a so-called *apparent viscosity coefficient*. For blood with a normal hematocrit, the apparent viscosity is from 3 to 4 times the viscosity of water, and the latter equals 0.01 dyne s/cm^2 = 0.01 poise = 0.001 N s/m^2.

Flow in a cylindrical vessel can be described as concentric shells with different velocities varying parabolically from zero at the wall to maximal in the center, as depicted in Figure 4-1. The velocity at the wall must be zero because of the *no-slip condition,* which is the

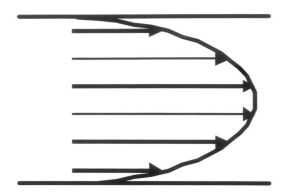

FIGURE 4-1. Parabolic flow profile in a straight tube far enough away from the tube entrance.

consequence of cohesive forces between the molecules of the fluid and the vessel wall. According to Eq. 1, the shear stress is highest at the vessel wall and zero in the center of the vessel. The parabolic velocity profile results in a relationship between flow, Q, and pressure drop, ΔP, over a vessel segment with length L, which is known as *Poiseuille's law:*

$$\Delta P = \frac{128 \, \mu L}{\pi D^4} Q \qquad \text{Eq. 2}$$

where D is the diameter of the vessel segment. Note that ΔP is related linearly to the length of the vessel segment, whereas it is inversely related to the fourth power of the radius.

Flow and average cross-sectional velocity, v_m, are related by

$$v_m = \frac{Q}{A} = \frac{4Q}{\pi D^2} \qquad \text{Eq. 3}$$

where A is the cross-sectional area of the vessel.

For a parabolic velocity profile, the maximum velocity, v_{max}, occurs at the center of the tube and is given by

$$v_{max} = 2v_m \qquad \text{Eq. 4}$$

Guidewires equipped with a Doppler-flow sensor measure maximal velocity in the vessel just distal to the wire tip. Equations 3 and 4 relate this maximal velocity to flow. Equations 2 and 4 apply only to straight vessels with a sufficient entrance length for the characteristic parabolic velocity profile to develop.

Coronary vessels are curved, which introduces skewing of the velocity profile, which in turn induces so-called *secondary flows,* resulting in helical flow patterns along the coronary vessels. Similarly, deviations from parabolic velocity profiles are induced at branch points. Depending on the branching angle, flow disturbances may be generated at such a location. In order to prevent too much interference with these factors it is advisable to measure velocity some distance away from branch points. Very good representations of predicted flow fields for several physiological and pathophysiological states can be found on the Internet (eg, \URL\http://www.imaging.robarts.ca/~steinman/).

【 】 TURBULENT FLOW

Flow in a vessel can become unstable when average velocity increases. The structure of moving laminae is broken up and the velocity field becomes disorganized, which is denoted as turbu

lence. A dimensionless number, called the *Reynolds number, R_e,* can predict the transition from laminar to turbulent flow:

$$R_e = \frac{\rho \, vD}{\mu} \qquad \text{Eq. 5}$$

where ρ is the density of the fluid. There is no strict numeric value for the critical Reynolds number above which transition to turbulence occurs. A value below 2100 is considered indicative of laminar flow. However, this value depends on several factors, such as the roughness of the vessel wall, and hence, in nonsteady flow, critical values for Reynolds numbers calculated from peak velocities may be much greater than 2100. Turbulence must also develop and, at Reynolds numbers greater than about 4000, the entire flow field becomes turbulent. In general, one may assume that arterial blood flow is laminar and that turbulence is absent under normal physiologic circumstances in a healthy body, except at peak systolic flow in the largest arteries, such as the ascending aorta or main pulmonary artery just past the valves.

Turbulence in a vessel segment adds to pressure drop calculated on the basis of Poiseuille flow because the average shear stress in the vessel increases, which results in an increased energy loss by heat dissipation. In addition, the velocity profile becomes more flat and the shear stress at the wall increases with turbulence. Flow may be turbulent in the core of a vessel, but there is always a thin boundary layer with laminar flow because of the no-slip condition at the wall. Hence, the distance over which velocity must decrease from mean center velocity in the turbulent area to zero at the wall is much smaller than in the absence of turbulence, which results in higher wall shear stress values and increased overall resistance in the vessel segment.

【 】 UNSTEADY LAMINAR FLOW

Unsteady flow and pressure in the arterial system have been extensively studied by Womersly (1957) and later by McDonald (1960). The theories developed by these scientists form the foundations for the analysis of pulsatile flow and pressure in the arterial system. Only the basic principles are elucidated here such that some fundamental fluid dynamic principles can be understood.

When flow is not steady but varies periodically with time, pressure drop over a vessel segment is not only related to viscous losses as described by Poiseuille's law. First, a term must be added describing the pressure gradient in relation to acceleration or deceleration of flow. Second, the viscous losses described by Eq. 2 must be modified to take into account the deviations from a parabolic velocity profile that is induced by the acceleration and deceleration of blood. One may achieve insight into the dynamic relation between spatial pressure and rate of change of flow from the following equation:

$$\frac{\delta P}{\delta z} = - K_1 \frac{128 \mu Q}{\pi D^4} - K_2 \, \rho \, \frac{\delta Q}{\delta t} \qquad \text{Eq. 6}$$

where K_1 and K_2 are coefficients whose values depend on the frequency of flow and pressure pulsations.

When pressure and flow oscillate, the pressure gradient increases and becomes out of phase with the gradient in flow. This additional pressure gradient depends on the specific mass of the fluid.

The constants K_1 and K_2 are factors depending on the deviations of the velocity profile in the artery from parabolic. For low frequencies the profile is parabolic and $K_1 = 1$, and the first term in Eq. 6 follows directly from Poiseuille's law. However, for low frequencies K_2 approaches two thirds, because with a parabolic profile accelerations of blood are maximal at the centerline but decrease toward the wall. For increasing frequencies, the velocity profile becomes flatter. This increases the viscous losses because the shear stress concentrates closer to the wall. K_1 steadily rises with frequency. However, the contribution of the layers of blood to the dynamic component of pressure gradient becomes uniform over the vessel cross-section, and $K_2 = 1$.

Note that the pressure gradient can be opposite to the direction of flow. In other words, flow may be forward while the pressure gradient is backward. In physiology, this phenomenon of pressure gradient reversal at continuing forward flow is well known across the aortic valve in the last part of the systole. Ventricular pressure decreases below the aortic pressure level because of deceleration of blood flow in the aortic root.

[ ] WAVES IN THE CORONARY SYSTEM

Because the vessel wall is elastic, its diameter increases when coronary pressure increases and energy is stored in the wall. This stored energy is released when pressure decreases. The combination of the dynamic pressure gradient as a result of pulsatile flow as described by Eq. 6 and the elasticity of the wall results in pressure waves propagating through the vascular system. The wave speed in the coronary arteries is between 4 m/s and 11 m/s under normal conditions.

Coronary wave transmission has been studied in larger animals.[12,13] Changes in transmission of the incisura in the aortic pressure wave at valve closure to the coronary artery have been used to quantify the effect of coronary stenosis.[14] About 1990,[15–17] the method of wave intensity analysis was introduced to describe the pressure and flow waves in the arterial system.[15–17] This method is now also being applied to study waves in the coronary arteries of animals.[18,19] It should be noted that a proper analysis of pressure and velocity waves in the coronary system requires the combined measurement of these quantities, either directly or indirectly, at the same location.

[ ] WALL SHEAR STRESS

Wall shear stress has become a most important fluid dynamic property for vascular and coronary medicine. The physical stress sensed by the endothelial cells stimulates them to produce nitric oxide, which is important for many vascular functions, but in this context, its role in flow-induced reduction of vascular tone is important. Although flow-induced vasodilation of the resistance vessels obviously has a large effect on overall coronary resistance, the ability of the endothelium to react to shear at the vessel wall is considered to be an important parameter of health of the vascular bed in general.[20]

The problem with wall shear stress is that it cannot be measured. It is a quantity calculated from viscosity near the wall and velocity gradients assumed to hold at the wall. Clearly, wall shear stress is determined by boundary layer properties. The endothelial

cells are covered by a gel-like layer, the glycolcalyx, which is a highly hydrated mesh of membrane-associated proteoglycans, glycosaminoglycans, glycoproteins, and glycolipids.[21] This glycocalyx interacts with blood cells, plasma proteins, and other substrates.[21–25] From a fluid dynamics point of view, both the thickness and porosity of this layer are important. The thickness may reach 2 μm in healthy vessels but it may be absent in diseased vessels. Because it is very difficult to measure velocity close to the vessel wall, the velocity profile is often extrapolated to the wall from a measurement of velocity over the vessel diameter. The thickness of the glycocalyx is therefore a factor of uncertainty in wall shear stress calculations. The porosity is an important factor because the no-slip condition does not hold at the interface between a porous medium and fluid, as fluid within the porous medium may interfere with measuring the velocity profile near the wall as well.

Wall shear stress may vary greatly in a vascular tree, and especially at branch points or in curved vessels; the induced secondary flows may result in low shear stress at one side of the wall and high shear stress at the other side. These differences are important, because locations with low wall shear stress are associated with atherosclerosis.[26–28]

CORONARY FLUID DYNAMICS

The coronary circulation is exceptional compared to other vascular beds because the heart impedes its own blood supply during systole. Thus, in contrast to all other circulatory subsystems, blood flow to the heart during systole is less than during diastole despite higher systolic input pressure.

Coronary blood flow is pulsatile and is conducted through a curved, tree-like structure that consists of shorter and longer branch segments with highly variable branching angles,[29–31] and is deformed during every heartbeat. In addition, the vessel wall is elastic, with the consequence that local vessel diameters are not constant, but vary with pressure over time. Although the epicardial vessels mainly serve as conductance channels for blood flow, the intramural vessels not only distribute blood flow within the myocardium, but also have distinctive functions for coronary blood flow control.

Most of the coronary vasculature is embedded within the cardiac wall, where it is subjected to the periodical compression and shear forces exerted by the contracting myocardium. The pressure and flow signals in the outer epicardial vessels are determined to a large degree by events within the myocardium. In an exception to the general rule that most blood volume is stored in the venules and smaller veins,[32] most of the coronary blood volume is located within the capillary bed. This high capillary volume is the result of the dense capillary network needed for the supply of oxygen and substrates to the myocytes.[33] Under normal conditions, most of the coronary vascular resistance stems from the small arteries with a diameter of 400 μm or less, and from the arterioles. The distribution of resistance in the coronary tree and its control is discussed in a different section. In this section, we focus on the effect of heart contraction on coronary flow and on coronary arterial pressure–flow lines.

Many of the experiments discussed here were performed on animals with the use of an external perfusion system. The advantage of this approach is that the coronary arterial system is perfused independently from the systemic circulation. This allows the study of coronary physiology by interventions that are hardly possible in humans.

【 】 CORONARY VOLUME

Total intramural blood volume can be on the order of 10%–15% of cardiac tissue volume, but it is highly variable. Estimates of intramural blood volume were derived from a variety of techniques such as tracer dilution curves for the normal beating heart, remaining blood volume after the heart has been taken out, and volume calculations from casts.[32] The intramural blood volume depends on the frequency and force of contraction of the heart and on microvascular distending pressure. A good demonstration of the magnitude of possible intramural blood volume variations is provided by an experiment with a heart that was artificially paced after the bundle of His was destroyed, and where an external system was used to perfuse the coronary main stem. Arterial flow and venous flow velocity were measured continuously.[34] The coronary perfusion was stopped with the heart still beating, allowing intramural blood to be expelled through the veins. Then the heartbeat was halted by cessation of pacing. After a few seconds, the arterial inflow was restored. A typical result is shown in Figure 4-2, which demonstrates some important features of coronary dynamics.

After restoration of arterial perfusion, it takes about 3 s before venous outflow is fully restored to the original level. In a period where outflow is lower than inflow, intramural volume must increase. The arterial blood volume flowing into the myocardium without any venous outflow is called the *unstressed intramyocardial volume* and amounts to 4 mL/100 g. It is difficult to estimate the volume increase in the later phase of flow restoration because venous velocity and flow may not be related by a constant factor. However, if that is the case, about an additional 2 mL/100 g tissue is restored in this second phase. Hence, during the maneuver depicted in Figure 4-2, intramural blood volume varied by about 6 mL/100 g. The second important observation is that arterial inflow rather quickly returns to a steady level with only a little

overshoot. One would expect a higher overshoot in arterial inflow because increasing microvascular pressure as a result of restoration of intramural blood volume would progressively hamper inflow. The absence of such a strong overshoot in arterial flow is discussed in more detail later.

CORONARY COMPLIANCE

By definition, compliance of a compartment is the ratio of the change in its volume divided by the change of pressure responsible for this volume change. All blood vessels demonstrate compliance because of the elastic nature of their walls. The distensibility of a vessel is defined as the ratio of the relative change in cross-sectional area induced by a change of pressure. The compliance of a vascular compartment is therefore simply the product of distensibility and volume of that compartment under the prevailing conditions.[32]

A fundamental property of the blood vessel wall is its nonlinear elasticity. When a vessel is fully dilated, the slope of the passive pressure–diameter relation decreases with increasing pressure. Coronary diameter is thus more affected by variations at lower pressures. This is due to the stretching of collagen fibers up to or over their slack length.[35] Pressure–diameter relations of small arteries have practically all the same shape when normalized to their diameter at a pressure of 100 mm Hg. A typical relation between distending pressure and diameter is provided in Figure 4-3.

Figure 4-3 also demonstrates that in the presence of tone, the diameter of vessel may decrease upon an increase in pressure.[7,36] These myogenic constrictive responses are rather slow. Although for slow variations in pressure the direction of change of diameter is opposite to that of pressure, diameter variations follow pressure variations when the frequency is close to that of heart rate (HR). Hence, also in the presence of tone, compliance remains positive, whereas one may consider the steady-state compliance negative.[37]

Chilian and Marcus[38] measured coronary diameter continuously at different mean aortic pressures and found that the area change caused by the pulse pressure was three times less at pressures above 125 mm Hg than at pressures between 30 mm Hg and 75 mm Hg, indicating decreased coronary compliance at higher pressures. Epicardial artery compliance was found to decrease from 0.009 to 0.003 mL/mm Hg with increasing mean pressure. These values are an order of magnitude smaller than those found for the myocardial vascular bed, which is in the order of 0.07 mL/mm Hg/100 g.[32]

There are two important reasons why compliance in the coronary microcirculation is larger than in the larger coronary arteries. First, pressure is lower in the microcirculation so that this compartment is operating on a steeper slope of the pressure–diameter relation. Second, the volume in the capillary bed is much larger.

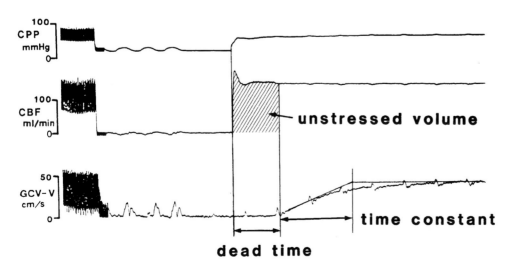

FIGURE 4-2. Change in intramural blood volume after restoration of coronary arterial flow during a long diastole. *(Redrawn from Kajiya et al., 1987.[6])*

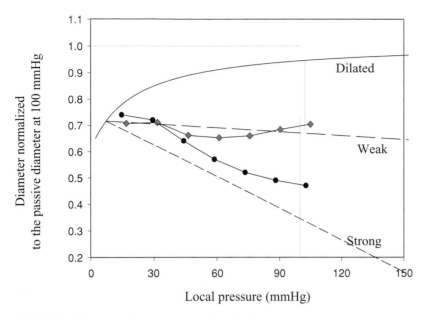

FIGURE 4-3. Pressure diameter relationship of isolated coronary resistance arteries, without and with tone. The constriction is spontaneous and called *myogenic tone*. (Redrawn from Cornelissen et al., 2000[5]; data points on active tone from Kuo, Davis, and Chilian, 1988,[7] and from Liao and Kuo, 1997.[8])

【 】 PULSATILITY OF CORONARY BLOOD FLOW: THE INTRAMYOCARDIAL PUMP

Coronary arterial and venous flows are phasic, but their waves are almost 180° out of phase. Arterial flow is high in systole, but venous flow is practically zero, and arterial flow is low in systole when venous flow is high. From the law of conservation of mass it follows that intramural blood volume is lower in systole and higher in diastole. These volume variations may be in the order of 1 mL/100 g under normal conditions, but as high as 3 mL/100 g at vasodilation. Many effects play a role in the relationship between cardiac squeeze and the arterial and venous flow waves. Vessel diameters change, affecting their resistance; the stiffness of myocytes surrounding the intramural vessels changes, thereby affecting the vascular compliance; and the local geometry of the myocardium is altered, which may induce additional changes in local resistance. The best starting point to understand these effects both conceptually and in practical terms is the intramyocardial pump concept.[4]

The intramyocardial pump model is depicted in Figure 4-4. All intramural vessels are assumed to be represented by the compliant "balloon," which is surrounded by a medium that can compress it. The overall resistance of the system is split into inflow and outflow parts. When its volume changes for whatever reason, blood flows out of the balloon, and the rate at which this happens is dV/dt, where V is the intramyocardial blood volume. A flow related to a change in volume is termed *capacitive flow*. Because of the conservation of mass, the capacitive flow must equal the difference between inflow and outflow. The inflow and outflow resistances impede the inflow and outflow, respectively. These resistances need not be constant, but may vary because of the effects of cardiac contraction as explained previously, and because of perfusion pressure variations as a result of vessel distensibility. In the normal situation with autoregulation present, the inflow resistance is also dependent on the level of oxygen consumption of the heart.

An important conclusion following from this model is that normally arterial and venous flow variations are uncoupled. The intramyocardial compliance is so large that a steady-state between arterial and venous flow requires seconds to be established, which was also demonstrated in Figure 4-2. These slow volume variations also occur after a change in arterial pressure[39] and during brief periods of cardiac arrest.[40]

In linear system analysis, it is very useful to separate signals into their time averages and dynamic variations around these average values. In the intramyocardial pump concept, mean coronary flow is related to the time-averaged difference between arterial and venous pressure divided by the sum of the two resistances. The phasic behavior of arterial flow is then related to the difference between pressure generated within the compliance and arterial pressure divided by only the inflow resistance.

The model was tested in a coronary perfusion experiment in which the main stem was perfused at constant pressure. However, the perfusion line of the perfusion source contained an adjustable flow resistance. Pressure at the source was manipulated to compensate for the pressure drop over the perfusion source resistance, such that mean arterial pressure equal to pressure distal of the source resistance remained constant. It was found that mean flow remained practically constant when mean pressure remained constant, but that the increase in perfusion source resistance increased pressure pulsations on the arterial pressure signal and simultaneously decreased the pulsations in coronary flow signal.

Figure 4-5 depicts the magnitude of coronary pressure pulsations as a function of the magnitude in coronary flow pulsations is plotted for four different levels of mean coronary arterial pressure. The relationships are reasonably linear and intercept the pressure axis at similar values. These relationships are known as *load lines for the intramyocardial pump*. The intercept of each load line with the pressure axis can be interpreted as the source pressure and the slope as the internal inflow resistance of the intramyocardial pump. The sum of the two resistances can be calculated from the

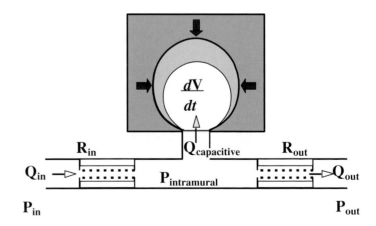

FIGURE 4-4. Intramyocardial pump model. All compliance of the microcirculation is believed to be concentrated in one blood compartment subjected to compressive forces. Flow in, Q_{in}, and flow out, Q_{out}, of the compartment is impeded by resistance in, R_{in}, and resistance out, R_{out}, and may differ by an amount equal to capacitive flow, dV/dt.

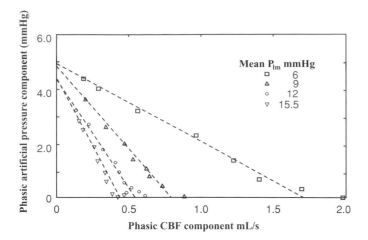

FIGURE 4-5. Load line analyses of amplitudes of pulsatile pressure and flow at different constant mean perfusion pressures obtained by varying stenosis degree on the perfusion line and adjusting pressure proximal to the stenosis. *(Redrawn from Spaan, Breuls, and Laird, 1981.[4])*

mean pressure difference and mean flow, and in this way, the outflow resistance can also be calculated.

From Figure 4-5 it can be concluded that the pressure generated by the intramyocardial pump is rather independent of mean arterial pressure, but that the inflow resistance is not. Lowering mean pressure results in vasodilation because of autoregulation, and this causes a reduced impediment to phasic flow.

The intramyocardial pump model is extremely relevant for the interpretation of the coronary pressure and flow velocity signals obtained in the catheterization room. In the presence of a stenosis, the stenosis resistance becomes part of the inlet resistance. As a result, the distal pressure wave becomes uncoupled from the aortic pressure wave and more closely resembles a left ventricular pressure wave, albeit with reduced pulsation amplitude. Also, the pulsations in coronary flow become reduced. In contrast to the experiments discussed previously, the pressure drop across the stenosis in patients is not compensated by an increase in proximal pressure, and hence, mean distal pressure is reduced. This in turn triggers distal vasodilation, thus reducing the inflow resistance of the coronary vascular bed.

It is difficult to predict from this graph how pulsatility of flow and pressure changes with increasing stenosis degree in patients because the pulsations in flow and pressure are also determined by microvascular resistance, which depends on cardiac work. The general observation is that flow pulsations in a stenosed vessel are smaller than in a non-stenosed vessel.[41,42]

【 】 VARYING ELASTANCE AS GENERATOR OF PULSATILE CORONARY FLOW

The intercept of the load lines on the pressure axis amounted to about half of the magnitude of left ventricular pressure, which was in concordance with the then prevailing concept that intramyocardial pressure is coupled to left ventricular pressure. Calculations of intramyocardial tissue pressure (IMP) by mechanical models[43] as well as by direct measurements of tissue pressure via the insertion of small pressure probes into the ventricular wall[44] had shown that IMP decreases from ventricular pressure at the subendocardium to intrathoracic pressure at the subepicardium.

However, simple coupling of IMP to left ventricular pressure would predict that coronary flow is not pulsatile in an empty beating heart. However, measurements on isolated rat hearts in the fully dilated state revealed that the magnitude of coronary flow pulsations was rather independent of diastolic–systolic left ventricular pressure variations.[45,46] This was confirmed in dogs and, more importantly, it was demonstrated that subendocardial perfusion as measured by microspheres was similar in an empty beating heart compared to a pumping heart.[47] The rat heart perfusion experiments by Krams et al.[48] further demonstrated that pulsations of flow in a dilated coronary bed were related to the filling of the intramural vascular bed. These findings lead to the elastance concept for the coronary circulation to explain coronary blood flow pulsatility, as formulated by Westerhof.[49] Basically, the intramyocardial pump holds as a model explaining flow pulsations in the coronary arteries, but the pressure generator of the pump is more complicated than the tissue pressure concept originally assumed.

The elastance model of the coronary circulation is based on the elastance model of Suga and coworkers[2] for left ventricular function as is outlined in Figure 4-6. As in the left ventricular function diagrams according to Suga et al.,[2] one can discern a diastolic and endsystolic pressure–volume curve. A heart cycle is described by a P-V loop. In diastole, the intramural vessels are filled up to their enddiastolic volume, which is determined by the rate of filling of the intramural vessels and the onset of contraction. Contraction then expels volume from the intramural vessels to the coronary arteries (reduction of coronary arterial flow) and to the veins (increase of venous outflow). Because of inlet and outlet valves in the ventricles, the heart chambers have isovolumic phases, and because valves are lacking in the coronaries, these phases are absent in the coronary P-V loops. However, similar to the ventricles, blood is expelled until intramural blood volume reaches the end-systolic pressure–volume relation. During relaxation and the subsequent diastole, the intramural

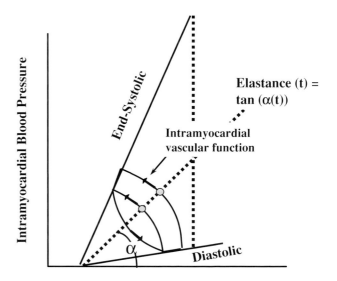

FIGURE 4-6. Elastance model relating changes in intramural blood volume to changes in elastance induced by cardiac contraction. The theory is similar to the elastance model by Suga, Sagawa, and Shoukas, 1973,[2] for ventricular function. Note that as a result of the absence of valves in the coronary system, no isovolumic phases (as in ventricular function curves) exist.

vascular volume increases again and the cycle is closed. In Figure 4-6, the elastance as function of time is indicated by the slope of the dotted line, which rotates at a fixed position on the volume axis and intercepts the volume-pressure relation of the intramural vessels.

As explained previously, mechanics of the ventricle as well as of intramural vessels can be described by a time-varying elastance. The actual course of the P-V loop for the intramural vascular space is determined by the factors responsible for the rate of filling and emptying of this space, such as the coronary arterial pressure, the compliance of the vascular bed at the different moments in time, and the inlet and outlet resistances. With increasing coronary arterial pressure and constant inlet and outlet resistances, the intramural volume increases, thereby causing the P-V loop to shift to the right, generating larger volume and intramural pressure variations. Obviously, there are limits to this interpretation of coronary flow mechanics, as we discuss next.

【 】 INTERACTION OF TISSUE PRESSURE AND TIME-VARYING ELASTANCE

From a mechanical point of view, tissue pressure is assumed to be in balance with the radial wall stress in the myocardium. On a macroscopic scale, this is obviously true. However, at the scale of capillaries, other small blood and lymph vessels, and the interstitium, this concept is too simple. These compartments can be considered to be fluid pockets enclosed by muscle fibers and connective tissue structures, and the orientation of their interfaces with the environment is random. In addition, the mechanical stiffness of tissue in which all these compartments are embedded varies over time. The stiffness is much higher in systole than in diastole. Moreover, during contraction, the geometry of these pockets changes as a result of shortening and thickening of muscle fibers. In fact, it has been demonstrated that capillaries in a heart fixated in systole have a larger diameter than when fixated in diastole.[50] This finding is difficult to tie to any concept of cardiac contraction based on systolic squeezing of blood vessels.

In the past, tissue pressure was measured by inserting pressure transducers into the heart muscle. However, these insertions create their own fluid pockets around the sensors that strongly affected the measurements. The size of the pressure transducer is important as well. Moreover, when solid-state sensors were applied, the strength of the signal depended on the direction of the sensor surface with respect to the muscle fiber orientation, which clearly indicated that direct loading of the sensor by tissue structures occurred. Pressure is a scalar and not a vector, and should therefore be independent of direction of the sensor surface, at least when the dynamic pressure component is small, and therefore measured IMP should be independent of direction of pressure transducer. The interplay between tissue pressure and elastance becomes clear when considering pressure in epicardial lymph vessels, which are in open connection with the interstitium. It was found that left ventricular pressure had a strong effect on lymph pressure throughout diastole, but only in the beginning of systole.[51] A typical result is shown in Figure 4-7. Please note that the end-diastolic waves in left ventricular and epicardial lymph pressure are of the same magnitude. Lymph pressure starts to increase concomitantly with left ventricular pressure, 2, but then abruptly takes a different course and exhibits a second wave, 3. This second wave ends at the end

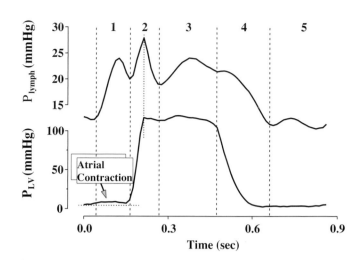

FIGURE 4-7. Stop-flow pressure measured in a cannulated epicardial lymph vessel and left ventricular pressure. (See text for interpretation.)

of systole and the lymph pressure is again dominated by changes in left ventricular pressure. In diastole, 5,1, the tissue has hardly any stiffness and behaves like a plastic water bag in which pressure is transmitted easily. However, in the middle of systole, 3, the wall has become stiff, and this stiffness protects the fluid pockets from further compression by pressure transmitted from the left ventricle. Apparently, left ventricular pressure rises ahead of its stiffness, such that left ventricular pressure is still transmitted in the very beginning of systole. After stiffness has increased in midsystole, lymph pressure has become independent of left ventricular pressure. It still increases as a result of mechanical loading of the interstitial pockets, but to a much lesser extent than when P_{LV} would have had free play in determining midsystolic compression.

As is clear from this discussion, both tissue pressure and elastance of the myocardium give rise to a systolic flow level lower than in diastole. However, the stiffer myocardium prevents the left ventricular pressure from being fully transmitted, and in that sense protects the intramural vessels from further collapse.[52,53]

【 】 CORONARY PRESSURE AND FLOW VELOCITY SIGNALS

Some important features in the pressure and velocity signals are demonstrated in Figure 4-8. The top panel is the maximal velocity signal in a reference coronary vessel of one of the patients in baseline conditions. The coronary pressure signal is quite similar to the aortic pressure and coronary flow velocity is pulsatile, being higher in diastole than in systole. In this case, the systolic velocity waveform shows fewer details of the different phases within systole than the lymph pressure signal of Figure 4-7. In order to see those details, a constant perfusion pressure source is needed.[52] The bottom panel depicts signals measured distal of a stenosis during adenosine-induced hyperemia. The systolic–diastolic differences in flow velocity disappear, and the distal pressure signal deviates from the aortic signal, not only because the mean is lower but especially the shape of the signal. Note that the initial rise in distal pressure in systole precedes the initial rise in aortic pressure. The systolic distal pressure wave is more dominated by the left ventricular pressure wave than by the aortic pressure wave.

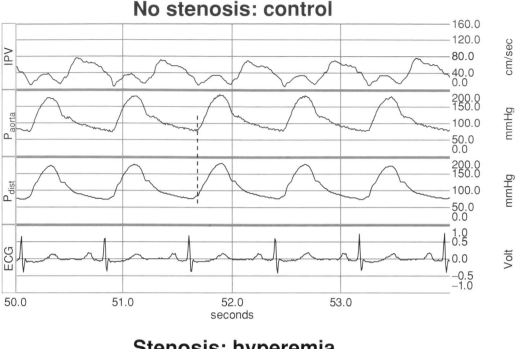

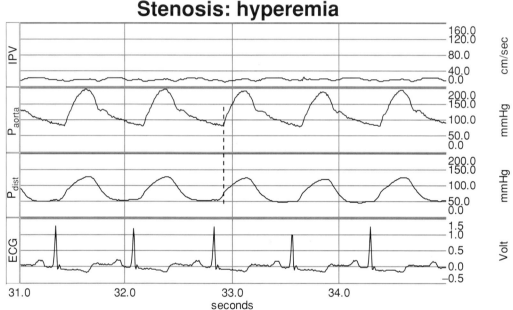

FIGURE 4-8. Phasic tracings demonstrating the damping effect of a stenosis on the distal coronary velocity, IPV, and how the stenosis alters the distal coronary pressure, P_{dist}, from aortic pressure, P_{aorta}, to a pressure signal dominated by left ventricular pressure.

【 】 CORONARY PRESSURE FLOW-LINES AND THE DEFINITION OF CORONARY RESISTANCE

In this section we limit ourselves to pressure–flow lines at full vasodilation. These lines lack an autoregulatory plateau, which is discussed in a later section of this chapter (eg, Figure 4-13). Typical pressure–flow lines as measured in a cannulated coronary preparation are depicted in Figure 4-13, which is redrawn from Downey and Kirk's[1] classic paper. The two curves were obtained by applying a constant flow pump. The flow was set at a certain level, and the perbeat average of coronary pressure was measured before and after

a short cardiac arrest induced by vagus stimulation. At higher pressures, the two curves appear to be rather straight, with a parallel shift to the right of the curve for the beating heart. This shift between beating and arrested pressure–flow lines amounts to approximately half of the difference in mean left ventricular pressure.

This parallel shift was considered proof of the waterfall model, which was the prevailing model for interpretation of coronary flow mechanics before the intramyocardial pump model.[4] The waterfall model is not discussed in detail here (see Hoffman and Spaan[54] for review), but the original curves depicted in Figure 4-9 are used to illustrate some features of coronary pressure–flow lines and to discuss the problems related to the definition of coronary resistance.

As explained previously, resistance, R, of a vascular compartment is defined by the equivalent of Ohm's law for an electrical resistance:

$$R = \Delta P/Q \qquad \text{Eq. 7}$$

where ΔP is the drop in pressure over that compartment and Q is the flow. Comparison with Eq. 2 relates blood viscosity and vessel dimensions to resistance in this definition. In order to calculate coronary resistance from a pressure–flow line, which provides information only for the arterial input pressure, one must agree on the downstream outlet pressure of the compartment. The most obvious choice for the downstream pressure of the coronary bed is the coronary venous pressure, p_v. Resistance at a certain arterial pressure, p_A, is then the slope of the line connecting the point of $P = P_v$ on the pressure axis with the data point on the pressure–flow line for that P_A. Two of these help-lines are depicted in Figure 4-9 for $P_A = 100$ mm Hg for the heart in the beating state and for arrest.

If one accepts that venous pressure acts as the backpressure, one must accept not only that coronary resistance is increased by the beating of the heart, but also that the resistance is pressure dependent. Both these conclusions agree well with two basic physiologic principles: (1) cardiac contraction impedes coronary blood flow at full vasodilation, and (2) all vessels are distensible and increase in diameter on an increase in pressure. The notion of a constant coronary resistance at maximal vasodilation is in conflict with these principles.

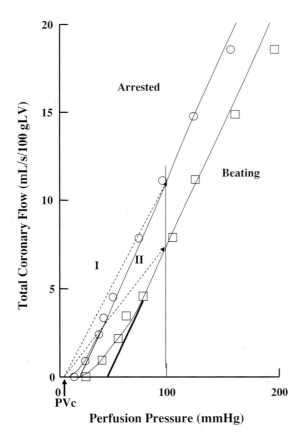

FIGURE 4-9. Pressure–flow relations at full vasodilation in the left anterior descending (LAD) artery during beating and cardiac arrest. Data points are from Downey and Kirk, 1975,[1] and the fitted curves are found by a nonlinear intramyocardial pump model. The gray lines demonstrate the intercepts of the extrapolations of the linear parts of the curves to the x-axis. The slopes of the broken lines I and II represent the conductance (1/resistance) of the LAD at a perfusion pressure of 100 mm Hg. Note that resistance is both pressure- and HR-dependent.

The alternative to assuming venous pressure as coronary backpressure is to assume that vessels at some location in the coronary circulation collapse and form a waterfall, and that the external collapse pressure equals the backpressure for arterial inflow.[1,55] However, several observations put the validity of this assumption into question. Although vessel collapse has been observed in the coronary microcirculation, this has never been shown for conditions where arterial pressure was in a normal range. Moreover, the relative diameter variations of endocardial small arteries and veins throughout the cardiac cycle become smaller with smaller average diameters, which is in contrast to the assumption that small vessels would collapse periodically within the heart cycle.[56] In addition, the high mean pressure measured in small epicardial veins of about 100-μm diameter makes collapse in the presence of flow at realistic arterial pressures unlikely.[3]

The pressure–dependence of coronary resistance is clearly supported by a number of observations. Microvascular studies demonstrate that the diameter of resistance vessels at full dilation changes with pressure as to be expected from isolated vessel studies. The input impedance of the septal circulation of the non-beating dog heart demonstrated a clear pressure dependence of the resulting transfer functions.[57] It is unlikely that these input transfer functions in the frequency range around 1 Hz are dominated by events distal of the capillary bed. Also, experiments with a constant difference between P_A and P_v at varying mean pressure, achieved by changing both pressures to different levels, clearly demonstrated the pressure dependence of coronary resistance in the nonbeating heart.[58]

The linear part of the pressure–flow line presents a strong temptation for extrapolation to the pressure axis, as indicated by the gray lines in Figure 4-9. The intercept of such extrapolation with the pressure axis has been termed "zero-flow pressure, P_{ZF}." The slope of the linear part is then referred to as coronary resistance. Based on this approach coronary resistance would be constant (constant slope) and heart contraction would result in an increase in P_{ZF}. Such an approach may be valid if one is interested only in mathematically describing the pressure–flow relation at higher pressures. However, serious problems arise when relating extrapolated pressure–flow relations to other biophysical phenomena, such as changes in diameter of resistance vessels with pressure, pressure dependence of input impedance, and changes induced in intramural volume both by changes in arterial pressure and by heart rate.

It should be noted that the pressure–flow relations in the dilated coronary bed can be described very well by a model in which the resistance of vessel compartments depends on compartmental blood volume, and vascular compression by cardiac contraction is described by the intramyocardial pump principle.[59] In fact, the two curved lines in Figure 4-9 fitting the data come from such a model. Hence, there is no need for a rather artificial assumption of microvascular collapse that is not supported by evidence from microvascular studies, and of a constant coronary resistance, while observations have demonstrated clearly that vessel diameters, and thus their resistance, vary with pressure.

STENOSIS HEMODYNAMICS

A stenosis represents a focal narrowing of the flow channel that develops by atheromatous thickening of the arterial wall. The residual lumen of the lesion may be circular, elliptical, or slitlike, and the plaque may be positioned circumferentially or eccentrically. Several pathologic studies indicate that about 75% of coronary atherosclerotic plaques are eccentric as a result of the curved nature of the epicardial vessels.

The laws of fluid dynamics discussed previously also apply to the stenosis, but there are some additional factors to consider. The most important one is that fluid flowing into a narrowed channel is accelerated, and then decelerated when it leaves the stenosis. The second factor arises from the geometric characteristics of the stenosis. Especially when the stenosis is asymmetric, the remaining flow channel is partly surrounded by normal vessel wall, and the channel geometry is not fixed but varies in response to changes in vasomotor tone or to changes in intraluminal pressure induced by flow.

[ ] PRESSURE LOSS WITHIN AND ACROSS A STENOSIS

The undesired pressure drop across a stenosis is governed by two fluid dynamic mechanisms. The first is because of viscous friction according to Poiseuille's law (Eq. 2), and the second is because of convective acceleration of blood within the narrowed flow channel. The fluid dynamic events determining the pressure drop over a stenosis are depicted in Figure 4-10. In the vessel proximal to the stenosis the pressure drop per unit length is negligible. However, within the stenosis the diameter is much smaller, such that the viscous pressure loss per unit length may become considerable according to the inverse fourth-power relationship between pressure gradient and diameter. Distal to the stenosis this term becomes negligible again.

The second cause for pressure drop is even more important. Velocity is inversely proportional to cross-sectional area (Eq. 3). Because of conservation of mass, blood flow accelerates when it enters the narrow part of the stenosis, thereby increasing its kinetic energy. This happens at the expense of potential energy, which is pressure. The relation between these two terms is described by Bernoulli's law:

$$P + \tfrac{1}{2}\rho v^2 = \text{constant} \qquad \text{Eq. 8}$$

where P is pressure, ρ is mass density of blood, and v is velocity. This law expresses the conservation of energy for inviscid flow, with pressure representing a potential energy and $\tfrac{1}{2}\rho v^2$ a kinetic

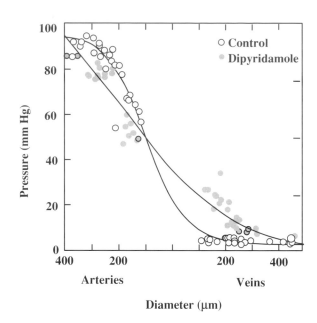

FIGURE 4-11. Gradual drop of pressure in the coronary arterial system and its alteration by vasodilation indicates that all small arteries with a diameter less than 400 μm play a role in coronary flow control. *(Data from Chilian et al., 1989.[3])*

energy per unit volume. The term $\tfrac{1}{2}\rho v^2$ is often referred to as *dynamic pressure.**

In a normal coronary artery, velocity varies between 10 cm/s and 75 cm/s, but may exceed 1 m/s during vasodilation (Figure 4-11). For the example of a velocity of 1 m/s, the dynamic pressure for blood is approximately 500 Pa, which corresponds to about 3.3 mm Hg. Hence, under normal conditions dynamic pressure is not seriously high. However, in a 75% area stenosis, velocity is a factor of 4 higher that in the proximal vessel segment and dynamic pressure is 16 times higher. Hence, for the example velocity of 1 m/s in the nonstenotic vessel, static pressure drops because of an increase of dynamic pressure by be 52.8 mm Hg in the stenosis. This pressure drop is much more serious than a pressure drop as the result of viscous losses in such a stenosis of 1 cm length.

The pressure energy as a result of the increase in dynamic pressure within the stenosis is not entirely lost, because deceleration of flow at the diameter expansion converts some kinetic energy back to static pressure. However, static pressure is not fully recovered because of eddies that are caused by the expanding jet just distal of the stenosis, and the resulting energy loss because of heat dissipation. The pressure drop relating to these energy losses is also known as *exit losses.*

The pressure drop over a stenosis is thus the sum of viscous and exit losses

$$\Delta p = \Delta p_v + \Delta p_e$$
$$= A \cdot v + B \cdot v^2 \qquad \text{Eq. 9}$$

Coefficients A and B relate to geometric factors of the stenosis and density and viscosity of blood.

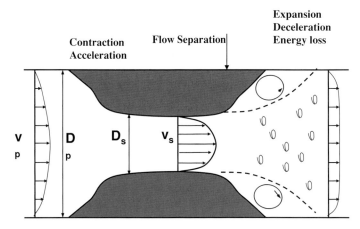

FIGURE 4-10. Illustration of convective acceleration of blood flowing into a narrowing. When leaving the narrowing, blood flow is decelerated, but eddies are created that absorb energy as well.

---

* The wings of airplanes are designed such that airspeed is higher on the top of the wing than airspeed at the bottom of the wing, resulting in a difference between dynamic pressure. Because the sum of static and dynamic pressure must be equal, the static pressure under the wing is higher and provides the lift force for the plane.

Because resistance is by definition equal to the pressure drop divided by flow, Eq. 9 results in the following relation between stenosis resistance, R_{sten}, and flow:

$$R_{sten} = R_{visc} + BQ \qquad \text{Eq. 10}$$

The first term on the right side of the equation is the viscous resistance, and the second term is the result of the exit losses of the stenosis. Hence, resistance of a stenosis is not constant, but depends linearly on flow through the stenosis. Note that B is constant for a given stenosis geometry.

【 】 STENOSIS PRESSURE–FLOW RELATIONSHIP IN HUMANS

In the past, the curvilinear pressure gradient–flow relationships of a stenosis have been determined in vitro as well as in animal experiments. At present, these seminal studies still form the basis for interpretation of pressure gradient–flow relations of stenosis in humans. With the availability of sensor-equipped guidewires, it is now possible to measure the pressure gradient–flow velocity relation of a coronary artery stenosis in patients. A typical result is demonstrated in Figure 4-12.

The data depicted in Figure 4-12 were obtained at different stages during treatment of the lesion: pretreatment, after balloon inflation, and after stent placement. Flow was increased by inducing maximal vasodilation of the downstream resistance vessels via a bolus of adenosine. With each treatment step, the stenosis became less severe and the maximally obtainable flow increased while the pressure drop for a given flow decreased. The solid curves represent a quadratic least-squares fit to the data and validate the shape predicted by the theories underlying the pressure drop–velocity relationship for the human situation. The dotted lines are drawn from the origin to the endpoint of the fitted pressure drop–velocity curves. The slopes of these curves indicate the stenosis resistance at full vasodilation. The implication and use of these relationships for clinical decision making are discussed next.

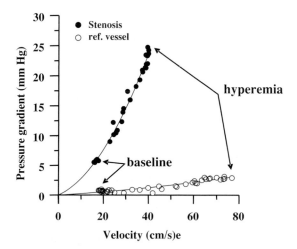

FIGURE 4-12. Measurement of pressure–flow velocity relationship of a stenosis compared to that of a reference vessel. Note the quadratic nature of the stenosis pressure–velocity relationship.

CONTROL OF CORONARY BLOOD FLOW

Earlier we discussed coronary pressure–flow lines at full dilation. However, the coronary circulation rarely operates under these conditions. The vasodilation of the coronary bed is a reference state used in the clinical situation to indicate the range of flow that the coronary system has available to allow for increased cardiac work, and in physiology to discuss the effect of cardiac contraction and arterial pressure on coronary resistance. Normally, coronary blood flow is well controlled and adapted to the needs of the heart. If cardiac work becomes so high that maximal dilatation is obtained, the heart operates on the verge of ischemia.

【 】 CHARACTERIZATION AND LOCALIZATION OF CORONARY BLOOD FLOW CONTROL

Coronary blood flow normally adapts to myocardial oxygen demand when arterial pressure is also constant. This adaptation to oxygen consumption is denoted as *metabolic flow adaptation* as well as *functional hyperemia*. The constancy of flow at constant oxygen consumption despite changes in pressure is denoted *autoregulation*. Although metabolic adaptation and autoregulation are defined separately, both are probably the result of the same feedback mechanism. An autoregulation curve is depicted schematically in Figure 4-13.

Isolated hearts also demonstrate metabolic flow adaptation and autoregulation. These processes are thus based primarily on local feedback, although central neural and humoral factors interact with this control system. The local nature of flow control in the coronary system is important for heart transplantation, where no direct neural pathways between the donor heart and the recipient's central nervous system exist. Animal experiments demonstrated that denervation affects the rate of the coronary resistance response to changes in the workload of the heart, but not the steady state flow control properties.[30]

A simple way to understand the relationship among flow, coronary arterial pressure, and oxygen consumption is to assume that tissue oxygen pressure is the controlled variable. Tissue oxygen pressure is then assumed to affect arteriolar resistance in such a way that a decrease in oxygen pressure results in dilation and an increase in oxygen pressure results in constriction. Tissue oxygen pressure can be reduced by increasing oxygen consumption or by decreasing perfusion pressure. In these conditions, vasodilation results in an increase of blood flow or a restoration of tissue oxygen pressure, respectively. The control of blood flow, or tissue oxygen PO_2 for that matter, is the result of different interacting mechanisms that are discussed later in the chapter. However, it is not clear which molecule is responsible for the signaling between tissue PO_2 and vasomotor tone.

It is important to recognize that flow is controlled not just by a single vessel type, but that all arteries smaller than approximately 400 μm are contributing. This conclusion is drawn from pressure distribution measurements in the coronary arterial tree. In the beating cat heart, pressure pipettes were inserted in small arteries and veins, which was made possible by high-frequency ventilation of the cat at the heart frequency, and image freezing by applying a stroboscope, allowing the visualization of the epicardium at a fixed moment in the cardiac cycle. Results of this study are provided in Figure 4-11. The figure shows that with tone intact, the pressure starts to drop in vessels of 300 μm in diameter and is already reduced to 40 mm Hg

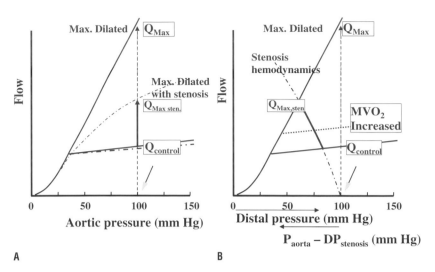

FIGURE 4-13. Schematic pressure-flow diagrams elucidating the effects of a coronary stenosis on coronary flow reserve. (**A**) The resistance of the stenosis is added to the baseline and hyperemic resistance of the microcirculation. Flow at a given aortic pressure decreased because of the pressure drop over the stenosis. (**B**) The flow-dependent pressure drop over the stenosis, $\Delta P_{stenosis}$, is separated from the coronary pressure–flow diagram. The x-axis represents pressure, being the distal pressure when applied to the microcirculation with zero at the origin of the axis system and stenosis pressure drop being zero at zero flow, but increases more than proportional with increasing flow.

at the level of 100 μm arterioles. The remaining pressure drop is over the part of the tree that was not accessible for the pressure measurement. With vasodilation, the pressure starts to drop at vessels of 400 μm. Note also the pressure increase in the small veins with vasodilation, which implies that capillary pressure increased tremendously as a result of the vasodilation. Because pressure decreases gradually along vessels from 400 μm down, all these vessels must be involved in local control of blood flow. This raises the question of how the control actions of all these segments are tuned. Before discussing this issue, we describe some essential mechanisms involved in the control of smooth muscle tone.

【 】 MECHANISMS OF SMOOTH MUSCLE TONE CONTROL IN CORONARY RESISTANCE ARTERIES

Responses of resistance vessels to vasoactive stimuli are generally studied either in isolated cannulated vessels where pressure and flow can be controlled independently or by direct observations of epicardial or endocardial arteriolar diameter in the beating heart. Obviously, direct in vivo observations are very important but their interpretation is hampered by the interaction of responses by vessels not under observation. These interpretation problems are not present when studying isolated vessels in vitro; however, it is always the question of what is changed by removing the vessel out of its "networking" environment. Later we discuss results from both types of experiments. Only a limited amount of mechanisms are discussed and the choice is made by the purpose to demonstrate interaction of control mechanisms in the coronary circulation. For a more detailed review, the reader is referred to a review article on this topic.[60]

Myogenic tone

When smooth muscle is fully relaxed and at full vasodilation, the shape of the pressure diameter relation is fully dominated by the

extracellular matrix, with elastin and collagen as the major components. However, this is not the normal state of the vascular wall. The normal state is that smooth muscle has a basal tone and maintains the diameter of the vessel below that at full vasodilation. This basal tone increases when pressure increases, and this may even result in a decrease of vascular diameter. The constriction and resulting increase in resistance induced by an increase of pressure is denoted *myogenic response*.

Obviously, the myogenic response helps establish autoregulation of an organ. Autoregulation requires an increase in resistance with increasing coronary pressure. However, the myogenic response by itself cannot fully account for autoregulation, because it misses the link to a metabolic signal. A major role of the myogenic response is to compensate for the destabilizing effect described by Laplace's law, which relates wall tension to pressure and diameter

$$P = \sigma \, R/d \qquad\qquad \text{Eq. 11}$$

where σ is wall stress, d is wall thickness, and R is radius. Hence, when at a certain pressure the radius of a vessel increases, the wall tension becomes smaller, which results in an increase of the radius and further reduction in wall tension. This is a phenomenon we all recognize from inflating a balloon, which takes less effort as the balloon increases in volume. This increasing ease of inflation is concomitant to an increasing stress in the wall of the balloon. Without myogenic tone the vessels would always be maximally dilated or must be replaced by a different pressure-induced constrictor mechanism. Hence, myogenic tone is needed for stabilization of vessel diameter at a certain pressure. The myogenic tone is independent of the endothelium.[61,62]

In general, tone increase is related to an increase in intercellular calcium, but the myogenic tone requires a much smaller increase in calcium than other stimuli for the development of tone.[63] A complicating factor is that addition of a pulsatile component to the pressure signal reduces the myogenic tone.[64]

Flow-dependent dilation

Increasing blood flow through arteries resulting in vasodilation was first observed in larger arteries in 1933.[65] However, it was more than 50 years later that the role of the endothelium in this response was established by varying the viscosity of the perfusion medium in isolated artery preparations, thereby demonstrating that shear stress was an important factor.[66–68] Shear stress leads to an increased NO-synthase activity in these cells, which in turn enhances the production of NO from L-arginine. NO diffuses to the adjacent smooth muscle cells in the media, where it mediates the transformation of guanosine triphosphate into cyclic guanosine monophosphate, which in turn leads to a decrease in intracellular Ca^{2+}, causing vasodilation by relaxing the smooth muscle tone. Flow-dependent dilation interacts with the myogenic response,[62] and its strength depends on the size of the blood vessel.[8] Also, flow-dependent dilation cannot by itself fulfill the conditions of a control system. An increase of flow would result in a reduced resistance, which causes an increased flow, which would result in further dilation.

There is also a difference between the effect of steady and pulsatile shear stress. Oscillating shear stress by itself generates oxygen radicals that scavenge NO, and does not result in vasodilation.[69] There is evidence that NO release is mediated by the glycocalyx covering the endothelium.[70,71] Enzymatic destruction of this layer diminishes the production of NO by shear, although acetylcholine still induces NO release by the endothelium.

Adenosine

Adenosine has been proposed as the link between metabolism and smooth muscle tone. It was thought that interstitial adenosine concentrations would increase following an increase in ATP phosphorylation.[72] Adenosine concentrations in venous blood and interstitial fluid indeed increased with increasing oxygen consumption, but administration of adenosine deaminase reduced these adenosine levels considerably without affecting the characteristics of flow control.[73,74] It was later considered that adenosine was being compartmentalized at sufficient local concentrations to affect tone in resistance vessels without being detectable in venous blood or interstitial fluid. However, detailed theoretical modeling of the fate of adenosine revealed that adenosine concentrations remain below a level at which it actively affects smooth muscle tone.[75,76]

Adenosine certainly plays a role during ischemia. Blockage of adenosine production results in a diminished reactive hyperemic response.[73] There are many other important functions of adenosine, for example, in ischemia reperfusion, but these are not related to physiologic flow control.

Endothelin is a vasoconstrictor, and one wonders why a vasoconstrictor would be important for metabolic control, because this is generally considered a vasodilatory response to an increase in metabolism. However, one needs constriction in order to have vasodilation. Endothelin may very well be the required endogenous vasoconstrictor. However, this implies that the level of preconstriction is an important factor in setting the level of tone from which metabolic vasodilators act as modulators dependent on metabolism. Evidence indicates that endothelin is modulated by alpha-adrenergic receptors, linking the preconstrictor level to the neural system.

K_{ATP}-*channels* have been implicated in the control of coronary blood flow. Blocking of these channels results in higher levels of oxygen extraction by the heart, but flow remains, changing with oxygen consumption.[77,78] Blockage of these channels reduced the rate by which smooth muscle adapts to changes in metabolic conditions or pressure by a factor of 4.[79]

Endothelial-Dependent Hyperpolarizing Factor

It was found that smooth muscle hyperpolarization can be achieved by shear stress, which results in vasodilation. This so-called EDHF is not NO-mediated, but is H_2O_2-mediated, and may be used as a backup system for flow-mediated dilation under conditions where the NO-related system fails.[80]

Neural and Humoral Factors

Beta-receptor stimulation results in a rapid coronary flow increase and it is believed that this acts as a feed-forward mechanism, increasing coronary blood flow in the expectation that the oxygen consumption will rise.[81,82] It should also be noted that in local flow control the dilatory responses are faster than the constrictor responses.[83,84]

[ ] INTERACTION OF MECHANISMS OF VASCULAR TONE

Coronary resistance is controlled by small arteries and arterioles with diameters between 400 μm and 10 μm. Under normal circumstances these vessels have a significant pressure drop, and they respond differently to many different stimuli. In isolated vessels, the myogenic response is the strongest in vessels of about 90 μm,[7,8] and it is less in smaller and larger vessels. Flow-dependent dilation is stronger in the larger than in the smaller vessels, and in vessels taken from the subendocardium, flow-dependent dilation is larger than in epicardial vessels.[69] Casting studies demonstrated that the smaller arterioles are in close contact with the myocytes and capillary bed,[33] in contrast to the larger resistance arteries. From these observations, the picture emerges on how smaller and larger resistance vessels interact to form an integral flow-control system.

A prerequisite for a resistance vessel to contribute to flow control is the presence of constrictive tone. Myogenic tone acts as in the larger resistance vessels, but is not strong enough in the smallest vessels because the stimulus for constriction, pressure, is too small. Endothelin acts as a constrictor, but there may be several other factors. The smallest vessels sense the metabolic signal or combination of signals. On a dilatory response of the smallest vessels, flow increases in all vessels proximal to it along the flow pathway. The increased flow in these larger vessels then contributes to the flow control by further vasodilation.[85,86] Hence, flow-dependent dilation acts as an amplifier of the metabolic signal, which affects only the smallest resistance vessels.[87] These interactions between smaller and larger resistance vessels have been studied both experimentally and theoretically. Observations on the epicardial small vessels in a dog heart preparation demonstrated that blocking the endothelial NO production by LNAME results in vasoconstriction of the proximal resistance vessels and compensatory vasodilation in vessels smaller than 200 μm.[85] In a theoretical model, the resistance distribution over the arterial tree was represented by a series of 10 adjustable resistances, each corresponding to a certain class of arterial diameters. Each compartment was assigned flow-dependent and myogenic properties, and their interaction was studied.[87] The resulting findings underlined the need for constrictor activity in the smaller resistance vessels in order to modulate the tone in these vessels by a metabolic signal. Furthermore, these studies demonstrated that the myogenic response alone results in autoregulation behavior of the model, which is then being annihilated by flow-dependent dilation.[5] The myogenic response to a change in arterial pressure was strongest in vessels of 190-μm diameter, whereas myogenic strength in response to local pressure was distributed according to the measured values from isolated vessels, and therefore was strongest in vessels of 90 μm. This apparent shift of location of maximal sensitivity is caused by myogenic vessel segments in series. A change in perfusion pressure induces myogenic changes in all vessel segments, thereby altering the pressure distribution over these segments. In the 190-μm segment, the combination of myogenic sensitivity and pressure change is larger than in the 90-μm segments. This highlights the important role of the network structure itself, in addition to the control properties of single vessels.

【 】 DRUGS AND CORONARY FLOW REGULATION

Knowledge of mechanisms of flow control is also important to understand the action of drugs. Often a drug is administered and the flow response is measured, whereby an increase in flow is considered to be an indication of vasodilation. Such an interpretation is much too simple. One must realize that coronary blood flow is the result of such interacting factors as coronary arterial pressure, diastolic ventricular pressure, diastolic time fraction, and oxygen consumption. A drug may result in vasodilation in an indirect way, for example, by increasing oxygen consumption.[88,89]

The beneficial role of a beta-blocker is generally explained by its reduction in oxygen consumption because of a reduced heart rate. However, the reduction in heart rate also increases diastolic time fraction, which is the major determinant for subendocardial perfusion when coronary reserve is exhausted.

EFFECT OF A STENOSIS ON CORONARY FLOW

A coronary stenosis not only limits the flow rate at maximal vasodilation, but also alters several parameters of the coronary flow control system. Analysis of the interaction of a stenosis with the physiologic responses of the coronary circulation is complicated by the flow-dependent pressure drop over the stenosis.

【 】 STENOSIS AND LIMITATION OF CORONARY RESERVE

Ischemia is induced when coronary flow is not sufficient to match oxygen demand. Because the coronary circulation usually has a large reserve and may accommodate an increase in oxygen demand by a factor of 4, a stenosis need not be an immediate threat to the myocardium. The coronary microcirculation responds with vasodilation to compensate for the pressure drop over the stenosis, but this diminishes its capacity to dilate further in order to increase flow when needed for an increased oxygen demand. These effects are illustrated in Figure 4-13 by two different diagrams, each elucidating the same stenosis effect but in a different way. In both cases it is assumed that aortic pressure equals 100 mm Hg. The case without stenosis is identically sketched in both panels by the heavy lines. At maximal dilation, the pressure-flow line is straight in the physiologic pressure range but curvilinear at lower pressures (see also Figure 4-11). In the case of autoregulation, the pressure–flow line has a slightly upward-sloping plateau. Flow increases with pressure, but much less than with the fully vasodilated case.

The principles of coronary perfusion in the absence and presence of a stenosis as outlined previously are best visualized in Figure 4-13B where the stenosis and microvascular hemodynamics are separated. The vertical line at P = 100 mm Hg indicates the no-stenosis case and is depicted for reference. The curve representing stenosis pressure drop as function of flow (Eq. 9) is drawn to the left of this line. The combined system of stenosis and microcirculation must fulfill the rules for stenosis hemodynamics and microvascular circulation. During control, this is the case at the intersection of the stenosis curve with the autoregulatory plateau:

at maximal vasodilation, at the intersection with the line representing full dilation. Note that for a given stenosis, distal pressure decreases nonlinearly with increasing flow. Hence, despite a constant aortic pressure, as in this example, the pressure distal of the stenosis is not a constant, but depends on oxygen demand. In this diagram, it is not so difficult to further analyze what happens when stenosis degree or hyperemic resistance changes by factors discussed earlier. An increase in stenosis severity increases the pressure drop for a given flow rate, and the stenosis curve intersects the coronary pressure–flow line at vasodilation at a lower flow rate. An increase in hyperemic coronary resistance causes a decrease in the slope of the pressure–flow line at vasodilation, and thereby leads to a decrease in maximal flow for a given perfusion pressure. Both events combined can seriously impede adequate perfusion of the cardiac muscle tissue, leading to ischemia or infarction.

Figure 4-13A considers the stenosis and microvascular resistance to be a series of compartments, and relates flow to the aortic input pressure on the horizontal axis. In this case, the coronary pressure–flow line at maximum vasodilation is no longer a straight line, but its slope decreases with increasing flow, because stenosis resistance increases with flow (see Eq. 10). Moreover, the autoregulatory curve in the presence of a stenosis deviates from the curve obtained without, although the difference is small. The advantage of this representation is that it is easier to see how coronary reserve is reduced by the presence of a stenosis, but does not provide insight into the level of perfusion pressure distal of the stenosis and how this decreases with oxygen demand.

【 】 STENOSIS AND MICROVASCULAR TONE

In Figure 4-5, we discussed that pulsatility of intracoronary pressure and flow depends on the degree of a stenosis. The pressure pulse changes into a left ventricular pressure signal and the flow pulsations become smaller. It is difficult to predict these changes in pressure and flow at the level of resistance vessels, because these depend on the position of the resistance vessel within the myocardium. Pulsatility of flow and vascular transmural pressure are normally larger in the subendocardium than in the subepicardium. However, these patterns change in the presence of a stenosis. Most likely, the variations at the subendocardium decline in the presence of a stenosis because reverse flow is impeded by the stenosis. At the same time, pulsatility of flow and vascular transmural pressure at the subepicardium increases as a result of the interaction with the subendocardium. There are indications that these alterations result in a significant net reduction of the dilatory response of the subendocardial arterioles after a decrease in coronary arterial perfusion pressure.[90]

EVALUATION OF CORONARY BLOOD FLOW VELOCITY AND PRESSURE IN THE CATHETERIZATION LABORATORY

Some indication of coronary flow can be obtained from the rate at which contrast medium advances within a major coronary artery or spreads over the myocardium. However, the ability to make use of the physiologic principles discussed previously in humans came with the introduction of sensor-equipped guidewires. First, a wire with a crystal to measure Doppler velocity was developed, which was followed by a guidewire that incorporated a pressure transducer. More recently, guidewires combining both pressure and velocity measurement are being developed.[91] Each technique introduced its own model to quantify the impact of a stenosis on the perfusion of the heart, and with a cut-off value for the resulting index that indicated whether treatment of the stenosis was imperative or could be deferred. Demonstration of inducible ischemia by noninvasive tests such as SPECT has been used as the gold standard for most of these studies.

We discuss these indices in light of these physiologic studies and compare their predictions on theoretic and experimental grounds.

【 】 CORONARY FLOW VELOCITY IS MORE THAN JUST A SURROGATE FOR FLOW

Physiologic experiments in animals have focused on the measurement of flow in coronary arteries, and especially on flow per unit weight. The reason for this is simply that in order to balance oxygen supply with oxygen demand, one needs flow instead of velocity. However, when coronary artery flow is measured in absolute units, one must also know the amount of tissue that is perfused by the artery. The diameter of an epicardial artery correlates well with perfused area,[92] and therefore flow may be low because of a smaller amount of tissue perfused by the artery and not because of impediment by a stenosis. Because the perfused tissue mass is not easy to determine in a clinical setting, it is not always useful to strive for an absolute measure of volume flow.

Blood-flow velocity may be a valuable signal in its own right. For example, if one is interested in estimating wall-shear stress, an estimate of velocity is more useful than an estimate of flow. Moreover, in healthy coronary vessels, velocity is rather independent of the location of measurement in the epicardial arteries[93] or of the amount of perfused mass.[92] One could say that velocity is related to the flow scaled by mass, as has been found for normal arteries under resting conditions. However, this relation no longer holds in diseased arteries as a result of the geometric changes induced by the vascular disease process. Because tone affects diameter and thus velocity for a given volume flow, it is advisable to administer intracoronary nitroglycerine to minimize tone in the larger epicardial arteries. When two conditions at different arterial pressures are compared, one must be aware of the fact that the diameter is pressure dependent in the absence of tone as well. Volume flow in a vessel is frequently estimated from the product of mean cross-sectional velocity and vessel area (Eq. 3). However, several possible errors are introduced when determining flow in this way. The Doppler sensor measures maximal velocity in the vessel lumen, and this has a fixed relationship only to the average cross-sectional velocity (Eq. 4) when the velocity profile has a parabolic shape. The curvature of the coronary vessels and the pulsatile nature of the flow reduce the applicability of this fixed relationship. Moreover, although vessel diameter can readily be measured from an angiogram to determine the cross-sectional area, the vessel has not always a circular shape at the site of measurement. As mentioned earlier, vessel diameter at the site of measurement may vary because of variations in tone induced by neural, humoral, or pharmacologic stimuli. In addition, vessel diameter

changes continuously as a function of pulsatile pressure, and one must measure vessel diameter under the same conditions and during the same phase of the cardiac cycle as velocity. Frequently, peak velocity averaged over a cardiac cycle is used together with end-diastolic vessel diameter, which introduces an underestimation of the calculated volume flow.

【 】 CORONARY FLOW VELOCITY RESERVE

In the earlier physiology literature, coronary flow reserve was defined as difference between control blood flow and hyperemic blood flow at the same aortic pressure. This difference indicates the extra amount of flow that is available for cardiac work at the prevailing control condition, as illustrated in Figure 4-13. The cardiology oriented literature introduced *coronary flow reserve (CFR)* as the ratio of hyperemic flow to control flow, which was considered to be a more practical index. With the development of intracoronary devices measuring flow velocity instead of volume flow, the concept of *coronary flow velocity reserve (CFVR)* was introduced as the ratio of maximal to baseline flow velocity. Vessel diameter changes at the location of velocity measurement induced by local change of vascular tone may be prevented by administration of nitroglycerine, but pressure distal of a stenosis decreases after the administration of a microvascular vasodilator such as adenosine. This reduction in pressure leads to a smaller diameter, and thus to a higher value of hyperemic velocity than would be measured without this passive diameter decrease. Hence, CFVR may overestimate CFR because of this reason. However, because the values of CFVR are interpreted in their clinical context without translation to volume flow reserve, it is not always necessary to consider these differences.

The physiologic idea behind application of reserve is that pharmacologic dilation resulting in an increase of flow by a certain factor indicates a possible equivalent exercise hyperemia of the same level. Clinical studies where CFVR was compared to noninvasive measures of inducible ischemia as estimated by SPECT resulted in a cut-off value of 2 or 2.5. Problems with the application of CFR and CFVR relate to the fact that it is an integral measure of both the status of the microcirculation and of the impairment by the stenosis. By definition, their values depend on the magnitude of flow (or velocity) at baseline conditions, which in turn depends on the oxygen consumption at the time of measurement. Furthermore, hyperemic flow (or velocity) depends on pressure and, as discussed earlier, microvascular tone is influenced by several other factors that cannot always be controlled during the catheterization procedure.

【 】 RELATIVE CORONARY FLOW VELOCITY RESERVE

In order to overcome the difficulties with respect to basal flow in the target vessel, *relative coronary flow reserve (RCFR)* was introduced. It was originally defined as the ratio between the hyperemic flow in an artery with stenosis and the hyperemic flow in the same artery without stenosis,[94] which makes this parameter independent of basal flow, and thereby eliminates one factor of uncertainty associated with CFR in assessing the hemodynamic severity of a stenosis. Because it is not possible in the clinical setting to assess CFR in the target vessel without the stenosis, CFR measured in a perfusion area supplied by an undiseased reference vessel is substituted, assuming that the hyperemic state of the microcirculation is homogeneous over the heart muscle and at least part of the myocardium can function as reference. RCFR can then be determined from imaging technologies such as *positron emission tomography (PET)*.

The concept of relative coronary flow reserve has been extended to the application with flow velocity wires as well. The ratio of CFVR in the diseased vessel compared to that in the reference vessel is denoted *relative coronary flow velocity reserve (RCFVR)*. In a small set of selected patients this method worked rather well,[95] but in a larger cohort, the method appeared not to have a better predictive value than flow velocity reserve by itself.[96]

【 】 FRACTIONAL FLOW RESERVE

As a practical extension of the previously described concept, one can assess the reduction in maximal flow as the result of a stenosis in an indirect way by a pressure measurement distal to a stenosis under hyperemic conditions. The *pressure-derived myocardial fractional flow reserve (FFR)* was originally defined as the ratio of distal pressure to aortic pressure during maximal hyperemia, assuming that venous pressure can be regarded as zero,[97]

$$FFR = \frac{Q_s}{Q_n} = \frac{(P_d - P_v) \cdot R_{m,n}}{(P_a - P_v) \cdot R_{m,s}} \approx \frac{P_d}{P_a} \qquad \text{Eq. 12a}$$

Note that this equivalence is true only under the assumption that microvascular resistance in the dilated myocardial vascular bed distal to a normal ($R_{m,n}$), and to a diseased ($R_{m,s}$) artery is the same.

A cut-off value of 0.75 was derived based on clinical studies where FFR was compared to a number of noninvasive indices of reversible ischemia. This simply means that at an aortic pressure of 100 mm Hg, a pressure of 75 mm Hg or higher distal of the stenosis during hyperemia is regarded as sufficient to guarantee adequate blood supply of the coronary microcirculation during maximal flow. The applicability FFR for decision making in diagnosis and treatment evaluation has been established in a number of clinical trials.[98,99] The practical application of this concept of FFR by pressure measurement is illustrated by the model depicted in Figure 4-14, where the coronary circulation is represented by a stenosis resistance, R_s, is in series with the microvascular resistance distal to the stenosis, R_m, during maximal hyperemia. Such a schematic is known in engineering as a voltage (pressure) divider, which relates FFR to the ratio between microvascular resistance and total resistance as follows:

$$FFR = \frac{P_d - P_v}{P_a - P_v} = \frac{Q \cdot R_m}{Q \cdot (R_s + R_m)} = \frac{R_m}{R_s + R_m} \qquad \text{Eq. 12b}$$

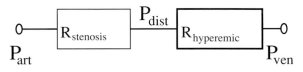

FIGURE 4-14. Model for FFR considering the stenosis resistance in series with the coronary microvascular resistance during maximal hyperemia.

Expressed this way, FFR becomes significant (< 0.75) when coronary microvascular resistance is less than three times the stenosis resistance during hyperemia.

The advantage of FFR is that it focuses on the reduction of maximal possible flow at full dilation and is independent of baseline conditions with tone present. Another strong advantage of FFR is that the measurement of pressure is more stable than that of flow velocity because it does not depend on the orientation of the sensor to the flow field. Furthermore, it has a definite normal value of 1 in case of no stenosis (ie, in the absence of a pressure gradient). However, it is important to realize that FFR is not strictly a stenosis-specific parameter, because according to Eq. 12b, it is a function not only of stenosis resistance, but also of hyperemic microvascular resistance distal to the stenosis, which may vary with hemodynamic conditions at the time of measurement and is subject to changes caused by disease processes. Owing to the flow dependence of stenosis resistance and the pressure dependence of the microcirculation at maximal vasodilation, it can be appreciated that FFR is theoretically not independent of aortic pressure and factors that affect hyperemic microvascular resistance.[100] The combined effect of hemodynamic changes on FFR depends on their relative influence on stenosis and microvascular resistance. It is therefore difficult to demonstrate the hemodynamic dependence of FFR in vivo, more so because interaction of hemodynamic effects on alteration of a single parameter such as aortic pressure or heart rate cannot be avoided. In a patient study, administering norepinephrine to manipulate aortic-pressure FFR appeared to be rather constant.[101] However, further experimental evaluation using a wide variation of conditions is warranted, bearing attention to the separate influence on stenosis and microvascular resistance.

【 】 HYPEREMIC VELOCITY-BASED STENOSIS RESISTANCE INDEX

The combined measurement of pressure drop across a stenosis and distal flow velocity allows the calculation of a velocity-based stenosis resistance index under hyperemic conditions, HSR

$$HSR = \frac{\Delta P}{v} \qquad \text{Eq. 13}$$

This index aims at quantifying the impediment to maximal flow caused exclusively by the stenosis. In a clinical study involving a large patient population where HSR was compared to SPECT outcomes, a value of 0.8 mm Hg/cm/s was found as the threshold for prediction of reversible ischemia.[102]

As discussed earlier, stenosis resistance is flow dependent, and flow through a given stenosis depends on microvascular resistance. Thus, HSR is still dependent on microvascular resistance, but to a lesser extent than FFR or CFVR because it is a ratio of pressure gradient and velocity, which change in the same direction during induced vasodilation. Therefore, HSR is less sensitive to achieving maximal vasodilation (minimal microvascular resistance) than FFR or CFVR. One can predict this effect from the model of stenosis resistance in series with microvascular resistance as given in Figure 4-14. Applying this circuit and using average pressure gradients and flow velocities at rest and hyperemia, we calculated the relative change in these parameters for stenoses with the top 25 HSRs in our study (avg. HSR = 3.63 mm Hg/cm/s). For a 10%

and 25% decrease in maximal flow, the resulting change for FFR was +15% and +35%, for CFVR −12% and- −27%, and for HSR −2% and −6%, respectively. Therefore, achievement of maximal vasodilation is not as critical for evaluation of stenosis severity by HSR as it is for either FFR or CFVR.[102]

【 】 FFR, CFVR, SR_v AND THE PREDICTION OF ISCHEMIA BY SPECT

In a group of 181 patients, FFR, CFVR, SR_v, and SPECT were determined,[103] which allows the comparison of these techniques in predicting ischemia. Using SPECT as the gold standard and applying the ROC analysis we found the highest accuracy for SR_v, 87%, and for CFVR as well as FFR the accuracy rate was 75%. Hence, the highest accuracy was obtained for the index that quantifies the stenosis with the least influence of microvascular resistance. In order to clarify the results obtained by the three intracoronary indices, their concomitantly obtained values in the same patients are compared later in the chapter.

The comparison between the respective thresholds for clinical decision-making FFR and CFVR is depicted in Figure 4-15, which also contains division lines at FFR = 0.75 and CFVR = 2. Although the scatter between the two parameters is considerable, the suggestion for treatment or deferral was concordant in about three quarters of the cases. However, it is especially important to understand the disparity between the two indices in those quadrants where conflicting conclusions are suggested. If FFR was 0.75 or more and CFVR less than 2, the FFR measurements suggest deferral of treatment, whereas CFVR demands it; if FFR was less than 0.75 and CFVR was 2 or more, it is the opposite, with FFR demanding treatment and CFVR suggesting that treatment be deferred. These discordant outcomes were found in 27% of the cases, which is a considerable fraction.

It was found that hyperemic microvascular resistance was different in these two discordant groups. It was significantly higher in the quadrant where FFR was above the threshold but CFVR below (lower right) the threshold, compared to the quadrant where FFR

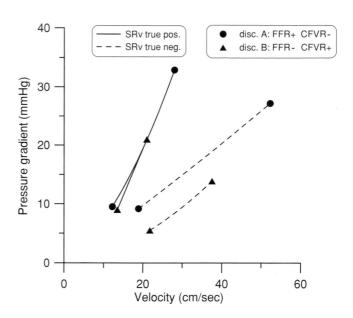

FIGURE 4-16. Stenosis pressure gradient–velocity curves obtained in coronary arteries of patients. SR_v correctly predicted the absence (dashed line) or presence (solid line) of reversible ischemia, whereas FFR and CFVR had discordant outcomes. Hyperemic microvascular resistance was significantly lower in group A than in group B.

was below and CFVR above its respective threshold (upper left). According to the model shown in Figure 4-14 and Eq. 12, it can be understood why a lower microvascular resistance results in a higher FFR for the same stenosis. Lower microvascular resistance results in a higher flow through the stenosis and therefore higher-pressure drop over the stenosis.

The role that microvascular resistance plays with respect to the three intracoronary indices is illustrated in Figure 4-16. It shows the average stenosis pressure drop-velocity curves (see Figure 4-12) for the two discordant groups in FFR and CFVR, grouped according to their prediction of inducible ischemia as determined by SPECT. These curves show the quadratic pressure drop-velocity relationships connecting the average baseline date in each subgroup with corresponding hyperemic data. True positive results in HSR (inducible ischemia) have a steeper pressure drop-velocity relationship (solid curves) reflecting a higher stenosis resistance and true negative results (absence of ischemia) have curves with a lower slope (dashed curves). The curves for group B (triangles) are shorter due to a higher microvascular resistance during hyperemia resulting in reduced hyperemic flow velocities compared to group A (circles).

At a low microvascular resistance (group A, circles), FFR predicted ischemia despite a low stenosis resistance (dashed curve) due to the higher pressure drop induced by a high hyperemic velocity, whereas CVFR gives a too optimistic view of blood supply for a high stenosis resistance (solid curve), since the ratio between hyperemic and basal flow remained above the threshold due to the low value of baseline flow velocity (lower circle). Similarly, at a higher microvascular resistance (group B, triangles), FFR failed to predict inducible ischemia for a more severe stenosis (solid curve) because hyperemic velocity is reduced, resulting in a lower pressure gradient. And CFVR is false positive in the presence of a low stenosis resistance (dashed curve) due to a higher level of basal flow velocity (lower triangle) combined with a lower hyperemic flow velocity (upper triangle).

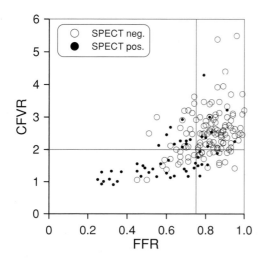

FIGURE 4-15. FFR versus CFVR. In 27% of these cases, there was discordance between the outcomes of these parameters. Agreement with SPECT outcomes was 75% for both parameters.

Stenosis resistance index also fails to predict reversible ischemia in about 10% of the cases. Partly this is the result of the imperfection of the gold standard, but that holds true for the other two indices as well. More important is the question of how it is that the stenosis resistance index predicts ischemia so well. One would expect that a certain stenosis resistance corresponds with ischemia in the presence of high microvascular resistance, but not in the presence of a low microvascular resistance, and the variability in microvascular resistance should be more reflected by a worse prediction of ischemia. It appears that the stenosis resistance index reflects the progression of vascular disease in its impact on oxygen supply to the myocardium. More studies, especially long-term studies, concerning the effects of stenosis on microvascular resistance are needed to come to a better understanding of the role of HSR.

【 】 PRESSURE GRADIENT–VELOCITY RELATIONSHIP FOR EVALUATION OF STENOSIS HEMODYNAMICS

The dual-sensor guidewire with combined measurement of pressure and velocity distal to a lesion allows for the construction of stenosis pressure gradient–velocity relationships in humans. These relationships provide a comprehensive visualization of the improvement in stenosis hemodynamics achieved by percutaneous coronary intervention[91] as illustrated in Figure 4-17. With each step of stenosis dilation (ballon angioplasty and stent placement), this effect was reflected by a clockwise lowering of the pressure drop-velocity relationship.

It is not yet clear whether the measurement of these curves results in a better prediction of reversible ischemia, than that already obtained by the hyperemic stenosis resistance index, as discussed previously. HSR is represented by the endpoint of the pressure drop-velocity relationship. However, visualization of these curves provides a much better insight into the hemodynamic behavior of the lesion under study during treatment.

In addition, compliant coronary lesions can be identified with this approach, because their geometric severity increases during the decrease in intraluminal pressure (according to Bernoulli's law) induced by increased flow after distal vasodilation. The typical curvilinear relationship for a fixed stenosis then changes into an open loop, which reflects the continuous geometric changes of a partially compliant stenosis throughout the hyperemic response to adenosine.

【 】 FUTURE DEVELOPMENTS

The work on combined measurement of pressure and velocity demonstrates the importance of a separate quantification of stenosis and microvascular resistance. At present, this is possible with a guidewire combining solid-state technology for measuring pressure and blood velocity independently.[91] It is also attempted to measure coronary flow indirectly by a pressure sensor–equipped guidewire by exploiting the thermal of the sensor and applying it in the thermodilution principle. At present, no absolute flows are measured with this technique, but it is the focus of measuring FFR and a ratio of mean transit times reflecting CFVR with a single pressure wire.[104,105] This method improves the analysis of stenosis severity in the conditions that FFR and CFVR provide a concordant outcome. It is, however, not clear how this method will improve the clinical decision making when these parameters are discordant.

This chapter has restricted itself to the analysis of single lesions, whereas many patients have multiple lesions in a coronary artery. Then it is important to quantify the relative resistances of the different diseased sites. An important step in this direction has been taken by measuring pullback pressure profiles in the coronary arteries, providing insight into the relative contribution of each lesion to the overall pressure drop over the diseased vessel.[106,107]

PERFUSION DISTRIBUTION

Flow and pressure signals in the epicardial arteries reveal essential physiologic mechanisms determining coronary blood flow and allow the quantification of vascular disease, but it is difficult to relate these measurements to distribution of perfusion over the myocardial wall. Yet, it is important that these distributions be understood, not only because they are of importance for understanding signals in the coronary artery, as in the case of collateral flow, but also for the cause of infarction, as in the case of subendocardial perfusion. This section does not analyze perfusion distribution in depth, but indicates the most important features.

【 】 SPATIAL HETEROGENEITY OF MYOCARDIAL PERFUSION

Measurements of flow by the microsphere technique led to the insight that perfusion is distributed heterogeneously over the myocardium during control and during maximal dilation.[108] Correlations between distribution of flow and metabolic factors suggest a strong relation between these two variables.[109] There exists, however, an important difference between the perfusion characteristics of the subendocardium and subepicardium. This difference becomes especially apparent during vasodilation, and

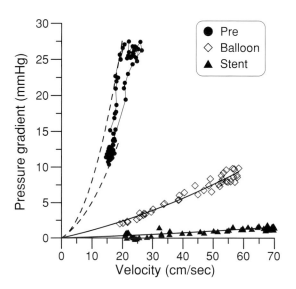

FIGURE 4-17. Example of development of pressure–velocity relations during treatment: untreated stenosis (Pre), after balloon deflation (Bal), and placement of a stent (Stent). Note that the relationship shows hysteresis pretreatment.

has the consequence that in the presence of a stenosis, subendocardial perfusion falls more rapidly than subepicardial perfusion.[110] This has to do with the more dominant effect of cardiac contraction on the subendocardial vessels. At a resting heart rate, the perfusion distribution between subepicardium and subendocardium is about even, but at a heart rate of 180 bpm and at full vasodilation, perfusion at the subendocardium is only half that of the subepicardium when perfusion pressure is maintained, and even lower when perfusion pressure is decreased by a stenosis.

【 】 COLLATERAL FLOW

In ischemic heart disease, the developments of collaterals form the rescue of tissue otherwise at risk. In humans, the collaterals are believed to be preexisting, but remodel during ischemia under the influence of several factors. Some publications demonstrate important roles for factors as VGEF,[111] and ICAM-1 and CD44,[112,113] while biophysical properties like shear stress also play an important role.

Collateral flow can be visualized by contrast injections at reduced pressure in the contralateral vessel, but may also be quantified by flow wires because flow in the epsilateral vessel increases on a balloon occlusion of the contralateral vessels.[114,115]

In many studies on the evaluation of the significance of a stenosis, cases are selected where collateral flow is not very significant. Collateral flow requires a pressure gradient, which is maximal if the contralateral bed is dilated and the epsilateral vessel is not. The flow through the contralateral bcd is the sum of the flow through the feeding artery and the collaterals. The flow in the contralateral artery is therefore an underestimate of the microvascular perfusion in that part of the vascular bed. Because this effect is stronger at vasodilation, that control collateral flow results in an underestimate of CFVR. In the presence of collaterals, the pressure drop over the stenosis is less without collaterals because of the flow reduction in the contralateral vessel, and therefore results in an overestimate of FFR.[116] A practical index for the collateral flow is the wedge pressure distal of the stenosis measured during angioplasty.[117] With more developed collateral flow, the wedge pressure is higher. Some caution is required because wedge pressure is higher than venous pressure in the absence of collaterals and is dependent on mechanical factors as well, especially diastolic left ventricular pressure, which may rise after a coronary occlusion of some duration.[118]

Theoretically, the stenosis resistance index is only marginally dependent on collateral flow. The only effect is that the range of velocity over which the stenosis pressure–velocity relation is measured is reduced, and the nonlinear behavior of the pressure–velocity relation causes a somewhat lower value of hyperemic resistance index than without collaterals. The estimate of this effect on the resistance index goes along the same lines as with a limited vasodilation discussed previously.

CONCLUSIONS AND SUMMARY

Coronary flow is the result of many interacting mechanisms of biophysical and biochemical nature. The intracoronary measurements of pressure and velocity bridge the clinical diagnosis to physiologic principles that until recently could only be studied in animals and by theoretical models. Bridging this gap between basic research and clinical diagnosis may prove to be very important in directing basic research into clinically relevant areas as well. In cases of arterial disease with single lesions, the combined measurement of pressure and velocity has been demonstrated to be very powerful. What is required is a better integration of physiological measurement with other information that is obtainable by other techniques like SPECT, QCA, and, in the future, MRI. These techniques are not only important for the diagnosis of stenosis severity, but also in evaluating new therapies directed to revascularization or stimulated collateral development.

REFERENCES

1. Downey JM, Kirk ES. Inhibition of coronary blood flow by a vascular waterfall mechanism. *Circ Res.* 1975;36:753.
2. Suga H, Sagawa K, Shoukas AA. Load independence of the instantaneous pressure-volume ratio of the canine left ventricle and effects of epenephrine and heart rate on the ratio. *Circulation.* 1973;32:314.
3. Chilian WM, Layne SM, Klausner EC et al. Redistribution of coronary microvascular resistance produced by dipyridamole. *Am J Physiol.* 1989; 256:H383.
4. Spaan JA, Breuls NP, Laird JD. Diastolic–systolic coronary flow differences are caused by intramyocardial pump action in the anesthetized dog. *Circ Res.* 1981;49(3):584.
5. Cornelissen AJ, Dankelman J, VanBavel E et al. Myogenic reactivity and resistance distribution in the coronary arterial tree: a model study. *Am J Physiol Heart Circ Physiol.* 2000;278(5):H1490.
6. Kajiya F, Tsujioka K, Ogasawara Y et al. Analysis of flow characteristics in poststenotic regions of the human coronary artery during bypass graft surgery. *Circulation.* 1987;76(5):1092.
7. Kuo L, Davis MJ, Chilian WM. Myogenic activity in isolated subepicardial and subendocardial coronary arterioles. *Am J Physiol.* 1988;255:H1558.
8. Liao JC, Kuo L. Interaction between adenosine and flow-induced dilation in coronary microvascular network. *Am J Physiol.* 1997;272(4 Pt 2):H1571.
9. Ladisa JF, Jr., Guler I, Olson LE et al. Three-dimensional computational fluid dynamics modeling of alterations in coronary wall shear stress produced by stent implantation. *Ann Biomed Eng.* 2003;31(8):972.
10. Gross ER, Ladisa JF, Jr., Weihrauch D et al. Reactive oxygen species modulate coronary wall shear stress and endothelial function during hyperglycemia. *Am J Physiol Heart Circ Physiol.* 2003;284(5):H1552.
11. Wentzel JJ, Janssen E, Vos J, et al. Extension of increased atherosclerotic wall thickness into high shear stress regions is associated with loss of compensatory remodeling. *Circulation.* 2003;108(1):17.
12. Nerem RM, Rumberger JA, Jr., Gross DR, et al. Hot-film anemometer velocity measurements of arterial blood flow horses. *Circ Res.* 1974;34(2):193.
13. Rumberger JA, Jr., Nerem RM, Muir WW, III. Coronary artery pressure development and wave transmission characteristics in the horse. *Cardiovasc Res.* 1979;13(7):413.
14. Brosh D, Higano ST, Kern MJ et al. Pulse transmission coefficient: a nonhyperemic index for physiologic assessment of procedural success following percutaneous coronary interventions. *Cathet Cardiovasc Interv.* 2004;61(1):95.
15. Parker KH, Jones CJ. Forward and backward running waves in the arteries: analysis using the method of characteristics. *J Biomech Eng.* 1990;112 (3):322.
16. Jones CJ, Sugawara M. "Wavefronts" in the aorta–implications for the mechanisms of left ventricular ejection and aortic valve closure. *Cardiovasc Res.* 1993;27(11):1902.
17. Wang JJ, O'Brien AB, Shrive NG et al. Time-domain representation of ventricular–arterial coupling as a windkessel and wave system. *Am J Physiol Heart Circ Physiol.* 2003;284(4):H1358.
18. Sun YH, Anderson TJ, Parker KH, Tyberg JV. Effects of left ventricular contractility and coronary vascular resistance on coronary dynamics. *Am J Physiol Heart Circ Physiol.* 2004;286(4):H1590.
19. Sun YH, Anderson TJ, Parker KH, Tyberg JV. Wave-intensity analysis: a new approach to coronary hemodynamics. *J Appl Physiol.* 2000;89(4):1636.
20. Bonetti PO, Lerman LO, Lerman A. Endothelial dysfunction: a marker of atherosclerotic risk. *Arterioscler Thromb Vasc Biol.* 2003;23(2):168.

21. van den Berg BM, Vink H, Spaan JA. The endothelial glycocalyx protects against myocardial edema. *Circ Res.* 2003;92(6):592.

22. Constantinescu AA, Vink H, Spaan JAE. Endothelial Cell Glycocalyx Modulates Immobilization of Leukocytes at the Endothelial Surface. *Arterioscler Thromb Vasc Biol.* 2003;23(9):1541.

23. Van Haaren PM, VanBavel E, Vink H, Spaan JA. Localization of the permeability barrier to solutes in isolated arteries by confocal microscopy. *Am J Physiol Heart Circ Physiol.* 2003;285:H2848.

24. Vink H, Duling BR. Identification of distinct luminal domains for macromolecules, erythrocytes, and leukocytes within mammalian capillaries. *Circ Res.* 1996;79(3):581.

25. Vink H, Constantinescu AA, Spaan JA. Oxidized lipoproteins degrade the endothelial surface layer: implications for platelet-endothelial cell adhesion. *Circulation.* 2000;101(13):1500.

26. Schwenke DC, Zilversmit DB. The arterial barrier to lipoprotein influx in the hypercholesterolemic rabbit. 2. Long-term studies in deendothelialized and reendothelialized aortas. *Atherosclerosis.* 1989;77(2–3):105.

27. Neumann SJ, Berceli SA, Sevick EM et al. Experimental determination and mathematical model of the transient incorporation of cholesterol in the arterial wall 2. *Bull Math Biol.* 1990;52(6):711.

28. Berceli SA, Warty VS, Sheppeck RA et al. Hemodynamics and low density lipoprotein metabolism. Rates of low density lipoprotein incorporation and degradation along medial and lateral walls of the rabbit aorto-iliac bifurcation. *Arteriosclerosis.* 1990;10(5):686.

29. VanBavel E, Spaan JAE. Branching patterns in the porcine coronary arterial tree. Estimation of flow heterogeneity. *Circ Res.* 1992;71(5):1200.

30. Kassab GS, Rider CA, Tang NJ, Fung YC. Morphometry of pig coronary arterial trees. *Am J Physiol.* 1993;265(1 Pt 2):H350.

31. Zamir M, Phipps S, Langille BL, Wonnacott TH. Branching characteristics of coronary arteries in rats. *Can J Physiol Pharmacol.* 1984;62(12):1453.

32. Spaan JA. Coronary diastolic pressure–flow relation and zero flow pressure explained on the basis of intramyocardial compliance. *Circ Res.* 1985;56(3):293.

33. Bassingthwaighte JB, Yipintsoi T, harvey rb. Microvasculature of the dog left ventricular myocardium. *Microvasc Res.* 1974;7(2):229.

34. Kajiya F, Tsujioka K, Goto M, et al. Functional characteristics of intramyocardial capacitance vessels during diastole in the dog. *Circ Res.* 1986;58(4):476.

35. VanBavel E, Siersma P, Spaan JA. Elasticity of passive blood vessels: a new concept. *Am J Physiol Heart Circ Physiol.* 2003;285:H1986.

36. VanBavel E, Giezeman MJ, Mooij T, Spaan JA. Influence of pressure alterations on tone and vasomotion of isolated mesenteric small arteries of the rat. *J Physiol.* 1991;436:371.

37. Giezeman MJMM, VanBavel E, Grimbergen CA, Spaan JAE. Compliance of isolated porcine coronary small arteries and coronary pressure–flow relations. *Am J Physiol.* 1994;267(3 Pt 2):H1190.

38. Chilian WM, Marcus ML. Effects of coronary and extravascular pressure on intramyocardial and epicardial blood velocity. *Am J Physiol.* 1985;248 (2 Pt 2):H170.

39. Chilian WM, Marcus ML. Coronary venous outflow persists after cessation of coronary arterial inflow. *Am J Physiol.* 1984;247:H984.

40. Vergroesen I, Noble MIM, Spaan JAE. Intramyocardial blood volume change in first moments of cardiac arrest in anesthetized goats. *Am J Physiol.* 1987;253:H307.

41. Gould KL. Pressure–flow characteristics of coronary stenoses in unsedated dogs at rest and during coronary vasodilation. *Circ Res.* 1978;43(2):242.

42. Ofili EO, Kern MJ, Labovitz AJ, et al. Analysis of coronary blood flow velocity dynamics in angiographically normal and stenosed arteries before and after endolumen enlargement by angioplasty. *J Am Coll Cardiol.* 1993;21(2):308.

43. Arts T, Reneman RS. Interaction between intramyocardial pressure (IMP) and myocardial circulation. *J Biomech Eng.* 1985;107(1):51.

44. Heineman FW, Grayson J. Transmural distribution of intramyocardial pressure measured by micropipette technique. *Am J Physiol.* 1985;249:H1216.

45. Krams R, Sipkema P, Zegers J, Westerhof N. Contractility is the main determinant of coronary systolic flow impediment. *Am J Physiol.* 1989;257: H1936.

46. Krams R, Sipkema P, Westerhof N. The varying elastance concept may explain coronary systolic flow impediment. *Am J Physiol.* 1989;257:H1471.

47. VanWinkle DM, Swafford AN, Downey JM. Subendocardial coronary compression in beating dog hearts is independent of pressure in the ventricular lumen. *Am J Physiol.* 1991;261:H500.

48. Krams R, Sipkema P, Westerhof N. Coronary oscillatory flow amplitude is more affected by perfusion pressure than ventricular pressure. *Am J Physiol.* 1990;258:H1889.

49. Westerhof N. Physiological hypotheses–intramyocardial pressure. A new concept, suggestions for measurement. *Basic Res Cardiol.* 1990;85:105.

50. Borg TK, Caulfield JB. The collagen matrix of the heart. *Fed Proc.* 1981;40:2037.

51. Han Y, Vergroesen I, Goto M, et al. Left ventricular pressure transmission to myocardial lymph vessels is different during systole and diastole. *Pflügers Arch.* 1993;423:448.

52. Kouwenhoven E, Vergroesen I, Han Y, Spaan JA. Retrograde coronary flow is limited by time-varying elastance. *Am J Physiol.* 1992;263(2 Pt 2):H484.

53. Spaan JA. Mechanical determinants of myocardial perfusion. *Basic Res Cardiol.* 1995;90(2):89.

54. Hoffman JIE, Spaan JAE. Pressure–flow relations in coronary circulation. *Physiol Rev.* 1990;70:331.

55. Klocke FJ, Mates RE, Canty JM, Jr., Ellis AK. Coronary pressure–flow relationship: controversial issues and probable implications. *Circ Res.* 1985; 56:310.

56. Yada T, Hiramatsu O, Kimura A, et al. In vivo observation of subendocardial microvessels of the beating porcine heart using a needle-probe videomicroscope with a CCD camera. *Circ Res.* 1993;72(5):939.

57. Spaan JAE, Cornelissen AJM, Chan C, et al, inventors. Dynamics of flow, resistance and intramural vascular volume in canine coronary circulation. *Am J Physiol Heart Circ Physiol* 2000;278:H383.

58. Hanley FL, Messina LM, Grattan MT, Hoffman IE. The effect of coronary inflow pressure on coronary vascular resistance in the isolated dog heart. *Circ Res.* 1984;54(6):760.

59. Bruinsma P, Arts T, Dankelman J, Spaan JAE. Model of the coronary circulation based on pressure dependence of coronary resistance and compliance. *Basic Res Cardiol.* 1988;83:510.

60. Komaru T, Kanatsuka H, Shirato K. Coronary microcirculation: physiology and pharmacology. *Pharmacol Ther.* 2000;86(3):217.

61. Kuo L, Chilian WM, Davis MJ. Coronary arteriolar myogenic response is independent of endothelium. *Circ Res.* 1990;66:860.

62. Kuo L, Chilian WM, Davis MJ. Interaction of pressure and flow-induced responses in porcine coronary resistance vessels. *Am J Physiol.* 1991;261: H1706.

63. VanBavel E, Wesselman JPM, Spaan JAE. Myogenic activation and calcium sensitivity of cannulated rat mesenteric small arteries. *Circ Res.* 1998;82(2):210.

64. Goto M, VanBavel E, Giezeman MJ, Spaan JA. Vasodilatory effect of pulsatile pressure on coronary resistance vessels. *Circ Res.* 1996;79(5):1039.

65. Schretzenmayr A. Ueber kreislaufregulatorische vorgange an den groben arterien bei der muskelarbeit. *Pflügers Arch.* 1933;232:743.

66. Khayutin VM, Melkumyants AM, Rogoza AN et al. Flow-induced control of arterial lumen. *Acta Physiol Hung.* 1986;68:241.

67. Hull SS, Jr., Kaiser L, Jaffe MD, Sparks HV, Jr. Endothelium-dependent flow-induced dilation of canine femoral and saphenous arteries. *Blood Vessels.* 1986;23(4-5):183.

68. Pohl U, Herlan K, Huang A, Bassenge E. EDRF-mediated shear-induced dilation opposes myogenic vasoconstriction in small rabbit arteries. *Am J Physiol Heart Circ Physiol.* 1991;261:H2016.

69. Sorop O, Spaan JA, sweeney te, VanBavel E. Effect of steady versus oscillating flow on porcine coronary arterioles: involvement of NO and superoxide anion. *Circ Res.* 2003;92(12):1344.

70. Mochizuki S, Vink H, Hiramatsu O, et al. Role of hyaluronic acid glycosaminoglycans in shear-induced endothelium-derived nitric oxide release. *Am J Physiol Heart Circ Physiol.* 2003;285(2):H722.

71. Florian JA, Kosky JR, Ainslie K, et al. Heparin sulfate proteoglycan is a mechanosensor on endothelial cells. *Circ Res.* 2003;93(10):e136.

72. Rubio R, Berne RM. Release of adenosine by the normal myocardium in dogs and its relationship to the regulation of coronary resistance. *Circ Res.* 1969;25(4):407.

73. Saito D, Steinhart CR, Nixon DG, Olsson RA. Intracoronary adenosine deaminase reduces canine myocardial reactive hyperemia. *Circulation.* 1981;49:1262.

74. Hanley FL, Grattan MT, Stevens MB, Hoffman JIE. Role of adenosine in coronary autoregulation. *Am J Physiol.* 1986;250:H558.

75. Kroll K, Feigl EO. Adenosine is unimportant in controlling coronary blood flow in unstressed dog hearts. *Am J Physiol.* 1985;249:H1176.

76. Kroll K, Deussen A, Sweet IR. Comprehensive model of transport and metabolism of adenosine and S-adenosylhomocysteine in the guinea pig heart. *Circulation.* 1992;71:590.

77. Zhang J, From AH, Ugurbil K, Bache RJ. Myocardial oxygenation and high-energy phosphate levels during K_{ATP}-channel blockade. *Am J Physiol Heart Circ Physiol.* 2003;285(4):H1420.

78. Ishibashi Y, Duncker DJ, Zhang J, Bache RJ. ATP-sensitive K+ channels, adenosine, and nitric oxide-mediated mechanisms account for coronary vasodilation during exercise. [Review]. *Circulation*. 1998;82(3):346.

79. Dankelman J, Van der Ploeg CPB, Spaan JAE. Glibenclamide decelerates the responses of coronary regulation in the goat. *Am J Physiol*. 1994;266(5 Pt 2):H1715.

80. Miura H, Bosnjak JJ, Ning G, et al. Role for hydrogen peroxide in flow-induced dilation of human coronary arterioles. *Circ Res*. 2003;92(2):e31.

81. Miyashiro JK, Feigl EO. A model of combined feedforward and feedback control of coronary blood flow. *Am J Physiol*. 1995;268(2 37-2):H895.

82. Mohrman DE, Feigl EO. Competition between sympathetic vasoconstriction and metabolic vasodilation etc. *Circ Res*. 1978;42:79.

83. Dankelman J, Spaan JAE, Stassen HG, Vergroesen I. Dynamics of coronary adjustment to a change in heart rate in the anaesthetized goat. *J Physiol (London)*. 1989;408:295.

84. Dankelman J, Vergroesen I, Han Y, Spaan JA. Dynamic response of coronary regulation to heart rate and perfusion changes in dogs. *Am J Physiol*. 1992;263(2 Pt 2):H447.

85. Jones CJ, Kuo L, Davis MJ, Chilian WM. Regulation of coronary blood flow: coordination of heterogeneous control mechanisms in vascular microdomains. *Cardiovasc Res*. 1995;29(5):585.

86. Jones CJH, Kuo L, Davis MJ, Chilian WM. Myogenic and flow-dependent control mechanisms in the coronary microcirculation. *Basic Res Cardiol*. 1993;88:2.

87. Cornelissen AJ, Dankelman J, VanBavel E, Spaan JA. Balance between myogenic, flow-dependent, and metabolic flow control in coronary arterial tree: a model study. *Am J Physiol Heart Circ Physiol*. 2002;282(6):H2224.

88. Vergroesen I, Kal JE, van WH. Coronary vasodilating drug effects or normal coronary blood flow regulation?. *J Cardiothorac Vasc Anesth*. 1998;12(4):450.

89. Vergroesen I, Kal JE, Spaan JAE, Van Wezel HB. Myocardial oxygen supply:demand ratio as reference for coronary vasodilatory drug effects in humans. *Heart*. 1997;78(2):117.

90. Merkus D, Vergroesen I, Hiramatsu O et al. Stenosis differentially affects subendocardial and subepicardial arterioles in vivo. *Am J Physiol Heart Circ Physiol*. 2001;280(4):H1674.

91. Siebes M, Verhoeff BJ, Meuwissen M, et al. Single-wire pressure and flow velocity measurement to quantify coronary stenosis hemodynamics and effects of percutaneous interventions. *Circulation*. 2004;109(6):756.

92. Anderson HV, Stokes MJ, Leon M, et al. Coronary artery flow velocity is related to lumen area and regional left ventricular mass. *Circulation*. 2000;102(1):48.

93. Ofili EO, Labovitz AJ, Kern MJ. Coronary flow velocity dynamics in normal and diseased arteries. *Am J Cardiol*. 1993;71(14):3D.

94. Gould KL, Kirkeeide RL, Buchi M. Coronary flow reserve as a physiologic measure of stenosis severity. *J Am Coll Cardiol*. 1990;15(2):459.

95. Baumgart D, Haude M, Goerge G, et al. Improved assessment of coronary stenosis severity using the relative flow velocity reserve. *Circulation*. 1998;98(1):40.

96. Chamuleau SA, Meuwissen M, Eck-Smit BL, et al. Fractional flow reserve, absolute and relative coronary flow velocity reserve in relation to the results of technetium-99m sestamibi single-photon emission computed tomography in patients with two-vessel coronary artery disease. *J Am Coll Cardiol*. 2001;37(5):1316.

97. Pijls NH, De Bruyne B, Peels K, et al. Measurement of fractional flow reserve to assess the functional severity of coronary–artery stenoses. *N Engl J Med*. 1996;334(26):17C3.

98. De Bruyne B, Baudhuin T, Melin JA, et al. Coronary flow reserve calculated from pressure measurements in humans. Validation with positron emission tomography. *Circulation*. 1994;89(3):1013.

99. De Bruyne B, Pijls NH, Bartunek J, et al. Fractional flow reserve in patients with prior myocardial infarction. *Circulation*. 2001;104(2):157.

100. Siebes M, Chamuleau SA, Meuwissen M, et al. Influence of hemodynamic conditions on fractional flow reserve: parametric analysis of underlying model. *Am J Physiol Heart Circ Physiol*. 2002;283(4):H1462.

101. De Bruyne B, Bartunek J, Sys SU, et al. Simultaneous coronary pressure and flow velocity measurements in humans. Feasibility, reproducibility, and hemodynamic dependence of coronary flow velocity reserve, hyperemic flow versus pressure slope index, and fractional flow reserve. *Circulation*. 1996;94(8):1842.

102. Meuwissen M, Siebes M, Chamuleau SA, et al. Hyperemic stenosis resistance index for evaluation of functional coronary lesion severity. *Circulation*. 2002;106(4):441.

103. Meuwissen M, Chamuleau SA, Siebes M, et al. Role of variability in microvascular resistance on fractional flow reserve and coronary blood flow velocity reserve in intermediate coronary lesions. *Circulation*. 2001;103(2):184.

104. Barbato E, Aarnoudse W, Aengevaeren WR, et al. Validation of coronary flow reserve measurements by thermodilution in clinical practice. *Eur Heart J*. 2004;25(3):219.

105. De Bruyne B, Pijls NH, Smith L, et al. Coronary thermodilution to assess flow reserve: experimental validation. *Circulation*. 2001;104(17):2003.

106. De Bruyne B, Hersbach F, Pijls NH, et al. Abnormal epicardial coronary resistance in patients with diffuse atherosclerosis but "normal" coronary angiography. *Circulation*. 2001;104(20):2401.

107. Pijls NH, De Bruyne B, Bech GJ, et al. Coronary pressure measurement to assess the hemodynamic significance of serial stenoses within one coronary artery: validation in humans. *Circulation*. 2000;102(19):2371.

108. Austin RE, Aldea GS, Coggins DL, et al. Profound spatial heterogeneity of coronary reserve. Discordance between patterns of resting and maximal myocardial blood flow. *Circulation*. 1990;67:319.

109. Loncar R, Flesche CW, Deussen A. Coronary reserve of high- and low-flow regions in the dog heart left ventricle. *Circulation*. 1998;98(3):262.

110. Canty JM, Jr. Coronary pressure–function and steady-state pressure–flow relations during autoregulation in the unanesthetized dog. *Circ Res*. 1988;63(4):821.

111. Matsunaga T, Warltier DC, Weihrauch DW, et al. Ischemia-induced coronary collateral growth is dependent on vascular endothelial growth factor and nitric oxide. *Circulation*. 2000;102(25):3098.

112. Van Royen N, Voskuil M, Hoefer I, et al. CD44 regulates arteriogenesis in mice and is differentially expressed in patients with poor and good collateralization. *Circulation*. 2004;109(13):1647.

113. Hoefer IE, Van Royen N, Rectenwald JE, et al. Arteriogenesis proceeds via ICAM-1/Mac-1-mediated mechanisms. *Circ Res*. 2004;94:1179.

114. Piek JJ, Koolen JJ, Metting van Rijn AC, et al. Spectral analysis of flow velocity in the contralateral artery during coronary angioplasty: a new method for assessing collateral flow. *J Am Coll Cardiol*. 1993;21(7):1574.

115. Piek JJ, van LR, Koch KT, et al. Pharmacological modulation of the human collateral vascular resistance in acute and chronic coronary occlusion assessed by intracoronary blood flow analysis in an angioplasty model [see comments]. *Circulation*. 1997;96(1):106.

116. Pijls NH, van SJ, Kirkeeide RL, et al. Experimental basis of determining maximum coronary, myocardial, and collateral blood flow by pressure measurements for assessing functional stenosis severity before and after percutaneous transluminal coronary angioplasty. *Circulation*. 1993;87(4):1354.

117. Pijls NH, Bech GJ, el Gamal MI, et al. Quantification of recruitable coronary collateral blood flow in conscious humans and its potential to predict future ischemic events. *J Am Coll Cardiol*. 1995;25(7):1522.

118. Spaan JA, Piek JJ, Hoffman JI, Siebes M. Physiological basis of clinically used coronary hemodynamic indices. *Circulation*. 2006;113:446.

CHAPTER 5

Physiological Evaluation of Renal Artery Stenosis: A Hemodynamic Approach

Rajesh Subramanian, MBBS, and
Christopher J. White, MD

Impairment of renal blood flow as a result of renal artery stenosis (RAS) may manifest clinically as systemic hypertension, ischemic nephropathy (leading to end-stage renal disease), and cardiac destabilization syndromes including decompensated heart failure ("flash" pulmonary edema), and acute coronary syndromes.[1,2] Revascularization by surgical or percutaneous methods often corrects the clinical manifestations of RAS.[3–6]

RENAL BLOOD FLOW REGULATION

The pathophysiology of renovascular hypertension involves renin–aldosterone–angiotensin activation. Renal blood flow autoregulation occurs through changes in renal vascular resistance primarily via an intrinsic myogenic mechanism at the level of the afferent arteriole.[7] In addition, vasoactive local factors such as nitric oxide, prostaglandins, and kinins play a role in renal blood flow autoregulation.[8] This autoregulation is maintained until the perfusion pressure falls below 70–80 mm Hg. Although hypoperfusion of the kidney is the pathophysiologic mechanism stimulating renin–aldosterone–angiotensin activation, its precise relationship with stenosis severity and hemodynamic renal blood flow alterations is unknown. Most investigators agree that a narrowing of at least 70% diameter stenosis reduces renal blood flow; however, lesser degrees of stenosis have also been associated with impaired renal blood flow.[9]

ASSESSMENT OF RENAL ARTERY STENOSIS

Clinically significant RAS is often diagnosed after response to revascularization.[10] Prospective identification of clinically significant RAS allows for the appropriate utilization of resources to maximize benefit of revascularization procedures. Although angiography remains the gold standard for the detection of RAS, it often provides insufficient information regarding its clinical significance. The angiographic appearance of "string-of-beads" suggests fibromuscular dysplasia, and is associated with a high likelihood of clinical success following percutaneous revascularization.[11] However, fibromuscular dysplasia accounts for 10%–15% of cases of RAS. Atherosclerosis, which accounts for the 85%–90% of RAS, predominantly affects the ostium and the proximal segment of the main renal artery. The aorto-ostial segment represents a challenging region to evaluate angiographically as a result of the difficulty in obtaining orthogonal views.[12] Also, angiography provides no functional information regarding the impact of a stenosis on kidney perfusion.

A host of invasive and noninvasive tests have been used to determine the clinical significance of RAS with disappointing results. Renal vein renin levels and captopril scintigraphy have failed to distinguish responders and nonresponders to revascularization among patients with RAS.[13] Doppler-ultrasound has been used to evaluate the intraparenchymal renal blood flow patterns, and an index of severity, the renal resistive index (RI), has been measured.[14] The ability of RI to predict responders to revascularization has been challenged.[15]

HEMODYNAMIC ASSESSMENT

The relationship between arterial obstruction and organ perfusion has been well studied in the coronary circulation. A coronary stenosis with diameter restriction of less than 40% does not significantly affect blood flow and cardiac perfusion under conditions of rest or increased physiologic or pharmacologic demand. Increasing stenosis severity initially affects blood flow during conditions of increased demand, with additional increases in stenosis severity affecting resting blood flow.[16] The physiologic consequences of arterial obstruction and coronary ischemia may be assessed noninvasively using stress testing with or without additional imaging modalities, or invasively by assessing the coronary fractional flow reserve (FFR). We postulate that similar invasive techniques may be useful in evaluating RAS.

【 】 PRESSURE GRADIENTS

Invasive hemodynamic assessment can be performed with pressure gradients representing one end of the spectrum and determination of flow and flow reserve representing the other end. The resistance to flow offered by a stenosis in a conduit artery results in a pressure drop distal to the obstruction. This pressure gradient offers a measure of the severity of the stenosis and is obtained by measuring the pressure proximal and distal to the stenosis. Pressure gradient determinations are attractive in large-diameter arteries such as the renal arteries, but they have limitations related to the method of acquisition, which may affect their physiologic significance. Pressure gradients have been determined using catheters.[17] These catheters may introduce errors in the measurement because of their profile.[18] The larger the catheter, the more likely the gradient is related to obstruction by the catheter itself. Pressure gradients are best measured using a 0.014-inch diameter pressure wire, as this is the smallest profile device available.

Pressure gradients may be inadequate measures of stenosis severity because of physiologic factors. Organ (renal) perfusion is related to the absolute distal pressure and not to the gradient across the stenosis.[19] Pressure gradients are dependent on factors that affect blood flow, such as cardiac output, systemic blood pressure, and the vasodilatory state of the renal microvasculature. This principle is illustrated when pressure gradients are measured at rest and following administration of a vasodilator, wherein the same stenosis is associated with differing pressure gradients (the resting pressure gradient and the hyperemic pressure gradient).

【 】 VASODILATORS

Studying the effects of stenosis on blood flow is best done under conditions of maximum hyperemia, ensuring the hemodynamic measures obtained are not dependent on blood flow. Hyperemia is obtained following the administration of pharmacologic stimuli (vasodilators), which can be classified by the mechanism of action (endothelium-dependent versus endothelium-independent) or by the location of action (conduit versus capacitance vessel). Acetylcholine represents the prototypical endothelium-dependent vasodilator requiring an intact endothelium to effect its action, whereas papavarine is the prototypical endothelium-independent

vasodilator that causes vasodilation with either an intact or a diseased endothelium. Nitroglycerine and nitroprusside represent the conduit-vessel and capacitance-vessel vasodilators, respectively. The ideal vasodilator to study the renal circulation induces predictable vasodilation in the renal circulation in both normal and diseased states without producing systemic hypotension or other local or systemic adverse effects.

Adenosine has been used extensively to study the hemodynamic alterations of coronary stenosis and cardiac ischemia. Adenosine has been shown to increase renal blood flow in hypertensive patients, but causes a reduction in renal blood flow in normal patients and in patients with chronic heart failure.[20,21] Therefore, adenosine is not an optimal agent for studying the renal circulation because of its variable actions in different disease states.

Acetylcholine causes vasodilation by releasing nitric oxide from intact endothelium. There are differences in bioavailability in nitric oxide in the renal vasculature in essential hypertension and RAS, with acetylcholine producing differential effects on blood flow in the stenotic kidney compared to the nonstenotic kidney.[22] Acetylcholine-mediated changes in renal blood flow are not uniform, and therefore not optimal for the study of the renal circulation.

Papavarine causes vasodilation as a direct vascular smooth muscle relaxant, and acts on the renal microcirculation. Papavarine has been used successfully to study the renal circulation in hypertensive and RAS patients.[23,24] One caveat is that papavarine forms a precipitate in contact with heparinized solutions, and care must be taken because of the common use of heparinized solutions in the angiographic suite.

【 】 RENAL FLOW AND RENAL FLOW RESERVE

Renal blood flow is affected by disease states, and measuring renal blood flow may provide insight into the pathophysiology of ischemic renal dysfunction. The absolute renal blood flow velocity can be measured using a Doppler-tipped angioplasty guidewire (Doppler-wire).[25] Used with the vessel's cross-sectional area, measured by quantitative vascular angiography (QVA) or intravascular ultrasonography (IVUS), one can calculate the absolute renal blood flow. When renal blood flow is measured following vasodilation, one can assess the renal blood flow reserve. Doppler-wire measured renal blood flow in normal patients demonstrates significant interkidney (intrapatient) and interpatient variability.[26] There is also significant interpatient variability in renal blood flow reserve in hypertensive patients without RAS.[23] This variability in renal blood flow and renal blood flow reserve limits the clinical utility of Doppler-wire measures of flow. Although renal blood flow and flow reserve can be used in the hemodynamic evaluation of renal artery stenosis, the presence of microvascular disease may limit its utility.

【 】 RENAL FRACTIONAL FLOW RESERVE

The limitation of Doppler-derived parameters of flow in discerning the effects of the large-vessel obstruction to flow may be overcome by determining the pressure-derived fractional flow reserve (FFR). Pressure-derived FFR was initially developed and its clinical utility established in the coronary circulation. Coronary FFR has been demonstrated effective in assessing the functional significance of a coronary stenosis.[27]

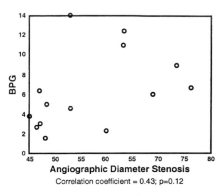 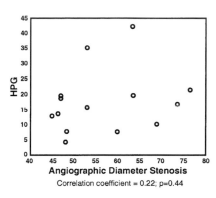 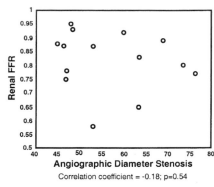

FIGURE 5-1. The correlation of quantitative angiographic diameter stenosis (angiographic diameter stenosis) with baseline mean translesional pressure gradient (BPG) (**A**), hyperemic mean translesional pressure gradient (HPG) (**B**), and renal FFR (**C**). *(Subramanian R, White CJ, Rosenfield K, et al. Renal circulatory physiology at rest and hyperemia: inducing hyperemia with papavarine and measuring pressure-derived renal fractional flow reserve in renal arteries with moderate stenosis. Cathet Cardiovasc Intervent. 2005;64:480.)*

Blood flow across a vascular bed is proportional to the pressure across the vascular bed and inversely proportional to the vascular resistance. The pressure is the driving pressure in the conduit artery, and is the aortic pressure in the absence of a stenosis in the conduit artery and the pressure distal to the stenosis in the presence of a stenosis in the conduit artery. In a state of maximum vasodilation, the resistance offered by the microvasculature is at a minimum and is constant. Under these conditions, the factor-limiting theoretical maximum flow is a stenosis in the conduit artery. FFR, a pressure-derived hemodynamic measure of stenosis severity, obtained at maximum hyperemia is the ratio between the maximum blood flow in the conduit artery with a stenosis compared to the maximal blood flow in the absence of a stenosis. In a state of maximum vasodilation, the FFR is proportional to the ratio of the pressure proximal and distal to the stenosis.[28] The pressure proximal and distal to the stenosis is measured using a 0.014-inch pressure guidewire.

As renal FFR reflects the extent of reduction in blood flow because of the stenosis, it may be the best hemodynamic measure of the consequences of main renal artery stenosis. Coronary FFR is an established measure to determine the clinical effects of epicardial coronary stenosis. Similar information is lacking in RAS. We have measured renal FFR in renal arteries with aorto-ostial stenosis following vasodilation using intrarenal papavarine.

〔 〕 EXPERIMENTAL RENAL FFR RESULTS

We performed hemodynamic assessments in patients with aorto-ostial renal artery stenosis while determining the range and optimal dose of intrarenal papavarine to achieve maximum hyperemia.[23] Intravascular pressures (aorta and renal artery) were measured using a 0.014-inch pressure guidewire (Pressurewire XT, Radi Medical Systems, Uppsala, Sweden). Intra-arterial papavarine was administered selectively to the renal artery to achieve hyperemia. Papavarine was administered into the renal artery, distal to the stenosis in 8-mg increments (8–40 mg) via a low-profile infusion catheter or the lumen of a balloon dilation catheter to minimize systemic vasodilation. Technical considerations during the procedure include the avoidance of mixing papavarine with heparinized saline (papavarine precipitates with heparin) and the avoidance of measuring pressure during pressure damping by the

catheter used to administer papavarine. The latter is achieved by withdrawing the infusion catheter from the renal artery and into the aorta during the pressure measurements.

Thirteen patients and 14 arteries with mild to moderate RAS (visually estimated diameter stenosis of 50%–90%) were studied. The renal arteries studied had a visual diameter stenosis of 74.9 ± 11.5% (range: 50–90%) with corresponding quantitative angiographic diameter stenosis of 56.6 ± 10.8% (range: 45–76%). The baseline (resting) mean translesional pressure gradient was 6.3 ± 3.9 mm Hg (range: 1.5–14 mm Hg).

Papavarine administration was well tolerated without systemic hypotension at a mean final dose of 26.9 ± 8.7 mg, with maximum hyperemia being achieved at 24 or 32 mg in most patients. The average hyperemic mean translesional pressure gradient following vasodilation was 17.5 ± 10.3 mm Hg (range: 4–42 mm Hg). The renal FFR ranged from 0.58 to 0.95.

Simple linear regression analysis was performed using the angiographic and hemodynamic measures of lesion severity. There was a poor correlation between the quantitative angiographic diameter stenosis and the hemodynamic measures of baseline mean translesional pressure gradient ($r = 0.43$, $p = 0.12$), hyperemic mean translesional pressure gradient ($r = 0.22$, $p = 0.44$) and renal FFR ($r = -0.18$, $p = 0.54$) (Figure 5-1). Renal FFR provided a good measure of lesion severity, with a good correlation being obtained between the baseline (resting) mean translesional pressure gradient ($r = -0.76$, $p = 0.0016$) and the hyperemic mean translesional pressure gradient ($r = -0.94$, $p = < 0.0001$) (Figure 5-2).

CONCLUSION

Hemodynamic assessment of the renal circulation provides information in addition to that obtained noninvasively and at angiography. Among the hemodynamic measures, renal FFR appears to provide the best measure of physiologic severity of anatomic obstruction because of a stenosis of the main renal artery. Identification of likely "responders" to renal artery revascularization in patients with clinical manifestations of RAS allows only those patients likely to benefit from treatment to be exposed to the

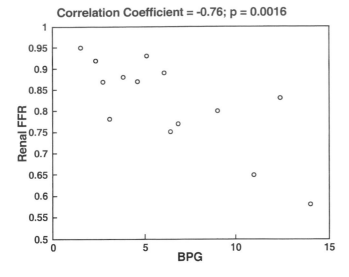

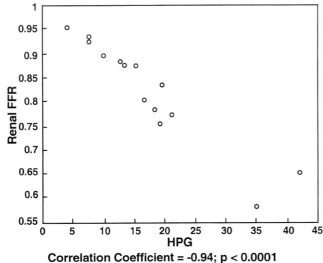

FIGURE 5-2. The correlation of renal FFR with the baseline mean translesional pressure gradient (BPG) (**A**) and hyperemic mean translesional pressure gradient (HPG) (**B**). *(Subramanian R, White CJ, Rosenfield K, et al. Renal circulatory physiology at rest and hyperemia: inducing hyperemia with papavarine and measuring pressure-derived renal fractional flow reserve in renal arteries with moderate stenosis. Cathet Cardiovasc Intervent. 2005;64:480.)*

risk of invasive therapy, and avoids performing procedures on patients unlikely to benefit. Longer-term assessment of clinical outcomes and larger studies are required to better understand the utility of these hemodynamic measures.

REFERENCES

1. Safian RD, Textor SC. Renal-artery stenosis. *N Engl J Med.* 2001;344:431.
2. Zierler RE, Bergelin RO, Davidson RC, et al. A prospective study of disease progression in patients with atherosclerotic renal artery stenosis. *Am J Hypertens.* 1997;9:1055.
3. Khosla S, White CJ, Collins TJ, et al. Effects of renal artery stent implantation in patients with renovascular hypertension presenting with unstable angina or congestive heart failure. *Am J Cardiol.* 1997;80:363.
4. White CJ, Ramee SR, Collins TJ, et al. Renal artery stent placement: utility in lesions difficult to treat with balloon angioplasty. *J Am Coll Cardiol.* 1997;30:1445.
5. Nordmann AJ, Woo K, Parkes R, Logan AG. Balloon angioplasty or medical therapy for hypertensive patients with atherosclerotic renal artery stenosis? A meta-analysis of randomized controlled trials. *Am J Med.* 2003;114:44.
6. Watson PS, Hadjipetrou P, Cox SV, et al. Effect of renal artery stenting on renal function and size in patients with atherosclerotic renovascular disease. *Circulation.* 2000;102:1671.
7. Stein JH. Regulation of renal circulation. *Kidney Int.* 1990;38:571.
8. Campbell WB, Henrich WL. Endothelial factors in the regulation of rennin release. *Kidney Int.* 1990;38:612.
9. Schoenberg SO, Knopp MV, Bock M, et al. Renal artery stenosis: grading of hemodynamic changes with cine phase-contrast MR blood flow measurements. *Radiology.* 1997;203:45.
10. de Leeuw PW. On the significance of renal vein renins in renovascular hypertension. *J Hypertens.* 2002;20:843–845.
11. Tegtmeyer CJ, Selby JB, Hartwell GD, et al. Results and complications of angioplasty in fibromuscular disease. *Circulation.* 1991;83[suppl I]:155.
12. Cameron A, Kemp HG, Fisher LD, et al. Left main coronary artery stenosis: angiographic determination. *Circulation.* 1983;68:484.
13. Vasbinder GBC, Nelemans PJ, Kessels AGH, et al. Diagnostic tests for renal artery stenosis in patients suspected of having renovascular hypertension: a meta-analysis. *Ann Intern Med.* 2002;135:401.
14. Radermacher J, Chavan A, Bleck J, et al. Use of Doppler ultrasonography to predict the outcome of therapy for renal artery stenosis. *N Engl J Med.* 2001;344:410.
15. Zeller T, Muller C, Frank U, et al. Stent angioplasty of severe atherosclerotic ostial renal artery stenosis in patients with diabetes mellitus and nephrosclerosis. *Cathet Cardiovasc Intervent.* 2003;58:510.
16. Uren NG, Melin JA, De Bruyne B, et al. Relationship between myocardial blood flow and severity of coronary stenosis. *N Engl J Med.* 1994;330:1782.
17. Nahman NS, Maniam P, Hernandez RA et al. Renal artery pressure gradients in patients with angiographic evidence of atherosclerotic renal artery stenosis. *Am J Kid Dis.* 1994;24:695.
18. Colyer WR, Cooper CJ, Burket MW, Thomas WJ. Utility of a 0.014" pressure-sensing guidewire to assess renal artery translesional systolic pressure gradients. *Cathet Cardiovasc Intervent.* 2003;59:372.
19. Pijls NHJ, van Son JA, Kirkeeide RL, et al. Experimental basis of determining maximum coronary, myocardial and collateral blood flow by pressure measurements for assessing functional stenosis severity before and after percutaneous transluminal balloon angioplasty. *Circulation.* 1993;86:1354.
20. Wierema TKA, Postma CT, Houben AJHM, et al. Adenosine-induced renal vasodilation is prolonged in renal artery stenosis. *J Hypertens.* 1998;16:2109.
21. Marraccini P, Fedele S, Marzilli M, et al. Adenosine-induced renal vasoconstriction in man. *Cardiovasc Res.* 1996;32:949.
22. Wierema TKA, Houben AJHM, Kroon AA, et al. Nitric oxide dependence of renal blood flow in patients with renal artery stenosis. *J Am Soc Nephrol.* 2001;12:1836.
23. Beregi JP, Mounier-Vehier C, Devos P, et al. Doppler flow wire evaluation of renal blood flow reserve in hypertensive patients with normal renal arteries. *Cardiovasc Intervent Radiol.* 2000;23:340.
24. Subramanian R, White CJ, Rosenfield K, et al. Renal circulatory physiology at rest and hyperemia: inducing hyperemia with papavarine and measuring pressure-derived renal fractional flow reserve in renal arteries with moderate stenosis. *Cathet Cardiovasc Intervent.* 2005;64:480.
25. van der Hulst VPM, van Baalen J, Kool LS, et al. Renal artery stenosis: endovascular flow wire study for validation of Doppler US. *Radiology.* 1996;200:165.
26. Savader SJ, Lund GB, Osterman FA. Volumetric evaluation of blood flow in normal renal arteries with a Doppler Flow Wire: a feasibility study. *J Vasc Intervent Radiol.* 1997;8:209.
27. Bech GJW, De Bruyne B, Pijls NHJ, et al. Fractional flow reserve to determine the appropriateness of angioplasty in moderate coronary stenosis: a randomized trial. *Circulation.* 2001;103:2928.
28. Pijls NHJ, De Bruyne B. Coronary pressure measurements and fractional flow reserve. *Heart.* 1998;80:539.

CHAPTER (6)

VALVULAR PATHOPHYSIOLOGY

Blasé A. Carabello, MD

The cardiac valves permit efficient forward blood flow while preventing backflow, in turn creating unidirectional forward cardiac output. Valve disease leads either to reduction in orifice area (stenosis), impeding forward flow, or to incompetence, permitting either regurgitant flow or a combination of these effects. Valve stenosis exerts a pressure overload on the ventricle behind the stenotic valve because that chamber must generate increased pressure to drive the blood stream past the narrowed orifice. Valve incompetence exerts a volume overload on the affected ventricle, which must enlarge to compensate for the forward flow that is lost to regurgitation. The effects of these overloads on ventricular function and geometry are dealt with in subsequent chapters. This chapter focuses on the evaluation of valve lesion severity and the effects of valve disease on hemodynamics.

VALVULAR STENOSIS

【 】 MITRAL STENOSIS

Usually in early diastole there is a small gradient across the mitral valve that initiates filling and then rapidly dissipates (Figure 6-1A).[1] Indeed, the normally opened mitral orifice is 4–5 cm², which creates a functionally single chamber of left atrium and left ventricle (LV) during diastole; thus, pressures in both chambers are equal. Mitral stenosis, which is usually caused by rheumatic heart disease, reduces orifice area, in turn causing a gradient between left atrium and left ventricle. Mitral stenosis eventually leads to pronounced hemodynamic effects, although little hemodynamic disturbance develops until orifice area is compromised to less than half its normal size. As stenosis worsens, the pressure gradient between left atrium and left ventricle becomes larger and longer in duration (Figure 6-1B). This gradient is added to normal

left atrial pressure, causing left atrial hypertension, and eventually leading to pulmonary congestion. As mitral stenosis worsens further, reduced valve aperture impairs LV filling, limiting cardiac output. Thus, despite usually normal LV muscle function, the hemodynamics are those of LV failure. Although left atrial contraction assists late atrial emptying, most transmitral flow occurs early in diastole, and much of the propellant force creating the pressure driving blood across the valve ultimately is derived from the right ventricle. Therefore it is this chamber that is pressure overloaded by the disease. Still further stenosis of the mitral valve causes secondary pulmonary vasoconstriction, reinforcing and worsening pulmonary hypertension and right ventricular pressure overload.

【 】 ASSESSING STENOSIS SEVERITY

Because transvalvular gradient is flow dependent, a measure of stenosis severity that incorporates both flow and gradient is helpful in assessing stenosis severity. Valve area has become the most widely used of these measures.[2] Flow (F) is the product of orifice area (A) and stream velocity (V) ($F = A \times V$). Rearranging the terms, $A = F/V$. When using Doppler echocardiography to assess orifice area, velocity is measured directly. In using invasive hemodynamics to assess stenosis severity, the transvalvular pressure gradient is measured and converted to velocity using the formula $V = \sqrt{2}\,gh$, where g is the acceleration as a result of gravity (980 m/sec) and h = the mean pressure gradient. Thus, valve area equals $F/44.3\sqrt{h}$. Because flow normally tends to stream through the center of an orifice, physiologic valve area is smaller than actual anatomic valve area. This property is corrected using a constant of orifice contraction, C_c. Because not all of the pressure gradient is converted to flow (some energy is lost to friction) another constant, that of velocity loss (C_v), is used. In 1951, Richard Gorlin and his father[2] proposed the following equation for calculation of

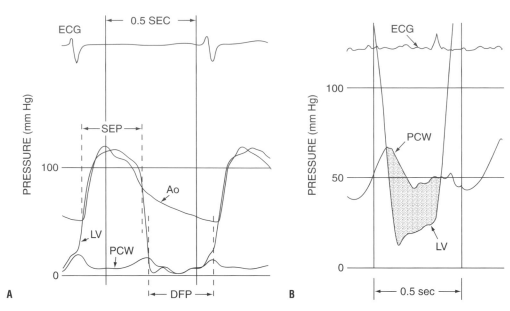

FIGURE 6-1. (A) Simultaneous normal left ventricular (LV), aortic (Ao), and pulmonary capillary wedge pressure (PCW) tracings are shown. SEP = systolic ejection period; DFP = diastolic filling period. *(Reproduced with permission from Carabello BA, Grossman W. Calculation of stenotic valve orifice area. In: Grossman's Cardiac Catheterization, Angiography, and Intervention, 6th ed. Baim DS, Grossman W, eds. Lippincott, Williams & Wilkins, 2000;193–209.)* **(B)** Simultaneous LV and PCW tracings from a patient with mitral stenosis are shown. The shaded area represents the transmitral gradient. *(Reproduced with permission from Connolly HM, Oh JK, Schaff HV, et al. Severe aortic stenosis with low transvalvular gradient and severe left ventricular dysfunction: result of aortic valve replacement in 52 patients. Circulation. 2000;101:1940.)*

valve area:

$$A = F/C_c \cdot C_v \cdot 44.3\sqrt{h}$$

Flow is expressed as cardiac output during the time in diastole that the mitral valve is open (diastolic filling period, dfp). Thus the final formula is

$$MVA = CO/HR \cdot dfp$$

where CO equals cardiac output in l/min and HR is heart rate.

The Gorlins were unable to develop the constants for the equation. Instead, they compared their calculated results to actual valve areas from autopsy and surgical specimens and applied an empiric constant of 0.85 to the denominator. By doing so, the recalculated valve areas came to within 0.2 cm^2 of the actual valve areas. Even as newer noninvasive methods have become available for quantifying mitral valve area, the Gorlin formula has remained a gold standard for valve area determination.

WHEN INVASIVE DETERMINATION OF MITRAL VALVE AREA IS DESIRABLE

As noted previously, several noninvasive methods have been developed for the determination of mitral valve area. The two most commonly used are the pressure–half time method and direct planimetry.[3,4] In general, these methods are adequate for clinical decision making. However, in some cases there is a discrepancy between clinical and laboratory assessment of stenosis severity; in such cases the additional information from invasive evaluation is helpful in making a final decision regarding the severity of a given patient's mitral stenosis and its management. The usual cause of

discordance between clinical and noninvasive assessment of the severity of mitral stenosis occurs in the patient who manifests ambiguous symptoms of heart failure while valve area is calculated to be in the mild to moderate range. Here, an invasive evaluation of hemodynamics can settle the issue. Evaluation of left atrial pressure (pulmonary capillary wedge pressure, PCWP), cardiac output, and pulmonary artery pressure at rest and during exercise is usually very illuminating. Regardless of calculated valve area, if wedge pressure and transvalvular gradient are either significantly increased at rest or more likely provoked to increase with exercise, the hemodynamics explain the patient's symptoms and suggest that mechanical relief of obstruction will lead to clinical improvement. If exercise does not provoke significant hemodynamic abnormalities, causes other than the patient's mitral stenosis should be sought to explain the patient's symptoms. Unfortunately, in today's busy interventional catheter laboratories, careful assessment of hemodynamics, especially with exercise, has become a rarity.

PITFALLS IN THE INVASIVE ASSESSMENT OF MITRAL STENOSIS

【 】 MEASURING THE GRADIENT

In the absence of transseptal puncture, left atrial pressure is estimated from the PCWP. There is much debate concerning whether this is a reliable left atrial pressure surrogate.[5,6] In fact, the PCWP is or is not reliable, depending on the technique used to measure it. Apart from noting that the catheter appears to be wedged and has (in sinus rhythm) typical a and v waves, it is crucial to confirm that the catheter is truly wedged by removing highly oxygen-saturated (>90%) blood from the catheter while in the wedged position.[1,6] Failure to perform this confirmatory step often results in recording a pressure that is hybrid between PCWP and pulmonary artery pressure, in turn overestimating both the PCWP and the transvalvular gradient, often by as much as 5 mm Hg. In addition, the transducers measuring both the left ventricular and PCW pressures must be properly calibrated and zeroed. Although recording device internal standards for calibration have improved over the years, there is no substitute for mercury calibration, considering that errors of just a few mm Hg may have an impact on assessment of stenosis severity of the mitral valve, where a gradient of just 15 mm Hg is often consistent with severe disease.

[ ] ASSESSING MITRAL FLOW

The transmitral flow period used in calculating the valve area is the entire time the valve is open in diastole. This period is measured (Figure 6-1B) from the time the LV pressure tracing falls below PCWP in early diastole (valve opening) to where LV pressure exceeds PCWP in early systole (valve closing). However, the use of the PCWP to measure left atrial pressure causes an 80-msec delay from the actual pressure event in the left atrium and its recording as PCWP. Because the LV pressure is recorded directly, the two pressures become nonsimultaneous. This problem is corrected by tracing the PCWP recording on paper and reimposing it on the LV tracing using the correct timing of the actual pressure events. Failure to make this maneuver leads to substantial overestimation of the transvalvular gradient and inaccurate measurement of the dfp.

Mitral regurgitation adds a second error in assessing valve area. The pressure gradient is produced by the total flow crossing the valve. The cardiac output determination measures only forward flow, thus underestimating total flow, and, as a result, underestimates mitral valve area.

Finally and obviously, the cardiac output must be measured accurately. Although the gold standard for this determination is the Fick method, thermodilution is often substituted. Whereas this technique is usually accurate, accuracy diminishes in the presence of tricuspid regurgitation and low cardiac output, conditions commonly present in patients with mitral stenosis.[7,8] In some catheterization laboratories a "pseudo-Fick" approach is used, in which oxygen consumption is assumed from tables of normals adjusted for height and weight. Because patients with mitral stenosis are hardly normal with respect to cardiac physiology, this technique is fraught with error, and should be avoided.[9]

AORTIC STENOSIS

As with mitral stenosis, little hemodynamic disturbance occurs from aortic stenosis until the valve orifice area is reduced to less than half its normal 3.0 to 4.0 cm^2. Serious clinical consequences usually do not occur until aortic valve area is reduced to less than 1.0 cm^2 when the classic symptoms of angina, syncope, and heart failure develop, presaging sudden death.[10,11] As with mitral stenosis, aortic stenosis severity is usually assessed accurately noninvasively. An abundance of comparison studies show remarkable concordance between gradient measured invasively and gradient measured using Doppler echocardiography. Likewise, there is excellent concordance between invasively derived valve areas and those derived noninvasively using the continuity equation.[12,13] Thus in many catheterization laboratories coronary arteriography is only performed prior to contemplated aortic valve replacement with stenosis severity assessed noninvasively prior to catheterization.

[ ] INVASIVE ASSESSMENT OF AORTIC STENOSIS

Invasive assessment of aortic stenosis, like that of mitral stenosis, uses the Gorlin formula. Systolic ejection period is substituted for diastolic filling period (Figure 6-1A).[1] However, unlike mitral stenosis, the Gorlins had no data to compare calculated to actual valve area because at the time it was considered malpractice to cross the aortic valve with a catheter. Thus an empiric constant was never developed for the aortic valve area calculation.[14] Both the invasively derived and the noninvasively derived areas for the aortic valve are flow dependent, varying directly with flow.[15,16] Two explanations are usually given for this phenomenon. First, it may be that as flow through the valve is increased, the orifice truly opens wider. Second, there is speculation that the absence of knowing the discharge coefficient (or empiric constant) affects the calculation. In fact, there are data to support both points of view.[17,18]

[ ] WHEN INVASIVE DETERMINATION IS REQUIRED

Invasive assessment of aortic stenosis can be helpful in at least three situations. First, invasive assessment is useful when the clinical impression of the patient's symptoms and lesion severity do not agree with the noninvasive data; for example, in a patient with a angina, a physical exam consistent with severe disease but with an echo-Doppler exam that shows a gradient of only 20 mm Hg. Second, invasive evaluation is helpful when features of the noninvasive exam are inconsistent with one another; that is, the aortic valve opens well, yet there appears to be a large transvalvular gradient. Third, the invasive approach is often helpful in assessing the very difficult patient with low output and low gradient. This group of patients has advanced left ventricular dysfunction and both a high operative and late mortality rate (Figure 6-2).[19,20] However, patients in this group who augment their gradient and forward output during dobutamine stress show inotropic reserve and have a relatively good outcome following aortic valve replacement, whereas patients who fail to augment their gradient and forward output during dobutamine stress have a very poor prognosis (Figure 6-3).[21,22] Although dobutamine is often administered in the echo lab, administration during catheterization allows pre-analysis of the coronary anatomy. This is potentially important, because patients with severe coronary disease might fail to augment during dobutamine infusion, not because they lack inotropic reserve, but because dobutamine-induced ischemia from coronary disease precludes an increase in cardiac output.

Another aspect of managing this group of patients is a condition sometimes referred to as "pseudo-stenosis."[23] In this condition, a severely stenotic orifice area is calculated at rest. However, when output is increased, gradient fails to increase very much, resulting

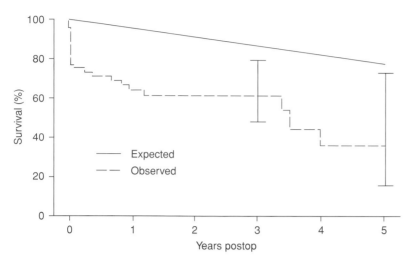

FIGURE 6-2. Postoperative survival for 52 patients with low gradient (<30 mm Hg) and low ejection fraction (<.35) is shown. Operative risk was 21%. *(Reproduced with permission from Connolly HM, Oh JK, Schaff HV, et al. Severe aortic stenosis with low transvalvular gradient and severe left ventricular dysfunction: result of aortic valve replacement in 52 patients. Circulation. 2000;101:1940.)*

in a much larger valve area.[21,24] Presumably, in such patients the aortic valve is only mildly or moderately stenotic, but incapable of being opened by a severely diseased left ventricle until inotropy is increased by dobutamine. Because in such cases it is primarily ventricular rather than valvular disease that is operative, it seems unlikely that such patients would improve with aortic valve replacement, although this issue has not been clearly resolved.

【 】 PITFALLS IN THE INVASIVE ASSESSMENT OF AORTIC VALVE AREA

Measuring the Gradient

The most common source of error in the invasive assessment of aortic valve area is made in measuring the transvalvular gradient.

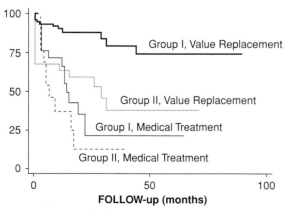

FIGURE 6-3. Survival for low ejection fraction, low gradient patients according to the presence of inotropic reserve. Group I consisted of 92 patients with inotropic reserve (>20% increase in stroke volume during dobutamine infusion). Group II consisted of 44 patients who failed to have inotropic reserve. *(Reproduced with permission from Monin JL, Quere JP, Monchi M, et al. Low-gradient aortic stenosis: operative risk stratification and predictors for long-term outcome. A multicenter study using dobutamine stress hemodynamics. Circulation. 2003;108:319.)*

Simultaneous measurement of ventricular and aortic pressures is preferred, and necessary if the patient is in atrial fibrillation. However, a gradient measured at pullback is acceptable, as long as reentering the left ventricle is not anticipated. As with mitral stenosis, proper gradient measurement begins with two properly balanced and zeroed pressure transducers. Confirmation of proper transducer fidelity is made by placing both catheters side by side in the ascending aorta (fluoroscopic confirmation) and recording perfectly matched pressures. After successfully crossing the aortic valve, the ventricular catheter must be confirmed as residing in the body of the left ventricle. This step is important because in almost all cases of aortic stenosis, there are really two gradients, one just beneath the valve and a second proximal to the outflow tract.[25,26] The subvalvular gradient is not to the result of true subvalvular stenosis, but rather occurs as blood accelerates into the relatively (compared to the body of the LV) narrow outflow tract.

In an effort to avoid using a second arterial puncture to admit a second catheter, some laboratories use a femoral sheath to record the distal arterial pressure. This technique simply does not work.[27] First, there can be no simultaneous recording of left ventricular and arterial pressure, because ventricular and femoral artery events do not occur simultaneously. Second, by the time the pressure wave reaches the femoral artery, there has been substantial pressure recovery as turbulent flow is converted back to laminar flow as velocity decreases away from the orifice narrowing. Pressure recovery can result in an extreme reduction in total gradient. Although pressure recovery is reflective of femoral hemodynamics, the same phenomenon interferes with proper measurement of the true transvalvular gradient.[28] Differences in pressure recording between proper and improper technique are demonstrated in Figure 6-4.[29]

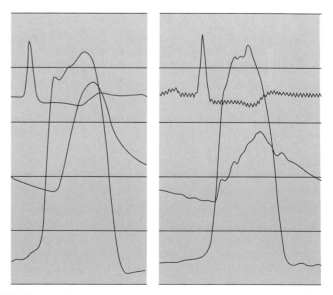

FIGURE 6-4. The transaortic valve gradient recorded properly with the left ventricular (LV) catheter in the body of the LV and the distal catheter in the aorta (**A**) is compared with the false low gradient recorded from LV outflow tract and femora artery (**B**). *(Reproduced with permission from Carabello BA. The timing of valve surgery. In: Cardiovascular Therapeutics, 2nd ed. Colucci WS, Gotto AM, Josephson ME, Loscalzo J, Oparil S, Popma JJ, eds. WB Saunders, 2002:975–993.)*

VALVULAR REGURGITATION

Although both the noninvasive and invasive assessments of valvular stenosis are quite accurate using modern technology, the assessment or valvular regurgitation as commonly practiced leaves much to be desired. In both the noninvasive and invasive arenas, excellent methods for quantifying the amount of left-side regurgitation present are available, but often ignored. The result is that the "eyeball technique" for assessing severity is often used. Here, the visual appearance of either the regurgitant jet at echocardiography or the opacification of the receiving chamber during contrast angiography is used to estimate the severity of regurgitation. Although no hard data exist, this method probably leads to significant errors in clinical judgment about the severity of the regurgitation present in about 20% of cases.

【 】 INVASIVE ASSESSMENT OF VALVULAR REGURGITATION

Waveforms

Although rarely used definitively to assess severity of valvular regurgitation, intracardiac pressures and their waveforms may give useful clues to regurgitant severity. In both mitral and aortic regurgitation, the volume overload on the left atrium (MR) and left ventricle (AR) leads to increased pressure in those chambers. It should be noted that chamber enlargement and enhanced chamber compliance can yield normal filling pressures even in the face of severe regurgitation. However, increased filling pressure, when present, helps support the presence of severe regurgitation. Increased left atrial pressure in mitral regurgitation is often but not always accompanied by a large v wave in the left atrial (pulmonary capillary wedge) pressure tracing.[30] In severe aortic regurgitation, a rapid rise in the left ventricular diastolic pressure, a femoral artery systolic pressure that is 40 mmHg or more higher than left ventricular systolic pressure (Hill's sign), and diastasis of left ventricular and aortic pressures add evidence that the aortic regurgitation is severe (Figure 6-5).[23] In tricuspid regurgitation, the right atrial pressure tracing may become ventricularized; that is, as the tricuspid valve becomes progressively less competent, the right ventricular pressure is transferred progressively more to the right atrium, so that right atrial and right ventricular pressures take on similar characteristics.

Angiography

In the noninvasive assessment of valvular regurgitation, the color-Doppler image observed is that of jet velocity, not of actual flow, one of the confounders in assessing regurgitant severity from jet characteristics. Contrast angiography (although still limited in assessing regurgitation) visualizes the actual flow of contrast from the initiating chamber to the receiving chamber through the regurgitant valve. This visualization, in turn, is used to estimate the amount of regurgitant flow using a semi-quantitative grading scale.

Quantitative Angiography

The best way of assessing the amount of regurgitation present would be to know actual regurgitant flow, which then could be represented as an absolute number or as a percentage of the total flow pumped by the left ventricle (regurgitant fraction). It is generally believed that a total regurgitant flow of more than 60 cc per beat or a regurgitant fraction exceeding 0.5 represents regurgitation severe enough to cause symptoms, ventricular damage, and death.

$$RF = sv_t - fsv$$

where RF is regurgitant flow, sv_t is total left ventricular stroke volume, and fsv is forward stroke volume. Regurgitant fraction is

$$RF/sv_t$$

Total stroke volume is determined by quantitative left ventriculography as end diastolic volume minus end systolic volume. These volumes are determined by the area–length or Simpson's rule methods. Forward stroke volume is forward cardiac output (Fick or thermodilution methods) divided by heart rate.

【 】 WHEN INVASIVE ASSESSMENT OF VALVULAR REGURGITATION SHOULD BE EMPLOYED

In usual practice, the estimation of regurgitant severity is made noninvasively. The validity of this assessment should be challenged when the clinical impression of lesion severity is at odds with the echocardiographic assessment. The most frequent error made is failing to take the apparent amount of regurgitation into the context of the ventricular geometry present. If severe regurgitation has

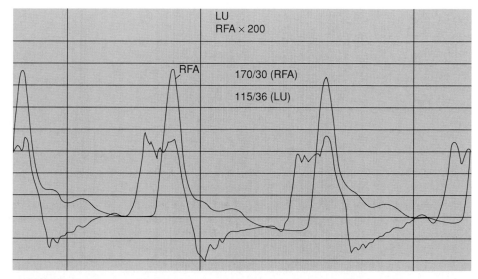

FIGURE 6-5. Left ventricular (LV) and femoral artery pressure tracings from a patient with severe aortic regurgitation. The femoral artery systolic pressure is substantially higher than the LV pressure (Hill's sign). Other features of severe aortic regurgitation include the rapid rise in the LV diastolic pressure and diastolic equalization of femoral and LV pressures (diastasis). *(Reproduced with permission from Carabello BA, Ballard WL, Gazes PC. Cardiology Pearls. Hanley & Belfus, 1994:142.)*

been present chronically and the patient is asymptomatic, adequate forward output at noncongestive filling pressure is implied. For this to occur, the left ventricle must enlarge in order to provide enough total stroke volume to make up for that which is lost to regurgitation.[31] In addition, in mitral regurgitation, the left atrium must enlarge to accommodate the regurgitant volume at normal filling pressure. If both chambers are normal in size, it implies that the regurgitation is not severe or is acute, in which case the patient should be symptomatic. Thus when the diagnosis of severe valvular regurgitation is made in the presence of normal left ventricular and/or left atrial volume, severity should almost always be confirmed invasively.

Pitfalls

As with the stenotic lesions, if the pressure measurements are to be useful, they must be obtained from properly calibrated and zeroed transducers. In addition, because wave contour is also a factor to be considered, proper damping of the recording system is essential. Confirmation that proper damping is present is an assessment made from experienced observers analogous to judging that an artist used the proper shade of blue in painting the sky. This art form seems to be waning as less attention is paid to proper pressure recording.

In performing contrast angiography, the most common error is the injection of too little dye into the initiating chamber. Because contrast must fill both the initiating and receiving chambers, which are enlarged to begin with, at least 60 cc of contrast should be injected. Smaller injections may lead to poor opacification of the receiving chamber, in turn causing significant underestimation of the amount of regurgitation present. In addition, in mitral regurgitation, ventricular ectopy, which by itself may cause mitral regurgitation, must be avoided, which requires careful placement of the left ventricular angiographic catheter and a test injection free of ectopy.

SUMMARY

Current noninvasive assessment of the severity of valvular heart disease is usually quite accurate. Further knowledge is added to noninvasive assessment by the ability of the technique to help establish valve pathoanatomy. Nonetheless, noninvasive assessment and clinical assessment are at odds with each, often enough that refined invasive assessment is necessary to arrive at a clinical decision. It is especially important in this case that attention be paid to the proper hemodynamic principles that are so crucial in making the correct clinical judgment.

REFERENCES

1. Carabello BA, Grossman W. Calculation of stenotic valve orifice area. In: *Grossman's Cardiac Catheterization, Angiography, and Intervention,* 6th ed. Baim DS, Grossman W, eds. Lippincott, Williams & Wilkins, 2000;193–209.
2. Gorlin R, Gorlin G. Hydraulic formula for calculation of area of stenotic mitral valve, other cardiac values, and central circulatory shunts. *Am Heart J.* 1951;41:1.
3. Hatle L, Brubakk A, Tromsdale A, et al: Noninvasive assessment of pressure drop in mitral stenosis by Doppler ultrasound. *Br Heart J.* 1978;40:131.
4. Martin RP, Rakowski H, Kleiman JH: Reliability and reproducibility of two-dimensional echocardiographic measurement of the stenotic mitral valve orifice area. *Am J Cardiol.* 1979;43:560.
5. Nishimura RA, Rihal CS, Tajik AJ, Holmes DR Jr. Accurate measurement of the transmitral gradient in patients with mitral stenosis: a simultaneous catherization and Doppler echocardiographic study. *J Am Coll Cardiol.* 1994;24:152.
6. Lange RA, Moore DM, Cigarroa RG, Hillis LD. Use of pulmonary capillary wedge pressure to assess severity of mitral stenosis: is true left atrial pressure needed in this condition? *J Am Coll Cardiol.* 1989;13:825.
7. Visscher MB, Johnson JA. The Fick principle: analysis of potential errors in the conventional application. *J Appl Physiol.* 1953;5:635.
8. van Grondelle AV, Ditchey RV, Groves BM, et al. Thermodilution method overestimates low cardiac output in humans. *Am J Physiol.* 1983;245:H690.
9. Dehmer GJ, Firth BG, Hillis LD. Oxygen consumption in adult patients during cardiac catheterization. *Clin Cardiol.* 1982;5:436.
10. Ross J Jr, Braunwald E. Aortic stenosis. *Circulation.* 1968;38SupplV:V-61-7.
11. Otto CM, Burwash IG, Legget Me, et al. A prospective study of asymptomatic valvular aortic stenosis: clinical, echocardiographic, and exercise predictors of outcome. *Circulation.* 1997;95:2262.
12. Ohlsson J, Wranne B. Noninvasive assessment of valve area in patients with aortic stenosis. *J Am Coll Cardiol.* 1986;7:501.
13. Teirstein P, Yeager M, Yock PG, Popp RL. Doppler echocardiographic measurement of aortic valve area in aortic stenosis: a noninvasive application of the Gorlin formula. *J Am Coll Cardiol.* 1986;8:1059.
14. Carabello BA. Advances in the hemodynamic assessment of stenotic cardiac valves. *J Am Coll Cardiol.* 1987;10:912.
15. Burwash IG, Thomas DD, Sadahiro M, et al. Dependence of Gorlin formula and continuity equation valve areas on transvalvular volume flow rate in valvular aortic stenosis. *Circulation.* 1994;39:827.
16. Cannon JD, Jr, Zile MR Crawford FA, Jr, Carabello BA. Aortic valve resistance as an adjunct to the Gorlin formula in assessing the severity of aortic stenosis in symptomatic patients. *J Am Coll Cardiol.* 1992;20:1517.
17. Tardif JC, Rodrigues AG, Hardy JF, et al. Simultaneous determination of aortic valve area by the Gorlin formula and by transesophageal echocardiography under different transvalvular flow conditions: evidence that anatomic aortic valve area does not change with variations in flow in aortic stenosis. *J Am Coll Cardiol.* 1997;29:1296.
18. Voelker W, Reul H, Nienhaus G, et al. Comparison of valvular resistance, stroke work loss and Gorlin valve area for quantification of aortic stenosis: an in vitro study in a pulsatile aortic flow model. *Circulation.* 1995;91:1196.
19. Carabello BA, Green LH, Grossman W, Cohn LH, Koster JK, Collins JJ, Jr. Hemodynamic determinants of prognosis of aortic valve replacement in critical aortic stenosis and advances congestive heart failure. *Circulation.* 1980;62:4208.
20. Connolly HM, Oh JK, Schaff HV, et al. Severe aortic stenosis with low transvalvular gradient and severe left ventricular dysfunction: result of aortic valve replacement in 52 patients. *Circulation.* 2000;101:1940.
21. Nishimuara RA, Grantham JA, Connolly HM, Schaff HV, Higano ST, Holmes DR. Low-output, low-gradient aortic stenosis in patients with depressed left ventricular systolic function: the clinical utility of the dobutamine challenge in the catherization laboratory. *Circulation.* 2002;106:809.
22. Monin JL, Quere JP, Monchi M, et al. Low-gradient aortic stenosis: operative risk stratification and predictors for long-term outcome. A multicenter study using dobutamine stress hemodynamics. *Circulation.* 2003;108:319.
23. Carabello BA, Ballard WL, Gazes PC. *Cardiology Pearls.* Hanley & Belfus, 1994:142.
24. deFilippi CR, Willett DL, Brickner ME, et al. Usefulness of dobutamine echocardiography in distinguishing severe from nonsevere valvular aortic stenosis in patients with depressed left ventricular function and low transvalvular gradients. *Am J Cardiol.* 1995;75:191.
25. Pasipoularides A. Clinical assessment of ventricular ejection dynamics with and without outflow obstruction. *J Am Coll Cardiol.* 1990;15:859.
26. Laskey WK, Kussmaul WG. Subvalvular gradients in patients with valvular aortic stenosis: prevalence, magnitude, and physiological importance. *Circulation.* 2001;104(9):1019.
27. Folland ED, Parisi AF, Carbone C. Is peripheral arterial pressure a satisfactory substitute for ascending aortic pressure when measuring aortic valve gradients? *J Am Coll Cardiol.* 1984;4:1207.
28. Assey Me, Zile MR, Usher BW, Karavan MP, Carabello BA. Effect of catheter positioning on the variability of measured gradient in aortic stenosis. *Cathet Cardiovasc Diagn.* 1993;30:287.
29. Carabello BA. The timing of valve surgery. In: *Cardiovascular Therapeutics,* 2nd ed. Colucci WS, Gotto AM, Josephson ME, Loscalzo J, Oparil S, Popma JJ, eds. WB Saunders, 2002:975–993.
30. Fuchs RM, Heuser RR, Yin FCP, et al. Limitations of pulmonary wedge V waves in diagnosing mitral regurgitation. *Am J Cardiol.* 1982;49(4):849.

CHAPTER (7)

Arterial Disease

Frederick G. P. Welt, MD, Campbell Rogers, MD, and Daniel I. Simon, MD

ATHEROSCLEROSIS

There is increasing understanding of the molecular and cellular pathophysiology of the vascular responses to injury, whether from the sustained effects of hyperlipidemia leading to atherosclerosis, or from the sudden impact of placement of a stainless steel stent under high pressure leading to restenosis. A common thread that links these events is an inflammatory response to injury, and it is increasingly appreciated that the inflammatory process not only initiates these lesions, but often dictates their clinical presentation as well. A fundamental knowledge of these processes is necessary to understand the natural history of the disease processes that affect the patients who present to the catheterization laboratory, as well as to understand the consequences of the therapies used during coronary intervention. This chapter is therefore designed to describe the known pathophysiology of atherosclerosis, the conversion of stable atherosclerotic plaques to ones that cause acute coronary syndromes, the pathophysiology of restenosis emphasizing the differences between balloon- and stent-induced injury, and to describe how vascular remodeling influences these processes.

【 】 ATHEROSCLEROSIS: A RESPONSE TO INJURY

Atherosclerosis is a chronic inflammatory disease initiated and sustained by injury to the vascular wall.[1] Several injurious processes have been identified, largely through extensive epidemiologic studies (Table 7-1). These include metabolic conditions such as sustained exposure to low-density lipoprotein (LDL), hyperglycemia associated with diabetes, and hyper-homocysteinemia. However, other factors, including physical (hypertensive changes in shear stress), environmental (tobacco smoke), and possibly infectious (*Chlamydia pneumoniae*) processes, have also been implicated. The common thread of injury to the vessel wall is an inflammatory response that involves a complex and still incompletely understood sequence of interactions between endothelial and smooth muscle cells (SMCs), leukocytes, and platelets. These cells and their secreted growth factors and cytokines combine with lipid and components of the vessel wall to eventually form the mature atherosclerotic plaque. The central role of inflammation in the pathogenesis of atherosclerosis is evidenced by numerous epidemiologic studies that demonstrate a correlation between circulating markers of inflammation (eg, fibrinogen, C-reactive protein (CRP), serum amyloid protein, myeloperoxidase) with subsequent risk of coronary events.[2,3]

【 】 ATHEROSCLEROSIS: PATHOGENESIS

There are several key biologic events involved in atherogenesis: extracellular lipid accumulation, leukocyte recruitment, foam cell formation, neointimal growth as a result of SMC migration and proliferation and extracellular matrix deposition, and vessel remodeling (Figure 7-1).

Extracellular and Intracellular Lipid Accumulation

The key event in the creation of the incipient atherosclerotic lesion is the accumulation of lipoproteins within the intima. These lipoproteins may subsequently be modified by processes such as oxidation, and glycation in the presence of aging and hyperglycemia. The modification of these lipoproteins helps elicit a cascade of molecular and cellular events, including the stimulation of growth factor and cytokine production from endothelial and SMCs. These early events lead to recruitment of leukocytes and eventually to SMC proliferation and migration, all of which act to form the mature atherosclerotic plaque. Of central importance is the understanding that hyperlipidemia is an inflammatory state.

TABLE 7-1

Causes of Vascular Injury

Metabolic
    Hyperlipidemia
    Hyperglycemia
    Hyperhomocysteinemia

Physical
    Shear forces (hypertension)
    Laminar vs. nonlaminar flow (ie, bifurcations)

Environmental
    Tobacco Smoke

Infectious
    Chlamydia
    Herpes simplex
    Cytomegalovirus

The interaction between inflammation and hyperlipidemia is evident in the presence of foam cells, the hallmark of the fatty streak, the initial lesion of atherosclerosis. The foam cell is a macrophage named for the abundance of lipid within the cell. Macrophages bind and internalize modified lipoprotein particles via a number of "scavenger receptors," including scavenger receptor–A family members, CD36, and macrosialin. Foam cells are able to further modify lipoproteins. In addition, lipoproteins can prove toxic to macrophages, leading to necrotic debris as well as free-cholesterol clefts and ester within the lesion. This necrotic debris, along with the expression of tissue factor and other molecules, leads to a very pro-thrombotic environment within the plaque, and is a serious threat to local blood flow in the setting of loss of integrity of the barrier between plaque and blood stream.

Leukocyte Recruitment

Leukocytes, especially macrophages, play pivotal roles in atherosclerosis through their release of critical cytokines and growth factors that influence not only atherogenesis, but processes of plaque rupture and thrombosis as well. The process of leukocyte recruitment, attachment, and migration into the plaque is under the influence of a variety of molecules. As a response to injury, such as the accumulation of lipoproteins, endothelial cells express certain adhesion molecules (CAMs), such as E-selectin, that interact with ligands on the surface of circulating leukocytes to begin a process of loose association and rolling along the surface of the vessel.[4] Subsequent tight binding mediated by the integrin class of adhesion molecules stops the leukocyte prior to the process of diapedesis. Although their pathologic role is uncertain, soluble forms of CAMs can be found in plasma. Human studies demonstrate that plasma levels of ICAM-1 and E-selectin correlate with clinical manifestations of coronary atherosclerosis.[5]

Also central to the recruitment of leukocytes to areas of vascular injury, chemokines are a group of chemoattractant cytokines produced by a variety of somatic cells, including SMCs, endothelial cells, and leukocytes. One important chemokine of the C-C class,

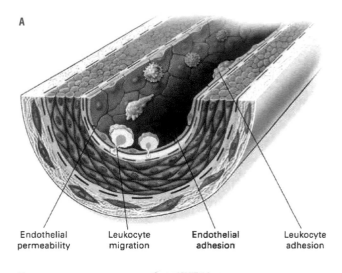

A

| Endothelial permeability | Leukocyte migration | Endothelial adhesion | Leukocyte adhesion |

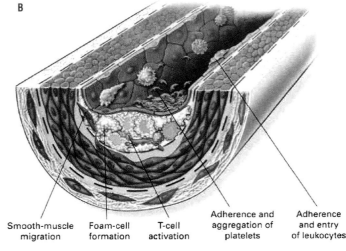

B

| Smooth-muscle migration | Foam-cell formation | T-cell activation | Adherence and aggregation of platelets | Adherence and entry of leukocytes |

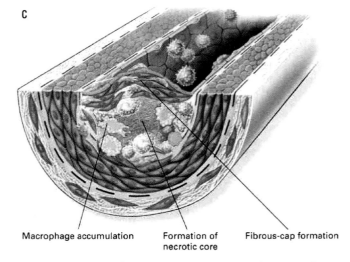

C

| Macrophage accumulation | Formation of necrotic core | Fibrous-cap formation |

FIGURE 7-1. Stages of atherosclerotic plaque growth. (**A**) Initial stage of atherosclerosis involves injury to the vessel wall with subsequent expression of inflammatory adhesion molecules, which leads to leukocyte recruitment. (**B**) Intermediate lesions involve macrophages imbibing oxidized LDL leading to foam cell formation. There is continued leukocyte recruitment, formation of an early lipid core, and smooth muscle cell (SMC) proliferation and migration. (**C**) The advanced or mature atherosclerotic plaque consists of a necrotic lipid core with foam cells, necrotic debris, and free cholesterol esters. In addition, there is a fibrous cap consisting of SMCs and extracellular matrix. (*Reproduced with permission from Ross R. The pathogenesis of atherosclerosis–an update. N Engl J Med. 1986;314:488.*)

monocyte chemoattractant protein-1 (MCP-1), participates in the recruitment of monocytes in particular.[6] Also critical is the C-X-C chemokine interleukin-8 (IL-8), which participates in the recruitment of leukocytes to areas of vascular injury. IL-8 has been extensively documented in the recruitment of neutrophils,[7] and more recent evidence suggests that the murine analog of IL-8, KC also plays a critical role in the recruitment of monocytes to injured areas.[8]

Several types of leukocytes that can be identified within advanced human plaques include macrophages and T-lymphocytes. However, the monocyte is thought to be the first leukocyte recruited to the incipient atheroma. As lesions mature, there tends to be excess accumulation of leukocytes at the "shoulder" regions of plaques, where the eccentric plaque merges with the more normal architecture of the vessel. This clustering is thought to make these shoulder regions more vulnerable to the consequences of atherosclerosis.[9] In addition, it has long been observed that atherosclerotic lesions develop preferentially at areas of bifurcations within the coronary tree. This likely is related to disturbances in flow patterns and resultant areas of flow separation and altered shear stress, leading to preferential areas of up-regulation of adhesion molecules and increased leukocyte recruitment.

Smooth Muscle Migration, Proliferation, and Extracellular Matrix Deposition

Smooth muscle cells and their products are responsible for giving structure to the mature atherosclerotic plaque, which is, at first, little more than a collection of lipids and foam cells. Under the influence of growth factors and chemoattractants such as platelet-derived growth factor (PDGF) and thrombin, SMCs migrate out from the media into the neointima where they begin to proliferate. In addition, SMCs produce extracellular matrix constituents including collagen, proteoglycans, elastin, fibrin, fibrinogen, fibronectin, and vitronectin. These proteins often account for a substantial volume of the plaque, and are important in determining the structural integrity of the fibrous cap. In some patients, an additional process of mineralization of the atherosclerotic plaque occurs with deposition of calcium and osteopontin. Although of uncertain biologic and prognostic significance, mineralization is of particular interest to the interventional cardiologist, as it may influence technical aspects of the procedure.

Plaque Angiogenesis

A newly emerging area of interest is the potential role of angiogenesis in plaque growth and in the pathogenesis of atherosclerotic complications.[10] New vasculature, under the influence of angiogenic growth factors, may grow from the vaso vasorum within the adventitia into the plaque. These vessels may be disrupted and cause plaque hemorrhage independent of plaque rupture. In addition, analogous to tumor growth, these vessels may stimulate plaque growth. There is experimental evidence demonstrating inhibition of plaque growth by angiogenic inhibitors in a mouse model of atherosclerosis.[10]

Mature Atherosclerotic Plaque

Mature atherosclerotic plaque is therefore made up of several components, including a fibrous cap consisting of SMCs and extracellular matrix proteins overlying a necrotic lipid core consisting of free cholesterol esters, foam cells, other leukocytes such as T-cells, and necrotic debris of dead foam cells (Figure 7-1). These plaques commonly are eccentric in nature, and there is heterogeneity in terms of the thickness of the cap as well as distribution of leukocytes, which tend to cluster in shoulder regions. Both of these features have potential importance in terms of propensity of plaques to cause acute coronary syndromes.

Vascular Remodeling

Although angiography remains the mainstay of diagnosis in coronary artery disease, its major limitation is that it provides information only on luminal encroachment of lesions, not on architecture of the vessel wall. Use of intravascular ultrasound (IVUS) provides a much broader understanding of the nature of atherosclerosis by allowing systematic investigation of plaque architecture not only at sites of flow-obstructing lesions, but also throughout the vessel. Although the interventional cardiologist is most concerned with focal obstructive lesions in proximal portions of the vessel, it is important to realize that it is now recognized that atherosclerosis is almost always universally present throughout the coronary tree. The amount of impingement of the plaque on the lumen is controlled not only by the growth of plaque volume, but also by vascular remodeling, which involves restructuring of cellular or noncellular components of the wall, and can occur under a variety of stimuli.[11] For instance, under situations of hypertension, muscle mass of the vessel wall can increase in order to normalize wall stress. In atherosclerosis, remodeling may consist of compensatory enlargement of the vessel to preserve luminal area (Figure 7-2). Central to the process of vascular remodeling are the matrix metalloproteinases (MMPs), a family of zinc-dependent proteases that have been demonstrated to be up-regulated in areas of vessel wall remodeling and are thought to play a central role in plaque rupture as well.[12]

【 】 CLINICAL SEQUELAE OF ATHEROSCLEROSIS

A convenient way of thinking about coronary artery disease is as a spectrum of syndromes, from stable angina at one end, associated

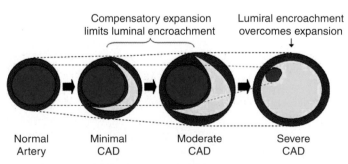

Figure 7-2. Schematic of vascular remodeling. As the atherosclerotic lesion progresses, initial enlargement of the entire vessel allows preservation of luminal area. As atherosclerosis becomes severe, enlargement is overcome by progression of the atherosclerotic plaque, and luminal area is compromised. (*Adapted from Glagov S, Weisenberg, Zarins CK, et al. Compensatory enlargement of human atherosclerotic coronary New Engl J Med. 1997;317:1371*).[11a]

with exertional angina and relatively benign outcomes, to ST segment elevation MI at the other end, associated with sudden complete thrombotic occlusion of an epicardial blood vessel and high rates of morbidity and mortality. The intermediate syndromes of unstable angina and non-q-wave myocardial infarction exist between these two extremes. However, unstable angina, non-q-wave MI, and ST-segment elevation MI are collectively termed the "acute coronary syndromes" because of their similar pathophysiology and worse prognosis in comparison to stable angina. This is explained by the fact that complications from atherosclerosis can result from two related but distinct mechanisms: (1) simple luminal narrowing can lead to an imbalance between supply and demand for blood, typically resulting in stable exertional angina; or (2) atheromatous plaques may rupture, resulting in a thrombus of varying degrees of occlusion.[13] Critical to the understanding of coronary disease is the knowledge that the propensity for thrombotic complications depends on a variety of vascular biologic factors, not the degree of stenosis.

Progressive Lumen Encroachment and Stable Angina

As atherosclerotic lesions grow in size and depending on the amount of compensatory vascular remodeling that occurs, they may gradually encroach on the lumen of the vessel (see Figure 7-2). As a response to reduction in flow, there is vasodilation of the distal microcirculation to increase in flow. This reduces coronary vascular reserve, or the ability of the coronary circulation to increase blood flow in response to demand, which typically leads to exertional angina, which is short in duration and relieved by rest. At what point luminal encroachment causes symptoms depends on many factors, including the severity of the lesion, the demand of the distal cardiac bed, and the oxygen-carrying capacity of the blood stream. However, in general, lesions begin to produce symptoms when they reach a diameter of approximately 60%–70% stenosis. Modern techniques of interrogating intracoronary hemodynamics with flow and pressure wires teach the interventional cardiologist that lesions with the same degree of angiographic stenosis may have very different hemodynamic consequences.[14]

Plaque Rupture and Thrombosis and the Acute Coronary Syndromes

The historical view of the conversion of stable to acute coronary syndromes held that atherosclerotic lesions impinged on the lumen of the vessel until some critical point was reached, at which either vasospasm or thrombosis in-situ developed to cause infarction. Considerable debate ensued as to whether thrombus found at autopsy was a pre- or postmortem phenomenon, despite the fact that James Herrick published his findings of thrombus as the predominant cause of sudden coronary obstruction in 1912.[15] The pivotal work was performed by DeWood and colleagues in their landmark 1980 paper,[16] where it was demonstrated angiographically that ST-segment elevation was associated with occlusion of epicardial vessels (Figure 7-3), and made the observation that thrombosis was present at the time of infarct. There is now considerable data to confirm this, including autopsy studies (Figure 7-4), as well as the use of angioscopy, which reveals the presence of visible thrombus associated with both unstable angina and acute myocardial infarction (MI).

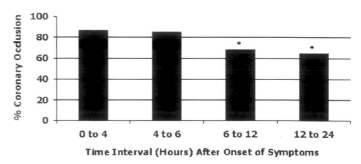

FIGURE 7-3. Percentage of patients with a totally occluded coronary artery in patients presenting after acute myocardial infarction as a function of time after onset of symptoms. *(Adapted from DeWood MA, Spores J, et al. Prevalence of total coronary occlusion during the early hours of transmural myocardial infarction. New Engl J Med. 1980;303:897.)*

Data from the early thrombolytic trials was instrumental in setting the stage for our modern understanding of acute coronary syndromes. As part of the design of these trials, patients presenting with acute MI underwent mandated angiography after randomization to either placebo or thrombolytic therapy. The angiograms revealed an unexpected finding, namely that the majority of lesions responsible for MI were less than 50% stenosed in diameter.[17] In addition, data from angiographic studies performed in patients before and after infarction show that mild and moderate stenoses may progress to cause MI in a matter of weeks to months. In analysis of four serial angiographic studies, only about 15% of acute MIs were found to arise from lesions with degrees of stenosis greater than 60% on an antecedent angiogram[18](Figure 7-5). The implication of these data is that the vascular biologic state of the lesion is responsible for its propensity to cause an infarct, not

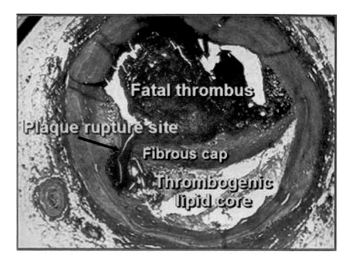

FIGURE 7-4. Histologic cross-section of coronary artery showing ruptured plaque at shoulder region and resultant fatal thrombosis. *(Reproduced with permission from Constantinedes, P: Plaque hemorrhages, their genesis and their role in supra-plaque thrombosis and atherogenesis. In Pathology of the Human Atherosclerotic Plaque, Glagov, S, Newman, WP III, Schaffer SA, eds. Springer-Verlag, 1990:393–411.)*

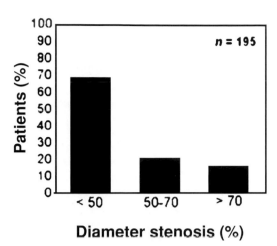

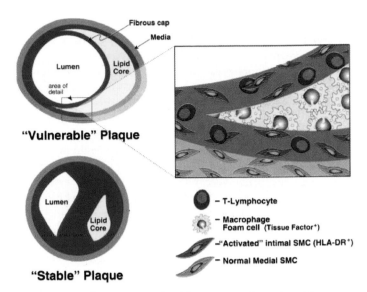

FIGURE 7-5. Data compiled from four thrombolytic trials showing that the majority of underlying lesions responsible for acute myocardial infarction are less than 50% diameter stenosis. *(Reproduced with permission from Smith SC, Jr. Risk-reduction therapy: the challenge to change. Presented at the 68th scientific sessions of the American Heart Association, November 13, 1995, Anaheim, California. Circulation. 1996;93:2205.)*

FIGURE 7-6. Characteristics of stable as opposed to vulnerable plaques. Vulnerable plaques have thinner fibrous caps and larger, more inflammatory cell—rich lipid cores. *(Reproduced with permission from Libby P. Molecular bases of the acute coronary syndromes. Circulation. 1995;91:2844.)*

the severity of stenosis. These data should not be misinterpreted to suggest that lesion severity is correlated with danger of infarction. Rather, noncritical lesions represent a larger population than critical lesions. In addition, as described previously, compensatory enlargement of the vessel often accompanies atherosclerosis. Therefore, even mildly stenotic lesions may represent large plaques by volume. In summary, thrombosis, often on a noncritical stenosis, caused by lesion disruption causes the majority of myocardial infarctions.

The proximate event leading to thrombosis at a lesion is plaque rupture (or, less commonly, endothelial denudation), leading to exposure of blood to highly thrombotic subendothelial components of the plaque. Histologic studies have identified several features that appear to be associated with plaques more vulnerable to rupture. These include a thin fibrous cap, a large lipid core, and an abundance of inflammatory cells largely concentrated at the shoulder regions of the plaque[9] (Figure 7-6). It is thought that inflammation is the key regulator of the structural integrity of the plaque.

The structural integrity of the plaque is dependent on a balance between two components: SMC mass and extracellular matrix content. In turn, SMC mass is a balance between migration of cells from the media and subsequent proliferation in the neointima on the one hand, and cell death on the other. There is evidence to suggest that cytokines released from inflammatory cells control apoptosis, or programmed cell death.[19] Extracellular matrix content is a balance between production from SMCs and degradation by a variety of proteases (Figure 7-7). Production of extracellular matrix content is dependent on both the number of cells present and their activity. Activated T-cells in the plaque secrete interferon-γ (IFN-γ), an inhibitor of SMC collagen synthesis. Inflammatory cells in atherosclerotic plaques also produce enzymes, such as matrix metalloproteinases and cathepsins, that are

capable of degrading important constituents of the extracellular matrix (eg, collagens, elastin).[9] Therefore, inflammatory cells can contribute to plaque weakening by decreasing SMC mass, decreasing extracellular matrix content, and increasing extracellular matrix degradation.

How and why plaques rupture when they do is a subject of increasing study. It has long been observed that there is a circadian variation in presentation of MI, with a peak in the early morning hours.[20] In addition, MI rates are known to be effected by events that produce population-wide stress, as was observed after the Northridge earthquake in Southern California in 1994.[21] These observations have led researchers to suggest that cortisol and adrenaline levels may have an impact on plaque rupture through their effects on systemic hemodynamic parameters. On a smaller scale, biomechanical studies using finite element analysis indicate

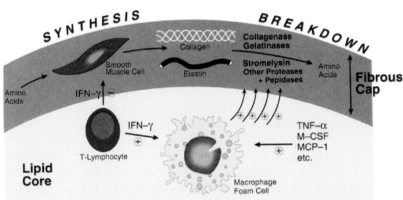

FIGURE 7-7. Thickness of the fibrous cap is a balance between synthesis of extracellular matrix proteins by SMCs and the breakdown of these products by degradative enzymes. These processes are largely under the influence of inflammatory cells. *(Reproduced with permission from Libby P. Molecular bases of the acute coronary syndromes. Circulation. 1995;91:2844.)*

that rupture sites coincide with highest circumferential biomechanical forces, which are highest at the shoulder regions of plaques.[22] Therefore, there is an interesting combination of both biochemical and biophysical characteristics that make rupture at the shoulder regions of plaques most likely. This is supported by histologic studies of coronary arteries of patients who died secondary to MI.

Although frank plaque rupture is the major antecedent cause of thrombotic complications of the acute coronary syndromes, other processes may also be responsible. Local superficial denudation of endothelial cells (perhaps secondary to apoptosis) may expose the internal elastic membrane representing an important thrombotic substrate. There is some evidence to suggest that these endothelial erosions occur more frequently in women and in diabetics. Mechanical injury during percutaneous coronary intervention is another source of local plaque disruption that may lead to thrombotic complications.

The final pathway through which either plaque rupture or endothelial denudation leads to alterations in flow is through thrombosis. Exposure of blood to the lipid core is a potent stimulus for thrombus formation, largely on the basis of exposure to tissue factor associated with lipid-laden and necrotic macrophages. There is a balance between procoagulant–anticoagulant and fibrinolytic–antifibrinolytic factors in the blood stream that likely predetermines the consequence of any given plaque disruption. In the presence of an intact and robust fibrinolytic system, a mural thrombus might undergo rapid lysis, limiting its clinical consequences to unstable angina or non-q-wave MI. Similarly, patients on antiplatelet agents such as aspirin obviously are protected to some degree. In the presence of prothrombotic factors such as elevated levels of fibrinogen or plasminogen activator inhibitor-1 (PAI-1), growth of a thrombus to occlusion may occur more frequently. Nonocclusive mural thrombus may be incorporated into the plaque during the process of healing, providing a mechanism for plaque growth.

There are numerous trials of antiplatelet therapy that corroborate the thrombotic paradigm of the acute coronary syndromes. Trials of lipid-lowering therapy have similarly demonstrated an interesting corroboration of theories of plaque vulnerability. These trials demonstrate marked reductions in subsequent coronary events associated with lipid lowering with essentially no change in lesion severity.[18] As stated previously, the hypothesis is that lipids within the plaque provide the critical initiating and sustaining inflammatory stimulus to plaque growth and rupture, and the beneficial actions of "statin" lipid-lowering agents may be derived in part from the reduction of inflammation, leading to stabilization of the fibrous cap and reduced thrombogenicity of the inner core. There is increasing evidence to support lipid-lowering therapy as a vital adjunct to acute as well as chronic therapy for patients presenting with acute coronary syndromes.

A more complete understanding of the mechanisms of plaque rupture and the development of novel strategies to stabilize lesions represents a major goal of vascular biologists and clinical cardiologists. Complicating the clinical situation is the fact that many different lesions of varying vulnerable potential may coexist in a vessel or throughout the coronary tree. Considerable interest exists in imaging techniques on both macroscopic and molecular levels to identify plaques most vulnerable to rupture in order to better prognosticate and direct therapy most effectively.

RESTENOSIS

Gruntzig et al.[23] ushered in the modern era of management of obstructive coronary artery disease with the introduction of coronary angioplasty. Yet, even in their first report on the subject (their 1979 landmark publication, "Non-operative dilatation of coronary-artery stenosis"), they found that 6 of 32 patients undergoing successful initial angioplasty suffered restenosis, a rate of 19%.[23] Large-scale registries have since documented a restenosis rate closer to 33%.[24] The clinical parameters most closely associated with restenosis are final vessel diameter, lesion length, and presence of diabetes. Understanding of the pathophysiology of restenosis has evolved considerably over time. Studies of human autopsy specimens revealed a fibrocellular response at sites of prior balloon angioplasty,[25] although early animal studies revealed initial endothelial denudation, medial dissection, and platelet deposition as an immediate response to balloon injury, and described late restenosis as a consequence of SMC migration and proliferation, as well as organized intraluminal thrombosis.[26,27] Synthesizing the results of these studies and studies of wound healing, Forrester et al.[28] proposed a paradigm for restenosis suggesting three phases in the process: (1) an inflammatory phase; (2) a granulation or cellular proliferation phase; and (3) a phase of remodeling involving extracellular matrix protein synthesis. As with atherogenesis, studies reveal a critical role for inflammatory cells in the restenotic process. In addition, the thrombotic response to vascular injury imposed by coronary intervention appears to play a critical role in the initial recruitment of inflammatory cells. Coronary stenting, now performed in the majority of cases, has a profound impact on the vascular biologic response to coronary intervention, particularly the impacts on the inflammatory response and vascular remodeling.

[ ] NEOINTIMAL GROWTH AND REMODELING IN STENT AND BALLOON ANGIOPLASTY RESTENOSIS

Given the difficulty obtaining human restenotic tissue, our understanding of the pathophysiology is heavily dependent on imaging techniques, such as IVUS, and animal models. Mintz et al.[29] used IVUS to determine the contributions of neointimal hyperplasia and negative remodeling after balloon angioplasty. They found that, although both negative remodeling (as measured by external elastic membrane area) and neointimal hyperplasia (as measured by plaque plus media cross-sectional area) contributed to restenosis, negative remodeling contributed substantially more. In contrast, angiographic analysis of the first two large-scale studies of coronary stents in humans (the STRESS[30] and BENESTENT[31] studies) revealed distinct differences between the pathophysiology of restenosis in balloon-injured and stented arteries. Arteries that received a stent experienced a much larger initial lumen gain, presumably as a result of the rigid scaffolding provided by the stent,

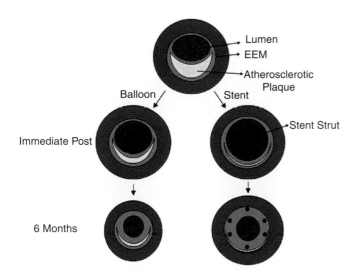

FIGURE 7-8. Illustration of differences in mechanisms of restenosis between plain balloon angioplasty and stenting. In balloon angioplastied vessels, restenosis is caused by a combination of neointimal growth and negative remodeling. Stented arteries have lower rates of restenosis despite incurring greater neointimal growth due to their ability to achieve a larger initial lumen size, and the elimination of negative remodeling. (Adapted from Welt FGP, Sobieszczsk PS. Coronary artery stents: design and biologic considerations. Cardiology Special Edition. 9:9.)[31a]

which prevents acute elastic recoil. At six-month follow-up, luminal area was greater and binary restenosis was less than balloon-angioplastied arteries. However, late loss (lumen immediately post minus lumen at follow-up) was actually greater in stented arteries. Therefore, stents cause greater neointimal growth, with their eventual benefit in restenosis attributable to their larger initial lumen gain and prevention of remodeling (Figure 7-8). This was confirmed with a serial IVUS study conducted by Hoffman and coworkers.[32]

【 】 MECHANISMS OF LEUKOCYTE RECRUITMENT AND INFILTRATION

Expansion of a balloon or placement of a stent causes injury within the vessel wall including dissection, crush injury of SMCs, and de-endothelialization. Leukocyte recruitment and infiltration occur at these sites of injury where platelets and fibrin have been deposited. Within areas of injury such as atherosclerotic and postangioplasty restenotic lesions, and in areas of ischemia-reperfusion injury, in vivo studies show that leukocytes and platelets are deposited together. For the inflammatory response after angioplasty, this interaction between platelets and leukocytes appears to be important.[33,34]

This interaction is explained by Diacovo et al.,[35] who put forth a paradigm of leukocyte attachment to surface-adherent platelets followed by transmigration. As with atherosclerosis, the initial loose association of leukocytes is mediated through the selectin class of adhesion molecules (particularly by platelet P-selectin[36]) followed by their firm adhesion and transplatelet migration, processes that are dependent on the integrin class of adhesion molecules.[35] The β_2 integrin molecule Mac-1 (CD11b/CD18) is present on both neutrophils and monocytes, and appears to be of central importance in leukocyte recruitment following vascular injury. In addition to promoting the accumulation of leukocytes at sites of vascular injury, the binding of platelets to neutrophils amplifies the inflammatory response by inducing neutrophil activation, up-regulating cell adhesion molecule expression, generating signals that promote integrin activation and chemokine synthesis. These processes of activation may be mediated through the release of soluble CD40 ligand, a proinflammatory molecule stored most abundantly in platelets. Bolstering these data, both neutrophil–platelet and monocyte–platelet aggregates have been identified in the peripheral blood of patients with coronary artery disease, and may be markers of disease activity and prognosis.[37,38]

【 】 EVIDENCE FOR A ROLE OF INFLAMMATION IN RESTENOSIS

Restenosis does not appear to be a case of accelerated atherosclerosis but rather a distinct temporal and pathophysiologic process. However, inflammation is an important common link between atherogenesis and restenosis. Observations in regard to restenosis have been hampered by the difficulty of obtaining human restenotic tissue. Farb et al.[39] investigated stented arteries from pathologic samples of 116 stents from 87 patients more than 90 days postprocedure. They found a statistically significant association between extent of medial damage, inflammation, and restenosis. Also linking leukocytes and restenosis, Moreno et al[40] present data from tissue retrieved from directional atherectomy at the time of angioplasty. They found a strong positive correlation between the number of macrophages present in the tissue at the time of angioplasty and subsequent risk of restenosis.

Systemic markers of inflammation following angioplasty have also provided insight into the mechanisms of restenosis. Neumann et al.[41] investigated systemic inflammation using a technique in which they collected blood samples both proximal to and just distal to the site of balloon dilatation in humans. Using flow cytometry to determine the expression of the neutrophil adhesion molecules L-selectin and CD11b, they found an up-regulation of these markers of leukocyte activation after angioplasty measured as a gradient between distal and proximal specimens. Mickelson et al.[42] were able to document up-regulation of CD11b on both neutrophils and monocytes using systemic venous specimens from patients undergoing angioplasty. They found that levels of CD11b had a positive correlation with adverse clinical events. Inoue et al.[43,44] confirmed these data, demonstrating that elevated levels of neutrophil CD11b are predictive of future propensity for restenosis after balloon angioplasty[43] and stenting[44] (Figure 7-9). Pietersma et al.[45] showed that interleukin-1 production by stimulated monocytes isolated from blood preangioplasty was correlated positively with late luminal loss, although activation of granulocytes measured by CD66 levels was inversely correlated with late loss. Cipollone et al.[46] demonstrated up-regulated levels of MCP-1 following percutaneous intervention in humans and found that MCP-1 levels correlate with risk for restenosis. Gaspardone et al.[47] showed a positive correlation between the nonspecific inflammatory marker C-reactive protein following stent placement and propensity for restenosis.

Animal models have been invaluable in elucidating basic cellular and molecular mechanisms of restenosis. In several experimental animal models, cell adhesion molecules critical for leukocyte

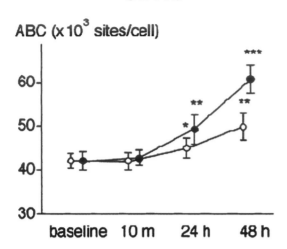

FIGURE 7-9. Serial changes in antibody-binding capacity (ABC) of CD11b after coronary stenting. Those patients with restenosis exhibit higher levels. * = p <0.05, ** = p <0.01, *** = p <0.001. (Reproduced with permission from Inoue T, Uchida T, Yaguchi I, Sakai Y, Takayanagi K, Morooka S. Stent-induced expression and activation of the leukocyte integrin Mac-1 is associated with neointimal thickening and restenosis. Circulation. 2003;107:1757.)

recruitment have been found to be up-regulated by an atherogenic diet,[48–50] induction of diabetes,[51] and increased shear stress.[52] After balloon endothelial denudation in a rabbit model, vascular cell adhesion molecule-1, ICAM-1, and MHC class II antigens were shown to be up-regulated in a sustained fashion.[53] A particularly potent inflammatory stimulus appears to be the implantation of a chronic indwelling endovascular stent, leading to a brisk early inflammatory response with abundant surface adherent leukocytes of both monocyte and granulocyte lineage.[54,55] Days and weeks later, macrophages invade the forming neointima and are observed clustering around stent struts, often forming giant cells. Evidence of the importance of monocytes comes from studies using blockade of early monocyte recruitment with antiinflammatory agents that result in reduced late neointimal thickening.[54,56,57] In the stented rabbit iliac artery, a strong correlation exists between tissue monocyte number and neointimal area, suggesting a causal role for monocytes in restenosis.[54] Activated macrophages may influence vascular repair through a variety of mechanisms, including production of a variety of mediators, including members of the interleukin family, tumor necrosis factor, monocyte chemoattractant protein-1, and growth factors such as platelet-derived growth factors, basic fibroblast growth factor, and heparin-binding epidermal growth factor.[58]

Several studies also show infiltration of neutrophils within the arterial wall following vascular injury.[59–61] As with macrophages, a concomitant reduction in neutrophil number and smooth muscle proliferation can be seen with administration of antiinflammatory agents, resulting in less neointimal growth.[55] The mechanisms by which neutrophils may affect vascular repair are not as fully understood as those for monocytes/macrophages. Although neutrophils are not typically thought to secrete growth factors, they can contribute to tissue injury through the release of reactive oxygen species and proteases.[58] In addition, it has been reported that rabbit vascular smooth cells are stimulated to proliferate when cocultured with neutrophils or neutrophil-conditioned media.[62] Neutrophils are also known to secrete cytokines, including IL-1, TNF-alpha, and IL-6.[63]

〖 〗 DIFFERENCES BETWEEN BALLOON AND STENT INJURY

Systematic investigation in both human and animal studies suggests important differences between vascular biologic responses to balloon- and stent-induced injury. Inoue et al.[64] used flow cytometry to measure CD11b (a member of the integrin family of adhesion molecules) expression on neutrophils following percutaneous coronary intervention, and found substantially higher levels on neutrophils from patients undergoing stent implantation as compared to patients undergoing balloon angioplasty alone. This increased inflammatory response may help to explain the larger neointimal growth seen in stented arteries.

Animal studies have also demonstrated differences in response to vascular injury between balloon-angioplastied and stented arteries. Heparin, an archetypal modulator of vascular repair in animal models, has long been known to reduce neointimal growth following vascular injury.[65,66] Heparin is equally effective at reducing neointimal hyperplasia following balloon injury or stent implantation.[67,68] Studies show that heparin, the archetypal modulator of vascular repair following vascular injury, maximally inhibits neointimal hyperplasia in stented rabbit iliac arteries only when given in prolonged fashion (14 days), whereas maximal inhibition of balloon-injured arteries requires only transient early heparin therapy (3 days).[68] An explanation of this difference is suggested by immunohistologic and molecular studies. Data demonstrate that there is a distinct pattern of leukocyte infiltration that distinguishes the superficial injury associated with simple balloon-induced de-endothelialization from the deep chronic injury associated with stent implantation. In a rabbit iliac artery model, balloon injury is associated with early and transient infiltration of neutrophils without monocyte accumulation, although stent implantation is associated with an early influx of neutrophils, followed by sustained recruitment of monocytes over days to weeks. These differences are mirrored by molecular studies in which mRNA levels of the monocyte chemokine MCP-1 and the neutrophil chemokine IL-8 at sites of vascular injury were determined using semi-quantitative reverse transcriptase polymerase chain reaction. In balloon injury, there is only transient (hours) expression of MCP-1 and IL-8. In contrast, in stented arteries, there was sustained expression of IL-8 and, more prominently, MCP-1 as late as 14 days.[69]

〖 〗 AN INTEGRATED VIEW OF THE PATHOPHYSIOLOGY OF RESTENOSIS

When a balloon and stent are inflated at the site of a mature atherosclerotic plaque, a series of events is initiated (Figure 7-10). The first is a predominant inflammatory phase. The initial consequences

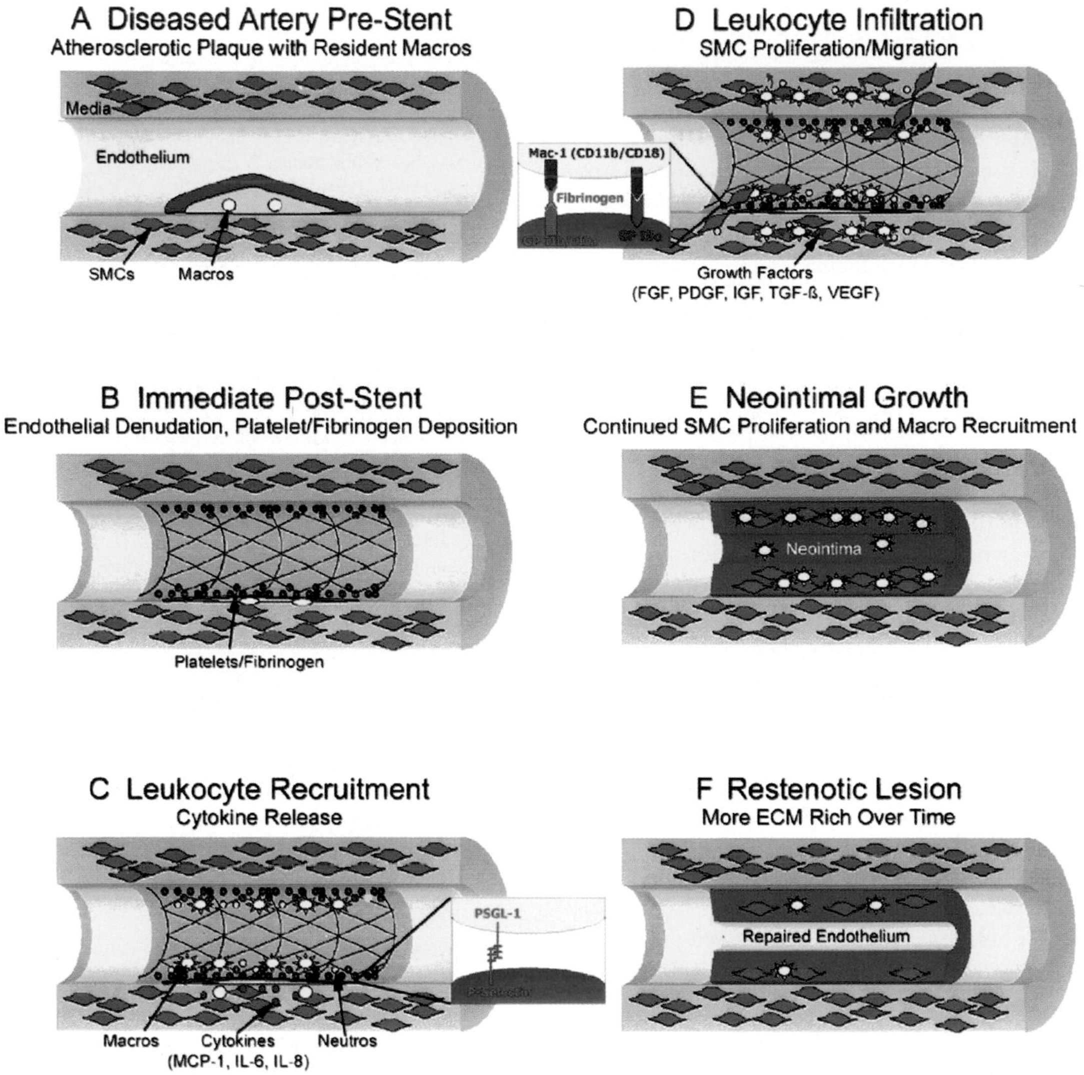

A Diseased Artery Pre-Stent
Atherosclerotic Plaque with Resident Macros

Media

Endothelium

SMCs   Macros

D Leukocyte Infiltration
SMC Proliferation/Migration

Mac-1 (CD11b/CD18)

Fibrinogen

GP IIb/IIIa   GP Ibα

Growth Factors
(FGF, PDGF, IGF, TGF-ß, VEGF)

B Immediate Post-Stent
Endothelial Denudation, Platelet/Fibrinogen Deposition

Platelets/Fibrinogen

E Neointimal Growth
Continued SMC Proliferation and Macro Recruitment

Neointima

C Leukocyte Recruitment
Cytokine Release

PSGL-1

P-selectin

Macros   Cytokines   Neutros
(MCP-1, IL-6, IL-8)

F Restenotic Lesion
More ECM Rich Over Time

Repaired Endothelium

FIGURE 7-10. (A) A mature atherosclerotic plaque prior to intervention. **(B)** The immediate result of stent placement with endothelial denudation and platelet/fibrinogen deposition. **(C, D)** Leukocyte recruitment, infiltration, and SMC proliferation and migration in the days following injury. **(E)** Neointimal thickening in the weeks following injury, with continued SMC proliferation and monocyte recruitment. **(F)** The long-term (weeks to months) change from a predominantly cellular to a less cellular and more ECM-rich plaque. *(Reproduced with permission from Welt FGP, Rogers C. Inflammation and restenosis in the stent era. Arterioscler Thromb Vasc Biol. 2002;22:1769–1776.)*[69a]

immediately following stent placement are de-endothelialization; crush of the plaque, often with dissection into the tunica media and occasionally adventitia; and stretch of the entire artery. A layer of platelets and fibrin are deposited at the injured site. Activated platelets on the surface expressing adhesion molecules such as P-selectin and GP Ibα attach to circulating leukocytes via platelet receptors such as P-selectin glycoprotein ligand (PSGL-1) and begin a process of rolling along the injured surface. Leukocytes then bind tightly to the surface and stop rolling mediated through the leukocyte integrin (ie, Mac-1) class of adhesion molecules via direct attachment to platelet receptors such as GP 1bα and through crosslinking with fibrinogen to the GP IIb/IIIa receptor. Migration of leukocytes across the platelet-fibrin layer and diapedesis into the tissue is driven by chemical gradients of cytokines released from SMCs and resident leukocytes. Next is a granulation, or cellular proliferation phase. Growth factors are subsequently released from platelets, leukocytes, and SMCs, which stimulates proliferation and migration of SMCs from the media into the neointima. The resul-

tant neointima consists of SMCs, extracellular matrix, and macrophages recruited over a period of time lasting several weeks. Over longer periods of time, the artery enters a phase of remodeling involving extracellular matrix protein degradation and resynthesis. Accompanying this phase is a shift to less cellular elements and greater production of extracellular matrix. In the balloon-angioplastied artery, this leads to shrinkage of the entire artery and negative remodeling. In the stented artery, this phase has less impact as a result of the rigid scaffolding of the stent, which prevents negative remodeling. In both balloon-angioplastied and stented arteries, there is eventual re-endothelialization of at least part of the injured vessel surface.

[ ] CLINICAL SEQUELAE OF RESTENOSIS

Although inflammation is a common link between atherogenesis and restenosis, there are distinct differences between the two processes that manifest in clinical presentation. In terms of the temporal pattern, atherogenesis is a process that occurs over decades, although multiple studies have revealed that restenosis is a process that occurs predominantly during the first 6 months after angioplasty whether a stent is implanted or not. Restenotic lesions typically lack the complex architecture of mature atherosclerotic plaque consisting mainly of SMCs and extracellular matrix as well as numerous leukocytes. As such, the clinical sequelae of restenotic lesions are usually not plaque rupture and acute thrombosis, but more typically progressive exertional angina.

【 】 IMPLICATIONS FOR ANTI-RESTENOTIC THERAPY

Anti-restenotic therapy has largely focused on either direct antiproliferative strategies or antiinflammatory strategies. Interestingly, many of the proved and most promising therapies share both antiproliferative and antiinflammatory features. For example, sirolimus, which has shown remarkable efficacy against restenosis in a coated stent design,[70] is an inhibitor of cell cycle progression, but also possesses important antiinflammatory properties, as evidenced by its initial development as an antifungal agent and its current use as an immunomodulatory agent in the treatment of renal transplant rejection.[71] Furthermore, in a porcine model of stent injury, sirolimus-coated stents have been shown to down-regulate vessel wall protein expression of the cytokines MCP-1 and IL-6 compared to bare metal stents.[72] Also, the microtubule stabilizer paclitaxel, a promising therapy for restenosis, is known to interfere with SMC proliferation and migration through its effect on microtubules.[71] However, there is also data to suggest that paclitaxel effects leukocyte function. This has been suggested to be at least in part mediated through the interference with cytoskeletal interactions with the integrin class of adhesion molecules.[73]

The data also suggest that there are important differences in the temporal and spatial pattern of inflammation between stent and balloon injury that must be taken into account when antirestenotic therapies are conceived. Specifically, the inflammatory response engendered by a stent is prolonged and contains more cells of the monocyte/macrophage lineage. Therefore, it may be necessary for antiinflammatory therapies to be delivered over a prolonged period of time, and be directed against macrophages in particular.

CONCLUSIONS

Over the past century, the molecular and cellular pathophysiology of atherosclerosis and related arteriopathies has been studied extensively. It has been confirmed that inflammation plays a central role in these processes. Important differences exist, however, between these processes, likely as a result of the injury imposed on the artery, which helps determine the clinical consequences of these processes. A more thorough knowledge of these processes has led to increasingly effective therapies for the treatment of atherosclerosis and the acute coronary syndromes, as well as restenosis. However, much remains to be determined regarding the molecular mechanisms of atherosclerosis, identification of plaques prone to rupture, and more effective and economic methods to treat restenosis.

REFERENCES

1. Ross R. The pathogenesis of atherosclerosis–an update. *N Engl J Med.* 1986; 314:488.
2. Ridker PM, Rifai N, Rose L, Buring JE, Cook NR. Comparison of C-reactive protein and low-density lipoprotein cholesterol levels in the prediction of first cardiovascular events. *N Engl J Med.* 2002;347:1557.
3. Brennan ML, Penn MS, Van Lente F, et al. Prognostic value of myeloperoxidase in patients with chest pain. *N Engl J Med.* 2003;349:1595.
4. Cybulsky MI, Gimbrone, MA, Jr. Endothelial expression of a mononuclear leukocyte adhesion molecule during atherogenesis. *Science.* 1995;251:788.
5. Ridker PM. Intercellular adhesion molecule (ICAM-1) and the risks of developing atherosclerotic disease. *Eur Heart J.* 1998;19:1119.
6. Rollins BJ. Chemokines. *Blood.* 1997;90:909.
7. Webb LMC, Ehrengruber MU, Clark-Lewis I, Baggiolini M. Binding to heparan sulfate or heparin enhances neutrophil responses to interleukin 8. *Proc Natl Acad Sciences U S A.* 1993;90:7158.
8. Huo Y, Weber C, Forlow SB, et al. The chemokine KC, but not monocyte chemoattractant protein-1, triggers monocyte arrest on early atherosclerotic endothelium. *J Clin Invest.* 2001;108:1307.
9. Libby P. Molecular bases of the acute coronary syndromes. *Circulation.* 1995;91:2844.
10. Moulton KS. Plaque angiogenesis and atherosclerosis. *Curr Atherosl Rep.* 2001;3:225.
11. Gibbons GH, Dzau VJ. The emerging concept of vascular remodeling. *N Engl J Med.* 1994;330:1431.
11a. Glagov S, Weisenberg, Zarins CK, et al. Compensatory, enlargement of human atherosclerotic coronary arteries. *N Engl J Med.* 1997;317:1371.
12. Galis ZS, Khatri JJ. Matrix metalloproteinases in vascular remodeling and atherogenesis: the good, the bad, and the ugly. *Circ Res.* 2002;90:251.
13. Fuster V, Badimon L, Badimaon JJ, Chesebro JH. The pathogenesis of coronary artery disease and the acute coronary syndromes. *N Engl J Med.* 1992;326:242.
14. Kern MJ. Coronary physiology revisited: practical insights from the cardiac catheterization laboratory. *Circulation.* 2000;101:1344.
15. Herrick JB. Clinical features of sudden obstruction of the coronary arteries. *JAMA.* 1912;59:2015.
16. DeWood MA, Spores J, Notske R, et al. Prevalence of total coronary occlusion during the early hours of transmural myocardial infarction. *N Engl J Med.* 1980;303:897.
17. Ambrose JA, Winters SL, Arora RR, et al. Coronary angiographic morphology in myocardial infarction: a link between the pathogenesis of unstable angina and myocardial infarction. *J Am Coll Cardiol.* 1985;6:1233.
18. Smith SC, Jr. Risk-reduction therapy: the challenge to change. Presented at the 68th scientific sessions of the American Heart Association, November 13, 1995, Anaheim, California. *Circulation.* 1996;93:2205.
19. Seshiah PN, Kereiakes DJ, Vasudevan SS, et al. Activated monocytes induce smooth muscle cell death: role of macrophage colony-stimulating factor and cell contact. *Circulation.* 2002;105:174.
20. Muller JE, Stone PH, Turi ZG, et al. Circadian variation in the frequency of onset of acute myocardial infarction. *N Engl J Med.* 1985;313:1315.
21. Leor J, Kloner RA. The Northridge earthquake as a trigger for acute myocardial infarction. *Am J Cardiol.* 1996;77:1230.
22. Lee RT, Schoen FJ, Loree HM, Lark MW, Libby P. Circumferential stress and matrix metalloproteinase 1 in human coronary atherosclerosis. Implications for plaque rupture. *Arterioscler Thromb Vasc Biol.* 1996;16:1070.
23. Gruntzig AR, Senning A, Siegenthaler WE. Nonoperative dilatation of coronary-artery stenosis: percutaneous transluminal coronary angioplasty. *N Engl J Med.* 1979;301:61.
24. Bourassa MG, Wilson JW, Detre KM, Kelsey SF, Robertson T, Passamani ER. Long-term follow-up of coronary angioplasty: the 1977–1981 National Heart, Lung, and Blood Institute registry. *Eur Heart J.* 1989;10(SupplG):36.
25. McBride W, Lange RA, Hillis LD. Restenosis after successful coronary angioplasty. Pathophysiology and prevention. *N Engl J Med.* 1988;318:1734.
26. Faxon DA, Weber VJ, Haudenschild C, Gottsman SB, McGovern WA, Ryan TJ. Acute effects of transmural angioplasty in three experimental models of atherosclerosis. *Arteriosclerosis.* 1982;2:125.
27. Faxon DP, Sanborn TA, Weber VJ, Haudenschild C, Gottsman SB, McGovern WA, Ryan TJ. Restenosis following transluminal angioplasty in experimental atherosclerosis. *Arteriosclerosis.* 1984;4:189.
28. Forrester JS, Fishbein M, Helfant R, Fagin J. A paradigm for restenosis based on cell biology: clues for the development of new preventive therapies. *J Am Coll Cardiol.* 1991;17:758.

29. Mintz GS, Popma JJ, Pichard AD, et al. Arterial remodeling after coronary angioplasty: a serial intravascular ultrasound study. *Circulation*. 1996;94:35.

30. Fischman DL, Leon MB, Baim DSet al. A randomized comparison of coronary artery-stent placement and balloon angioplasty in the treatment of coronary artery disease. *N Engl J Med*. 1994;331:496.

31. Serruys PW, de Jaegere P, Kiemeneij F, et al. A comparison of balloon-expandable-stent implantation with balloon angioplasty in patients with coronary artery disease. *N Engl J Med*. 1994;331·489.

31a. Welt FGP, Sobieszczsk PS. Coronary artery stents: design and biologic considerations. Cardiology Special Edition. *9:9*.

32. Hoffmann R, Mintz GS, Dussaillant GR, et al. Patterns and mechanisms of in-stent restenosis. A serial intravascular ultrasound study. *Circulation*. 1996;94:1247.

33. Marcus AJ. Thrombosis and inflammation as multicellular processes: significance of cell-cell interactions. *Semin Hematol*. 1994;31:261.

34. Libby P, Simon DI. Inflammation and thrombosis: the clot thickens. *Circulation*. 2001;103:1718–20.

35. Diacovo TG, Roth, SJ, Buccola, JM, Bainton, DF, Springer, TA. Neutrophil rolling, arrest, and transmigration across activated, surface-adherent platelets via sequential action of P-selectin and the beta 2-integrin CD11b/CD18. *Blood*. 1996;88:146.

36. Yeo EL, Sheppard JA, Feuerstein IA. Role of P-selectin and leukocyte activation in polymorphonuclear cell adhesion to surface adherent activated platelets under physiologic shear conditions (an injury vessel wall model). *Blood*. 1994;83:2498.

37. Ott I, Neumann FJ, Gawaz M, Schmitt M, Schomig A. Increased neutrophil-platelet adhesion in patients with unstable angina. *Circulation*. 1996;94:1239.

38. Furman MI, Benoit SE, Barnard MR, et al. Increased platelet reactivity and circulating monocyte–platelet aggregates in patients with stable coronary artery disease. *J Am Coll Cardiol*. 1998;31:352.

39. .Farb A, Weber DK, Kolodgie FD, Burke AP, Virmani R. Morphological predictors of restenosis after coronary stenting in humans. *Circulation*. 2002;105:2974.

40. Moreno PR, Bernardi VH, Lopez-Cuellar J, et al. Macrophage infiltration predicts restenosis after coronary intervention in patients with unstable angina. *Circulation*. 1996;94:3098.

41. Neumann F-J, Ott I, Gawaz M, Puchner G, Schomig A. Neutrophil and platelet activation at balloon-injured coronary artery plaque in patients undergoing angioplasty. *J Am Coll Cardiol*. 1996;27:819.

42. Mickelson JK, Lakkis NM, Villarreal-Levy G, Hughes B, Smith CW. Leukocyte activation with platelet adhesion after coronary angioplasty: a mechanism for recurrent disease. *J Am Coll Cardiol*. 1996;28:345.

43. Inoue T, Sakai Y, Morooka S, Hayashi T, Takayanagi K, Takabatake Y. Expression of polymorphonuclear leukocyte adhesion molecules and its clinical significance in patients treated with percutaneous transluminal coronary angioplasty. *J Am Coll Cardiol*. 1996;28:1127.

44. Inoue T, Uchida T, Yaguchi I, Sakai Y, Takayanagi K, Morooka S. Stent-induced expression and activation of the leukocyte integrin Mac-1 is associated with neointimal thickening and restenosis. *Circulation*. 2003;107:1757.

45. Pietersma A, Kofflard M, de Wit LEA, et al. Late lumen loss after coronary angioplasty is associated with the activation status of circulating phagocytes before treatment. *Circulation*. 1995;91:1320.

46. Cipollone F, Marini M, Fazia M, et al. Elevated circulating levels of monocyte chemoattractant protein-1 in patients with restenosis after coronary angioplasty. *Arterioscler Thromb Vasc Biol*. 2001;21:327.

47. Gaspardone A, Crea F, Versaci F, et al. Predictive value of C-reactive protein after successful coronary-artery stenting in patients with stable angina. *Am J Cardiol*. 1998;82:515.

48. Cybulsky MI, Gimbrone MAJ. Endothelial expression of a mononuclear leukocyte adhesion molecule during atherogenesis. *Science*. 1991;251:788.

49. Li H, Cybulsky M, Gimbrone MA, Libby P. An atherogenic diet induces VCAM-1, a cytokine-regulatable mononuclear leukocyte adhesion molecule, in rabbit endothelium. *Arterioscler Thromb*. 1992;13:197.

50. Li H, Cybulsky MI, Gimbrone Jr. MA, Libby P. Inducible expression of vascular cell adhesion molecule-1 by vascular smooth muscle cells in vitro and within rabbit atheroma. *Am J Pathol*. 1993;143:1551.

51. Richardson M, Hadcock SJ, DeReske M, Cybulsky MI. Increased expression in vivo of VCAM-1 and E-selectin by the aortic endothelium of nor-

52. Walpola PL, Gotlieb AI, Cybulsky MI, Langille L. Expression of ICAM-1 and VCAM-1 and monocyte adherence in arteries exposed to altered shear stress. *Arterioscler Thromb Vasc Biol*. 1995;15:2.

53. Tanaka H, Sukhova GK, Swanson SJ, et al. Sustained activation of vascular cells and leukocytes in the rabbit aorta after balloon injury. *Circulation*. 1993;88:1788.

54. Rogers C, Welt FGP, Karnovsky MJ, Edelman ER. Monocyte recruitment and neointimal hyperplasia in rabbits: Coupled inhibitory effects of heparin. *Arterioscler Thromb Vasc Biol*. 1996;16:1312.

55. Welt FGP, Edelman ER, Simon DI, Rogers C. Neutrophil, not macrophage, infiltration precedes neointimal thickening in balloon-injured arteries. *Arterioscler Thromb Vasc Biol*. 2000;20:2553.

56. Rogers C, Edelman ER, Simon DI. A mAb to the beta$_2$-leukocyte integrin Mac-1 (CD11b/CD18) reduces intimal thickening after angioplasty or stent implantation in rabbits. *Proc Natl Acad Sci U S A*. 1998;95:10134.

57. Mori E, Komori K, Yamaoka T, et al. Essential role of monocyte chemoattractant protein-1 in development of restenotic changes (neointimal hyperplasia and constrictive remodeling) after balloon angioplasty in hypercholesterolemic rabbits. *Circulation*. 2002;105:2905.

58. Libby P, Schwartz D, Brogi E, Tanaka H, Clinton S. A cascade model for restenosis. *Circulation*. 1992;86:III47.

59. Jorgensen L, Grothe AG, Groves HM, Kinlough-Rathbone RL, Richardson M, Mustard JF. Sequence of cellular responses in rabbit aortas following one and two injuries with a balloon catheter. *Br J Exp Pathol*. 1988;69:473.

60. Richardson M, Hatton MW, Buchanan MR, Moore S. Wound healing in the media of the normolipemic rabbit carotid artery injured by air drying or by balloon catheter de-endothelialization. *Am J Pathol*. 1990;137:1453.

61. Kockx MM, De Meyer GR, Jacob WA, Bult H, Herman AG. Triphasic sequence of neointimal formation in the cuffed carotid artery of the rabbit. *Arterioscler Thromb*. 1992;12:1447.

62. Cole CW, Makhoul RG, McCann RL, O'Malley MK, Hagen PO. A neutrophil derived factor(s) stimulates [3H]thymidine incorporation by vascular smooth muscle cells in vitro. *Clin Invest Med*. 1988;11:62.

63. Lloyd AR, Oppenheim JJ. Poly's lament: the neglected role of the polymorphonuclear neutrophil in the afferent limb of the immune response. *Immunol Today*. 1992;13:169.

64. Inoue T, Sohma R, Miyazaki T, Iwasaki Y, Yaguchi I, Morooka S. Comparison of activation process of platelets and neutrophils after coronary stent implantation versus balloon angioplasty for stable angina pectoris. *Am J Cardiol*. 2000;86:1057.

65. Clowes AW, Clowes MM. Kinetics of cellular proliferation after arterial injury. II. Inhibition of smooth muscle cell growth by heparin. *Lab Invest*. 1985;52:611.

66. Clowes AW, Clowes MM. Kinetics of cellular proliferation after arterial injury: IV. Heparin inhibits rat smooth muscle cell mitogenesis and migration. *Circ Res*. 1986;58:839.

67. Rogers C, Edelman ER. Controlled release of heparin reduces neointimal hyperplasia in stented rabbit arteries: Ramifications for local therapy. *J Intervent Cardiol*. 1992;5:195.

68. Edelman ER, Karnovsky MJ. Contrasting effects of the intermittent and continuous administration of heparin in experimental restenosis. *Circulation*. 1994;89:770.

69. Welt FG, Tso C, Edelman ER, et al. Leukocyte recruitment and expression of chemokines following different forms of vascular injury. *Vasc Med*. 2003;8:1.

69a. Welt FGP, Rogers C. Inflammation and restenosis in the stent era. *Arterioscler Thromb Vasc Biol*. 2002;22:1769–1776.

70. Morice MC, Serruys PW, Sousa JE, et al. A randomized comparison of a sirolimus-eluting stent with a standard stent for coronary revascularization. *N Engl J Med*. 2002;346:1773.

71. Oberhoff M, Herdeg C, Baumbach A, Karsch KR. Stent-based antirestenotic coatings (sirolimus/paclitaxel). *Cath Cardiovasc Interv*. 2002;55:404.

72. Suzuki TM, Kopia GP, Hayashi S-iM, et al. Stent-based delivery of sirolimus reduces neointimal formation in a porcine coronary model. *Circulation*. 2001;104:1188.

73. Zhou X, Li J, Kucik DF. The microtubule cytoskeleton participates in control of beta2 integrin avidity. *J Biol Chem*. 2001;276:44762.

molipemic and hyperlipemic diabetic rabbits. *Arterioscler Thromb*. 1994;14:760.

CHAPTER 8

Ventricular Pathophysiology

Michael J. Lim, MD

The fundamental role of the cardiovascular system is to provide blood flow–carrying nutrients, especially oxygen, to the organs and tissues of the body while returning waste products, including carbon dioxide (CO_2), back to the pulmonary tissue for exchange. The process is dependent on forward flow, which is critically related to left ventricular (LV) function. Left ventricular dysfunction may occur in the setting of impairment of systolic performance, diastolic performance, and/or abnormal hemodynamic loading conditions. Although an in-depth understanding of LV mechanics does not directly translate into improved day-to-day clinical practice for the interventional cardiologist, a general understanding of the factors with an impact on LV performance remains imperative to appropriate therapeutic decisions.

VENTRICULAR MECHANICS

【 】 PRESSURE–VOLUME RELATIONSHIPS

A great deal of work has been done in evaluating the interdependence of the multiple factors affecting overall LV performance. The earliest means to understanding left ventricular pump function was the assessment of the LV pressure-volume (P-V) loop (Figure 8-1).[1,2] The lower portion of this loop (from left to right) illustrates ventricular filling from the opening of the mitral valve (D) to end-diastole (A). A steep increase in pressure occurs from end-diastole to the opening of the aortic valve (B), and this is represented on the right side of the loop. The top of the loop begins at aortic valve opening (right to left) and ends at aortic valve closing (C), representing the stroke volume. The left side of the loop represents isovolemic relaxation between the closure of the aortic valve and the opening of the mitral valve.

The area of the P-V loop represents LV stroke work, which remains a good surrogate for LV systolic function under the loading conditions present when the pressure-volume curve was obtained.[3] One of the main drawbacks in using stroke work as an estimate for LV function is that loading conditions do not remain constant outside the experimental laboratory. Furthermore, stroke work represents a global estimate of LV performance, and as such does not take into account regional differences in function that are frequently present in patients with established coronary artery disease.

The end-systolic pressure–volume relation (ESPVR) has also been established as a marker of the overall contractile state of the ventricle.[4–6] This relationship is constructed by producing multiple P-V loops over varying loading conditions. A line can be drawn that connects the upper left portion of each loop (Figure 8-2), and the slope of this line represents the ESPVR. In general, a shift in the ESPVR to the left with an increased slope is associated with an increase in contractility, and a decrease in slope with a rightward shift to the line is associated with decreased contractility.

Left ventricular diastolic function can also be readily appreciated by looking at the lower portion of the pressure-volume loop (see Figure 8-1).[7,8] With an increase in LV stiffness the curve shifts upward, and with an increase in ventricular compliance the curve moves downward along the *y*-axis.

【 】 VENTRICULAR LOADING CONDITIONS

Left ventricular systolic function is tied intimately to loading conditions. *Preload* represents the load that stretches the ventricular myofibrils during diastole, and it has been quantified in the patient as the LV end-diastolic pressure. Increasing preload tends to increase the LV diameter, whereas its effects on overall function depend on the ventricle's ability to accommodate this stretch. This ability to distend can be estimated by evaluating the ventricular

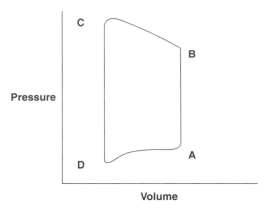

FIGURE 8-1. A representation of a left ventricular pressure (on y-axis) volume (on x-axis) loop. End-diastole is seen at point A and end-systole at point C. Diastole occurs between points D and A while systole occurs between points B and C. The total of the loop is representative of left ventricular stroke work.

diameter and extrapolating the concepts derived from the Frank Starling curve (Figure 8-3).

Afterload represents the force that resists the systolic contraction of the ventricle. The calculation of systolic wall stress by Laplace's law:

$$\text{stress} = \text{pressure} \times \text{chamber radius}/(2 \times \text{wall thickness})$$

is generally thought to represent ventricular afterload. One caveat that applies is that this wall stress varies during systole.[9,10] Therefore, the end-systolic wall stress remains as the best representative of afterload. Increasing afterload, in general, tends to decrease the stroke volume.

The intrinsic property of the myocardium to eject blood forcefully and do work is represented by the term *contractility*. Classically, contractility is independent of preload and afterload. However, from a practical standpoint, it is difficult to evaluate

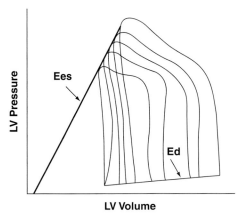

FIGURE 8-2. Multiple pressure volume-loops from the same ventricle under varying loading conditions or inotropic states can be drawn. The line that intersects all end-systolic points (Ees) is the end-systolic pressure volume relationship (ESPVR). The greater the slope of the line, the greater the contractility of the ventricle. *(Reproduced with permission from Chen CH, Nakayama M, Nevo E, et al. Coupled systolic–ventricular and vascular stiffening with age: implications for pressure regulation and cardiac reserve in the elderly. J Am Coll Cardiol. 1998;32: 1225.[38])*

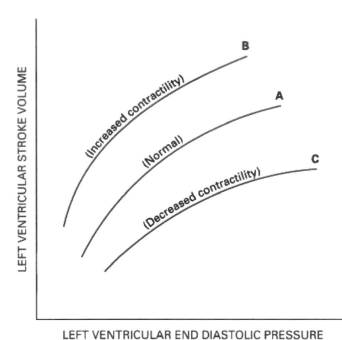

FIGURE 8-3. The relationship between preload (left ventricular end-diastolic pressure) and stoke volume is depicted here. Three separate Frank Starling curves are drawn representing ventricles with normal, decreased, or increased contractility. *(Reproduced with permission from Little WC. Assessment of normal and abnormal cardiac function in heart disease. In Brunwald E, Zipes D, Libby P, eds. A Textbook of Cardiovascular Medicine, 6th ed. WB Saunders, 2001.[39])*

these parameters independently. Contractility, also described as *inotropy*, is affected by circulating catecholamines or pharmacologic agents (eg, dobutamine, beta-blockers). The maximal rate of rise in LV systolic pressure per unit time (dP/dt) remains the best estimate of contractility.[11] Increases in dP/dt are seen with exercise, norepinephrine, and isoproterenol.[12] Although dP/dt remains an excellent marker of ventricular contractility, its measurement in the catheterization laboratory requires a micromanometer catheter capable of high frequency–signal differentiation, an impractical situation in the clinical laboratory, where fluid-filled catheters coupled to electric-strain gauges are in daily use. Thus dP/dt is therefore not assessed routinely.

GLOBAL VENTRICULAR FUNCTION

【 】 CONTRAST VENTRICULOGRAPHY

In the cardiac catheterization laboratory, ventricular pathophysiology is most frequently recognized by the performance of LV wall motion seen on the left ventriculogram. The left ventriculogram visually portrays the relationship between the stroke volume and the end-diastolic volume and, either quantitatively or qualitatively, an ejection fraction is determined. Universally, ejection fraction has been accepted as an estimate of the global LV contractile state. Furthermore, an assessment of regional LV function by wall motion on ventriculography has become an essential part of every cardiac catheterization.[13]

Qualitative assessment of LV function rests on the visual appreciation between stroke volume and end-diastolic volume. An increase in end-diastolic volume (ie, dilated LV chamber size) is commonly seen in patients with volume overload states (eg, aortic insufficiency). However, stroke volume (ie, the difference between end-diastolic and end-systolic volumes, also known as *ejection fraction*) is dependent on the myocardial contractile state and, in part, loading conditions. A reduction in the ventricular contractile state may be secondary to intrinsic myocardial disease (ie, nonischemic cardiomyopathy), or may be secondary to coronary artery disease and its associated regional wall motion abnormalities.

Depressed regional wall motion, defined as *hypokinesis,* reflects a decrease in the contractile state of a particular region of the left ventricle. Noncontraction of a region (akinesis) or outward contraction of a segment during systole (dyskinesis) may reflect the occurrence of a prior myocardial infarction (MI).[14] Commonly, the left ventricle is imaged in a right anterior oblique (RAO) projection giving good assessment of the anterobasilar, anterolateral, apical, diaphragmatic, and posterobasilar segments (Figure 8-4). In select cases involving the lateral LV wall, the left anterior oblique (LAO) projection is used to estimate the lateral, posterior, and septal walls. Assessment of regional wall motion is critical to risk stratification and management of patients with coronary artery disease.

Several methods are available to quantify the measurement of ejection fraction by on-line software. One method is the so-called *area–length method.* This method assumes an ellipsoid shape to the ventricle. Calculations of ventricular volume are made from the end-systolic and end-diastolic frame using the dimensional measurements of the ventricle. Regression equations correct for the overestimation of the calculated volume to the true volume.[15,16] A second method, the center-line method,[17] has also been used because of its ability to quantify both regional wall motion and ejection fraction. This method does not assume a geometric configuration of the ventricle, and measures the shortening fractions of 100 chords that are constructed perpendicular to a center line, which is drawn midway between the end-diastolic and end-systolic contours.

【 】 NONINVASIVE ASSESSMENT OF LEFT VENTRICULAR FUNCTION

With the advances in noninvasive imaging of the heart, some catheterization laboratories do not perform ventriculography routinely, especially in patients with impaired renal function or other situations where the increased amount of intravenous contrast required to perform a ventriculogram poses increased risk to the patient. Transthoracic echocardiography has become a well-accepted tool for the assessment of LV function. As with cardiac ventriculography, echocardiography allows the assessment of global LV function as well as regional wall motion in the three-dimensional chamber. Furthermore, it has the ability to better assess coexistent valvular disease, especially for aortic and mitral pathology. In addition, assessment of the tricuspid regurgitation jet permits an estimate of the right ventricular pressure and systolic function, which can alert the clinician to impaired hemodynamics that may require further evaluation.

Radionuclide ventricular imaging also possesses the ability to measure LV volume, ejection fraction, and regional wall motion by the adaptation of gated image acquisition techniques. By the same token, recent advances in contrast computed tomography (CT) and magnetic resonance imaging (MRI) technologies provide these noninvasive imaging techniques with the ability to evaluate LV size and function.

【 】 CORONARY ARTERY DISEASE AND LEFT VENTRICULAR DYSFUNCTION

Coronary artery disease remains the most prevalent diagnosis among patients requiring cardiac catheterization. As previously discussed, coronary artery disease usually manifests itself in regional ventricular wall motion abnormalities. In an acute setting, the wall motion abnormality may give early clues to the coronary artery involved as well as the location of the offending lesion. Severe degrees of LV dysfunction may represent the etiology of cardiogenic shock, in which the heart is unable to maintain enough forward-perfusing pressure to supply blood.

Mechanical complications of acute MI or acute coronary syndromes that make up LV function can be detected by left ventriculography, most notably, the occurrence of mitral regurgitation secondary to papillary muscle dysfunction and/or papillary muscle rupture, ventricular pseudoaneurysm formation, ventricular free-wall rupture, and ventricular septal defects. Although the incidence of these complications is rare, it is important to recognize its existence. Early surgical intervention decreases the morbidity and mortality associated with these conditions.[18–21] Although left ventriculography per se may not routinely be performed in all patients presenting with acute MI and/or acute coronary syndromes, the

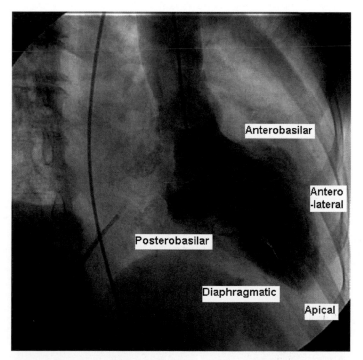

FIGURE 8-4. An end-diastolic frame taken from a right anterior oblique ventriculogram. The commonly interpreted myocardial segments of the left ventricle from this view are labeled (poseterobasilar, diaphragmatic, apical, anterolateral, and anterobasilar).

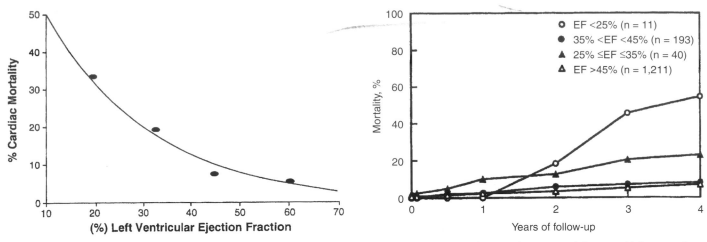

FIGURE 8-5. Graph showing the striking relationship overall ventricular function (ejection fraction) and cardiac mortality in patients following an acute myocardial infarction. *(Reproduced with permission from Gottlieb S, Moss AJ, McDermott M, et al. Interrelation of left ventricular ejection fraction, pulmonary congestion and outcome in acute myocardial infarction. Am J Cardiol. 1992;69:977.[40])*

FIGURE 8-6. Figure showing the impact of decreased left ventricular ejection fraction on mortality, despite successful percutaneous revascularization. *(Reproduced with permission from Holmes DR Jr, Detre KM, Williams DO, et al. Long-term outcome of patients with depressed left ventricular function undergoing percutaneous transluminal coronary angioplasty. The NHLBI PTCA registry. Circulation. 1993;82:21.[41])*

assessment of LV function remains one of the strongest predictors of short- and long-term survival in patients. Therefore, it is of critical importance to obtain either an angiographic or an echocardiographic assessment of global and regional LV function in all patients under these conditions. Furthermore, with the complex nature of myocardial necrosis with myocardial stunning, follow-up assessment of regional and global LV function also becomes paramount in the estimate of overall survival after primary reperfusion strategies (Figure 8-5).[22]

The patients presenting with angina-like symptoms and/or an abnormal stress test represent the most common presentation to the cardiac catheterization laboratory. The determination of their coronary anatomy with the goal of improving myocardial perfusion is either by coronary artery bypass grafting (CABG) or percutaneous coronary intervention (PCI). Ventricular performance weighs heavily in the decision-making process of revascularization techniques (Figure 8-6).[23–25]

As suggested by the Bypass Angioplasty Revascularization Investigation (BARI) study,[26] diabetic patients with LV dysfunction associated with two- or three-vessel coronary artery disease remain best treated by CABG compared to PCI (Figure 8-7). Furthermore, decreased LV function has been proved to be an independent negative risk predictor for patients undergoing percutaneous revascularization or CABG.

Many times in the assessment of stable coronary artery disease patients, chronic total occlusions of the coronary arteries are found. Although there is some debate as to whether a totally occluded vessel should be reopened by percutaneous techniques or bypass grafting surgery, it is indisputable that if there is no significant wall motion abnormality associated with coronary lesion in question, there must be sufficient viability and collateral flow to maintain the myocardium. However, if there is a significant wall motion abnormality despite the fact that the vessel seems to fill well with collaterals, a viability assessment of the myocardium in

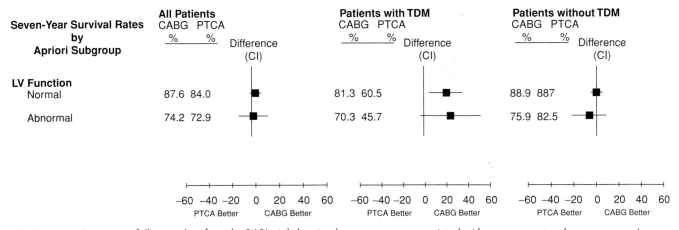

FIGURE 8-7. Seven year follow-up date from the BARI trial showing better outcomes associated with coronary artery bypass surgery in patients with impaired left ventricular function. *(Reproduced with permission from The BARI Investigators. Seven-year Outcome in the Bypass Angioplasty Revascularization Investigation (BARI) by treatment and diabetic status. J Am Coll Cardiol. 2000;35:1122.[42])*

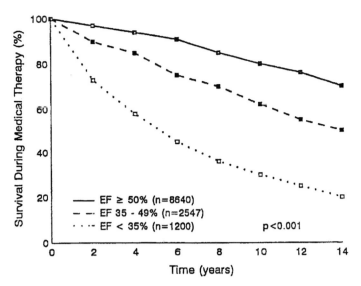

FIGURE 8-8. Survival curves from the CASS registry showing the impact of decreasing left ventricular ejection fraction on mortality on medically treated patients. *(Reproduced with permission from Edmond M, Mock MB, Davis KB, et al. Long-term survival of medically treated patients in the Coronary Artery Surgery Study (CASS) registry. Circulation. 1994;90:2645.[43])*

diac patients. It is especially evident in patients with coronary artery disease in whom LV dysfunction is manifest in congestive heart failure symptomatology. The Coronary Artery Surgery Study (CASS) registry firmly established that benefits of CABG surgery were more pronounced in most patients with moderate-to-severe depression of global ejection fractions (Figure 8-8).[27] In fact, in this patient population, upward of 40% of the patients have significant improvements in their ejection fraction over time following coronary vascularization, presumably secondary to the presence of "hibernating" but viable myocardium.[28–30] Given these findings, all patients with coronary artery disease and severe LV dysfunction are evaluated for possible revascularization. A key step in this revascularization process is the assessment of myocardial viability.

Myocardial Viability

Many modalities are now available to assess the presence of viability, including dobutamine echocardiography (DSE), magnetic resonance imaging (MRI), gated single-photon emission computed tomography (SPECT) with thallium or technetium tracers, and positron emission tomography (PET). Each of these modalities has potential for identifying the presence of underperfused myocardium with ischemia as well as the presence of myocardial tissue that is hibernating and may become functional once revascularized. Overall accuracy of these imaging modalities for predicting recovery of regional LV function after revascularization is similar, with 83% positive predictive value for PET and DSE and 68% for thallium SPECT. However, negative predictive value of thallium SPECT is about 90%, whereas PET and DSE both have negative predictive value of around 83% (Figure 8-9).[31]

question with dobutamine echo or perfusion studies should be performed before undertaking an intervention with its inherent risk.

Systolic LV function (ie, LV ejection fraction) has been well established as a strong independent predictor of outcomes in all car-

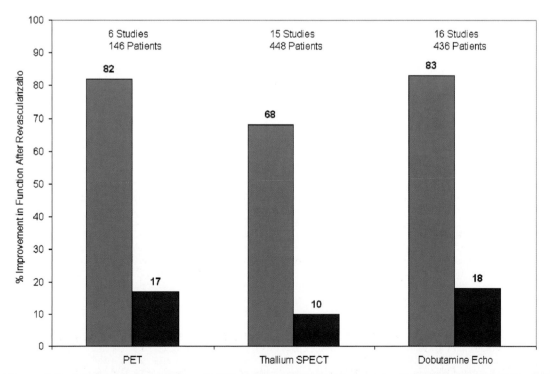

FIGURE 8-9. Summary of the data for viability assessment by PET, Thallium SPECT, and Dobutamine Echo and each test's ability to predict improved left ventricular function after revascularization. *(Reproduced with permission from Eitzman D, Al-Aeuar Z, Kauter HL, et al. Clinical outcome of patients with advanced coronary artery disease after viability studies with position emission tomography. J Am Coll Cardiol. 1992;20:559.[44])*

Dobutamine echocardiography may represent the more straightforward of the imaging techniques used to determine myocardial viability and ischemia. Experienced observers are able to evaluate regional wall motion abnormalities at rest, and then again while increasing doses of dobutamine are administered. Augmentation of regional wall motion with low-dose dobutamine is evidence for viability, although a decrement in function from the low-dose images represents ischemia. The specificity of DSE is markedly improved with respect to recovery of function after revascularization, if a biphasic response is found with dobutamine infusion.[32,33] That is, a regional wall motion abnormality that exists at rest and augments with low-dose dobutamine while subsequently deteriorating at higher doses, LV functional recovery is likely.

PET scanning involves the use of 18 F-fluorodeoxyglucose (FDG) to evaluate myocardial metabolism. Viable myocardium is indicated by uptake of FDG, which is indicative of myocardial metabolism, whereas images obtained with the perfusion tracer are able to determine if there is perfusion or relative underperfusion. Those patients with an FDG: blood-flow mismatch by PET imaging have been shown to have markedly diminished 1-year mortality if revascularized as compared to patients who do not have this mismatch.[34,35]

SPECT imaging with thallium or technetium perfusion tracers relies on the fact that myocardial membranes must be intact in order for the uptake of the tracer to occur. This is secondary to the fact that regional uptake and retention of this tracer relies on an entity-dependent cation-exchange mechanism. The uptake of these tracers is indicative of viable myocardium.[36,37]

New modalities include contrast echocardiography, which uses microbubble contrast agents to assess microvascular perfusion. Early studies suggested that with the use of these agents, it is possible to predict myocardial viability and assess microvascular integrity. Furthermore, advanced and improved MRI methods can now evaluate the regional differences in contrast uptake. Several centers have documented the utility of contrast-enhanced MRI to detect viable myocardium with similar degrees of sensitivity and specificity as more traditional methods of viability.

REFERENCES

1. Sagawa K, Mangham L, Suga H, Suragawa K. *Cardiac Contraction and the Pressure Volume Relationship.* Oxford University Press, 1988.
2. Kass DA. Clinical ventricular pathophysiology: a pressure volume view. In Warltier DC, ed. *Ventricular Function.* Williams & Wilkins 1995:131.
3. Suragawa K, Maugham WL, Sagawa K. Optimal arterial resistance for the maximal stroke work studied in isolated canine left ventricle. *Circ Res.* 1985;56:586.
4. Nemoto S, DeFreitas G, Mann DC, Carabella BA. Effects of changes in left ventricular contractility on indexes of contractility in mice. *Am J Physiol Heart Circ Physiol.* 2002;283:H2504.
5. Kass DA, Mangham WL. From "Emax" to pressure-volume relations: a broader view. *Circulation.* 1988;77:1203.
6. Little WC, Chang CP, Peterson T, Vinten-Johnsen J. Response of the left ventricular end systolic pressure–volume relation in conscious dogs to a wide range of contractile states. *Circulation.* 1988;78:736.
7. Grossman W. Diastolic dysfunction in congestive heart failure. *N Eng J Med.* 1991;325:1557.
8. Gilbert JC, Glantz SA. Determinants of left ventricular filling and of the diastolic pressure volume relations. *Circ Res.* 1989;64:827.
9. Regen DM, Anversa P, Capasso JM. Sequential calculation of left ventricular wall stress. *Am J Physiol.* 1993;264:M1411.
10. Regen DM, Calculation of left ventricular wall stress. *Circ Res.* 1990;67:245.
11. Little WC. The left ventricular dp/dt_{max} end diastolic volume relation in closed chest dogs. *Circ Res.* 1985;56:808.
12. Kass DA, Manghan WL, Guo ZM, et al. Comparative influence of load versus inotropic states on indexes of ventricular contractility: experimental and theoretical analysis based on pressure volume relationships. *Circulation.* 1987;76:1422.
13. Pomerantseu EV, Stertzer SH, Shaw RE. Quantitative left ventriculography: methods of assessment of the regional contractility. *J Am Coll Cardiol.* 1995;7:11.
14. Grossman W. Assessment of regional myocardial function. *J Am Coll Cardiol.* 1986;7:327.
15. Dodge HT, Sandler H, Ballew DW, Lord JD. The use of biplane angiocardiography for the measurement of left ventricular volume in man. *Am Heart J.* 1960;60:762.
16. Wynne J, Green LH, Mann T, et al. Estimation of left ventricular volumes in man from biplane cineangiograms filmed in oblique projections. *Am J Cardiol.* 1978;41:726.
17. Sheehan FH, Bolson EL, Dodge HT, et al. Advantages and applications of the centerline method for characterizing regional ventricular function. *Circulation.* 1986;74:293.
18. Wei JY, Hutchins GM, Bulkley BH. Papillary muscle rupture in fatal acute myocardial infarction: a potentially treatable form of cardiogenic shock. *Am Intern Med.* 1979;90:149–52.
19. Ryan TJ. For Acute ACC/AHA. Guidelines for the management of patients with acute myocardial infarction. *J Am Coll Cardiol.* 1999;34:890–911.
20. Park WM, Connery CP, Hochman JS, et al. Successful repair of myocardial free wall rupture after thrombolymic therapy for acute infarction. *Am Thorac Surg.* 2000;70:1345–9.
21. Lopez-Senden J, Gonzales A, Lopez de So E, et al. Diagnosis of subacute ventricular wall rupture after acute myocardial infarction: sensitivity and specifically of clinical hemodynamic and echocardiographic criteria. *J Am Coll Cardiol.* 1992;19:1145–53.
22. Gottlieb S, Moss AJ, McDermott M, et al. Interrelation of left ventricular ejection fraction, pulmonary congestion and outcome in acute myocardial infarction. *Am J Cardiol.* 1992;69:977–84.
23. Holmes DR Jr, Detre KM, Williams DO, et al. Long-term outcome of patients with depressed left ventricular function undergoing percutaneous transluminal coronary angioplasty. The NHLBI PTCA registry. *Circulation.* 1993;87:21–9.
24. Kohli RS, DiSciancio G, Cowley MJ et al. Coronary angioplasty in patients with severe left ventricular dysfunction. *J Am Coll Cardiol.* 1990;16:807–11.
25. Reynes K, Kunker B, Gransser R, et al. Percutaneous transluminal coronary angioplasty in patients with severely depressed left ventricular function. *Cardiology.* 1993;83:358–66.
26. The BARI Investigators. Seven-year outcome in the Bypass Angioplasty Revascularization Investigation (BARI) by treatment and diabetic status. *J Am Coll Cardiol.* 2000;35:1122.
27. Edmond M, Mock MB, Davis KB, et al. Long-term survival of medically treated patients in the Coronary Artery Surgery Study (CASS) registry. *Circulation.* 1994;90:2645–57.
28. Rozanski A, Bernard D, gray R, et al. Preoperative prediction of reversible myocardial asynergy by post exercise radionuclide ventriculography. *N Engl J Med.* 1982;307:212–3.
29. Brundage BH, Massie BM, Botvinick EH. Improved regional ventricular function after successful surgical revascularization. *J Am Coll Cardiol.* 1984;3:902–8.
30. Elefteriades JA, Tolis G Jr, Levi E, et al. Coronary artery bypass grafting in severe left ventricular dysfunction: excellent survival with improved ejection fraction and functional state. *J Am Coll Cardiol.* 1993;22:1411–17.
31. Bonow Ro, Identification of viable myocardium. *Circulation.* 1996;94:2674–80.
32. Chen C, Li L, Chen LL, et al. Incremental doses of dobutamine induce a biphasic response in dysfunctional left ventricular regions subtending coronary stenosis. *Circulation.* 1995;92:756–66.
33. Afrid: 1, Kleinman NS, Raizner AE, et al. Dobutamine echocardiogrpahy in myocardial hibernation: optimal dose and accuracy in predicting recovery of ventricular function after coronary revascularization. *Circulation.* 1995;91:663–70.
34. Eitzman D, Al-Aeuar Z, Kauter HL, et al. Clinical outcome of patients with advanced coronary artery disease after viability studies with position emission tomography. *J Am Coll Cardiol.* 1992;20:559.
35. Di Carli MF, Davidson M, Little R, et al. Value of metabolic imaging with positron emission tomography for evaluating prognosis in patients with coronary artery disease and left ventricular dysfunction. *Am J Cardiol.* 1994;73:527.

36. Zimmermann R, Mall G, Ranch B, et al. Residual 201T1 activity in irreversible defects as a marker of myocardial viability: clinicopathological study. *Circulation.* 1995;91:1016.

37. Medrano R, Lowry RW, Young JB, et al. Assessment of myocardial viability with Tc-99m sestamibi in patients undergoing cardiac transplantation: a scintigraphic/pathogical study. *Circulation.* 1996;94:1010.

38. Chen CH, Nakayama M, Nevo E, et al. Coupled systolic-ventricular and vascular stiffening with age: implications for pressure regulation and cardiac reserve in the elderly. *J Am Coll Cardiol* 1998;32:1221.

39. Little WC. Assessment of normal and abnormal cardiac function in heart disease. In Braunwald E, Zipes D, and Libby P, eds. *A Textbook of Cardiovascular Medicine,* 6th ed. WB Saunders, 2001.

40. Gortlieb S, Moss AJ, McDermott M, et al. Interrelation of left ventricular ejection fraction, pulmonary congestion and outcome in acute myocardial infarction. *Am J Cardiol* 1992;69:977.

41. Holmes DR, Detre KM, Williams DO, et al. Long-term outcome of patients with depressed left ventricular function undergoing percutaneous transluminal coronary angloplasty. The NHLBIPTCA registry. *Circulation* 1993;82:21.

42. The BARI investigators. Seven-year outcome in the Bypass Angioplasty Revascularization Investigation (BARI) by treatment and diabetic status. *J Am Coll Cardiol* 2000;35:1122.

43. Edmond M, Mock MB, Davis KB, et al. Long-term survival of medically treated patients in the Coronary Artery Surgery Study (CASS) registry. *Circulation* 1994;90:2645.

44. Eitzman D, Al-Aeuar Z, Kauter HL, et al. Clinical outcome of patients with advanced coronary artery disease after viability studies with positron emission tomography. *J Am Coll Cardiol* 1992;20:559.

PART 2 Equipment: Construction and Performance

CHAPTER (9)

Equipment for PCI

Fumiaki Ikeno, MD, and Alan C. Yeung, MD

GUIDEWIRE

The wire manipulation is the most important part of percutaneous coronary intervention (PCI).

In the first percutaneous transluminal coronary angioplasty (PTCA) performed by Andreas Gruentzig in 1977,[1] a 2–3 cm short wire fixed at the tip of balloon was used. In 1982, Simpson and coworkers[2] developed an over-the-wire system that made wire manipulation in coronary arteries easier and contributed to initial results improvement of PCI. Since this innovation, the current type of PTCA guidewire has been used. At the beginning of the history of the guidewire-based balloon delivery era, the guidewire was 0.018 in. in diameter, but now, because of the development of the lower-profile balloon catheter, almost all guidewires are 0.014 in. in diameter and only one length (300 cm). Recently, the rapid-exchange system has become more common, as has the shorter wire (180-cm length).

Current indications for PCI have increased as a result of the evolution of new devices, such as stents, rotablators, and so on, so the wire lineup should be more variable. The important points for Guidewire selection points are as follows: torque response, tip flexibility, stiffness and durability, transition of tip and shaft, shaft stiffness, durability, and affinity with devices. According to these requirements, culled from daily clinical practice, industries have been developing new types of PTCA wire technology.

In this chapter, wire characteristics are discussed from the aspect of device technology. The trackability, the stiffness of the tip and shaft, coating technology, and radiopacity have been considered, and manufacturers are developing new types of PTCA wire technology.

【 】 WIRE CHARACTERISTICS BY STRUCTURE

We can classify the guidewire structure into two types. One is a spring-tip wire made from stainless steel and wound around the tip of the spring coil wire. The other is a plastic wire in which a tapered wire tip is glued directly to the polymer sleeve and has hydrophilic coating.

Spring-Tip Wire

There are two kinds of spring-tip wires. (See Table 9–1). One consists of just a stainless steel shaft (Figure 9-1A). The other is a Nitinol tip jointed to a stainless steel shaft (Figure 9-1B). The Nitinol combined type is superior in shape retention and wire-tip durability because of the characteristics of Nitinol. The spring-tip wires are used not only in usual PCI applications but also in more complex lesions, including chronic total occlusion, because of their steerability.

The support wires have a stiff shaft without interstitial coil construction. The shaft is extended to the tip and longitudinal pushability is increased. This wire is used deliver the devices in more tortuous vessels (Figure 9-1C).

Plastic Wire

Plastic wires (Figure 9-2) have a hydrophilic coating that meets very little resistance when they come into contact with the irregular lumen, so they cross penetrate the tissue quite easily. (See Table 9–1). These wires provide good maneuverability in tortuous vessels and, compared with the coil wires, can be easier to choose the true lumen immediately after a sharp bend. However, the operator must be careful, because it is easy to find the way down a false lumen. Generally, these wires do not have the greatest torquability, and

TABLE 9-1

The Characteristics of the Wires

SPRING-TIP WIRE

	MANUFACTURER	DISTAL CORE MATERIAL	PROXIMAL CORE MATERIAL	DISTAL COATING
Standard use				
Route	Asahi Intec	Stainless	Stainless	Hydrophilic
HI-TORQUE BALANCE	GUIDANT	Nitinol	Stainless	Hydrophilic
Support wire				
Gradslam	Asahi Intec	Stainless	Stainless	Silicon

	PROXIMAL COATING	WIRE LENGTH (cm)	TIP STIFFNESS	TIP RADIOPACITY (cm)
Standard use				
Route	PTFE	175	0.8 g	3.0
HI-TORQUE BALANCE	PTFE	190, 300		3.0
Support wire				
Gradslam	Silicon	175, 300	0.7 g	4.0

PLASTIC WIRES

	MANUFACTURER	DISTAL CORE MATERIAL	PROXIMAL CORE MATERIAL	DISTAL COATING
HI-TORQUE WHISPER	GUIDANT	Nitinol	Stainless	Hydrophilic
PT series	Boston Scientific	Nitinol	Nitinol	Hydrophilic
Crosswire family	TERUMO	Nitinol	Nitinol	Hydrophilic

	PROXIMAL COATING	WIRE LENGTH (cm)	TIP STIFFNESS	TIP RADIOPACITY (cm)
HI-TORQUE WHISPER	PTFE	190,300		3.0
PT series	PTFE	185,300		2.0
Crosswire family	hydrophilic	180	Floppy (1.0 g)	3.0

STIFF-TIP WIRES

	MANUFACTURER	DISTAL CORE MATERIAL	PROXIMAL CORE MATERIAL	DISTAL COATING
Miracle family	Asahi Intec	Stainless	Stainless	Silicon or hydrophilic
Tapered-tip				
Confianza family	Asahi Intec	Stainless	Stainless	Silicon or hydrophilic
HI-TORQUE CROSS-IT	GUIDANT	Stainless	Stainless	hydrophilic

	PROXIMAL COATING	WIRE LENGTH (cm)	TIP STIFFNESS	TIP RADIOPACITY (cm)
Miracle family	PTFE	175	3,6,9,12 g	11.0
Tapered-tip				
Confianza family	PTFE	190,300	9 g, 12 g	3.0
HI-TORQUE CROSS-IT	PTFE	175	100 (2.8 g), 200 (4.3 g) 300 (6.8 g), 400 (8.7 g)	20.0

Asahi Intec (Nagoya, Aichi, Japan), GUIDANT (Santa Clara, CA, Japan). Boston Scientific (Natick, MA, USA), TERUMO (Shibuya, Tokyo, Japan). PTFE 2-5 polytetrafluoroethylene.

Spring-Tip Wire

A. Stainless steel type

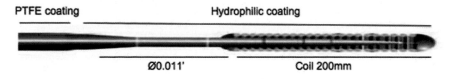

B. Nitinol combined type

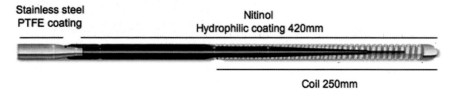

C. Support Wire

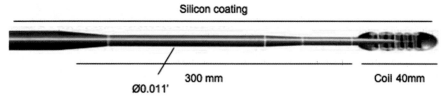

FIGURE 9-1. (**A**) Spring-tip wire (Nitinol combined type): Proximal part is made of stainless steel; distal part is made of Nitinol. The balance is made of middle weight (Guidant; Santu Clara, CA, USA). (**B**) Spring-tip wire (stainless-steel type): proximal and distal parts are made of stainless steel. Route (Asahi Intec; Nagoya, Aichi, Japan). (**C**) Support wire: Grand Slam (Asahi Intec).

they are not as easy to steer as coil wires. Plastic wires have very little friction with the vessel wall, and are very useful for severe tortuous lesions and severe stenosis with heavy calcification.

【 】 WIRE CHARACTERISTICS BY PURPOSE

There are four groups, classified by purpose. The first group is the standard-use guidewire, which is used for usual PCI cases (see previous section). The second group is stiff-tip wire, used especially for chronic total occlusion. The third group is tapered-tip wire, used for chronic total occlusion. Tapered tip wire is intended to clear chronic total occlusion, especially for those cases which require penetration through a hard, fibrous cap. The fourth group is the support wire, which is used as a support to cross devices over lesions with strong back-up force. Support wires are specific-use wires, such as Rota wire for Rotablator and marker wire.

Stiff-Tip Wire

Stiff-tip wires (Figure 9-3A) are usually used for opening the chronic total occlusion (See Table 9–1). Stiff-spring tip wires tend to encounter more resis-

tance inside the lumen than do plastic wires, but the stiff-spring tip wires have been developed for good torquability, even inside hard tissue of coronary total occlusion (CTO). The tip responds well to the operator's precise handling. The harder the wire tip, the greater the torquability of the wire; the less resistance to the tip felt by operator, the easier it is for the tip to go into the false lumen. Furthermore, because spring-tip wire meets resistance, the selectivity for the small channel is less than that for plastic wire, so the risk of finding the false lumen is higher.

Tapered Tip Wire

Tapered wire (Figure 9-3B, C) tends to select and slip into and the very narrow channel easier than coil wire, and these wires are also useful to penetrate the fibrous cap.[3] (See Table 9–1.) However, they can enter the false lumen after the bend of the vessel, and can easily cause perforation in the vessel wall.

BALLOON DILATATION CATHETER

Before stents, the balloon dilatation catheters were used alone to dilate the stenotic lesion of the artery for percutaneous coronary intervention (PCI). In this stent era, balloon dilatation catheters are still the main device as a predilatation

Plastic Wire

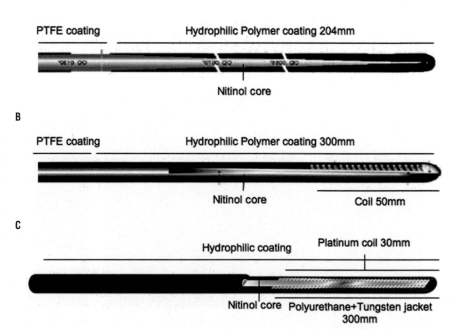

FIGURE 9-2. Plastic wire. (**A**) Choice PT (Boston Scientific; Natick, MA). (**B**) Whisper (Guidant; Santa Clara, CA, USA). (**C**) Crosswire (Terumo; Shibuya, Tokyo, Japan).

and postdilatation tool for stent deployment in PCI.

In 1964, Dotter and Judkins[3] succeeded in dilating the femoral artery with several different sizes of dilatation catheters. After Dotter and Judkins' success, angioplasty dilatation catheters for peripheral artery disease were developed in Europe.[4,5] In 1974, Gruentzig and coworkers developed 2-lumen balloon dilatation catheter for peripheral artery disease and because of this, the angioplasty for peripheral artery became safer and the success rate higher. In 1977, Gruentzig performed the first angioplasty for coronarty artery disease with his fixed wire balloon dilatation catheter[1] (Figure 9-4A). In 1981, Simpson and coworkers[2] invented the over-the-wire type balloon dilatation catheter (Figure 9-4B) which has a center lumen of catheter for a movable wire and this made the coronary angioplasty procedure safer and easier. Now the main type for PCI_3 is the monorail balloon dilatation catheter with shorter wire lumen for the single operator use.

The balloon dilatation catheter is still an important device after a quarter of a century has passed since its invention; therefore it is important to be familiar with its structure, type, and performance for PCI procedure.

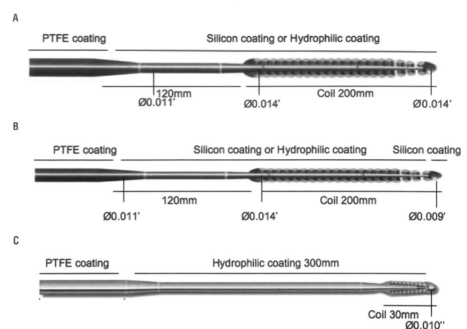

Stiff -Tip Wire

FIGURE 9-3. Stiff-tip wire. (**A**) Miracle Family (Asahi Intec; Nagoya, Aichi, Japan). (**B**) Tapered-tip wire: Confianza Family (Asahi Intec). (**C**) Cross-It Family (Guidant; Santa Clara, CA, USA).

【 】 BALLOON DILATATION CATHETER CHARACTERISTICS BY STRUCTURE

We can classify the balloon dilatation catheter into 4 groups. One is on-the-wire (fixed-wire) type that has the short spring coil wire fixed on the tip of the balloon catheter. The second is the over-the-wire type which has the wire lumen at the center of catheter for the mobilization of steerable guide wire. The third one is the monorail (rapid-exchange) type in which the wire lumen is shorter than the over-the-wire type and which makes the procedure easier for a single operator. Last are the miscellaneous types, such as cutting and perfusion balloons.

On-the-Wire (Fixed-Wire) Type (Figure 9-5A)

The length of 1–2 cm coil spring wire is attached at the tip of the balloon catheter. This configuration makes the catheter profile smaller and this makes it possible to cross the tortuous vessel and rigid vessel that the other type of catheters cannot cross. However, it is impossible to leave the wire in the lesion after balloon dilatation, therefore if the dissection happens after balloon dilatation, the wire must be recrossed for the bail out, which is not ideal in current practice. For this reason, the on-the-wire

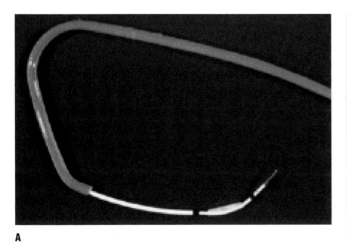

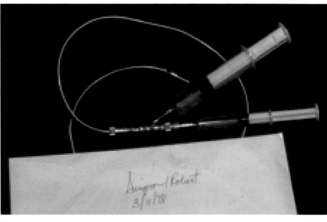

FIGURE 9-4. (**A**) On-the-wire balloon catheter developed by Dr. Gruentzig. (**B**) Simpson-Robert over-the-wire catheter. (*Courtesy of Dr. John B. Simpson.*)

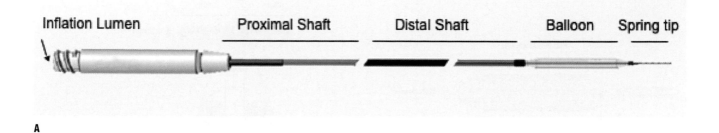

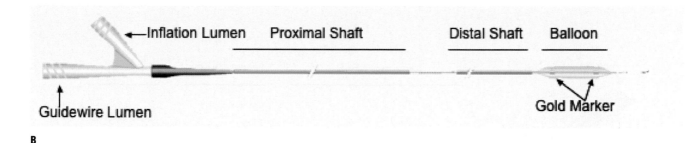

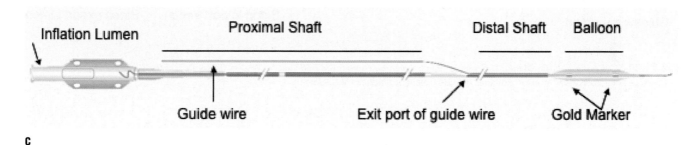

FIGURE 9-5. (**A**) On-the-wire balloon catheter ACE balloon catheter (Boston Scientific, Natrick, MA, USA). (**B**) Over-the-wire balloon catheter; MAVERICK Over-The Wire Balloon Catheter (Boston Scientific, Natrick, MA, USA). (**C**) Monorail (rapid exchange) balloon catheter; MAVERICK2 Monorail Balloon Catheter (Boston Scientific, Natrick, MA, USA).

balloon catheter is not often used now, and only a few such catheters are available.

Over-the-Wire Type (Figure 9-5B)

This type has both inflation and guide wire lumens in the catheter shaft. This type allows manipulation of the guide wire freely independent of the catheter. And also the guide wire can be pulled out when the catheter is in the artery and it is possible to change the shape of the guide wire tip and exchange to a different guide wire. It is possible to leave the guide wire inside the artery during the exchange of the catheter; however, two operators and a long guide wire (300 cm) are usually necessary.

Monorail (Rapid Exchange) Type (Figure 9-5C)

The guide wire lumen is only about 20–30 cm proximal from the tip. This type makes it possible to manipulate by a single operator, and a short guide wire (180 cm) can be used. The shaft of the catheter in smaller which makes it easier to use the smaller guide catheter in complex procedures, such as the kissing balloon technique. For convenience, the monorail balloon dilatation catheter is popular in daily clinical practice.

Miscellaneous (Figure 9-5D, E)

The cutting balloon dilatation catheter (Flextome, Boston Scientific Corporation, Natick, MA, USA) has a 3-4 stainless steel blade called an Atherotome. The blades are wrapped by balloon material at deflation, and once the balloon is inflated, they are exposed and cut the plaque. This concept helps to dilate the vessel avoiding the large dissection with 3-4 blades that can make sharp cuts in the atheroma. The benefit is less vessel injury for the vessel wall compared with balloon angioplasty; however, the large catheter profile makes it more difficult to cross the tortuous vessel and tight lesions.

The perfusion balloon dilatation catheter has inflow lumens proximal to the balloon and export lumens at the tip of the catheter to allow the blood to perfuse the artery during balloon inflation. This balloon is now used for sealing the ruptured vessel.

【 】 BALLOON DILATATION CATHETER CHARACTERISTICS BY MATERIAL

The balloon dilatation catheter has several different characteristics for the treatment of coronary artery disease. The compliance, the

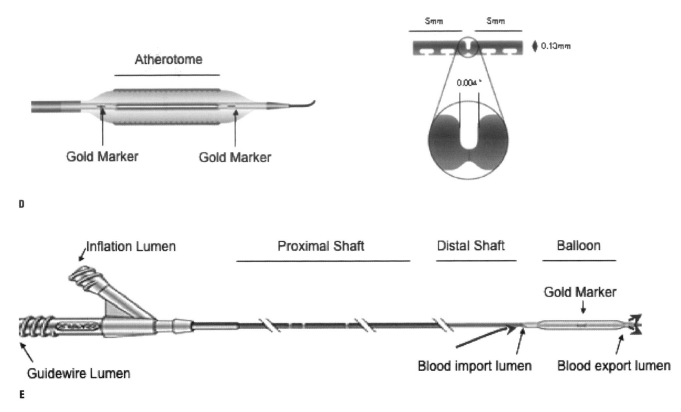

FIGURE 9-5. *(Continued)* (**D**) Cutting balloon catheter; Fletxome Cutting Balloon Device (Boston Scientific, Natrick, MA, USA). (**E**) Perfusion balloon catheter; Surpass Perfusion catheter (Boston Scientific, Natick, MA, USA).

size, and the length of the balloon are important for various types of atherosclerotic lesions. The balloon shaft material is also important for delivery into stenotic lesions.

Balloon Characteristics

There are three classifications of balloon compliance. One is the compliant balloon, the second is the semi-compliant balloon, and the last is the noncompliant balloon. The compliant balloon is made of soft material like polyolefin copolymer (POC), and with higher pressure, the balloon becomes 20% bigger in diameter than the labeled balloon size. When this type is used for the treatment of a hard lesion, both edges of the balloon become bigger compared with the midpart of the balloon and may cause dissection at the edge of the balloon.[6]

On the other hand, the noncompliant balloon is made of hard material like polyethylene terephtalate (PET). The balloon diameter does not change much even when inflated by high pressure, so this type of balloon has high power to dilate the lesion. Therefore, this type is used for the hard calicified plaque and the postdilatation of the stent. However, the ability for crossing the lesion is lower than the other types of balloon and the rewrap of the balloon is not good.

The semi-compliant balloon ranks between the compliant and the noncompliant balloon. This type is made of polyether block-amide (PEBAX), Nylon, and polyurethane elastomer. This type of balloon is mostly used in PCI because of its better trackability and the wide range of size control by pressure.

There are different diameter sizes of the balloons. The small size of balloon is used for chronic total occlusion to create the first canal after wire crossing. The big size balloon is used for bigger vessels, such as left main or saphenous vein graft intervention. Usually, each balloon catheter has a quarter or half millimeter step-up in size.

The balloon length is also variable. The shorter balloon is used for a short lesion and postdilatation after stenting. The longer balloon is used for a longer lesion.

Catheter Shaft Characteristics

For the over-the-wire balloon catheter, the wire is in the balloon shaft, so its pushability is better. However the monorail balloon catheter does not have wire lumen in most of the shaft, so two different kinds of materials are used for the shaft. One is a hypotube made of stainless steel. The hypotube shaft has a small profile and strong pushability. The other is the core wire shaft that has stiff wire inside the shaft made of polyamide or plastic. The core of the wire shaft is flexible, but the profile is bigger than the hypotube shaft.

GUIDING CATHETER

The selection of the guiding catheter is most important in order to perform PCI successfully. The selection of the tip shape will be explained in another section. In this section, the constitution of the guiding catheter is discussed.

TABLE 9-2

The Size of Guiding Catheters Needed for Various Devices

SIZE ID (inch)	5-Fr (0.058–0.059)	6-Fr (0.070–0.073)	7-Fr (0.078–0.081)	8-Fr (0.088–0.090)	9-Fr (0.098–0.101)
Balloon	○	○	○	○	○
Stent	△	○	○	○	○
Cutting balloon	△ (≤2.5 mm)	○	○	○	○
Perfusion Balloon	×	○	○	○	○
Kissing Balloon	×	△	○	○	○
Rotablator	×	≤1.75 mm	≤2.00 mm	≤2.25 mm	≤2.5 mm
DCA	×	×	×	○	○
IVUS	×	○	○	○	○

○ = possible. △ = partial possible. × = Impossible. ID: inner diameter, Fr = French, DCA: directional coronary atherectomy, IVUS: intravascular ultrasound
(Courtesy of Masahiko Ochial: Logical Analysis and Re-construction of Percutaneous Coronary Interventions. Tokyo: Chyugaiigakusya.)

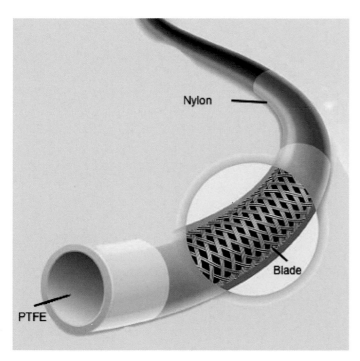

FIGURE 9-6. Constitution of guiding catheter; PTFE = polytetrafluoroethylene.

Labels: Nylon, Blade, PTFE

[ ] CONSTITUTION OF GUIDING CATHETER

Material of Guiding Catheter (Figure 9–6)

The guiding catheter should have precise torque response. This enhances maneuverability and engagement of coronary arteries. Backup support is also important for guiding catheters to deliver devices into the lesion especially in complex cases. To satisfy these requirements, the guiding catheter is made of several parts. The guiding catheter has the blade made of stainless steel, and this provides the high torque, kink resistance, and strong backup support.

The inner layer is made of PTFE (polytetrafluoroethylene), and this material has a smooth and lubricious surface to facilitate the passage of the device.

Size of Guiding Catheter Recently, the guiding catheters with larger inner lumen diameters have been used, and they provide improved dye flow for better visualization. Larger inner lumen diameters offer the device compatibility needed for multiple treatment options and clinical scenarios. (See Table 9–2.)

On the other hand, the small-sized of the guiding catheter avoids entry-site complications and decreases patient ambulation time.[7,8] Technology has developed smaller sizes, with larger inner diameter guiding catheters and high torquability. The larger inner lumen 6-Fr guiding catheter can support ordinary PCI procedures; however, the technique for complex cases, such as kissing balloon, stents, DCA (directional coronary atherectomy), and large-sized rotablators, requires a larger guiding catheter.

REFERENCES

1. Gruentzig AR. Percutaneous transluminal coronary angioplasty. Semin Roentgenol 1981;16:152.
2. Simpson JB, Baim DS, Robert EW, et al. A new catheter system for coronary angioplasty. Am J Cardiol 1982;49:1216.
3. Dotter CT, Judkins MP. Transluminal treatment of arteriosclerotic obstruction. Description of a new technic and a preliminary report of its application. Circulation 1964;30:654.
4. Zeitler E, Schoop W, Zahnow W. The treatment of occlusive arterial disease by transluminal catheter angioplasty. Radiology 1971;99:19.
5. Wierny L, Plass R, Porstmann W. Long-term results in 100 consecutive patients treated by transluminal angioplasty. Radiology 1974;112:543.
6. Bach RG. Dog bones, dumbbells, and dissections: sizing up angioplasty balloons. Cathet Cardiovasc Diagn 1994;32:310.
7. Talley JD, Mauldin PD, Becker ER. A prospective randomized trial comparing the benefits and limitations of 6Fr and 8Fr guiding catheters in elective coronary angioplasty: clinical, procedural, angiographic, and economic end points. J Interv Cardiol 1995;8:345.
8. Metz D, Meyer P, Touati C, et al. Comparison of 6F with 7F and 8F guiding catheters for elective coronary angioplasty: results of a prospective, multicenter, randomized trial. Am Heart J 1997;134:131.

CHAPTER (10)

Design and Construction of Stents

Michael S. Williams, BA, and Campbell Rogers, MD

As the understanding of vascular disease and restenosis has advanced, so has the understanding of stent design. This chapter focuses on cardiovascular stent design and how vascular biology and pathophysiology directly influence design factors, including geometry and materials. As the sophistication and understanding of cardiovascular disease increases, so will the sophistication of the designs and uses of stents. Certain lesions may benefit from very flexible, highly compliant stents, whereas other lesions may require more rigid, less compliant devices. Various drugs alone or multiple drug combinations in one stent will be available as well. There will likely evolve a matrix or toolbox of combinations of all stent properties that provide the user with an armamentarium well suited for most, if not all, clinical situations.

Stent design encompasses a wide range of interrelated variables. Although no variable is truly independent of another, in order to address clearly each variable in this chapter, each variable is delineated independently. The reader should remember that variable interrelationships cross over among mechanics, biology, materials, and performance, and that the sum of these interrelationships equals the difference between a well-designed stent and a less effective device.

Variables of stent design discussed in this chapter include diameter, length, flexibility, surface area, radiopacity, and radial strength. Materials and general processing methods are also addressed.

DIAMETER

The diameter of a stent is important to the designer for several reasons. The most obvious is that appropriate sizing of a stent to the vessel size is a critical factor in the vascular response to the device.

Providing an adequate spectrum of diameters to meet physician needs for coronary applications has been standardized to 0.25 mm–0.5 mm increments, starting at 2.0-mm diameter and ranging more than 5.0 mm.

To the designer, stent diameter is a key determinant of stent radial strength. Stents are often designed and manufactured to allow the achievement of multiple sizes from one base geometry. Post deployment strut angle (where in general, increased strut angle equals increased radial strength) varies from one diameter to another. In order for maximum strength to be obtained at any given diameter, the strut angle must be designed to fall within approximately 5% of the ideal maximum, typically a 46° included angle. The user must establish a usable and functional range to accommodate custom sizing. Such sizing is required to ensure that the device is seated securely against the vessel wall. Clinically, it has been shown that immediate post deployment luminal geometry induced by larger stent diameters provides greater acute procedural diameter gain and larger ultimate lumen size. The generally accepted user standard for appropriate sizing into a vessel wall is a 1.1: 1 stent-to-artery ratio.[1] This is typically measured from the proximal end of the stent, often with slightly greater stent-to-artery ratio at the distal end of the stent because of natural vessel tapering. The 1.1: 1 ratio is a general rule of thumb, because vascular morphology plays an important role in appropriate vessel sizing. For example, an oversized stent may dissect a vessel (especially a highly atherosclerotic lesion), whereas an undersized device may result in downstream migration or thrombosis of the stent. Excessive oversizing also may contribute to the degree of restenosis a lesion develops over time, related to increased injury associated with IEL (inner elastic lamina) rupture and medial injury.[2–4]

In most stent designs as the diameter increases during expansion, the length shortens. This foreshortening can occur as struts are reoriented via plastic deformation during deployment from a generally longitudinal orientation to a generally radial orientation. The designer knows that if the change in length during deployment is too great, the stent may not cover the targeted lesion adequately or accurately. This loss of accuracy is one of the primary reasons why self-expanding braid designs have not been more universally adopted. In balloon expandable designs, this phenomenon can be controlled in several ways, including by the number of crowns, by the end strut angle of the crowns (which, as mentioned earlier, has a major impact on the radial strength of a stent), and by longitudinal connectors oriented so as to maintain spacing between adjacent rings.

Another related aspect of stent diameter design is elastic recoil. Recoil is a function of strut angle design, thickness, and width of struts and material properties. Measured immediately after expansion in air, recoil of approximately 10% is typical for most steel stents. The *elastic modulus of a metal* is defined as the slope of a stress strain curve describing the degree to which, when stress is removed, the metal returns toward its original shape. (See Figure 10-1.) During deployment, stress is applied and focalized at the apex of each strut, causing the strut to undergo deformation or strain. As both stress and strain are increased, a metal eventually reaches its *yield point,* which is defined as the plastic or elastic limit. When a material under a load (stress) reaches its elastic limit, it will not return to its original orientation because the grain structure of the metal has been reoriented beyond recovery.

By thoroughly understanding the interrelationships of factors such as radial strength, foreshortening, elastic recoil, appropriate sizing, and vascular response to injury, the designer can balance a design that meets user and clinical needs. The interrelationship of these variables emphasizes the importance of stent diameter on the outcome of successful device implantation.

LENGTH

Stent length is a design parameter clearly defined by the interventional cardiologist. Physicians generally prefer to implant stents that exceed lesion length by several millimeters. In the era of drug-eluting stents, ever-greater stent to lesion length ratios are gaining popularity. This ensures that the lesion is completely covered and allows a safety factor accounting for misalignment as a result of misinterpretation of the fluoroscopic image, as well as scaffolding of minor atherosclerotic plaques at the margins of more severe narrowings. Most stents comprise a series of repeating units referred to as *elements, segments, rings, cells,* or *struts.* Elements are connected with various geometric patterns designed to enhance flexibility and strength. The element connections can also maintain interstrut distance, which may be challenged in tortuous vasculature thus preventing strut splay on the

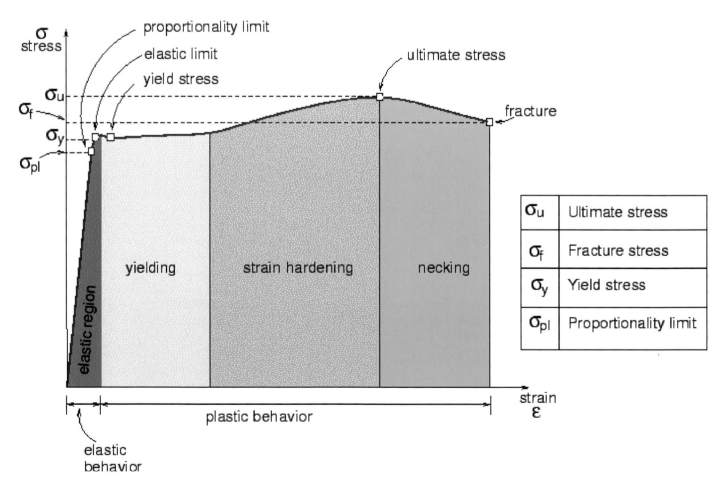

FIGURE 10-1. Typical Stress-Strain Curve.

outside (major) curvature of the stent, and strut compression and overlap on the inside (minor) curvature of the stent. If splay is too great, tissue prolapse through the strut and into the lumen may occur, resulting in poor rheologic outcomes, which may lead to thrombosis or restenosis.[5,6] The sum length of these repeating elements and connections equal the total length of the device.

FLEXIBILITY

Flexibility is a clinically important design element. Stents must be flexible in their preexpansion form in order to allow delivery to distal and tortuous anatomic targets. The historical development of stents has clearly demonstrated that improvements in flexibility have allowed a marked increase in successful lesion access.

Once implanted, stent flexibility after expansion is also important, as a device's conformability to varied vascular geometries may have a significant impact on clinical outcomes. One of the most important aspects of an implanted stent's flexibility is stent-end compliance and its relationship to compliance of the vessel. Physicians typically select stents that are longer than the target lesion in which they are implanted. Thus, there is overlap of the device with nondiseased regions of the vessel. This region of overlap, where there is high variance between stent compliance and vessel compliance, may represent a prime stimulus for vascular injury and adverse tissue responses. Furthermore, vascular responses may be heightened in this region as a result of a process similar to metallic fretting, where continuous motion between two surfaces results in wearing of those surfaces. In a stented artery, this continual wear is exacerbated by the extreme dissimilarity of physical properties between the implant and the vessel, and is aggravated by the continual motion of the artery and the heart. The fretting phenomenon is not a singular event, but rather a chronic problem induced and sustained to a different degree depending upon a device's flexural modulus.

The resultant trauma caused to the native tissue by this compliance mismatch can be reduced by designing stents with different mechanical properties on the ends of their working length. This can be justified and rationalized by the fact that this region, which extends into nondiseased vessel, is not a therapeutic or scaffolding region of the device, and therefore does not carry the same mechanical requirements as the working region of the stent. From the designer's perspective, the ideal stent has compliant and flexible end elements that more closely resemble the natural properties of healthy arterial tissue. Design variables for improved end compliance include combinations of geometry, length of transition, material property modifications, and material choice.[7,8]

Connection design, material thickness, material properties, and element length are design variables that influence flexibility. Controlling the pre- and post-deployment length and geometry of connecting elements influences device function. In many designs, as the stent is expanded, the strut element length decreases as the connecting element length increases (eg, a diamond shape, which becomes narrower as it elongates).

Varying strut thickness is also a useful method of enhancing flexibility, although biologic ramifications of changing strut thickness are not completely understood.[9,10] In general, thinner stents or stent regions produce more flexibility. Designers vary strut element and connector element thickness in order to cause preferential bending, thus enhancing overall flexibility. It should be noted that such variations in thickness are not simple manufacturing processes, but are dependent upon the material and method of production used, and therefore may not be readily implemented into just any device.

Clearly, material choice has an impact on a stent designer's ability to influence flexibility. Most cardiovascular stents are made from a variation of 316 L stainless steel. Other materials such as MP35N, Elgiloy, nickel titanium (NiTi) and polymers are used, although to a lesser extent. Characteristics of each of these materials are discussed later in the chapter.

SURFACE AREA

Stent surface area, of paramount importance in stent design, has an impact on a cascade of biologic events. The origin of this cascade is initial vascular injury induced by trauma to the vessel during stent deployment. It has been demonstrated that increased surface area, independent of vascular injury, plays a key role in the extent of neointimal formation within a stented vessel (the cause of in-stent restenosis). Injury is related to vessel sizing and, perhaps more important, to stent geometry. Assuming that the material selected for a design is "biocompatible," an increase in material surface area results in decreased biologic response. This reduced response is the result of an increase in surface area of the device, or "footprint," that distributes the load across a greater surface, thus minimizing the vascular strain at any given point of contact. In addition, increased surface area contributes to the acute circularity of the vessel. There is evidence that, subject to manipulation, stented arteries remodel to restore a circular cross-section, and if this can be augmented by a stent, it may increase the rate of normalization and healing of the vessel by reducing strain and improving flow dynamics.[10]

One potential drawback of increasing stent surface area is the increased mass of the device. The negative significance of increased mass of the device is a correlative increase in the biologic response to the implant. All materials induce some level of biologic response; hence, even "biocompatible" materials provoke a response. For example, although stainless steel is known for its biocompatibility and hemocompatibility, it still elicits a degree of biologic response that can lead to a substantial neointimal thickening. Surface coatings of drug or drug loaded polymer films (usually less than 5 microns thick) are intended as therapeutic tools to treat restenosis. A secondary benefit of these drug coatings (depending on their specific mechanism of action) may also be to nullify some of the biological response to the implant thus making the trade-off of increased surface area more palatable.

Surface area is perhaps most critical as a design element in drug-delivery stents. Increased surface area means that more drug can be loaded onto a device's surface and that the distribution of drug is more homogeneous over the vascular surface. This results in a more controllable pharmacokinetic profile, important in a dynamic environment characterized by high flow and variable morphology.

RADIOPACITY

Stent radiopacity (ie, fluoroscopic visibility) is key to successful implantation and future detection of a device's location within a coronary artery. Stent radiopacity is controlled by two primary variables. The first, control of material thickness, is the most common method a designer uses to increase or decrease radiopacity. However, increasing material thickness can have obvious negative impact on such other design parameters as thrombogenicity, delivery profile, flexibility, and degree of vascular injury. The second method for modifying radiopacity is material selection. For example, MP35N, a high-cobalt alloy material, allows the designer to create thinner stents without sacrificing radiopacity or strength. Other means of improving radiopacity include coating with radiodense materials such as gold or other metals, or use of gold or platinum markers at the ends of steel stents. However, the biologic effects of adding a radiopaque material to the surface of stents may not always be benign.[11-13] In purely polymeric stents, where radiopacity is not an inherent property, use of markers may be of even greater importance.

RADIAL COMPRESSIVE STRENGTH

The ability of a stent to withstand radial compressive forces exerted by a vascular wall is commonly termed *radial* or *hoop strength*. Radial compressive forces can be exacerbated by such pathophysiologic conditions as vascular spasm in acute or subacute postinterventional stages, which can produce a compressive force of 300 mm Hg and last minutes to hours. Vascular remodeling as a result of adventitial and medial inflammation and fibrosis is a second pathophysiolgic source of radial compression.[14,15] External impetus of radial forces onto a stent include loads applied in bending of a joint, during normal respiration, and during normal cyclic motion of the heart. In peripheral vascular devices such as popliteal stents, compression forces are exerted during normal bending of the knee or in external loads applied from contact or trauma.

Radial compressive strength is "designed in" by increasing strut thickness, using higher-modulus materials, and optimizing post deployment strut geometry. In general, as a stent deploys, the generally longitudinal orientation of struts transitions into a preferably radial (or perpendicular) orientation. Often, a trade-off is made between hemocompatibility or flexibility and postexpansion strength. This strengthening orientation is achieved during expansion of the device. Balloon expansion induces plastic deformation of the strut at designed locations. Plastic deformation increases the strength of a metal by cold-working, which results in reorientation of the grain structure. This microscopic material orientation compliments the geometric orientation described earlier.

When designing shape memory devices out of, for example NiTi, the preferred molecular grain structure is achieved during the manufacturing process. The device is "set" in the desired configuration, heated to temperatures in the 500° C range for a time, and then cooled. Once removed from the form fixture, the device must be restrained in its delivery configuration until use, when it is deployed into its set configuration. It should be noted that shape memory stents (eg. NiTi devices) always achieve their final set designed diameter. Depending on the morphology of the lesion this process may not be an acute phenomenon but rather a gradual process. Therefore, predicting final stent sizing is critical. The physician must be certain that the final diameter does not over exceed the native vessel diameter to the extent that further vessel injury or perforation occurs.

CONSTRUCTION OF STENTS

Stent construction methods and technologies are varied depending on the base material and design of the device. 316L stainless steel is the most commonly used stent manufacturing material. 316L stainless steel has many amenable attributes for implantable stents. It is machinable, heat treatable, lasable, polishable, plastically deformable, radiopaque, and biocompatible. Other materials used for stent manufacturing are Elgiloy, NiTi and MP35N. Elgiloy is characterized by high strength, temperature resistance and corrosion resistance. Elgiloy is a well known spring material. This property allows the stent designer to create an elastic device that stores energy when compressed and recovers to its basic form when released. Nickel Titanium (NiTi)(Nitinol) is in a unique class of materials known as shape memory alloys. A thermoelastic martensitic phase transformation in the material is responsible for its extraordinary properties including the shape memory effect and superelasticity. The properties of Nitinol can be modified to a great extent by changes in alloy composition and in secondary operations such as mechanical working and heat treatment. NiTi is most commonly used in peripheral and carotid stents. MP35N alloy is a nickel-cobalt based alloy with a unique combination of properties. MP35N alloy's toughness, high strength, resistance to stress cracking and ductility makes the alloy exceptional stent material. Additionally, MP35N has outstanding corrosion resistance and is highly radiopaque which allows for decreased wall thickness and thus lower delivery profiles.

There are many means by which to manufacture stents. Following is an example of the process a designer/manufacturer goes through in order to produce a standard stainless steel device for intravascular applications:

1. Design device using computer software such as AutoCad or SolidWorks and create drawing files.

2. Create a drawing exchange file (.dxf) from drawing files and download into *computer-aided manufacturing* (CAM) program.

3. Use .dxf file to create a cutting-tool path in the CAM profile.

4. Download tool path program onto a LASER computer that directs a physical operating system called *computerized numerical control (CNC)*.

5. Mount stent hypotubing material blank onto a retaining mandrel and load into the LASER, whereby it is motor driven, rotated and indexed as directed by the tool path to cut the designed geometry.

6. Remove the device from the mandrel.

7. Tumble the device to remove slag and break sharp edges.

8. Anneal the device to relieve stresses and to preferentially size and orient the physical grain structure.

9. Polish the device via electrolysis. This step leaves the stent with rounded edges and a smooth, hemocompatible surface.

10. Load stent onto a delivery system where it is secured by various means, including forming of the polymeric balloon or by mechanical attachment.

FUTURE DIRECTIONS IN STENTS

Stents have become mainstream in cardiovascular therapeutics, and are uniformly accepted as safe devices for the treatment of vascular disease. As it is with the life cycle of most medical-device technologies, stents are rapidly moving into the next frontier of scientific, engineering, and clinical development.

Advances in materials technology and in the understanding of vascular disease are enabling the redefinition of interventional intravascular medicine. Stents have become more than simple mechanical scaffolds. They are now being used as physical vectors for pharmaceutic and biologic therapeutics. One of the principal benefits of using stents as drug-delivery vehicles is that they allow for targeted site–specific delivery; thus concentrating therapeutic or regenerative therapy locally and avoiding the negative toxic effects associated with systemic delivery.

Although the mechanical aspects of stents continue to make incremental improvements, most current efforts are focused on selecting appropriate drugs and polymers and solving how to attach them to the device. There are several drug-delivery stent technologies being developed. The current state of the art is either drug-only or drug/polymer–coated metallic stents. These systems use standard stent substrates that have a covalently bound drug applied directly to the surface of the device or drug/polymer matrices that conform to cover the surface of the device. In general, these devices use a solvent-based drug/polymer mixture that is applied to the device either by a dipping or by a spray-coating process. In the case of the drug/polymer coating, it is important to use a solvent that is compatible with both entities and has a high vapor pressure to enhance solvent removal. Solvent removal is often accomplished by use of a low temperature vacuum oven. A general benchmark is a residual solvent level of less than 100 ppm. Low temperature is important, because many pharmaceutics and biologics are highly sensitive to heat. Too high a temperature denatures the therapeutic agent, rendering it ineffective.

The next generation of drug-delivery stents may use standard stent substrates that have been modified to carry greater volumes of drug and polymer by the addition of wells or increased surface area. These designs may be able to transport greater amounts of drug and even multiple drugs, if necessary. The questions surrounding these types of devices revolve around the uniformity and adequacy of pharmacokinetic dispersion of drug, the impact of surface anomalies on device thrombosis, durability, and potential trauma to the vessel wall from depleted drug reservoirs. All of these challenges, like so many design challenges, must be thoroughly understood and defined through theoretic and empiric experimentation. Clearly a critical component to the successful design and manufacture of pharmaceutical or biologic stents relies on the drug or biologic selected; however, this discussion extends beyond the intended scope of this chapter.

Although not a new concept,[16–19] perhaps the most promising new practical advancement in intravascular targeted drug delivery is the development of the 100% bioerodible polymeric stent. New and rapid advances in biomaterials and engineering technology have reinvigorated this decade-old idea.

Some of the theoretic advantages of fully erodible polymeric drug delivery stents are:

- High-volume pharmacologic or biologic loading capacity.
- Improved pharmacokinetics.
- Multiple drug loading capability.
- Staged release profiles.
- Nonpermanent implanted device.
- Improved vascular compliance.
- MR and CT compatibility.

There are numerous challenges to developing fully polymeric stents and the designer is constantly faced with difficult choices distinct from those facing a metal stent designer. For example, to increase the radial strength of a device with fixed cross-sectional geometry x. one logical step would be to increase the molecular weight and, more important, the percentage crystallinity of the polymer. However, in doing so, the designer must then weigh the benefit of strength gained against the loss of flexibility, increased degradation time, and the changes in release pharmacokinetics.

Decisions such as these are common, but most are not insurmountable and can be solved by logical mechanical design principles and by applying advances in materials science and technology, such as secondary processing. *Secondary processing of polymers or polymeric stents* refers to physical changes that are imparted on the material or device that improve its mechanical, biologic, or clinical therapeutic performance. One example of applying secondary processing to improve a mechanical property such as radial strength of a device is to modify the physical orientation of the molecular chains.

Material selection for polymeric stents is an interesting challenge. The designer must ask important questions such as the following:

- What are the geometric limitations of the device?
- What is the desired mechanism of deployment?
- For what length of time must the device maintain its mechanical strength?
- What is the desired erosion rate?
- How will the drug be loaded?
- Can it be sterilized by conventional means?
- What are the thermal limits of the drug and polymer?
- What is an acceptable amount of residual monomer, catalyst, solvent?
- What is the regulatory status of the drug and polymer?

Understanding the fundamental building blocks of the material and how it is made are crucial, beginning with the synthesis of the polymer. For example, polymer synthesis and the selection of catalysts have proved to be fundamental in material biocompatibility. In general it has been learned that zinc (Zn)-based catalysts have improved biocomaptibility over tin (Sn)-based catalysts. Also

TABLE 10-1

Candidate Bioresorbable Polymer Materials for Stents and Stent Coatings

poly (l-lactic acid) (L-PLA)

poly (dl-lactic acid) (DL-PLA)

poly glycolic acid (PGA)

epsilon poly (caprolactone) (PCL)

Copolymers of the above

Poly (anhydride)

Poly (dioxanone)

Poly (orthoester)

Poly (esteramide)

Poly (hydroxybutyrate-valerate)

important is solvent and thermal compatibility of materials as well as residual monomer levels.

There are several bioerodible polymeric materials to choose from, but by the time the designer filters out candidates based on factors such as, but not limited to, the mechanism of the design, mechanical properties over time, drug loading and release kinetics, sterilization compatibility, FDA history, and so on, the choices become fairly limited. Table 10-1 shows some examples of bioerodible polymers that have been or are being considered as materials for bioerodible vascular stents.

The same processes described earlier can achieve drug loading into or onto erodible stents. Downstream manufacturing steps of these devices can affect many factors that contribute to the outcome and functionality of the device. Special packaging is required for most erodible and drug-delivery combination products. Polymers that degrade by hydrolysis and ultimately end up as CO_2 and water byproducts via the Krebs cycle must be packaged in argon- or nitrogen-purged moisture-barrier pouches. These pouches also serve to protect photosensitive drugs.

The last, but not least, important step is sterilization of the device. Most designers choose ethylene oxide, as there is less loss of molecular weight than in gamma or e-beam processes.

Polymeric stents have great promise. There are many design and development challenges associated with these devices, many of which (but not all) have been touched on herein. These unique platforms provide the foundation for the next new frontier in interventional medicine.

Also under development are degradable metal stents. These magnesium (Mg)-based devices have very short degradation profiles which may be beneficial in certain types of lesions. Early work has shown promise in this variation of bioabsorbable stent design.

As with all new technologies there remain many questions but the promise of meaningful solutions to unmet medical needs will continue to push these and other new, disruptive, and exciting technologies forward.

REFERENCES

1. Colombo A, Hall P, Nakamura S, et al. Intracoronary stenting without anticoagulation accomplished with intravascular ultrasound guidance. *Circulation.* 1995;91:1676.
2. Schwartz RS, Huber KC, Murphy JG, et al. Restenosis and proportional neointimal response to coronary artery injury: results in a porcine model. *J Am Coll Cardiol.* 1992;19:267.
3. Schwartz RS, Holmes DH, Topol EJ. The restenosis paradigm revisited: an alternative proposal for cellular mechanisms. *J Am Coll Cardiol.* 1992;20:1284.
4. Rogers C, Edelman ER. Endovascular stent design dictates experimental restenosis and thrombosis. *Circulation.* 1995;91:2995.
5. Hoffman R, Mintz GS, Haager PK, et al. Relation of stent design and stent surface material to subsequent in-stent intimal hyperplasia in coronary arteries determined by intravascular ultrasound. *Am J Cardiol.* 2002;89:1360.
6. Hoffmann R, Mintz GS, Dussaillant GR, et al. Patterns and mechanisms of in-stent restenosis: a serial intravascular ultrasound study. *Circulation.* 1996;94;1247.
7. Squire JC, Rogers C, Edelman ER. Measuring arterial strain induced by endovascular stents. *Mol Biol Eng Comp.* 1999;37:692.
8. Rogers C, Tseng DY, Squire JC, Edelman ER. Balloon–artery interactions during stent placement: a finite element analysis approach to pressure, compliance, and stent design as contributors to vascular injury. *Circ Res.* 1999;84:378.
9. Kastrati A, Mehilli J, Dirschinger J, et al. Intracoronary stenting and angiographic restenosis results: strut thickness effect on restenosis outcome (ISAR-STEREO) trial. *Circulation.* 2001;103:2816.
10. Garasic JM, Edelman ER, Squire JC, Williams MS, Seifert P, Rogers C. Stent and artery geometry determine intimal thickening independent of arterial injury. *Circulation.* 2000;101:812.
11. Kastrati A, Schomig A, Dirshinger J. Increased risk of restenosis after placement of gold-coated stents. Results of a randomized trial comparing gold-coated with uncoated steel stents in patients with coronary artery disease. *Circulation.* 2000;101:2478.
12. Edelman ER, Seifert P, Groothuis A, Morss A, Bornstein D, Rogers C. Gold-coated NIR stents in porcine coronary arteries. *Circulation.* 2001;103:429.
13. Silber S, Reifart N, Morice M-C. The NUGGET trial (NIR ultimate gold-gilded equivalency trial): 6 month post-procedure safety and efficiency results. *Circulation.* 2001;104:II.
14. Post MJ, Borst C, Kuntz RE. The relative importance of arterial remodeling compared with intimal hyperplasia in lumen renarrowing after balloon angioplasty. *Circulation.* 1994;89:2816.
15. Anderson HR, Maeng M, Thorwest M, Falk E. Remodeling rather than neointimal formation explains luminal narrowing after deep vessel wall injury. *Circulation.* 1996;93:1716.
16. Murphy JG, Schwartz RS, Edwards WD, Camrud AR, Vlietstra RE, Holmes DRJ. Percutaneous polymeric stents in porcine coronary arteries. *Circulation.* 1992;86:1596.
17. Holmes DR, Camrud AR, Jorgenson MA, Edwards WD, Schwartz RS. Polymeric stenting in the porcine coronary artery model: differential outcome of exogenous fibrin sleeves versus poyurethane-coated stents. *J Am Coll Cardiol.* 1994;24:525.
18. van der Giessen WJ, Lincoff M, Schwartz RS, et al. Marked inflammatory sequelae to implantation of biodegradable and nonbiodegradable polymers in porcine coronary arteries. *Circulation.* 1996;94:1690.
19. Yamawaki T, Shimokawa H, Kozai T, et al. Intramural delivery of a specific tyrosine kinase inhibitor with biodegradable stent suppresses the restenotic changes of the coronary artery in pigs in vivo. *J Am Coll Cardiol.* 1998;32:780.

CHAPTER (11)

Adjunctive Devices: Atherectomy, Thrombectomy, Embolic Protection, IVUS, Doppler and Pressure Wires

Laura Mauri, MD, and Scott Kinlay, PhD

Rapidly advancing technology has led to an explosion in the number of devices available in the cardiac catheterization laboratory beyond balloons and stents. Remaining current with both the procedural technique required for each new device as well as the evidence base for their use requires dedication to both. In this chapter we review the principles of use of several adjunctive devices that are available in current practice, several of which have been shown to decrease adverse events significantly during percutaneous intervention.

INTERVENTIONAL DEVICES

【 】 ATHERECTOMY DEVICES

Rotational Atherectomy

Rotational atherectomy (Boston Scientific, Natick, MA, USA) was developed as a method to diminish plaque volume by abrasion, as opposed to fracturing plaque radially.[1] Rotational atherectomy has proved to be particularly useful in the treatment of calcified lesions.[2,3]

The rotational atherectomy system consists of four main components: guidewire, advancer, diamond-coated burr catheter, and control console system. Performance of rotational atherectomy requires a 0.009-in. wire, available in either a floppy version with a long, tapered shaft or an extra support version. The advancer supports the air turbine that drives rotation and contains the advancer knob that allows independent control of burr movement along the guide wire. Burrs are available from 1.25 mm to 2.50 mm in diameter, the 1.25-mm and 1.5-mm burrs fitting in a large-lumen 6-Fr guide.

Most rotational atherectomy is currently performed as an adjunct to either angioplasty or stenting in order to either debulk (bifurcation lesions)[4] or modify plaque (resistant or calcified lesions)[2] in stenotic native coronary arteries. In the era of stenting, rotational atherectomy, by modifying plaque morphology, may facilitate full-stent expansion in resistant lesions, or stent delivery across calcified segments (Figure 11-1). Attempts to translate the different mechanism of action of rotational atherectomy to lower restenosis rates, however, have been unsuccessful in large randomized trials, as the main determinant of restenosis risk, postprocedure minimum lumen diameter, is not different than with angioplasty.[5,6] More aggressive burr-sizing strategies (burr-to-artery ratios of >0.7) do not appear to overcome this limitation.[7,8]

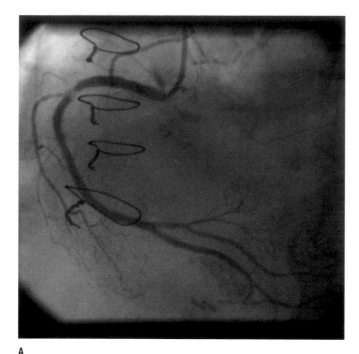
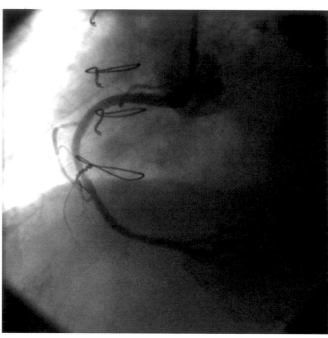

A   B

FIGURE 11-1. A 75-year-old woman on chronic hemodialysis with serial calcified stenoses of the ostial and proximal right coronary artery (RCA) (**A**). This patient was treated successfully with rotational atherectomy (1.5-mm burr over extra support Rota wire) followed by drug-eluting stent placement (**B**).

Several potential risks of rotational atherectomy can be minimized by judicious technique. First, a stepped-burr approach of increasing burr sizes by no more than 0.5 mm at a time to a maximum burr to artery ratio of 0.7 is recommended. Larger burr-to-artery ratios may be associated with higher rates of no-reflow phenomenon and higher periprocedural cardiac enzyme release. During rotational atherectomy, the revolutions per minute (rpm) should be monitored closely (recommended platform speeds of 160,000–180,000 rpm for 15–45 s) in order to avoid decelerations of more than 5000 rpm. Large decelerations associated with heat generation from undue resistance to burr passage should be avoided by releasing forward pressure on the burr when they occur, and considering use of a smaller-size burr.

Transient bradycardia may occur, particularly during rotational atherectomy of the right coronary artery; therefore, venous access to allow transvenous pacing is recommended for right coronary artery procedures.

Wire bias is a phenomenon observed when rotational atherectomy is performed in tortuous vessels, in which the wire and burr tend to have greater force at the inner curvature of a lesion.[9] This may be of benefit if the lesion is located eccentrically in this inner curvature. However, wire bias can also predispose to dissection or perforation. Use of the extra support wire enhances the effect of wire bias. Myocardial depression may occur with rotational atherectomy, and for this reason its use for "last remaining vessel" cases is not generally recommended, and if necessary, ventricular support is recommended (Figure 11-2). Finally, although rotational atherectomy can be helpful in treating stent restenosis, if rotational atherectomy into a jailed side branch is considered, it is important to confirm that this side branch has been balloon

dilated after stenting to avoid entrapment as only the distal half of the burr is diamond coated.

Directional Coronary Atherectomy

Directional coronary atherectomy (DCA), in contrast to angioplasty, which displaces plaque radially and longitudinally, is a method to excise atheroma. By physically removing atheroma from the coronary lumen, it was hoped that it would achieve larger postprocedure lumen diameters and result in lower restenosis rates. However, with the common application of stenting that achieves minimal residual stenosis in the majority of lesions, directional atherectomy is now most frequently used in settings where debulking would be anticipated to lessen the adverse effect of plaque shift, such as ostial left anterior descending (LAD) artery or bifurcation lesions.[10] Occasionally directional atherectomy may be useful when a pathologic sample of the atheroma is of interest.[11]

Directional coronary atherectomy can be performed in native coronary arteries or vein grafts, and should be restricted to non-calcified lesions.

Several atherectomy devices exist; the Flexi-cut device (Guidant Corporation, Santa Clara, CA, USA) is approved by the US Food and Drug Administration (FDA) for use in native coronary artery interventions and is available in 2.5–2.9-mm, 3.0–3.4-mm, and 3.5–3.9-mm sizes, compatible with a minimum guide internal diameter of 0.087 in. Guide choice is important; a gentle curve and adequate support facilitate delivery of the nose cone. The Flexi-cut wire is a 0.014-in. polytetrafluoroethylene (polytef, PTFE)-coated wire. The atherectomy device consists of the balloon catheter for vessel apposition, the cutter in its housing unit,

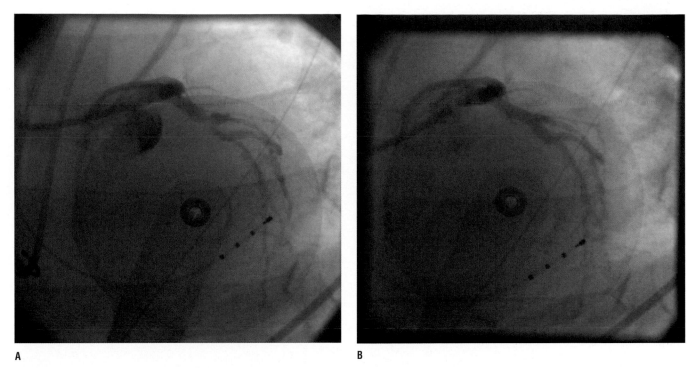

A   **B**

FIGURE 11-2. A 67-year-old man with severely reduced systolic function and persistent ischemia and cardiogenic shock after recent primary angioplasty for anterior myocardial infarction despite intraaortic balloon pump placement. The RCA was occluded ostially, and the LCX subtotally occluded and calcified (**A**). Successful rotational atherectomy and stenting of the LCX was performed while using femorofemoral bypass support in the cardiac catheterization laboratory (**B**).

and the attached motor-drive unit. After accessing the lesion with the Flexi-cut wire, the atherectomy catheter and motor-drive unit are advanced as a unit, with the cutter in the forward position. Coaxial guide engagement is important. Gradual rotation of the catheter facilitates advancement into the coronary lesion. At the lesion, the cutter track is visible as a concave shadow and can be directed to bulkiest part of the plaque. The balloon is inflated to 5 psi, the motor-drive unit turned on, the cutter retracted, the pressure increased to 10–50 psi, and the cutter advanced. Care should be taken that the cutter is fully advanced and remains advanced any time the balloon is not inflated. Next, the motor-drive unit is turned off, the balloon is deflated, and the unit may be redirected and the sequence repeated. For a concentric lesion, our usual approach is to perform four cuts at 90° separation before removing the catheter to assess the result. The excised plaque can be retrieved from the removed catheter by flushing the nose cone. If the goal lumen diameter is not achieved (<15% residual stenosis), repeat cuts may be performed at gradually increasing inflation pressures (eg, by 5 psi increments, up to a maximum of 50 psi).

Directional coronary atherectomy can be useful in ostial (Figure 11-3) or bifurcation *de novo* or restenotic lesions. As a general approach, however, in spite of promising trials in which optimal DCA was performed by experienced operators, multicenter randomized controlled trials comparing DCA with angioplasty[12,13] and with stenting[14] have failed to show lower restenosis rates.

Potential pitfalls for DCA include the incidence of creatine kinase elevation, perforation, and distal embolization. DCA should be avoided in calcified lesions, tortuous vessels, distal- or small-vessel (<2.5 mm) lesions, and degenerated saphenous vein grafts.

Thrombectomy

Visualization of thrombus by angiography is associated with increased rates of distal embolization and no-reflow phenomenon. Rheolytic thrombectomy with the AngioJet catheter (Possis Medical, Inc., Minneapolis, MN, USA) uses high-velocity saline jets to produce a vacuum for thrombus aspiration. This strategy has been useful to decrease thrombus burden during percutaneous interventions in both native coronary arteries and vein grafts.[15,16] A large randomized trial (AiMI), however, failed to demonstrate that the routine use of thrombectomy during primary angioplasty has a beneficial effect on infarct size.[17]

The AngioJet device consists of a tapered stainless-steel catheter attached to a driving unit, with a piston pump generating high-pressure pulsed flow. Three saline jets at the distal catheter tip are directed retrograde, creating a vacuum effect for thrombus aspiration. This device is compatible with 6-Fr guide catheters and is available in over-the-wire and monorail systems.

After crossing the thrombotic area with a standard 0.014-in. angioplasty wire, the AngioJet catheter is advanced distal to the thrombus. The pump unit is activated, and the catheter is withdrawn over the wire at a rate of 0.5 mm/s. Repeat passes can be performed until there is no further change in the visualized thrombus. Because most thrombotically occluded vessels are the result of acute plaque rupture, thrombectomy is generally followed by angioplasty and coronary stenting.

Bradyarrythmias are common, and prophylactic placement of a temporary pacing wire is helpful, particularly when the treatment location is a dominant right coronary artery. Other potential complications include no-reflow phenomenon, distal embolization,

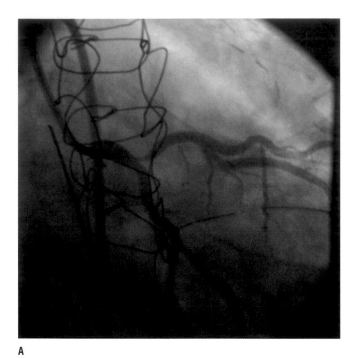

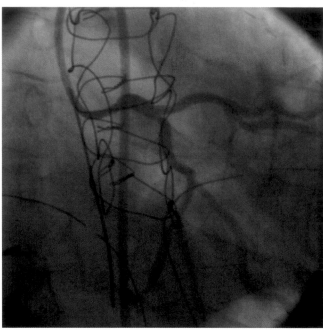

A   B

FIGURE 11-3. A 43-year-old man with ostial left anterior descending (LAD) artery stenosis initially referred for coronary artery bypass graft (CABG). The patient developed chest pain and ST elevation 1 day postoperatively. Emergency cardiac catheterization showed the distal LIMA anastomosis to be occluded (**A**). Successful directional coronary atherectomy of the ostial LAD stenosis was performed using the 3.5 mm–3.9 mm FlexiCut device at up to 20-psi balloon inflation pressure (**B**).

and perforation. The use of AngioJet in vessels less than 2-mm in diameter is not recommended.

The combination of the use of the AngioJet with embolic protection devices has been reported in small series, but has not yet been evaluated in larger trials.

【 】 EMBOLIC PROTECTION

Saphenous vein graft interventions are plagued by high rates of acute major adverse cardiac events (MACE), particularly as a result of distal embolization of degenerated vein graft material and its complications.[18,19] The FDA approval of the first embolic protection device was based on reduction in MACE rates by 42% in a large randomized trial using the GuardWire device (Medtronic Vascular, Minneapolis, MN, USA).[20] Subsequent generations of devices have attempted to achieve the same benefit with various technical designs. The FilterWire EX Randomized Evaluation (FIRE) trial demonstrated the FilterWire device (Boston Scientific-EPI, Santa Clara, CA, USA) to be noninferior to the GuardWire in the treatment of saphenous vein graft stenoses.[21]

Balloon-Type Occlusion Device

The GuardWire device is a 0.014-in. hollow-core wire with a fixed compliant balloon at the distal end, used to occlude flow in vessels 3-mm -to 6-mm in diameter. After dilation and stenting are performed, an Export catheter is used to aspirate particulate matter from the vessel before perfusion is reestablished. Multiple sequences of occlusion and aspiration may be performed if more than one dilation is required.

In the saphenous vein graft angioplasty free of emboli randomized (SAFER) trial, GuardWire use was associated with a decrease in MACE from 15% to 9%.[20] Although across all risk groups patients benefited from distal embolic protection, the risk of MACE was shown to correlate with the burden of saphenous vein graft disease, as measured by estimated plaque volume.[22] There was no additional beneficial effect of glycoprotein IIbIIIa inhibitor use in this setting. Aorto-ostial lesions were excluded from the SAFER trial because of the theoretic possibility of aortic embolization of debris.

Another distal balloon-type occlusion device has since been FDA-approved for use in saphenous vein grafts: the Triactiv system (Kensey Nash, Exton, Pennsylvania) based on the results of the PRIDE (Protection During Saphenous Vein Graft Intervention to Prevent Distal Embolization) Trial.[22a]

Filter Type

The FilterWire (Boston Scientific/EPI, Boston, MA, USA) consists of a 0.014-in. guidewire with a distal loop to which a long polyurethane bag with 110 micron pores is attached, designed to capture debris in vessel diameters of 3.5 mm to 5.5 mm. A 6-Fr compatible delivery–retrieval sheath is used to collapse the filter during delivery and retrieval after stenting. The filter design allows continued perfusion and visualization during the stenting procedure. When it is not possible to cross the lesion primarily, a buddy-wire technique is often helpful (Figure 11-4). In the FIRE trial, the FilterWire was shown to be noninferior to the GuardWire distal protection device in the treatment of saphenous vein graft stenoses, with major adverse cardiac event rates of 9.9% and 11.6%, respectively.[21]

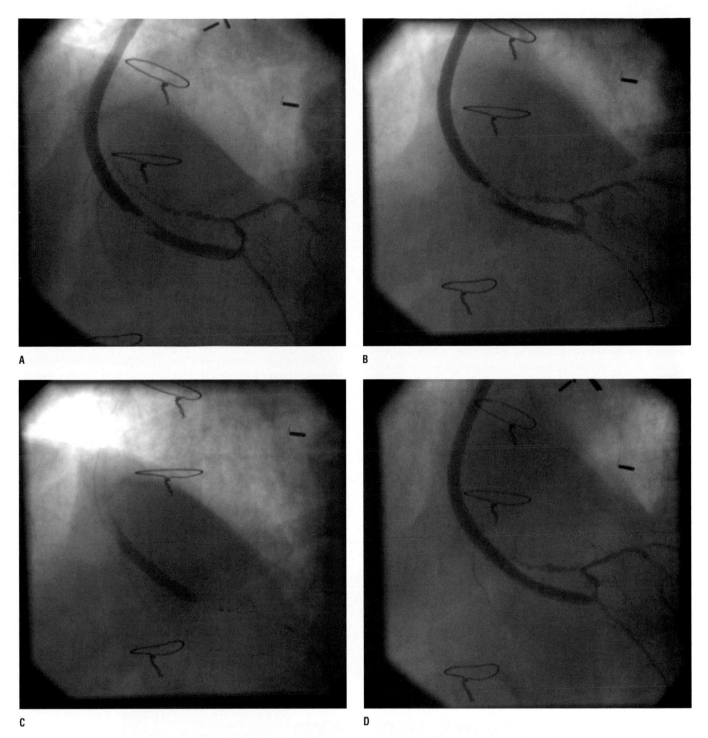

FIGURE 11-4. A 71-year-old who had had CABG performed 15 years prior and presented with a non-ST elevation myocardial infarction. A saphenous vein graft (SVG) to an occluded RCA had a high-grade, bulky, eccentric stenosis (**A**). The lesion was crossed with a Balanced Middle Weight wire, used as a buddy wire to deliver the FilterWire (**B**, **C**). Successful stenting of the vein graft was performed, with subsequent removal of atheromatous debris (**D**).

Several newer-generation filter devices are under evaluation, including the Interceptor (Medtronic Vascular, Minneapolis, MN, USA), with size ranges allowing treatment of both larger- and smaller-caliber vessels.[23] Interestingly, comparison of particulate retrieved with occlusive balloons or filters has shown that in saphenous vein graft (SVG) settings, the volume and size-range of particulate retrieved is roughly equivalent.[24,25]

The SAFER trial established embolic protection as the standard of care in SVG intervention. The fact that additional MACE persists (9%), even with the use of embolic protection, and the inability to use these devices when certain anatomic features are present (ostial lesions for GuardWire, <20-mm landing zone for FilterWire) are incentives to continue to develop improved and complementary devices for these high-risk lesions. It has been postulated that some distal embolization may occur during the first cross of the wire. A third variation on the embolic protection devices, proximal occlusion devices, may have an advantage in this regard (Proxis, Velocimed, Minneapolis, MN,

USA). This type of device also allows protection of multiple branches downstream of the treated lesion, rather than the single branch in which a distal protection device (balloon or filter) would be placed. This device consists of a 6-Fr balloon-tipped catheter advanced through a conventional 7-Fr or 8-Fr guide to a point proximal within the target vessel. After Proxis balloon-inflation interrupts distal flow, guidewires, balloon, and stents are used. Blood and embolic debris can be evacuated from the distal vascular bed by aspirating and reversing flow through the guiding catheter. This approach may permit protection of side branches proximal and distal to the lesion. The pivotal randomized trial, Proximal Protection During Saphenous Vein Graft Intervention Using the Proxis Embolic Protection System (PROXIS), demonstrated noninferiority in comparison to FDA-approved embolic protection devices.[26]

Uses of Embolic Protection Under Investigation

Acute Myocardial Infarction in Native Coronary Arteries.
Because distal embolization is also a challenging problem during stenting for acute myocardial infarction (MI), there is a potential benefit to the use of embolic protection devices in this setting. Although a nonrandomized study of FilterWire use in acute MI was promising in its demonstration of improvements in late left ventricular function compared to matched controls,[27] a randomized controlled trial using the GuardWire system in acute MI was disappointing, with no change in measures of infarct size.[28]

Non-Coronary Artery Stenting.
The use of embolic protection in stenting of carotid or vertebral arteries is a logical extension, where their use could diminish the risk of periprocedural stroke. The Accunet (Guidant, Santa Clara, CA, USA) and the Emboshield (Abbott Mednova, Abbott Park, IL, USA) devices are approved by the FDA in the setting of carotid artery stenting based on results of the ARCHER (Acculink for revascularization of carotids in high risk patients)[29] and SECURITY (Registry Study to Evaluate the Neuroshield Bare Wire Cerebral Protection System) trials.[29a] The Angioguard (Cordis, Miami Lakes, FL, USA) is another filter device designed for carotid artery stenting (expandable to 4-mm to 8-mm in diameter on an 0.014-in. guidewire). Studied in the recent SAPPHIRE (stenting and angioplasty with protection in patients at high risk for enderectomy) trial, carotid artery stenting with the Angioguard for embolic protection was demonstrated to be noninferior to carotid endarterectomy in high-risk patients.[30]

ADJUNCTIVE DIAGNOSTIC TOOLS

【 】 INTRAVASCULAR ULTRASOUND

Intravascular ultrasound (IVUS) is used primarily for intravascular imaging of the coronary arteries. However, new applications for this technology include imaging of peripheral arteries and structures within the heart chambers, particularly during electrophysiology studies.

Intravascular ultrasound uses catheters to obtain a cross-sectional or tomographic view of arterial and other structures (Figure 11-5).[31] The images are obtained by the catheters emitting and receiving ultrasound perpendicular to the long axis of the catheter.

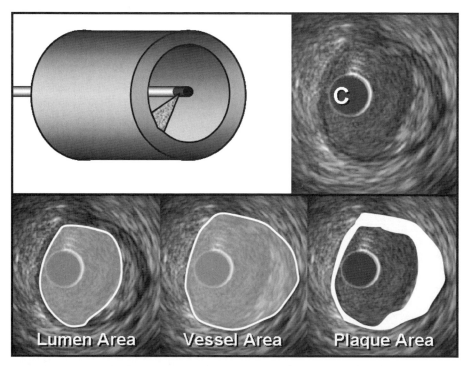

FIGURE 11-5. Intravascular ultrasound (IVUS) uses ultrasound to provide cross-sectional images of the artery that can be divided into lumen area, vessel area, and plaque area. C is the IVUS catheter. *(Reproduced with permission from Kinlay S. What has intravascular ultrasound taught us about plaque biology? Curr Atheroscler Rep. 2001;3:260.)*

IVUS offers real-time two-dimensional imaging that can provide a "third plane" perpendicular to the two-dimensional images obtained from angiography. Offline analysis can also provide three-dimensional rendering of the structures interrogated by a pullback through structures. Cross-sectional images of arteries can provide diagnostic information that guides the need and success of percutaneous interventions. IVUS is also used to identify the structures within the heart chambers, including the coronary sinus, and the atrial septum, which can assist catheter placement in electrophysiologic studies and percutaneous valvotomy.

There are two basic designs that permit image acquisition by this technique. These include the mechanically rotating single ultrasound crystal or sequential "firing" from multiple crystals arranged around the distal end of the catheter (Figure 11-6). Both designs rely on a guidewire for the safe delivery of the catheter into the artery or structure that is being imaged. Successive iterations have lead to miniaturization of the catheters and improvements in software that permit greater spatial resolution.

For small arteries and structures that are close to the catheter, small catheters approximately 1 mm in diameter are used (<3-Fr) and are compatible with 6-Fr guiding catheters. These catheters use high-frequency ultrasound that offers improved spatial resolution, but at a cost of less depth penetration. In larger arteries or the heart chambers, structures of interest may be of relatively greater distance from the catheter, and lower-frequency ultrasound is often used to obtain the necessary penetration to see distant structures. IVUS catheters for imaging larger structures such as the aorta use smaller frequencies and require 8-Fr or 9-Fr sheaths.

The catheters are connected to computer platforms that contain software and a user interface to adjust the imaging characteristics and allow measurement of pertinent structures. The platforms permit entry of patient details next to the images and allow the image runs to be recorded for later review.

Both catheter designs require connection of the catheter to an interface unit that may be coupled with a mechanical pullback sled. These sleds pull the catheter through the artery at a constant speed (usually 0.5 mm/s or 1.0 mm/s) and can be used to estimate the length of a lesion as well as permit a more accurate three-dimensional rendering of the region of interest.

The two main catheter designs have their pros and cons, although the potential differences in image quality of each design are decreasing with improvements in hardware and software. Both designs have artifacts very close to the catheter called *ring-down effect*, which consists of small rings or blossoming of the ultrasound (white appearance) around the central black catheter artifact. Ring down can interfere with near-field imaging (images close to the ultrasound crystal) and tends to be more noticeable with the nonmechanical multiple crystal catheters, especially if the catheter rests against the artery wall. This is partly because the mechanical catheters have an outer sheath that keeps the crystal away from the artery wall. The nonmechanical catheters use software to subtract the ring down digitally to reduce this artifact, and more recent advances in software and catheter design have improved near-field imaging. Nonuniform rotation deformity is another artifact specific to mechanical catheters. If the inner core of a mechanical catheter spins unevenly in the shaft (eg, in tortuous arteries), a nonuniform rotation deformity (NURD) of the image can occur. As the catheter speeds up and slows down as a result of uneven spinning, the IVUS image appears smeared in sectors where the catheter rotation is faster, and appears compressed in those sectors where the catheter spin is slower. Improvements in the design of the mechanical catheters have reduced the NURD compared to older catheter designs.

All catheters can give misleading or distorted images if the catheter is not coaxial to the long axis of the artery (eg, on bends where oval images can occur), or show equally spaced rings because of heavy calcification. The longitudinal reconstructions artificially straighten out curved arteries, may have a saw-tooth appearance with fluttering of the catheter (particularly over the cardiac cycle), and may give misleading length measurements if the pullback speed varies.

【 】 BOSTON SCIENTIFIC MECHANICALLY ROTATING INTRAVENOUS ULTRASOUND CATHETER

Boston Scientific has two IVUS catheters approved by the FDA for human use. These include the 2.6-Fr Atlantis catheter, primarily used for coronary and other small artery imaging, and a larger Atlantis PV peripheral imaging catheter for imaging larger peripheral arteries and other cardiac structures. Both catheters use a single rotating crystal to emit and receive ultrasound.

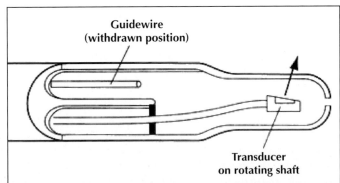
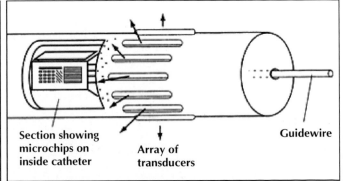

FIGURE 11-6. Current IVUS catheters use a mechanically rotating ultrasound crystal (**A**) or an array of ultrasound crystals around the catheter (**B**). *(Adapted from Atlas of Cardiac Imaging, by RT Lee and E Braunwald, eds, Current Medicine, Philadelphia, 1998, p. 6.1.)*

The catheter contains two key parts—an outer sheath, and an inner core that contains the ultrasound crystal at its tip (Figure 11-6). The inner core rotates within the outer sheath by a motor-drive unit between the catheter and the user interface or platform. The inner core rotates at approximately 30 rpm, providing images up to 30 frames per second.

The outer sheath protects the artery from the rotating inner core and is flushed by saline to allow the transmission of ultrasound between the crystal and the sheath. Any air between the inner core and the sheath dramatically reduces ultrasound transmission and image quality.

The 6-Fr compatible catheter has a short monorail design, allowing the tip of the catheter to be introduced over a 0.014-in. guidewire into the artery. The 8-Fr compatible peripheral catheter is introduced over a 0.035-in. guidewire. The proximal end of the catheter is attached to the motor-drive unit, which may be mounted on a disposable pullback sled for mechanical pullback of the artery once it is placed distal to the region of interest. The motor-drive unit is attached to a cable that inserts into the user interface of a platform that contains controls to adjust the image quality and to start and stop the rotation of the inner core of the catheter.

The most important part of preparing the 6-Fr Atlantis catheter for use is flushing the outer sheath with saline. A 10-mL syringe of saline is connected via a three-way stopcock to a smaller 2-mL flushing syringe and attached to the proximal hub of the outer sheath. The 10-mL syringe is used as a flush reservoir to fill the 2-mL syringe, and the 2-mL syringe is used to flush space between the outer sheath and the inner core to eliminate air. This is important, because air transmits ultrasound poorly and must be removed to improve image quality. A good flush is also required because any air left in the catheter could embolize into the artery and impair coronary blood flow. A pulsing flush is often used, and usually between 6 mL and 10 mL of saline is required to flush the catheter fully. The proximal hub of the catheter is connected to the motor drive, and the distal end is threaded onto a guidewire that is directed into the artery via a guiding catheter.

Using standard interventional cardiology practice, the patient is anticoagulated to prevent thrombus formation on the guidewire or ultrasound catheter. Once the IVUS catheter is placed distal to the artery of interest, the catheter is activated to start the inner core rotating and ultrasound imaging. This may be started from the motor drive or the user interface/platform.

The motorized pullback sled is a disposable device that interacts with the motor drive. An assistant hands the operator a sterile plastic bag, and the motor drive is placed into the bag to allow the operator to manipulate it and maintain sterility. The bagged motor drive with the IVUS catheter is clipped into the sled, and a digital readout on the motor drive is set to zero. Catheter imaging begins, and the mechanical pullback is started by pressing a specific button on the motor drive. The sled pullback speed can be set to 0.5 mm or 1.0 mm per second.

( ) BOSTON SCIENTIFIC USER INTERFACE (GALAXY PLATFORM)

The Boston Scientific user Galaxy interface (Figure 11-7) is relatively new, and a substantial improvement on the older Clearview interface. The Galaxy interface has controls to adjust image size, contrast, and brightness, as well as controls to start and stop imaging and recording. The Galaxy stores image runs digitally in a proprietary DICOM format on to one of two linked hard drives that can store up to 8 hours of imaging. The runs can also be recorded on VHS videotape. Digitally stored studies can be archived to CD or DVD, or directly via an Ethernet connection to another source, such as a hospital archive.

The Galaxy interface also allows previously recorded runs to be reviewed and structures on images to be measured. This includes linear measurements and area measurements from user-defined distances and areas, as well as computer-assisted area measurements (curvilinear areas defined by dots marked on the image by the user). Relative area and diameter stenoses from two different measurements are also calculated automatically. A longitudinal pullback reconstruction of the artery is also available by assembling adjacent IVUS images and slicing them along the longitudinal axis of the artery. If used with the mechanical pullback device, this can give accurate measurements of the length of an arterial lesion.

The Galaxy interface recognizes the different Boston Scientific IVUS catheters automatically when they are inserted into the motor-drive unit, and adjusts the scale used for measurements for each catheter.

( ) VOLCANO THERAPEUTICS INTRAVENOUS ULTRASOUND CATHETER

Volcano Therapeutics (Rancho Cardovo, CA, USA) is a relatively new device company that bought the Jomed IVUS catheter technology and Pressure and Flow wire technologies (in turn bought from Endosonics, Inc.). Volcano has three IVUS catheters, a 2.9-Fr coronary catheter a 3.4-Fr peripheral catheter, and an 8.2-Fr peripheral artery catheter. All catheters are nonmechanical and have an array of ultrasound crystals around the distal end of the catheter that are used to generate a two-dimensional IVUS image. As there are no moving parts, there is no image distortion as a result of nonuniform rotational deformation.

The Volcano Eagle Eye catheter replaces the Avanar IVUS catheter but shares many similar features. It is a 2.9-Fr nonmechanical design consisting of a long monorail catheter with 64 ultrasound crystals arranged radially around the tip of the catheter. The 64 crystals are "fired" off sequentially to obtain a "rotating" ultrasound signal, and several crystals are used to interrogate the returning ultrasound signals to create a tomographic image. The nominal frequency of the ultrasound is a mean 20 MHz, but the returning ultrasound is integrated by several crystals to offer a spatial resolution that is better than 20-MHz single crystal technology. Although the catheter offers a slightly lower spatial resolution compared to the higher-resolution 40-MHz catheters, this is offset by the greater penetration, allowing this catheter to be used in many peripheral applications. The Eagle Eye has improved near-field imaging compared to the Avanar catheter.

The Eagle Eye can be used for many peripheral artery applications. However, for large arteries, the 3.4-Fr catheter (0.018-in. guidewire) can be used. Greater depth and field of vision can be obtained with the Visions PV catheter, which is compatible with up to a 0.038-in. guidewire and requires a 9-Fr introducer. It uses an over-the-wire technology that allows flushing from a proximal guidewire port.

As there are no moving parts to this catheter, there is no need for an outer sheath and no regions where air may be trapped. The proximal end of the catheter is flushed with saline from a syringe before mounting onto a guidewire placed in the artery that is to be imaged. The distal end is connected to a patient interface unit that is attached to the user interface.

Using standard interventional cardiology practice, the patient is anticoagulated to prevent thrombus formation on the guidewire or ultrasound catheter. The Volcano IVUS catheter has a more noticeable ring-down, partly because of the lack of an outer sheath. However, the ring-down can be subtracted digitally once the IVUS tip is outside the guiding catheter in a large structure, such as a large left main artery or the aorta, using the following approach. The IVUS catheter is placed at the tip of the guiding catheter and ultrasound imaging is started from the user interface/platform. The ring-down subtraction is performed by pressing a button on the user interface, and once satisfactory, imaging of the artery or region of interest can commence.

The motorized pullback device is disposable and sterile and fits around the IVUS catheter near the O-ring that attaches to the guiding catheter. There is no need to place a sterile plastic bag around the catheter. The mechanical pullback is started by pressing a button on the pullback device. The sled pullback speed can be set to 0.5 mm or 1.0 mm per second. A longitudinal pullback reconstruction of the artery is also available, by assembling adjacent IVUS images and slicing them along the longitudinal axis of the artery. If used with the mechanical pullback device, this can give accurate measurements of the length of an arterial lesion.

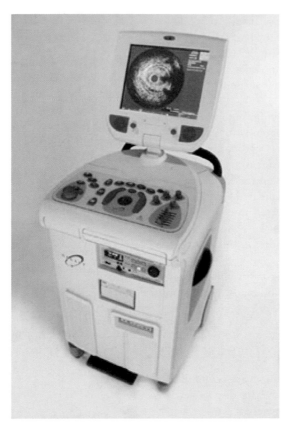 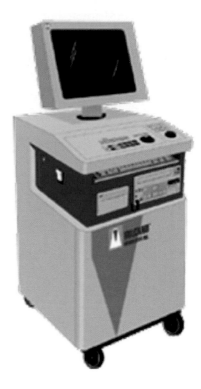

FIGURE 11-7. (**A**) Galaxy IVUS Interface produced by Boston Scientific. (**B**) In-Vision Gold Interface produced by Volcano Therapeutics.

【 】 VOLCANO THERAPEUTICS USER INTERFACE (IN-VISION GOLD PLATFORM)

The Volcano Therapeutics user interface contains an array of controls to regulate the image size, contrast, and brightness, as well as controls to start and stop imaging and recording (Figure 11-7). The Volcano Platform stores image runs digitally in a proprietary DICOM format. The runs can also be recorded on VHS videotape. Digitally stored studies can be archived to CD or directly via an Ethernet connection to another source, such as a hospital archive.

The Volcano user interface also includes an option to display blood flow as a red image overlying the two-dimensional IVUS image (ChromaFlo). The software identifies flowing blood by comparing adjacent IVUS frames to find differences in the position of echogenic blood particles. This can be used to help delineate blood—tissue borders, for example, small dissections.

More recently, Volcano acquired software that uses the raw radiofrequency signal from ultrasound to define different tissue characteristics in the artery wall. Using ex-vivo models, differences in the amplitude and frequency shifts of reflected ultrasound have been related to fibrous, calcified, and lipid-rich regions within plaques.[32] These plaque components are colorized and displayed adjacent to an IVUS gray-scale image. This technology may be useful in identifying structures that are related to plaque vulnerability, in addition to area measurements of lumen narrowing and plaque area.

The Volcano interface also allows previously recorded runs to be reviewed and structures on images to be measured. This includes linear and area measurements from user-defined distances and areas, as well as computer-assisted areas (curvilinear areas defined by dots marked on the image by the user). Area and diameter stenoses from two different measurements are also calculated automatically. A longitudinal pullback reconstruction of the artery is also available by assembling adjacent IVUS images and slicing them along the longitudinal axis of the artery. If used with the mechanical pullback device, this can give accurate measurements of the length of an arterial lesion.

【 】 INDICATIONS AND EVIDENCE FOR USE OF INTRAVENOUS ULTRASOUND

IVUS is indicated primarily where there is angiographic doubt about the details of a case. This may be doubt about the severity or cause of a lesion on angiography, or doubt about the success of an intervention.

Compared to ex-vivo samples and models of known dimensions, IVUS provides reliable information on linear and area dimensions.[33,34] IVUS is able to give only crude information on plaque structure. Specifically, it is able to distinguish calcified from noncalcified tissue, but other tissue characteristics (lipid and fibrous tissue) are poorly distinguished.[35,36] Calcium reflects virtually all ultrasound so that it demonstrates a characteristically bright echogenic signal with a dark acoustic shadow on the far side.

IVUS is particularly useful for identifying important vascular abnormalities, particularly when angiography is unclear. For example, in cases where a narrowing in a coronary artery is of dubious significance, a lumen cross-sectional area of less than 4 mm^2 is indicative of a significant flow-limiting lesion that may cause angina.[37] Although not as well validated, the equivalent cutoff for a left main lesion is probably <5 mm to 7 mm.[38,39] IVUS can also distinguish if the causes of hazy areas on angiography may be because of stenosis, dissection, thrombus, or eccentric calcium.[40]

IVUS is also useful after percutaneous interventions where it may identify poorly expanded stents or unopposed stent struts, which may predispose to stent thrombosis or restenosis.[41,42]

【 】 PITFALLS OF INTRAVENOUS ULTRASOUND

The main pitfalls of intravenous ultrasound are economic and concern costs as a result of the time and extra disposable costs. IVUS can add 10–20 minutes to the catheterization, but is justified if it answers uncertainties raised by angiography. Each IVUS catheter is designed for a single use at a cost of approximately US$600–$700 each. The disposable pullback devices and equipment are an extra US$50–$100 each.

The risks of IVUS are very small. Older catheter designs that were larger and stiffer were associated with arterial damage, such as dissection or perforation, in less than 1% of cases.[43] However, serious complications are likely to be substantially fewer with the current equipment. The most important guideline to prevent arterial damage is to avoid pushing excessively on the IVUS catheter. If the catheter does not track easily into an artery or around a lesion, then it is prudent to avoid forcing the catheter.

PRESSURE WIRE

Pressure-wire technology uses a small pressure-detecting device incorporated into the distal end of a 0.014-in. guidewire. This tool is well validated in the coronary artery bed for assessing the severity of coronary artery lesions.

The principle behind pressure-wire assessment is to compare the ratio of mean intraarterial pressure distal to a lesion to that proximal to the lesion (usually in the aorta from the guiding catheter) at maximum coronary blood flow induced by giving intracoronary or IV adenosine. This ratio is the fractional flow reserve (FFR), and in most patients is related to the ratio of myocardial blood flow at peak flow rates compared to myocardial flow if there were no coronary artery lesion. Lesions with an abnormal FFR (<0.75) are more likely to impair blood flow significantly at exercise and correlate with perfusion defects on noninvasive imaging.[44] In contrast, lesions with a normal FFR (>0.75) can have interventions safely deferred, as they are unlikely to lead to patients requiring revascularization in the next year or so.[45] The FFR can also be used to assess whether stents are adequately expanded. An FFR higher than 0.94 or greater suggests optimal stent expansion and a lower need for reintervention than does a lower FFR.[45]

【 】 RADI PRESSURE AND TEMPERATURE WIRE

The RADI Pressurewire has a small, pressure-sensing unit at the transition point of the 0.014-in. wire that gives a high-fidelity pressure signal more accurate than similar size fluid-filled catheters.

The RADI wire is advanced into an artery in the same fashion as an interventional guidewire. It is attached to a connector and user interface that is calibrated before introduction into the guide catheter, and gives a real-time graphic display of the pressure and automatic calculation of the FFR (Figure 11-8). The wire pressure is also transmitted to the catheterization laboratory pressure-monitor screens that display the guide pressure and ECG.

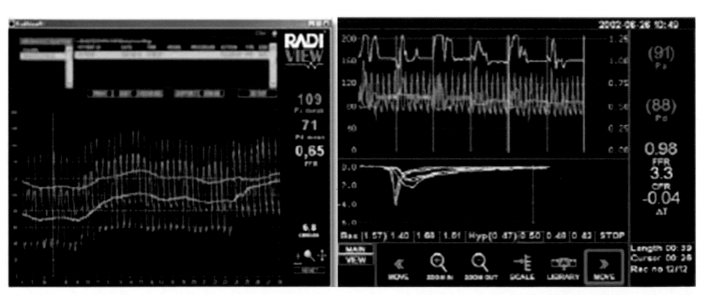

FIGURE 11-8. The RADI Pressure and Flow Recordings. **(A)** An abnormal pressure gradient with an FFR of 0.65. **(B)** Thermodilution curves yielding a CFR of 3.3 (the FFR is 0.98).

The user interface is connected to the pressure-monitoring system used in the cardiac catheterization laboratory. The pressures from the guiding catheter and the pressure wire are calibrated and zeroed. Using standard interventional cardiology practice, the patient is anticoagulated to prevent thrombus formation on the pressure wire. The wire is then advanced until the transition point of the wire (the pressure transducer) is just outside the guiding catheter. At this point, the guide pressure and the wire pressure are equalized to eliminate any differences as a result of variations in the height of the guide manifold transducer. The wire is advanced so that the transition point (and pressure transducer) is beyond the artery lesion.

The microvascular dilator adenosine is given by the intracoronary or intravenous route to induce maximal coronary blood flow. Generally, bolus doses of least 24 µg to −36 µg in the left coronary system and 18 µg to −24 µg in the right coronary artery are required to induce maximal coronary flow. Intravenous adenosine is used at 140 µg/kg/min and 180 µg/kg/min for 2 min each to achieve a similar affect.

Intracoronary adenosine tends to be asymptomatic, but lasts only 10–20 s and may lead to errors in calculating FFR if the mean guide pressure takes a longer time to stabilize after delivery. Intravenous adenosine leads to a more steady-state maximal blood flow, but may induce systemic hypotension and chest discomfort (not related to myocardial ischemia). The FFR is calculated at maximal blood flow by either technique.

[ ] VOLCANO THERAPEUTICS WAVE WIRE

The Volcano Therapeutics Pressure wire uses a pressure transducer at the transition point of a 0.014-in. guidewire. It is introduced into the coronary artery in the same fashion as an interventional guidewire, and the proximal end is connected to a user interface that gives a digital readout of the FFR and pressure. The wire pressure is transmitted to the catheterization laboratory pressure-monitor screens that also display the guide pressure and ECG.

A procedure similar to the RADI pressure wire is followed. The user interface is connected to the catheter laboratory pressure equipment, and the guide and wire pressures zeroed.

[ ] INDICATIONS AND EVIDENCE FOR USING THE PRESSURE WIRE AND FRACTIONAL FLOW RESERVE

The FFR is used when there is doubt about the angiographic interpretation of a suspicious lesion. The FFR uses guidewire technology familiar to the interventional cardiologist. The FFR cutpoints for defining a clinically significant lesion and optimal stent deployment are well defined,[44] and the number is easier to interpret than IVUS for those unfamiliar with IVUS images.

[ ] PITFALLS OF THE PRESSURE WIRE AND FRACTIONAL FLOW RESERVE

The pitfalls relate to the extra time and cost of this procedure, but like IVUS, they must be compared to the costs and risks of unnecessary interventions or delaying interventions.

Serial lesions are more difficult to interpret, although an abnormal FFR means that any or all lesions proximal to the pressure transducer are abnormal. In this situation, a pullback with the O-ring closed can identify regions that have abnormal FFR from proximal regions that are not significantly impaired.

It is also possible that complex or unstable lesions that may have a high likelihood of thrombotic occlusion will not be identified by FFR if they are not flow limiting. However, the angiographic appearance of ulceration or thrombus usually helps to distinguish these lesions.

The FFR may also be artificially high (false positive) in patients with high right-heart filling pressures (eg, heart failure) as this impairs myocardial perfusion and maximal flow rates. Similarly, arteries supplying infarcted areas will not dilate to adenosine and lead to higher FFR values. However, in this setting, revascularization is unlikely to reduce ischemic symptoms, which are probably caused by impaired flow to viable regions elsewhere.

CORONARY BLOOD FLOW

In the healthy state, coronary blood flow is regulated by myocardial oxygen demand that changes microvascular resistance and, to a lesser extent, by mean arterial pressure. The ability to augment coronary blood flow is regulated primarily by changes in microvascular resistance. However, in coronary artery disease, stenoses of the conduit coronary arteries impair the augmentation of coronary blood flow. Providing the coronary artery diameter remains the same, the ability to augment coronary blood flow velocity is also impaired by stenoses.

The ratio of maximal coronary blood flow or flow velocity induced by adenosine to basal resting coronary blood flow or velocity is called the *coronary flow reserve (CFR)*. The normal CFR is 2.0 or more. An abnormal CFR below 2.0 suggests a flow-limiting stenosis, and correlates with abnormalities on perfusion imaging, such as thallium.[46] However, less frequently, abnormalities in the coronary microcirculation may also impair CFR. Abnormalities in the microcirculation include myocardial infarction, microvascular angina, and other vasculopathies.

There are two methods used to commonly assess coronary blood flow. Although old techniques relied on coronary thermodilution catheters, these were relatively large and used mainly in the coronary sinus. For many years, the Volcano Therapeutics Doppler flow wire (FloWire) was the main method of assessing CFR. More recently, RADI have developed software that uses their Pressurewire to measure CFR by thermodilution. The Doppler technique gives instantaneous coronary flow velocity measurements, whereas the thermodilution method gives an average flow rate over several seconds.

[ ] RADI CORONARY BLOOD FLOW WIRE

The RADI wire is the same pressure wire described earlier. This wire has a high-fidelity distal sensor that measures pressure and temperature. The proximal shaft of the wire monitors temperature-dependent electric resistance and acts as a proximal thermistor. Additional software allows the FFR interface to measure temperature at both

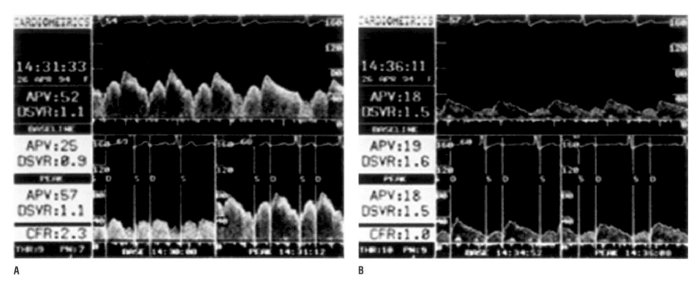

FIGURE 11-9. Recordings from the Volcano The therapeutics FloWire. (**A**) Instantaneous coronary flow velocity (top spectral display), baseline flow (bottom left) and normal hyperemic flow (bottom right) (CFR = 2.3). (**B**) No augmentation of flow with adenosine (bottom right) in an abnormal response (CFR =1.0).

sites on the wire and the time taken for a 3-mL bolus of room-temperature saline to run between the two sensors.

Coronary blood flow can then be calculated according to indicator dilution theory. CFR is determined by measuring coronary blood flow at hyperemia (induced by adenosine) compared to coronary blood flow at rest. Coronary blood flow is measured from 3–5 bolus injections of room-temperature saline (3-mL each bolus). The measurement is independent of the temperature of the saline bolus as long as it is cooler than blood. The thermodilution curves are displayed on the interface screen along with the CFR (Figure 11-9).

Maximal blood flow is induced with intracoronary or intravenous adenosine as described for FFR. Intravenous adenosine is probably easier to administer, as several estimations of coronary blood flow should be used to estimate CFR.

Thermodilution CFR is correlated with CFR obtained by Doppler wire technology.[47] Comparisons of CFR and severity of stenoses or clinical outcomes have mainly used CFR measured by the Doppler wire technique (see later).

[ ] VOLCANO THERAPEUTICS FLOWIRE

The Volcano FloWire is a 0.014-in. coronary guidewire with an ultrasound crystal at the tip of the guidewire. When introduced into an artery, ultrasound is emitted from the tip in a 45° arc and is reflected off moving blood cells. The velocity of the blood is calculated from the Doppler shift of the ultrasound from the moving blood cells. The output is a Doppler flow velocity pattern, which is an instantaneous readout of velocity (see Figure 11-9).

Using standard interventional cardiology practice, the patient is anticoagulated to prevent thrombus formation on the wire. The wire is introduced into the artery, and the user interface records average peak velocity (APV) and several other parameters from the tracings. Coronary blood flow can be calculated from APV and the cross-sectional area (usually estimated from the coronary diameter at the tip of the FloWire).

$$\text{Coronary blood flow} = \text{CSA} \times \text{APV}/2$$

Hyperemia is induced by intracoronary (or intravenous) adenosine. Assuming the cross-sectional area of the artery is unchanged, the CFR is the ratio of the APV at hyperemia versus the APV at rest.

CFR measured by Doppler is correlated with myocardial perfusion imaging[46,48,49] and with outcomes. In one study, patients with a CFR of more than 1.7 had a good outcome with deferred angioplasty[50]; however, a value greater than 2.0 is generally considered a normal response.

[ ] PITFALLS OF MEASURING CORONARY FLOW AND CORONARY FLOW RATE

Increased variability in the measurement of CFR measured by thermodilution may occur if the wire position is different in the resting and hyperemic states, adenosine leads to epicardial dilation (some advocate this test after giving intracoronary nitroglycerin), or if the sensor is placed within 6 cm of the guide tip. A distance of less than 6 cm may not allow adequate mixing of the indicator bolus with blood.

CFR measured by Doppler is dependent on the position of the Doppler wire, and can vary with changes in direction that do not capture the central stream of blood flow. This technique has improved by increasing the arc of ultrasound from earlier designs.

Because CFR also incorporates microvascular abnormalities, it is less specific for evaluating epicardial stenoses than is FFR.[51]

REFERENCES

1. O'Neill WW. Mechanical rotational atherectomy. *Am J Cardiol.* 1992;69:12F.
2. Ellis SG, Popma JJ, Buchbinder M, et al. Relation of clinical presentation, stenosis morphology, and operator technique to the procedural results of rotational atherectomy and rotational atherectomy-facilitated angioplasty. *Circulation.* 1994;89:882.

3. Teirstein PS, Warth DC, Haq N, et al. High speed rotational coronary atherectomy for patients with diffuse coronary artery disease. *J Am Coll Cardiol.* 1991;18:1694.

4. Dauerman HL, Higgins PJ, Sparano AM, et al. Mechanical debulking versus balloon angioplasty for the treatment of true bifurcation lesions. *J Am Coll Cardiol.* 1998;32:1845.

5. Dill T, Dietz U, Hamm CW, et al. A randomized comparison of balloon angioplasty versus rotational atherectomy in complex coronary lesions (COBRA study). *Eur Heart J.* 2000;21:1759.

6. Mauri L, Reisman M, Buchbinder M, et al. Comparison of rotational atherectomy with conventional balloon angioplasty in the prevention of restenosis of small coronary arteries: results of the Dilatation vs Ablation Revascularization Trial Targeting Restenosis (DART). *Am Heart J.* 2003;145:847.

7. Safian RD, Feldman T, Muller DW, et al. Coronary angioplasty and Rotablator atherectomy trial (CARAT): Immediate and late results of a prospective multicenter randomized trial. *Catheter Cardiovasc Interv.* 2001;53:213.

8. Whitlow PL, Bass TA, Kipperman RM, et al. Results of the study to determine rotablator and transluminal angioplasty strategy (STRATAS). *Am J Cardiol.* 2001;87:699.

9. Reisman M, Harms V. Guidewire bias: potential source of complications with rotational atherectomy. *Cathet Cardiovasc Diagn.* 1996;Suppl 3:64.

10. Airoldi F, Di Mario C, Stankovic G, et al. Clinical and angiographic outcome of directional atherectomy followed by stent implantation in de novo lesions located at the ostium of the left anterior descending coronary artery. *Heart.* 2003;89:1050.

11. Virmani R, Liistro F, Stankovic G, et al. Mechanism of late in-stent restenosis after implantation of a paclitaxel derivate-eluting polymer stent system in humans. *Circulation.* 2002;106:2649.

12. Baim DS, Cutlip DE, Sharma SK, et al. Final results of the Balloon vs Optimal Atherectomy Trial (BOAT). *Circulation.* 1998;97:322.

13. Baim DS, Cutlip D, Ho KK, Popma JJ, Senerchia C, Kuntz RE. Acute results of directional coronary atherectomy in the Balloon versus Optimal Atherectomy Trial (BOAT) pilot phase. *Coron Artery Dis.* 1996;7:290.

14. Stankovic G, Colombo A, Bersin R, et al. Comparison of directional coronary atherectomy and stenting versus stenting alone for the treatment of de novo and restenotic coronary artery narrowing. *Am J Cardiol.* 2004;93:953.

15. Kuntz RE, Baim DS, Cohen DJ, et al. A trial comparing rheolytic thrombectomy with intracoronary urokinase for coronary and vein graft thrombus (the Vein Graft AngioJet Study [VeGAS 2]). *Am J Cardiol.* 2002;89:326.

16. Rinfret S, Katsiyiannis PT, Ho KK, et al. Effectiveness of rheolytic coronary thrombectomy with the AngioJet catheter. *Am J Cardiol.* 2002;90:470.

17. Ali A. AIMI Trial. Presented at *Transcatheter Therapeutics.* Washington, DC: 2004.

18. Hong MK, Mehran R, Dangas G, et al. Creatine kinase—MB enzyme elevation following successful saphenous vein graft intervention is associated with late mortality. *Circulation.* 1999;100:2400.

19. Webb JG, Carere RG, Virmani R, et al. Retrieval and analysis of particulate debris after saphenous vein graft intervention. *J Am Coll Cardiol.* 1999;34:468.

20. Baim DS, Wahr D, George B, et al. Randomized trial of a distal embolic protection device during percutaneous intervention of saphenous vein aortocoronary bypass grafts. *Circulation.* 2002;105:1285.

21. Stone GW, Rogers C, Hermiller J, et al. Randomized comparison of distal protection with a filter-based catheter and a balloon occlusion and aspiration system during percutaneous intervention of diseased saphenous vein aortocoronary bypass grafts. *Circulation.* 2003;108:548.

22. Giugliano GR, Kuntz RE, Popma JJ, Cutlip DE, Baim DS. Determinants of 30-day adverse events following saphenous vein graft intervention with and without a distal occlusion embolic protection device. *Am J Cardiol.* 2005;95:173.

22a. Carrozza JJ, Mumma M, Breall J, Fernandez A, Heyman E, Metzger C. Randomized evaluation of the TriActiv balloon-protection flush and extraction system for the treatment of saphenous vein graft disease. *J Am Coll Cardiol.* 2005;46:1677.

23. Young JJ, Kereiakes DJ, Rabinowitz AC, Ammar R, Boucher FL, Rogers C. A novel, low-profile filter-wire (Interceptor) embolic protection device during saphenous vein graft stenting. *Am J Cardiol.* 2005;95:511.

24. Rogers C, Huynh R, Seifert PA, et al. Embolic protection with filtering or occlusion balloons during saphenous vein graft stenting retrieves identical volumes and sizes of particulate debris. *Circulation.* 2004;109:1735.

25. Quan V, Huynh R, Seifert PA, Chen WH, Sutsch G, Rogers C. Embolic protection devices: morphometric analysis of particulate debris extracted by four different embolic protection devices from coronary arteries, aortocoronary saphenous vein conduits, and carotid arteries. *Am J Cardiol.* 2005;95:1415.

26. Roger C. Proximal trial presentation. *Transcatheter. Therapeutics* Washington DC. 2005. abstract.

27. Limbruno U, Micheli A, De Carlo M, et al. Mechanical prevention of distal embolization during primary angioplasty: safety, feasibility, and impact on myocardial reperfusion. *Circulation.* 2003;108:171.

28. Stone GW, Webb J, Cox DA, et al. Distal microcirculatory protection during percutaneous coronary intervention in acute ST-segment elevation myocardial infarction: a randomized controlled trial. *JAMA.* 2005;293:1063.

29. Gray W. ARCHER Trials. Presented at the *American College of Cardiology.* New Orleans: 2004.

29a. Whitlow PL. Stenting and angioplasty with protection in patients at high risk for endarterectomy. Washington, DC: *Transcatheter Therapeutics* 2003, abstract.

30. Yadav JS, Wholey MH, Kuntz RE, et al. Protected carotid-artery stenting versus endarterectomy in high-risk patients. *N Engl J Med.* 2004;351:1493.

31. Kinlay S. What has intravascular ultrasound taught us about plaque biology? *Curr Atheroscler Rep.* 2001;3:260.

32. Nair A, Kuban BD, Tuzcu EM, Schoenhagen P, Nissen SE, Vince DG. Coronary plaque classification with intravascular ultrasound radiofrequency data analysis. *Circulation.* 2002;106:2200.

33. Nishimura RA, Edwards WD, Warnes CA, et al. Intravascular ultrasound imaging: in vitro validation and pathologic correlation. *J Am Coll Cardiol.* 1990;16:145.

34. von Birgelen C, van der Lugt A, Nicosia A, et al. Computerized assessment of coronary lumen and atherosclerotic plaque dimensions in three-dimensional intravascular ultrasound correlated with histomorphometry. *Am J Cardiol.* 1996;78:1202.

35. Tobis JM, Mallery J, Mahon D, et al. Intravascular ultrasound imaging of human coronary arteries in vivo. Analysis of tissue characterizations with comparison to in vitro histological specimens. *Circulation.* 1991;83:913.

36. Di Mario C, The SH, Madretsma Set al. Detection and characterization of vascular lesions by intravascular ultrasound: an in vitro study correlated with histology. *J Am Soc Echocardiogr.* 1992;5:135.

37. Abizaid AS, Mintz GS, Mehran R, et al. Long-term follow-up after percutaneous transluminal coronary angioplasty was not performed based on intravascular ultrasound findings: importance of lumen dimensions. *Circulation.* 1999;100:256.

38. Fassa AA, Wagatsuma K, Higano ST, et al. Intravascular ultrasound-guided treatment for angiographically indeterminate left main coronary artery disease: a long-term follow-up study. *J Am Coll Cardiol.* 2005;45:204.

39. Jasti V, Ivan E, Yalamanchili V, Wongpraparut N, Leesar MA. Correlations between fractional flow reserve and intravascular ultrasound in patients with an ambiguous left main coronary artery stenosis. *Circulation* 2004; 110: 2831.

40. Grewal J, Ganz P, Selwyn A, Kinlay S. Usefulness of intravascular ultrasound in preventing stenting of hazy areas adjacent to coronary stents and its support of support spot-stenting. *Am J Cardiol.* 2001;87:1246.

41. Moussa I, Di Mario C, Reimers B, Akiyama T, Tobis J, Colombo A. Subacute stent thrombosis in the era of intravascular ultrasound-guided coronary stenting without anticoagulation: frequency, predictors and clinical outcome. *J Am Coll Cardiol.* 1997;29:6.

42. Hoffmann R, Mintz GS, Mehran R, et al. Intravascular ultrasound predictors of angiographic restenosis in lesions treated with Palmaz—Schatz stents. *J Am Coll Cardiol.* 1998;31:43.

43. Hausmann D, Erbel R, Alibelli-Chemarin MJ, et al. The safety of intracoronary ultrasound. A multicenter survey of 2207 examinations. *Circulation.* 1995;91:623.

44. Pijls NH, De Bruyne B, Peels K, et al. Measurement of fractional flow reserve to assess the functional severity of coronary-artery stenoses. *N Engl J Med.* 1996;334:1703.

45. Pijls NH, Klauss V, Siebert U, et al. Coronary pressure measurement after stenting predicts adverse events at follow-up: a multicenter registry. *Circulation.* 2002;105:2950.

46. Miller DD, Donohue TJ, Younis LT, et al. Correlation of pharmacological 99mTc—sestamibi myocardial perfusion imaging with poststenotic coronary flow reserve in patients with angiographically intermediate coronary artery stenoses. *Circulation.* 1994;89:2150.

47. De Bruyne B, Pijls NH, Smith L, Wievegg M, Heyndrickx GR. Coronary thermodilution to assess flow reserve: experimental validation. *Circulation.* 2001;104:2003.

48. Joye JD, Schulman DS, Lasorda D, Farah T, Donohue BC, Reichek N. Intracoronary Doppler guide wire versus stress single-photon emission computed tomographic thallium-201 imaging in assessment of intermediate coronary stenoses. *J Am Coll Cardiol.* 1994;24:940.

49. Heller LI, Cates C, Popma J, et al. Intracoronary Doppler assessment of moderate coronary artery disease: comparison with 201Tl imaging and coronary angiography. FACTS Study Group. *Circulation.* 1997;96:484.

50. Kern MJ, Donohue TJ, Aguirre FV, et al. Clinical outcome of deferring angioplasty in patients with normal translesional pressure-flow velocity measurements. *J Am Coll Cardiol.* 1995;25:178.

51. de Bruyne B, Bartunek J, Sys SU, Pijls NH, Heyndrickx GR, Wijns W. Simultaneous coronary pressure and flow velocity measurements in humans. Feasibility, reproducibility, and hemodynamic dependence of coronary flow velocity reserve, hyperemic flow versus pressure slope index, and fractional flow reserve. *Circulation.* 1996;94:1842.

PART 3

Principles and Catheter Laboratory Equipment

CHAPTER (12)

X-Ray Cinefluorographic Systems

Jack T. Cusma, PhD

X-ray fluoroscopic imaging is at the core of interventional cardiology. The dramatic developments of the capability of interventional cardiovascular procedures since the mid-1980s would not have been possible without a parallel development and refinement of the capabilities of x-ray fluoroscopic imaging systems.

X-ray fluoroscopic image generation generally falls into two classes:

1. Fluoroscopic imaging used for continuous monitoring of device positioning and depiction of patient anatomy.

2. Angiographic (or acquisition) imaging used to acquire and store a lasting record following injection of contrast agent into the vasculature of interest.

Fluoroscopy originated with the very first discovery of x-rays. The term is used to describe methods for viewing of structures in real-time, ie, visualization of dynamic events as they happen. Over time, a succession of methods has been introduced to record these dynamic images. These methods fall under the general term *fluorography*. Some of these latter methods for acquisition—and storage for later review—are discussed later in the chapter. They include the familiar use of 35-mm movie (cine) film, leading to the introduction of the term *cinefluorography*, typically shortened to *cine*. Although, strictly speaking, elimination of the cine camera as the recording device might logically result in the adoption of other more accurate descriptions, the term remains widely used to refer to any acquisition method. Currently, the most precise term used to describe these image-recording modes is *acquisition*.

Fluoroscopic imaging is generally performed at an x-ray input dose that is at least 10-fold lower than that used for acquisition imaging. The principal consequence of this difference familiar to interventionalists is the greater image noise in images produced in the fluoroscopy mode. This noise, resulting from the statistical fluctuations in x-ray intensity at the detector, is one of several parameters used to characterize the overall *quality* of an image. Other parameters used to characterize the images include the amount of *contrast* between the object of interest and other objects in the background and the *spatial resolution*—how well fine details and sharp edges are visualized.

The evolution of interventional cardiology created a radiation safety issue for both patients and operating personnel. The increasing complexity of interventional cardiovascular procedures led to the need for significantly longer fluoroscopic durations than were necessary for solely diagnostic procedures. In addition to the longer amounts of fluoroscopy time required, the need for higher-quality fluoroscopic images for positioning of low-contrast wires, balloons, and stents produces pressures to increase the fluoroscopic x-ray dose. Thus, forces exist that have the potential to increase both patient and operating personnel radiation exposure.

This chapter reviews the basic physics of x-ray fluorographic image formation. It also reviews the design and theory of operation of an x-ray cinefluorographic unit.

SOURCES OF X-RAYS

The starting point for studying the factors that affect the quality of an x-ray image is the process of generating x-rays. The intensity and energy distribution of the x-rays incident on a given patient determine the image signal and noise as well as the radiation dose delivered to the patient and staff. The clinical demands of modern interventional cardiology have fueled a prodigious engineering effort to develop and refine x-ray sources that can deliver greater amounts of x-rays while limiting the exposure to the patient.

【 】 X-RAY TUBE

The source of the x-rays incident on the patient is the *x-ray tube*, a complex assembly depicted schematically in Figure 12-1. X-rays are

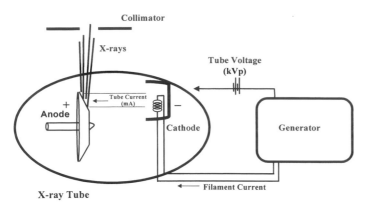

FIGURE 12-1. Schematic diagram of the major components of an x-ray tube with associated electronics.

produced by bombarding a tungsten "target" with a beam of high-energy electrons. The target—or *anode*—is set to a positive electrical voltage relative to the electron source—the *cathode*—so that electrons emitted from the cathode are accelerated toward the target. After collision with the target, the high-velocity electrons lose most of their energy as heat, with a small fraction of energy transformed into x-rays.

The energy of the x-rays varies over a range of values because, as the electrons slow down or "brake" in the tungsten target, they lose energy to a varying degree, depending on the number and strength of interactions they have with atoms of the target material. Overall, roughly 1% of the total energy carried by the electron beam is transformed to x-rays whereas the other 99% is deposited in the anode as heat. When all of an electron's initial energy is lost in a single interaction, the resultant emitted x-ray has the highest possible energy, equivalent to the voltage applied across the tube. This is referred to as the kVp, or *peak kilovoltage (kV)*, of the emitted x-rays. Typical x-ray tube voltages range from 60 kV to 120 kV. For example, if the voltage across the tube were 80,000 volts, or 80 kV, the x-ray beam would be characterized as an *80-kVp beam*. It would contain a spectrum of x-ray photon energies up to the peak value of 80 kV. A sample of the spread or spectrum of the x-ray energies produced by an x-ray tube is shown in Figure 12-2, referred to as the *Bremsstrahlung x-ray spectrum* (from the German word for "braking radiation").

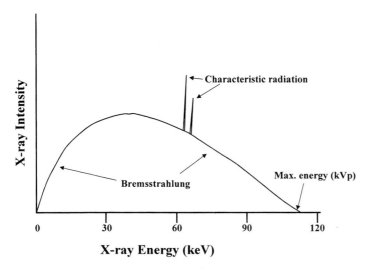

FIGURE 12-2. Representative spectrum of x-rays produced within an x-ray tube. The actual shape is dependent on the actual tube voltage (kVp) and current (mA).

The number of electrons per second that arc across the gap from the cathode to the anode is the *tube current*, measured in milliamperes (mA). The more electrons that strike the target, the more x-ray photons are produced.

Thus, an x-ray beam is characterized both by its photon energy spectrum (kVp) and its photon flux (mA).

Modern x-ray tubes do not generate continuous beams of x-rays. Instead, x-rays are generated in pulses that are synchronized with the rest of the fluoroscopic system (the video camera and/or the cine camera). The number of x-ray photons emitted per pulse is also determined by the duration of time that electrons strike the target—the *pulse width*, measured in milliseconds (msec). For a given tube voltage V, the intensity of the x-rays per image formed is proportional to the product of the milliamperes and the pulse width.

Anode

The design of the x-ray tube target is one of the main factors that affects how intensely an x-ray system can be operated during a long, complex procedure. The anode is a disk made of tungsten, used because its very high melting point enables it to withstand the high temperatures produced when high-energy electrons constantly bombard it. During a typical cineangiographic procedure, representative factors of 80 kVp and 800 mA result in energy deposited in the target at a rate of 64,000 W, or 64 kW. Because 99% of this energy is absorbed by the target as heat, that heat must be removed to avoid melting the target. To improve the heat-handling capabilities, the anode is rotated at speeds up to 10,000 rpm so that the area on the target bombarded by the relatively small beam of electrons is actually a circular track rather than a single point.

The small area on the anode toward which the electrons are accelerated and from which the x-rays are emitted is called the *focal spot*. Because the anode is rotating, this spot is actually a circular track on the rotating disk. The focal spot affects image quality in several ways:

1. A smaller focal spot yields sharper images because there is less overlap of x-rays from different parts of the focal spot area.

2. A larger focal spot absorbs more power and, thus, produces more x-rays.

3. The focal spot area is actually angled relative to the axis of the emitted x-ray beams to provide a compromise between the desire for a small size and the need to spread the energy over a larger area.

4. The angle of tilt of the anode, known as the *target angle*, determines the maximum field of view over which x-rays can be directed.

Typical configurations for cardiac angiography use two focal spots (eg, 0.6 mm and 0.9 mm in diameter) to provide users a choice between higher resolution at lower power or more x-ray intensity to penetrate larger patient thicknesses. A representative target angle is about 9°, capable of a maximum field-of-view of 12 in. (30 cm).

There are three fundamental performance-determining factors for an x-ray tube:

1. The amount of energy that can be deposited in the anode in a single exposure. The measure of this capability is the *instantaneous* heat rating of the tube.

2. The total heat that can be deposited over a long series of exposures and over the multiple series required during a diagnostic or interventional procedure.

3. The rate at which the x-ray tube assembly can dissipate heat. The heat generated in the anode is transferred to the surrounding housing, from which it must be dissipated. The rate of heat dissipation is determined by the total heat that can be accommodated by the housing and the dissipation efficiency. This housing heat capacity can be about 2 million to 3 million Heat Units (HU), and the rate at which power can be dissipated from the system can range from 800 W to more than 3000 W.

In practical terms, higher ratings translate to the ability to provide imaging for longer periods of time, with greater penetration and potential for lower patient exposures, without the need for delays while the tube cools to a usable range.

Cathode

The cathode is a tungsten wire (filament) that is the source of the electrons accelerated towards the anode. Current is passed through the cathode to heat it to a high temperature. The wire is maintained at a large negative voltage relative to the target and, as electrons are "boiled off" the filament, they are accelerated toward the target by the voltage difference, reaching their maximum energy of 60 kV to 120 kV just before they collide with the target. In cardiac fluoroscopy systems, there are generally two filaments of different sizes, in turn producing different-size beams of electrons corresponding to the two focal spots at the target referred to earlier.

X-RAY SPECTRUM AND BEAM FILTERING

As noted earlier, the spread in energies in the x-ray beam is the result of the braking process that the electrons undergo after collision with the target. The spikes superimposed on this continuous distribution are known as the *characteristic radiation*, a reference to the fact that an incident electron's energy has matched exactly one of the characteristic energy levels of tungsten atoms. Figure 12-2 shows that a substantial fraction of the x-rays produced have low photon energies (ie, <25–30 keV). These x-rays, if allowed to reach the patient, would be completely absorbed in the superficial portion of the patient. As they would not be able to penetrate the patient completely, they would not provide useful diagnostic information, but contribute to the patient's radiation exposure. To remove these low-energy x-rays from the beam, all x-ray tubes have metal filtering material placed in the beam exit port that absorbs photons selectively from this region of the energy spectrum. This filtration, specified in equivalent thickness of aluminum (eg, 3.0 mm), is mandated by regulatory requirements and is provided through use of metal in addition to the tube and housing materials. This approach can be extended by using additional thicknesses of metal to further shape the spectrum of the beam filtering out a greater fraction of low energy photons.

Beam filtration is of value for two reasons:

1. To reduce the exposure to the patient.

2. To improve the contrast of structures of interest for the imaging task.

Modern systems typically use filters constructed of copper ranging in thickness from 0.2 mm to as much as 0.9 mm. The consequence of adding absorbing material in the beam path is that its removal of x-rays from the beam means that fewer x-rays are available to form an image. This requires increased tube output (which in turn requires greater x-ray tube loading and, consequently, heat dissipation). However, if this is accomplished successfully (requiring a higher power x-ray tube), there is greater output in the energy range of interest.

COLLIMATORS

Collimators are used to adjust the shape and size of the x-ray field emerging from the tube. Collimators are constructed from lead shutters that completely absorb the x-ray beam. They provide a crucial component for limiting exposure to the patient only to the region of interest. This, in turn, reduces unnecessary exposure to the procedure room staff as a result of radiation scatter from the patient.

X-RAY GENERATORS AND EXPOSURE CONTROL

The electric power required to heat the cathode filament, turn the x-ray pulses on and off, and accelerate the electrons toward the target is provided by the x-ray generator. The clinical demands of cardiac angiography require a generator that can deliver up to 100 kW of power to the tube at all voltages in the diagnostic range. The generator automatically adjusts the tube voltage, tube current, and x-ray pulse width as needed to maintain constant brightness at the image receptor—the output of an image intensifier or flat panel detector, for example—as the patient thickness changes because of panning or angulation. X-ray generators have preset modes for fluoroscopy, along with various acquisition modes that determine the ranges of factors, including the focal spot to be used.

The exposure control is a critical piece of the generator circuitry. This provides the mechanism for adjusting the exposure parameters as the demands of the imaging situation change with time. The mechanisms of exposure modulation vary among vendors, but, in general, the image brightness at the output of the imaging chain is sampled rapidly and its value is sent back to the generator, where it is used to modulate the pulse width, tube current, or voltage to achieve the desired imaging chain output signal brightness. The combination and order of adjustment varies among different kinds of equipment, but the list of parameters that can be changed is a short one:

1. Tube current—mA.

2. Tube voltage—kVp.

3. Exposure duration or pulse width—msec.

4. Camera aperture—allowing more or less light into the imaging camera.

5. Electronic amplification gain.

Traditionally, the exposure during both fluoroscopy and angiography—cine or digital—is calibrated to deliver the same amount of x-rays to the detector for each image. The x-ray tube output is adjusted so that the same amount of x-rays is transmitted to the detector. In the fluoroscopic mode, the tube output is limited to a maximum value determined by regulatory bodies. During acquisition, the output can increase as much as necessary (until the capacity of the generator or tube is reached). In recent developments, the feedback algorithms have added the capability for actually varying the number of x-rays used in each image, depending on the relative signal and noise in that specific frame.

INTERACTIONS OF X-RAYS WITH MATTER

A useful x-ray image is formed when the spatially varying intensity of x-rays transmitted through an object of interest is detected and converted into a visible light display that can be detected by the human eye. The intensity of the incident beam directed toward the patient is assumed to be uniform (ie, the same number of x-rays—on the average—is incident per unit area at the input surface of the patient). The intensity of the beam that exits from the patient is modulated by processes of x-ray absorption in the patient. This process is similar to the formation of a shadow of a solid object when illuminated by visible light—with the important difference that the degree of darkness in the shadow forming an x-ray image is determined by the energy of the x-rays incident on the object, the thickness of the object, and the elemental makeup of the object.

X-rays are removed from the incident beam through a number of physical absorption processes. In the diagnostic energy range, an x-ray photon can interact with matter in one of two ways:

1. The photoelectric effect.

2. Compton scattering.

The photoelectric effect is the principal process for differentiation between structures. It varies with the atomic number of the absorbing material through which the x-rays travel. Another characteristic of the photoelectric effect is that the probability for the absorption of an x-ray photon by an atom is strongly dependent on the energy of the incident photon. This probability is higher when the photon's energy matches one of the discrete energies required to eject an electron from the atom; when that happens, the photon is completely removed from the beam.

Compton scattering, which does not depend strongly on the makeup of the absorbing material, results in a change in the direction of an x-ray photon as it passes through the patient. The scattered photon either does not reach the detector at all, or, if it does, it strikes a different location from a different angle. As a result, at the detector where the image is formed, deflected x-rays from different locations in the patient can contribute to the signal at the same image location. The net effect is a reduction in contrast of the object of interest. Other deflected x-rays are the source of the radiation to the personnel in the laboratory.

The removal of x-rays from a beam as a function of material thickness follows the familiar exponential relationship, where the properties of the material are characterized by the linear attenuation coefficient. An important concept in understanding differential attenuation is the *half-value layer (HVL)*, defined as the thickness of a particular absorbing material that removes exactly one-half of the x-ray intensity from the beam. For x-ray energies used in cardiovascular angiographic imaging, the HVL of several materials of interest are

1. Muscle—3.2 cm.

2. Bone—1.5 cm.

3. Iodine (100%)—0.01 cm.

4. Lead—0.01 cm.

These values are calculated for x-rays with the same energy as described earlier. In a typical diagnostic x-ray beam there is actually a spread in energies, and the calculation of the HVL is more complicated, but, empirically, the same concept applies—the amount of material that cuts the intensity in half.

X-RAY IMAGE FORMATION

〖 〗 PARAMETERS THAT CHARACTERIZE X-RAY IMAGES

Geometric Magnification. The x-rays leaving the tube can be considered to be originating from approximately a single point and diverging as they travel toward the patient on their way to the image detector. This divergence, or *spread of the beam,* produces a magnified image as shown in Figure 12-3, where the magnification at the image intensifier is given by the ratio

$$M = SID/SOD$$

SID is the source-to-image distance and SOD is the source-to-object distance (ie, the distance between the x-ray source and the patient). Increasing the magnification can be achieved either by decreasing the SOD or by increasing the SID; in the former case, this also increases the exposure to the patient; in the latter case, this places a greater demand on the x-ray generator to deliver the necessary exposure at the receptor. The reason for increasing the magnification is to make small objects appear larger in the images, but doing so also affects the other parameters in the image: contrast, noise, and sharpness.

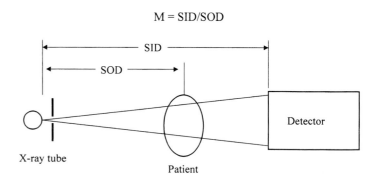

SOD = source-object-distance
SID = source-image-distance

FIGURE 12-3. Block diagram depicting the geometric magnification produced in a cardiac angiographic system. The amount of magnification is a function of the distance from the x-ray tube to the patient (SOD) and from the x-ray tube to the detector (SID).

Image Resolution. As noted earlier, the ability of an imaging system to reproduce sharp edges and small objects is specified by its spatial resolution, usually referred to simply as resolution. Resolution is measured in units of "spatial frequency," typically line pairs per millimeter (lp/mm), a measure of how many alternating cycles of dark and light can be distinguished over a distance of 1 mm. In basic terms, to visualize objects about 0.2 mm requires a system that can image spatial frequencies of at least 2.5 lp/mm. If a state-of-the-art system has a limiting resolution of 3.0 lp/mm to 3.5 lp/mm, it is capable of resolving high-contrast objects as small as 0.15 mm. It should be noted that other factors in a particular clinical procedure or patient might make it difficult to delineate objects that small.

Characteristics of each component of the imaging chain can affect the overall system's spatial resolution. Patient characteristics are further superimposed on the intrinsic properties of the system to affect overall image quality. These include

1. X-ray tube focal-spot size.

2. X-ray pulse duration.

3. Characteristics of the image detector.

4. Characteristics of the digital image sampling and processing system.

The finite size of the focal spot affects sharpness with increased focal-spot size, causing increased image blur (geometric unsharpness). The system components used to convert x-rays to an electronic signal can themselves blur the image, reducing the ability to resolve small objects in the image at the system output. A principal determinant of this phenomenon is the thickness of the phosphor on the image detector (discussed later in the chapter). In the case of digital images, the size of the sampling interval when creating digital images can affect image blur. This phenomenon is particularly important in circumstances of subject motion, such as the normal movement of the heart. This causes imaged objects to move during the imaging process. In this circumstance, x-ray pulse duration (or width) is an important determinant of the degree of blur. The degree of motion blurring is determined by the velocity and extent of the motion and the duration of the x-ray pulses used to generate the images. One context in which to interpret this relationship is to consider that a 5-msec pulse width is equivalent to a 1/200-sec shutter speed for a camera.

Image Contrast. Diagnostic imaging information consists of differential image brightness caused by varying attenuation of x-rays by structures in the patient that have different absorption characteristics for x-rays in the diagnostic energy range. For our purposes, we consider that absorption of x-rays in cardiac angiograms takes place in a small variety of materials:

1. Tissue (fat, muscle, and blood).

2. Air.

3. Bone.

4. Contrast agent (iodine).

In Figure 12-4, the absorption of x-rays is illustrated schematically for tissue and iodine over a range of x-ray energy. It is evident from the figure that the amount of absorption varies with x-ray energy, that the absorption for the same amount of iodine is

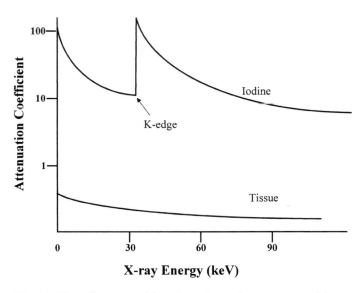

FIGURE 12-4. Illustration of the relationship with x-ray energy of the attenuation coefficient of tissue and iodine. The discontinuity in the neighborhood of 30 keV results from a K-edge of iodine. This represents the attenuation for x-rays of a given energy; in the case of angiography, the output of an x-ray tube will instead have a spread of energies as shown in Figure 12-2.

greater than for tissue, and that there are several x-ray energies where the absorption of iodine is much greater. This last effect occurs when an x-ray's energy exactly matches an atomic energy level of iodine. This is referred to as a *K-edge effect* when the energy is equal to a transition from a K electron shell of the iodine atom. X-ray photon energies in this range have a maximal differential absorption between iodine-containing contrast agent and surrounding tissue.

The K-edge effect dictates that an imaging system designed to maximize the contrast between iodine and surrounding tissue should try to deliver a large fraction if its x-rays at an energy just above K-edge, approximately 33 kV. This is not possible in practice because the x-ray beam contains a spread of energies and only a small proportion have energy at the K-edge for iodine. If one had an unlimited number of x-rays, one could use filter materials to cut out the lower- and higher-energy x-rays and leave only those that deliver the maximum contrast. In practice, the tube output is limited, and an imaging system designer must compromise between getting enough transmission through the patient to make a bright image, enough of the middle-energy x-rays to get a high degree of contrast, and eliminating the lowest energy x-rays that would be almost completely absorbed in the first layers of a patient's skin.

Scatter Radiation. The discussion so far assumes that x-rays travel in a straight line through the patient from the focal spot on their way to the detector, and that only x-rays along the line of travel are absorbed in the patient or transmitted to the corresponding point on the detector. In fact, the Compton scattering process described earlier allows scattered x-ray photons to reach the detector from points in the patient that did not lie on the original straight-line path. These x-rays are referred to as *scatter radiation.* If they contribute to the image formed at the detector, they reduce image contrast as much as 45%–50% compared to that in the absence of scatter radiation. Scatter radiation also leaves the

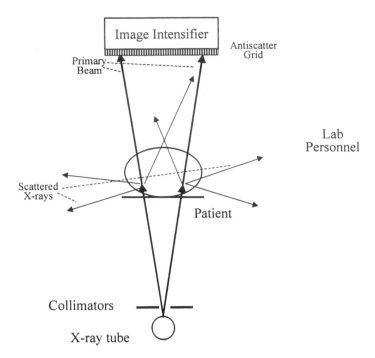

FIGURE 12-5. Schematic diagram illustrating the origin of scattered x-rays within the patient and their directional distribution compared to the primary beam, which provides the desirable diagnostic information. It can be seen that the scatter radiation contributes to the signal at the image intensifier and also is the source of radiation exposure by lab personnel.

patient traveling in all directions, and is the main source of exposure to personnel, as can be seen from Figure 12-5.

The effect of scatter on image contrast can be minimized with the use of an *antiscatter grid* on the face of the detector. This device blocks a high proportion of the x-rays coming in at an angle from reaching the detector point. Although this is a desirable objective from an image-quality perspective, the grid also absorbs some primary-beam x-ray photons. As a result, fewer x-rays are available to brighten that point in the image. This requires a greater x-ray output, which increases the patient exposure (as well as scatter radiation to the surrounding personnel).

Other methods are also useful for reducing the amount of scatter radiation to the image plane. As can be seen in Figure 12-6, by increasing the *air gap* between the patient and the detector, the scattered photons at the steeper angles miss the image detector and cannot contribute to the image intensity. However, increasing the source-to-image distance also affects the image quality by increasing the magnification, and requires an increase in the x-ray intensity incident on the patient. If the tube cannot deliver more x-rays at the desired energy range, this in turn forces a shift to higher kVp, which may lead to reduced contrast as a result of the lower absorption at the higher x-ray energies. An obvious method for reducing scatter radiation to the surrounding areas as well as to the detected image is through the limitation of the irradiated volume with the use of collimators.

Image Noise. Even when we have the desirable degree of resolution and sufficient contrast to see the desired object, there is one remaining image parameter that can obscure the object—noise in the image. Image noise arises from the fact that x-rays are discrete or individual particles, and many of them are needed at a location to "build up" the desired information at that location. At the x-ray exposures used in typical fluoroscopic and low-to-moderate exposures used during acquisition, the quantum noise or *quantum mottle* is (and, in fact, should be) visible in the image. Rather than a perfectly uniform intensity of x-rays, the amount of x-rays incident on the same amount of area actually varies randomly about a mean value. The fluctuation of the number of x-rays is apparent to the observer as a "grainy" appearance of the image. When the degree of fluctuations is on the order of the contrast produced by a small object such as a guidewire, it becomes difficult to differentiate the object from background graininess.

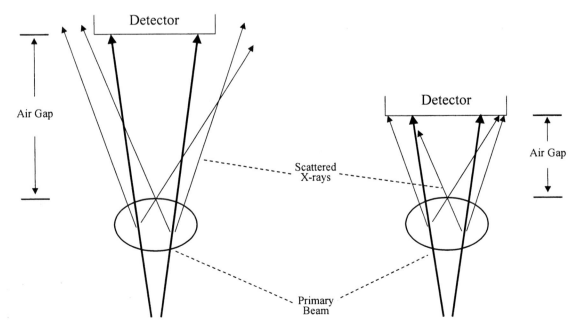

FIGURE 12-6. The effects of air gap—the distance from the patient to the detector—on the contribution of scatter radiation to the image. Reducing the amount of scattered x-rays that reach the detector results in improved contrast but most likely requires an increase in the tube output.

There are mathematical techniques that can be applied to reduce the noise in an image, but they can also smooth out desired objects, eliminating fine detail of features and making them difficult to visualize.

Using an x-ray beam with a higher proportion of high-energy x-rays also produces a noisier image because fewer high-energy x-rays are needed to produce the same image brightness level. Another major source of image noise can be found in the electronic circuits that convert the signal from the detected x-ray image to an electric signal that can be displayed and recorded. A well-designed system includes electronics whose noise cannot be seen compared to the fluctuations of the x-ray intensity. In addition, some image processing methods such as those that enhance the edges of arteries can add to the noise in an image, and there is a tradeoff between the desired degree of edge sharpness and the tolerable degree of noise.

IMAGE DETECTION

【 】 IMAGE INTENSIFIER

The spatial distribution of x-ray intensity information leaving the patient contains the anatomic (and, through temporal changes, physiologic) information necessary to make a clinical diagnosis and perform an interventional procedure. However, that information is not detectable by human senses. Thus, it must be converted to a visible light image that the physician can observe.

The first stage in that process is the transformation of the x-ray intensity to a form that can be converted into an electric signal. For many years, this step was performed using the *image intensifier (II)*. The development of the II made x-ray fluoroscopically guided procedures possible, and thus is the x-ray system component most responsible for the evolution of current interventional cardiology.

Recently, new technologies have been introduced to replace this process. It would be safe to say, however, that the II remains the detector used in the vast majority of fluoroscopic systems used in interventional laboratories. Accordingly, an effort to understand its role in the image formation process is warranted.

The function of the image intensifier is to convert the x-ray intensity information at its input into a visible light image that can be used to expose photographic film or illuminate a video camera. The II, shown schematically in Figure 12-7, is enclosed within a metallic or glass container from which the air has been removed and which contains electrostatic components for focusing and accelerating electrons similar to processes found in a cathode ray tube (CRT) used for a video or computer monitor. The input face, ranging up to 16 in. in diameter, is coated with a phosphor made of cesium iodide (CsI), which emits several thousand light photons for each x-ray photon that it absorbs. These light photons in turn eject electrons from a photocathode immediately adjacent to the phosphor. The ejected electrons are accelerated toward the output phosphor at the other (top) end of the II. When these fast electrons collide in the output phosphor, a fluorescent visible light image is produced that is then focused on a video camera or cine film.

The electrostatic components in the II can operate in several modes, enabling multiple magnification modes for a given device,

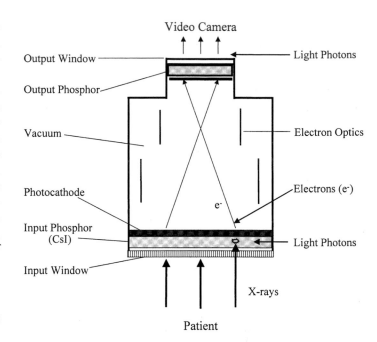

FIGURE 12-7. Schematic diagram illustrating the stages of an image intensifier (II) used to convert the x-ray intensity information exiting to the patient into a visible image.

depending on the desired field of view at the input face. Typically, the field of view is selected from one of three (eg, 4.5-in., 6-in., and 9-in., where the dimension refers to the diameter of the region of the input face that is imaged on the output face). Because the size of the image on the output face–1-in. diameter is typical—remains the same, selection among the modes changes the amount of magnification in the image; going from 9 in. to 6 in. means that objects are magnified by a factor of 1.5, compared to the larger size. This also reduces the field of view within the patient. In most cardiac angiographic systems, selection of a smaller field of view also increases the number of x-ray photons needed to form the image, resulting in greater load on the x-ray tube and higher exposure to the patient.

【 】 VIDEO CAMERA

In traditional systems, the visible light image generated on the output phosphor of the II is focused onto the target surface of a video camera. The signal generated by the video camera can be displayed directly on a television monitor but, in most modern systems, it undergoes digital processing before display. This pathway is also the source of the digital image data that makes up the fluorographic record in the majority of digital fluoroscopy systems.

The x-ray image is formed during the short pulse during which the tube current is on—about 1 msec to 10 msec. After the x-ray exposure is terminated, the signal is read off the camera target line by line and processed. The most common number of lines used to form the image is either 525 or 1050 (of active video data).

There are two main types of cameras: those based on pickup tube technology and those based on solid-state charge-coupled device (CCD) image sensors. The CCD device is a relatively recent development, whereas pickup tube cameras have been used since the first use of IIs in the catheterization laboratory.

The pickup tube camera used in fluoroscopic systems can also take several variations depending on the material used to convert the input light signal to an electric signal. A circular target 1 in. or more in diameter receives light from the output surface of the II and produces a distribution of charge on the target proportional to the incident light intensity (and, working backward, the original x-ray intensity exiting the patient). A scanning beam of electrons scans the target from upper left to lower right, resulting in a voltage that varies from location to location, again, proportional to the x-ray intensity. This time-varying voltage can be used as the input to standard video monitors, or it can be converted into numbers as described next.

A CCD camera receptor is a two-dimensional array of discrete elements that form "cells" of charge whose magnitude depends on the amount of incident light. The array of elements, typically 1024 rows by 1024 columns, is read off as, again, a time-varying voltage and processed in a manner similar to that of the pickup tube. There are a number of advantages of the CCD camera: They are much more compact than a pickup tube with potential for longer effective lifetime, and the sensors have a much more linear response to light input over a wider range. It should be noted that the output of the CCD camera is an analog signal, just as with the pickup tube, and a similar digital conversion is required to convert the signal to an array of numbers.

【 】 VIDEO MONITOR

A necessary component in every x-ray fluorographic system is a monitor used to display the x-ray image produced by the imaging chain, either continuously during fluoroscopy or on playback of a digitally recorded acquisition sequence. In most cases, these are standard analog video monitors operating at either 525 or 1050 lines of video with a refresh rate of 30 frames/sec. More recently, newer systems use workstation monitors that operate at higher resolutions and higher refresh rates.

There are two video monitor display modes—interlaced and progressive. Standard video monitors (ie, those refreshing the display 30 times a second) operate in an interlaced display, where the image is divided in two by alternating the number of lines and sorting the halves into two fields. The fields are sent to the monitor a time interval of 1/60th of a second apart, so that adjacent lines are actually separated in time by 1/60th of a second, and the complete pair is refreshed at an interval of 1/30th of a second. This is done to avoid the image flicker that takes place when the eye detects a scene change at 30 refresh cycles a second; instead, the scene is changing at 60 times per second, which the eye cannot detect. The lines in the image formed at the input to the video camera are acquired sequentially over a time interval of 1/30th second. On the way to the display on the video monitor, the video signal is processed by a scan converter that interweaves the lines so that they can be displayed on a standard monitor running in an interlaced mode. This approach is standard practice in modern systems, and its use during fluoroscopy, combined with pulsed exposures, avoids the possibility of motion blurring and provides options for managing exposure versus image quality during fluoroscopy compared to the older continuous fluoroscopy systems. Its use was a requirement for the development of digital angiography, where pulsed exposure was already used for cine recording in parallel.

Many newer systems use a progressive scan display, in which sequential lines are shown one after another. This type of display requires a refresh rate of at least 50 times a second to eliminate perceptible image flicker.

DIGITAL IMAGING FUNDAMENTALS

The development and refinement of digital imaging systems is one of the most valuable technologic developments for the practice of interventional cardiology. Digital imaging systems are able to record high-quality cine images and provide them for review immediately, eliminating the delay associated with processing of cine film. Furthermore, film-based systems require compromise between the light requirements of the 35-mm film cine camera and the digital video camera. Often, optimizing image characteristics for one camera compromises the image quality produced by the other.

Clinical practice has evolved to the point where virtually all new angiographic equipment is delivered as primarily a digital imaging system and, even when cine film is produced in parallel, the assessment of cardiac anatomy and function during and immediately following the procedure is achieved using digital images. Recent innovations have expanded the scope of capabilities available to the interventionalist, and an understanding of the basic process involved in the formation of digital x-ray images is of value.

【 】 ANALOG-TO-DIGITAL CONVERSION

The phenomena of interest for any medical imaging application reside in the real or analog world. The information we wish to turn into an image—whether viewed from film or a workstation monitor—corresponds to a representation of physical interactions between the x-ray photons entering the patient and structures of interest. With the image intensifier imaging chain, for example, this information could be represented mathematically as a distribution in space, whether of x-ray particles, electrons in the II, visible light at the output face of the II, or as an electric signal in a video camera.

A digital image is produced from this physical phenomenon when the information is converted into an array of distinct numbers. Such an image is represented using a fixed number of values, and the values are distributed over a limited or discrete set of coordinates. This contrasts with a film image, where there is a continuous range of intensity values and the precision with which we are able to identify a position in the image is not inherently limited.

In order to produce a digital image, a conversion step is required from an analog to a digital representation. In traditional II systems, the analog signal typically used is the electric signal leaving the video camera. This continuously time-varying voltage is fed to an *analog-to-digital converter* (ADC), which samples the signal at regular time intervals (eg, every 100 nanoseconds [nsec], or 10 million times a second). During each sample, the ADC converts the input voltage to an integer value (typically between 0 and 255). In the case of a maximum value of 255, the output of the ADC can only take the values 0, 1, 2, 3, . . . 254, 255, and the system is calibrated so that the maximum brightness in the image maps to 255, whereas the darkest level maps to 0. Each video line is sampled (eg, 512 times), converting the signal to its discrete equivalent, and the process is repeated for a total of 512 video lines before it starts over again for the next frame of video, which comes along 1/30th second later—following another x-ray pulse.

In the example described here, the digitized image has an image matrix of 512 × 512 picture elements, or *pixels,* and each pixel is digitized to 256 gray scales. Because in digital systems numbers are represented using combinations of 1s and 0s, called *bits,* and it requires 8 bits to represent the range of 0–255, this digital image is said to have a *bit depth* of 8 bits, or 1 *byte.* Each digital image consists of a total of 262,144 bytes, or 1/4 *megabyte (MB)* (in the binary number scheme used in digital systems, *kilo* refers to 1024, and *mega* refers to the product of 1024 × 1024), and a repeat of the process 30 times a second results in a total data rate of 30 × 1/4 MB, or 7.5 MB/s. Other common variations on the example provided here are image matrices of 1024 × 1024 pixels and bit depths of 10 bits (values of 0–1023) or 12 bits (0–4095). As a result of the ADC process, the digital image can be thought of as a square array of values, where each pixel is a much smaller square, whose size, projected back to the object of interest in the patient, depends on the magnification mode of the II and the geometric magnification. For a II operating in the 6-in. mode and with an optical magnification of 1.2, this would lead to a pixel size of approximately 0.25 mm on each side. At first glance, the sampling process results in a limit on the smallest object that can be displayed—in this case, 0.25 mm—and this process may be the ultimate limiting factor in the system, determining the spatial resolution of the system for a particular geometry and magnification mode.

【 】 FLAT-PANEL DETECTORS

In recent years, a truly new component has been introduced into the fluoroscopic imaging chain with the replacement of the image intensifier and video camera with a *flat-panel detector* using thin-film transistor (TFT) arrays. In general, flat-panel detectors used in radiographic systems belong to two classes referred to as *direct* or *indirect detectors.* In fluoroscopy to date, indirect detectors have been used primarily, and the following discussion focuses on their principles of operation.

A fluoroscopic flat-panel x-ray detector consists of several components shown schematically in Figure 12-8. The use of the term *indirect* refers to the fact that the detector elements (each is a combination of an amorphous silicon photodiode and a TFT) are not themselves sensitive to x-rays, but, rather, to visible light. If a visible light photon encounters a flat-panel detector element, it is absorbed and produces a buildup of charge proportional to the amount of light captured. Because the flat-panel element is not sensitive to x-rays, an intermediate step is required to convert x-ray photons to visible light—thus the indirect nature of the process. The method chosen in fluoroscopic systems is the same technology used as the first stage in the image intensifier: a CsI phosphor layer. The resulting visible light photons are absorbed in the amorphous silicon photosensitive detector element.

After the flat panel is exposed to a single short x-ray pulse, the result is a two-dimensional array of electric signals captured as voltages in the discrete flat-panel elements. A panel for use in cardiac applications typically contains 1024 × 1024 elements over a rectangular area covering a common field of view (eg, 20 cm²). The transistor component of each picture element serves as a switch synchronized with the driving "readout" electronics. The readout process requires that the million discrete values be read out and the detector prepared for a new exposure, within 33 msec in a typical catheterization laboratory configuration. In some ways, the output of the flat-panel detector resembles the operation of the CCD camera used in II systems. For a brief time, the CCD camera sensor also represents a two-dimensional array of voltages, but the CCD readout is performed as a continuously time-varying signal and the discrete nature is lost in this process. In contrast, each flat-panel element's voltage signal is converted one-by-one from an analog voltage to a digital representation. Thus, the digital conversion of the flat-panel detector image can be considered figuratively to take place *at the detector,* whereas with a video camera, an analog signal is transmitted along standard electric cables to the digitization electronics hardware. It should be emphasized, however, that the signal at each flat-panel element remains analog until the digital conversion occurs, as is the case with CCD or, for that matter, pickup tube cameras. The discrete nature of the detector elements should not lead to the misunderstanding that the detector itself is any more inherently digital than the comparable components in the image-intensifier imaging chain. There are significant obvious differences between the way that digital images are produced with flat-panel detectors compared to image intensifiers, but it should be emphasized that there are many more similarities in other aspects of the overall imaging chain. As a result, many of the issues discussed earlier and in the following text apply to images produced with both types of detectors.

【 】 IMAGE PROCESSING

As noted previously, early adoption of digital imaging technology in cardiovascular cinefluorography was facilitated by the availability of the angiographic record immediately after completion of the x-ray exposures during a contrast injection. The sequence of images—in final form—is available for review, and decisions regarding the need for further views or further intervention can be made with no processing delay. Once the image data is stored as an array of numbers, it can also be processed using complex computational methods. Among the types of processing that are most familiar are *spatial-filtering* or *edge-enhancement* algorithms that sharpen the edges of vessels and wires in the images. The brightness and contrast of the images can be changed dynamically in

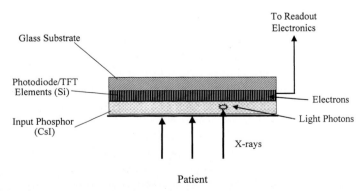

FIGURE 12-8. Schematic diagram illustrating the imaging stages of an indirect detection flat-panel detector.

order to better visualize particular areas of interest, and images can be zoomed and panned to magnify the display and enlarge objects of interest. Other types of image processing include temporal filtering to reduce the amount of noise in relatively low-exposure images, and digital subtraction methods that remove background structures from an image. Another class includes *dynamic range reduction* methods that process image intensity values in such a manner that brighter areas in the original image are shifted lower, avoiding the "blooming" that was common in cine film and video images when thinner regions of the patient were included in the same view with denser regions. The use of digital images also facilitates the application of quantitative analysis methods such as QCA, left ventricular analysis, and even physiologic function measurements and three-dimensional reconstruction of the coronary vasculature.

[ ] IMAGE FORMATS AND STANDARDS

Among the advantages of digital imaging technology is the ability to make exact copies of the image for review and exchange between laboratories and hospitals. The accepted standard for organizing the image data in order to enable other image users to translate the information accurately is known as the DICOM standard (Digital Imaging Communications in Medicine). DICOM, now used by all major vendors, allows the image results to be displayed at other locations after storage and writing on removable media (eg, a recordable compact disk [CD-R]; over a digital computer network). Details of systems for performing these review, transmission, and archival tasks are included elsewhere in this volume. (See Chapter 18 for a more detailed discussion.)

RADIATION EXPOSURE AND OPERATIONAL SAFETY

The patient and operating personnel radiation exposure levels associated with cardiovascular x-ray fluoroscopically guided procedures are among the largest associated with medical imaging. The mechanisms and effects of tissue damage produced by x-rays are discussed in Chapter 13, along with general methods for reduction of exposure to the patient and staff.

A core principle of the use of x-radiation in medicine is to use only levels of radiation that are *as low as reasonable achievable* (*ALARA*). Another priority for a catheterization procedure is to produce image data of satisfactory quality. In general, image quality improves as radiation dose increases because of the reduction of image noise. Thus, in equipment selection and calibration, it is important to strike an appropriate balance between image quality and dose.

Methods for exposure reduction fall into two basic categories.

1. Equipment factors that reduce the radiation that enters the patient.

2. Procedural factors that can reduce the exposure to the operator and support staff.

The equipment factors are discussed later in the chapter, whereas other procedural factors are discussed in Chapter 13.

[ ] EQUIPMENT PARAMETERS

Detector Dose

The number of x-rays that are required by the system to produce a single image of sufficient diagnostic quality is a general setting for a piece of x-ray equipment and is "hard-coded" when the system is calibrated. This required detected dose has been determined empirically from generally accepted levels of noise tolerance. Reduction of the acceptable detected dose directly reduces all exposure measurements in all situations at the cost of increased image noise. Alternatively, equipment can be equipped with multiple modes that use different amounts of detected dose, depending on the degree of detail required. Operator knowledge of the situation and the degree of detail required allow the operator to switch to other modes as warranted.

For the image intensifier, the higher the efficiency of the conversion process from x-rays to visible light, the fewer the number of x-rays that are required. Newer image intensifiers are more efficient than older models and have higher conversion factors than do older models. Image intensifier x-ray detection efficiency declines with time. Thus, regular monitoring is necessary to detect when a significant increase in the input x-ray exposure is required for satisfactory light output. One of the theoretic advantages of flat-panel detectors is that this degradation process is not inherent, but this remains to be proved.

Detector Magnification Mode

The image intensifier magnification mode chosen for an x-ray acquisition in most modern systems also affects the amount of radiation required to form an image. In general, selection of a higher magnification mode increases the required detected dose because a smaller area is available for formation of the image, and the exposure control sends a signal to the generator to increase the incident radiation. Going to the next highest magnification mode can increase the input exposure up to a factor of 2, in turn increasing the exposure to the patient and the staff by the same factor (if everything else stays the same). Newer systems are more flexible and use of variable apertures in front of the video camera can be used to keep the exposure rate the same in different magnification modes. Again, flat-panel detectors are hypothetically not subject to this behavior, but it remains to be seen which configurations will be found acceptable for this technology.

Acquisition Frame Rate

In the absence of cine film, operators have more flexibility with regard to the image-framing rate, and this directly affects the amount of exposure required. Use of lower frame rates during cine angiography—and even fluoroscopy—reduce the exposure rate approximately proportionally with no other changes in the image dose requirements. Newer systems have the ability to perform fluoroscopy at rates of 15 or 7.5 frames/sec—or slower—and these modes may still provide useful information in appropriate situations. Angiographic recording at 15 frames per second is also common in many laboratories, significantly reducing the exposure. It should be noted that the approaches described here require less x-ray tube loading, reducing the delays that may take place because of heat buildup during a complex procedure in a heavier patient and, at the same time, extending the life of an x-ray tube. Another technical factor in newer systems is the use of spectral filtration as described earlier; these techniques can reduce the patient exposure by 20% to 70%, maintaining other parameters.

SUMMARY

The state-of-the-art in x-ray imaging systems for use in cardiovascular interventions continues to evolve, incorporating the most advanced developments in x-ray production technology, together with automated control procedures to produce the highest quality images with the minimum possible radiation exposure. Algorithms that change the appearance of the images produced during the procedure have the potential for significantly improving the ability to detect low-contrast objects and structures. Like all tools, an understanding of these sophisticated capabilities allows the interventional cardiologist to select the optimal techniques to guide the diagnostic or therapeutic procedure.

CHAPTER (13)

Operational Radiation Management for Patients and Staff

Louis K. Wagner, PhD

Fluoroscopic radiation is a carcinogen that can also cause severe injury ("radiation burns") to patients and practitioners. Figures 13-1 -through 13-4[1–4] illustrate the severe effects of radiation. All effects pictured were caused by radiation associated with fluoroscopy. The author knows of at least 200 cases of injury, and more are suspected. Many have been reported in the medical literature.[4–9] When fluoroscopy is well managed, the likelihood that these severe effects could occur is extremely low. However, when it is not well managed, the carcinogenic risk to both personnel and patient becomes higher than necessary, and the risk for injury to the patient increases.[5] The goal of this chapter is to discuss factors involved in the proper management of fluoroscopic and fluorographic radiation.

Figure 13-1[1] is a breast cancer caused by a fluoroscopically guided interventional procedure performed to cure pulmonary tuberculosis in the mid-twentieth century. Chronic radiation dermatitis is also readily apparent in this picture, taken in the 1960s, approximately 10–15 years after exposure to the radiation. Figure 13-2[2] shows the residual scarring in a 17-year-old girl who had undergone two procedures for electrophysiologic ablation. She also had difficulty raising her right arm, and has been placed at elevated risk for breast cancer as a result of the direct and indirect radiation doses to her breasts.

Medical practitioners who have accumulated considerable radiation doses have been shown to have developed radiation-induced cancer, cataracts, or skin injury.[10–13] The interventional radiation environment creates conditions conducive to the accumulation of high doses in personnel. Attention to rigorous radiation abatement measures is therefore warranted and required.[14]

Interventionalists are also at risk for subtle changes in the ocular lens.[15] Although these changes are detectable, their impact on vision is not presently known. In other words, radiation may have subtle unknown effects, and only careful attention to radiation management practices can avoid them or reduce their severity.

Figures 13-3[3] and 13-4[4] are skin injuries in patients who underwent fluoroscopically guided invasive cardiologic procedures. The patient in Figure 13-3 underwent coronary angioplasty and stent placement involving 63 minutes of fluoroscopy and about 5000 frames of cine fluorography. The affected skin area required a full-thickness graft. The patient in Figure 13-4 underwent three electrophysiologic and ablation procedures for WPW syndrome, accumulating more than 300 minutes of fluoroscopy on-time. At last follow-up, the lesions on the back resolved into a scarred area, whereas the injury to the arm required grafting. Both cases involved x-ray irradiation with the x-ray beams oriented in a fixed trajectory for long periods of time, resulting in very high doses to the affected areas.

The first radiation injury related to interventional cardiology occurred in 1990.[16] By September 1994, the United States Food and Drug Administration (FDA) issued a warning to physicians and healthcare providers about occasional but severe radiation injuries in patients undergoing certain fluoroscopically guided interventional procedures.[17] The warning described the nature of these injuries and provided numerous recommendations on how to avoid them. In the years since, hundreds of very serious radiation-induced injuries occurred. Many, but not all, of those recommendations are addressed in this chapter. The complete FDA warning is provided as an appendix at the end of this chapter.

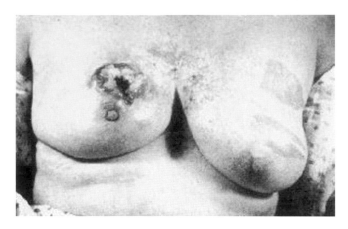

FIGURE 13-1. Breast cancer and skin injuries induced by fluoroscopically guided intervention for pulmonary tuberculosis. *(Adapted with permission from MacKenzie I. Breast cancer following multiple fluoroscopies. Br J Cancer. 1965;19:1-8.)*

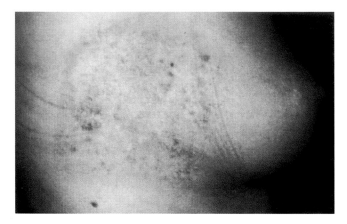

FIGURE 13-2. Skin changes on right side of thorax and breast following two attempts at cardiac ablation procedure in 17-year-old patient. Dose ~11–15 Gy. Patient has difficulty raising right arm. *(Adapted with permission from Vañó E, Arranz L, Sastre JM, et al. Dosimetric and radiation protection considerations based on some cases of patient skin injuries in interventional cardiology. Br J Radiol. 1998;71:510-6.)*

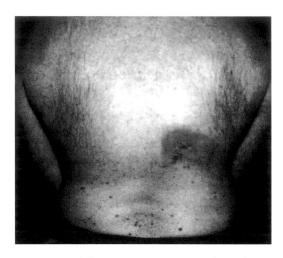

FIGURE 13-3. Injury following percutaneous transluminal coronary angioplasty (PTCA) and stent placement involving 63 minutes of fluoroscopy and nearly 5000 frames of cine. This left anterior oblique (LAO) view with cranial tilt resulted in a large entrance dose build-up in the lower right back. The injury required grafting. *(Adapted with permission from Wagner LK. Radiation dose management in interventional radiology. In: Interventional Brachy Therapy—Fluoroscopically Guided Interventions (American Association of Physicists in Medicine Monograph #28). Balter S, Chan R, Shope T, eds. Medical Physics Publishing, 2002;195–218.)*

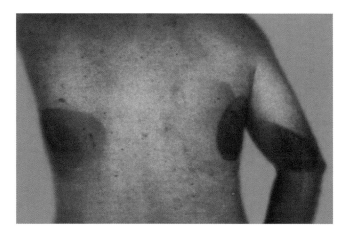

FIGURE 13-4. Injuries from electrophysiologic ablation. This patient had three bi-plane electrophysiologic and ablation procedures within about 4 months, with a cumulative total of 372 minutes of fluoroscopy. The lesions on the back healed, leaving a discolored scarred area. The arm required grafting. *(Adapted with permission from Vlietstra RE, Wagner LK, Koenig T, Mettler F. Radiation burns as a severe complication of fluoroscopically guided cardiological interventions. J Interven Cardiol. 2004;17:131.)*

UNDERSTANDING MEASURES OF RADIATION

No discussion of radiation management is meaningful without an understanding of descriptors used to discuss radiation levels. In particular, a facile understanding and use of the concepts of air kerma, absorbed dose, equivalent dose, and effective dose are essential. Table 13-1 summarizes the relevant quantities.[18]

【 】 ABSORBED DOSE

Absorbed dose is the concept used to assess the potential risk to specific tissues for stochastic and deterministic effects. *Absorbed dose* is the concentration of radiation energy absorbed by a particular tissue. Specifically, as x-rays pass through tissues they interact with the biologic matter, and this transfers energy that causes molecular changes. These changes can potentially lead to biologic effects. Assessing the concentration of energy deposited in the specific tissue provides a measure of the amount of biochemical disruption, and thus a measure of risk for biologic effects. The special unit of absorbed dose is *gray (Gy)*, and 1 Gy is the same as 1 joule of energy concentrated in 1 kilogram of tissue. It is important to emphasize that a gray represents a quantity of radiation, not a dose rate.

【 】 EQUIVALENT DOSE

Equivalent dose is the quantity usually quoted in radiation safety reports for doses to the hands or to the eyes of personnel. *Equivalent*

TABLE 13-1

Relevant Radiation Quantities

QUANTITY	UNITS OF MEASUREMENT	WHAT IT IS	WHAT IT MEASURES	WHY IT IS USEFUL	CONVERSION BETWEEN OLD AND NEW UNITS
Absorbed dose	Gray (Gy) or milligray (mGy) (rad or millirad [mrad])	The amount of energy locally deposited in tissue per unit mass of tissue	Measures concentration of energy deposition in tissue	Assesses the potential biologic risk to that specific tissue	1 rad = 10 mGy
Effective dose	Sievert (Sv) or millisievert (mSv) (rem or millirem [mrem])	An attributed whole-body dose that produces the same whole-person stochastic risk as an absorbed dose to a limited portion of the body	Converts any localized absorbed or equivalent dose to a whole-body risk factor	Permits comparison of risks among several exposed individuals, even though the doses might be delivered to different sets of organs in these individuals	1 rem = 10 mSv
Air kerma[a]	Gray (Gy) or milligray (mGy) (rad or millirad [mrad])	The sum of initial kinetic energies of all charged particles liberated by the x-rays per mass of air	Measures the amount of radiation at a point in space	Assesses the level of hazard at the specified location[b]	1 rad = 10 mGy
Equivalent dose[c]	Sievert (Sv) or millisievert (mSv) (rem or millirem [mrem])	A dose quantity that factors in the relative biologic damage caused by different types of radiations	Provides a relative dose that accounts for increased biologic damage from some types of radiations	The most common unit used to measure radiation risk to specific tissues for radiation protection of personnel[c]	1 rem = 10 mSv

[a]The physician should be aware that air kerma can be presented in two separate ways. *Incident air kerma* is the kerma to air from an incident x-ray beam measured on the central beam axis at the position of the patient and excludes backscattered radiation. *Entrance surface air kerma* is the kerma to air from an incident x-ray beam measured on the central beam axis at the position of the patient with backscattered radiation included. The two may differ from each other by as much as 40%.

[b]Exposure and air kerma are both used for the same purpose. Exposure used to be the most common measure, but with the switch to international units, air kerma is the preferred unit.

[c]For x-rays, gamma rays, and electrons, there is no difference between absorbed dose and equivalent dose (ie, 1 mGy = 1 mSv). This is not the case for neutrons and alpha particles, but these radiation types are not relevant to x-ray exposure. The important issue is that cardiologists recognize that for their interests, there is no practical difference between a measurement of mGy and that of mSv.

Reprinted from Hirshfeld JW, Balter S, Brinker JA, et al. ACCF/AHA/HRS/SCAI clinical competence statement on optimizing patient safety and image quality in fluoroscopically guided invasive cardiovascular procedures: A report of the American College of Cardiology/American Heart Association/American College of Physicians Task Force on Clinical Competence (ACCF/AHA/HRS/SCAI Writing Committee to Develop a Clinical Competence Statement on Fluoroscopy). J Am Coll Cardiol. 2004;44:2259.

dose is an estimate of the biologic potency that a particular radiation might have for an absorbed radiation dose. Equivalent dose is related to absorbed dose, but is also determined by other properties of the absorbed radiation. Thus for radiations other than xrays, equivalent dose can be different even though the absorbed dose is equal to that of x rays. Because cardiologists do not apply other types of radiation during interventional work, this term is of little use other than to communicate radiation safety doses. The unit of measure for this quantity is *sievert (Sv)*. For our purposes in interventional cardiology, 1 Sv is equivalent to 1 Gy. (It should be remembered that this is not true for other specialties, like radiation therapy, where neutron radiation might be used.) Thus, *equivalent dose* is a radiation safety term that, for our purposes, carries the same risk as the absorbed dose in gray.

[ ] EFFECTIVE DOSE

Effective dose is used to relate the potential for stochastic risk from an exposure to radiation, regardless of the spatial non-uniformities of the exposure. For example, interventionalists wear lead aprons to protect themselves. When an interventionalist is exposed in the laboratory, the arms, legs, and head are not as well protected from radiation as are the internal organs under the apron. Therefore, the spatial distribution of the radiation throughout the interventionalist's body is very non-uniform. This is permitted because the exposed limbs and head are not as radiosensitive as the internal organs. The risk associated with such an exposure is, therefore, not well specified by absorbed dose, because low-sensitivity limbs receive a much higher dose than sensitive organs. Effective dose removes this complexity in risk assessment. Effective dose is a hypothetic dose that would have to be delivered uniformly to an interventionalist's entire body in order to yield the same risk for stochastic effects as the non-uniform dose actually delivered. Thus, as a hypothetic uniform whole-body dose, *effective dose* is a risk descriptor that permits us to compare any type of non-uniform exposure to that of any other non-uniform exposure. How effective dose is derived from the non-uniform exposure is complex, and not within the scope of this chapter. (For a more complete description, see the National Council on Radiation Protection and Measurements. Limitation of Exposure to Ionizing Radiation. NCRP Report No. 116, from the National Council on Radiation Protection and Measurements, Bethesda, Maryland, 1993.[19]) The important thing to know is that effective dose allows assessment of stochastic risks from non-uniform dose deliveries. The special unit of effective dose is the sievert (Sv). In cardiology, any effective dose in sievert (Sv or mSv) may be considered the same as a whole-body absorbed dose of uniformly delivered x-rays given in units of gray (Gy or mGy).

[ ] AIR KERMA

The previous terms all relate to absorbed dose and biologic effects. However, it is often necessary to describe how much radiation is present at a specific location. This requires a different descriptor known as *air kerma*. The presence of x rays at any location can be measured by analyzing the ionization they produce in air at that location. Because energy transfer is required to create ions in air, *air kerma* is defined as the concentration of energy released by the x rays in air. The special unit of air kerma is the gray (Gy). One gray of air kerma is the same as 1 joule of energy released in 1 kilogram of air.

[ ] RATES AND ACCUMULATION OF RADIATION

All of the previous dose and kerma descriptors can be assessed as an instantaneously delivered amount, as an amount accumulated over time, or as a delivered rate, as, for example "air kerma rate" in units of milligray per minute (mGy/min). These concepts should be clear in the context of any discussion on dose or kerma.

RADIATION EFFECTS

Health effects of radiation are commonly separated into two categories—stochastic and deterministic.

[ ] STOCHASTIC RISKS

Stochastic effects involve changes in single cells that render them adversely functional. These changes involve alterations of important macromolecules and can conceivably result from a single interaction with radiation. Therefore, these effects can probably occur at any radiation dose level, although they are extremely unlikely to occur at very minimal levels. The two prominent stochastic effects are radiation-induced neoplasm and heritable changes in reproductive cells. The likelihood of their occurring increases as dose increases, and induced cancer becomes measurable in exposed adult populations at doses in excess of about 100 mSv.[20] In children and in the fetus, lower doses have been implicated as carcinogenic.[21]

[ ] DETERMINISTIC RISKS

Deterministic effects are the result of damage to many cells. Examples are skin erythema, depilation, and vision-impairing cataract. Because the effect results from changes in multiple cells, a certain minimal level of radiation insult is necessary before the effect can occur. This is referred to as the *threshold dose*. As dose increases beyond the threshold, the severity of the effect increases. The most familiar example of this is effects in the skin. Table 13-2[22] lists

TABLE 13-2

Threshold Skin Entrance Doses for Different Skin Injuries

EFFECT SINGLE DOSE	THRESHOLD (Gy)	ONSET
Early transient erythema	2	Hours
Main erythema	6	~10 d
Late erythema	15	~6 – 10 wk
Temporary epilation	3	~3 wk
Permanent epilation	7	~3 wk
Dry desquamation	14	~4 wk
Moist desquamation	18	~4 wk
Secondary ulceration	24	>6 wk
Ischemic dermal necrosis	18	>10 wk
Dermal atrophy (1st phase)	10	>14 wk
Dermal atrophy (2nd phase)	10	>1 yr
Induration (invasive fibrosis)	10	a
Telangiectasia	10	>1 yr
Late dermal necrosis	>12?	>1 yr
Skin cancer	Not known	.5 yr

aNo estimate available.

d = day(s); Gy = Gray; wk = week(s); yr = years(s).

Data from Wagner LK, Eifel PJ, Geise RA. Potential biological effects following high x-ray dose interventional procedures. JVIR. 1994;5:71; and personal communication with J.W. Hopewell, 1999.

various effects of large doses to the skin. Note how the severity increases as dose increases. The threshold doses listed in this table are to be regarded as guidelines, and not as well-defined risk barriers. Variations on sensitivities occur for different skin sites, and there are also variations among individuals as a result of, for example, differences in health of the skin, among other factors.[23–25]

TEMPORAL PATTERNS OF RADIATION EFFECTS

For both stochastic effects and for deterministic effects, there is a delay between irradiation and the detection of a change. For malignancies, delays may be as short as 2 years or as long as many decades. For deterministic effects in the skin, the delay is typically many days to weeks before erythema develops, and is likely to be weeks to months before inflammation or necrosis develop. The delays provided in Table 13-2 are relevant to effects occurring following acute threshold doses. Delays vary depending on skin sensitivity, dose level, and rate of accumulation of dose. The transient form of erythema can occur within 24 hours, but this does not always occur and usually goes unnoticed. It may sometimes be confused with erythemas resulting from improperly attached electrosurgic pads.

An important fact is that a fluoroscopy-related "burn" is markedly unlike that of a thermal burn. Thermal insults are readily recognized by conscious individuals and immediate measures can be taken by them to defend against further injury. With medical radiation, there is no sensation that forewarns of an injury; the first signs that an injury was induced do not occur until the procedure has been long over. Therefore, physicians cannot rely on any signal from the patient that a burn is occurring. In addition, and much unlike a fluoroscopy burn, the progression of a thermal burn occurs within a short time after the injury (days), and the extent of medical care necessary for treatment can be readily determined. For a fluoroscopic radiation injury the progression of the injury is slow (months), and early interventions often fail because of residual injury that has yet to manifest itself. Proper radiation management with fluoroscopic equipment therefore requires a knowledgeable application of the radiation and use of effective radiation monitoring devices.

STRATEGIES TO LIMIT EXPOSURE TO RADIATION

There are four basic methods of radiation dose abatement that are applicable for personnel. Time, intensity, distance, and shielding (TIDS) describes management of radiation exposure by minimizing the *time* to which one is exposed to the radiation, by minimizing *intensity* of the radiation that is deployed, by maximizing *distance* from the source, and by *shielding* personnel from the radiation. Personnel assisting in a procedure must know how to limit their exposure to radiation and must apply this knowledge routinely. The physician–fluoroscopist must also know to apply radiation in a conservative manner in order to limit exposures to the patient and to personnel. Quite frequently, the two go hand-in-hand: What is good for the patient is also good for personnel. For example, by realizing that limiting the time that a fluoroscope is activated and by appropriately managing the intensity of the applied radiation, the operator limits radiation in the environment, and this saves exposure to all personnel in the room.

ROOM DESIGN

The primary feature of room design is space. Large rooms (~60 m² with ~15 m² control room) are preferred for many reasons, one of which is radiation management for personnel. Only a large room is conducive to maximal effective use of distance and shielding. Satisfactory space is required at ceiling level for suspended shields. At floor level, space is required for mobile shields that are often used to protect in-room personnel who remain positioned at one station during the procedure. Because dose decreases rapidly with distance, a large room provides the opportunity for personnel to attend to their duties at a healthy distance from the source of radiation, which is primarily the patient, while remaining readily available to attend the patient when necessary.

UNDERSTANDING EQUIPMENT

Cardioangiographic equipment is some of the most sophisticated and complex equipment used in medicine. To effectively perform procedures, at least three essential factors must be in place: (1) The equipment must be properly designed for the procedures; (2) the equipment must be well maintained; and (3) the users must be well trained in the sophisticated use of their specific equipment. Training is related both to the technical aspects for the efficient and effective completion of a procedure and to the proper deployment of available dose-management features. These features differ from machine to machine, and very important differences can exist, even for two machines that appear to be identical. Although we review general principles of operation of equipment, the specific manner of performance of a particular machine must be understood and be used effectively by the users of the equipment.

Fundamental Aspects of Image Production

The fluoroscopy system produces images by generating x-rays that emanate from a point source inside an x-ray tube. The x-rays fan out in all directions from the source, but the housing of the x-ray tube is designed to permit only those that travel toward the patient to escape their enclosure (Figure 13-5).[26] (A small number of x rays do escape the housing, but by regulation at 1 meter, this is

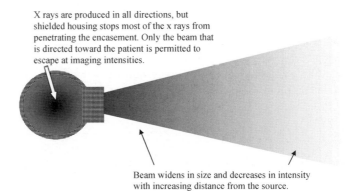

X rays are produced in all directions, but shielded housing stops most of the x rays from penetrating the encasement. Only the beam that is directed toward the patient is permitted to escape at imaging intensities.

Beam widens in size and decreases in intensity with increasing distance from the source.

FIGURE 13-5. X-ray production. X-ray photons are produced from a very small area (~1 mm²) inside the x-ray housing. The housing is shielded to keep radiation levels below those limits by regulation. The beam that emerges from the imaging port is made up of x rays that fan out in a diverging pattern, resulting in a beam that increasingly widens with distance and correspondingly decreases in intensity. *(Adapted with permission from Louis K. Wagner, PhD.)*

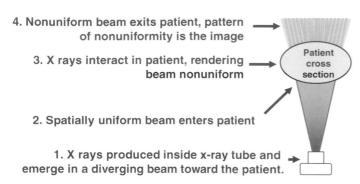

4. Nonuniform beam exits patient, pattern of nonuniformity is the image

3. X rays interact in patient, rendering beam nonuniform

Patient cross section

2. Spatially uniform beam enters patient

1. X rays produced inside x-ray tube and emerge in a diverging beam toward the patient.

FIGURE 13-6. Image production. Demonstrated is how the uniform x-ray beam is transformed into an x-ray image as the beam passes through the patient. *(Adapted with permission from Louis K. Wagner, PhD.)*

less than 1 mGy/hr at maximum continuous operation. The actual leakage is typically much less than this.)

X-ray radiations are individual particles of pure energy called *photons*. They travel at the speed of light and their path is a straight line, unless they interact with something in their way. Interaction is critical to the imaging process. Figure 13-6[26] shows that a beam of evenly distributed x rays enters the patient. There is no effective pattern to the xray beam at this point. As the beam passes through the patient, many of the x rays interact with atoms and molecules of the tissues. This interaction either removes them or redirects them away from their place in the beam. Interactions of other photons continue until there emerges from the patient a residual beam of undisturbed x-rays. At this point, because of the interactions that previously took place, the beam is now very non-uniform, and this non-uniformity is the x-ray image. Only a very small percentage (<1%) of the original beam makes it through to exit the typical adult patient.

Not all x-rays are the same; and, in fact, the x-ray beam is initially composed of a mix of useful and useless x-rays. The energy of an x-ray determines its usefulness because the energy determines the interaction processes that create the image. Only a small portion of the x-rays that are produced are appropriate for cardiologic procedures. The two major factors that control the energy characteristics of the x-ray beam are kVp and filtration. The kVp is the electric potential that determines the energies of the x rays. The filtration is composed of thin sheets of materials like aluminum or copper that selectively remove unnecessary x rays from the beam. Filtration occurs when the x-ray beam escapes through the x-ray-tube portal. The goal is to produce an x-ray beam that results in an excellent compromise between appropriate image quality and radiation dose. Some equipment does this better than others.

Filters

Filters are simple, small sheets of thin metal, usually copper or aluminum, that are placed at the port of an x-ray tube and through which the x-ray beam must pass. In passing through the filters, a good portion of the poorly penetrating, useless, low-energy x-rays are removed from the beam. Unfortunately, a smaller portion of the useful x rays is also removed. The result is an x-ray beam with a better mix of x-ray energies, but at a much-reduced intensity. To compensate for the reduced intensity, the x-ray tube must operate at higher production rates, and this stresses the tube. Manufacturers

therefore put a great deal of consideration into tube design so that tubes can withstand or circumvent the stress of well-filtered x-ray production. Some x-ray tubes are better engineered than others, and inevitably, good engineering adds to cost.

In addition to permanent filtration that is typically equivalent to about 3 mm of aluminum, all angiocardiologic equipment should use x-ray tubes with heavily filtered x-ray sources. An option of filters should be available, typically in tenths of millimeters of copper (eg, 0.1 mm, 0.2 mm, 0.3 mm). How the filters are used may differ among different machines and manufacturers. Many manufacturers incorporate filters into different dose-management schemes selectable by the user. The particular filter incorporated into a procedure is often decided by the dose-management option selected by the user, and is also based on the mass of tissue that the beam must penetrate for imaging. Typically, the thickest filters are reserved for small patients, whereas the thinnest filters are used on the largest patients. During cine fluorography, because high beam intensities are required for short exposure times, only thin filters are used. The user should specify at purchase that filtration options be available for equipment, and the user should understand what operational actions might affect the use of filters during a procedure.

Variable Pulsed Fluoroscopy

The dynamics of fluoroscopic and cinecardioangiographic imaging are familiar to many. The perception of motion is achieved by displaying in rapid succession a sequence of distinct still images, each of which represents the same scene at a progressively different moment in time. Each static image is separated from the previous image by a very short moment. The fidelity of the motion improves with shorter time intervals between images. This principle is applied to fluoroscopy as well as to cine.

Continuous motion is perceived by most people when about 30 images per second are displayed to mimic the motion. This rate has been a standard in the United States for the entertainment industry. However, in cardiology the goal is not to entertain, but to use the imaging system as a tool to advance a catheter along a lumen or to place a catheter tip at a specific node inside a ventricle. To accomplish these tasks, the necessary number of distinct images captured per second is variable. This is true for fluoroscopy as well as for such serial imaging as digital angiographic runs or cinefluorography. Choosing an adequately low-image capture rate is one of the most effective user-selectable ways to limit utilization of radiation.

In fluoroscopy, the image capture rate is often referred to as the *pulse rate*. For serial imaging, it is often called the frame rate. In all modern cardiology units, each fluoroscopic image is captured using a very short pulse of radiation (~3–10 ms). (The use of short pulses is necessary to stop the action in each image. Longer pulses would result in significant motion blur.) Each pulse of x-rays results in one image, and the pulse rate is therefore identical to the image capture rate. Between pulses, no radiation is produced. If 30 images are captured per second, fluidity in motion is perceived, but the radiation utilization might be excessive for the task. If the pulse rate is reduced to 15 images per second, the motion might no longer appear completely fluid, but it is likely adequate for the task, and the radiation utilization is potentially reduced by 50%. For interventional procedures, a reduction in dose by 50% is substantial and could mean the difference between a severe skin reaction and no skin reaction for long procedures in large patients. For this reason, cardiologists should use the lowest pulse rate option for both fluoroscopy and for any fluorography (serial imaging such as digital angiography or cine) that is adequate for the efficient and effective completion of a procedure. (A word of caution: Not all machines are set up for dose-reduction options when changing the pulse rates in fluoroscopy. Users must be well trained for their specific equipment to understand what occurs when different fluoroscopic pulse rate options are used.)

Dose-Rate Control

At the heart of all radiologic imaging tasks is the challenge to reach the best compromise in radiation dose delivery and image quality. Dose-rate control is achieved in many ways as, for example, by adjusting pulse frequency, pulse width, tube current (mA), x-ray beam energy (kVp), and filtration, only some of which are under the operator's control. Selecting a lower pulse rate, as described earlier, is a method of operator-based dose-rate control. However, that method affects the temporal image display and has only an indirect effect on the appearance of noise. The effects of noise are demonstrated in Figure 13-7. Pulse width, tube current (mA), x-ray beam energy (kVp), and filtration have a more direct effect on the noise characteristics of each image because they affect the radiation level that produces the image.

Most cardioangiographic machines, if not all, are designed to operate in different noise control modes. The temptation might be to use the dose-rate mode that produces the least noise, but this is inevitably the mode that results in the highest dose rate. The challenge to the cardiologist is to select the dose-rate mode that draws the most appropriate compromise between dose to the patient and adequate, but not excessive, image quality.

There are frequently at least two types of dose-rate controls. The first type provides a selection of dose rates, none of which allow the unit to exceed standard limits on fluoroscopy output. The other type is an option that allows the unit to operate at up to twice the standard limit, and sometimes more. These are explained next.

Standard-Limit Dose-Rate Options. The FDA places legal restrictions on the manufacture of fluoroscopes. For example, for angiographic equipment, the maximum output of the radiation in the standard fluoroscopic mode is restricted to less than 87.6 mGy air kerma per minute when tested at 30 cm from the image receptor. Standard dose-rate options that are selectable by the user all operate within this range. However, in a low dose-rate option, the output would be less than that of a mid-level dose-rate option. The mid-level dose rate should be less than an upper-level option. Cardiologists should familiarize themselves with these options and understand the consequences of each selection with regard to changes in dose rate as well as image quality. Select the option that provides the best balance between imaging needs and radiation use. Regardless of which level is selected, the output will not exceed the standard maximum.

High-Level Fluoroscopy. The FDA allows machines to be manufactured with a high-dose-rate option for fluoroscopy. This is a

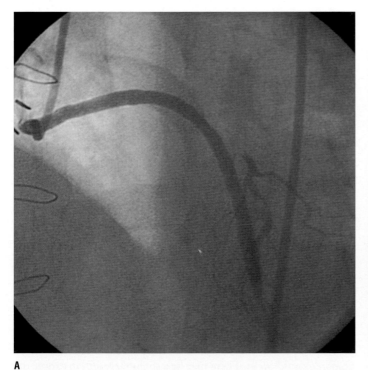
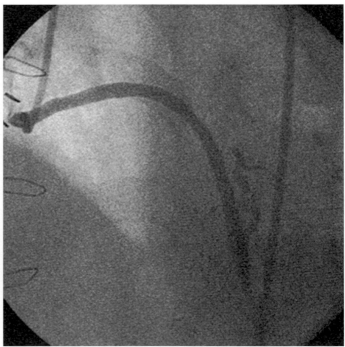

A   **B**

FIGURE 13-7. Simulation of the effects of dose rate on image noise. (**A**) The effects of the higher dose rate in reducing image noise. (**B**) An increase in noise and a decrease in image quality with lower dose rate. It is not possible to demonstrate the fact that the increased noise can be acceptable for the procedure because the noise is less apparent when the display is dynamic. The challenge for the physician is to limit the dose rate to that necessary to safely and efficiently complete the procedure. (*Adapted with permission from Louis K. Wagner, PhD.*)

particularly important option to understand because it can result in dangerously high radiation dose rates to patients. For this option, a special means of selection must be available and a special sound must warn the operator that the high-level mode is engaged. Sometimes this sound is barely audible to the user. Users therefore must be aware of this mode and know when it is engaged.

In machines manufactured before mid-1995, this option had no restrictions with regard to radiation output. In some cases machines were capable of exceeding dose rates of 2 Gy per minute to the patient. Such rates are dangerous and have been implicated in severe injuries to some patients.

Units manufactured after mid-1995 can still have a high-level option, but output is restricted to less than twice the standard maximum rate for fluoroscopy. This option can still result in dose rates in excess of 0.4 Gy per minute under some configurations of use. High-level control must be used on an infrequent basis when special imaging detail is momentarily necessary.

A Word About Governmental Regulation and Radiation Output.

One of the most common errors of logic is to assume that regulatory restrictions on radiation output render fluoroscopes safe for virtually unrestricted use. This is most certainly not true. In the United States, many are familiar with the concept that regulation restricts the standard output of a fluoroscopy unit to less than 87.6 mGy air kerma per minute and to less than 175 mGy per minute in high-level mode. This information alone is extremely misleading. The regulations apply only to a standard testing configuration that places the entrance skin surface at 30 cm from the face of the image receptor for angiographic devices. It also excludes the effects of scattered radiation in elevating the actual rates. Under normal cardioangiographic beam orientations, the skin of the patient where the beam enters is frequently much further away from the image intensifier, placing the patient closer to the source than what is assumed for compliance testing. This frequently means that the entrance air kerma at the true skin position can be in excess of 40% greater than that at the compliance testing position. The effects of scatter mean that an entrance air kerma rate renders an actual skin-dose rate that is another 30%–40% greater. The combined results of these two factors mean that the actual dose rates to the skin can be a factor of 2 or more higher than the regulatory air kerma limit, which means more than 175 mGy per minute in the standard mode and more than 350 mGy per minute in the high-level mode (for machines manufactured after mid-1995). At maximum rate, a necrosing skin injury can occur in 100 minutes of standard fluoroscopy on-time, and this does not take into account the additional dose from cine.

The same logic applies to cine output rates. The rates for standard testing are often quoted at the compliance testing point. Maximum cine air kerma rates in many systems can well exceed 1000 mGy per minute at the compliance point. The actual dose rate to the skin of the patient can be well in excess of 2000 mGy per minute. For twenty 6-sec cine runs, the skin dose from cine alone could be 4 Gy (4000 mGy). Under these circumstances, a procedure involving 80 minutes of fluoroscopy and twenty 6-sec cine runs focused over the same area could result in a skin necrosis. This is exactly what has occurred in many cases for which necrotic skin injury has been reported (eg, Figure 13-3).

PHYSICIAN–OPERATOR STRATEGIES TO LIMIT RADIATION RISK TO THE PATIENT

The important question now becomes, "So, what can I do about it?" There are many options the physician can decide among to limit radiation risk. Most essential is that the physician be properly trained and experienced enough for the procedure and for dose management. Inexperienced personnel typically use more radiation to complete a procedure than do veterans. The expeditious completion of a procedure is a primary factor in the conservative use of radiation.

Radiation management of the patient has three phases: before, during, and after the procedure.

【 】 BEFORE THE PROCEDURE

The first phase of patient management involves an assessment of the radiation risk for the patient. Small adult patients are at low risk for skin injury because of their size. Many factors work in their favor: image quality is usually high, radiation output rates are at their lowest, and good geometry is usually easier to achieve. Large patients with difficult lesions that require highly oblique beam orientations are at greatest risk for the opposite reasons.

Facilities should assess their procedures and decide under which conditions patient counseling on radiation risk should take place. This depends on the type of procedure, the size of the patient, the number of lesions, and perhaps on the anticipated difficulty in treating the lesions. A history of a previous interventional procedure should prompt a brief physical examination of the patient's skin, particularly the back, to determine if there might be some residual evidence of radiation effects. A previous procedure might result in a weakened skin structure that could elevate the risk of serious skin effects from additional irradiation. If residual effects are noted, the cardiologist can try to avoid the injured site, and should advise the patient of this increased risk. In addition, patients with certain diseases, patients taking medications, or patients receiving treatments for other problems may be at elevated risk for adverse and perhaps severe skin reactions. It is thought, for instance, that patients with connective tissue disease, such as discoid lupus erythematosis, scleroderma, mixed connective tissue disease, or perhaps even rheumatoid arthritis, can be at elevated risk depending on factors related to their disease at the time of the radiation exposure.[23] Patients with diabetes mellitus are also suspected to be at higher risk.[24] Patients homozygous for ataxia telangiectasia and patients with Fanconi's anemia, among other conditions, are known to be at high risk.[25]

As an example of counseling, a facility might decide that all patients undergoing electrophysiologic ablation should be counseled for radiation risks. The following is an example of counseling: "An electrophysologic ablation procedure uses x-rays, and in some cases, exposure can be prolonged. Although the vast majority of procedures do not demonstrate any adverse consequences associated with the radiation, there is a small risk that an adverse response could occur. There may be a slight elevation in cancer risk associated with this exposure. In addition, there is a risk that a skin rash may result from the radiation exposure. There is a very small risk that severe skin effects may occur, resulting in blistering, ulceration, and sores. These extremely rare events may require surgical correction."

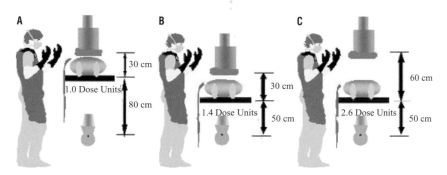

FIGURE 13-8. Dose rate and position of the x-ray tube and the image receptor. (**A**) The physician performs the procedure with the patient table elevated and the image intensifier close to the patient (total distance from the X-ray tube to the detector = 110 cm). In the center, the physician uses a lower table setting, but maintains the image intensifier close to the patient's chest (total distance from the x-ray tube to the detector = 80 cm). Because of the closer proximity to the x-ray tube, the dose rate to the patient at the beam entrance port is about 40% higher. (**B**) The physician uses a low table height but has elevated the image intensifier (total distance from the x-ray tube to the detector = 110 cm). The skin dose to the patient on the right is 260% that of the patient on the left. (The image generated by the configuration on the right is 40–50% larger because of geometric magnification caused by the elevated image intensifier.) If the procedure in (**A**) required a 3-Gy skin dose, the same procedure using the (**B**) configuration would result in a 4.2 Gy dose, whereas the procedure performed using the configuration in (**c**) would result in 7.8 Gy. (Adapted with permission from Wagner LK, Archer, BR. Minimizing Risks from Fluoroscopic X-rays, 4th ed. Partners in Radiation Management, Ltd., Co. 2004.)

〖 〗 DURING THE PROCEDURE

Besides using equipment-related factors of good radiation management, including minimizing fluoroscopy time and intensity and limiting the number and rate of serial imaging frames, other highly effective strategies can be used. These include considerations regarding beam orientation and patient set up, monitoring of dose, and a more subtle factor of avoiding the presence of unnecessary body parts in the beam.

The Importance of Positioning

Figure 13-8[26] demonstrates how dose rate to the patient can change with simple changes in the position of the patient relative to the image receptor and the x-ray tube. This occurs because the x-ray source originates in a diverging pattern from a small spot inside the x-ray tube. As with heat from a match, the radiation intensity increases rapidly as one gets closer to the source, and serious injury becomes more likely with closer proximities. Dose rates are properly managed by the application of two simple guidelines: (1) keep the entrance site of the patient's skin at a maximum practicable distance from the x-ray source; and (2) keep the image receptor as close as practicable to the skin where the beam exits the patient. The first rule avoids the high intensities of the beam associated with its diverging characteristic, and the second rule reduces the radiation output rate necessary to produce sufficient radiation at the input of the image receptor. The dose rate at the skin of the patient in Figure 13-8A is about 40% less than that in Figure 13-8B and 160% less than that of Figure 13-8C. These percentage differences translate into very large dose savings when procedures are prolonged.

The Ramifications of Patient Size and Beam Orientation

Large patients are inevitably the patients at greatest risk for skin injury. Their size generates a large amount of image-degrading scatter that reduces contrast. Because of their size, a high-energy beam must be used to penetrate the body mass adequately, reducing contrast even further. Beam pulse time might increase, which leads to motion blur. These imaging difficulties are obstacles that lead to an increase in procedure time. Also, as we discuss later, large size alone means that radiation output is markedly increased over that of a thin patient. When lesions prove difficult to treat, doses can be extremely high.

X-rays are a poorly penetrating radiation. As previously noted, less than 1% of the x-rays entering an average-size patient (~23-cm thick mediastinum) actually emerge from the patient to make an image. For large patients (~30-cm thick mediastinum), this percentage reduces to less than 0.3%. To compensate for this reduced penetration, large patients require entrance dose rates considerably greater than average or thin patients.

The patient-related factor most influential in determining how much radiation must be used to render a proper image is the mass of tissue that must be penetrated between the positions where the beam enters to where it emerges from the patient. Oblique and cranially or caudally tilted beam orientations result in the thickest tissue mass, and require markedly higher outputs than do simple posteroanterior orientations. Not only must the machine generate radiation at a higher rate to penetrate the mass, the geometry of the situation inevitably places the skin of the patient closer to the source, the combined effects of which greatly increase dose rate to the skin. This is demonstrated in Figure 13-9.[26] A necrotic injury resulted from 63 min of fluoroscopy and more than 5000 frames of cine in this gentleman, who has an unusually large chest. The thick body mass of the chest coupled with the oblique and cranially tilted beam resulted in high radiation dose rates to the skin and the rectangular skin injury. When doses are high and procedures prolonged, the physician may consider rotating the beam to a slightly different location so that a different skin area is irradiated.

The Ramifications of Extraneous Body Parts

We have just seen that thick patients are more difficult to manage for good reasons. Sometimes, extraneous body parts like the breasts and arms intercept the beam. This should be avoided because they increase the amount of tissue mass that the beam must penetrate. This drives up dose rates, reduces image quality, and places those tissues at elevated risks.

The young female breast (≤40 years of age) is known to be at substantively elevated risk for induced breast cancer; with older women there is less risk. Working diligently to keep the breasts out of the direct x-ray beam is a worthwhile task and has two potential advantages. By keeping extra tissue away from the beam, dose rates are lower, and by keeping breasts away from the direct beam, the dose to the glandular tissue is maintained at markedly lower levels. This is especially important for the breast in closest proximity to the x-ray source. For this breast, dose accumulations can be very substantive.

Arms in the direct beam are a known hazard. Figure 13-4 demonstrates injuries to arms during cardiologic procedures. Figure 13-10

Thick Oblique vs Thin PA geometry

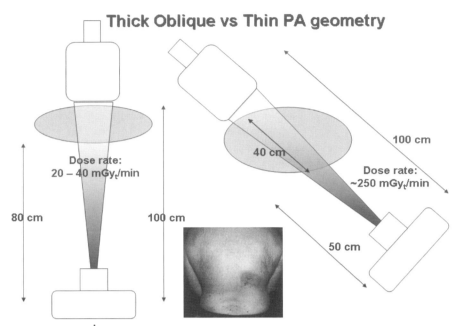

FIGURE 13-9. The problem of steep beam angles in large patients. Dose rates to the entrance skin surface are highest for oblique and cranially or caudally tilted beams in large patients, such as the one shown. This not only poses the difficulty of penetrating a very large mass of tissue, but it also forces the skin of the patient to be in closer proximity to the x-ray source, where the beam is more intense. The injury shown resulted in necrosis and involved 63 minutes of fluoroscopy and nearly 5000 frames of cine. *(Adapted with permission from Wagner LK, Archer, BR. Minimizing Risks from Fluoroscopic X-rays, 4th ed. Partners in Radiation Management, Ltd., Co. 2004 and Wagner LK. Radiation dose management in interventional radiology. In: Interventional Brachy Therapy—Fluoroscopically Guided Interventions (American Association of Physicists in Medicine Monograph #28), Balter S, Chan R, Shope T, eds. Medical Physics Publishing, 2002;195–218.)*

demonstrates the geometry of this procedure, along with a picture of a second case of arm injury. Efforts must be made to manage arms in a manner that is comfortable to the patient (maintaining good circulation) and that keeps them away from the direct path of the beam. This applies to both arms. Although the arm that is on the exit side of the beam receives only an exit dose, its presence adds tissue mass to the radiation path, thus driving up output and dose rate to the entrance skin site. The arm on the x-ray tube side is at greatest risk because it not only drives up output, it also experiences the more intense beam because of its proximity to the diverging x-ray source.

Monitoring Dose

Almost all modern cardioangiographic equipment has built-in monitors to help assess dose delivered to the patient. Even if no dose monitoring equipment is built-in, simple external and easy-to-use methods are available. Monitoring radiation doses to patients has many advantages. It provides useful information on the radiation risks to your patients from your procedures; it provides highly effective quality improvement data; and it can be applicable during a prolonged procedure, when dose build-up can be substantial, making it possible to take dose abatement steps, if necessary.

There are three main types of monitors—film-like monitors, monitors to measure cumulated air kerma at a standard point in the imaging system, and cumulated kerma-area product (KAP) monitors (also known as *dose-area product monitors,* or *DAP meters*).

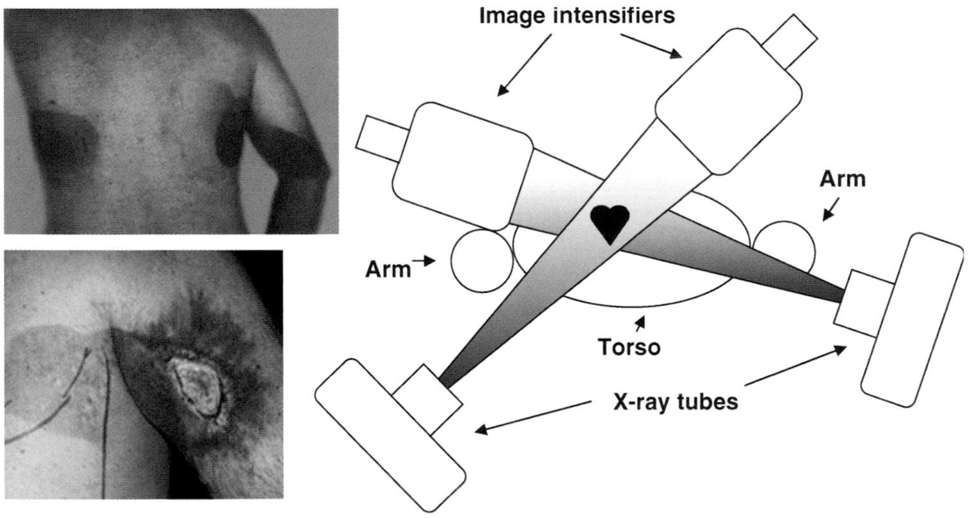

Film-Like Monitors. Figures 13-11 and 13-12 demonstrate use of a film-like monitor. The film is self-processing and is not readily sensitive to visible light. However, as x-rays pass through the film, the film turns darker. It is made of a low-density material and does not affect the radiation output in any adverse way, nor is it visible in the image. The film darkness is a direct measure of the radiation dose to the skin of the patient. The film is simply placed on the table under the patient in the general area where the beam enters. It can be used to assess dose during or after a procedure. In critically long procedures, if dose build-up is a concern, the film can be pulled out and examined to determine the potential skin dose. A simple measuring device is used to assess the darkness of the film, and this translates into dose. More generally, the "film" is examined after the procedure and the dose recorded in the patient's record and then entered into

FIGURE 13-10. Demonstration of arms subtending x-ray beam close the x-ray source. Two cases of injury to the right arm for separate patients undergoing fluoroscopically guided ablation procedures for arrhythmias. The diagram depicts a bi-plane fluoroscopic configuration illustrating how arms inadvertently placed in the x-ray beam can be seriously injured. *(Image in lower left reproduced with permission from Wong L, Rehm J. Radiation injury from a fluoroscopic procedure. N Engl J Med. 2004;350(25):e23. Copyright © 2004 Massachusetts Medical Society; all rights reserved. Image in the upper left reproduced with permission from Vlietstra RE, Wagner LK, Koenig T, Mettler F. Radiation burns as a severe complication of fluoroscopically guided cardiological interventions. J Interven Cardiol. (Blackwell Publishing) 2004;17:131-142. Diagram reproduced with permission from Wagner LK, Archer, BR. Minimizing Risks from Fluoroscopic X-rays, 4th ed. Partners in Radiation Management, Ltd., Co., The Woodlands, Texas, 2004.)*

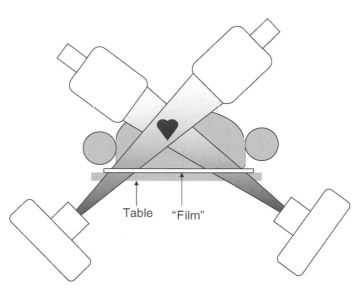

FIGURE 13-11. Demonstration of the use of a film-like dose monitor. The "film" inside a protective envelope lies flat on the table with the patient on top. The beam is directed from beneath the patient and must pass through the film before entering the patient. An example of an exposed film demonstrating the locations of the different x-ray beams and their collimation. *(Adapted with permission from Wagner LK, Archer, BR. Minimizing Risks from Fluoroscopic X-rays, 4th ed. Partners in Radiation Management, Ltd., Co. 2004)* (See also Figure 13-12.)

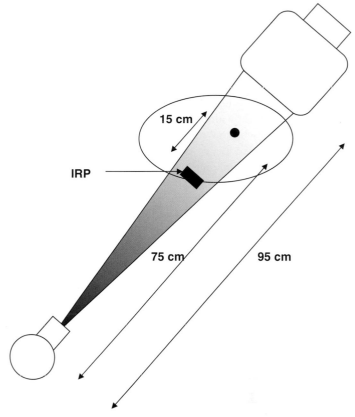

FIGURE 13-13. Location of the interventional reference point. This point is located along a line from the x-ray source to the image receptor and 15 cm from the isocenter of the C-arm in a direction toward the x-ray tube. As the C-arm is rotated, the interventional reference point (IRP) rotates with it. Although the IRP is representative of the entrance skin site, for some beam orientations and patient positions it is located a distance from the actual skin site. Thus the cumulative dose at the IRP might over- or underestimate the true cumulative skin dose. This dose reference must therefore be used with discretion to guide patient care, and not as an absolute measure of risk to the skin. *(Adapted with permission from Hirshfeld JW, Balter S. Barinker JA, et al. ACCF/AHA/HRS/SCAI clinical competence statement on optimizing patient safety and image quality in fluoroscopically guided invasive cardiovascular procedures: A report of the American College of Cardiology/American Heart Association/American College of Physicians Task Force on Clinical Competence (ACCF/AHA/HRS/SCAI Writing Committee to Develop a Clinical Competence Statement on Fluoroscopy). (J Am Coll Cardiol. 2004;44:2259.)*

the quality control log for evaluation at a future date. This very simple technique has the advantage that the dose recorded is a true skin dose because it records the dose at the skin site. It also demonstrates nicely the effect of collimation and beam reorientation on the dose. No other external monitor provides more useful and more easily obtained information. Its disadvantage is that its utility is restricted to posterior beams. It is more difficult to use with lateral beam projections or for overhead orientation of the source.

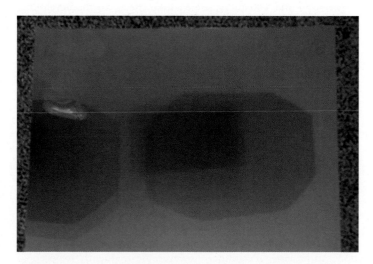

FIGURE 13-12. An exposed dosimetry film. The darkness of the exposed areas is proportional to the dose. A simple calibration film can be used for comparison to determine the skin dose delivered. Thus during a prolonged procedure the film could be removed to assess the skin dose and determine the benefit–risk of continuing the procedure. (International Specialty Products, Wayne, New Jersey.)

Cumulated Air Kerma at the Interventional Reference Point. Most modern machines have a built-in device that monitors the total accumulation of air kerma at a reference point. The interventional reference point is located 15 cm from isocenter along a line between the x-ray source and the isocenter of the C-arm (Figure 13-13). (The *isocenter* is the point in space about which the imaging system rotates, and an object at that point remains in the center of the image regardless of beam rotation.) The interventional reference point (IRP) approximates the position of the skin where the beam enters the patient. Figure 13-13 demonstrates this reference point. This measure of cumulated air kerma is highly useful as a quality control device and as a guide to manage procedures. Because it measures only the accumulation of air kerma, three things must be kept in mind when using it. First, as an accumulation monitor, it adds up the radiation from all beam orientations.

This results in overestimation of radiation dose to a single skin site. However, at any one skin site, the actual skin dose is about 40% greater than the cumulated entrance air kerma. Finally, the reference point is only an approximation of the position of the skin, and the true entry site might be closer to or further away from the x-ray tube. An appropriate judgment must be rendered as to whether the reference reading over- or underestimates the dose. Regardless of these difficulties, dose at the interventional reference point is a highly useful tool to assist the physician in patient skin-dose management and quality control.

For example, guidelines might be established to assist the physician. It might be useful, for example, to establish a 2-4-6-8 rule for management. If the reference accumulation air kerma reaches 2 Gy, then the physician is advised that dose is building and that this is an "FYI" so that the physician knows the pace of radiation build up. At 4 Gy, the physician is advised again and now knows that the threshold of erythema might be reached if the beam is not reoriented soon and if the IRP is inside the skin surface. At 6 Gy, the potential is higher, if and actions to abate the risk might be an important consideration. At 8 Gy, the risk of skin injury is considerable, especially if there was no beam reorientation earlier and the same skin site is being dosed. The purpose of this is to assist the physician in making the appropriate benefit–risk decisions for the patient, and in managing the patient after the procedure.

Kerma-Area Product and Dose-Area Product Meters. A full discussion of a kerma-area product (KAP) meter is beyond the scope of this chapter. KAP is the product of the air kerma at a position in space and the area of the beam at that position. With distance from the source, beam area naturally increases and air kerma naturally decreases in an identically compensating manner. The product of these two entities is, therefore, theoretically the same at all positions along the unobstructed accessible beam. It is primarily a quality control tool and is not a very useful monitor of dose to the skin of a patient, although that task is possible. A medical physicist is usually employed in any attempts to use such a device for management of skin doses to patients.

[ ] AFTER THE PROCEDURE

After a prolonged procedure in which the skin dose may have been high, the patient should be counseled about the complexity of the procedure and that a skin reaction could develop there within the next few weeks. The patient should be told the approximate location where this might occur, and to report any skin reaction to the physician's office. This information has many advantages. The first is that the patient is not surprised if it occurs. The second is that you now have feedback that your procedure did result in a reaction, and you can assess how frequently this occurs. You can use this knowledge to take any appropriate action to reduce this. The final advantage is that you can recommend that the patient see a dermatologist and the physician can call the dermatologist to let them know that the skin reaction might be due to x-ray radiation from the patient's previous cardioangiographic procedure. The dermatologist can then determine if the location is correct will not be puzzled by the rare event or by its delayed progression should it get worse.

Dose to the skin of the patient should also be recorded in the patient's record. This was recommended by the FDA in 1994[17] (see

Appendix). The information necessary to make a proper measure of skin dose is discussed next.

Recording of dose

Recording of skin dose and the location of the principally exposed area in the patient's chart has several benefits. The first is that dose can be reviewed when additional procedures are required. It could also become important if the patient requires radiation treatment at a later date. Each facility should decide for which types of procedures dose will be recorded. (See FDA guidelines in the Appendix.)

[ ] THE PREGNANT PATIENT

Periodically, a woman who is pregnant may require a cardiologic procedure. Pregnancy should not be considered an absolute contraindication for any needed cardiologic study. Dose to a baby from a cardiologic procedure can usually be well managed so as to avoid any radiation levels that would significantly place the conceptus at risk. For example, direct irradiation of the pelvis results in the most direct dose to an early pregnancy. However, in many cases, irradiation of the pelvis can either be completely avoided or be kept to a very short interval. When examining the cardiac system, the area of the beam should be collimated to the area of interest. The only radiation reaching the conceptus is scattered radiation that must penetrate many centimeters of the patient's abdomen before reaching the conceptus and is much reduced in intensity from that of the primary beam. For a conceptus more than 10 cm from the primary beam, this dose is less than 2% of the entrance skin dose. Typically, it is much less than this. A cumulative entrance skin dose of more, and usually much more, than 2.5 Gy would have to be delivered before dose to the conceptus would approach 50 mGy. At doses under 50 mGy, the only suspected risk to the child is a possibility of induced neoplasia. The risk for a 10-mGy dose is thought to be about 1 mortality in 1000 cases, and overall less than 4 cases of induced neoplasia.[21] The threshold dose for malformation is estimated at 100 mGy, but the magnitude and the likelihood depend on gestation age. Between 50 and 100 mGy, some subtle effects on the developing central nervous system might occur if development is between 8 and 15 weeks postconception. A complete discussion of these risks is beyond the scope of this chapter, and the reader is referred to other texts for a complete discussion.[25,27] Therefore, in evaluating a pregnant patient for a procedure, a benefit–risk decision is necessary. Well-executed dose-management practices can keep the potential risks to levels very acceptable in comparison to the benefits.

PERSONNEL SAFETY

One adage of good radiation management is, "What's good for the patient is usually very good for personnel." Patients are very infrequently exposed to radiation, but their doses during one intervention can be large. Personnel, however, are frequently exposed to radiation, but at low levels. Economic use of radiation in the patient helps circumvent unnecessary long-term build-up of high radiation doses to personnel. Therefore, practicing good radiation management for the patient has the added benefit of a safer working environment for personnel.

【 】 TIME

Previously we noted the importance of limiting beam-on time for the patient. This has the added benefit of also limiting exposure time for personnel.

To further reduce exposure time to personnel, only those who must be in the room with the patient should be there, and only when their services are needed. Otherwise, personnel should limit their time of exposure to radiation by leaving the procedure room or by remaining behind a fixed radiation barrier.

【 】 INTENSITY

This safety measure relates to the management of the intensity of radiation delivered to the patient as previously described for both fluoroscopy and for fluorography (cine and digital runoffs).

Another aspect relates to a savvy understanding of how radiation is distributed in the room. Figure 13-14 demonstrates how radiation is distributed in an interventional environment when the C-arm is in a left anterior oblique (LAO) orientation. Scattered radiation (also called *stray radiation*) results from interactions of x-rays with matter. From this, it follows that stray radiation is most intense closest to sites where the most interactions occur, which is always the site where the x-ray beam enters the patient. Generally speaking, stray radiation emanates in all directions from the site of interaction, but because of the patient's body, the scatter distribution around the patient is very lopsided, as shown in Figures 13-14A and 13-14B. At the exit surface of the patient the beam is markedly reduced in intensity (by about

a factor of 100 in most adult patients), and thus stray radiation from this site is much lower than that from the entrance site. At intermediate points around the patient from the entry site to the exit site, the stray intensity changes from its maximum to its minimum. Thus, personnel positioned near the entry site of the patient (near the x-ray tube) experience the most intense exposure to stray radiation, whereas those on the correspondingly opposite side experience the least. This is why the x-ray systems are usually oriented with the x-ray tube under the patient and the image receptor over the patient. In this orientation, the intense scatter off the posterior aspect of a supine patient is directed primarily at the floor. The scatter emanating from the anterior surface of an adult is much less, saving considerable radiation exposure to the face and hands. With the C-arm oriented in an LAO position with cranial tilt, the intense scatter field is directed at the feet and legs of personnel standing to the right of the supine patient. Thus, the legs and feet of cardiologists are at considerable risk to accumulate very large doses of radiation after years of work.

Figure 13-14A and 13-14B apply only to the LAO orientation. The distribution of stray radiation changes with different orientations. What workers must remember is that stray radiation is most intense on the side where the beam enters the patient and least intense on the opposite side where it exits the patient.

A Note on Equipment Design

There is a perceptually misleading circumstance for the worker who is on the exit side of the beam when the beam is oriented in a lateral manner. The individual near the image receptor can see the port of

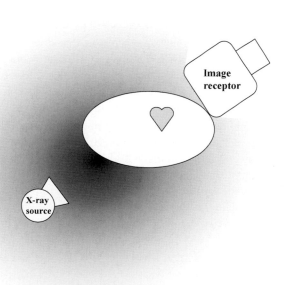

A

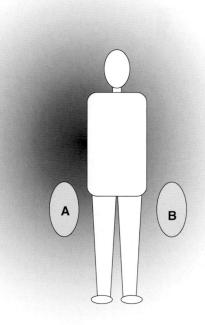

B

FIGURE 13-14. Depiction of stray radiation intensities from a patient in an interventional environment for a left anterior oblique beam orientation. (**A**) Patterns around the cross-section of the patient. (**B**) Patterns as viewed from above the patient. These patterns apply only to this orientation. In other orientations an analogous pattern is produced, with the greatest intensity emanating from the skin area where the beam enters. A person standing at position A receives about three times more radiation than a person at position B.

the x-ray tube and the collimator housing. Logically, the concern is that they are standing in the direct path of the x-ray beam. This should not be the case, and some simple tests, as listed next, can be applied to make sure that there is no direct beam exposing them.

1. The FDA requires that the x-ray beam that emerges from the x-ray port be directed at and confined to the area of the image receptor, regardless of any operating configuration. This should be verified by a medical physicist when the quality control survey is performed.

2. It is easy to verify that the beam is confined to the image receptor. Simply manipulate the collimators to assure that the edges of the blades are visible as shadows in the imaging field. If the collimators are visible in the image, the beam is confined to that area and must be inside the area of the image receptor.

3. By federal regulation, the image receptor is housed in a shielded container, and the small amount of radiation scattered through the shield is nearly unmeasurable. This can be verified by a medical physicist.

4. The x-ray tube and collimator housings are also well-shielded and well-regulated devices. These can be tested by a medical physicist.

【 】 DISTANCE

The use of distance to reduce radiation exposure is extremely effective. Commonly referred to as the *inverse square law,* radiation levels decrease rapidly with increasing distance from the source. Specifically, with each doubling of distance from the patient, scatter decreases by about a factor of 4. So, if you are standing at about 1 m from the patient, taking a 1-m step backward decreases the unshielded intensity by about a factor of 4. The working rule of thumb that "One should work at a practicable maximum distance from the irradiated area of the patient while in the room" is one that serves everyone well.

【 】 SHIELDING

Shielding materials are abundantly available. Generally speaking, shielding is any material that absorbs or deflect a substantial portion of the x-rays that strike it. Many forms of shielding are available and include lead aprons, leaded eyewear, thyroid shields, hanging shields to protect the upper body, floor shields or tableside shields to protect the legs, stand-up mobile barriers to protect the entire body, and flexible shields that are draped on the patient to stop scatter at its source. There is further shielding in the walls, ceiling, and floors to protect people outside the room. Regarding the use of shields, the following are some guidelines:

1. Verify that there is sufficient shielding in the walls, floor, and ceiling to protect people who are outside the room. In 1 full year, no secretary, clerk, or other member of the public should receive more than 1 mSv effective dose from man-made radiation.

2. Radiation levels behind the barrier of a control booth should not exceed 5 mSv per year.

3. Barriers suspended from the ceiling, the table, or standing on the floor should be a minimum of 0.5-mm of lead equivalent (ie, equivalent to the same protection provided by 0.5 mm of lead). Some shields are equivalent to 1.0 mm of lead or more.

4. Barriers suspended from the ceiling must be readily accessible and should be designed so as to block radiation from the oval contour of the patient. This can be achieved with a drape or by purchasing a specially contoured hard shield. Flexible shields that lie over the patient might also be useful to reduce scatter.

5. Protective eyewear is optional in most cases. Eyewear should be equivalent to about 0.5 mm of lead (and usually are much more) and should fully cover the eyes, wrapping around the sides to cover the entire eye. Goggles that also provide splash protection should be considered. Standard glasses are not satisfactory for this purpose.

6. Thyroid shields are an option. They should be comfortable to wear. (The adult thyroid of the average person is not a highly radiosensitive organ, but protection is always recommended as a precaution.)

7. Lead aprons must be comfortable. Many states require by regulation that they be 0.5-mm lead equivalent in the front. This blocks about 95% of the radiation. Protection should wrap around the sides. Rear torso protection of at least 0.15-mm is also recommended for personnel working in close proximity to the patient and for personnel who might have to work with their backs sometimes toward the patient. Support belts that distribute the weight between the shoulders and hips are recommended, and a two-piece blouse-plus-skirt design is preferred by some.

8. Radiation monitors must be worn at all times during procedures to measure the amount of radiation incident on personnel. Some regulatory bodies require that the monitor be worn under the lead apron, whereas others require that it be outside the lead apron, and some require that two monitors be worn, one under the apron and one outside. These varying points of view often confuse workers and are the result of a conflict on the need to monitor for safety versus the need to monitor as a matter of regulatory mandate. For safety purposes, I recommend that one monitor be worn outside the lead apron near the collar and on the side of the body that is closest to the x-ray source. This adequately monitors the exposure to the unprotected areas of the head and neck and provides sufficient information to assure adequate safety measures can be taken when necessary. The dose under a 0.5-mm lead equivalent apron is about 5% of that dose. My goal for heavy users of radiation is that the annual readings not exceed 50 mSv. I never recommend that only one under-the-apron monitor be worn because this renders a false sense of security and ignores potentially high doses to important unprotected body parts.

9. Cardiologists should consider monitoring, periodically at least for several months, the doses to their legs and hands. This is achieved by attaching a monitor to the pant leg and a ring badge to the dominantly exposed finger. This provides important information on the adequacy or inadequacy of protection for these areas. Extra shielding, or better attention to using the shielding, should be considered if doses to these sites exceed 50 mSv in 1 year.

【 】 THE PREGNANT EMPLOYEE

Radiation exposure to an employee who is or might become pregnant must be managed so as to adequately protect the conceptus while not interfering with the individual's ability to execute her duties. To do this, I recommend that preparations for pregnancy be taken before any employee becomes pregnant, and that certain actions be taken once her pregnancy becomes known.

Preferably, before or at the commencement of employment, the worker should be advised of policies regarding radiation and pregnancy. This should be conducted for both men and women so that all employees are familiar with the policies. It must be made clear that extra protective measures cannot be initiated until the radiation safety staff is apprised of a pregnancy. It is therefore incumbent on the employee to advise the radiation safety officer (RSO), preferably in writing, when she first becomes aware of her pregnancy. Her options regarding safe practices can then be reviewed and extra precautions initiated.

I recommend that all female employees of childbearing potential who are required to have a whole-body dosimeter also be provided a specially marked "belly badge" dosimeter. The special marking helps ensure that the badges do not get confused. Although the whole-body badge should be worn at the collar outside the lead apron, the belly badge should be worn under all protective devices at the level of the belt. The readings of these badges should be reviewed by the radiation safety officer to assure that they do not exceed 0.25 mGy per month. This limit assures that any would-be conceptus would receive less than half that of the maximum recommended by professional agencies (recommended maximum dose to the conceptus is 0.5 mGy per month).[19] If the readings do exceed 0.25 mGy, action should be taken to determine the cause and corrective measures should be initiated.

Once an employee advises the RSO that she is pregnant, the following should be considered:

1. Review the belly badge history. This should demonstrate that current practices are sufficient to protect the baby. If not, corrective actions are necessary.

2. Provide the employee with the option of wearing an additional pelvic shield. This could be as simple as a small lap apron that can be 0.25 or 0.5 mm of lead equivalent material. This further reduces any potential exposure to the child.

3. Continue to provide the belly badge and switch it to monthly readouts if the present exchange is bimonthly. In some cases, employees might also want to wear a real-time dose monitor under their protective apron. This provides daily feedback about the radiation exposure under the apron, rather than having to wait for the badge report at monthly intervals.

4. Provide the employee with duties involving less exposure to radiation, if necessary.

CONCLUSION

Radiation can be both friend and foe. To remain a friend, it must be treated with respect. Developing respectful habits that appropriately protect patient and personnel is the goal of all radiation management training.

REFERENCES

1. Mackenzie I. Breast cancer following multiple fluoroscopies. *Br J Cancer.* 1965;19:1.

2. Vañó E, Arranz L, Sastre JM, et al. Dosimetric and radiation protection considerations based on some cases of patient skin injuries in interventional cardiology. *Br J Radiol.* 1998;71:510.

3. Wagner LK. Radiation dose management in interventional radiology. In: *Interventional Brachy Therapy—Fluoroscopically Guided Interventions* (American Association of Physicists in Medicine Monograph #28), Balter S., Chan R., Shope T., eds. Medical Physics Publishing, 2002;195.

4. Vlietstra RE, Wagner LK, Koenig T, Mettler F. Radiation burns as a severe complication of fluoroscopically guided cardiological interventions. *J Interven Cardiol.* 2004;17:131.

5. International Commission on Radiological Protection. Avoidance of radiation injuries from medical interventional procedures. ICRP Publication 85. *Ann ICRP.* 2000;30:7.

6. Koenig TR, Wolff D, Mettler FA, Wagner LK. Skin injuries from fluoroscopically guided procedures. Part 1: Characteristics of radiation injury. *Am J Roentgenol.* 2001;177:3.

7. Koenig TR, Mettler FA, Wagner LK. Skin injuries from fluoroscopically guided procedures. Part 2: Review of 73 cases and recommendations for minimizing dose delivered to the patient. *Am J Roentgenol.* 2001;177:13.

8. Mettler FA Jr, Koenig TR, Wagner LK, Kelsey CA. Radiation injuries after fluoroscopic procedures. *Semin Ultrasound CT MR.* 2002;23(5):428.

9. Wong L, Rehm J. Images in clinical medicine: radiation injury from a fluoroscopic procedure. *N Engl J Med.* 2004;350:e23.

10. Matanoski GM, Sartwell P, Elliott E, et al. Cancer risks in radiologists and radiation workers. In: Boice JD, Fraumeni JF Jr (eds.), *Radiation Carcinogenesis: Epidemiology and Biological Significance.* Raven Press. 1984:83.

11. Vañó E, Gonzalez L, Beneytez F, Moreno F. Lens injuries induced by occupational exposure in nonoptimized interventional radiology laboratories. *Br J Cancer.* 1998;71:728.

12. Kassabian MK. *Röntgen Rays and Electro-Therapeutics with Chapters on Radium and Phototherapy,* 2nd ed. JB Lippincott Company, 1910.

13. Yoshinaga S, Mabuchi K, Sigurdson, AJ, Doody MM, Ron E. Cancer risks among radiologists and radiologic technologists: Review of epidemiologic studies. *Radiology.* 2004;233:313.

14. Wagner LK. Overconfidence, overexposure, and overprotection. Editorial. *Radiology.* 2004;233:307.

15. Interventional radiology carries occupational risk for cataracts. *RSNA News,* June 2004.

16. Shope TB. Radiation-induced skin injuries from fluoroscopy. *RadioGraphics.* 1996;16:1195.

17. United States Food and Drug Administration. *Public Health Advisory: Avoidance of serious x-ray-induced skin injuries to patients during fluoroscopically-guided procedures.* Center for Devices and Radiological Health, 1994.

18. Hirshfeld JW, Balter S, Brinker JA, et al. ACCF/AHA/HRS/SCAI clinical competence statement on optimizing patient safety and image quality in fluoroscopically guided invasive cardiovascular procedures: A report of the American College of Cardiology/American Heart Association/American College of Physicians Task Force on Clinical Competence (ACCF/AHA/HRS/SCAI Writing Committee to Develop a Clinical Competence Statement on Fluoroscopy). *J Am Coll Cardiol.* 2004;44:2259.

19. National Council on Radiation Protection and Measurements. *Limitation of Exposure to Ionizing Radiation.* NCRP Report No. 116. National Council on Radiation Protection and Measurements, 1993.

20. Pierce DA, Preston DL. Radiation-related cancer risks at low doses among atomic bomb survivors. *Radiat Res.* 2000;154:178.

21. National Academy of Sciences. *Biological Effects of Ionizing Radiations (BEIR VII).* In press.

22. Wagner LK, Eifel PJ, Geise RA. Potential biological effects following high x-ray dose interventional procedures. *JVIR.* 1994;5:71.

23. Wagner LK, McNeese MD, Marx MV, Siegel EL. Severe skin reactions from interventional fluoroscopy: case report and review of the literature. *Radiology.* 1999;213:773.

24. Herold DM, Hanlon AL, Hanks GE. Diabetes mellitus: a predictor for late radiation morbidity. *Int J Radiat Oncol Biol Phys.* 1999;43:475.

25. Hall EJ. *Radiobiology for the Radiologist,* 5th ed. Lippincott, Williams & Wilkins, 2000:178.

26. Wagner LK, Archer, BR. *Minimizing Risks from Fluoroscopic X-rays,* 4th ed. Partners in Radiation Management, Ltd., Co. 2004.

27. Wagner LK, Lester RG, Saldana LR. *Exposure of the Pregnant Patient to Diagnostic Radiations: A Guide to Medical Management,* 2nd ed. Medical Physics Publishers, 1997:93.

28. Annals of the International Commission on Radiological Protection. *Pregnancy and Medical Radiation.* Pergamon, 2000.

29. Balter S. *Interventional Fluoroscopy: Physics, Technology, Safety.* Wiley-Liss, 2001.

APPENDIX 13-1

Avoidance of Serious X-Ray-Induced Skin Injuries to Patients During Fluoroscopically Guided Procedures

Warning: FDA has reports of occasional but at times severe radiation-induced burns to patients from fluoroscopically guided, invasive procedures. This communication describes the nature of these injuries and provides recommendations for avoiding them.

Procedures Resulting in Injuries

An increasing number of invasive procedures, primarily therapeutic in nature and involving use of devices under fluoroscopic guidance, are becoming accepted medical practice. Examples of such procedures are listed in Table 13A-1. These procedures are performed by a variety of medical specialists and may provide significant advantages over alternative therapies in terms of improved clinical outcome and reduced overall patient risk. *However, physicians performing these procedures should be aware of the potential for serious radiation-induced skin injury caused by long periods of fluoroscopy occurring with some of these procedures.* Such injuries have recently been reported as a result of radiation exposure during some of these procedures[1-3] due to long fluoroscopic exposure times, high dose rates or both.

Types of Injuries

The types of injuries to skin and adjacent tissues which result from x-ray radiation are summarized in Table 13A-2 along with the typical absorbed dose in the skin required to produce the injury. (See below for a discussion of radiation quantities and units.) Each of these injuries has recently been observed as a result of fluoroscopically guided procedures. These "threshold doses" are typical of the absorbed dose in skin required to cause the effect, since appearance of the injury is dependent on a number of variables other than the cumulative dose in the skin, such as: the rate of delivery of the radiation; the fractionation of the absorbed dose; the age and characteristics of the person exposed; and the site on the skin of the exposure.

Absorbed Doses to Skin from Fluoroscopy

The absorbed dose rate in the skin from the direct beam of a fluoroscopic x-ray system is typically between 0.02 and 0.05 Gy/min (2 and 5 rad/min), but may range from 0.01 to more than 0.5 Gy/min, depending on the mode in which the fluoroscopic equipment is operated and the size of the patient. The times required to deliver the typical "threshold doses" shown in Table 13A-2 are for fluoroscopic dose rates of 0.02 Gy/min (third column) and 0.2 Gy/min (fourth column) in that portion of the skin irradiated by a *stationary*, continuous fluoroscopic x-ray beam. These dose rates are, respectively, the usual or typical dose rate for normal fluoroscopy for an average-size patient and a dose rate near the maximum which will be permitted for high-level control mode of operation under a recently established Federal limit.[5-7] *Thus, even typical dose rates can result in skin injury after less than one hour of fluoroscopy.* For comparison, the absorbed dose to the skin from a typical diagnostic x-ray examination is hundreds to thousands of times smaller than the threshold doses for skin injuries given in Table 13A-2.

It should be noted that many fluoroscopic x-ray systems used for invasive procedures have modes of operation which result in dose rates which significantly exceed the usual dose rate of 0.02 Gy/min used as an example in Table 13A-2. Many systems currently in use are capable of dose rates which are higher than 0.2 Gy/min. In addition, many fluoroscopically guided procedures involve image recording (fluorography) using film or digital means to permanently record images. *The recording modes typically involve much higher dose rates than fluoroscopy and the contributions from fluorography must also be included in assessing total absorbed dose to the skin.* Fluoroscopic systems which are improperly adjusted or have dose rates increased to compensate for degraded performance can also result in unnecessarily high absorbed dose and consequent injury from very long exposure times.

Other Risks

Procedures of the type described here may also increase the risk for late effects such as radiation-induced cancers in other tissues and organs. The potential for such late effects should not be disregarded in risk/benefit considerations, especially for individuals with many decades of expected life remaining, such as pediatric and young adult patients, or for procedures involving absorbed dose to radiosensitive tissues such as the breast. These interventional procedures can also result in increased occupational exposure to physicians and staff, and efforts to reduce the exposure to patients will result in reductions in the exposure to those conducting the procedures.

TABLE 13A-1

Procedures Typically Involving Extended Fluoroscopic Exposure Time

Radiofrequency cardiac catheter ablation
Percutaneous transluminal angioplasty (coronary and other vessels)
Vascular embolization
Stent and filter placement
Thrombolytic and fibrinolytic procedures
Percutaneous transhepatic cholangiography
Endoscopic retrograde cholangiopancreatography
Transjugular intrahepatic portosystemic shunt
Percutaneous nephrostomy, biliary drainage or urinary/biliary stone removal

From Food and Drug Administration. Important Information for Physicians and Other Health Care Professionals September 9, 1994.

TABLE 13A-2

Radiation-Induced Skin Injuries

EFFECT	TYPICAL THRESHOLD ABSORBED DOSE (Gy)*	HOURS OF FLUORO. "ON TIME" TO REACH THRESHOLD+ AT:		TIME TO ONSET OF EFFECT++
		USUAL FLUORO. DOSE RATE OF 0.02 Gy/min (2 rad/min)	HIGH-LEVEL DOSE RATE OF 0.2 Gy/min (20 rad/min)	
Early transient erythema	2	1.7	0.17	hours
Temporary epilation	3	2.5	0.25	3 wk
Main erythema	6	5.0	0.50	10 d
Permanent epilation	7	5.8	0.58	3 wk
Dry desquamation	10	8.3	0.83	4 wk
Invasive fibrosis	10	8.3	0.83	
Dermal atrophy	11	9.2	0.92	>14 wk
Telangiectasis	12	10.0	1.00	>52 wk
Moist desquamation	15	12.5	1.25	4 wk
Late erythema	15	12.5	1.25	6–10 wk
Dermal necrosis	18	15.0	1.50	>10 wk
Secondary ulceration	20	16.7	1.67	>6 wk

*The unit for absorbed dose is the gray (Gy) in the International System of Units. One Gy is equivalent to 100 rad in the traditional system of radiation units. Fluoro. = fluoroscopic.

+Time required to deliver the typical threshold dose at the specified dose rate.

++Time after single irradiation to observation of effect.

Table adapted from Ref. 4.

Delayed Symptoms

Complicating the assessment of the magnitude of the problem of injuries from fluoroscopy is the fact that the injuries are not immediately apparent. Typical times to onset or appearance of the effect are given in Table 13A-2. Other than the mildest symptoms, such as transient erythema, the effects of the radiation may not appear until weeks following the exposure. Physicians performing these procedures may not be in direct contact with the patients following the procedure and may not observe the symptoms when they occur. Missing the milder symptoms in some patients can lead to surprise at the magnitude of the absorbed doses delivered to the skin of other patients when more serious symptoms appear. For this reason, it is recommended that information be recorded in the patient's record which permits estimation of the absorbed dose to the skin. This is especially important for patients who may receive a significant fraction of a threshold dose, such as from an hour of fluoroscopy or from a large number of recorded images, or who may be subject to repeated treatments using fluoroscopy. Consideration should be given to counseling such patients on the possible symptoms and risks from these procedures.

Because of these concerns and reported injuries, the following advice is provided for physicians performing fluoroscopically guided procedures. The goal is to avoid such injuries without adversely affecting the clinical objectives of the procedure.

General Principles and Recommendations for Facilities in which Invasive Procedures are Performed

1. Establish standard operating procedures and clinical protocols for each specific type of procedure performed. The protocols should address all aspects of the procedure such as patient selection, normal conduct of the procedure, actions in response to complications and consideration of limits on fluoroscopy exposure time.

   • Include all fluoroscopic system modes of operation used, including image recording.

   • Strive for clinically adequate images with minimum fluoroscopic exposure.

   • Assure appropriate credentials and training for physicians performing fluoroscopy.

   • Minimize exposure duration.

   • Collimate the radiation beam.

   • Communicate and enforce protocols.

2. Know the radiation dose rates for the specific fluoroscopic system and for each mode of operation used during the clinical protocol.

   • All operators of the system must be trained and understand system operation, including the implications for radiation exposure from each mode of operation.

- Have a quality assurance program for the x-ray system supervised by a qualified medical physicist.
- Calibrate and document radiation output.
- Record information permitting estimation of the absorbed dose to skin in the patient's medical record.

3. Assess the impact of each procedure's protocol on the potential for radiation injury to the patient.

- Facilities should ensure that physicians performing fluoroscopic procedures have education so they may, on a case-by-case basis, assess risks and benefits for individual patients, considering variables such as age, beam location and direction, tissues in the beam and previous fluoroscopic procedures or radiation therapy.
- Counsel patients regarding the symptoms and risks of large radiation exposures and address risks from radiation in the consent form.
- Justify and limit the use of high dose rate modes of operation.

4. Modify the protocol, as appropriate, to limit the cumulative absorbed dose to any irradiated area of skin to the minimum necessary for the clinical tasks, and particularly to avoid approaching cumulative doses that would induce unacceptable adverse effects. Use equipment which aids in minimizing absorbed dose with such features as:

- Indication of cumulative fluoroscopic exposure time.
- Indication of cumulative absorbed dose to the skin or a related quantity such as dosearea product.
- Real-time indication of dose rate or related quantity.
- "Last image hold" or "freeze frame" image display.
- Optimum beam filtration, removable grids, variable optical aperture, and radiation efficient automatic brightness control algorithms.

5. Enlist a qualified medical physicist to assist in implementing these principles in such a manner as not to adversely affect the clinical objectives of the procedure.

Reporting Requirements

Healthcare practitioners who are aware of fluoroscopy or radiation related deaths or injuries are asked to notify FDA. The Safe Medical Devices Act of 1990 (SMDA) requires hospitals and other facilities to report death, serious illness and serious injury associ-ated with the use of medical devices. The reporting procedures established by each medical facility to comply with the mandatory reporting requirements should be used. Practitioners who become aware of any medical device related adverse event or product problem/malfunction should inform their designated Medical Device User Facility reporter. To reinforce the point that second degree burns requiring medical treatment, along with other serious injuries, resulting from use of a medical device are reportable under the SMDA, the FDA is considering a proposal to make this requirement explicit in the medical device user facility reporting regulations. FDA encourages these reports now. In addition, any issues concerning the quality or performance of a medical device can be reported directly to the MedWatch program. Anonymous reports are accepted. Please submit your reports to MedWatch, the Medical Product Reporting Program, by phone at 1-800-FDA-1088 (you may also use this number to request MedWatch information); by FAX at 1-800-FDA-0178; by modem at 1-800-FDA-7737; or by mail to MedWatch, HF-2, Food and Drug Administration, 5600 Fishers Lane, Rockville, MD 20857.

Radiation Quantities and Units

The quantity which is used to assess the energy deposited in tissue from radiation is absorbed dose. In the current International System the unit of absorbed dose is the joule/kilogram with the special name of gray (Gy) (in honor of the radiobiologist L. H. Gray). An absorbed dose of one Gy is 100 times the magnitude of the older unit of absorbed dose, the rad. Thus, a dose rate to skin of 0.02 Gy/min is equivalent to 2 rad/min.

REFERENCES

1. Food and Drug Administration Mandatory Device Reporting System. Report Nos. 241641, 275018, 275019, 298419, 298423, 487999.
2. Private communication, LG Smith, May 16, 1994.
3. Davidson County Circuit Court, Nashville, Tennessee. Case No. 93C-1916, 1993.
4. Wagner LK, Eifel PJ, Geise RA. Potential Biological Effects Following High X-ray Dose Interventional Procedures. *J Vas Interv Rad* 1994; 5:71.
5. National Council on Radiation Protection and Measurements. Quality assurance for diagnostic imaging equipment. NCRP Report No. 99, Bethesda, MD, 1988.
6. American College of Radiology. Proceedings of the ACR/FDA Workshop on Fluoroscopy: Strategies for Improvement in Performance, Radiation Safety and Control, October 16, 17, 1992, Washington, DC.
7. FEDERAL REGISTER, Vol. 59, No. 96. May 19, 1994, p 26402.

CHAPTER (14)

General Principles of Coronary Artery Brachytherapy

Paul E. Wallner, DO, and Peter Bloch, PhD

In-stent restenosis (ISR) following coronary angioplasty and stenting is a particularly thorny problem for interventional cardiology. Treatment with conventional balloon dilation is plagued by unsatisfactory rates of recurrent stenosis. The mechanisms and incidence of restenosis following coronary artery angioplasty alone, or subsequent to angioplasty with percutaneous stent placement, have been well described.[1-3] As the use of coronary angioplasty has increased, the incidence of ISR has increased concomitantly.

Numerous interventions have been investigated in attempts to reduce the frequency of ISR, but none was highly effective until the introduction of a variety of radiation (brachytherapy) techniques. Initial interest in these techniques was prompted by a presumption that the pathogenesis of postangioplasty ISR had features in common with the development of keloids in the skin.

Shortly after the introduction of radium brachytherapy and external beam radiation for the management of cancer in the early 1900s, anecdotal reports described the secondary effects of radiation on wound healing. In the 1940s and more recently, a body of literature described a variety of radiation techniques in the management of benign keloids and the general impact of radiation on wound healing.[4-6] External radiation beams or intersititial implants of radioactive sources, known as *brachytherapy*, were explored. Brachytherapy technique limits the radiation dose to tissues close to the implant. The core concept was that the biologic effect of radiation would impair the normal healing response activation of fibroblastic activity within the radiated segment. Mature keloids contain relatively few fibroblasts in an admixture of dense and disorganized hyalinized collagen fibers. Prophylactic radiation was found to be quite effective in preventing or delaying keloid recurrence after removal, but also caused delayed normal wound healing.

In the early 1990s, investigators began to consider the analogies between postangioplasty/stent placement ISR, wound healing, and keloid formation, especially as related to the neointimal proliferation responsible for ISR, and reports began to appear from studies in animal models using external beam and brachytherapy radiation to suppress postangioplasty/stent placement neointimal proliferation and remodeling.[7-11] After the first intracoronary study in humans was reported by Candado and coworkers in 1997,[12] remarkable interest in the modality was generated.

TERMINOLOGY

A variety of terminology has been used for radiation therapy to the coronary arteries, including

- Coronary artery radiation therapy (CART)
- Coronary radiation therapy (CRT)
- Vascular brachytherapy (VBT)
- Endovascular brachytherapy (EVB)
- Intravascular brachytherapy (IVB)
- Intracoronary artery brachytherapy (IAB)

For precision and consistency, the term *coronary artery radiation therapy (CART)* is used for this discussion.

PHYSICAL AND BIOLOGIC PRINCIPLES

The interaction of radiation in tissue results in both direct ionization and production of chemically reactive radicals. If the ion track traverses a DNA molecule within the intimal subendothelial space surrounding the vessel wall, a single or double strand break may occur that would inhibit mitosis and, thus, neointimal proliferation. The chemical radicals can also produce lesions within the DNA.

The precise mechanism of radiation-related retardation of restenosis remains uncertain, but other factors have been described. Injury to the adventitial microvasculature with subsequent angiogenesis may be produced by balloon dilatation of a coronary artery. It is known that radiation may exert an antiangiogenic effect and, therefore, an antiproliferative effect.[23] It has also been postulated that the radiation target may be migrating adventitial fibroblasts or proliferating smooth muscle cells in the media and adventitia with the development of radiation-induced apoptosis.[21–23]

The success of brachytherapy is critically dependant on the magnitude of the delivered radiation dose. Either too small or too large a dose will have a detrimental rather than a beneficial effect. The theory for calculating dosimetry for planar and volume interstitial implants of radioactive sources has been developed extensively and used for cancer therapy.[13] Various configurations of the radioactive sources have been used clinically to obtain the desired dose distribution within the target volume of tissue. The dosimetry for intravascular brachytherapy is different because usually only a single point or line radioactive source is used to deliver a radiation dose to the vessel wall. However, the vessel wall may be very near the radioactive source (<1 mm), whereas for cancer therapy the dose to tissue is typically prescribed for a planar implant or for a single linear radioactive implant 5–10 mm from the target tissue. The prescription point for a volume implant may differ between radiation oncologists; however, it is always greater than 5 mm from any source.

An extensive review of dosimetry calculations for intravascular brachytherapy is contained in Task Group Report No. 60 prepared by the Radiation Therapy Committee of the American Association of Physicist in Medicine.[14] The reader is referred to this report for a thorough discussion of the history, available equipment, dosimetric characteristics, quality assurance and safety of intravascular brachytherapy. This discussion is limited to some of the unique aspects of the dosimetry of intravascular brachytherapy as it relates to interpreting the clinical outcome.

In CART, the short distance between the radioactive source and the vessel wall results in large dose gradients near the sources that lead to technical difficulties in performing accurate measurements. However, analytical and Monte-Carlo calculations of the dose distribution at mm distances from various radioactive sources such as ^{192}Ir (Iridium), ^{125}I (Iodine), ^{103}Pd (Palladium), ^{32}P (Phosphorus), and ^{90}Sr (Strontium) have been used and verified by linear extrapolation from measurements at greater distances (5–10 mm) from the source.[13,15,16]

The steep dose gradients are primarily associated with geometric fall-off of dose with distance from the source. Geometric dose gradients occur for both gamma and beta radiation sources; however, because of the different tissue-penetrating properties of beta and gamma rays, the dose gradients for beta radiation are considerably steeper than for gamma radiation. As discussed later, this property confers both advantages and shortcomings. The large dose gradient surrounding the source creates a particular compli-

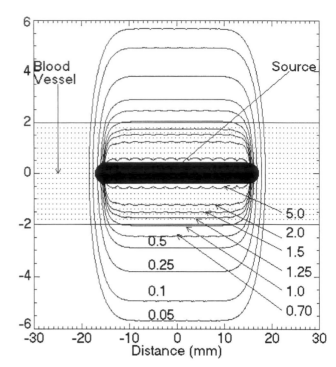

FIGURE 14-1. Calculated dose distribution about a 30-mm long ^{90}Sr source train centered in a coronary artery 4 mm in diameter. The dose is normalized at the prescription point at the center of the source train 0.1 mm from the vessel wall.

cation in the dosimetry of CART implants if eccentric placement of the source in the lumen of the vessel occurs. Figure 14-1 demonstrates the calculated dose distribution surrounding a catheter centered in the lumen containing a beta source train consisting of 12 ^{90}Sr seeds, each 2.5 mm in length. The dose was normalized to the prescription point at the center of the implant and 0.1 mm outside the vessel wall. The calculations were performed using a Monte Carlo–derived dose deposition kernel for a single ^{90}Sr seed.[17,18] When the source train was offset 0.5 mm from the center of the lumen the calculated dose (Figure 14-2) to one wall of the vessel was 0.7 times lower than the prescribed dose for a centered source and 1.5 times higher to the opposite wall. Eccentric placement of the source train thus results in nonuniform irradiation of the vessel wall during intravascular brachytherapy.

In CART, the region of interest for radiation represents the thin arterial wall consisting of intima, media, and adventitia. This target may be, at most, several millimeters from the artery lumen. These short distances and other factors—the steep dose gradients of various types of radiation sources, impact of low energy secondary radiation, complicated effects of specific source, applicator, and stent design, and complicated issues of patient geometry (eg, plaque thickness and vessel curvature)—have engendered significant discussion and opinion.

The debate regarding the relative advantages of gamma versus beta radiation has also been heated. Gamma radiation can provide improved penetration and reduce dose perturbations. Beta radiation enables the safe delivery of large doses to confined volumes, with an important advantage both in the achievable dose rate and the safety of operating personnel. In clinical practice, the differences remain uncertain.[19] CART following percutaneous transluminal

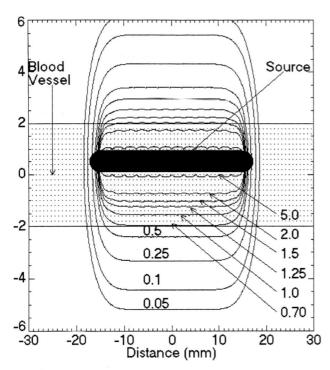

FIGURE 14-2. Calculated dose distribution for the source train in Figure 14-1 that is offset 0.5 mm from the center of the blood vessel.

coronary angioplasty (PTCA) of occluded and previously stented coronary arteries has also been shown clinically to inhibit restenoses without special care to center the source in the lumen.

A core radiation therapy principle for cancer is that all of the diseased tissue should be uniformly irradiated to a high dose. However, a uniform dose to the vessel wall is not required to inhibit restenosis. Therefore, the principles of vascular brachytherapy require some modification from the principles of radiation oncology.

DELIVERY SYSTEMS AND TECHNICAL CONSIDERATIONS

A variety of radiation delivery techniques have been explored that do not achieve high rates of clinical success or commercial viability. These include radioactive stents, external beam radiation, and radioactive liquid–filled balloons.[24] Although three systems that use sealed radioactive sources for delivery of CART ultimately received FDA approval and were commercialized in the United States, only one continues to be marketed. Clinical results with these systems are reported elsewhere in this text.

The systems differ in the three basic functional CART components:
- Storage/transport/delivery device (STD).
- Radioactive source.
- Delivery catheter design.

Various factors that differentiate the systems have an impact on their clinical efficacy and, therefore, drive user selection. Some of these variables include
- Required source dwell (treatment) time.
- Attendant personnel exposure.
- Dose uniformity and distribution.
- Ease of handling.
- Presence or absence of source-centering catheters.
- Source replacement.

BETA RADIATION SYSTEMS

The Beta-Cath 3.5-Fr System (Best Vascular, Springfield, VA, USA) uses a combination radioactive source of ^{90}Strontium/^{90}Yttrium with a principal beta particle radioactive decay scheme. The maximum beta particle energy emitted by ^{90}Sr and ^{90}Y are 0.55 and 2.27 MeV (million electron volts), respectively. The maximum range of the beta particle from the decay of ^{90}Y is 11 mm in tissues and much less for the lower-energy beta particles from the decay of ^{90}Sr. The dose to tissues at a distance beyond the range of the beta particles is negligible. In addition, the beta system produces no significant exposure to personnel in the catheterization laboratory when the source is covered with a material having a thickness greater than the range of the beta particle, which is approximately 11 mm of water or 1 mm of lead. Because of relatively low shielding requirements for beta-emitting isotopes, the STD device is lightweight and hand-held. The radioactive sources are supplied as seeds, and delivery of the source train through the mono-Rail Delivery Catheter is by hand-applied hydraulic pressure. Currently available source-train lengths are 30 mm (12 sealed sources) and 40 mm (16 sealed sources). As with all available systems, the catheters are closed-end and designed for single use, and the mono-Rail Delivery Catheter passes through a guide catheter with an internal diameter of 7-Fr or more. The catheters are guidewire compatible ($\leq$0.014 in.), and an open-lumen guide wire traverses the distal segment. The catheter has a 135-cm working length. Current dose recommendations are to deliver 18.4 Gy to lesions on arteries with reference vessel diameter (RVD) of between 2.7 and 3.35 mm, and a greater dose of 23.0 Gy to lesions on larger-diameter vessels with RVD of more than 3.35 but no larger than 4.0 mm. The delivery catheter is not designed for source centering. Inactive radiopaque markers within the delivery catheter and at either end of the source train facilitate catheter and source positioning. The principal advantage conferred by the short path length of the beta radiation is that the source can be made safely at a very high specific activity level. This minimizes the necessary dwell time needed to deliver the therapeutic dose.

Typical treatment times average approximately 3–4 min. The half-life of the radiation source nucleides is sufficiently long that a source has sufficient activity to be clinically useful for more than a month.

The GALILEO Intravascular Radiotherapy System (Abbott Vascular, Redwood City, CA, USA) is no longer marketed but used a pure beta-particle source consisting of Phosphorus 32 (^{32}P), which has a half-life of 14.3 days and emits a maximum energy beta particle of 0.69 MeV. The STD device is automated for dosimetry dwell time and source delivery/withdrawal, and a helical balloon is designed to center and stabilize the source wire. Catheters are currently available in 2.5, 3.0, and 3.5 mm diameters with radiopaque markers to facilitate positioning. Usable length of the catheter is 145 cm, and the diameter is compatible with a 7-Fr or larger guiding catheter. This source similarly has sufficient activity to permit treatment times averaging approximately 4 min. The source similarly has a shelf life of approximately 1 month.

GAMMA RADIATION SYSTEMS

The CHECKMATE Intravascular Brachytherapy System (Cordis Corp., Miami, FL, USA) is no longer marketed but used radioactive Iridium 192 (^{192}Ir) with a half-life of 73.83 days. The energies of the gamma rays emitted by ^{192}Ir are between 0.136 and 1.06 MeV, which is considerably greater than the mean x-ray energies of 0.03–0.04 MeV obtained from conventional diagnostic x-ray systems (approximately 80–120 KeV [thousand electron volts]). The radiation shielding in the catheterization lab, which is adequate for diagnostic x-ray procedures, is inadequate for radiation protection of personnel involved with a brachytherapy procedure using a gamma-ray intravascular source. Greater local shielding of the gamma intravascular system is provided by having a free-standing lead shield on wheels. The radioactive sources of 6, 10, or 14 seed ribbons, measuring 23 mm, 39 mm, and 55 mm, respectively, are fed into a single-lumen catheter by hand-applied pressure. The catheter is compatible with a guide catheter of 7-Fr or greater. Because of the high ambient radiation levels that accompany gamma brachytherapy, the specific activity of the source is, by design, lower. Thus, treatment times average approximately 30 min. The substantial shielding required to contain radiation from the ^{192}Ir source requires that the device containing the source be considerably larger. This poses additional problems in storage and shipping. The shelf life of the source is approximately 1 month.

INDICATIONS, CONTRAINDICATIONS, AND AFTERCARE

The Beta-Cath System (Best Vascular, Springfield, VA, USA) is currently approved for the treatment of ISR in native coronary arteries with discrete lesions. A lesion smaller than 20 mm in length is treated with a 30-mm long source train, a 30-mm long lesion with a 40-mm long source train, and a 40-mm long lesion with a 60-mm long source train. The reference vessel diameter may range between 2.7 mm and 4.0 mm. Patients excluded from CART for safety and effectiveness considerations are those who

- are undergoing or having prior chest radiation.
- are unable to tolerate that recommended dwell time of the source train in the delivery catheter, reference vessels smaller than 2.7 mm.
- require revascularization methods other than balloon angioplasty.
- require directional and rotational atherectomy and excimer laser for revascularization of ISR.
- vessel or lesion morphologies that would preclude revascularization or placement of the β-Rail 3.5-Fr delivery catheter
- present with thrombotic lesions.

- multiple vessel lesions.
- vein graft segments.
- overlapping stents.
- myocardial infarction less than or equal to 72 hours prior to the procedure.
- ejection fraction less than 30%.
- have received a heart transplant.
- are women of childbearing potential who are pregnant or suspect pregnancy.

The GALILEO III Intravascular Radiotherapy System (Abbott Vascular, Redwood City, CA, USA) was currently approved for the treatment of ISR in native coronary arteries with an injured length of no more than 47 mm in a reference vessel with a diameter from 2.4 mm to 3.7 mm. Precautions are similar to those listed previously, with the addition of lack of safety and effectiveness information for

- coronary artery sites previously treated with radiotherapy.
- bifurcation lesions.
- aorto-ostial lesions.
- patients with previously diagnosed autoimmune diseases, such as rheumatoid arthritis, scleroderma, and systemic lupus erythematosis (SLE).

The Checkmate System (Cordis Corp., Miami, FL, USA) approval was similar to that of the Beta-Cath device, with the exception that treated lesions might be up to 45 mm in length.

Current contraindications of all systems are limited to unprotected left main disease (>50% narrowing) and individuals in whom antiplatelet or anticoagulant agents are contraindicated.

IMPORTANCE OF ANTIPLATELET THERAPY

In the initial experience, following the CART procedure, the incidence of site thrombosis within 270 days after the index procedure was up to 9%, with a higher incidence in patients who underwent concomitant stent placement in the treated site. This highly adverse phenomenon was promptly recognized by clinical investigators and was found to be attributable to delayed regrowth of endothelium at the treated site, leaving it with a longer prothrombotic potential. It is now accepted that dual antiplatelet therapy with aspirin and with a thienopyridine (ticlopidine or clopidrogel) should be initiated immediately after completion of CART and continued for 6–12 months.[25,26] This practice has greatly reduced the frequency of late site thrombosis.

EFFICACY

Overall, brachytherapy at an appropriate dose clearly inhibits the neointimal proliferation that causes restenosis. However, at acceptable doses, its ability to inhibit neointimal growth is only partial. Thus, all of the clinical studies that compare brachytherapy to placebo show an approximately 50% reduction in the rate of

TABLE 14-1

Comparison of CART Systems

MANUFACTURER	TRADE NAME	RADIATION SOURCE	RADIOACTIVE DECAY	HALF-LIFE
Best Vascular, Springfield, VA	BetaCath	Strontium 90/Yttrium 90	Beta	28.5 years
Cordis Corp. Miami, FL	CHECKMATE	Iridium 192	Gamma	73.83 days
Abbott Vascular, Redwood City, CA	GALILEO III	Phosphorus 32	Beta	14.28 days

clinically significant restenosis.[27–29] Thus, coronary artery brachytherapy found its best niche in the treatment of diffuse ISR. Diffuse ISR has a 75% recurrence rate following treatment by conventional balloon angioplasty. Administration of coronary brachytherapy reduces this rate to 35%—a substantial beneficial effect, but certainly not a cure.

These results made brachytherapy the standard of care for ISR between 2001 and 2004. In 2002, more than 50,000 coronary brachytherapy procedures were performed in the United States. In 2004, the frequency of brachytherapy procedures decreased markedly as enthusiasm built for the use of drug-eluting stents for the treatment of ISR. At present, the market penetration and demonstrated effectiveness of drug-eluting stents has dramatically limited the role of CART, and precise future indications are under investigation.

REGULATORY ISSUES

The CART systems that were commercially available used either by-product material or radiation from by-product material, and as such are regulated by the US Nuclear Regulatory Commission (NRC) or by the various states (Agreement States) that have previously established agreements with the NRC to regulate these materials independently. In most instances, individual state requirements parallel those of the NRC.

The NRC regulations regarding these materials and procedures are specified in the Code of Federal Regulations (CFR), Title 10 (NRC Regulations), Part 35 (Medical Use of By-Product Materials), sub-parts F (Manual Brachytherapy) and J (Training and Experience Requirements).[30]

Current regulations are such that an "authorized user" must supervise the materials and brachytherapy portions of the procedure. This individual, specified as a physician, may delegate this supervision to a qualified physicist, but continues to have overall responsibility for handling, safety, and regulatory requirements.

REFERENCES

1. Bittl JA. Advances in coronary angioplasty. *N Engl J Med.* 1996;335:1290.
2. Fischman DL, Leon MD, Baim DS, et al. A randomized comparison of coronary-stent placement and balloon angioplasty in the treatment of coronary artery disease. Stent Restenosis Investigators. *N Engl J Med.* 1994;331:496.
3. Serruys PW, de Jaegere P, Kiemeneij F, et al. Comparison of balloon-expandable-stent implantation with balloon angioplasty in patients with coronary artery disease. BENESTENT Study Group. *N Engl J Med.* 1994;331:489.
4. Dewing SB. *Radiotherapy of Benign Disease.* Charles C. Thomas, 1965;pp 228–229.
5. Order SF, Donaldson SS. *Radiation Therapy of Benign Diseases.* Springer-Verlag, 1990:147–153.
6. Cox JD. *Moss' Radiation Oncology: Rationale, Techniques, Results.* Mosby-Year Book, Inc. 1994:853–854.
7. Wiedermann JG, Marboe C, Amols H, et al. Intracoronary irradiation markedly reduces restenosis after balloon angioplasty in a porcine model. *J Am Coll Cardiol.* 1994;23:1491.
8. Shefer A, Eigler NL, Whiting JS, et al. Supression of intimal proliferation after balloon angioplasty with local beta radiation in rabbits. *J Amer Coll Cardiol.* 1995;142:212.
9. Mayberry MR, Shimotakahara S. Radiation inhibition of intimal hyperplasia after arterial injury. *Rad Res.* 1995;142:212.
10. Maryianowski MH, Robinson K, Crocker IR. Comparison of endovascular and external beam irradiation in the prevention of restenosis. In Waksman R. (ed.), *Vascular Brachytherapy*, 2nd ed. Futura Publishing Co., 1999:221–230.
11. Hehrlein C, Stintz M, Kinscherf R, et al. Pure beta-particle emitting stents inhibit neointima formation in rabbits. *Circulation.* 1996;93:641.
12. Candado A, Gurdicl O, Espinoza R. Percutaneous transluminal angioplasty (PTCA) and intracoronary radiation (ICRT): a possible new modality for the treatment of coronary restenosis. A preliminary report of the first 10 patients treated with intracoronary radiation therapy. *J Amer Coll Cardiol.* 1995; 25(Suppl):228A.

TABLE 14-2

Comparison of Dose/Depth Profiles

SOURCE	CATHETER SURFACE DOSE[a]	DOSE[a] @ 1 mm	DOSE[a] @ 2 mm	DOSE[a] @ 3 mm
Sr-90/Y-90	53	16	8	3
Ir-192	12	12	8	6
P-32	67	27	8	2

[a]All doses indicated in gray (Gy).

13. Amols HI, Zaider M, Weinberger J, Ennis R, Schiff PB, Reinstein LE. Dosimetric consideration for catheter-based beta and gamma emitters in the therapy of neointimal hyperplasia in human coronary arteries. *Int J Radia Oncol Biol Phys.* 1996;36:913.

14. Nath R, Anderson LL, Luxton G., Weaver KA, Williamson JF, Meigooni AS. Dosimetry of interstitial brachytherapy sources: recommendation of the AAPM Radiation Therapy Committee Task Group No. 43. *Med Phys.* 1995;2:209.

15. Williamson JF. Measurement and calculated dose rates in water near ^{125}I and ^{192}Ir seeds. *Med Phys.* 1991;18:776.

16. Nath R, Amols H, Coffey C, et al. Intravascular brachytherapy physics: report of the AAPM Radiation Therapy Committee Task Group 60. *Med Phys.* 1999;26,119.

17. Bloch P, Wallner P, Lobdell J. Display of dose distribution on cine/fluoro images acquiring during IVBT. 44th Annual Meeting AAPM, Montreal Canada, July 2002. *Med Phys.* 2002;29:1225.

18. Bloch P, Wallner P, Lobdell J. Image-guided coronary intravascular brachytherapy treatment planning. Biomedical Imaging Research Opportunities Workshop p39, Bethesda, MD; Jan 2003.

19. Li XA, Yu, C, Suntharalingam M. Beta versus gamma for catheter-based intravascular brachytherapy: dosimetric perspective in the presence of metallic stents and calcified plaques. *Int J Radiat Oncol Biol Phys.* 2000;44(4):1043.

20. Kollum M, Cottin Y, Chan RC, et al. Decreased adventitial neovascularization after intracoronary irradiation in swine: a time course study. *Int J Rad Oncol Biol Phys.* 2001;50(4):1033.

21. Tripuraneni P. Intravascular brachytherapy. *Adv Rad Onc.* 2000;3:31.

22. Brenner D, Miller RC, Hall EJ. The radiobiology of intravascular irradiation. *Int J Radiat Oncol Biol Phys.* 1996;36(4):805.

23. Kim H-S, Chan RC, Kollum M, et al. Effects of ^{32}P radioactive stents on in-stent restenosis in a double stent injury model of the porcine coronary arteries. *Int J Radiat Oncol Biol Phys.* 2001;5(4):1058.

24. Razavi M, Rege S, Zeigler W, et al. Feasibility of external beam radiation for prevention of resentosis following balloon angioplasty. *Int Jour Radiat Oncol Biol Phys.* 1999;44:363.

25. Hoffman R, Mintz GS. Coronary in-stent restenosis—predictors, treatment and prevention. *Euro Heart J.* 2000;21:1739.

26. Leon MB, Teirstein PS, Moses JW, et al. Localized intracoronary gamma-radiation to inhibit the recurrence of restenosis after stenting. *N Engl J Med.* 2001;344(4):250.

27. Waksman R, Raizner AE, Yeung AC, et al. Use of localised intracoronary radiation in treatment of in-stent restenosis: the INHIBIT randomized controlled trial. *Lancet.* 2002;359:551.

28. Waksman R, Ajani AE, White RL, et al. Intravascular radiation for in-stent restenosis in saphenous-vein bypass grafts. *N Engl J Med.* 2002;346:1194.

29. Waksman R, Cheneau E, Ajani A, et al. Intracoronary radiation therapy improves the clinical and angiographic outcomes of diffuse in-stent restenotic lesions. Results of the Washington Radiation for In-Stent Restenosis Trial for Long Lesions (Long WRIST) Studies. *Circulation.* 2003;107:1744.

30. Code of Federal Regulations, Title 10, Part 35, Sub-parts F and J.

CHAPTER (15)

X-Ray Computed Tomography and Magnetic Resonance Imaging of the Coronary Arteries

Victor A. Ferrari, MD, Daniel K. H. Thomas, MD, and Harold I. Litt, MD, PhD

X-ray coronary angiography has been the predominant technique for assessing the extent of severity of coronary artery disease (CAD) in the clinical setting. However, concerns related to complications from the invasive nature of the procedure, as well as safety-associated risks of x-ray and intravenous contrast agent exposure have stimulated the search for noninvasive imaging alternatives for CAD visualization. The two leading technologies are magnetic resonance coronary angiography (MRCA) and computed tomographic angiography (CTA). Advances in both techniques have created great interest in the clinical application of these methods, and clinical studies highlight the benefits and limitations of the various approaches to their implementation. The purpose of this chapter is to review the technical and clinical aspects of these techniques and to compare and contrast the performance of the methods as applied to detection of CAD.

PART I

Imaging of the Coronary Arteries Using Magnetic Resonance Imaging

Technical Aspects of Coronary Magnetic Resonance Coronary Angiography

BASIC PRINCIPLES OF MAGNETIC RESONANCE IMAGING

Clinical magnetic resonance imaging (MRI) is based on the detection of signals from fat and water protons in the body in a three-dimensional manner. Hydrogen molecules (H^1) have one proton and no neutron, which results in the spinning of this proton about its axis, thereby creating a small magnetic field. Under normal circumstances, these magnetic fields point in random directions, so that the net magnetization in the body equals zero. If subjected to a large static magnetic field, the protons align along the z-axis of the field (head to toe in conventional scanners). Under these conditions, they not only spin about themselves, but also about the axis of the external field. This wobbling angular spin is referred to as *precession*. The frequency of the precession spin (cycles/s or Hz) is given by the Larmor equation,

$$0 = \gamma \cdot \beta_0$$

where 0 is the precessional frequency, γ is the gyromagnetic ratio, B_0-strength of external magnetic field (1.5 Tesla in conventional clinical scanners).

As the spins precess randomly along the z-axis of the magnetic field, they are out of phase with one another. The magnetic components that point along the x- or y-axis of the magnetic field cancel each other out, such that there is only a net magnetic component along the z-axis.

In an MRI scanner, an applied radiofrequency (RF) pulse oriented in the direction of the x-axis and matching precisely the resonance frequency of the H^1, causes the protons to precess perpendicular to the z-axis. This resonance results in the RF pulse adding energy to the protons. The application of the RF pulse not only flips the protons, but also aligns them and causes them to precess in phase with one another. The *flip angle,* which describes the fractional angle of a single precession cycle, corresponds to the angle that the flipped magnetization vector makes with the z-axis. It is proportional to the duration of the RF pulse, its strength, and the gyromagnetic ratio. On cessation of the applied RF pulse, an oscillating magnetic field, caused by the flipped precessing spins as they relax, can be detected. This corresponds to the emitted MR signal, which is detected and reconstructed to produce an image. The protons gradually realign with the z-axis of the static magnetic field and return to their lowest energy state. This relaxation occurs mainly as the result of two processes that result in tissue-specific relaxation times. The *T1-time,* or *longitudinal relaxation time,* refers to the rate at which the magnetization along the z-axis recovers to its initial state. It corresponds to the *spin-lattice relaxation,* which means the release of energy to the environment. The *T2-time,* or *transverse magnetization time,* characterizes the rate at which the transverse (along the x–y axis) magnetization decays. It corresponds to the spin–spin relaxation, which is determined by proton–proton interaction. Approximate T1 and T2 times at 1.5 T for myocardium are 880 and 75 ms, respectively.

The spatial distribution of signal intensity is used to create a three-dimensional map of proton density, which forms the basis for the MR image. Lung tissue, with fewer protons per square centimeter, has a lower signal intensity than fat, which has an abundant number of protons. The signal itself has amplitude, frequency, and phase. A fourth value—spatial localization—is needed to fulfill the requirement for image reconstruction. Therefore, a combination of magnetic gradients is applied after initial application of the RF pulse. Typically, the first gradient applied is the *slice-selective gradient.* It is applied perpendicular to the imaged slice. The gradient causes a slight variation in precession frequency along the gradient field, as defined by the Larmor equation. By choosing an appropriate RF pulse, only spins of a given frequency and slice position are excited. Next, during the echo readout, a *frequency-encoding gradient* (also called a *readout gradient*) is applied in the direction of the x-axis. As a result, all tissue or spins along that gradient have a different frequency that provides spatial information along the x-axis. To derive spatial information along the y-axis, a third gradient is applied. This is called the *phase-encoding gradient,* which is applied at any time between the RF pulse and the readout gradient. This gradient introduces a phase shift to the spins, so that at the echo time (TE), the protons all have a distinct frequency and phase, which encode for the x and y coordinates. It is important to recognize that the phase-encoding step is the time-consuming process with MRI scanning. This step must be repeated n times until full collection of data for an image with an n-matrix size in the y-direction ($n = 256$ for a 256×256 matrix

size). By using a different phase-encoding step per RF pulse, each of the signals acquired from the slice has a different phase shift. Each signal fills one row of the image dataset, which, after application of a 2-D Fourier transform, is referred to as *k-space.* The *k*-space data contains all of the spatial, spectral, and intensity data needed to reconstruct the final image. Each point in k-space contains information about the entire slice, because signals from the entire slice are sampled. For reasons that are beyond the scope of this chapter, the central portion of *k*-space contains data that are more motion sensitive but have the greatest signal, whereas data at the edges of *k*-space contribute to the fine details of the image. These concepts relate to the potential limitations in temporal and spatial resolution using current MRI techniques.

All the pulse sequences used in MRCA are based on these fundamental principles. The pulse sequences and strategies to collect the phase-encoded data are discussed in more detail later in the chapter.

MAGNETIC RESONANCE IMAGING: HARDWARE

The standard clinical MRI scanners used for cardiac imaging are superconducting magnets operating at a static field strength of 1.0 to 1.5 Tesla (T), with the majority cooled by helium. The use of high-field scanners operating at 3T is currently the subject of intense clinical investigation. The capacity of modern scanners is limited by both hardware and software issues. Typical parameters determining a scanner's capabilities are the *gradient capacity* (how large a gradient is produced over a given distance) and the *slew rate* (how quickly the gradients can be changed). Typical values for gradient capacity and slew rate are 30–40 mT/m and 130–200m T/m/s, respectively. Within the scanner, the generated signals are measured with an RF coil. In general, the same RF coil can be used for signal transmission and detection. Because of greater signal-to-noise ratio (SNR) and RF penetration, a combination of a *body transmit* (which is integrated into the scanner) and phased-array surface coils are frequently used for cardiac imaging. With the patient supine, these surface coils have 2–3 coil elements positioned under the patient's back, and 2–3 coil elements positioned on the patient's chest. The signal is transmitted from the coil to an RFamplifier, and then Fourier-transformed so that the final image may be reconstructed and displayed on the scanner console.

【 】 PATIENT PREPARATION

The use of a large, static magnetic field and rapidly switching gradients prohibits the examination of patients with pacemakers, internal cardiac defibrillators (ICDs), or with certain implanted ferromagnetic materials (although more recent work shows that modern pacemakers and even ICDs can tolerate noncardiac MRI scans). Irregular rhythms such as atrial fibrillation or frequent ectopy reduce scan quality, prolong scan time, or make it unrealistic to scan a patient with these problems. Another contraindication to MRI scanning is claustrophobia, which results in unsuccessful exams in 1%–2% of patients. Gentle sedation can increase the success rate of MRI in this patient group. A single imaging session is typically 1 hr, depending on the exam. Specific patient preparation is not needed before the exam, unless a stress study is planned, in which the preparation is comparable to that for a stress echo or adenosine nuclear perfusion study—specifically, holding beta-blockers for dobutamine studies or withholding caffeine for 24 hr for an adenosine study.

[ ] CHALLENGES TO MAGNETIC RESONANCE CORONARY ANGIOGRAPHY

Spatial Resolution

The proximal coronary arteries are less than 6 mm in diameter in normal adults. Current MRCA techniques can achieve a maximum resolution of 0.7–1.0 mm in plane, but only 1.5–2 mm slice thicknesses can be achieved. Thus, the resolution is well below that achieved using conventional coronary angiography (0.3–0.5 mm). Two factors inhibit the use of a higher resolution: the first is SNR, which is inversely correlated with the resolution. Optimization of cardiac coil design represents one attempt to improve SNR. The

closer the coil is to the heart, the greater the signal. In addition, imaging at a higher magnet field strength, as discussed later in this chapter, offers an inherently greater SNR. The second limiting factor is that each increase in resolution in the phase-encoding direction is associated with one additional phase-encoding step, which, as previously discussed, increases imaging time. Of note, the potential for blurring increases with an increasing number of phase-encoding steps, because each phase-encoding step is acquired at a different time. The image acquisition is timed to end-diastole, but the data for each image must be acquired over many cardiac cycles. Thus, slight variations in cardiac position are possible, even at the same time in diastole. (See Table 15-1.)

Cardiac Motion

With cardiac magnetic resonance imaging (CMR), the image acquisition is usually gated to end-diastole to avoid motion artifacts, unless the aim is to acquire a cine study. To understand the principle of timing of data acquisition, we use the term *acquisition window*. Within the context of CMR, the *acquisition window* is

TABLE 15-1

Meta-Analysis of Magnetic Resonance Coronary Arteriography Versus X-ray Angiography: Subgroup Analyses of Valuable Segments–Random Effects Estimates and 95% Confidence Intervals

SUBGROUPS	STUDIES (n)	WEIGHTED SENSITIVITY (%)	WEIGHTED SPECIFICITY (%)
Acquisition technique			
2-dimensional	4 (605)	80 (65–90)*	91 (76–97)*
3-dimensional	23 (4,223)	72 (67–76)*	86 (80–90)*
Respiratory motion compensation			
Breath holding	9 (1,546)	78 (69–84)*	91 (84–95)*
Retrospective navigator	13 (2,000)	71 (65–77)*	80 (71–87)*
Prospective navigator	5 (1,074)	70 (54–82)*	89 (69–96)*
Publication year			
≥2001	12 (2,112)	71 (63–77)*	83 (74–89)*
≤2000	15 (2,508)	74 (68–80)*	88 (80–93)*
Non-CAD subjects			
Included	18 (3,272)	71 (64–78)*	88 (82–93)*
Not included	9 (1,348)	74 (69–79)*	79 (66–88)*
Distal segments			
Considered	5 (568)	64 (46–79)*	93 (88–96)*
Not considered	22 (4,052)	74 (70–78)*	83 (77–88)*
Blinding stated			
Test and clinical data	12 (1,648)	71 (65–77)*	80 (71–87)*
Test only	10 (1,604)	75 (67–83)*	91 (81–96)*
None	5 (1,368)	72 (59–82)*	84 (67–93)*
Sample size			
≥200 segments	7 (2,302)	76 (69–82)*	83 (70–91)*
<200 segments	20 (2,318)	71 (65–77)*	87 (80–91)*

*Statistically significant (P < .10) between study heterogeneity.

CAD = coronary artery disease; CI5 confidence interval.

(Modified from Danias et al. J Am Coll Cardiol. 2004; 44:1867.)

referred to as the time within each cardiac cycle during which data is collected. As previously discussed, the time-consuming process is the phase encoding. Therefore, the acquisition window is determined by the number of phase-encoding steps per cardiac cycle. The time it takes to perform one phase encoding is determined by the repetition time (TR) time of a sequence. By choosing the number of phase-encoding steps per cardiac cycle, one can vary the acquisition window of a pulse sequence. The higher the image resolution in the phase-encoding direction, the longer the total image acquisition time. For example, if one wishes to acquire an image with a 256 × 256 matrix, a total of 256 phase-encoding steps must be performed. In order to keep scanning time as short as possible, more than one phase-encoding step per cardiac cycle is performed. Depending on the heart rate, the relative "quiescent" period of the cardiac cycle—in which image acquisition can occur with a minimum of motion artifacts—varies between 70 ms and 330 ms. In order to keep errors to a minimum, the acquisition window should be approximately 70–100 ms. With a typical TR of 7–10 ms for a standard gradient echo sequence for MRCA, one could acquire between 7 and 10 phase-encoding steps per cardiac cycle. Thus, with a TR of 7 ms, 10 phase-encoding steps per cardiac cycle and a resulting acquisition window of 70 ms, an entire image with a matrix size of 256 × 256 could be acquired within 26 heart cycles. This concept of filling several lines of *k*-space during one cardiac cycle is also referred to as *segmented k-space acquisition.*

Because cardiac motion may be different in each patient, more recent studies suggest acquiring a cine scout sequence orthogonal to the right coronary artery (RCA), so that the quiescent period of the coronary can be assessed individually and the acquisition window chosen accordingly. This approach has been shown to be superior to protocols using a fixed acquisition window. Correct placement of the ECG electrodes is very important, because faster gradient switching can interfere with the ECG signal. Newer developments, such as the vector–ECG and optical ECG signal transmission, can overcome these problems.

Coronary Anatomy

Given the imaging time constraints for MRCA, it is desirable to plan a scan using as few slices as possible. This is particularly true with 2D imaging, because the duration of breath-holding for respiratory compensation is an important factor. Slice planning must be carefully performed because of the tortuous course of the coronary arteries. A low-resolution scout scan that covers the entire volume containing the coronary vasculature is acquired first. The scout scan is used to prescribe the high-resolution scans that map the course of the coronary vessels. One tool that facilitates the planning of the high resolution scans is the *3-point planscan tool.*[1] The RCA is marked at its origin and at the middle and distal segment along its course. Subsequently, the program calculates a slice position with the center of the plane traversing the 3 points. Similarly, slice positions can be calculated for the left anterior descending (LAD) and the circumflex coronary arteries. Another approach, suggested by Wielopolski et al.,[2] prescribes very thin volume coronary arteriography with targeted scans (VCATS) along the course of the coronary arteries using very thin 3D-volumes and the breath-hold technique.

Respiratory Motion: Breath-Hold and Free-Breathing Techniques

Breath-Hold Technique. Motion artifacts encountered with MRCA are the result not only of cardiac motion, but also of respiratory motion. Diaphragmatic motion can be 1–2 cm, even during shallow breathing; thus, some form of respiratory compensation is needed. Breath-holding was proposed for first-generation MRCA, whereby stacks of 2D-sequences were acquired during repeated breath-holds (Figure 15-1A-D). This approach was appealing because the entire dataset was rapidly acquired, but despite promising results in healthy volunteers, it was not well suited for patients. Breath-hold duration can become unacceptably long, as it is dependent on the physical condition of the patient, the scan resolution chosen, and the heart rate. In addition, it has been observed that the diaphragm can move even during a breath-hold ("diaphragmatic drift"), and that the end-expiratory or end-inspiratory position of the diaphragm can vary between breath-holds. The use of patient visual feedback systems can address the latter issue, but not the former. However, the most important concern is the limited spatial resolution achievable using breath-hold techniques. This holds true for the use of even small 3D-VCATS (ie, acquiring multiple small 3D-volumes with a slightly higher resolution, and covering the entire vasculature using multiple breath-holds).[3] When higher spatial resolution is chosen, the SNR decreases significantly, which can be overcome in part by acquiring a thicker 3D volume. However, both approaches result in an increased acquisition time, rendering the sequence unsuitable for a breath-hold acquisition scheme.

Free-Breathing. Free-breathing techniques are advantageous because minimal cooperation is required from the patient. The data acquisition is not limited by the patients' ability to hold their breath, thus, the acquisition of large 3D-datasets becomes possible.[4] As described later, various approaches to free-breathing have been implemented, with the current "gold standard" (in terms of spatial resolution and documented clinical value) being the prospective navigator method with slice following technique.[1,5] However, all approaches follow a similar scheme in that patient breath-holding is not necessary and respiratory motion is monitored (breathing belt, navigator echo). The information from the monitoring device is used to reconstruct the data retrospectively or prospectively using only the data acquired during a given breathing period. Early attempts to oversample the data and thus average breathing artifacts have not been accurate and have largely been abandoned.

Although a respiratory belt is easy to implement, the development of the navigator echo technique was a revolutionary event for the field of coronary MRA.[6,7] This technique uses a pencil-beam-like excitation pulse that is placed on the lung–liver interface at the dome of the right hemidiaphragm (Figure 15-2). Respiratory excursion is monitored and displayed on a separate console window. An acceptance range or "window" (usually 3–5 mm), for data acquisition is chosen prior to scanning. Once scanning commences, an end-expiratory reference navigator is acquired during the preparatory phase of the scan. Following image acquisition, only data acquired when the position of the diaphragm is within the acceptance window is used for reconstruction.

The navigator echo sample volume may be placed in several locations, such as above the left hemithorax or on the heart.

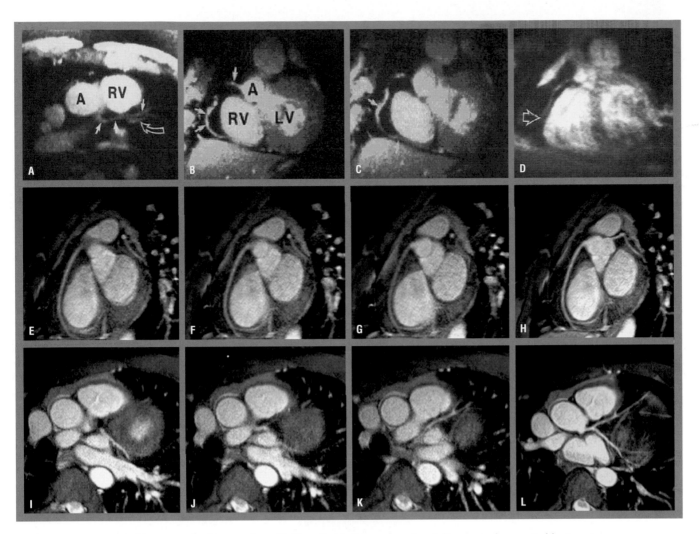

FIGURE 15-1. Breath-hold images of subjects without (**A–C**) and with (**D**) coronary heart disease as documented by invasive coronary angiography. *(Reprinted with permission from Manning WJ, Li W, Edelman RR. N Engl J Med. 1993;328:828.)* The resolution of this early MRCA sequence was 1.4–1.9 mm × 0.9 mm in plane with a slice thickness of = mm. Images **E–G** and **I–K** represent the current gold standard in magnetic resonance coronary angiography (MRCA) acquired with a 3D sequence using prospective navigator gating with the slice-following technique. Images **H** and **L** are multiplanar reformatted images.

However, the right lung–liver interface at the dome of the right hemidiaphragm has been shown to yield optimal image quality.

Retrospective Gating

Retrospective gating implies that the imaging data is acquired continuously. The respiratory pattern is monitored (using a belt or navigator echo) during the entire data acquisition, so that retrospectively only the data from a given respiratory period is used for image reconstruction. Reasonably good image quality may be obtained using this gating technique; however, it is not comparable to the quality of the high-resolution scans obtained using the prospective navigator technique.[8]

Prospective Navigator with Real-Time Slice-Following Technique

The prospective navigator with real-time slice-following technique processes the navigator information in real time (Figures 15-2, 15-3). Within each cardiac cycle, the navigator data and image data are collected simultaneously. The image data are processed only if the

diaphragm position is within the predefined acceptance window. Therefore, the concept of the *slice-following* or *tracking* navigator was introduced.[9,10] It refers to the ability of the navigator (software) to account for the cardiac motion by repositioning the imaging slab within each heartbeat adaptively.

Using an acceptance window of 5 mm and the slice-following technique, a navigator efficiency of about 50% has been reported.[1,9] Some factors, like the change of the end-expiratory position of the diaphragm over time compared to the reference navigator at the beginning of the sequence ("diaphragmatic drift"), can render the image acquisition very long. In fact, the navigator efficiency can drop to zero such that the acquisition must be repeated.

【 】 BASIC IMAGING SEQUENCES

Black-Blood Techniques

The "black-blood" techniques have been given their name because the blood pool appears black compared to the surrounding tissues[11] (Figure 15-4C). These are typically spin-echo (SE) or

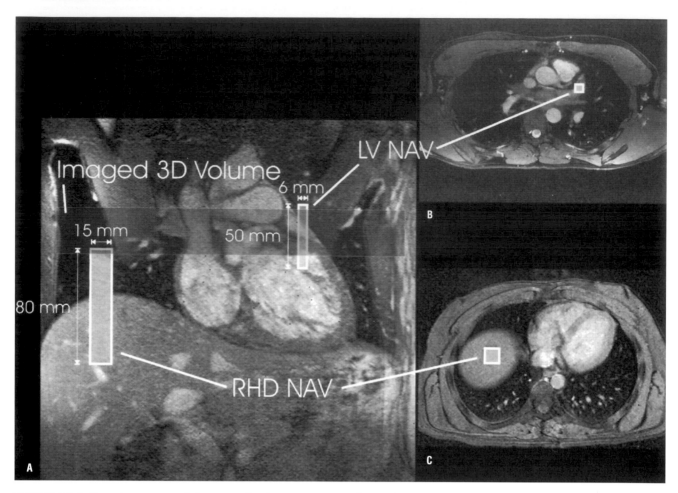

FIGURE 15-2. Typical positions and dimensions for the 2D navigator pulse: on the lung–liver interface at the dome of the right hemidiaphragm (RHD) and on the left ventricle (LV). Positioning the navigator on the RHD yields better image quality. *(Reprinted with permission from Stuber M, Botnar RM, Danias PG, et al. Radiology. 1999;212:579.)*

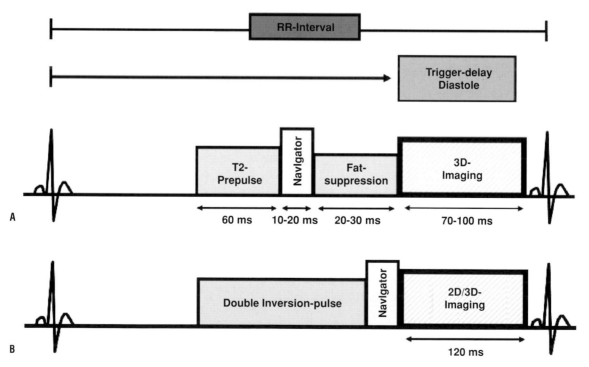

FIGURE 15-3. Two pulse diagrams depicting the typical sequence setup of current MRCA sequences. The imaging portion of the sequence is delayed to diastole. The resting period during diastole can be determined empirically or by choosing a subject-specific trigger delay, after acquiring a scout timing sequence. The navigator should be positioned as close to the imaging portion as possible to avoid changes in diaphragmatic position between the navigator and the imaging block. For GRE sequences (**A**), also called *bright-blood imaging*, the navigator is preceded by the T2-preparatory pulse and followed by the prepulses for fat-signal suppression. In current black-blood sequences (**B**), a double-inversion pulse to null the signal from blood is implemented before the navigator.

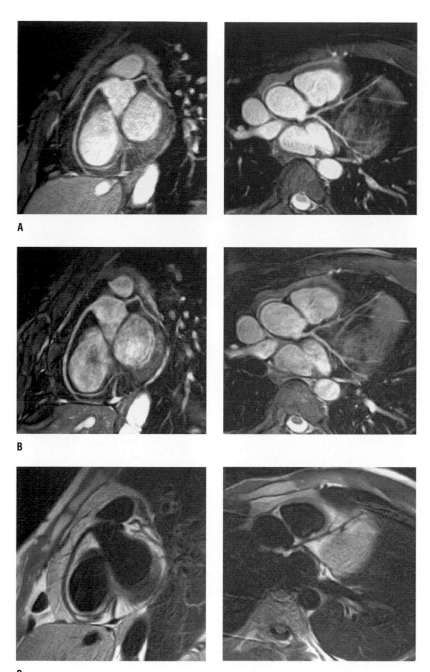

FIGURE 15-4. (A–C) Multiplanar reformatted images of the right and left coronary systems. All right coronary images were acquired in one subject, and all left anterior descending (LAD)/circumflex coronary artery (LCX) images were acquired in another subject. All images were acquired using a prospective navigator with slice-following technique. **(A)** Conventional GRE images, which can be regarded as the standard acquisition scheme. **(B)** The SSFP sequence was used with the same prepulses as in **(A)**. Both are bright-blood images. **(C)** Typical black-blood (TSE) images of the same volunteers. Instead of the T2-prepulse, a double-inversion recovery prepulse was used for enhanced black-blood properties of the sequence.

turbo-spin-echo (TSE) sequences, the latter being ultra-fast sequences that acquire several lines of *k*-space within one heartbeat and with one 90° excitation pulse, similar to the earlier described segmented *k*-space acquisition scheme. In SE, the blood typically gives no signal, because the signal is not acquired after an initial 90° pulse but after the application of a 180° refocusing pulse. The moving spins in the blood pool are exposed to only one

of either of the pulses so that they do not contribute to the signal. Therefore, these techniques offer an inherently good contrast between the coronary vessels and the surrounding fat, which appears bright. Contrast between the dark blood pool and the rather dark myocardium is not as good. Although the first SE coronary attempts allowed depicting the origin of the coronary arteries, newer TSE techniques in combination with the navigator technique yield good image quality and are able to depict long portions of the coronaries up to the distal segments. However, because of slow blood flow, the blood can still appear bright in standard SE or TSE sequences. Thus, implementation of the double inversion-pulse (Figure 15-3) has increased the black-blood properties of these sequences.[12,13] A first nonselective prepulse inverts the magnetization in the entire imaging slab. Subsequently, a slice-selective second inversion pulse cancels the effect of the first pulse. The blood that enters the imaging slice at the time of the excitation pulse has experienced only the first pulse, so that it cannot be excited by the RF pulse.

However, clinical studies using a black-blood sequence for assessment of coronary stenosis have not been published to date. This technique also yields reduced image quality compared to gradient-echo techniques when choosing a comparably high-image resolution.[14]

Bright-Blood Technique

In gradient-echo sequences (GREs), the blood pool appears generally bright, giving the sequence its name. In this sequence, the flip angle is lower than in SE and TSE imaging. In a typical GRE acquisition, the fast repeated RF pulses (with no refocusing pulses in between) lead to a quick saturation of the tissue in a slice, because the spins do not have sufficient time to relax back to equilibrium state between the RF pulses. Thus, tissue with a very short T1 (eg, fat) appear brighter compared to tissue with a longer T1 (eg, muscle). Inflowing blood appears rather bright in GRE sequences, because it has not experienced the preceding RF pulses. In the first generation breath-hold MRCA sequences, typically 2D-sequences were used, taking full advantage of the inflow effect. However, because the 3D-acquisition scheme is typically used for coronary MRA and its resulting saturation effects, this inflow effect is usually less prominent.

Because the coronaries are embedded in the bright epicardial fat tissue and also in close proximity to the myocardium, different prepulses are typically used to increase the tissue contrast in state-of-the-art MRCA.

Most important, the signal from epicardial fat is being saturated using a frequency selective (spectral) prepulse or, alternatively, a spatial-spectral RF pulse that excites water selectively (Figure 15-4). Both techniques make use of the frequency shift of the fat protons compared to the water protons (-220 Hz at 1.5T).

Typical prepulses to enhance contrast between the coronary arteries and the myocardium are known as *T2 preparation*[4,15] or magnetization transfer contrast (MTC).[16] The T2 preparatory

No T2prep   **T2prep**

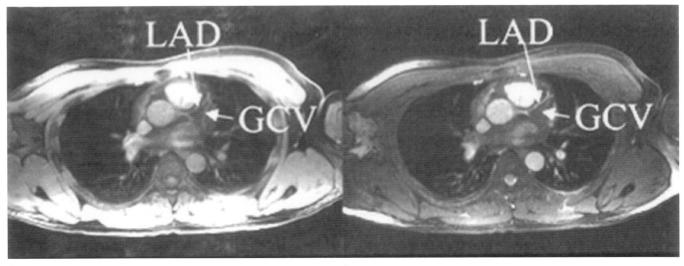

A   B

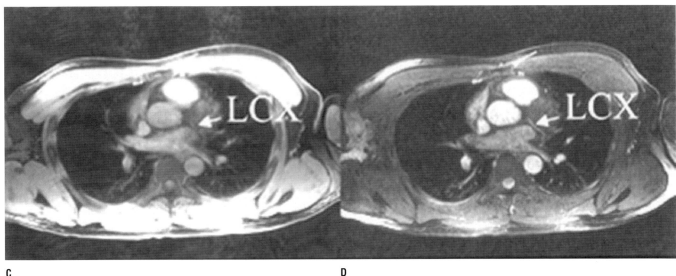

C   D

FIGURE 15-5. (A,C) The LAD and the LCX using a fat-saturated transversal 3D GRE sequence. As can be clearly seen on **B** and **D**, the application of the T2 preparatory pulse increases the contrast between the bright vessels and the darker myocardium. The signal in the greater cardiac vein (GCV) is suppressed as well. *(Reprinted from Botnar RM, Stuber M, Danias PG, et al. Improved coronary artery definition with T2-weighted, free-breathing, three-dimensional coronary MRA. Circulation. 1999;99:3139, with permission.)*

pulse takes advantage of the different T2 times of myocardium (≈ 50 ms) and arterial blood (≈ 250 ms). As a consequence of this pulse, the myocardial signal is suppressed as compared to the blood pool (Figures 15-3, 15-5). Another favorable effect of this pulse is the suppression of the signal from the cardiac veins (T2 of ≈ 35 ms because of the paramagnetic deoxyhemoglobin), which run adjacent to the left anterior descending artery and to the circumflex artery (see Figure 15-5).

The use of a segmented GRE sequence in combination with a prospective navigator and slice-following technique is regarded as the current gold standard for coronary MRA. This technique has also been evaluated in larger clinical studies, incorporating more than 100 patients.[5,17] This approach does not require the administration of contrast agents, but vessel definition relies solely on

the inflow effect, as well as the fat-saturation prepulse and the T2 preparatory pulse.

In addition to the prepulses, the administration of intravenous contrast agents can improve the vessel contrast in GRE sequences by reducing the T1 time. Because of this T1 shortening, the blood signal recovers rapidly between RF pulses, thereby yielding a strong signal independent of the inflow effect in the standard GRE sequence. Again a prepulse (inversion pulse) can be used to maximize the effect of the contrast agent by flipping the longitudinal magnetization (Figure 15-6). If the image is acquired while the myocardial magnetization is going through the zero crossing, it yields no signal while the RF pulse is applied. Because of the short T1, the blood has already recovered most of the longitudinal magnetization at that time.

T2Prep   ## B22956

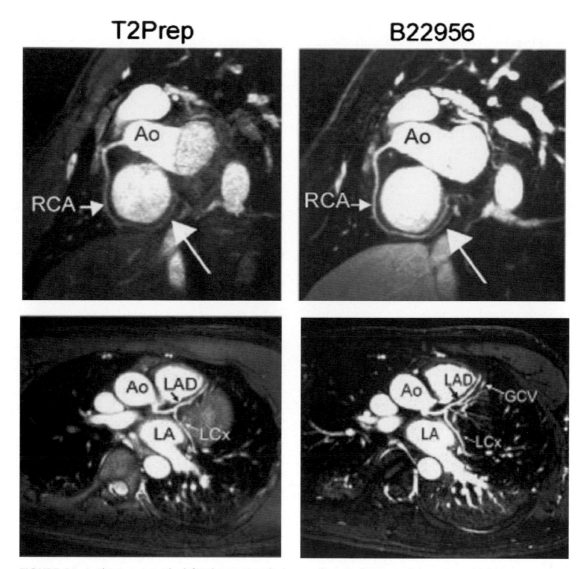

FIGURE 15-6. The images in the left column are multiplanar reformatted images of the right and left coronary systems acquired without a contrast agent. Images on the right were acquired after applying an inversion pulse and following intravenous application of B-22956, a gadolinium-based intravascular contrast agent. A significant increase in signal-to-noise ratio (SNR), contrast-to-noise ratio (CNR), and vessel sharpness was observed compared to standard T2-prepared gradient-echo MRCA. *(Reprinted from Paetsch I, Huber ME, Bornstedt A, et al. Improved three-dimensional free-breathing coronary magnetic resonance angiography using gadocoletic acid (B-22956) for intravascular contrast enhancement. J Magn Reson Imag. 2004;20:288, with permission).*

The major drawback of this approach is that the current FDA-approved contrast agents are extravascular contrast agents. Because they leave the intravascular space rapidly, data acquisition must be accomplished during the first pass. This implies that a very fast acquisition scheme is used for data acquisition. This can be achieved only with a breath-hold scan at a lower resolution, with all its disadvantages, as discussed previously.

Newer intravascular contrast agents have all the advantages of the extravascular agents. However, because they are restricted to the blood pool, the acquisition of the data is not limited to the first pass. These properties permit the use of 3D high-resolution imaging in combination with prospective navigator gating or other free-breathing methods (see Figure 15-6). Two different kinds of intravascular contrast, Gd-chelates[18–21] (EPIX Medical, Cambridge, MA, USA; and B-22956, Bracco Diagnostics,

Princeton, NJ, USA) and iron-oxide-based agents[22,23] (NC100150, Nycomed Amersham, Oslo, Norway), are currently under investigation. First studies in animals and healthy volunteers yielded promising results and an image quality superior to that achievable using the current gold standard.[19–24]

【 】 NEW TECHNIQUES

Alternative *k*-Space Sampling–EPI, Spiral, and Radial Acquisition Scheme

Echo-planar imaging (EPI) uses rapidly switching gradients to fill several lines of *k*-space after a single RF pulse. Even though this readout method improves acquisition speed, the technique is limited by prominent flow and susceptibility artifacts. Combining the EPI approach (eg, 5–9 EPI readouts) with a segmented *k*-space acquisition (eg, 2–4 RF pulses) scheme may limit these artifacts. Compared to the standard, as described earlier, this technique did not become widely accepted.

The spiral *k*-space sampling strategy has many theoretical advantages over Cartesian *k*-space sampling, where one line in *k*-space is acquired after the other with varying phase encodes.[25] This acquisition scheme has an intrinsically high SNR, is less sensitive to flow and motion artifacts, and is faster than conventional *k*-space sampling. However, spiral imaging is very sensitive to off-resonance effects associated with image blurring. Indeed, initial promising results in volunteers, showing advantages compared to standard 3D-MRCA, have not yet been translated into clinical studies.[26] The implementation of a radial acquisition scheme in combination with a steady-state free-precession GES has been reported to yield superior image quality compared to the standard 3D-MRCA.[27,28] Using a radial acquisition scheme, the susceptibility for motion artifacts can be similarly reduced. This leads to less vessel blurring and has shown to improve vessel definition and contrast-to-noise ratio (CNR) compared to conventional *k*-space sampling. Further investigation is warranted to prove the clinical value of these alternative acquisition schemes.

Steady-State Free Precession

Since 2001, steady-state free precession (SSFP) sequences have been studied extensively regarding their potential for coronary MRA[14,29–34] (Figure 15-4B). SSFP is basically a GRE sequence in which the residual transverse magnetization after each RF pulse is not spoiled, as with conventional GRE imaging, but refocused by using balanced gradients. Compared to conventional sequences, the image contrast is not T1 weighted but depends on the T2/T1 ratio of tissues. Blood signal does not depend on inflow of unsaturated spins with this technique, and therefore provides an increased SNR and CNR. The SSFP sequence is sensitive to magnetic field homogeneity, however. Thus, in addition to a strict requirement for a homogeneous magnetic field—achieved by the shimming abilities of the scanner—a high-performance gradient system is also needed to keep the TR short. Indeed, despite a number of studies showing the superiority of the SSFP approach over the conventional GRE approach at lower resolution,[31,33,35] a disadvantage is demonstrated if a very high spatial resolution is chosen.[14] However, as with the newer *k*-space acquisition schemes, the clinical value of this approach has yet to be shown.

Parallel Imaging—SMASH and SENSE

Compared to the previously mentioned acquisition schemes and techniques, *parallel imaging* is a technique that undersamples *k*-space.[36,37] This technique is independent of gradient performance, and requires the use of phased array coils. Depending on the number of coil elements integrated into the phased array coil, the acceleration factor (usually 2–4) can be chosen. Both techniques require the acquisition of an initial scan, not for image acquisition but to obtain a sensitivity profile of each surface coil (or element). Subsequently, the surface coil sensitivity variation can be used for complementary spatial encoding information, in addition to traditional *k*-space encoding. Although with simultaneous acquisition of spatial harmonics (SMASH) the missing *k*-space lines are reconstructed directly before the Fourier transform (FT) and the image generation, with sensitivity encoding (SENSE), the receiver coil sensitivity profiles are used to "unwrap" the image information, subject to aliasing, and derived from both coils after the FT.

The advantage of this technique is an enormous increase in imaging time, but because fewer profiles are sampled, the SNR is reduced by at least the square root of the acceleration factor.[38] Thus, even though successfully implemented for coronary imaging at 1.5T, the technique is more valuable with imaging at 3T, which has a higher intrinsic SNR[39] (Figure 15-7).

Newer Generation Scanners—3 Tesla

As discussed previously, the current sequence design in coronary imaging is a compromise between imaging time and a goal of higher spatial resolution, which is mainly limited by the SNR. Imaging at 3T offers an inherently greater SNR because of increased polarization of the spins. Even though cardiac imaging at 3T is associated with undesirable effects such as susceptibility artifacts, RF nonhomogeneity, and compromised RF penetration,[40,41] preliminary data suggest an advantage over conventional coronary MRA.[42] The higher SNR shows clear advantage if parallel acquisition schemes are used. Huber and coworkers[39] report that with a SENSE factor of 2, high-quality images of the coronaries can be acquired with a dramatically reduced scanning time (Figure 15-7). Alternatively, the decrease in acquisition time can be used to increase spatial resolution without compromising SNR.

PART II

Imaging of the Coronary Arteries Using X-ray Computed Tomography

EQUIPMENT

Computed tomography (CT) uses x-rays to create tomographic slices of objects. This is accomplished by rotating an x-ray beam around the object and measuring the transmission of x-rays through the object at many angles, called *projections*. This function of x-ray transmissions versus projection angle can be transformed using a mathematical reconstruction technique called *filtered back projection* to create an image in which the value at each pixel represents the x-ray density of the object at that location. These densities are represented in what are called *Hounsfield units* (HU) after Sir Godfrey Hounsfield, one of the developers of the CT scanner. HU are generally scaled from −1024 to +1024; in a properly calibrated scanner, air measures −1024 HU, water 0 HU, and bone +1024. An extended Hounsfield scale, with values up to +3096, is currently implemented on most scanners to allow quantification of densities higher than bone, such as metal. HU measurements are directly comparable across machine platforms, regardless of manufacturer.

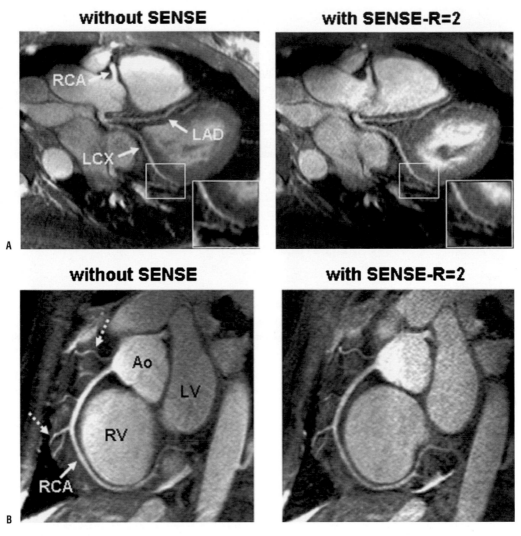

without SENSE   **with SENSE-R=2**

without SENSE   **with SENSE-R=2**

FIGURE 15-7. Images of the left **(A)** and right **(B)** coronary system of a healthy subject, acquired with and without SENSE (factor 2) on a 3T system. As is evident, the image quality is only slightly compromised. Small side branches can still be seen when using SENSE; however, the scan time has been reduced by one-half compared with the scan time without SENSE. *(Reprinted from Huber ME, Kozerke S, Pruessmann KP, et al. Sensitivity-encoded coronary MRA at 3T. Magn Reson Med. 2004;52:221, with permission.)*

CT imaging may be performed using either axial or helical acquisition. In the axial or "step-and-shoot" technique, the x-ray beam rotates around a fixed position in the object, acquiring one or more slices, then the table moves to another object position, at which another set of slices is acquired. In the helical or spiral technique, the x-ray beam is on continuously during the acquisition, and the object moves continuously through the x-ray beam as it rotates. The resultant trajectory of the x-ray beam through the object traces out a helix or spiral. Although axial images can be reconstructed only at the fixed positions at which they were obtained, helically acquired data sets can be reconstructed at any point along the spiral trajectory, and with any desired degree of overlap. For example, 3-mm thick slices can be reconstructed at every 1-mm interval. Overlapping reconstructions can be useful for visualization of small objects and creation of multiplanar reformatted (MPR) images.

Two technologies are currently available for CT imaging of the coronary arteries: electron beam CT and multidetector mechanical gantry CT.

【 】 ELECTRON BEAM CT

Electron beam CT (EBCT), also known as *ultrafast CT,* operates without motion of a mechanical x-ray source around the patient. In this technology, a magnetic field controls the direction of an electron beam, sweeping it across a fixed target ring that extends around a portion of the circumference of the gantry. A fan beam of x-rays is produced at each point on the target ring on which the electron beam is incident. These x-rays sweep across a fixed detector ring on the opposite side of the gantry from the target ring. Because there are no mechanical parts, the x-ray beam can rotate around the patient very rapidly, allowing a slice acquisition time of 50–100 msec, making cardiac imaging the predominant use for EBCT. Cardiac studies performed with EBCT scanners use prospective cardiac triggering (ie, data are acquired at fixed points in the cardiac cycle; Figure 15-8A). Images may be acquired at multiple times during the cardiac cycle ("cine" or "movie" mode) to obtain left ventricular functional measurements, but this is less common than with multidetector CT.

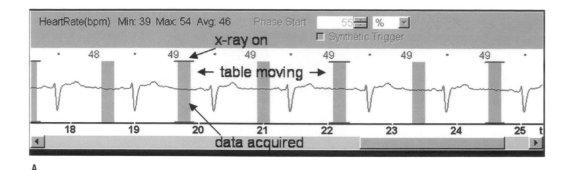

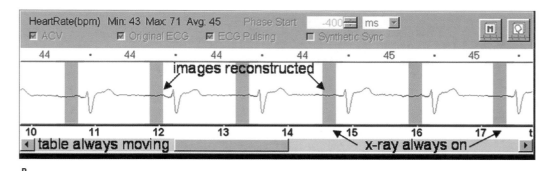

FIGURE 15-8. (**A**) Schematic of an ECG-triggered coronary CT acquisition used in EBCT and some MDCT applications. The x-ray beam is turned on during only a portion of the cardiac cycle (pink lines). Images can be reconstructed only when data is acquired (gray boxes), in this case in late diastole. The table position is fixed during each acquisition and moves between acquisitions. (**B**) In an ECG-gated MDCT acquisition, the x-ray beam remains on throughout the cardiac cycle (pink and blue lines–pink denotes a full x-ray dose, blue denotes a reduced dose; see section on Radiation Exposure) and the table is moving continuously. Images can be reconstructed retrospectively at many points (gray boxes), in this case in late diastole.

【　】 MULTIDETECTOR CT

Mechanical gantry systems, in which the entire x-ray tube and detector spin around the patient, were first introduced in the 1970s. However, the development of 4-slice multidetector CT (MDCT) in 1998—also called *multichannel* or *multislice CT*–permitted practical CT examinations of the heart with a widely available technology. The increased volumetric coverage of 16-, 32-, and now 64-slice MDCT, in combination with ECG-synchronized reconstruction, enables the acquisition of examinations of the coronary arteries in a single breathhold, with isotropic submillimeter spatial resolution and temporal resolution of less than 200 msec.[43] Cardiac studies performed with MDCT scanners use retrospective cardiac gating (ie, data are acquired throughout the cardiac cycle and reconstructions may be obtained at multiple points during the cardiac cycle). Thin-slice images are usually reconstructed in mid- to late-diastole because the proximal coronary arteries are relatively stable in position, and this generally produces images with the least motion artifacts. Other points in the cardiac cycle may be reconstructed as needed for coronary visualization, or to allow functional measurements such as calculating ejection fraction and wall-motion analysis. The use of multisector reconstruction, in which data from more than one heartbeat are combined to reconstruct an image at a particular point in the cardiac cycle, may allow improvement in temporal resolution to near 50 msec. However, this technique is sensitive to even small beat-to-beat variations in heart rate and may provide benefits only in certain circumstances.

【　】 DIGITAL FLAT-PANEL CT

Recent developments in MDCT technology focus on a steadily increasing number of thinner detectors, which permit acquisition of a greater number of thinner cardiac slices and coverage of a greater volume per gantry rotation. One natural path in this evolution would be the use of digital flat-panel detectors for CT, in which the entire volume of the heart could be acquired in one gantry rotation at very high isotropic spatial resolution.[44] Several manufacturers have constructed such machines for research purposes; commercialization is currently limited by slow detector response times and lack of contrast resolution compared to conventional CT detectors. This results in unacceptably long gantry rotation times ($\approx$ 10 seconds) for cardiac imaging applications. Nevertheless, these high-resolution tomographic devices are currently used for coronary imaging research, as described next.

【　】 EBCT VERSUS MDCT

Table 15-2 summarizes the technical performance of EBCT and different generations of MDCT scanners compared to digital flat-panel catheter angiography and to future digital flat-panel CT systems. In general, EBCT still has superior temporal resolution, but at the cost of decreased spatial resolution, thicker slices, and longer breath-holds compared to MDCT.[45] EBCT scanners are not widely available, as they are produced by only one manufacturer,

TABLE 15-2

Technical Specifications of EBCT and Successive Generations of MDCT for Coronary CTA Compared to Digital Flat-Panel Catheter Angiography (Theoretical Performance of a Digital Flat-Panel Area Detector CT System is Also Included)

TECHNOLOGY	EBCT	SINGLE SLICE	4-SLICE	16-SLICE	64-SLICE	AREA DETECTOR	DIGITAL FLAT-PANEL CATHETER ANGIOGRAPHY
Year introduced	1984	1990	1998	2001	2004	Future	2000
Gating mode	Prospective	—	Retrospective	Retrospective	Retrospective	Unknown	None
Gantry rotation time	50–100 msec	1 sec	0.5 sec	0.37 sec	0.33 sec	Currently ≈ 10 sec but improving	—
Temporal resolution single-sector/2-sector reconstruction (msec)	50	—	250	185/93	165/83 (83/42 msec for dual source)	—	33
Spatial resolution (mm)	0.8	0.6	0.6	0.5	0.3	0.15	0.15
Slice thickness for coronary imaging (mm)	3	—	1	0.5–0.75	0.4	0.15	—
Time for cardiac exam	30–40 sec	—	30–40 sec	15–20 sec	5–12 sec	1 rotation	—
Radiation dose (mSv)	1.5–2	—	10–15	7–10 (4–6 mSv with ECG pulsing)	5–20 (4–15 mSv with ECG pulsing)	Unknown	—

and have not been implemented widely outside of cardiac imaging because of limitations in tube output, which abdominal and other types of CT imaging are dependent on. Current MDCT scanners with 16- or 64-slice technology can acquire volumetric datasets with isotropic resolution of less than 0.5 mm in a breath-hold time achievable for most patients, but at the cost of decreased temporal resolution and increased radiation dose compared to EBCT. Despite technical improvements resulting in greater temporal resolution for coronary MDCT examinations, image quality is optimum when the heart rate is relatively slow and regular, and most centers administer beta-blockers (usually 50–100 mg of oral metoprolol, although some use intravenous medications for rapid onset) to patients with heart rates higher than 60–70 bpm prior to imaging.

SPECIFIC APPLICATIONS

[ ] CORONARY CALCIUM SCORING

Acquisition and Processing Technique

The amount of calcium contained in the pericoronary artery areas, known as the *coronary calcium score,* has been shown to have predictive value for risk of future cardiac events in large population based studies. The technical aspects of the score as measured by EBCT, including interscan and interreader variability, have been studied extensively.[46] No large studies have yet been performed using MDCT, as concerns were raised regarding reliability and measurement variability when single-slice and early MDCT units were used for coronary calcium scoring. However, several more-recent studies demonstrate similar performance of MDCT (especially 16-slice) and EBCT for determination of coronary calcium score, in terms of delineation of small calcifications, accuracy and reproducibility.[47,48] A review of the coronary calcium study databases of the MESA and CARDIA trials suggested that either EBCT or MDCT would be appropriate if a standardized protocol is used.[49]

Coronary calcium imaging is performed with prospective ECG-triggering when using EBCT and either prospective triggering or retrospective gating when using MDCT. Generally, 3-mm slices are obtained without intravenous contrast, although thinner slices are possible when using MDCT. Images are evaluated using software that thresholds images to display pixels with density greater than 130 HU. Deposits of calcium in the coronary arteries are manually selected by the operator and quantified automatically using a threshold or seed-growing operation. Figure 15-9 shows a coronary calcium scoring session using one vendor's software, although most are quite similar.

The amount of coronary calcium has traditionally been expressed using the *Agatston score*, which multiplies the area of a calcium deposit by a weighting factor reflecting the maximum density (in HU) of the calcium. More recently, coronary calcium quantification was performed using the calcium volume score and calcium mass. The calcium volume score is determined by multiplying the number of pixels with HU greater than 130 by the volume of each pixel. Calcium mass reflects the equivalent mass of

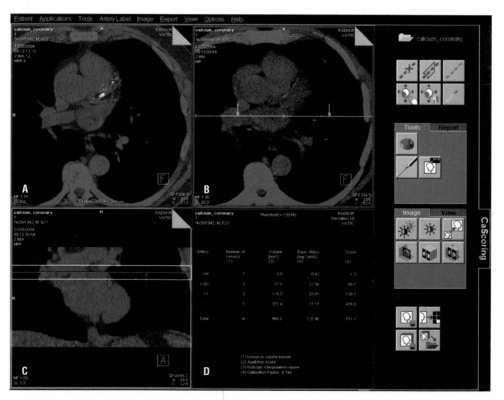

FIGURE 15-9. Coronary calcium scoring software. Pixels measuring more than 130 HU are displayed in purple (**B,C**); the user assigns calcifications to a specific vessel (**A**), and the volume, mass, and Agatston scores are calculated automatically (**D**). A reporting module that provides percentiles for a specific patient based on normative databases is also available.

calcium hydroxyapatite in a calcium deposit, and is measured by calibrating to a sample with known hydroxyapatite concentration. Although most normative data relating coronary calcium to cardiac risk are presented relative to Agatston score, recent studies suggest that the volume and mass scores may be more reproducible than the Agatston score. These measures may be adopted for coronary calcium quantification when large population databases using them are available.

Performance and Utility

Coronary calcium scoring has been applied in several different settings, including risk stratification, evaluation of symptomatic patients, and monitoring of therapy for and progression of atherosclerosis. Although several large studies demonstrate the correlation between elevated coronary calcium score and risk of future cardiac events,[50] prospective studies show variable results concerning the additional benefit of calcium scoring over traditional risk factor assessment.[51–53] However, the negative predictive value of a zero calcium score for the presence of significant obstructive coronary artery disease is well documented, as is the association between high coronary calcium score and the presence of obstructive coronary disease. This power has been used in several studies applying calcium scoring to evaluation of patients with chest pain, in which a negative test was used to exclude coronary artery disease as an explanation for the patients' symptoms.[54] Other studies also demonstrate the ability of calcium scoring to follow patients being treated for atherosclerosis with statins or other therapies.[55] In addition, coronary calcium scoring has been suggested as a method to select asymptomatic patients for further evaluation or treatment.[56] A high coronary calcium score in an asymptomatic patient with intermediate risk factors may be used as motivation for preemptive aggressive lifestyle modification or justification for medical therapy, whereas a low score may encourage continuation of a healthy lifestyle.

[ ] CORONARY ANGIOGRAPHY

Acquisition Techniques

Catheter-based coronary angiography has long been recognized as the gold standard for evaluation of coronary artery disease. However, an accurate noninvasive method for visualization of coronary artery stenosis would have great utility. In addition, the tomographic nature of CT allows for more than just a lumenographic view of the coronary arteries and permits some degree of visualization and characterization of atherosclerotic plaque.

Regardless of whether one performs coronary CT angiography using EBCT or MDCT, imaging is performed during rapid intravenous injection (3–5 ml/sec) of 80–120 ml of high iodine concentration (300–400 mg) non-ionic contrast. The timing of imaging with respect to the contrast injection can be determined using a small test bolus of 15–20 ml of contrast and imaging the passage of the bolus at a single level, usually every 1–2 seconds in the ascending or descending thoracic aorta. The computed tomographic angiography (CTA) acquisition begins at or just before the peak aortic enhancement time as measured using the test bolus. This method is used for all prospectively triggered exams and in many centers for retrospectively gated exams. An alternative for helical retrospectively gated exams is *bolus tracking* (known by

different names for different vendors). In this method, imaging is performed at a fixed level in the ascending or descending aorta during the injection of the main contrast bolus. The CTA scan is triggered when the enhancement in the aorta reaches a specific threshold, usually 120–140 HU. A flush of 40–60 ml of saline is usually given after the contrast to remove concentrated contrast from the superior vena cava (SVC) and right atrium, which can lead to streak artifacts, especially in the region of the RCA. High-quality coronary studies generally show most of the contrast bolus localized in the left side of the heart and systemic arterial system, with less opacification of the right-side chambers. Of note, this is not the desired distribution of contrast for noncoronary exams of cardiac anatomy and function, where equal opacification of both sides of the heart is of greater use.

The EBCT technique for coronary angiography is similar to that for calcium scoring. Imaging is prospectively triggered in mid-to-late diastole, and 3-mm slices are acquired axially. Coverage of the entire heart usually takes 30–40 seconds. Again, technical parameters are summarized in Table 15-2.

MDCT coronary acquisition protocols use retrospective gating and depend on the number of detectors and volume coverage per gantry rotation of the particular scanner being used. The x-ray beam is on throughout the entire acquisition, and the ECG is recorded to allow image reconstruction at specific points after study acquisition. This is in contrast to prospective triggering, in which the ECG signal is used to determine when to turn on the x-ray beam during the exam, but is not used afterward. In general, examinations are performed with a very low pitch, which is the ratio of table motion per gantry rotation to the volume of slices acquired. For example, if the table moves 18 mm per gantry rotation, while acquiring 16 × 0.75-mm slices (12-mm volume coverage), the pitch is 1.5. Typical pitch settings for 16-detector coronary CTA exams are 0.3–0.4, compared to 1–2 for noncardiac CT. This low pitch is necessary to ensure that the table motion per heartbeat is not greater than the volumetric coverage gantry rotation, which would result in the inability to reconstruct a completely continuous cardiac volume at a fixed point in the cardiac cycle. The pitch must be further decreased for patients with very low heart rates, usually less than 50 bpm. The length of the exam is directly proportional to the pitch, and it is the major reason for the greater radiation doses associated with MDCT coronary exams. The greater volumetric coverage of the 64-detector machines may allow higher pitches, resulting in shorter exams and perhaps decreased radiation doses.

Images are acquired using the thinnest detector collimation of the scanner, ranging from 0.5 mm to 0.75 mm, and are reconstructed at 0.4- to 1.0-mm slice thickness with some overlap. Isotropic submillimeter resolution is preferable. The current generation of 64-slice machines feature different acquisition characteristics: one manufacturer emphasizes thinner slices, and others acquire thicker slices but cover more volume of the heart per rotation. It is not yet clear which of these two factors is more important for coronary CTA. Although thinner slices may be useful for improved visualization of calcified and noncalcified plaque and in-stent evaluation, shorter acquisition times lessen the effects of heart rate changes during the acquisition. Typical acquisition times range from 5 to 12 seconds for 64-slice machines to 15 to 20 seconds for 16-slice scanners.

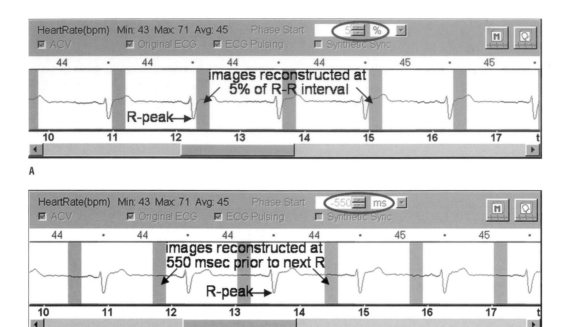

FIGURE 15-10. Two methods for reconstruction window positioning with respect to the R-peak. **(A)** Forward percentage method—window centered at a percentage of the R–R interval after the R-peak. **(B)** Absolute reverse method—window centered at a fixed time before the next R-peak, a more reproducible point in the presence of a variable heart rate.

Postprocessing, Visualization, and Analysis Techniques

After data acquisition in MDCT coronary angiography, images can be reconstructed at any point in the cardiac cycle. The location of the center of the reconstruction window, the width of which defines the temporal resolution of the image, is placed at the desired position in the cardiac cycle. This location can be represented either as a percentage of the R-R interval or an absolute time after the previous R-peak or before the next R-peak (Figure 15-10). The absolute reverse method uses a fixed time before the next R-peak, which has been demonstrated to be a more reproducible location in the cardiac cycle in the presence of variations in heart rate compared to the absolute forward or relative percentage methods. Images are usually reconstructed in mid-late diastole, which is a period of relatively stable position of the heart in patients with lower heart rates. For slower 4-slice machines, a separate set of images was usually reconstructed earlier in diastole, as this was the time of least motion for the RCA; however, a separate right coronary reconstruction is usually not necessary with newer machines. In patients with very high heart rates, peak systole may be the period of least motion, and images reconstructed at that time may be the most diagnostic. A typical reconstruction at a single point in the cardiac cycle has 150–300 images, depending on slice thickness and volume of coverage. Additional reconstructions can be performed at regular intervals throughout the cardiac cycle to obtain functional measurements such as ejection fraction, as discussed later in this chapter. Many centers routinely reconstruct as many as 10 points at the time that the scan is performed, as it may be logistically difficult to reconstruct them off-line at the time of study interpretation.

An image can be reconstructed from data acquired during a 180° gantry rotation, or 165–250 msec for currently available scanners. For slower heart rates (eg, < 75 bpm for a fast 16-slice machine), the late diastolic period is long enough to reconstruct motion-free images at a given location using 180° worth of data from only a single heartbeat. For higher heart rates, the diastolic period may be too short for a motion-free 180° rotation window. In this case, one can combine data from two adjacent heartbeats to reconstruct an image, using 90° worth of data (one fourth of a gantry rotation) from each. This method is called *multisector reconstruction,* and effectively doubles the temporal resolution of the image; however, the data from the two adjacent beats may not be consistent if there is any beat-to-beat variation in heart rate or cardiac position, and leads to motion artifacts. This technique can be extended to three or more adjacent heartbeats or sectors, but artifacts also increase. Most vendors provide the option of allowing the scanner to decide automatically whether to use single or multisector reconstruction; both techniques can be used within a single study if the heart rate varies over the acquisition.

After reconstructing images at the desired points, the visualization and analysis steps are performed. Evaluation of the large number of images generated in a coronary CTA exam precludes the use of film for study interpretation, and most studies are reviewed on postprocessing workstations. Many different workstations are available, both from CT scanner manufacturers and independent companies. These workstations display coronary CTA data differently, including axial viewing (Figure 15-11A), multiplanar reformatting (MPR) (Figure 15-11B), curved MPR (Figure 15-11C), maximum intensity projection (MIP) (Figure 15-12A), and volume rendering (VR) (Figure 15-12B). Most workstations have automated methods for processing and analysis, including vessel

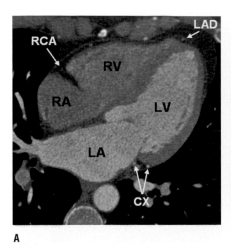
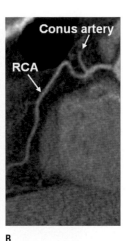

FIGURE 15-11. Methods for display of coronary CTA studies. (**A**) Axial source images are useful for visualization of noncardiac structures. (**B**) Multiplanar reformatted (MPR) can be used to create cardiac views such as this four-chamber view. Cardiac chambers and mid-distal coronary branches are marked. (**C**) Curved MPR can lay out the entire course of a vessel, such as the right coronary artery (RCA).

segmentation, centerline calculation, and quantitative stenosis analysis (Figure 15-13). Only one 4-slice study has evaluated which visualization or analysis methods are superior,[57] finding that all postprocessing methods were generally equivalent, and less accurate than viewing axial source images. It is generally accepted that one must at least initially evaluate the imaging volume tomographically at full resolution, and that viewing of VR images alone is not sufficient for accurate diagnosis.

Figures 15-11 through 15-13 are examples of normal coronary CTA studies, whereas Figures 15-14 through 15-16 demonstrate visualization of coronary stenosis, intraluminal thrombus, noncalcified plaque in the absence of luminal stenosis, and calcified stenoses, repectively, all performed using 16-slice scanners. Figure 15-17 shows a study performed using a newer 64-slice machine.

Performance and Utility

Several studies have evaluated the performance of EBCT coronary angiography, finding sensitivities for detection of stenoses greater than 50% to 74%–92%.[58,59] Similar values were also found for 4-slice MDCT with slightly higher values for 8-slice CT.[60] However, as described later, a greater percentage of the coronary segments were judged to be unevaluable for 4- and 8-slice MDCT compared to EBCT. Single center trials recently evaluated the accuracy of 16-slice coronary CTA in patients suspected of having coronary artery disease, with results for sensitivity and specificity for detection of stenoses more than 50% to 89%–93%, and much lower rates of unevaluable excluded coronary segments. The negative predictive value for hemodynamically significant stenosis was found to be quite high, at approximately 97%. When subjects with very high coronary calcium were excluded, sensitivity improved to 98%.[61]

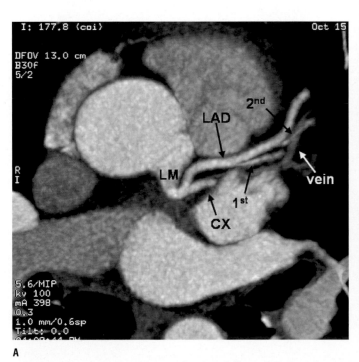

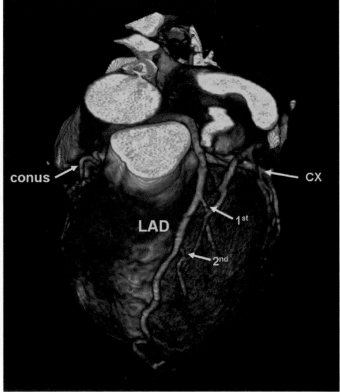

FIGURE 15-12. Other methods for display of coronary CTA studies. (**A**) Maximum intensity projection (MIP) images show the brightest pixel in a volume slab and are useful for showing portions of one or more vessels. Here the left main (LM), proximal and mid-left anterior descending (LAD) artery, first and second diagonal branches, and proximal circumflex (CX) are seen; however, veins are also visualized. (**B**) Volume rendered (VR) view of another patient with normal coronary arteries (*arrowhead* = left main coronary artery).

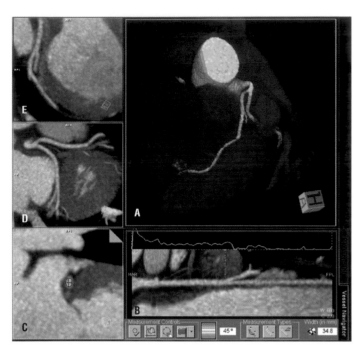

FIGURE 15-13. Quantitative vessel analysis software applied to a normal circumflex artery. (**A**) Segmented VR view; (**B**) straightened curved MPR or "ribbon" view with vessel area plot; (**C**) view perpendicular to vessel center line used for area calculation. (**D, E**) Thin-slab MIP images showing distal circumflex and '"spider" view of proximal LAD and circumflex.

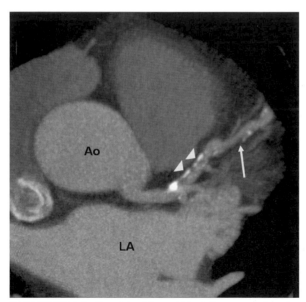

FIGURE 15-14. Thin-slab oblique MIP of the proximal and mid-LAD in a patient who had previously undergone angioplasty shows mixed calcified (*arrowheads*) and noncalcified plaque (*arrow*), resulting in moderate stenosis. (Ao = aorta).

Although promising, these results have not yet been confirmed in multicenter trials, or using the latest 64-slice technology, and not all studies evaluated side branch disease. In addition, these studies were performed in patients scheduled to undergo catheter coronary angiography—in whom there may be referral bias—and not in a screening population or other groups in which CTA may have the most benefit.

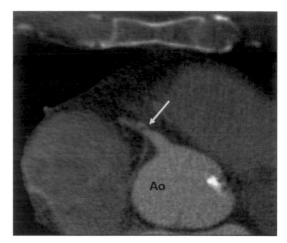

FIGURE 15-15. Axial image showing intraluminal thrombus in the proximal RCA (Ao = aorta). The distal vessel curves out of the image plane, and is therefore not shown on the present slice.

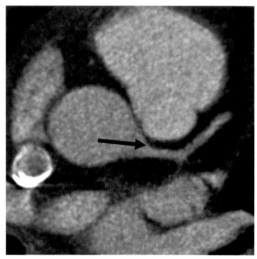

FIGURE 15-16. Mild, noncalcified lipid or "soft" plaque in the left main coronary artery (LMCA, *arrow*) by CTA, with no abnormality seen at catheter angiography.

One important limitation in determining the accuracy of CTA for detection of coronary stenosis is the use of catheter angiography as a gold standard. Catheter angiography visualizes only the caliber of the vessel lumen (a *lumenogram*), and may not accurately depict the degree of atherosclerosis, especially in the presence of positive arterial remodeling (*the Glagov phenomenon*). A preliminary 16-slice CTA study of patients who had "normal" catheter angiograms demonstrated atherosclerotic lesions in 20% of these subjects.[62]

OTHER APPLICATIONS

【 】 PLAQUE DETECTION AND CHARACTERIZATION

One advantage of a tomographic technique like CT versus catheter angiography is the ability to visualize the wall of a coronary artery

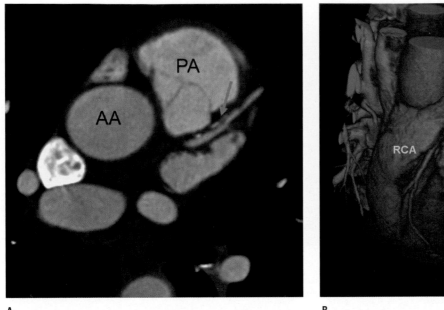
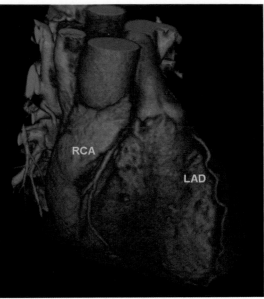

A   **B**

FIGURE 15-17. Images obtained using 64-slice machine with 0.4 mm slice thickness (Siemens Sensation64). (**A**) Axial source image showing mixed calcified and noncalcified plaque in the LAD (*arrow*), ascending aorta (AA), and pulmonary outflow tract (PA). (**B**) Volume-rendered image showing LAD and RCA. *(Images courtesy of Bernd Wintersperger, MD, University of Munich-Grosshadern.)*

and to characterize atherosclerotic plaque. Although the ability of unenhanced CT to demonstrate calcified plaque is well known, the presence and complex composition of atherosclerotic plaque can be evaluated by contrast-enhanced CTA because the different components have different x-ray attenuation properties. Preliminary studies comparing CT to intravascular ultrasound (IVUS) for evaluation of plaque components show that CT is able to accurately detect and characterize plaques as soft (predominantly lipid containing), intermediate, or calcified on the basis of their HU attenuation[63,64] (Figures 15-14 and 15-15), and also to detect positive remodeling.[65] CT performs less well when evaluating plaques with mixed constituency or plaques that are highly calcified. Continued improvements in spatial resolution will likely aid in this application; however, the ability of CT to detect soft plaque noninvasively is an important finding, given that these lesions may represent those predisposed to rupture. Ex-vivo studies of coronary artery specimens using MDCT, flat-panel CT, and micro-CT are being used to analyze the histologic structure of plaque. Coronary MRA has also been used for plaque characterization, given its superior soft-tissue contrast; however, it is technically more challenging at present.[66]

【 】 BYPASS GRAFT IMAGING

Imaging of coronary artery bypass grafts (CABGs) was an early application for both ungated CT and prospectively triggered EBCT, and demonstrated high accuracy for determination of patency or occlusion. Studies using gated MDCT likewise demonstrate accurate determination of graft patency, and studies are being initiated to evaluate in-graft stenosis[67–69] (Figure 15-18). Another useful application of gated MDCT is preoperative planning for

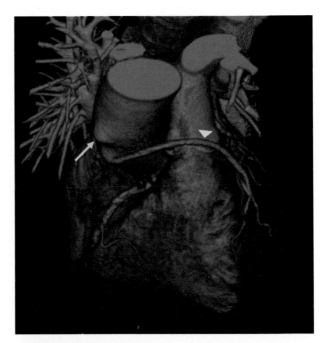

FIGURE 15-18. Volume-rendered image of patent bypass graft to LAD (*arrowhead*) and occluded graft origin (*arrow*). *(Image courtesy of Bernd Wintersperger, MD, University of Munich-Grosshadern.)*

minimally invasive bypass surgery. CTA can demonstrate the course of the internal mammary arteries and the location and size of touchdown vessels prior to surgery.[70,71] CTA may also be used prior to re-do CABG to determine the precise location and relationship of bypass grafts to the overlying osseous and soft-tissue anatomy.

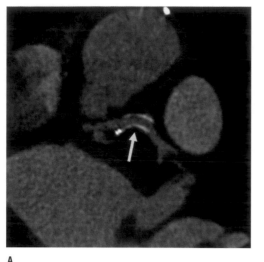 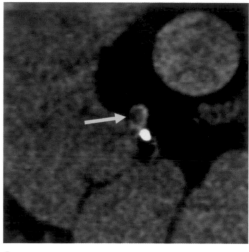

A   B

FIGURE 15-19. (A) Curved MPR showing lumen of stent in LMCA (*arrow*). **(B)** Cross-section perpendicular to vessel centerline shows in-stent stenosis, which was confirmed at catheter angiography (*arrow*).

【 】 STENT IMAGING

Stent imaging is a very challenging application for CT, as a 2- or 3-mm stent may encompass only a few pixels on an image, and artifacts from the metal in the stent may obscure the lumen.[72] However, noninvasive evaluation of in-stent stenosis remains an important goal for CT, and has been studied in-vitro and in-vivo using both EBCT and MDCT.[73,74] One study[75] demonstrated high accuracy for detection of stenosis in left main stents using 16-slice MDCT, with nondiagnostic visualization only in cases of heavy vessel calcification. In-vitro studies using flat-panel CT at 0.25-mm resolution show improved visualization of the stent lumen, and may be an important technique in the future[72] (Figure 15-19).

【 】 CORONARY ANOMALIES

Coronary MRA has often been used as a supplement to catheter angiography for evaluation of the presence and course of anomalous coronary vessels, and has come to be regarded as the gold standard for evaluation of the proximal course of anomalous coronary arteries.[76–80] However, EBCT has also been used in this setting. More recently, 16-slice MDCT was evaluated and its accuracy and utility as a supplement to catheter angiography for demonstrating both the origin and course of anomalous coronary vessels was demonstrated[81] (Figure 15-20).

【 】 IMAGING OF PATIENTS WITH IMPLANTED DEVICES

Implanted pacemakers or defibrillators, as well as several other types of devices, are generally considered to be contraindications to MR. Cardiac CT can be used safely in this setting for evaluation of cardiac structure and function, as well as coronary imaging (Figure 15-21). Artifacts from pacing leads are generally less problematic on newer-generation scanners.

【 】 ACUTE CHEST PAIN PROTOCOL

The enhanced volume coverage of 64-slice CT has led to the ability to perform an ECG-gated study of the entire chest in a reasonable breath-hold. This has prompted some to consider whether a single scan could be used for evaluation of the most common causes of acute chest pain (eg, pulmonary embolism, aortic dissection, acute coronary syndrome) as well as a diagnostic evaluation of the lungs. Preliminary investigations are currently being performed using both 16- and 64-slice technology to demonstrate the feasibility of this approach, which has also been referred to as the *triple rule-out*. Further studies must be performed to document the accuracy and cost effectiveness of this approach before it is widely adopted.

LIMITATIONS AND OTHER ISSUES

【 】 SPATIAL AND TEMPORAL RESOLUTION

Despite the promising performance of 16-slice coronary CTA in published trials, there are several important limitations that may hamper acceptance of this technique. The spatial resolution, even with 0.4-mm slices, may not be sufficient to delineate small side branches, particularly if they are stenotic. Current digital coronary angiography systems have a resolution of approximately 0.25 mm per pixel, which 64-detector or flat-panel systems may come closer to achieving in the future. Improved spatial resolution is also needed to move beyond qualitative detection of a "significant" stenosis to accurate quantification of percentage stenosis, which has not yet been attempted using CTA. Limited temporal resolution continues to be problematic as vessel visualization is highly dependent on heart rate, even using newer 16-slice technology,[82] necessitating beta-blockade for many patients. This has several effects on patients and exam throughput, including the

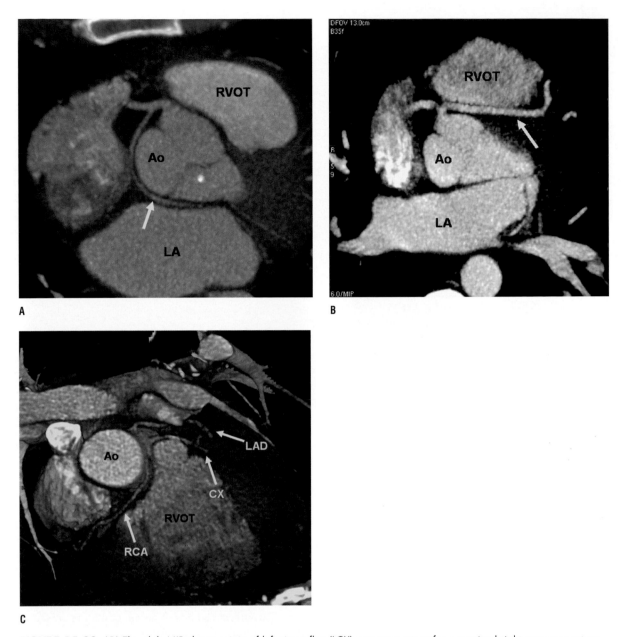

FIGURE 15-20. (A) Thin-slab MIP shows origin of left circumflex (LCX) coronary artery from proximal right coronary artery (RCA) with posterior course between aortic root (Ao) and left atrium (LA). **(B)** Origin of left coronary artery from proximal right coronary artery with course between aortic root and right ventricular outflow tract (RVOT). **(C)** Volume-rendered view (Siemens InSpace ver. VB10) shows separate origin of left anterior descending (LAD) and LCX from left coronary cusp and high origin of RCA from left cusp with interarterial course.

need for increased patient monitoring, decreased patient convenience, and exclusion of those in whom beta-blockers are contraindicated. Continued improvements in MDCT technology will ameliorate this problem, but it is unlikely that the temporal resolution of CT will ever reach that of catheter angiography. Multisector reconstruction shows improved coronary visualization for moderately elevated heart rates using older 16-slice technology, although it remains to be tested rigorously for newer machines. EBCT provides superior temporal resolution, but at the cost of spatial resolution and exam length. For 16- and 64-slice CT, the scan length is well within the breath-hold capacity of most patients.

[ ] CALCIFICATIONS

The presence of coronary calcification can significantly degrade diagnostic performance. Large, calcified plaques result in several types of artifacts that may limit visualization of the segment of interest, or of noncalcified plaques in adjacent coronary segments. Several studies show significant reductions in diagnostic accuracy in patients with markedly elevated coronary calcium,[61] and many centers will not perform examinations in patients with a large amount of coronary calcium (>600–1000 Agatston score). However, if evaluation of a heavily calcified vessel is required, investigations suggest that a stenosis is likely not to be high grade

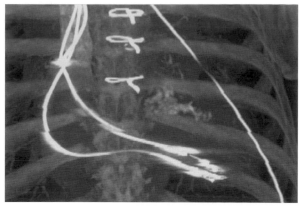

A

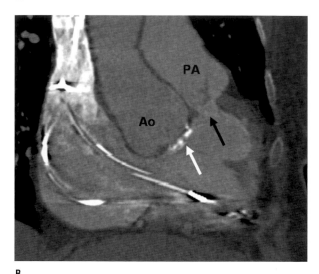

B

FIGURE 15-21. Thick slab MIP (**A**) and oblique coronal MPR (**B**) show one pacemaker lead in the RA and two in the RV. The patient was postrepair for tetralogy of Fallot; calcified VSD patch (*white arrow*) and subvalvular pulmonic stenosis (*black arrow*) are seen.

at catheter angiography if any residual lumen can be detected adjacent to a large calcification.[83] MRI is not affected to nearly the same degree as CT by the presence of calcified plaque, and coronary MRA may be preferable in this setting.

【 】 ARRHYTHMIA

Another significant limitation to CTA is the need for a regular heart rate to obtain high-quality images. Imaging of patients with frequent ectopy or atrial fibrillation with variable ventricular response is challenging, and premedication is often required. When using retrospective gating, one can edit the acquired ECG tracing to a limited degree, and data related to ectopic beats can be removed if ectopy is infrequent. Several studies demonstrate that the regularity of the heart rate is at least as important as the rate. In addition, a satisfactory ECG gating signal is required for any type of image reconstruction, which can be quite challenging to obtain in some patients. One alternative under investigation is to use the actual motion of the heart as the gating signal, referred to as *Kymogram gating* or *self-gating*. This technique is theoretically less sensitive to arrhythmia and does not require an electric gating signal.

【 】 THE "EXCLUDED SEGMENTS" PROBLEM

Limitations in spatial and temporal resolution, artifacts related to calcified plaques, and arrhythmia during acquisition may all lead to difficulty in evaluation of a particular coronary artery segment. Many of the studies cited earlier did not attempt to evaluate the presence of stenosis in a coronary segment if these artifacts limited visualization. These segments are reported as "unable to be evaluated," and were excluded from data analysis, which may lead to a falsely elevated accuracy compared to catheter angiography for detection of greater than 50% stenosis. Excluded segment values for EBCT coronary angiography ranged from 10% to 28%, similar to the 27% to 32% values reported for 4-slice MDCT. Figures improved considerably for 16-slice CT, with a recent study of the latest generation of 16-slice machine reporting 6.2% of arteries with diameter greater than 1.5 mm as not assessable. One study reports results for all segments, without exclusion, finding sensitivity and specificity of 95% and 86% for stenosis detection.[84]

【 】 RADIATION EXPOSURE

The radiation dose associated with coronary CTA performed using MDCT with retrospective gating (11 mSv) is considerably higher than EBCT (1.2 mSv), and is similar to or slightly higher than diagnostic catheter angiography (3–10 mSv) when performed using 16-slice machines.[85,86] The effective radiation dose in women is 25% greater than in men (8 vs. 10 mSv). Although doses may be lower with 64-slice scanners, dose reduction strategies are of major importance, and several methods are implemented on current scanners. Most vendors include a form of ECG-related dose modulation; this technique decreases the x-ray tube current by up to 80% during systole, when full detail is not needed, with the full nominal current present only during late diastole, when the majority of images are acquired.[87] This technique can decrease overall dose by as much as 40% to 50% in patients with lower heart rates, but current implementations are not flexible enough to account for arrhythmias or large changes in heart rate over the scan. Two other methods of dose modulation are currently in use; the first adjusts the x-ray tube current rapidly (up to 60 times/sec) as the beam rotates around the patient. The dose is decreased when the beam is traveling anterior to posterior, where most patients are thinner, and increased when traveling medial to lateral. The second method changes the tube current slowly as the patient moves through the gantry to maintain constant image quality throughout the scanned portions of the body. For example, because the lung does not attenuate x-rays as much as the heart, portions of the chest containing only lung receive a lower dose than the portion containing the heart.

【 】 CT VERSUS MR FOR CORONARY ARTERY IMAGING

The solution to many of these limitations may be found in coronary MRA, which does not use ionizing radiation or iodinated contrast and has superior temporal resolution to both EBCT and MDCT. However, coronary MRA is still very much a user- and vendor-dependent technique, and the largest and most successful trials have been published using only a single vendor's equipment and acquisition technique (Philips Navigator technique).[88] One study[89] evaluated 4-slice MDCT and coronary MRA compared to catheter angiography, finding higher sensitivity but lower specificity and overall accuracy for CTA compared to MR, but a high negative predictive value for both (93% for CTA and 90% for MRA). Studies comparing MRA to 16-slice or 64-slice CT directly have not yet been performed, but separate studies comparing both to catheter angiography show that MR has a higher excluded segment rate, although both have very high negative predictive values. Other disadvantages of MR for coronary imaging include longer acquisition times and inability to image patients with implanted devices. At times, MR has some difficulty visualizing calcified plaque, although image quality is not as degraded in the presence of calcified plaque.

FUTURE DEVELOPMENTS AND CONCLUSIONS

MDCT technology has evolved very rapidly in the years since its practical implementation in 1998, and the field of cardiac CT has accelerated significantly since the introduction of 16-slice machines in 2002. Technology will, no doubt, continue to develop, and most observers agree that the flat-panel area detector CT will most likely be the next large advance. This development, however, is still several years from commercial implementation, and in the interim there will likely be continuing progress in the "slice war." A recently introduced "dual-source" 64-slice system, with two x-ray tubes and detectors mounted on a single gantry, achieves a temporal resolution of 83 msec and may allow imaging of almost all patients without the use of beta-blockers.[90] Although initial reported trials using 64-slice technology show some improvement in performance for stenosis detection[91] and plaque evaluation[92] with increased reliability, it is still very new and undergoing testing to determine its incremental benefit. It is difficult to predict what the effect of another increase in volume coverage would mean for coronary imaging.

At this point, we can state that MDCT will be the dominant CT technology for CT coronary angiography, given its wide availability and the flexibility to use MDCT scanners for other types of CT imaging (eg, chest, abdomen). Despite its superior temporal resolution and much larger body of supporting evidence, EBCT will likely not find wide implementation in coronary CTA given its small installed user base. Coronary MRA will continue to improve and may supplant CTA in several years given the lack of ionizing radiation and iodinated contrast.

In the near future, large multicenter trials will be performed to determine both the accuracy of coronary CTA and MRA and their ultimate role in the diagnostic evaluation of patients with coronary artery disease. As noted earlier, one important potential application of CTA is the evaluation of patients presenting to emergency departments with acute chest pain, most of whom will be found not to have acute coronary syndrome. The availability of a rapid, relatively noninvasive test that can demonstrate coronary stenosis with high accuracy and find and characterize atherosclerotic plaque, even in the absence of stenosis, has the potential to change the evaluation and management of coronary artery disease profoundly.

REFERENCES

1. Stuber M, Botnar RM, Danias PG, et al. Double-oblique free-breathing high resolution three-dimensional coronary magnetic resonance angiography. *J Am Coll Cardiol.* 1999;34:524.
2. Wielopolski PA, van Geuns RJ, de Feyter PJ, et al. Breath-hold coronary MR angiography with volume-targeted imaging. *Radiology.* 1998;209:209.
3. van Geuns RJ, Wielopolski PA, de Bruin HG, et al. MR coronary angiography with breath-hold targeted volumes: preliminary clinical results. *Radiology.* 2000;217:270.
4. Botnar RM, Stuber M, Danias PG, et al. Improved coronary artery definition with T2-weighted, free-breathing, three-dimensional coronary MRA. *Circulation.* 1999;99:3139.
5. Kim WY, Danias PG, Stuber M, et al. Coronary magnetic resonance angiography for the detection of coronary stenoses. *N Engl J Med.* 2001;345:1863.
6. McConnell MV, Khasgiwala VC, Savord BJ, et al. Comparison of respiratory suppression methods and navigator locations for MR coronary angiography. *Am J Roentgenol.* 1997;168:1369.
7. Oshinski JN, Hofland L, Mukundan S, Jr., et al. Two-dimensional coronary MR angiography without breath holding. *Radiology.* 1996;201:737.
8. Du YP, McVeigh ER, Bluemke DA, et al. A comparison of prospective and retrospective respiratory navigator gating in 3D MR coronary angiography. *Int J Cardiovasc Imag.* 2001;17:287.
9. Danias PG, McConnell MV, Khasgiwala VC, et al. Prospective navigator correction of image position for coronary MR angiography. *Radiology.* 1997; 203:733.
10. McConnell MV, Khasgiwala VC, Savord BJ, et al. Prospective adaptive navigator correction for breath-hold MR coronary angiography. *Magn Reson Med.* 1997;37:148.
11. Edelman RR, Mattle HP, Wallner B, et al. Extracranial carotid arteries: evaluation with "black blood" MR angiography. *Radiology.* 1990;177:45.
12. Simonetti OP, Finn JP, White RD, et al. "Black blood" T2-weighted inversion-recovery MR imaging of the heart. *Radiology.* 1996;199:49.
13. Stuber M, Botnar RM, Kissinger KV, et al. Free-breathing black-blood coronary MR angiography: initial results. *Radiology.* 2001;219:278.
14. Thomas D, Krug B, Hackmann D, et al. MR- coronary angiography: comparison of SSFP and spoiled GRE sequence (bright blood technique) and a TSE sequence (black blood technique) in healthy volunteers. *Rofo.* 2004; 176:1589.
15. Brittain JH, Hu BS, Wright GA, et al. Coronary angiography with magnetization-prepared T2 contrast. *Magn Reson Med.* 1995;33:689.
16. Li D, Paschal CB, Haacke EM, et al. Coronary arteries: three-dimensional MR imaging with fat saturation and magnetization transfer contrast. *Radiology.* 1993;187:401.
17. Sommer T, Hofer U, Hackenbroch M, et al. [Submillimeter 3D coronary MR angiography with real-time navigator correction in 107 patients with suspected coronary artery disease]. *Rofo.* 2002;174:459.
18. Li D, Dolan RP, Walovitch RC, et al. Three-dimensional MRI of coronary arteries using an intravascular contrast agent. *Magn Reson Med.* 1998;39:1014.
19. Stuber M, Botnar RM, Danias PG, et al. Contrast agent-enhanced, free-breathing, three-dimensional coronary magnetic resonance angiography. *J Magn Reson Imag.* 1999;10:790.
20. Paetsch I, Huber ME, Bornstedt A, et al. Improved three-dimensional free-breathing coronary magnetic resonance angiography using gadocoleric acid (B-22956) for intravascular contrast enhancement. *J Magn Reson Imag.* 2004;20:288.
21. Huber ME, Paetsch I, Schnackenburg B, et al. Performance of a new gadolinium-based intravascular contrast agent in free-breathing inversion-recovery 3D coronary MRA. *Magn Reson Med.* 2003;49:115.
22. Klein C, Nagel E, Schnackenburg B, et al. The intravascular contrast agent Clariscan (NC 100150 injection) for 3D MR coronary angiography in patients with coronary artery disease. *Magma.* 2000;11:65.
23. Klein C, Schalla S, Schnackenburg B, et al. Improvement of image quality of non-invasive coronary artery imaging with magnetic resonance by the use of the intravascular contrast agent Clariscan (NC100150 injection) in patients with coronary artery disease. *J Magn Reson Imag.* 2003;17:656.
24. Taylor AM, Panting JR, Keegan J, et al. Safety and preliminary findings with the intravascular contrast agent NC100150 injection for MR coronary angiography. *J Magn Reson Imag.* 1999;9:220.
25. Meyer CH, Hu BS, Nishimura DG, et al. Fast spiral coronary artery imaging. *Magn Reson Med.* 1992;28:202.
26. Bornert P, Stuber M, Botnar RM, et al. Direct comparison of 3D spiral vs. Cartesian gradient-echo coronary magnetic resonance angiography. *Magn Reson Med.* 2001;46:789.

27. Spuentrup E, Katoh M, Stuber M, et al. Coronary MR imaging using free-breathing 3D steady-state free precession with radial *k*-space sampling. *Rofo.* 2003;175:1330.

28. Spuentrup E, Katoh M, Buecker A, et al. Free-breathing 3D steady-state free precession coronary MR angiography with radial *k*-space sampling: comparison with cartesian *k*-space sampling and cartesian gradient-echo coronary MR angiography—pilot study. *Radiology.* 2004;231:581.

29. Barkhausen J, Hunold P, Jochims M, et al. [Comparison of gradient-echo and steady state free precession sequences for 3D-navigator MR angiography of coronary arteries]. *Rofo.* 2002;174:725.

30. Deshpande VS, Shea SM, Chung YC, et al. Breath-hold three-dimensional true-FISP imaging of coronary arteries using asymmetric sampling. *J Magn Reson Imag.* 2002;15:473.

31. Deshpande VS, Shea SM, Laub G, et al. 3D magnetization-prepared true-FISP: a new technique for imaging coronary arteries. *Magn Reson Med.* 2001;46:494.

32. Shea SM, Deshpande VS, Chung YC, et al. Three-dimensional true-FISP imaging of the coronary arteries: improved contrast with T2-preparation. *J Magn Reson Imag.* 2002;15:597.

33. Spuentrup E, Buecker A, Stuber M, et al. Navigator-gated coronary magnetic resonance angiography using steady-state-free-precession: comparison to standard T2-prepared gradient-echo and spiral imaging. *Invest Radiol.* 2003;38:263.

34. Spuentrup E, Bornert P, Botnar RM, et al. Navigator-gated free-breathing three-dimensional balanced fast field echo (TrueFISP) coronary magnetic resonance angiography. *Invest Radiol.* 2002;37:637.

35. Giorgi B, Dymarkowski S, Maes F, et al. Improved visualization of coronary arteries using a new three-dimensional submillimeter MR coronary angiography sequence with balanced gradients. *Am J Roentgenol.* 2002;179:901.

36. Sodickson DK, Manning WJ. Simultaneous acquisition of spatial harmonics (SMASH): fast imaging with radiofrequency coil arrays. *Magn Reson Med.* 1997;38:591.

37. Pruessmann KP, Weiger M, Scheidegger MB, et al. SENSE: sensitivity encoding for fast MRI. *Magn Reson Med.* 1999;42:952.

38. Madore B, Pelc NJ. SMASH and SENSE: experimental and numerical comparisons. *Magn Reson Med.* 2001;45:1103.

39. Huber ME, Kozerke S, Pruessmann KP, et al. Sensitivity-encoded coronary MRA at 3T. *Magn Reson Med.* 2004;52:221.

40. Gutberlet M, Spors B, Grothoff M, et al. Comparison of different cardiac MRI sequences at 1.5 T/3.0 T with respect to signal-to-noise and contrast-to-noise ratios–initial experience. *Rofo.* 2004;176:801.

41. Schar M, Kozerke S, Fischer SE, et al. Cardiac SSFP imaging at 3 Tesla. *Magn Reson Med.* 2004;51:799.

42. Stuber M, Botnar RM, Fischer SE, et al. Preliminary report on in vivo coronary MRA at 3 Tesla in humans. *Magn Reson Med.* 2002;48:425.

43. Ferencik M, Moselewski F, Ropers D, et al. Quantitative parameters of image quality in multidetector spiral computed tomographic coronary imaging with submillimeter collimation. *Am J Cardiol.* 2003;92:1257.

44. Jaffray DA, Siewerdsen JH. Cone-beam computed tomography with a flat-panel imager: initial performance characterization. *Med Phys.* 2000;27:1311.

45. Lembcke A, Wiese TH, Schnorr J, et al. Image quality of noninvasive coronary angiography using multislice spiral computed tomography and electron-beam computed tomography: intraindividual comparison in an animal model. *Invest Radiol.* 2004;39:357.

46. Achenbach S, Ropers D, Mohlenkamp S, et al. Variability of repeated coronary artery calcium measurements by electron beam tomography. *Am J Cardiol.* 2001;87:210.

47. Horiguchi J, Yamamoto H, Akiyama Y, et al. Coronary artery calcium scoring using 16-MDCT and a retrospective ECG-gating reconstruction algorithm. *Am J Roentgenol.* 2004;183:103.

48. Stanford W, Thompson BH, Burns TL, et al. Coronary artery calcium quantification at multi-detector row helical CT versus electron-beam CT. *Radiology.* 2004;230:397.

49. Carr JJ, Nelson JC, Wong ND, et al. Calcified Coronary Artery Plaque Measurement with Cardiac CT in Population-based Studies: Standardized Protocol of Multi-Ethnic Study of Atherosclerosis (MESA) and Coronary Artery Risk Development in Young Adults (CARDIA) Study. *Radiology.* 2005;234:35.

50. Keelan PC, Bielak LF, Ashai K, et al. Long-term prognostic value of coronary calcification detected by electron-beam computed tomography in patients undergoing coronary angiography. *Circulation.* 2001;104:412.

51. Shaw LJ, Raggi P, Schisterman E, et al. Prognostic value of cardiac risk factors and coronary artery calcium screening for all-cause mortality. *Radiology.* 2003;228:826.

52. O'Malley PG, Greenberg BA, Taylor AJ: Cost-effectiveness of using electron beam computed tomography to identify patients at risk for clinical coronary artery disease. *Am Heart J.* 2004;148:106.

53. Greenland P, LaBree L, Azen SP, et al. Coronary artery calcium score combined with Framingham score for risk prediction in asymptomatic individuals. *JAMA.* 2004;291:210.

54. Raggi P, Callister TQ, Cooil B, et al. Evaluation of chest pain in patients with low to intermediate pretest probability of coronary artery disease by electron beam computed tomography. *Am J Cardiol.* 2000;85:283.

55. Achenbach S, Ropers D, Pohle K, et al. Influence of lipid-lowering therapy on the progression of coronary artery calcification: a prospective evaluation. *Circulation.* 2002;106:1077.

56. Guerci AD, Arad Y: Potential use of Ca++ scanning to determine the need for and intensity of lipid-lowering therapy in asymptomatic adults. *Curr Cardiol Rep.* 2001;3:408.

57. Vogl TJ, Abdolmaali ND, Diebold T, et al. Techniques for the detection of coronary atherosclerosis: multi-detector row CT coronary angiography. *Radiology.* 2002;223.

58. Achenbach S, Ropers D, Regenfus M, et al. Contrast enhanced electron beam computed tomography to analyse the coronary arteries in patients after acute myocardial infarction. *Heart.* 2000;84:489.

59. Nikolaou K, Huber A, Knez A, et al. Intraindividual comparison of contrast-enhanced electron-beam computed tomography and navigator-echo-based magnetic resonance imaging for noninvasive coronary artery angiography. *Eur Radiol.* 2002;12:1663.

60. Maruyama T, Yoshizumi T, Tamura R, et al. Comparison of visibility and diagnostic capability of noninvasive coronary angiography by eight-slice multidetector-row computed tomography versus conventional coronary angiography. *Am J Cardiol.* 2004;93:537.

61. Kuettner A, Trabold T, Schroeder S, et al. Noninvasive detection of coronary lesions using 16-detector multislice spiral computed tomography technology: initial clinical results. *J Am Coll Cardiol.* 2004;44:1230.

62. Fine JJ, Edelson RA. Multi-slice CT angiography identifies atherosclerosis missed by traditional catheter angiography. *Cardiovasc Imag.* 2004;89(P).

63. Inoue F, Sato Y, Matsumoto N, et al. Evaluation of plaque texture by means of multislice computed tomography in patients with acute coronary syndrome and stable angina. *Circ J.* 2004;68:840.

64. Komatsu S, Hirayama A, Omori Y, et al. Detection of coronary plaque by computed tomography with a novel plaque analysis system, "Plaque Map," and comparison with intravascular ultrasound and angioscopy. *Circ J.* 2005;69:72.

65. Achenbach S, Ropers D, Hoffmann U, et al. Assessment of coronary remodeling in stenotic and nonstenotic coronary atherosclerotic lesions by multidetector spiral computed tomography. *J Am Coll Cardiol.* 2004;43:842.

66. Nikolaou K, Becker C, Muders M, et al. Multidetector-row computed tomography and magnetic resonance imaging of atherosclerotic lesions in human ex vivo coronary arteries. *Atherosclerosis.* 2004;174:243.

67. Marano R, Storto ML, Maddestra N, et al. Non-invasive assessment of coronary artery bypass graft with retrospectively ECG-gated four-row multi-detector spiral computed tomography. *Eur Radiol.* 2004;14:1353.

68. Willmann JK, Weishaupt D, Kobza R, et al. Coronary artery bypass grafts: ECG-gated multi-detector row CT angiography–influence of image reconstruction interval on graft visibility. *Radiology.* 2004;232:568.

69. Schlosser T, Konorza T, Hunold P, et al. Noninvasive visualization of coronary artery bypass grafts using 16-detector row computed tomography. *J Am Coll Cardiol.* 2004;44:1224.

70. Herzog C, Dogan S, Diebold T, et al. Multi-detector row CT versus coronary angiography: preoperative evaluation before totally endoscopic coronary artery bypass grafting. *Radiology.* 2003;229:200.

71. Caimmi PP, Fossaceca R, Lanfranchi M, et al. Cardiac angio-CT scan for planning MIDCAB. *Heart Surg Forum.* 2004;7:E113.

72. Mahnken AH, Seyfarth T, Flohr T, et al. Flat-panel Detector Computed Tomography for the Assessment of Coronary Artery Stents: Phantom Study in Comparison with 16-Slice Spiral Computed Tomography. *Invest Radiol.* 2005;40:8.

73. Hong C, Chrysant GS, Woodard PK, et al. Coronary artery stent patency assessed with in-stent contrast enhancement measured at multi-detector row CT angiography: initial experience. *Radiology.* 2004;233:286.

74. Knollmann FD, Moller J, Gebert A, et al. Assessment of coronary artery stent patency by electron-beam CT. *Eur Radiol.* 2004;14:1341.

75. Gilard M, Cornily JC, Rioufol G, et al. Noninvasive assessment of left main coronary stent patency with 16-slice computed tomography. *Am J Cardiol.* 2005;95:110.

76. McConnell MV, Ganz P, Selwyn AP, et al. Identification of anomalous coronary arteries and their anatomic course by magnetic resonance coronary angiography. *Circulation*. 1995;92:3158.

77. Post JC, van Rossum AC, Bronzwaer JG, et al. Magnetic resonance angiography of anomalous coronary arteries. A new gold standard for delineating the proximal course? *Circulation*. 1995;92:3163.

78. White CS, Laskey WK, Stafford JL, et al. Coronary MRA: use in assessing anomalies of coronary artery origin. *J Comput Assist Tomogr*. 1999;23:203.

79. Klessen C, Post F, Meyer J, et al. Depiction of anomalous coronary vessels and their relation to the great arteries by magnetic resonance angiography. *Eur Radiol*. 2000;10:1855.

80. Bunce NH, Lorenz CH, Keegan J, et al. Coronary artery anomalies: assessment with free-breathing three-dimensional coronary MR angiography. *Radiology*. 2003;227:201.

81. van Ooijen PM, Dorgelo J, Zijlstra F, et al. Detection, visualization and evaluation of anomalous coronary anatomy on 16-slice multidetector-row CT. *Eur Radiol*. 2004;14:2163.

82. Hoffmann MH, Shi H, Manzke R, et al. Noninvasive Coronary Angiography with 16-Detector Row CT: Effect of Heart Rate. *Radiology*. 2005;234:86.

83. Sakuma T NM, Fukuda K, Yoshida S. Management of Severe Calcified Lesions on Coronary CT Angiography Using 16-slice Multidetector CT: Is Severe Calcified Lesion High-grade Stenosis or Not? *Proc RSNA Ann Mtg*. 2003:367(P).

84. Nieman K, Rensing BJ, van Geuns RJ, et al. Usefulness of multislice computed tomography for detecting obstructive coronary artery disease. *Am J Cardiol*. 2002;89:913.

85. McCollough CH. Patient dose in cardiac computed tomography. *Herz*. 2003;28:1.

86. Morin RL, Gerber TC, McCollough CH. Radiation dose in computed tomography of the heart. *Circulation*. 2003;107:917.

87. Jakobs TF, Becker CR, Ohnesorge B, et al. Multislice helical CT of the heart with retrospective ECG gating: reduction of radiation exposure by ECG-controlled tube current modulation. *Eur Radiol*. 2002;12:1081.

88. Kim WY, Danias PG, Stuber M, et al. Coronary magnetic resonance angiography for the detection of coronary stenosis. *N Engl J Med*. 2001;345:1863.

89. Gerber BL, Coche E, Pasquet A, et al. Coronary Artery Stenosis: Direct Comparison of Four-Section Multi-Detector Row CT and 3D Navigator MR Imaging for Detection—Initial Results. *Radiology*. 2005;234:98.

90. Achenbach S, Ropers D, Kuettner A, et al. Contrast-enhanced coronary artery visualization by dual-source computed tomography—initial experience. *Eur J Radiol*. 2006;57:331.

91. Mollet N, Cademartiri F, van Mieghem C, et al. High-resolution spiral computed tomography coronary angiography in patients referred for diagnostic conventional coronary angiography. *Circulation*. 2005;112:2318.

92. Leber A, Becker A, Knez A, et al. Accuracy of 64-slice computed tomography to classify and quantify plaque volumes in the proximal coronary system: a comparative study using intravascular ultrasound. *J Am Coll Cardiol*. 2006;47:672.

CHAPTER (16)

Intracardiac Echocardiography in the Catheterization Laboratory

Frank E. Silvestry, MD

Intracardiac echocardiography (ICE) is an intravascular ultrasound (IVUS) modality that provides diagnostic imaging of cardiac structures from within the heart, and has become widely used for guiding noncoronary interventions in the catheterization and electrophysiology laboratories. The first IVUS catheters used high-frequency transducers (20–40 Mhz) containing a single ultrasound crystal that rapidly rotated at the end of the catheter, produces a radial two-dimensional image.[1] This type of high-frequency IVUS transducer provides excellent spatial resolution in the near field, making it uniquely suited for imaging the coronary arteries and other small vessels. The main limitation of IVUS in this frequency domain, however, is the short imaging depth (several millimeters).[1,2] To accomplish ICE imaging from atria to apex, lower frequency transducers (5–12 MHz) have been miniaturized and mounted onto catheters capable of percutaneous insertion and manipulation within the heart.[1,3–7] These lower-frequency transducers are capable of greater tissue penetration and imaging depth, permitting high-resolution two-dimensional imaging of the whole heart.[2,8–11] The earliest reports of such low-frequency ICE catheters were described in the late 1970s and early 1980s.[3,4] More recently, with the introduction of the newest phased array transducers, full Doppler flow data can be obtained.

Two different types of ICE catheters are currently available for clinical use. A mechanical transducer, similar to that used with IVUS, has an ultrasound transducer that rotates as it is driven by a motor unit at the opposite end of the drive shaft, resulting in a 360° "radial" view that is perpendicular to the axis of the catheter. The second type is a fixed or phased array catheter-mounted transducer that uses electronically controlled multiple transducers mounted on one side of the catheter shaft, which results in a wedge-shaped 90° image sector similar to that of transthoracic or transesophageal echo probes.

Both types of catheters provide high-resolution, real-time images of anatomic structures and of other intracardiac devices and catheters. These catheters currently range between 6- and 10-French in diameter, and are typically introduced through a sheath into a femoral vein. Phased array catheters typically offer a large depth of field and add Doppler imaging capabilities, whereas mechanical catheters offer superior near-field resolution.

BENEFITS OF INTRACARDIAC ECHOCARDIOGRAPHY

ICE offers imaging that is comparable or, in some cases, superior in quality to transesophageal echocardiography (TEE). The additional anatomic imaging detail that ICE provides is a substantial adjunct to x-ray fluoroscopy for electrophysiologic ablation procedures and transcatheter atrial septal defect closure. ICE been shown to provide procedural benefits when used for radiofrequency ablation of atrial fibrillation and transcatheter atrial septal closure procedures,[12–26] and as such, ICE has become the "gold standard" for imaging during these procedures. Its major advantage over TEE that general anesthesia is not needed. In addition, if sufficiently skilled and knowledgeable, the operator performing the percutaneous closure can also manipulate the ICE catheter and interpret the images. In this setting, ICE has been shown to improve patient comfort and shorten both procedure and fluoroscopy time, at costs comparable to TEE-guided interventions when general anesthesia is used.[21,27,28] ICE is currently used as the primary imaging modality during percutaneous transcatheter closure (PTC) without the need for supplemental transthoracic echo (TTE) or TEE. ICE has also been shown to provide incremental diagnostic benefit over TTE and TEE. In one series of 94 patients undergoing PTC,[28] 32% had additional diagnoses made with ICE, the vast majority of whom had undergone both TTE and TEE prior to the PTC procedure. These diagnoses included additional atrial septal defects, atrial septal aneurysm, atrial septal redundancy, anomalous pulmonary venous return, pulmonary arteriovenous malformation, and pulmonary vein stenosis.

Additional interventional uses of ICE may include guidance of transseptal catheterization, placement of left atrial appendage occluder devices, placement of percutaneous left ventricular assist device cannula, performance of percutaneous mitral balloon valvuloplasty, and many others (Table 16-1).[29-43] Diagnostic intracardiac imaging may be used as an alternative to TEE in patients with contraindication (ie, esophagectomy), or to evaluate anatomic regions that TEE may not adequately visualize because of shadowing from other structures (ie, the ascending aorta, which is not well seen on TEE because of tracheal shadowing in the "TEE blind spot").[44-46] Similarly, ICE can readily evaluate native and prosthetic valves that are not invariably well visualized by TEE.

In the electrophysiology laboratory, use of ICE includes guidance of pulmonary vein radiofrequency isolation for focal atrial fibrillation ablation, sinus node modification, idiopathic ventricular tachycardia ablation (both located in the right ventricular outflow tract and the aortic cusps), left ventricular ablation procedures, and extraction of pacer and defibrillator leads.[13,47-50] In the electrophysiology laboratory, shorter procedure times, reduced rates of arrhythmia recurrence, and reduced risk of pulmonary vein stenosis have all been described with ICE guidance.[13-16,18,19,51]

[ ] AVAILABLE SYSTEMS

There are three currently commercially available ICE systems, each with unique features and advantages. The Boston Scientific UltraICE system uses a mechanical radial ICE imaging transducer, is not steerable, and does not provide Doppler-derived information. Both Siemens AcuNav and the newer EP Medsystems ImageMate use phased array transducers. These transducers are steerable and deflectable. They provide two-dimensional sector imaging and also have color and spectral Doppler capabilities. The ImageMate system has two directions of steering (anterior and posterior), whereas the AcuNav system has four (anterior, posterior, right, and left). All three systems use a single-use ICE imaging catheter, require 10- to 11-French venous access, and are relatively expensive, with costs ranging from approximately $800 to $2800. Recently released transducer catheters have been reduced in external diameter to 8-Fr.

> ### TABLE 16-1
>
> ### Current and Potential Uses of ICE

Interventional

- Percutaneous PFO and ASD closure
- Guidance of transseptal procedures
- Placement of left atrial appendage occlusion device
- Percutaneous ventricular septal defect closure
- Percutaneous left ventricular assist device cannula placement
- Pulmonary vein percutaneous transluminal venoplasty and stenting (after atrial fibrillation ablation)
- Percutaneous mitral repair (Evalve clip, coronary sinus device)
- Mitral and aortic balloon valvuloplasty
- Hypertrophic cardiomyopathy alcohol septal ablation
- Guidance of myocardial biopsy

Electrophysiologic

- Pulmonary vein isolation (atrial fibrillation ablation)
- Sinus node modification
- Aortic cusp ablation
- Right and left ventricular ventricular tachycardia ablation
- Extraction of pacer and defibrillator leads

Diagnostic intracardiac imaging

- Alternative to TEE in those with contraindication
- Aortic evaluation including arch ("TEE blind spot")
- Tricuspid and pulmonic prosthetic valve evaluation

[ ] LIMITATIONS OF ICE

Current limitations of ICE include the relatively high cost of the single-use catheters and their large shaft diameters (now less of an issue with the release of the 8-Fr catheters). They provide only single-plane imaging with a relatively narrow field of view. The risks of ICE are small, but include all of the traditional vascular access-related complications and perforation of the cava or cardiac chambers with tamponade (Table 16-2).

[ ] PRINCIPLES OF IMAGING

Images acquired with the newer phased-array steerable transducers such as the AcuNav catheter produce images that are similar to TEE images, except that they originate from within the heart and accordingly require that the interpreter become familiar with a different set of image orientations. The AcuNav transducer has lockable steering controls, so that a particular imaging plane may be set and held in a stable position. Typically, AcuNav images are presented

TABLE 16-2

Risks of ICE

Vascular trauma at groin site
Superficial cutaneous nerve palsy
Vascular bleeding and groin hematoma
Retroperitoneal hematoma
Perforation of venous structures
Pericardial effusion
Cardiac tamponade
Atrial arrhythmia
Thromboembolism

within a 90° sector originating from the cardiac chamber where the transducer is located. The AcuNav catheter is typically placed in a femoral vein. Advancing and withdrawing the catheter moves the screen images from side to side. Advancing moves the transducer to image structures that are more superior relative to the catheter; withdrawing moves the transducer to image those that are more inferior. A small marker placed outside the imaging sector represents the "operator end" of the catheter, and this display orientation can be changed using the right–left screen display switch on the keyboard of the ultrasound machine. The emerging convention is to place this marker on the left side of the sector, representing the more inferior aspect of the imaging sector. Image "families" are then derived by very small degrees of catheter rotation, with clockwise rotation imaging structures that are more leftward and counterclockwise more rightward. Imaging is typically performed with the transducer in the right atrium, although images can be obtained from any cardiac and vascular structure into which the transducer tip of the catheter can be manipulated. Currently, as virtually all imaging is done using systemic venous vascular access, the most common imaging locations include, in addition to the right atrium, the cavae, the right ventricle, and, on occasion, the left atrium—accessed transseptally. In contrast, with radial ICE imaging the catheter is typically placed in the right atrium or cavae, with a more limited range of motion, as these catheters are neither steerable nor deflectable.

RIGHT ATRIAL IMAGING VIEWS

The imaging sequence with AcuNav usually begins from the right atrium, with the catheter in a neutral position and the locking mechanism disengaged. In the default position, the ultrasound array is oriented vertically and outward toward the anterior right atrial wall. A small marker line on the handle indicates the direction the array is pointing. This is the default position, and all subsequent maneuvers are described relative to this starting point. The catheter is gently rotated approximately 15° to 30° clockwise from the default position to image the "home view" (Figure 16-1 A,B). This view provides excellent imaging of the mid-right atrium, tricuspid valve, right ventricle, and typically provides an oblique or short axis view of the aortic valve.

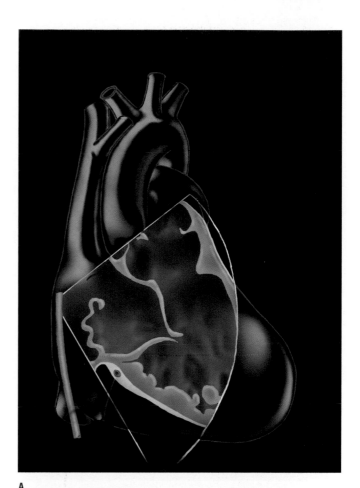

A

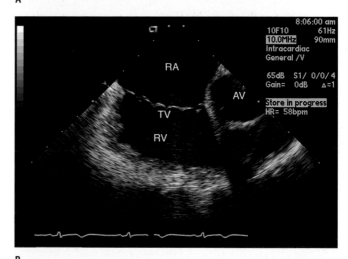

B

FIGURE 16-1. (**A**) Anatomic diagram indicating position of the AcuNav catheter in the right atrium with rotation to image the "home view." (Image courtesy of Siemens Medical Solutions. Used with permission. Medical Artist is Starr Kaplan.) (**B**) Corresponding echocardiographic image of the "home view." RA = right atrium; RV = right ventricle; AV = aortic valve; EV = Eustachian valve.

With continued rotation of the catheter in a clockwise direction to approximately 30°, the right ventricular outflow tract and pulmonic valve are seen. The aortic valve appears in a near short axis view (Figure 16-2 A,B). With continued rotation clockwise to approximately 45°, the left ventricle is seen in an

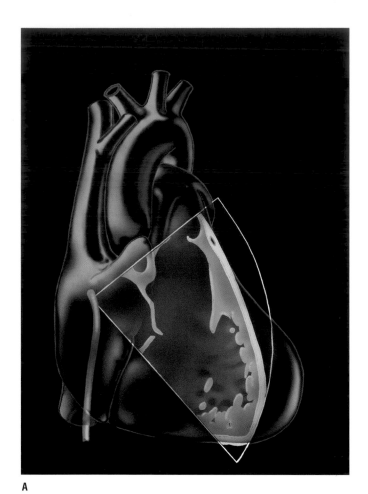

A

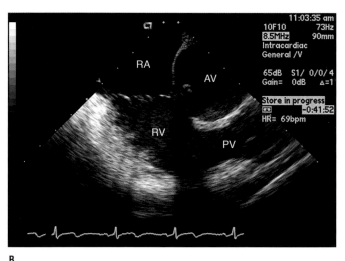

B

FIGURE 16-2. (A) Anatomic diagram indicating position of the AcuNav catheter in the right atrium with rotation to image the "RVOT view." (Image courtesy of Siemens Medical Solutions. Used with permission. Medical Artist is Starr Kaplan.) (B) Corresponding echocardiographic image of the "RVOT view." RA = right atrium; RV = right ventricle; AV = aortic valve; PV = pulmonic valve.

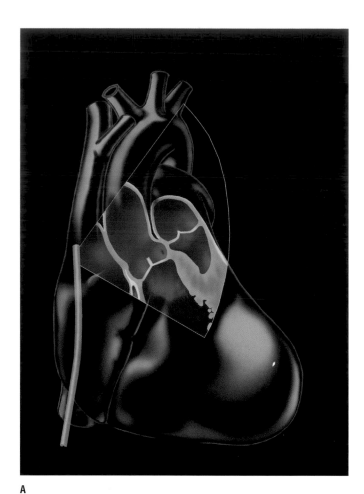

A

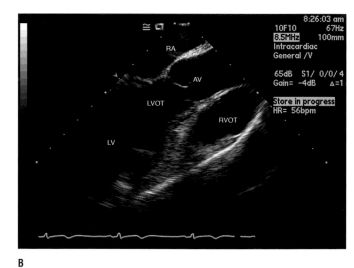

B

FIGURE 16-3. (A) Anatomic diagram indicating position of the AcuNav catheter in the "LVOT view." (Image courtesy of Siemens Medical Solutions. Used with permission. Medical Artist is Starr Kaplan.) (B) Corresponding echocardiographic image of the "LVOT view." RA = right atrium; LV = left ventricle; AV = aortic valve; Ao = aorta.

oblique long axis view with the apex down toward the bottom of the imaging sector, and the left ventricular outflow tract and aortic valve visualized (Figure 16-3 A,B). Color Doppler interrogation in the view may demonstrate aortic regurgitation if present (Figure 16-4).

As the catheter is rotated clockwise further to approximately 60°, a long axis view of the left ventricle (LV) and the mitral valve are seen (Figure 16-5 A,B). Often a small degree of anterior tilting toward the septum helps optimize the view of the LV. With continued rotation to approximately 70° to 80°, the interatrial septum

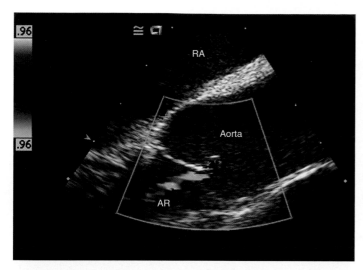

FIGURE 16-4. Echocardiographic image of the "LVOT view" demonstrating mild aortic regurgitation by color-flow Doppler. RA = right atrium; LV = left ventricle; AV = aortic valve; Ao = aorta.

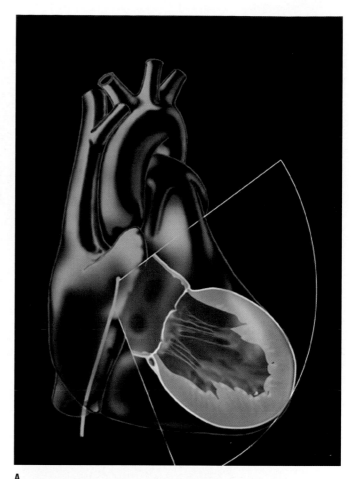

A

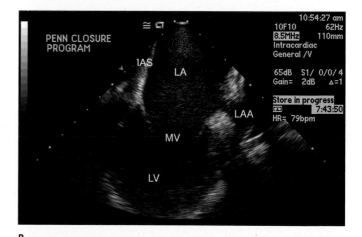

B

FIGURE 16-5. (A) Anatomic diagram indicating position of the AcuNav catheter in the "LV long axis view" (Image courtesy of Siemens Medical Solutions. Used with permission. Medical Artist is Starr Kaplan.) **(B)** Corresponding echocardiographic image of the "LV long axis view"; LA = left atriumLV = left ventricle; LAA = left atrial appendage.

(IAS) is visualized, with the left atrial appendage in the far field (Figure 16-6). With further clockwise rotation to approximately 90° to 100°, positioning the ICE transducer along the IAS demonstrates the left inferior and left superior pulmonary veins in the far field (Figure 16-7). Color Doppler and pulse-wave Doppler flow patterns help differentiate the left atrial appendage (LAA) from the left pulmonary veins. This view represents an optimal angle for Doppler interrogation of the left pulmonary veins, as the beam is aligned parallel with the direction of flow.

With continued rotation to approximately 150° to 180°, the right-sided pulmonary veins are visualized, as is the right atrial appendage (Figures 16-8 and 16-9) with continued rotation. These structures may be also visualized by counterclockwise rotation to 30° if they are among the primary imaging targets (ie, crista ablation, pulmonary vein isolation for atrial fibrillation). To image the superior vena cava (SVC) entry into the right atrium (RA), the catheter is rotated approximately 210° to 240° from neutral, with posterior tilting of the catheter to image superiorly (Figure 16-10)

LEFT ATRIAL IMAGING VIEWS

Imaging can also be performed from the left atrium (by passing the catheter through an atrial septal defect (ASD) or patent foramen ovale (PFO), as well as from other structures. Imaging from the left atrium (LA) provides excellent images of the LAA,[22] as well as of the mitral valve (Figures 16-11 and 16-12). Imaging from the SVC demonstrates the ascending aorta and arch (Figure 16-13). Imaging from the RV through the intrventricular septum (IVS) provides near long axis views of the LV and the mitral valve (MV) (Figure 16-14), as well as of the right ventricular outflow tract (RVOT) and pulmonic valve. Imaging from the aorta has also been performed and used to guide endovascular interventions and biopsy procedures.[46]

【 】 ICE DURING PERCUTANEOUS TRANSCATHETER CLOSURE PROCEDURES

The use of ICE in guiding PTC of ASD and PFO serves as a general model for the use of ICE in the catheterization laboratory. In guiding these procedures, images are typically obtained from the

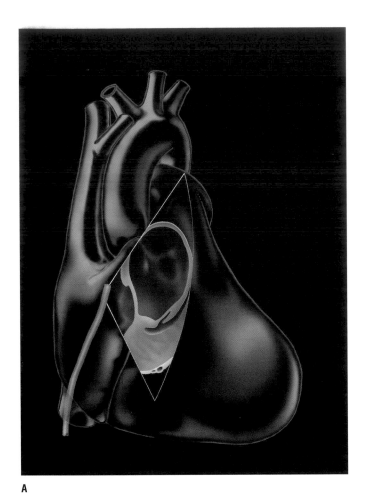

A

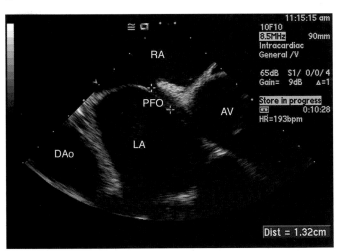

B

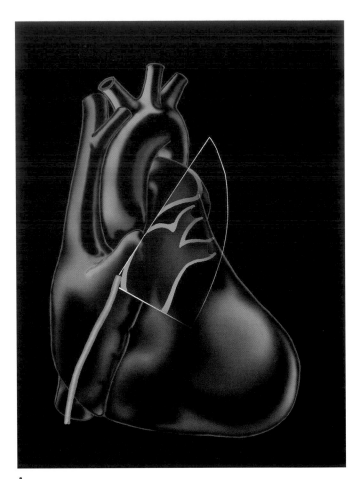

A

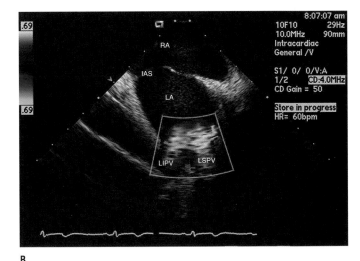

B

FIGURE 16-6. (A) Anatomic diagram indicating position of the AcuNav catheter in the "interatrial septal view." (Image courtesy of Siemens Medical Solutions. Used with permission. Medical Artist is Starr Kaplan.) **(B)** Echocardiographic image of the "interatrial septal view" in at patient with a PFO. RA = right atrium; LA = left atrium; AV = aortic valve; Dao = descending thoracic aorta; PFO = patent foramen ovale.

FIGURE 16-7. (A) Anatomic diagram indicating position of the AcuNav catheter in the "left pulmonary veins view." (Image courtesy of Siemens Medical Solutions. Used with permission. Medical Artist is Starr Kaplan.) **(B)** Corresponding echocardiographic image of the "left pulmonary veins view" with color-flow Doppler into the left atrium, with the color map demonstrating red flow moving toward the transducer. LA = left atrium; LSPV = left superior pulmonary vein; LIPV = left inferior pulmonary vein.

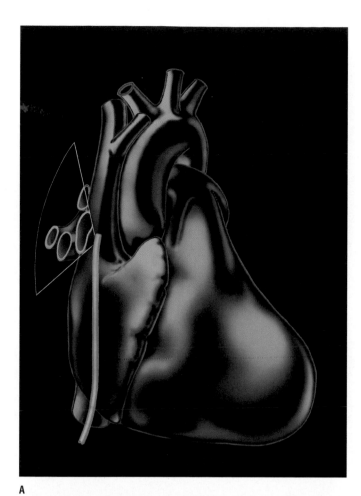

A

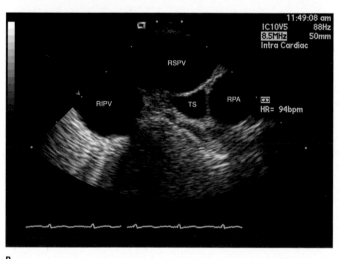

B

FIGURE 16-8. (A) Anatomic diagram indicating position of the AcuNav catheter in the "right pulmonary veins view." (Image courtesy of Siemens Medical Solutions. Used with permission. Medical Artist is Starr Kaplan.) **(B)** Corresponding echocardiographic image of the "right pulmonary veins view." RSPV = right superior pulmonary vein; RIPV = right inferior pulmonary vein; TS = transverse sinus; RPA = right pulmonary artery.

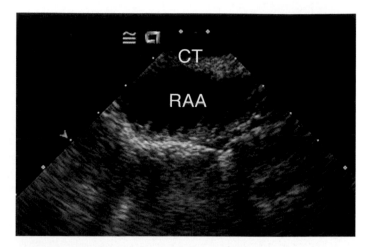

FIGURE 16–9. Echocardiographic image of the "right atrial appendage view." RAA = right atrial appendage; CT = crista terminalis.

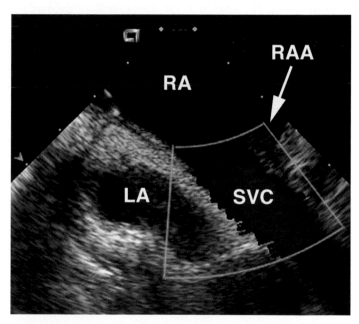

FIGURE 16-10. Echocardiographic image of the "SVC view." RA = right atrium; RAA = right atrial appendage; SVC = superior vena cava.

right atrium. With the steerable and deflectable catheters, placement in the mid-right atrium with posterior and rightward tilting of the transducer away from the IAS provides excellent imaging of the septum and surrounding structures. Posterior tilting increases the distance between the IAS and the ICE probe, and allows better spatial resolution for structures in the near field. This is particularly helpful in imaging the septum in the presence of an atrial septal aneurysm. Once set, sweeping through the desired imaging plane may be accomplished either by gently rotating the catheter through the desired imaging plane or by moving the right and left control wheel.

The preprocedural assessment of the IAS by ICE includes a complete evaluation of the entire IAS and its surrounding structures. A *patent foramen ovale (PFO)* is defined as a right-to-left communication through the fossa ovalis, in the anatomic region where septum primum overlaps the septum secundum (Figure 16-15). Right-to-left shunting can be demonstrated by the injection of agitated saline at rest and with provocative maneuvers such as Valsalva, coughing, or sniffing (Mueller's maneuver) (Figure 16-16). It is important to image the passage of contrast through the

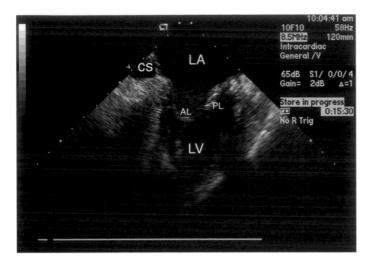

FIGURE 16-11. Echocardiographic image of the left atrium, left ventricle, and mitral valve after the catheter has been passed through an atrial septal defect. LA = left atrium; LV = left ventricle; AL = anterior mitral valve leaflet; PL = posterior mitral valve leaflet; CS = coronary sinus.

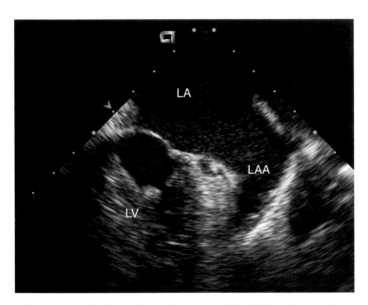

FIGURE 16-12. Echocardiographic image of the left atrial appendage from the LA after the catheter has been passed through an atrial septal defect. LA = left atrium; LV = left ventricle; LAA = left atrial appendage.

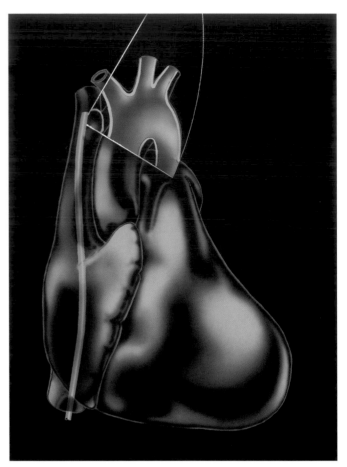

A

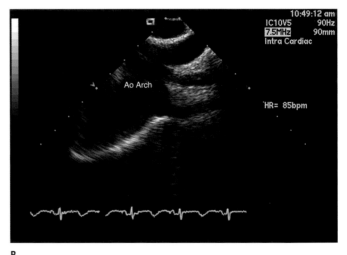

B

FIGURE 16-13. (**A**) Anatomic diagram indicating position of the AcuNav catheter in the SVC to image the aortic arch and great vessels. (Image courtesy of Siemens Medical Solutions. Used with permission. Medical Artist is Starr Kaplan.) (**B**) Corresponding echocardiographic image from the SVC of the aortic arch and great vessels.

foramen itself, as opposed to simply evaluating for the presence of contrast in the left heart. Intrapulmonary shunting as a result of pulmonary arteriovenous malformations or other right-to-left shunts may mimic PFO and present with positive contrast studies. When right atrial pressure exceeds left atrial pressure, resting or intermittent right-to-left color Doppler flow may be seen, although this finding is not invariably present in all patients with PFO. An *atrial septal aneurysm* is usually defined as greater than 15 mm of total movement of a 15-mm length of atrial septal tissue. This can be demonstrated with M-mode echo (Figure 16-17), and measurements of total peak-to-trough excursion made. A *stretched PFO* is defined as an interatrial communication at the fossa ovalis in the anatomic region where septum primum overlaps with septum secundum, with resting or intermittent left-to-right flow by

color Doppler imaging (Figure 16-18). This often results as a consequence of elevated left atrial pressure.

Associated abnormalities of the pulmonary veins, IVC, SVC, coronary sinus, and atrioventricular valves should be excluded. Careful evaluation of the pulmonary venous drainage should be performed to exclude anomalous drainage that would require

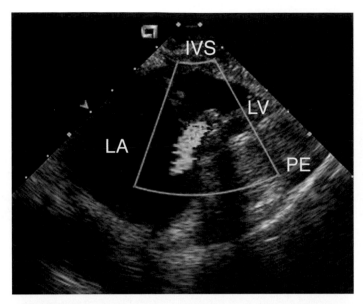

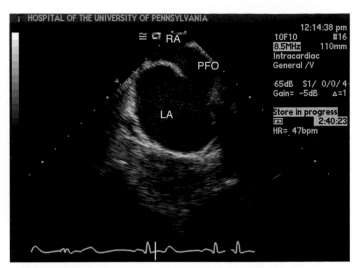

FIGURE 16-14. Imaging from the RV through the IVS provides near long-axis views of the LV and MV. RV = right ventricle; IVS = interventricular septum; AL = anterior mitral valve leaflet; PL = posterior mitral valve leaflet.

FIGURE 16-15. Imaging from the mid-RA demonstrating a patent foramen ovale; note the opening of the PFO tunnel with color Doppler demonstrating right-to-left flow

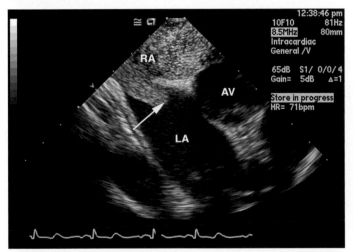

A

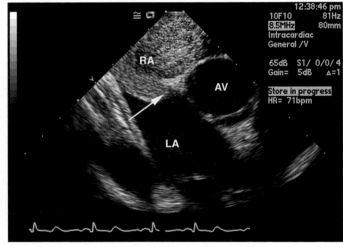

B

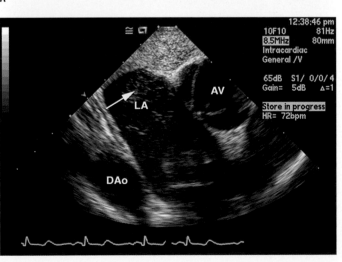

C

FIGURE 16-16. Imaging from the mid-RA during saline contrast (Bubble) with Valsalva maneuver demonstrating passage of right-to-left contrast consistent with PFO. Panel **A** demonstrates initial opacification of the right atrium (RA) and the foramen with saline microbubble contrast *(arrow)*. Panel **B** demonstrates initial contrast passage into the fossa *(arrow)* and left atrium (LA), and panel **C** demonstrates continued passage of saline microbubbles into the left atrium. Aortic Valve (AV), descending aorta (DAo).

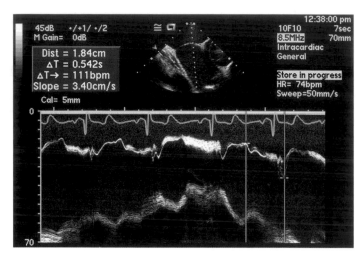

FIGURE 16-17. M-mode demonstration of characteristic hypermobility of the interatrial septum seen with atrial septal aneurysm.

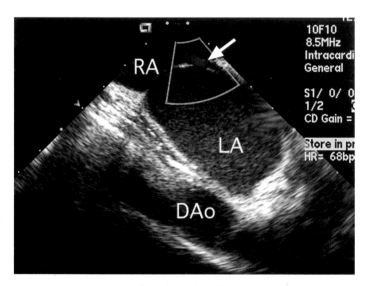

FIGURE 16-18. Imaging from the mid-RA demonstrating a "stretched PFO" with left-to-right color-flow Doppler.

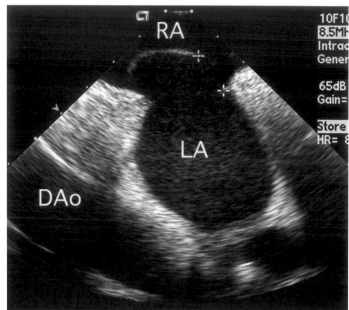

FIGURE 16-19. Imaging from the mid-RA demonstrating a prominent atrial septal aneurysm with a large ostium secundum atrial septal defect

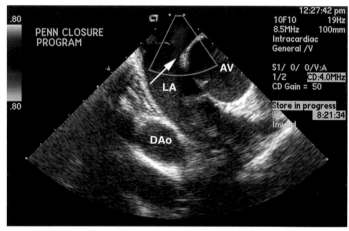

FIGURE 16-20. Imaging from the mid-RA, with posterior and rightward tilting applied. The catheter is then rotated toward the tricuspid valve to image the superior atrial septal rim of the septum secundum. A deficient (<5 mm) rim is seen.

surgical correction. Measurement of the largest static diameter of the atrial septal defect is performed using two-dimensional imaging (Figure 19-19). Consideration of the size of the atrial septal rim of tissue surrounding the defect is important in evaluating patients for successful PTC, and a rim of 5 mm is generally considered adequate (Figure 16-20). The inferior and superior rims may be particularly important for successful PTC, although small series have reported success in patients with deficient rims.

Balloon sizing of the ASD can be achieved by one of two methods. First, a "pulling technique" has been described, where a sizing balloon is inflated in the left atrium to a size larger than the ASD and pulled to occlude the defect (documented by lack of color Doppler flow). The balloon is then slowly deflated until it moves from the left atrium to the right atrium through the ASD. The amount of fluid inside the balloon at the time the balloon crosses the defect is measured, and once the balloon is removed it is compared with a sizing plate that corresponds to the diameter of the

defect. Alternatively, the simpler and more commonly used "stationary balloon" technique, involves the inflation of a soft, low-pressure balloon across the ASD while monitoring with ICE as well as fluoroscopy. When the defect is completely occluded, no color Doppler flow across the defect is seen, and a "waist" may appear in the balloon contour. The balloon waist diameter is measured by echocardiography as well as by fluoroscopy, and this size corresponds to the stretched diameter of the ASD (Figure 16-21).

The balloon is then removed leaving the guidewire in place (Figure 16-22), and the proper-size device delivery sheath is passed over the wire into the left atrium under ICE guidance (Figure 16-23). The closure device is then delivered through the sheath into the left atrium. The individual insertion technique varies at this point, but typically uses opening the left atrial disc or arms and pulling

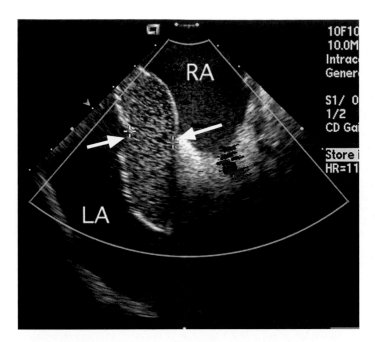

FIGURE 16-21. Imaging during balloon stretch sizing of an ostium secundum ASD. The arrows represent the "waist" of the balloon, corresponding to an average diameter of the defect.

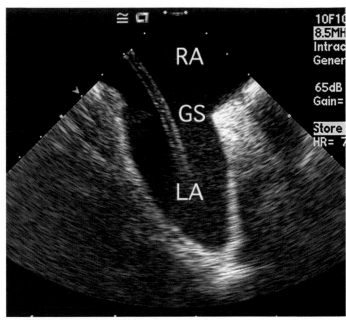

FIGURE 16-23. Image demonstrating the device delivery sheath passing from RA to LA through an ostium secundum ASD.

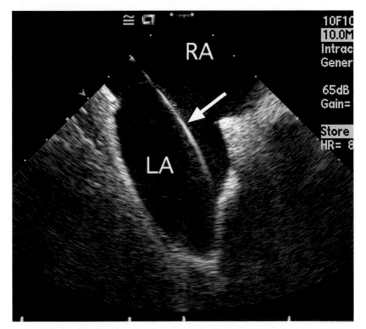

FIGURE 16-22. Image demonstrating the guidewire passing from RA to LA through the ASD.

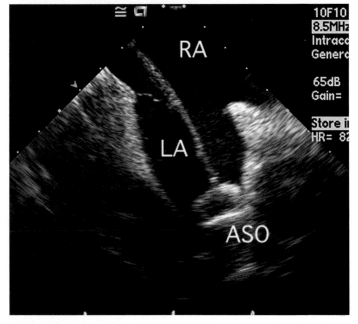

FIGURE 16-24. Image demonstrating the Amplatzer ASO disc opening in LA.

them back to the interatrial septum (Figure 16-24). Once the LA aspect of the device is in position, the RA aspect is opened, thereby "sandwiching" the septum. The arms of the device rest on the rims of atrial tissue surrounding the defect, and as such in ASDs associated with deficiencies in these rims, a stable position can be more difficult to achieve. A stable device position for certain devices (eg, Amplatzer Septal Occluder) is confirmed by moving the connecting cable (and thus the device attached to it) forward and backward (Figure 16-25).

When the device is confirmed to be in a satisfactory position, surrounding structures are evaluated prior to final release. Large ASD or PFO devices may compromise the patency of the right pulmonary veins, cavae, coronary sinus, and occasionally the function of the tricuspid and mitral valves. The device is then released, and re-imaged with echocardiography to assess for immediate ASD or PFO closure, as well as for position changes that often occur as a result of the release of traction from the connecting cable (Figure 16-26). In PFO closure, a contrast study is typically

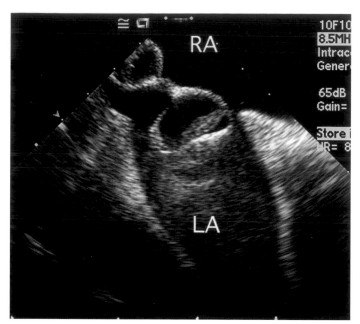

FIGURE 16-25. Image demonstrating the push–pull maneuver ("Minnesota Wiggle") to ensure stability of the Amplatzer device.

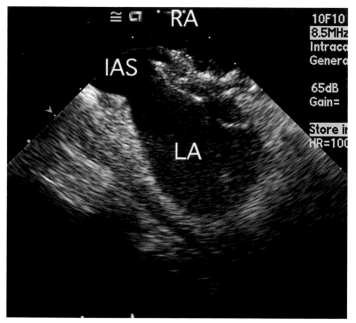

FIGURE 16-26. Image demonstrating the final Amplatzer position after release of the device.

performed to document the immediate postprocedural adequacy of closure.

FUTURE DIRECTIONS

Further refinement and miniaturization of ICE transducers, through continued technological progress, will make way for primary operator–controlled, integrated ultrasound–guided interventional devices. Smaller catheters are being developed that may offer greater degrees of freedom with regard to catheter rotation, as well

as the potential for decreased risk of vascular complications. Newer imaging modalities currently being developed include on-line real-time three-dimensional ICE, which offers the potential for additional advantages in the guidance of percutaneous noncoronary interventions. These modalities offer the advantage of being able to delineate the complex relationships among intracardiac anatomy, physiology, and device function, although they have not been evaluated systematically in these settings.

REFERENCES

1. Pandian NG, Weintraub A, Schwartz SL, et al. Intravascular and intracardiac ultrasound imaging: current research and future directions. *Echocardiography.* 1990;7(4): 377.
2. Pandian NG, Hsu TL. Intravascular ultrasound and intracardiac echocardiography: concepts for the future. *Am J Cardiol.* 1992;69(20):6H.
3. Syracuse DC, Gaudiani VA Kastl DC, Henry WL, Morrow AC. Intraoperative, intracardiac echocardiography during left ventriculomyotomy and myectomy for hypertrophic subaortic stenosis. *Circulation* 1978;58(3 Pt 2):I23.
4. GlassmanE, Kronzon I.Transvenous intracardiac echocardiography. *Am J Cardiol.* 1981;47(6):1255.
5. Schwartz SL, Pandian NG, Kusay R, et al. Real-time intracardiac two-dimensional echocardiography: an experimental study of in vivo feasibility, imaging planes, and echocardiographic anatomy. *Echocardiography.*1990;7(4):443.
6. Pandian NG, Kumar R, Katz SE, et al. Real-time, intracardiac, two-dimensional echocardiography: enhanced depth of field with a low-frequency (12.5 MHz) ultrasound catheter. *Echocardiography.* 1991;8(4):407.
7. PandianNG, Schwartz SL, Hsu TL, et al. Intracardiac echocardiography. Experimental observations on intracavitary imaging of cardiac structures with 20-MHz ultrasound catheters. *Echocardiography.* 1991;8(1):127.
8. PandianNG, Schwartz SL, Weintraub AR, Hsu TL, Konstam MA, Salem DN.Intracardiac echocardiography: current developments. *Int J Cardiac Imaging.*1991;6(3–4):207.
9. Schwartz SL, Gillam LD, Weintraub AR, et al. Intracardiac echocardiography in humans using a small-sized (6F), low frequency (12.5 MHz) ultrasound catheter. Methods, imaging planes and clinical experience. *J Am Coll Cardiol.* 1993;21(1):189.
10. Tardif JC, Cao QL, Schwartz SL, Pandian NC. Intracardiac echocardiography with a steerable low-frequency linear-array probe for left-sided heart imaging from the right side: experimental studies. *J Am Soc Echocardiogr.* 1995;8 (2):132.
11. Ren JF, Schwartzman D, Michele JJ, et al. Lower frequency (5 MHz) intracardiac echocardiography in a large swine model: imaging views and research applications. *Ultrasound Med Biol.* 1997. 23(6):871-7.
12. Cooper JM, Epstein LM. Use of intracardiac echocardiography to guide ablation of atrial fibrillation. [Erratum appears in *Circulation* 2002;105(10):1256]. *Circulation.* 2001;104(25):3010.
13. Hynes BJ, Mart C, Artman S, Pu M, Naccarelli GV. Role of intracardiac ultrasound in interventional electrophysiology. *Curr Opin Cardiol.* 2004;19(1):52.
14. Jongbloed MR, Bax JJ, de Groot NM, et al. Radiofrequency catheter ablation of paroxysmal atrial fibrillation; guidance by intracardiac echocardiography and integration with other imaging techniques. *Eur J Echocardiogr.* 2003;4 (1):54.
15. Mangrum JM, Mounsey JP, Kok LC, DiMarco JP, Haines DE. Intracardiac echocardiography–guided anatomically based radiofrequency ablation of focal atrial fibrillation originating from pulmonary veins. *J Am Coll Cardiol.* 2002;39(12):1964.
16. Marrouche NF, Martin DO, Wazni O, et al. Phased-array intracardiac echocardiography monitoring during pulmonary vein isolation in patients with atrial fibrillation: impact on outcome and complications. *Circulation.* 2003; 107(21):2710.
17. Martin RE, Ellenbogen KA, Lau YR, et al. Phased-array intracardiac echocardiography during pulmonary vein isolation and linear ablation for atrial fibrillation. *J Cardiovasc Electrophysiol.* 2002;13(9):873.
18. Saad EB, Cole CR, Marrouche NF, et al.Use of intracardiac echocardiography for prediction of chronic pulmonary vein stenosis after ablation of atrial fibrillation. *J Cardiovasc Electrophysiol.* 2002;13(10):986.
19. Schwartzman D, Bazaz R, Nosbisch J. Catheter ablation to suppress atrial fibrillation: evolution of technique at a single center. *J Interv Card Electrophysiol.* 2003;9(2):295.

20. Wood MA, Wittkamp M, Henry D, et al. RA comparison of pulmonary vein ostial anatomy by computerized tomography, echocardiography, and venography in patients with atrial fibrillation having radiofrequency catheter ablation. *Am J Cardiol.* 2004;93(1):49.

21. Boccalandro F, Baptista E, Muench A, Carter C, Smalling RW.Comparison of intracardiac echocardiography versus transesophageal echocardiography guidance for percutaneous transcatheter closure of atrial septal defect. *Am J Cardiol.* 2004;93(4):437.

22. Hijazi Z, Wang Z, Cao Q, Koenig P, Waight D, Lang R. Transcatheter closure of atrial septal defects and patent foramen ovale under intracardiac echocardiographic guidance: feasibility and comparison with transesophageal echocardiography. *Cathet Cardiovasc Interven.* 2001;52(2):194.

23. Koenig PR, Abdulla RI, Cao QL, Hijazi ZM.Use of intracardiac echocardiography to guide catheter closure of atrial communications. *Echocardiography.* 2003;20(8):781.

24. Onorato E Melzi G, Casilli F, et al. Patent foramen ovale with paradoxical embolism: mid-term results of transcatheter closure in 256 patients. *J Interven Cardiol.* 2003;16(1):43.

25. Zanchetta M, Rigatelli G, Onorato E. Intracardiac echocardiography and transcranial Doppler ultrasound to guide closure of patent foramen ovale. *J Invas Cardiol.* 2003;15(2):93.

26. Morton JB, Sanders P, Sparks PB, Morgan J, Kalman JM. Usefulness of phased-array intracardiac echocardiography for the assessment of left atrial mechanical "stunning" in atrial flutter and comparison with multiplane transesophageal echocardiography. *Am J Cardiol.* 2002;90(7):741.

27. Du ZD, Koenig P, Cao QL, Waight D, Heitschmidt M, Hijazi ZM. Comparison of transcatheter closure of secundum atrial septal defect using the Amplatzer septal occluder associated with deficient versus sufficient rims. *Am J Cardiol.* 2002;90(8):865.

28. Earing MG, Cabalka AK, Seward JB, Bruce CJ, Reeder GS, Hagler DJ. Intracardiac echocardiographic guidance during transcatheter device closure of atrial septal defect and patent foramen ovale. *Mayo Clin Proc.* 2004;79:24.

29. Cafri C, de la Guardia B, Barasch E, Brink J, Smalling RW.Transseptal puncture guided by intracardiac echocardiography during percutaneous transvenous mitral commissurotomy in patients with distorted anatomy of the fossa ovalis. *Cath Cardiovasc Interven.* 2000;50(4):463.

30. Calo L, Lamberti F, Loricchio ML, et al. Transseptal activation during left atrial pacing in humans: electroanatomic mapping using a noncontact catheter and the intracardiac echocardiography. *J Interven Card Electrophysiol.*2002; 6(2):149.

31. Daoud EG, Kalbfleisch SJ, Hummel JD. Intracardiac echocardiography to guide transseptal left heart catheterization for radiofrequency catheter ablation. *J Cardiovasc Electrophysiol.* 1999;10(3):358.

32. Epstein LM, Smith T, TenHoff H. Nonfluoroscopic transseptal catheterization: safety and efficacy of intracardiac echocardiographic guidance. *J Cardiovasc Electrophysiol.* 1998;9(6):625.

33. Hanaoka T, Suyama K, Taguchi A, et al. Shifting of puncture site in the fossa ovalis during radiofrequency catheter ablation: intracardiac echocardiography-guided transseptal left heart catheterization. *Japan Heart J.* 2003;44(5):673.

34. Hung JS, Fu M, Yeh KH, Chua S, Wu JJ, Chen YC. Usefulness of intracardiac echocardiography in transseptal puncture during percutaneous transvenous mitral commissurotomy. *Am J Cardiol.* 1993;72(11):853.

35. Hung JS, Fu M, Yeh KH, Wu CJ, Wong P. Usefulness of intracardiac echocardiography in complex transseptal catheterization during percutaneous transvenous mitral commissurotomy. *Mayo Clin Proc.* 1996;71(2):134.

36. Johnson SB, Seward JB, Packer DL. Phased-array intracardiac echocardiography for guiding transseptal catheter placement: utility and learning curve. *Pacing Clin Electrophysiol.* 2002;25(4 Pt 1):402.

37. Miyamoto N, Kyo S, Motoyama T, et al. Usefulness of intracardiac echocardiography for guidance of transseptal puncture procedure. *J Cardiol.* 1995;25(1):29.

38. Szili-Torok T, Kimman G, Theuns D, Res J, Roelandt JR, Jordaens LJ. Transseptal left heart catheterisation guided by intracardiac echocardiography. *Heart (Br Card Soc).* 2001;86(5):E11.

39. Nakai T, Lesh MD, Gerstenfeld EP, Virmani R, Jones R, Lee RJ. Percutaneous left atrial appendage occlusion (PLAATO) for preventing cardioembolism: first experience in canine model. *Circulation.* 2002;105(18):2217.

40. Schwartz SL, Pandian NC, Kumar R, et al. Intracardiac echocardiography during simulated aortic and mitral balloon valvuloplasty: in vivo experimental studies. *Am Heart J.* 1992;123(3):665.

41. Salem MI, Makaryus AN, Kort S, et al. Intracardiac echocardiography using the AcuNav ultrasound catheter during percutaneous balloon mitral valvuloplasty. *J Am Soc Echocardiol.* 2002;15(12):1533.

42. Mazur W, Parilak LD, Kaluza G, DeFelice C, Raizner AE. Balloon valvuloplasty for mitral stenosis. *Curr Op Cardiol.* 1999;14(2):95.

43. Das P, Prendergast B. Imaging in mitral stenosis: assessment before, during and after percutaneous balloon mitral valvuloplasty. *Expert Rev Cardiovasc Ther.* 2003;1(4):549.

44. Teragaki M, Takeuchi K, Toda I, et al. Potential applications of intracardiac echocardiography in the assessment of the aortic valve from the right ventricular outflow tract. *J Am Soc Echocardiog.* 1999;12(4):225.

45. Allan LD, Chita SK, Anderson RH, Fagg N, Crawford DC, Tynan MJ. Coarctation of the aorta in prenatal life: an echocardiographic, anatomical, and functional study. *Br Heart J.* 1988;59(3):356.

46. Zanchetta M, Rigatelli G, Pedon L, Zennaro M, Ronsivalle S, Maiolino P. Endovascular repair of complex aortic aneurysms: intravascular ultrasound guidance with an intracardiac probe. *Cardiovasc Interven Radiol.* 2003;26(5):448.

47. Kedia A, Hsu PY, Holmes J, Burnham D, West G, Kusumoto FM. Use of intracardiac echocardiography in guiding radiofrequency catheter ablation of atrial tachycardia in a patient after the senning operation. *Pacing Clin Electrophysiol.* 2003;26(11):2178.

48. Lesh MD, Kalman JM, Karch MR. Use of intracardiac echocardiography during electrophysiologic evaluation and therapy of atrial arrhythmias. *J Cardiovasc Electrophysiol.* 1998;9(8 Suppl):S40.

49. Olgin JE, Kalman JM, Chin M, et al. Electrophysiological effects of long, linear atrial lesions placed under intracardiac ultrasound guidance. *Circulation.* 1997;96(8):2715.

50. Ren JF, Schwartzman D, Callans D, Marchlinski FE, Gottlieb CD, Chaudhry FA. Imaging technique and clinical utility for electrophysiologic procedures of lower frequency (9 MHz) intracardiac echocardiography. *Am J Cardiol.* 1998; 82(12):1557.

51. Saad EB, Rossillo A, Saad CP, et al. Pulmonary vein stenosis after radiofrequency ablation of atrial fibrillation: functional characterization, evolution, and influence of the ablation strategy. *Circulation.* 2003;108(25):3102.

CHAPTER (17)

Cardiac Catheterization Laboratory Physiologic Recorders

John W. Hirshfeld, Jr., MD

Today's clinical cardiac catheterization laboratory evolved from facilities that were originally human hemodynamic research laboratories. In the 1940s and 1950s, these facilities worked out much of our current understanding of the pathophysiology of many cardiovascular disorders with a principal focus on cardiac valve disease. Catheterization laboratory physiologic recorders were developed to meet two needs of these endeavors:

1. The need to monitor the patient's condition during invasive procedures.

2. The need to make permanent analog recordings of physiologic signals from the patients.

The catheterization laboratory physiologic recorder evolved from the multichannel oscillographic physiologic recorders that had been developed for animal physiologic research in the first half of the twentieth century. The original physiologic recorders were ink-writing multichannel oscillographs.

The importance of displaying and recording multiple superimposed channels of physiologic signals was rapidly recognized. Thus, the first major development was the move from ink-writing oscillographs to multichannel oscilloscopic recorders. These instruments had the advantage of displaying multiple channels in real time on an oscilloscopic screen. The physician/operator could view the screen in order to monitor in real time both the data being obtained and the patient's condition. These instruments also incorporated photo-optical recorders that could record the oscilloscopic beams on light-sensitive paper, permitting permanent recordings of superimposed physiologic signals.

These instruments made the development of cardiac catheterization possible. However, the early instruments had many shortcomings. Since the early 1980s, progress in electronic instrumentation and computer capability has fostered an evolution of the cardiac catheterization laboratory recorder, refining its functionality and enabling it to incorporate additional information management and reporting capabilities. In addition to serving their original function, the recorders that are currently available also serve as front ends for clinical database management, hospital information system data, report generation, and laboratory inventory management.

ORIGINAL PURPOSES

The purpose of the original catheterization laboratory recorders was to receive, condition, and display various types of physiologic signals from the patient that were of value for monitoring the patient, as well as to record for analysis. These signals fall into three basic types:

1. Pressure signals from pressure transducers.

2. ECG signals.

3. DC voltage signals representing either voltages recorded from the patient, or signals from other instruments, such as flow meters or respiration probes.

The recorder had the capability to display these processed signals with appropriate gain in a variety of superimposition formats in order to present a comprehensive picture of the patient's condition and the relationships between the phenomena represented by the different signals. In addition, the recorder could produce a hard copy output on light-sensitive paper of selected signal recordings that were to be preserved for archiving and analysis.

EVOLUTION TO CURRENT UNITS

Several developments have refined the capabilities of physiologic recorders yielding the highly capable units that are in current use. These include the following:

1. The development of stable reliable solid-state electronics.

2. The refinement of displays to high-resolution multicolor flat-panel monitor units.

3. The application of computer technology for control, display archiving, and hard-copy output generation.

4. The evolution of cardiovascular and hospital information systems leading to the interface of these units with hospital information systems and cardiovascular databases.

The principal development in the evolution of the catheterization laboratory physiologic recorder is the incorporation of a computer for operational control. This has transformed the design of the recorder to become fundamentally a computer-run device. The physical recorder itself is now an assembly of generic computer, computer display, and output hardware. Its capabilities and the distinction among different units lie entirely in the software that operates it. The software generates the system's human interface and operates the system's components.

CAPABILITIES OF AND PERFORMANCE CRITERIA FOR CURRENT UNITS

【 】 CAPABILITIES

A current fully functional catheterization laboratory physiologic recorder should have the following capabilities and features:

1. Accept, condition, and display a minimum of eight physiologic signals from patient. These should include intravascular pressure from pressure transducers, 12-lead ECG, DC signals from other portable equipment such as flow meters, and other transducers that produce a DC output signal, pulse oximetry, noninvasive blood pressure, and respiration.

2. Display the analog signals and their numeric values on a color monitor available for the operating physician to view in order to monitor the patient during the procedure.

3. Record the physiologic signals both as a hard copy and as a digital archive that can be exported as a digital imaging and communications in medicine (DICOM) object to a laboratory archiving system.

4. Perform hemodynamic calculations such as valve orifice areas.

5. Interface with the hospital information system in order to read admissions/discharge/transfer (ADT) demographic data from the hospital information system as well as to export procedure utilization data back to it.

6. Maintain a time-stamped procedure log of the events of the procedure, including patient vital signs for the purposes of conscious-sedation monitoring.

7. Record supplies used during the procedure for inventory management and billing purposes.

8. Generate a final catheterization report, ideally integrated with the x-ray system so that it can incorporate angiographic images.

9. Archive the report on the laboratory archive as a DICOM object.

10. Export the report to the hospital information system to facilitate clinical information transfer.

【 】 CAPABILITIES PERFORMANCE CRITERIA

There are five performance criteria that should be assessed when judging a cardiac catheterization laboratory physiologic recorder.

1. The core performance criterion for any cardiac catheterization laboratory system is stability and reliability. These systems are computer applications that run on top of any one of several commercially available operating systems. The introduction of the computer into the cardiac catheterization laboratory recording system creates a new issue not previously present in earlier non-computer based units—the computer crash. This is particularly important because a computer crash could potentially render the system inoperable until the computer is successfully restarted and reinitialized. Current systems, although based on very fast computers, are also based on complex operating systems and complex applications. Thus, the "boot," or initialization time, for a computer to start up either from being shut off or to reinitialize after a crash can be unacceptably long. Consequently, these systems must have very robust code that is relatively crashproof. In addition, ideally, these systems should be isolated from the Internet so that they are at less risk of infection with computer viruses. This parameter may be difficult to achieve, as the system must interact with the hospital information system. Finally, these systems should have a "limp home" mode that permits them to continue to perform basic monitoring functions even if the main computer system has crashed or is in the process of being restarted. This capability provides for patient safety by continuing to provide patient monitoring during a restart, if necessary.

2. The user interface must be intuitive and easy to use. The recorder operator has multiple responsibilities in addition to actually operating the recorder. These include monitoring the patient and maintaining communication outside of the laboratory. As these systems have become more complex and have acquired additional capabilities, the demands of designing an intuitive graphical user interface (GUI) have increased. These systems now have many features and functions that are accessed through a GUI. The organization of that interface, including the design of menus, the design and placement of icons, and the overall screen layout, presents a major challenge to the interface designer. A good GUI has menus that contain functions organized logically according to typical catheterization laboratory workflow. This facilitates the performance of the "routine" procedure. In addition, however, it should be easy and straightforward to configure the recorder for an unusual circumstance.

3. The system must interface effectively with the hospital information system, the x-ray system, and the catheterization laboratory's database and DICOM archive. These interfaces have the potential to be problematic when different components are furnished by different vendors. It is important to verify prior to installation that the selected recorder is also compatible with the other systems that it must interface with.

4. The system must perform complex hemodynamic measurements and calculations according to valid algorithms in a manner that it is easy to verify. If a complex calculation such as a valve area is based on improper measurements of cardiac output or valve pressure gradient, it should be possible to assess the basis of the calculation and edit any of the parameters that went into the calculation so that the calculation may be revised, if necessary.

5. The system must generate a properly organized report constructed in such a manner that it effectively communicates the findings of the procedure and, in particular, can effectively report any unusual circumstances or findings. Particular care must be taken in the report design to allow adaptation to the exigencies of particular procedures so that the reports do not all come out with a generic quality to them.

CONCLUSION

Current cardiac catheterization lab physiologic recorders are sophisticated units with many valuable capabilities made possible by the sophisticated application of computer technology to the task of monitoring a patient and recording physiologic data. Nonetheless, the design of a well-executed system is a challenge that must satisfy multiple performance criteria successfully.

CHAPTER (18)

Digital Image Formats and Archiving Practices

Jonathan L. Elion, MD

THE BASICS OF DICOM DIGITAL IMAGE FILE STRUCTURE

The work to develop standards for the exchange of medical images began in 1982, when the American College of Radiology (ACR) and the National Electrical Manufacturers Association (NEMA) began working on standards for connecting digital imaging devices. Version 1.0 of the ACR-NEMA standard was published in 1985 and provided for connecting two devices directly ("point-to-point"), along with a set of rules for encoding information and a set of messages to initiate transactions. Version 2.0 of the ACR-NEMA standard followed in 1988, providing further enrichment of the rules by which messages are organized. In 1992, Version 3.0 of the standard was published, and its name changed to DICOM (Digital Imaging and Communications in Medicine). This version of the standard established interconnectivity using standard computer networks.[1]

Until digital imaging was developed, photographic film was the unique vehicle for recording, archiving, and exchanging medical image data. With the advent of digital imaging, a need for a common standard that would apply across different manufacturers and different items of equipment was essential in order to avoid total confusion in the exchange of medical image information. The DICOM standard has become a vital means of information exchange of digital image data. It permits the exchange of image data from one image acquisition and display system to another. It also has the potential to facilitate the filing and archiving of images in digital form according to a common standard.

【 】 ORGANIZATIONAL STRUCTURE

The organizational structure of the DICOM standard uses a complex information model.[2] For most imaging modalities, it can be simplified to just four levels:

1. Patient.
2. Study.
3. Series.
4. Images/Reports.

The patient is at the top of this hierarchy. Each patient can have one or more studies, typically consisting of everything that happens from the time the patient gets on the examination table until the time he/she gets off. Each study can have one or more series, the exact use of which is not specified, but is typically used to separate logical portions of an examination and portions performed with different equipment. Each series can have one or more images or one or more reports. In DICOM usage, "image" may mean a complete cine run, rather than a single frame of the run.

An array of data that contains information about an image is called a *DICOM Image Object*. There are more than 400 separate data items that can be included in a DICOM Image Object for an X-ray Angiographic (XA) study. Following is a partial listing of some of the categories of information, along with a few representative data items for each category:

- **Patient Information**
  - *General Patient Information*: Name, ID, birthdate, gender, ethnic group.

---

[1]http://www.rsna.org/IHE

- **Study Information**
  - *General Study Information*: Study date and time; study description.
  - *Patient Information* (at the time the study was performed): Admitting diagnoses; age; weight.
  - *Clinical Trial Identifiers*: Protocol name; site name; subject ID.
- **Series Information**
  - *General Series Information* (within a study): Modality; series date and time; performing physician name; body part examined.
  - *General Equipment Information*: Manufacturer; model; software version; location.
  - *Synchronization Information*: Time synchronization method.
- **Image Information**
  - *General Image Information*: Image acquisition date and time; indicator as to whether the image has undergone lossy compression; image icon.
  - *Image Pixel Data*: matrix size of the image; number of bits per pixel; actual pixel data.
  - *Contrast Agent Information*: Agent used; route; volume; rate; duration.
  - *Cine Image Information*: number of milliseconds between frames; recommended display rate.
  - *X-Ray Image Information*: Pixel intensity relationship (linear, logarithmic or ready to be displayed).
  - *X-Ray Acquisition Information*: KvP; x-ray tube current; exposure time; average pulse width; intensifier size; focal spot size.
  - *X-Ray Positioner Information*: Source to patient; source to detector; estimated radiographic magnification factor; positioner angles.
  - *Modality Lookup Table* (Required if the pixel intensity relationship is logarithmic; optional if it is ready to be displayed): Defines a transformation applied to stored pixel values to account for characteristics of the acquisition modality.
  - *Value of Interest Lookup Table*: Optional transformations applied to stored pixel values, such as "Window Width" and "Window Level."
  - *Basic Object Information*: Character set used; unique identifier of the object; date class of the object; time and date it was created; digital signature(s).

THE IMPORTANCE OF THE STANDARD IN IMAGE INTERCHANGE

Prior to 1995, there was little compatibility among the various commercial digital x-ray systems, making interoperability and image exchange problematic at best.[3] In 1992, the Cardiac Catheterization Committee of the American College of Cardiology became engaged in the DICOM standards process and helped develop the file formats and physical media exchange standards that would permit images to be freely exchanged and viewed.[4] This culminated in the first large-scale interoperability demonstration in 1995,[5] in which 29 vendors showed the ability

to exchange and view (XA) images using DICOM, establishing the common platform that helped usher in the digital imaging era in the cardiac catheterization laboratory.

Today, the DICOM standard is widely accepted and implemented, with many cardiac catheterization laboratories going completely digital and abandoning cine film altogether.[6] Recordable compact discs (CD-R) were used initially to exchange cineangiographic images between institutions, but as interventions became more prevalent and image resolution increased, recording media with greater capacity has become necessary. CD-R is therefore being supplanted by recordable DVD discs (DVD-R, DVD+RW, and similar variants).

DATA COMPRESSION IN CORONARY ANGIOGRAPHY

【 】 THE NEED FOR COMPRESSION

Coronary angiography is now often performed using a matrix of 1024^2 pixels for each frame, with each pixel having a numeric value between 0 and 4096 (requiring 2 bytes per pixel). Each frame therefore is 2 megabytes (MB) in size, requiring 60 MB to store each second of the image data at 30 frames per second. A short diagnostic coronary angiogram of only 60 s duration would require 3600 MB of computer storage, filling more than five CDs with image data (if no compression were used).

【 】 TYPES OF IMAGE COMPRESSION

Image compression refers to a transformation of the original set of picture elements ("pixels") to reduce its size and associated storage requirements. The process is termed *lossless* when the compression is done in a manner that allows it to be completely reversed (fully restoring the pixel data to its original values). Computer programs downloaded from the Internet are typically compressed by the sending system in this fashion to reduce the time it takes to be transmitted over a network and allowing them to be reconstituted to their original form by the receiver. The degree of compression is expressed as the ratio of the original file size to the compressed file size. The lossless compression used in DICOM for (XA) studies generally achieves a compression ratio between about 2.0 and 2.5. A relatively new alternative for lossless compression based on LOCO-I (Low Complexity Lossless Compression for Images) has been standardized as JPEG-LS[7] and has now been added to the DICOM standard (but not incorporated as an option for x-ray angiography written onto media). Lossless compression can achieve ratios up to 3.8:1 with this approach.

Lossy compression techniques are not completely reversible, as the image content after decompression is not identical to that in the original, but much higher compression rates can be achieved. This technique is particularly well suited to echocardiographic images,[8] where any compression artifacts that are introduced are obscured by the ultrasound speckle (noise) in the images.

The Joint Photographic Expert Group (JPEG) has defined standards for both lossy and lossless compression.[9] The latter has been less well known until its use in the DICOM standard. Another approach to lossy compression known as *wavelets* has been found to be highly effective when applied to medical images,[10–12] and recently was specified in a sufficiently standardized fashion as to permit its selection as another alternative compression technique that can be use in DICOM. This approach, now called *JPEG 2000*,[13] can achieve higher compression ratios with less data loss,[14] and has seen growing use in radiology applications. There is also a lossless version of JPEG 2000 that is just as effective as JPEG-LS, but the algorithm is slower and uses more computer resources. Efforts are continuing to improve and refine the levels of compression that can be achieved with both the original JPEG compression standard[15,16] and JPEG 2000.[17]

STUDIES OF COMPRESSION IN CORONARY ANGIOGRAPHY

In order to examine some of the issues regarding the use of JPEG image compression in coronary angiography, the American College of Cardiology, the European Society of Cardiology, and the DICOM Working Group for Cardiovascular Information ("Working Group 1") carried out a three-part study designed to examine some of the questions.[18] This International Angiographic Compression Study analyzed a large set of high-quality angiograms that were collected from systems from a variety of manufacturers. The angiograms were either reviewed in their original unprocessed state or after one of three levels of lossy compression had been applied (6:1, 10:1, and 16:1).

Phase 1 of these studies looked at the impact of JPEG compression on the ability to detect subtle diagnostic features in angiograms,[19] including filling defects (possible thrombus), dissection, calcification, and complex stenosis (multiple irregularities, overhanging edges, haziness or poorly seen edges). This study found that the JPEG compression used had no significant effect on feature detection at the 6:1 compression ratio, but there was a significant negative impact at the 16:1 compression ratio.

Phase 2 of these studies examined the effect of JPEG compression on quantitative coronary arteriography (QCA). A series of coronary lesions was analyzed at the same levels of compression. Compression had a significant impact on catheter calibration, coronary vessel measurements, and increased the variability of resulting measurements.

Phase 3 of these studies examined perceived image quality differences between compressed and uncompressed images that could be ascribed to the compression effects.[20] Compressed and uncompressed images were shown side by side on one monitor and readers were asked to assess quality differences. A small visual difference was present even at the lowest compression ratio (6:1) and became quite noticeable at the higher compression ratios. The increase in error rates for detecting subtle image features paralleled that seen in Phase 1 of the study.

In another study of the impact image compression has on lesion assessment, angiograms were reviewed (visually and quantitatively) before and after 15:1 JPEG compression.[21] They were also reassessed at a later sitting to examine intraobserver variability. This study showed that the variability of visual assessment was similar to that seen with cine film. However, unlike the International Compression Study, there was no significant impact on quantitative measures.

ANGIOGRAPHIC IMAGE COMPRESSION IN PERSPECTIVE

One should exercise caution in evaluating the impact of lossy compression on clinical practice. It is difficult to compare the findings of the various clinical studies that have been reported to date, as many of the important factors have been controlled differently in different studies, and some lack the statistical power to detect a difference, even if one were present. These factors include, but are not limited to: the selection of image sets to study; viewing conditions (ambient light, monitor quality and settings); the specific algorithms used for QCA; characteristics of the evaluators (eg, experience, potential biases, study-specific training, supervision); angiographic image quality; radiation dose and image noise; radiographic features studied; and number of angiographic labs providing images. There is also an important difference between the performance of observers for a particular diagnostic task, and ability to perceive a difference in quality or appearance.[22]

There is considerable debate over whether JPEG 2000 (or actually wavelets in general) actually does better than other lossy compression methods, except at relatively high rates of compression.[22] As a consequence, in the absence of a similar trial to the ACC JPEG study, the appropriateness of using JPEG 2000 for coronary angiography is undetermined.

There are many technical factors that influence the performance of lossy compression algorithms, and other factors may have an impact on the measures used to assess the diagnostic quality of the images:

- **Matrix Size:** The majority of studies that have been reported to date on the impact of lossy compression on coronary angiographic images can only be applied to $512^2 \times 8$-bit coronary angiograms. If a 16:1 compression is performed on a 1024^2 image, it results in the same file size as doing a 4:1 compression on a 512^2 image. The resulting image quality and feature distinctiveness may be expected to differ, and to date have not been compared.

- **Frequency Response:** The lossy JPEG compression that has been tested has been performed using the "baseline" JPEG algorithm. The various frequencies in the image are compressed differently, based on assumptions that have been derived from photographs. *Image frequency* refers to the abruptness of changes in image brightness with respect to spatial coordinates. The diaphragm, for example, has a gradual change in brightness across the image and is considered low-frequency information. The struts of a stent have rapid changes of brightness over a small area of the image, and are considered high-frequency information. New approaches to optimizing the JPEG algorithms are being developed[15] and have yet to be studied for coronary angiograms. It should be possible to analyze the frequency content of the image and preserve more of the information in the clinically relevant ranges, thereby achieving less content loss at higher compression ranges.

- **Compression Measures:** At a given compression ratio, an optimized JPEG compression algorithm may have better image fidelity than the baseline JPEG algorithm. Studies of 16:1 compression using the baseline JPEG process would not, therefore, be applicable to images with 16:1 compression with an optimized compression algorithm. Compression ratios alone are an incomplete measure of the impact on image content. Other ways to express effects of compression have been described, including the sum of absolute differences between matching pixels of compressed and uncompressed images, the sum of squared differences, and the peak signal-to-noise ratio (PSNR).[10] These measures have their own limitations, because they give assessment of the entire image and ignore local effects.

- **Image Quality:** There is a continuing effort to reduce radiation exposure to the patient and the operator, but with decreased radiation dose comes an increase in image noise. Because the noise represents high-frequency information, it is likely to have an impact on the efficiency of JPEG compression. Other characteristics of the image are also likely to affect results, including pixel depth (number of gray levels represented) and dynamic range.

- **QCA Algorithms:** There is a variety of algorithms used in quantitative arteriography. Their ability to detect and track vessel edges has evolved based on certain expected image characteristics. The various existing algorithms can be expected to be affected differently when faced with images that have been degraded through lossy compression.

Compression continues to be of interest both in radiology and in cardiology.[23] Lossy compression is generally considered, not because it is desirable, but rather because it is necessary to stretch the capabilities of the existing digital storage and networking technology.[24] Continuing advances in digital storage capacity and network speeds continue to reduce the need for lossy compression, especially in situations where the cardiologist viewing the images is using a system that is connected directly to the hospital network.

THE CHALLENGES OF IMAGE DISPLAY ACROSS SYSTEMS

The ACC/AHA Task Force describes the use of DICOM in the cardiac catheterization laboratory.[25] Despite a growing experience with the DICOM format, serious challenges remain in achieving the complete ubiquitous exchange of cardiovascular images. Many of these problems are caused by the omission of optional but useful data in the DICOM image files. The DICOM standard defines three levels of requirements for data elements in a DICOM file:

- **Type 1 Elements:** Data element must be present and must contain valid data.

- **Type 2 Elements:** The data element must be present, but the associated data field can be empty if the value is unknown to the creating system.

- **Type 3 Elements:** Not required.

One significant historical example of how the omission of data can affect interoperability happened when one vendor began to omit the contents of the "Basic Offset Table" used to assist review station software in finding any given image inside a stream of compressed data. Without it, it is not possible to jump to any requested frame for viewing. Instead, the software must read frames sequentially until the desired frame is found. The DICOM standard requires that the Basic Offset Table be present, but can be of zero length (that is, it may have no information in it). Viewing software had evolved to expect this table to contain valid data, as all XA DICOM files up to that point had contained the information. When XA images began to appear without the information in the Basic Offset Table, viewing applications were initially unable to handle and display the images. Even when the software was fixed to handle the missing data (eg, by building its own frame offset table while loading the entire set of frames), some degree of functionality was still missing (such as the ability to jump to any frame in the sequence or to quickly construct an icon image that represents the sequence).

Another example of optional data that would improve interoperability if it were guaranteed to be present is the use of "Window Level" and "Window Width." As a growing number of XA image files are greater than 8 bits (that is, they contain 10-bit or 12-bit image data), it is important to know how to set the Window Level (corresponding to the image brightness) and Window Width (corresponding to the image contrast) for viewing. This is typically known by the sending system, but it can cause a discrepancy between perceived image quality on the sending system and the receiving system if the viewing parameters are not transmitted and therefore do not match. More sophisticated viewing programs can perform a statistical analysis on the image pixels to determine appropriate default windows, but there is still no assurance that this will result in an image display that matches that seen on the originating system.

A similar problem exists with images that are meant for digital subtraction. This is more typically seen with peripheral angiography, where the original acquisition modality has information about how the images are to be subtracted optimally, but a complete set of this information is not required to be transmitted along with the images. When viewing the images on a different system, the information about optimal frames to be used for subtraction may be missing.

Current technology for image formation in an all-digital cardiac catheterization laboratory may involve a considerable amount of image processing for noise reduction, edge enhancement, and extending the effective dynamic range. The degree of image processing may differ between the in-room display and the DICOM images that are exported by the system, and the details of the image processing may not be made available because they may be considered by the vendors to be highly proprietary. This creates the opportunity to have significant inconsistencies in the degree to which transmitted images have been preprocessed, and may lead to the use of inappropriate image types for quantitative analysis. Because edge enhancement affects the performance of quantitative coronary analysis, every effort must be made to receive and store the images in their raw (unprocessed) format.[26] Further studies must be carried out to determine the magnitude of these differences, as well as to better characterize the impact of different matrix sizes and pixel depths on quantitative algorithms.[27] True consistency of image quality requires the use of calibrated display systems, a technology that is currently underused in the angiography world, in contrast to its acceptance for radiology PACS.

NETWORKS FOR IMAGE STORAGE AND REVIEW

Network storage and display architecture has evolved from simple systems serving one or two cath labs to more complex systems serving multiple modalities and multiple hospitals. Storage strategies have evolved as well.[28] Initially, the high cost of disk storage led to the deployment of multitiered storage architectures. Only the most recent images were stored on the highest-speed media ("online storage"). When available online storage runs low, studies are migrated to slower and less-expensive media ("nearline storage") such as digital tape, CD-R, and DVD-R. As the cost of disk storage has fallen, systems can be deployed effectively with a single-tier approach, in which all of the images are kept on fast disks and the slower, less-expensive media is used only for storing backup and recovery copies.

Regardless of the choice of hardware for disk storage, the format in which images are encoded and stored should be standardized, both on the disks themselves and on the backup media. This would facilitate recovery from disaster, especially when support from the vendor is no longer available, as well as enable migration to a new vendor or technology in the future. DICOM specifies only the way information is stored for interchange, and not for its format inside archives.

【 】 A SIMPLE IMAGING NETWORK

Initial image network design centered on a large central server that received, stored, and distributed images (Figure 18-1). This design met the requirements of even large-volume cardiac catheterization facilities, allowing them to abandon film altogether and go totally digital.[29] The main storage device is a redundant array of independent disks (RAID) that is attached directly to its host server. This type of "host-attached RAID" is fast and reliable, but difficult to upgrade when more storage is required. This makes it an inflexible choice in an institution whose needs may evolve over time. The RAID is typically configured to be large enough to hold all of the angiographic images that might be acquired for a given period of time. A database keeps track of the demographic information

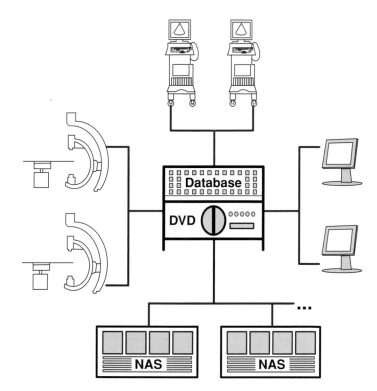

FIGURE 18-2. This large hospital-wide network expands on the concepts of the simple image network, but the inflexible host-attached RAID has been replaced by *network attached storage (NAS)*. Additional NAS devices can be added as needed to keep all of the studies online, reducing the architectural to one tier. DVDs are used for backup and disaster recovery.

about the patients and their studies and rapidly services queries from viewing stations. As the RAID fills up, older images are migrated to slower, less-expensive nearline storage. The different levels of storage can be managed either by a hierarchical storage management system[30] or be tracked directly by the database.

【 】 A LARGE HOSPITAL-WIDE NETWORK

The next major advance in storage systems was the advent of *network-attached storage (NAS)* (Figure 18-2). This innovation allowed a more flexible management strategy for online storage, as there was no longer the tight coupling between the disks and the host server. Additional NAS devices could be connected as needed on the network. NAS provides all of its file and storage services through standard network protocols, and when used with high-speed Ethernet, it can scale to a very high performance level. The fact that additional storage can be added as needed is also attractive, as storage requirements always seem to expand past initial predictions (because of higher-resolution systems coming online, as well as the performance of more complex interventional procedures with their attendant increase in the number of images taken).

As prices dropped, the strategy for balancing online and nearline storage also changed, as it became a technically feasible and economically sound decision to keep all cases online. Performance was also greatly enhanced, as the delays inherent in retrieving studies from nearline storage were eliminated. Less-expensive storage options (like DVD) are now relegated to keeping backup and disaster recovery copies.

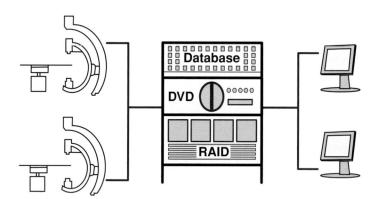

FIGURE 18-1. A simple imaging network showing two cardiac catheterization laboratories connected to a server with *host-attached RAID*. As the RAID fills up, studies are migrated to a DVD jukebox that functions as *nearline storage*. A database makes an index of the contents of the archive available to viewing stations.

【 】 ENTERPRISE-WIDE NETWORK DESIGNS

The most recent advance in network design has been the enterprise-wide system. Information services (IS) departments at hospitals looked for better solutions to the problem of supporting multiple distinct archives and archive interfaces (one in each department).[31] To solve this problem, they are implementing specialized high-speed networks dedicated to the storage of data known as *storage area networks (SAN)* (Figure 18-3). This allows for economy of scale, the use of one central facility for all of the departments in the hospital and on the hospital network. Image archives use a special-

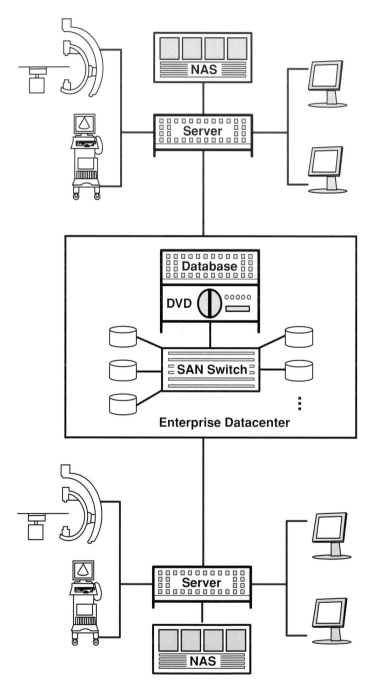

FIGURE 18-3. An enterprise-wide network showing two hospitals connected to an enterprise datacenter. By maintaining NAS storage at each hospital, the network load can be optimized while still leveraging large *storage-area network (SAN)* storage. By centralizing the database, studies can be searched and viewed anywhere in the enterprise.

ized high-speed connection to the SAN that relieves the archive system of much of the communications housekeeping that would be associated with a simple NAS. Files can be retrieved many times faster than when a simple NAS is used because of the greater speed of the SAN and the lower processor overhead of handling the data.

A SAN-based architecture also permits standardization of the data handling policies and reduces variations in data integrity. By continuing to use NAS locally, another level of redundancy is introduced that provides a level of backup in the case of network or central facility problems. It also enhances performance, as images can be fetched from the closest (and fastest) storage device. More sophisticated storage handling algorithms are required to keep track of the multiple online storage locations.

【 】 TELEMEDICINE APPLICATIONS

With the widespread availability of angiographic images in digital format, it has become possible to extend image exchange and viewing onto wide-area networks. This has been used to support low-risk *percutaneous coronary intervention (PCI)* at a community hospital with no cardiac surgery capabilities,[32] to review and select candidates for coronary artery bypass surgery,[33] and to support reference laboratories analyzing images from clinical trials of new interventional devices. As the cost of high-speed bandwidth decreases and broadband cable and digital subscriber line (DSL) networks become more prevalent, these telemedicine applications can be expected to proliferate.

【 】 DISASTER RECOVERY

Effective April 21, 2005, federal regulations in the United States required that all healthcare entities have a disaster recovery plan in effect. This requires that a copy of the images and associated data should be maintained in a location away from the primary storage facility, and that these copies can be used to rebuild the storage archive.[34] The disaster recovery options must provide copies of studies in a different building to avoid a "single point of failure."

Less well known is the fact that the same federal regulations require hospitals to have "downtime," or emergency procedures to be followed in the event of failure of a data center or network. Even though networks can be designed to be redundant and highly reliable, unforeseen circumstances can still intervene. Computer virus outbreaks have caused hospitals to voluntarily shut down the network, making central storage site design (without local redundancy) fail. The use of DVDs as a means for backup and disaster recovery has the additional benefit of fulfilling this need for downtime procedures, as a properly recorded and formatted DVD can be removed from its jukebox and taken to the point of care for emergency viewing.

THE FUTURE OF THE DICOM AND RELATED STANDARDS

【 】 DICOM STRUCTURED REPORTING

The DICOM standard continues to evolve and has now been extended to include standards for the transmission and storage of clinical documents using structured reporting (SR).[35] The SR specifications support both conventional unstructured ("free-text") reports as well as structured (coded) information. Structured data allows for precision and unambiguous clarity in specifying clinical information. Findings that can be expressed include text, codes, numeric measurements, coordinates of specific regions of interest in images, temporal coordinates in waveforms, and references to comparison objects (images, waveforms, and previous reports). Structured reporting helps bridge the gap between imaging and hospital information systems,[36] enabling the integration of image and patient record data.[37] Well-defined standards have already been created for information from hemodynamics systems, electrocardiogram reports, cardiac catheterization, procedure logs, quantitative coronary angiography and ventriculography, intravascular ultrasound, and echocardiography. This marks a big step toward the goal of being able to provide a comprehensive set of images and database-compatible information that can be sent electronically over networks or even written as a single "unit record" (for example, on DVD-R media) that can be transported with patients or sent through the mail or overnight courier.

The primary benefit of DICOM SR for cardiology is the distribution of quantitative information derived from images (eg, ventriculogram outlines, volume determinations, QCA measurements). It provides the technical foundation for the large-scale collection of structured data as would be needed for multicenter clinical trials and national data registries[38] such as the American College of Cardiology's National Cardiovascular Data Registry (NCDR).[39] Although DICOM SR can also be used to encode the full reports, it remains to be seen whether this proves to be a popular or useful format in that role, as compared to other existing digital standards or even the distribution of preformatted reports.

[ ] INTEGRATING THE HEALTHCARE ENTERPRISE

The latest advances have to do with the integration of the imaging networks with the hospital information systems, thereby merging patient demographics, medical records, and images.[40] This type of integration also provides a means whereby images can be stored directly into the online patient record.[41] This assists a healthcare enterprise in leveraging their existing infrastructure, especially the clinical information review stations that have already been installed in patient care areas.

There is an international effort underway to improve the overall levels of systems interoperability known as *Integrating the Healthcare Enterprise (IHE)*. This initiative brings together healthcare professionals and industry experts to coordinate the use of standards to enhance the ability of computer systems to share information in the healthcare setting.[42] IHE began by addressing structured workflow in radiology,[43] and has now expanded to include discrete efforts in information technology, laboratory, and, most recently, in cardiology. It identifies the components of the involved systems ("actors") and the messages that are exchanged ("transactions"). The IHE Technical Frameworks[1] provide a detailed description of how given clinical scenarios are to be handled, including the placement of orders, reconciliation of patient identifiers in multiple computer systems, the creation of a worklist for a modality, and the associated steps necessary to accomplish an ordered study. The IHE cardiology work addresses specifically the difficulties of the catheterization laboratory: integrating and synchronizing multiple modalities from multiple vendors, the frequent emergency cases, combined diagnostic and interventional cases (whether planned or not), and procedures that continue across several rooms in the catheterization suite.

Efforts are continuing to achieve the goal of full integration of patient information and images.[44] This will be facilitated by the adoption of the DICOM standards for structured reporting, as such devices as echocardiographs and hemodynamic systems begin to use this standard to communicate their findings in a standardized fashion. The IHE initiative provides a framework to assure better coordination of patient information across a broad range of computing systems and, before long, should start to help achieve this at the national and, it is hoped, the international level.

REFERENCES

1. Bidgood WD, Horii SC. Introduction to the ACR-NEMA DICOM Standard. *Radiographics.* 1992;12(2):345.
2. National Electrical Manufacturers Association, American College of Radiology. *Digital imaging and communications in medicine (DICOM).* 2003; National Electrical Manufacturers Association.
3. Nissen SE, Pepine CJ, Bashore TM, et al. Cardiac angiography without cine film: erecting a "tower of Babel" in the cardiac catheterization laboratory. *J Am Coll Cardiol.* 1994;24:834.
4. ACC/ACR/NEMA Ad Hoc Group. American College of Cardiology and industry develop standards for digital transfer of angiographic images. *J Am Coll Cardiol.* 1995;25:800.
5. Elion JL. DICOM media interchange standards for cardiology: initial interoperability demonstration. *Proc Annu Symp Comput Appl Med Care.* 1995;591.
6. Nissen SE. Evolution of the filmless cardiac angiography suite: Promise and perils of the evolving digital era. *Am J Cardiol.* 1996;78:41.
7. Weinberger M, Seroussi G, Sapiro G. LOCO-I lossless image compression algorithm: principles and standardization into JPEG-LS. *IEEE Trans Image Proc.* 2000;9:1309.
8. Karson TH, Chandra S, Morehead AJ, Stewart WJ, Nissen SE, Thomas JD. JPEG compression of digital echocardiographic images: impact on image quality. *J Am Soc Echocardiog.* 1995;8(3):306–18.
9. Pennebaker WB, Mitchell JL. *JPEG still image data compression standard.* 1992; Van Nostrand Reinhold.
10. Iyriboz TA, Zukoski MJ, Hopper KD, Stagg PL. A comparison of wavelet and Joint Photographic Experts Group lossy compression methods applied to medical images. *J Dig Imag.* 1999;12(2):14.
11. Puniene J, Punys V, Punys J. Medical image compression by cosine and wavelet transforms. *Stud Health Technol Inform.* 2000;77:1245.
12. Portoni L, Combi C, Pozzi G, Pinciroli F, Fritsch JP, Brennecke R. Angiocardiographic digital still images compressed via irreversible methods: concepts and experiments. *Int J Med Inf.* 1997;46(3):185.
13. Acharya T, Tsai PS. *JPEG 2000 standard for image compression concepts, algorithms and VLSI architectures.* 2004; Hoboken, NJ.
14. Sung MM, Kim HJ, Yoo SK, et al. Clinical evaluation of compression ratios using JPEG2000 on computed radiography chest images. *J Dig Imag.* 2002;15(2):78.
15. Onnasch DG, Prause GP, Ploger A. Objective methods for optimizing JPEG compression of coronary angiographic images. *Int J Card Imag.* 1995;11(3):151.
16. Brennecke R, Burgel U, Rippin G, Post F, Rupprecht HJ, Meyer J. Comparison of image compression viability for lossy and lossless JPEG and Wavelet data reduction in coronary angiography. *Int J Cardiovasc Imag.* 2001;17(1):1.
17. Zhang Y, Pham BT, Eckstein MP. Automated optimization of JPEG 2000 encoder options based on model observer performance for detecting variable signals in X-ray coronary angiograms. *IEEE Trans Med Imag.* 2004;23(4):459.
18. Nissen SE, Hirshfeld JW, Jr., Simon R. Introduction and background: the International Angiographic Compression study. *J Am Coll Cardiol.* 2000;35(5):1367.
19. Kerensky RA, Cusma JT, Kubilis P, et al. American College of Cardiology/European Society of Cardiology International Study of Angiographic Data Compression Phase I: The effect of lossy data compression on recognition of diagnostic features in digital coronary angiography. *J Am Coll Cardiol.* 2000;35(5):1370.

20. Brennecke R, Burgel U, Simon R, et al. American College of Cardiology/European Society of Cardiology International Study of Angiographic Data Compression Phase III: measurement of image quality differences at varying levels of data compression. *J Am Coll Cardiol.* 2000;35(5):1388.

21. Rigolin VH, Robiolio PA, Spero LA, et al. Compression of digital coronary angiograms does not affect visual or quantitative assessment of coronary artery stenosis severity. *Am J Cardiol.* 1996;78(2):131.

22. Proceedings of SPIE—Volume 3980. Medical Imaging 2000: PACS Design and Evaluation: Engineering and Clinical Issues. Blaine GJ, Siegel EL, eds. May 2000, pp 85–96. Available at: http://adsabs.harvard.edu/abs/2000SPIE.3980...85F

23. Andriole KP, Erickson BJ, Gould RG, Morin RL, Piraino DW, Reiner BI. *Irreversible Compression of Medical Images.* 2000; Society for Computer Applications in Radiology.

24. Elion JL, Whiting JS. Clinical use of lossy image compression in digital angiography. *Am J Cardiol.* 1996;78(2):219.

25. Bashore TM, Bates ER, Berger PB, et al. Cardiac catheterization laboratory standards: a report of the American College of Cardiology Task Force on Clinical Expert Consensus Documents. *J Am Coll Cardiol.* 2001;37:2170.

26. Reiber JHC, Koning G, Goedhart B. The effect of DICOM on QCA and clinical trials. *Int J Card Imag.* 1998;14:7.

27. Reiber JH, Goedhart B, Brand GJ, Schiemanck L, van der Zwet PM. Quantitative coronary arteriography: current status and future. *Heart Vessels.* 1997;Suppl12:209.

28. Dumery B. Digital image archiving: challenges and choices. *Radiol Manage.* 2002;24(3):30.

29. Cusma JT, Wondrow MA, Holmes DR. Replacement of cinefilm with a digital archive and review network—Initial experience of a large catheterization laboratory. *Int J Card Imag.* 1998;14(5):293.

30. Avrin DE, Andriole KP, Yin L, Gould RG, Arenson RL. A hierarchical storage management (HSM) scheme for cost-effective on-line archival using lossy compression. *J Dig Imag.* 2001;14(1):18.

31. Erickson BJ, Persons KR, Hangiandreou NJ, James EM, Hanna CJ, Gehring DG. Requirements for an enterprise digital image archive. *J Dig Imag.* 2001;14(2):72.

32. Ting HH, Garratt KN, Singh M, et al. Low-risk percutaneous coronary interventions without on-site cardiac surgery: two years' observational experience and follow-up. *Am Heart J.* 2003;145(2):278.

33. Bonvini RF, Caoduro L, Menafoglio A, Calanca L, von SL, Gallino A. Telemedicine for cardiac surgery candidates. *Eur J Cardiothorac Surg.* 2002;22(3):377.

34. Smith EM. Storage options for the healthcare enterprise. *Radiol Manage.* 2003;25(6):26.

35. Hussein R, Engelmann U, Schroeter A, Meinzer HP. DICOM structured reporting—Part 1. Overview and characteristics. *Radiographics.* 2004;24(3):891.

36. Csipo D, Dayhoff RE, Kuzmak PM. Integrating digital imaging and communications in medicine (DICOM)-Structured reporting into the hospital environment. *J Dig Imag.* 2001;14(2):12.

37. Munch H, Engelmann U, Schroter A, Meinzer HP. The integration of medical images with the electronic patient record and their web-based distribution. *Acad Radiol.* 2004;11(6):661.

38. Bidgood WD. Clinical importance of the DICOM structured reporting standard. *Int J Card Imag.* 1998;14(5):307.

39. Brindis RG, Fitzgerald S, Anderson HV, Shaw RE, Weintraub WS, Williams JF. The American College of Cardiology–National Cardiovascular Data Registry (ACC-NCDR): building a national clinical data repository. *J Am Coll Cardiol.* 2001;37(8):2240.

40. Creighton C. A literature review on communication between picture archiving and communication systems and radiology information systems and/or hospital information systems. *J Dig Imag.* 1999;12(3):138.

41. Kuzmak PM, Dayhoff RE. The use of digital imaging and communications in medicine (DICOM) in the integration of imaging into the electronic patient record at the Department of Veterans Affairs. *J Dig Imag.* 2000;13(2):133.

42. Carr CD, Moore SM. IHE: a model for driving adoption of standards. *Comput Med Imaging Graph.* 2003;27(2-3):137.

43. Moore SM. Using the IHE scheduled work flow integration profile to drive modality efficiency. *Radiographics.* 2003;23(2):523.

44. Boochever SS. HIS/RIS/PACS integration: getting to the gold standard. *Radiol Manage.* 2004 May;26(3):16.

PART 4 Pharmacology

CHAPTER (19)

Antithrombin Therapies

Anna Kalynych, MD

Coronary artery thrombosis, which occurs both during acute coronary syndromes and percutaneous coronary interventions (PCIs), results from complex interactions between the three main components of the hemostatic system: the vessel wall, plasma coagulation proteins, and platelets. These three components are interdependent, and thrombin plays a pivotal role their interactions (Figure 19-1). At sites of plaque disruption, tissue factor is exposed, triggering activation of the coagulation cascade with resultant generation of thrombin. Thrombin catalyzes the conversion of fibrinogen to fibrin. It amplifies the coagulation cascade by activating factors V, VII, VIII, and XI. It also activates factor XIII, which stabilizes the fibrin strands. Thrombin stimulates platelet aggregation and is one of the most potent platelet activators. The fibrin mesh provides the anchor for the platelet plug. Activated platelets in turn provide a surface for further thrombin generation. Thrombin also exerts effects on endothelial cells, resulting in changes in shape, permeability, cell surface molecule expression, and secretion of various factors. Endothelial cells activated by vascular injury also provide a surface for thrombin generation. In addition, thrombin also plays an important role in inflammation, activating monocytes, neutrophils, and smooth muscle cells.

Because of thrombin's central role in arterial thrombosis, antithrombotic therapy has been a mainstay in the treatment of patients with acute coronary syndromes as well as for use in patients undergoing PCI. Unfractionated heparin (UFH) has historically been the anticoagulant of choice, despite significant shortcomings. UFH requires the cofactor antithrombin (AT). It cannot inhibit thrombin bound to fibrin, fibrin degradation products, or subendothelial matrix. It exhibits nonspecific binding to other plasma proteins. It fails to prevent thrombin-mediated activation of platelets. It is inactivated by platelet factor 4. It may result in heparin-induced thrombocytopenia (HIT). Enoxaparin, a low-molecular-weight heparin (LMWH), overcomes some but not all of these shortcomings. LMWHs exhibit less protein binding than UFH. LMWHs cause less platelet activation than UFH, and they are not inactivated by platelet factor 4. There is a lower likelihood of HIT.

Direct thrombin inhibitors (DTIs) have many theoretical advantages over both UFH and LMWH. DTIs require no cofactors. They inhibit both circulating and clot-bound thrombin. They exhibit no nonspecific binding. DTIs prevent thrombin-mediated activation of platelets and are not inhibited by platelet factor 4. There is no risk of HIT. Despite their many theoretical advantages, DTIs have not been widely used clinically for the treatment of acute coronary syndrome (ACS) and during PCI. Until recently, evidence from large clinical trials supporting their use has been lacking. Larger trials are currently underway to help define the role of DTS in contemporary PCI.

UNFRACTIONATED HEPARIN

【 】 MECHANISM OF ACTION

AT is the major plasma protease inhibitor of thrombin. It also inactivates other coagulation factors, including factor Xa. Heparin binds to AT, causing a conformational change in AT. This change results in accelerated inactivation by AT of several coagulation factors, including Xa. To inactivate thrombin, heparin must simultaneously bind to AT and thrombin. This occurs only when the molecule is long enough. UFHs are a heterogeneous

---

A list of the clinical trials cited in Chapters 19 through 24 is presented in Appendix IV-1 at the end of Part IV.

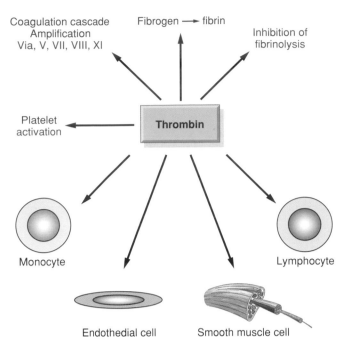

Coagulation cascade
Amplification
Via, V, VII, VIII, XI

Fibrogen → fibrin

Inhibition of
fibrinolysis

Platelet
activation

Thrombin

Monocyte

Lymphocyte

Endothedial cell

Smooth muscle cell

FIGURE 19–1. Multiple targets of thrombin.

group of molecules, and only about one third of molecules are of sufficient length to be active.

【 】 PHARMACOKINETICS

The pharmacokinetics of heparin are complex due to heparin's heterogeneity and nonspecific protein binding. Dosing is weight-based and can be monitored by either the activated partial thromboplastin time (aPTT) or the activated clotting time (ACT). In the catheterization laboratory, the ACT is usually used. No dosing adjustments are required for patients with renal or hepatic insufficiency.

INDICATIONS

The current American College of Cardiology (ACC)/American Heart Association (AHA)/Society for Cardiac Angiography and Interventions (SCAI) guidelines for PCI state that UFH should be administered to patients undergoing PCI (class IC recommendation).[1]

CLINICAL TRIALS

UFH has been used as the anticoagulant of choice during PCI since the earliest days of angioplasty, but the optimal level of anticoagulation has been inadequately defined. Data from the heparin control arms of 6 randomized, controlled trials of glycoprotein (GP) IIb/IIIa inhibitors or DTIs during PCI from the 1990s were pooled and analyzed for ischemic and bleeding complications.[2] Of the 6146 patients receiving UFH, 5216 (85%) had ACT data available at or

around the time of device activation. The minimum ACT at the time of device activation was used to assess ischemic complications at 7 days. Maximum ACTs were available in 5444 patients (89%), and the maximum ACT was used to assess bleeding complications. About 60% of patients had ACSs, and 15% received stents. Patients were divided into 25-second intervals of ACTs, with ranges of less than 275 seconds to greater than 476 seconds. The lowest composite ischemic event rate was 6.6%, which occurred at ACTs between 350 and 375 seconds. The relationship followed a U-shaped curve, with event rates of 11.1% at 275 to 300 seconds, 8.9% at 325 to 350 seconds, and 9.8% at 425 to 450 seconds. The higher rate of ischemic events at high ACTs was believed to be consistent with heparin–induced platelet activation. The same range was optimal for various subgroups, including patients with diabetes, patients receiving stents, and patients with ACS. The lowest rate of major or minor bleeding was 8.6%, which occurred at ACTs of 325 to 350 seconds; it was 12.4% at ACTs of 350 to 375 seconds. In the 4362 patients receiving abciximab, there was a prolonged plateau of ischemic events rates between ACTs of 250 to 375 seconds, ranging about 4.5% to 5%. There was no U-shaped curve, which suggested that heparin-induced platelet activation is overcome by GP IIb/IIIa inhibition. There was a steady increase in major and minor bleeding complications at ACTs greater than 275 seconds, with a substantial increase at ACTs greater than 375 seconds.

【 】 DOSING

Dosing of UFH depends on whether the patient is receiving concomitant GP IIb/IIIa inhibitors. According to the ACC/AHAI/SCAI[1] and ACCP[3] recommendations, for patients not receiving GP IIb/IIIa inhibitors, a bolus dose of 70 to 100 IU/kg is given intravenously to achieve a target ACT of 250 to 300 seconds with the HemoTec device and 300 to 350 seconds with the Hemochron device. The ACT may be checked 5 minutes after administration. If the ACT is less than 250 seconds, additional bolus doses of 2000 to 5000 IU can be given. For patients receiving GP IIb/IIIa inhibitors, a bolus of 50 to 70 IU/kg is given, with a target ACT of 200 seconds for either the HemoTec or Hemochron device. The sheath may be removed once the ACT is less than 150 to 180 seconds. Routine use of heparin after the PCI is no longer recommended because of lack of efficacy and increase in bleeding complications.

LOW-MOLECULAR-WEIGHT HEPARIN

【 】 MECHANISM OF ACTION

LMWHs are formed by either enzymatic or chemical depolymerization of UFH, forming molecules about one third the size of UFH. The molecule length is in general too short to bind to both AT and thrombin, but it can catalyze the inhibition of factor Xa by AT. Therefore, LMWHs are more potent inactivators of factor Xa than thrombin, and various LMWHs have different antifactor Xa:antifactor IIa activities. For enoxaparin, the ratio is 3.8:1. Although multiple LMWHs are available, enoxaparin has the most extensive data during PCI.

[ ] PHARMACOKINETICS

Enoxaparin pharmacokinetics are predictable. The peak effect occurs 3-5 hours after a subcutaneous (SQ) injection, with a duration of action of approximately 12 hours. The plasma half-life is 4.5 to 7 hours. There is little binding to plasma proteins. Metabolism is hepatic. Excretion is renal (40% of dose; 10% as active fragments). The aPTT and ACT cannot be used to monitor dosing, but monitoring is not generally necessary. Antifactor Xa activity can be measured, and levels of 0.8 to 1.8 IU/mL are therapeutic.

[ ] INDICATIONS

The current 2002 ACC/AHA guidelines state that LMWH or UFH should be added to antiplatelet therapy for patients with unstable angina or non–ST-segment elevation myocardial infarction (MI).[4] As a class IIa recommendation, the guidelines state that enoxaparin is preferable to UFH in the absence of renal failure and unless coronary artery bypass grafting is planned within 24 hours. Therefore, many patients arrive to the cardiac catheterization laboratory receiving enoxaparin. The seventh American College of Chest Physicians (ACCP) Conference on Antithrombotic and Thrombolytic Therapy recommendation suggests continuing enoxaparin therapy during PCI in patients on enoxaparin prior to arrival to the cardiac catheterization laboratory; the dosing recommendations are listed below. Small investigations and nonrandomized studies using enoxaparin de novo during PCI with or without GP IIb/IIIa suggest that these regimens are safe and effective.[5,6] These treatments have not yet been incorporated into the ACC/AHA or ACCP guidelines. However, the ACCP guidelines do state that enoxaparin "appears to be safe when used in combination with tirofiban or eptifibatide during PCI. A favorable outcome has been reported with the combination of dalteparin and abciximab in patients undergoing PCI." The use of LMWH after PCI does not appear to significantly reduce early ischemic events.

[ ] CLINICAL TRIALS

Multiple early studies have suggested that enoxaparin has a role throughout the broad spectrum of patients with ACS. It is likely superior to heparin in patients with ACS who are managed conservatively and not inferior in high-risk patients. In these trials, most patients did not undergo PCI. In the Thrombolysis in Myocardial Infarction (TIMI) IIB and Efficacy Safety Subcutaneous Enoxaparin in Non–Q-Wave Coronary Events (ESSENCE) trials, 445 patients of 7081 patients treated with either UFH or enoxaparin underwent PCI. The enoxaparin arm had a lower 1-year rate of death or MI but more bleeding complications, due mostly to minor bleeding.

In the Superior Yield of the New Strategy of Enoxaparin, Revascularization, and GP IIb/IIIa Inhibitors (SYNERGY) trial, 9978 patients with non–ST elevation ACS were randomized to enoxaparin versus UFH. GP IIb/IIIa inhibitors, aspirin, and clopidogrel were used at the discretion of the physician.[7] This was the first large study with enoxaparin in which patients were managed with an early invasive strategy. About 75% of patients had received some form of antithrombotic drug prior to randomization. Patients who received no treatment prior to randomization or those who did receive treatment but whose therapy was the same as that prior to randomization benefited from enoxaparin with respect to the primary end point of death or nonfatal MI at 30 days without an increase in bleeding. Changing the antithrombotic drug with randomization was associated with no treatment benefit but resulted in an increased risk of bleeding. Based on this study, changing the antithrombotic agent during the course of treatment in these patients cannot be recommended. In the Integrilin and Enoxaparin Randomized Assessment of Acute Coronary Syndrome Treatment (INTERACT) trial, 746 patients with non–ST-elevation ACS were treated with eptifibatide and either enoxaparin 1 mg/kg SQ BID or UFH.[8] Of these patients, 214 underwent PCI. The 30-day death or MI rate was lower in the enoxaparin group (5% vs 9%). Major bleeding was lower in the enoxaparin group, but minor bleeding was higher. In a study by Collet et al, 132 of 451 patients with ACS treated with enoxaparin for at least 48 hours underwent PCI within 8 hours of the last dose without any additional bolus.[9] In this subgroup, the 30-day death or MI rate was 3%.

Multiple small or nonrandomized studies have addressed the use of intravenous (IV) enoxaparin at the time of PCI with or without GP IIb/IIIa inhibitors. The Pharmacokinetics of Enoxaparin in PCI (PEPCI) study looked at the pharmacokinetics of IV enoxaparin dosing in 55 patients that had received SQ doses of enoxaparin.[10] Antifactor Xa levels were within therapeutic range in 98% of patients who had received the last dose of SQ enoxaparin 2 to 8 hours prior to the PCI. For patients whose last SQ dose was 8 to 12 hours prior to the intervention, an additional IV dose of 0.3 mg/kg resulted in antifactor Xa levels that were within the therapeutic range in 96% of patients at the time of PCI. In the Coronary Revascularization Using Integrilin and Single bolus Enoxaparin (CRUISE) study, 261 patients receiving eptifibatide were randomized to either enoxaparin 0.75 mg/kg IV bolus or UFH.[11] All patients underwent elective or urgent PCI. There were no differences in the primary endpoint of bleeding complications. The National Investigators Collaborating on Enoxaparin (NICE) pilot study randomized 60 patients to UFH or IV enoxaparin 1 mg/kg prior to PCI. In the NICE-1 trial, 828 patients underwent PCI with IV enoxaparin 1 mg/kg. In the NICE-4 trial, approximately 800 patients were treated with IV enoxaparin 0.75 mg/kg and abciximab. Sheaths were removed 4 hours after the bolus. These combinations appeared safe and effective when compared to historical controls. A small study involving 242 patients investigated low-dose (0.3 mg/kg) enoxaparin, but this dose is not recommended.

The Safety and Efficacy of Enoxaparin in Percutaneous Coronary Intervention Patients, an International Randomized Evaluation (STEEPLE) study compared 2 doses of IV enoxaparin (0.5 mg/kg or 0.75 mg/kg) versus UFH in patients undergoing nonemergent PCI.[12] The target ACT for the UFH group was 300 to 350 seconds with UFH alone and 200 to 300 seconds with a GP IIb/IIIa inhibitor. The primary end point was non–CABG-related major and minor bleeding at 48 hours. The secondary end points were (1) the percentage of patients achieving target levels of anticoagulation at the start and end of the procedure; and (2) a composite of death, recurrent MI, urgent target vessel revascularization, and major non–CABG-related major bleeding at 30 days. Forty-one percent of patients received GP IIb/IIIa inhibitors, and 85% received aspirin. Drug-eluting stents were used in 57%. There was a statistically significant reduction in the primary end point of major and minor bleeding, with enoxaparin 0.5 mg/kg (6.0%, $P =$.014 compared to UFH), and enoxaparin 0.75 mg/kg (6.6%, $P = $.052 compared to UFH) versus UFH (8.7%). Individually, there was a statistically significant difference in the major but not in the minor rates of bleeding. More patients receiving enoxaparin achieved the target level of anticoagulation. There was no statistically significant difference in the quadruple end point, death, MI, or urgent target vessel revascularization between the three groups at 30 days (7.2%, 7.9%, and 8.4%). Of note, patient enrollment in the low-dose enoxaparin arm was stopped near the end of the study because of concerns about a difference in mortality. This difference was not statistically significant in the 30-day analysis.

[ ] DOSING

Dosing of enoxaparin during PCI depends on the timing of the last SQ dose received prior to the PCI. Therapeutic levels are achieved 30 to 60 minutes after a SQ injection and minutes after an IV injection. If the last SQ dose of enoxaparin has been given 8 hours or less prior to the procedure, no additional anticoagulant is given. If the last dose has been given 8 to 12 hours prior to the procedure, a 0.3 mg/kg IV bolus is given. (An IV bolus given 8 to 12 hours after the last SQ dose gives antifactor Xa levels in the target range for at least 2 additional hours.) If the last dose has been given more than 12 hours prior to the procedure, either enoxaparin 0.75 to 1 mg/kg bolus intravenously or conventional anticoagulation can be used. Dosing in patients receiving a GP IIb/IIIa inhibitor is unclear but is being evaluated. A reasonable dose may be 0.75 mg/kg intravenously. Enoxaparin cannot be monitored by either the aPTT or the ACT. Because of its more predictable level of anticoagulation, monitoring of antifactor Xa activity has not been routinely performed. More recently, point-of-care testing for enoxaparin has become available.

Safe or optimal levels of antifactor Xa activity are evolving. A procedural antifactor Xa level of 0.8 to 1.8 IU/mL is suggested, which corresponds to a Rapidpoint ENOX time of 250 to 450 seconds. SQ dosing must be adjusted in patients with renal insufficiency. For enoxaparin, SQ doses of 1 mg/kg SQ bid for patients with normal renal function, 0.75 mg/kg SQ bid for patients with a creatine clearance (CrCl) of 30 to 60 mL/min, and 1 mg/kg once a day for patients with a CrCl of less than 30 mL/min are suggested. Dosing during PCI in patients with renal insufficiency is unclear, but monitoring of antifactor to Xa activity would be useful. For obese patients, no dose cap for enoxaparin has been recommended, although some institutions have placed a cap for the very obese. Monitoring antifactor Xa activity may be reasonable in these patients, particularly if the patient weight is greater than 150 kg. The sheath may be removed 6 to 8 hours after the last dose; in some studies, the sheath has been safely removed 4 hours after the last dose. A Rapidpoint ENOX time of less than 200 to 250 seconds has been recommended for sheath removal.[13]

DIRECT THROMBIN INHIBITORS

[ ] MECHANISM OF ACTION

Thrombin has one active site and two exosites. The active, or catalytic, site possesses the serine protease activity where fibrinogen is cleaved. Exosite 1 is the binding site for fibrinogen.

Three IV DTIs are currently available. No oral DTIs are approved, although many are in development. Hirudin (desirudin) and bivalirudin are bivalent inhibitors, and argatroban is a univalent inhibitor. Bivalent inhibitors bind to both the active site and to exosite 1. Univalent inhibitors bind only to the active site. Bivalent inhibitors are more selective than univalent inhibitors. Because the active site of thrombin is structurally similar to that of other serine proteases, univalent inhibitors may bind to other serine proteases.

Hirudin is a 65–amino acid polypeptide originally isolated from the saliva of the medicinal leech *Hirudo medicinalis.* Lepirudin, the approved form of hirudin, is produced by recombinant DNA technology and differs by two amino acids and one sulfate group. It binds to thrombin with a nearly irreversible 1:1 complex. There is no antidote.

Bivalirudin is a synthetic 20–amino acid polypeptide and an analog of hirudin, which also binds to both the active site and exosite 1 of thrombin in a 1:1 complex. Thrombin cleaves the active site portion of the bivalirudin molecule, leaving only the portion that binds to exosite 1. This binding is weaker, and competition for the binding site occurs. Thus, the inhibition is short-lived. It is postulated that this confers a safety advantage of bivalirudin over hirudin.

Argatroban is a small, synthetic univalent inhibitor and an analog of arginine, which binds to the active site of thrombin in a 1:1 complex. It binds with moderately high affinity. There is little interaction with other serine proteases.

[ ] PHARMACOKINETICS

Because the majority of data using DTIs in the cardiac catheterization laboratory involve bivalirudin and to a much lesser extent argatroban, the pharmacology discussion is limited to these two agents.

Bivalirudin is effective immediately following IV injection. It exhibits a linear dose-response relationship when administered intravenously. Drug metabolism is 80% degradation by peptidases in the blood and 20% active drug elimination via the kidney. The half-life is approximately 25 minutes in patients with normal renal function, 34 minutes in patients with moderate renal impairment (glomerular filtration rate [GFR], 30-59 mL/min), 57 minutes in patients with severe renal impairment (GFR, 10-29 mL/min), and 210 min in dialysis-dependent patients. It can be monitored by the aPTT and ACT. The international normalized ratio also becomes prolonged during the infusion. The anticoagulant effect returns to baseline 1 to 2 hours after the infusion is discontinued. Large amounts of the drug can be cleared by hemofiltration using pores of a large size or plasmapheresis. There is no pharmacodynamic interaction between heparin and bivalirudin.

Argatroban is effective immediately after IV administration. The drug is metabolized hepatically, and the metabolized products are eliminated via biliary excretion. Dosing adjustments are necessary in patients with hepatic dysfunction but not in patients with renal dysfunction. The infusion is monitored by the aPTT and ACT. The half-life is 40 to 50 minutes. There is no antidote.

[ ] INDICATIONS

Bivalirudin is approved for use in patients with ACS undergoing PCI. The ACC/AHA guidelines state that results from the Randomized Evaluation of Percutaneous Coronary Intervention Linking Angiomax to Reduced Clinical Events 2 (REPLACE-2) trial "established that bivalirudin is not a replacement for standard therapy, but appears to be a good alternative." The 2004 ACCP guidelines recommend bivalirudin:

- For patients undergoing PCI who are not treated with heparin or a GP IIb/IIIa inhibitor (grade 1A).

- For patients undergoing PCI who are at a low risk of complications, as an alternative to heparin as an adjunct to GP IIb/IIIa inhibitors (grade 1B).

- For patients undergoing PCI who are at high risk of bleeding, in place of heparin as an adjunct to GP IIb/IIIa inhibitors (grade 1B).

Argatroban is approved for anticoagulation in patients with HIT as well as for patients with or at risk of HIT who are undergoing PCI. Data for use during PCI are limited due to small studies.

Lepirudin is approved for patients with HIT. There is no approved indication in PCI.

[ ] CLINICAL STUDIES

The REPLACE-2 study was a randomized, double-blind active-controlled trial conducted among 6010 patients undergoing urgent or elective PCI who received bivalirudin (0.75 mg/kg IV bolus, then 1.75 mg/kg/h for the duration of the PCI; additional 0.3 mg/kg IV bolus for ACT < 225 seconds) with provisional GP IIb/IIIa usage or heparin (65 U/kg bolus) with planned GP IIb/IIIa inhibition (abciximab or eptifibatide).[14] The primary end point was the quadruple end point of death, MI, urgent revascularization, or in-hospital major bleeding at 30 days. The secondary end point was the triple endpoint of death, MI, or urgent revascularization. Major bleeding was defined as intracranial, intraocular, or retroperitoneal hemorrhage; clinically overt blood loss resulting in a decrease in hemoglobin or more than 3 g/dL; any decrease in hemoglobin of more than 4 g/dL; or transfusion of two or more units of packed red blood cells or whole blood. Bleeding was also characterized according to TIMI criteria.

The objective of the REPACE-2 study was to show that bivalirudin with provisional GP IIb/IIIa inhibition was superior to heparin alone and not inferior to heparin plus GP IIb/IIIa inhibition. The authors believed that a heparin monotherapy arm was unethical and therefore used a complex indirect computation comparing the bivalirudin group to the heparin control groups of the Evaluation of Platelet Inhibitor for Stenting (EPISTENT) and Enhanced Suppression of the Platelet IIb/IIIa Receptor with Integrilin Therapy (ESPRIT) trials. No bivalirudin plus GP IIb/IIIa arm was included. Fifty-six percent of patients had stable angina or an abnormal stress test. Patients with acute MI or unstable ischemic syndromes requiring empiric GP IIb/IIIa inhibition were excluded. Patients were also excluded if they had been treated with UFH within 6 hours of the procedure unless the aPTT was less than or equal to 50 seconds, the ACT was less than or equal to 175 seconds, or if they had received LMWH within 8 hours. Eighty-five percent of patients received stents. More than 85% of patients received thienopyridine prior to the PCI. Only 7.2% of patients in the bivalirudin had provisional GP IIb/IIIa use, evenly divided between abciximab and eptifibatide. The primary end point was reached in 9.2% of patients in the bivalirudin group versus 10% of patients in the heparin plus GP IIb/IIIa group (OR 0.92; 95% CI 0.77–1.09; $P = .32$). The imputed odds ratio for bivalirudin versus heparin alone was 0.62 (95% CI 0.47-0.82). The secondary end point was achieved in 7.1% of patients in the heparin plus GP IIb/IIIa group and 7.6% of patients in the bivalirudin group (OR 1.09; 95% CI 0.90–1.32; $P = .40$). The imputed odds ratio for bivalirudin relative to heparin was 0.61 (95% CI 0.44–0.83).

The authors concluded that bivalirudin plus provisional GP IIb/IIIa inhibition was not inferior to heparin plus planned GP IIb/IIIa inhibition with respect to ischemic endpoints and was associated with less bleeding. There was a 0.8% absolute increase in the rate of MI in the bivalirudin group, predominantly secondary to non–Q-wave MIs with a creatine kinase, myocardial bound (CK-MB) of five to ten times the upper limit of normal. Although this was not statistically significant, this finding cannot be ignored, especially because the significance of postprocedural CK-MB elevation continues to be debated. There was a 41% relative reduction in the incidence of major bleeding in the bivalirudin group, as defined by the study protocol, largely due to decreases in vascular access site bleeding and gastrointestinal bleeding. There was no difference in intracranial bleeding. When using the TIMI criteria, there was no significant difference in major bleeding between the two study groups. Using both the study and TIMI criteria for minor bleeding, there were excess events in the heparin plus GP IIb/IIIa group.

Of note, the median ACT 5 minutes after study drug administration was 358 seconds in the bivalirudin group and 317 seconds in the heparin plus GP IIb/IIIa group. The ACT at the end of the interventional procedure was about 345 seconds in the bivalirudin group and 275 seconds in the heparin plus GP IIb/IIIa group. Although the ACT was higher in the bivalirudin group, the ACC/AHA target ACT for UFH in PCI is 300 to 350 seconds and 200 seconds for patients treated with heparin plus GP IIb/IIIa. The ACT was proportionally higher than recommended in the heparin plus GP IIb/IIIa group than in the bivalirudin group, and this may have skewed the bleeding results in favor of bivalirudin.

At 6 months, the death, MI, or any revascularization rate in REPLACE-2 was 18.3% in the bivalirudin group and 17% in the heparin plus GP IIb/IIIa group ($P = .21$).[15] For death, it was 0.95% versus 1.35%, respectively ($P = .148$), and for death, MI, or urgent revascularization it was 11.1% versus 10.2%, respectively ($P = .25$). At one year, the mortality was 1.89% in the bivalirudin group and 2.46% in the heparin + GP IIb/IIIa group.

An economic analysis of the REPLACE-2 trial suggested a savings of $375 to $400 per patient due to lower costs of the anticoagulants as well as lower rates of bleeding complications and thrombocytopenia requiring treatment.[16]

In a meta-analysis of three early randomized trials of bivalirudin (Bivalirudin Angioplasty Trial [BAT], Comparison of Abciximab Complications with Hirulog for Ischemic Events Trial [CACHET], and REPLACE-1) involving PCI, the benefit of bivalirudin for ischemic and bleeding complications increased as the degree of renal insufficiency worsened.[17] In the BAT study, 4312 patients were randomized to receive either heparin or bivalirudin. Both heparin and bivalirudin dosing was higher than the current standards. No stents or GP IIb/IIIa inhibitors were used. In the CACHET trial, 280 patients were randomized to heparin plus abciximab or one of two bivalirudin dosing regimens in a 1:1:1 manner. Twenty-four percent of patients taking bivalirudin received provisional GP IIb/IIIa inhibitors. Eighty-eight percent of patients received stents. In the REPLACE-1 trial, 1034 patients were randomized to heparin or bivalirudin. Seventy-two percent of patients taking heparin and 71% of patients taking bivalirudin received a GP IIb/IIIa inhibitor. Eighty-five percent received stents. Baseline creatinine levels were measured in 88%, 100%, 98% of the patients, respectively. Of the 5035 patients, 39 patients had normal renal function (CrCl > 90 mL/min), and 1578, 2163, 1255 had mild (60–89 mL/min), moderate (30–59 mL/min) or severe (30 mL/min) renal dysfunction, respectively. Bivalirudin usage was associated with a lower triple end point of death, MI, or urgent revascularization (OR 0.75; 95% CI 0.59-0.94; $P = .018$). The relative risk reduction was similar for each group. Bivalirudin usage was associated with lower major bleeding complications in patients with normal (OR 0.45; 95% CI 0.21-0.96), mild (OR 0.40; 95% CI 0.09-1.86), and moderate renal dysfunction (OR 0.46; 95% CI 0.30-0.70). No patient in the severe group who received bivalirudin had a major hemorrhage. The absolute reduction in the quadruple endpoint in the bivalirudin group occurred in 2.2%, 5.8%, 7.7%, and 14.4% of patients respectively ($P = .041$). Of note, few patients in this analysis had severe renal insufficiency, and no patients were undergoing dialysis.

The Acute Catheterization and Urgent Intervention Triage strategY (ACUITY) trial is currently underway.[18] In this trial, 13,800 patients with moderate-to high-risk ACS are being randomized to one of four regimens: UFH, enoxaparin plus GP IIb/IIIa inhibition, bivalirudin plus GP IIb/IIIa inhibition, and bivalirudin plus provisional GP IIb/IIIa inhibition. All patients are to undergo coronary angiography within 72 hours, with PCI or CABG if appropriate. Patients assigned to GP IIb/IIIa inhibitors will be further randomized to upstream initiation versus administration during PCI only. The primary end point is a quadruple end point of death, MI, unplanned revascularization for ischemia, or major bleed at 30 days. This study will hopefully answer questions regarding the optimal choice of antithrombotic agents or combination of agents as well as their timing for moderate-to-high risk ACS patients.

DOSING

For bivalirudin, the ACCP guidelines recommend the REPLACE-2 dosing regimen of 0.75 mg/kg IV bolus plus 1.75 mg/kg/h for the duration of the PCI. Additional 0.3 mg/kg IV boluses of bivalirudin can be administered for ACTs of less than 225 seconds. The infusion should be reduced by 20% in patients with moder-

ate renal impairment and by 60% in patients with severe renal impairment. The infusion should be reduced by 90% in patients on dialysis. For patients arriving to the catheterization laboratory on heparin with an ACT of greater than 175 seconds, the bivalirudin dosing has not been determined. The ACCP guidelines recommend bivalirudin as an adjunct to GP IIb/IIIa inhibitors in patients who are at high risk of bleeding. The upfront use of bivalirudin and GP IIb/IIIa inhibitors is being evaluated in the ACUITY study. Bivalirudin dosing has not been established for patients that have received LMWH within 8 hours of the planned procedure.

For patients with type II HIT undergoing PCI, argatroban can be used with a bolus of 350 mg/kg given intravenously over 3 to 5 minutes then an infusion of 25 µg/kg/min. An ACT should be checked in 5 to 10 minutes. If the ACT is less than 300 seconds, then a bolus of 150 mg/kg is given and the infusion is increased to 30 µg/kg/min; if the ACT is greater than 450 seconds, then the infusion rate is decreased to 15 µg/kg/min. Argatroban should be avoided in patients with hepatic insufficiency.

OTHER TOPICS

[ ] HEPARIN-INDUCED THROMBOCYTOPENIA

Heparin-induced thrombocytopenia (HIT) occurs in approximately 1% of patients treated with heparin for 3 days and in up to 5% to 10% in patients treated for 5 or more days. It can also occur in patients receiving LMWH, although it much less likely. HIT typically occurs 4 to 10 days after initiation of therapy. Delayed-onset HIT may occur, even up to 19 days after the discontinuation of the drug. Antibodies are usually nondetectable after a median of 50 to 85 days. If antibodies persist, HIT may occur at a median time of 10.5 hours after reinitiating therapy. If antibodies are no longer detectable, brief reexposure to UFH may be safe. However, due to the longer half-life and lack of antidote, LMWH should not be readministered.

Once HIT is suspected clinically, the diagnosis can be confirmed by a serotonin release assay (sensitivity 100%, specificity 97%), heparin-induced platelet aggregation assays (sensitivity 80%, specificity >90%), or the solid phase immunoassay (sensitivity 91%, low specificity). HIT is best minimized or prevented by limiting heparin to short-term use, using LMWH or DTIs. Treatment requires discontinuation of the offending agent, including heparin flushes, and DTI therapy to prevent thrombotic complications. Fondaparinux and danaparoid are not Food and Drug Administration–approved for treatment of HIT, but data suggest that these drugs are safe and effective. Argatroban is approved for use during PCI in patients with HIT. Bivalirudin is not approved for HIT, although there are data supporting its use.

[ ] CARDIAC SURGERY

Heparin has long been the gold standard for antithrombin therapy in patients undergoing open-heart surgery. In small studies, bivalirudin has been shown to be feasible without a clinical increase in blood loss compared to UFH.[19]

[ ] POINT-OF-CARE MONITORS

Two point-of-care monitors are routinely used for measurement of the ACT, the Hemochron and the HemoTec devices. The ACT measured by the HemoTec device is 30 to 50 seconds lower than the ACT measured by the Hemochron device. ACC/AHA and ACCP guidelines take this difference into account when suggesting target ACTs.

The Rapidpoint ENOX (Pharmanetics Inc., Morrisville, North Carolina) has recently become available for measuring the degree of anticoagulation with enoxaparin. A time range of 250 to 450 seconds corresponds to a suggested procedural antifactor Xa level of 0.8 to 1.8 IU/mL.

CONCLUSIONS

Options for antithrombin therapy during PCI, historically limited to UFH, have expanded and now include heparin, LMWHs, and DTIs. The indications for each agent continue to be refined as data from randomized trials become available. This growth has occurred simultaneously with advances in antiplatelet therapies such as thienopyridines and GP IIb/IIIa inhibitors. The role of each single agent or combination of agents, as well as the timing of administration of the agents, for the treatment of stable and ACS patients continues to evolve.

REFERENCES

1. Smith SC Jr, Feldman, TE, Hirshfeld JW Jr, et al. ACC/AHA/SCAI 2005 guideline update for percutaneous coronary intervention: a report of the American College of Cardiology/American Heart Association Task Force on Practice Guidelines (ACC/AHA/SCAI Writing Committee to Update the 2001 Guidelines for Percutaneous Coronary Intervention). Available at: http://www.acc.org/clinical/guidelines/percutaneous/update/index_rev.pdf.
2. Chew DP, Bhatt DL, Lincoff AM, et al. Defining the optimal activated clotting time during percutaneous coronary interventions: aggregate results from 6 randomized, controlled trials. *Circulation.* 2001;1013:961.
3. Popma JJ, Berger P, Ohman EM, et al. Antithrombotic therapy during percutaneous coronary intervention: the Seventh ACCP Conference of Antithrombotic and Thrombolytic Therapy. *Chest.* 2004;126:576S.
4. Braunwald E, Antman EM, Beasley JW, et al. ACC/AHA guideline update for the management of patients with unstable angina and non-ST-segment elevation myocardial infarction-2002: summary article. a report of the American College of Cardiology/American Heart Association Task Force of Practice Guidelines (Committee on the Management of Patients with Unstable Angina). *Circulation.* 2002;106:1893.
5. Kereiakes DJ, Grines C, Fry E, et al. Enoxaparin and abciximab adjunctive pharmacotherapy during percutaneous coronary intervention. *J Invasive Cardiol.* 2001;13:272.
6. Bhatt D, Lee B, Casterella P, et al. Safety of concomitant therapy with eptifibatide and enoxaparin in patients undergoing percutaneous coronary intervention: results of the coronary revascularization using Integrilin and single bolus enoxaparin study. *J Am Coll Cardiol.* 2003;41:20.
7. The SYNERGY Trial Investigators. Enoxaparin vs. unfractionated heparin in high risk patients with non-ST-segment elevation acute coronary syndromes managed with an intended early invasive strategy: primary results of the SYNERGY randomized trial. *JAMA.* 2004;292:45.
8. Goodman SG, Fitchett D, Armstrong PW, et al. Randomized evaluation of the safety and efficacy of enoxaparin versus unfractionated heparin in high-risk patients with non-ST-segment elevation acute coronary syndromes receiving the GP IIb/IIIa inhibitor eptifibatide. *Circulation.* 2003;107:238.
9. Collet JP, Montalescot G, Lison L, et al. Percutaneous coronary intervention after subcutaneous enoxaparin pretreatment in patients with unstable angina pectoris. *Circulation.* 2001;103:658.
10. Martin JL, Fry ETA, Sanderlink G-JCM, et al. Reliable anticoagulation with enoxaparin in patients undergoing percutaneous coronary intervention: the pharmacokinetics of enoxaparin in PCI (PEPCI) study. *Catheter Cardiovasc Interv.* 2004;61:163.
11. Bhatt DL, Lee BI, Casterella PJ, et al. Safety of concomitant therapy with eptifibatide and enoxaparin in patients undergoing percutaneous coronary intervention: results of the coronary revascularization using Integrilin and single bolus enoxaparin study. *J Am Coll Cardiol.* 2003;41:20-25.
12. Montalescot G. Presented at the European Society of Cardiology Hot Line Session. 2005.
13. Moliterno DJ, Hermiller JB, Kereiakes DJ, et al. A novel point-of-care enoxaparin monitor for use during percutaneous coronary intervention. results of the evaluating enoxaparin clotting times (ELECT) study. *J Am Coll Cardiol.* 2003;42:1132.
14. Lincoff AM, Bittl JA, Harrington RA, et al. Bivalirudin and Provisional GP IIb/IIIa Blockade Compared With Heparin and Planned GP IIb/IIIa Blockade During Percutaneous Coronary Intervention: REPLACE-2 Randomized Trial. *JAMA.* 2003;289:853.
15. Lincoff AM, Kleinman NS, Kereiakes DJ, et al. Long-term efficacy of bivalirudin and provisional GP IIb/IIIa blockade vs heparin and planned GP IIb/IIIa blockade during percutaneous coronary revascularization: REPLACE-2 randomized trial. *JAMA.* 2004;292:696.
16. Cohen DJ, Lincoff AM, Lavelle TA, et al. Economic evaluation of bivalirudin with provisional GP IIb/IIIa inhibition versus heparin with routine GP IIb/IIIa inhibition for percutaneous coronary intervention: results from the REPLACE-2 trial. *J Am Coll Cardiol.* 2004;44:1792.
17. Chew DP, Bhatt DL, Kimball W, et al. Bivalirudin provides increasing benefit with decreasing renal function: a meta-analysis of randomized trials. *Am J Cardiol.* 2003;92:919.
18. Stone GW, Bertrand M, Colombo A, et al. Acute catheterization and urgent intervention triage strategy (ACUITY) trial: study design and rationale. *Am Heart J.* 2004;148:764.
19. Merry AF, Raudkivi PJ, Middleton NG, et al. Bivalirudin vs. heparin and protamine in off-pump coronary artery bypass surgery. *Ann Thorac Surg.* 2004;77:925.

CHAPTER 20

Antiplatelet Therapies in Contemporary Percutaneous Coronary Intervention

David E. Kandzari, MD

The practice of clinical medicine has rapidly evolved into a new era characterized by dramatic advances in the understanding of disease biology through the identification of receptors, agonists, and antagonists that enable the development of therapies targeted against specific biologic processes. The continuing rigorous evaluation of the safety and efficacy of antithrombotic therapies in cardiovascular disease reflects this changing approach to the development of novel pharmacologic agents modeled after our evolving understanding of the pathophysiology, therapeutic applications, and clinical outcomes of patients with cardiovascular disease.

The recognition that thrombosis is fundamental to the process of arterial injury associated with both acute coronary syndromes (ACSs) and percutaneous coronary intervention (PCI) has inspired the development of novel therapies to inhibit platelet aggregation and thrombus formation. Accordingly, several recent advances have been made in the management of patients undergoing percutaneous coronary revascularization to improve early and late clinical outcomes. The research efforts leading to these improvements in care have focused on inhibition of molecular targets within the coagulation cascade coupled with early invasive treatment options. In particular, the role of the glycoprotein (GP) IIb/IIIa receptor as the final common pathway for platelet aggregation and the need for adjunctive thrombin inhibition have led to extensive clinical investigation to evaluate new therapies; these treatments are intended not simply to treat broad populations of patients with cardiovascular disease but rather to tailor or refine

treatments for individual patients based on clinical risk. Ongoing clinical trials seek to refine treatment strategies for patients relative to individual risk presentation, the availability of facilities for invasive procedures, and the timing of revascularization. The purpose of this review is to provide a pathophysiologic rationale for antiplatelet therapies and PCI, examine the results of recent trials, and present future directions for clinical investigation.

PATHOPHYSIOLOGY OF THROMBOSIS: INTERPLAY OF PLATELET-MEDIATED INFLAMMATION AND AGGREGATION

The pathogenesis of coronary arterial thrombosis is characterized by atherosclerotic plaque rupture, platelet activation and aggregation, and resultant thrombus formation.[1,2] Whether plaque rupture occurs spontaneously or instead is the result of mechanical balloon angioplasty, platelets first adhere to the subendothelium by binding to class I GPs. The presence of thrombin or other agonists such as adenosine or epinephrine activates platelets, precipitating a conformational change in the GP IIb/IIIa receptor and platelet degranulation. These changes cause the release of serotonin, adenosine diphosphate (ADP), and other vasoactive substances that stimulate further platelet activation and recruitment. The conformational change in the GP IIb/IIIa receptor also allows cross-binding of fibrinogen and von Willebrand factor with other

---

A list of the clinical trials cited in Chapters 19 through 24 is presented in Appendix IV-1 at the end of Part IV.

TABLE 20-1

Pharmacological Properties of Food and Drug Administration (FDA)–approved platelet Glycoprotein IIb/IIIa Inhibitors

	ABCIXIMAB	EPTIFIBATIDE	TIROFIBAN
Chemical nature	Antibody	Peptide	Nonpeptide
Size	Large (48 kDa)	Small (1 kDa)	Small (<1 kDa)
Onset of effect	Rapid	Rapid	Rapid
Reversibility	Slow	Rapid	Rapid
Binds other integrins?	Yes	No	No
Antibody response?	Yes	No	No

Adapted with permission from Kandzari DE, Califf RM.[97]

platelets, resulting in platelet aggregation and clot formation. The subsequent clinical outcome is determined by whether the thrombotic mass is occlusive, partially occlusive, or nonobstructive, and the outcome is influenced by collateral flow, baseline left ventricular function, amount of jeopardized myocardium, diabetes, and other factors. Although ACS manifests as a heterogeneous combination of clinical symptoms, electrocardiographic changes, and biochemical markers of myocardial injury, treatment remains directed at the common underlying event of platelet activation and thrombus formation. Similarly, intentional vascular injury from balloon angioplasty creates an ideal opportunity for platelet inhibition and subsequent avoidance of thrombotic vascular occlusion.

Recognition that the GP IIb/IIIa receptor serves as the common denominator for mediating platelet aggregation made its inhibition a pivotal transition from bench work to clinical practice.[3–5] Aside from separate investigations with oral antiplatelet agents, including aspirin, dipyridamole, and thienopyridines, Coller and coworkers first reported in 1983 the production of a murine monoclonal antibody that irreversibly blocked the GP IIb/IIIa receptor.[6] These findings led to the engineering of a chimeric monoclonal antibody, abciximab (ReoPro), which was first studied in patients undergoing high-risk PCI (Table 20-1). Since then, several other inhibitors that mimic the arginine-glycine-aspartic acid binding sequences of the GP IIb/IIIa receptor have undergone extensive clinical investigation. These include the synthetic cyclic heptapeptide eptifibatide (Integrilin) as well as peptidomimetics such as tirofiban (Aggrastat) (see Table 20-1). Despite differences in pharmacodynamics and pharmacokinetics, the common mechanism of these drugs is to inhibit platelet aggregation by occupying the fibrinogen binding site.

In addition to new insights to the development of platelet inhibition, recent discoveries have also identified the contribution of platelets to systemic inflammation as a manifestation of thrombosis. Antiplatelet therapies that block platelet aggregation either through the GP IIb/IIIa or ADP receptor pathways may therefore also inhibit platelet-mediated inflammation. Aside from observations underlying the systemic nature of ACS that have identified multiple coronary plaque ruptures in patients with unstable coronary syndromes,[7,8] markers of platelet- and neutrophil-mediated inflam-

mation have been detected in blood, including soluble CD40 ligand (CD40L),[9,10] myeloperoxidase,[11] high-sensitivity C-reactive protein (CRP),[12] and interleukins.[13] Not only do platelet-mediated inflammatory markers such as CD40L reliably predict the future occurrence of adverse outcomes,[9,10] but they may also directly mediate the development of thrombosis, atherosclerosis, and restenosis following angioplasty.[10,14–16] A recent discovery, for example, found that platelet-derived CD40L was capable of binding to the GP IIb/IIIa receptor, thereby promoting thrombus formation and clot stabilization.[14] In a substudy of patients with non-ST-elevation (NSTE) and ACS in the Chimeric 7E3 Antiplatelet Therapy in Unstable Refractory Angina (CAPTURE) trial, escalating plasma levels of CD40L were independently predictive of death and myocardial infarction (MI) at both 30 days and 6 months (Figure 20-1).[9]

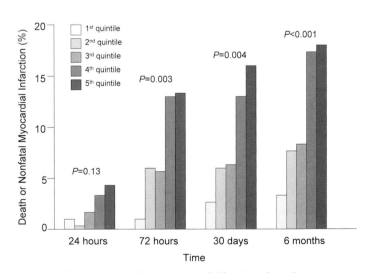

FIGURE 20-1. Relationship between soluble CD40 ligand concentration and the rate of adverse cardiac events among 544 patients with ACS receiving placebo in the CAPTURE trial. The patients were divided into quintiles according to the serum level of soluble CD40 ligand: first quintile, below; second quintile, 1.93 to 3.50 μg/L; third quintile, 3.51 to 5.00 μg/L; fourth quintile, 5.01 to 6.30 μg/L; and fifth quintile, above 6.30 μg/L. P values are for trend at each time point. (Modified with permission from Heeschen C, Dimmeler S, Hamm CW, et al.[9])

However, among patients with the highest levels of CD40L, treatment with the GP IIb/IIIa antagonist abciximab was associated with a risk reduction similar to those individuals having the lowest CD40L concentrations. Treatment with the thienopyridine clopidogrel also appears to attenuate elevations in CRP and platelet-derived soluble CD40L expression among patients undergoing PCI.[17,18]

INTRAVENOUS GLYCOPROTEIN IIB/IIIA INHIBITION IN PERCUTANEOUS CORONARY INTERVENTION

In the past decade, remarkable advances in both interventional drugs and devices have improved outcomes significantly for patients undergoing percutaneous coronary revascularization. Combined with both oral and intravenous antiplatelet therapy, stenting has reduced the incidence of abrupt vessel closure to less than 0.5% and the need for repeat revascularization by 30% to 50%.[19–21] In addition, several randomized trials have shown that GP IIb/IIIa inhibition during elective PCI reduces the composite incidence of death, nonfatal MI, or target vessel revascularization (TVR) at both 30 days and 6 months.[22,23] The synergy between PCI and GP IIb/IIIa blockade is especially prominent in patients with ACS without ST-segment elevation, although similar clinical benefit has been observed for patients with acute ST-elevation MI. Overall, investigations examining GP IIb/IIIa antagonists as adjunctive therapy to PCI in thousands of patients undergoing PCI in an array of clinical settings have shown markedly improved outcomes with a variety of GP IIb/IIIa inhibitors. In meta-analysis of more than 20,000 patients enrolled in randomized trials, two independent studies have reaffirmed the efficacy of these agents in PCI, demonstrating an approximate 25% reduction in 30-day mortality among those receiving treatment with GP IIb/IIIa inhibition (Figure 20-2).[24,25]

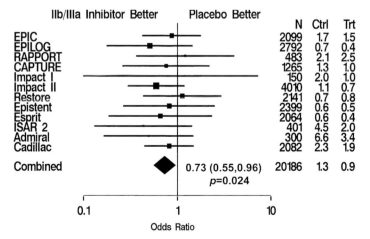

FIGURE 20-2. Odds ratios of 30-day survival in randomized trials evaluating glycoprotein (GP) IIb/IIIa antagonists in PCI. In meta-analysis, treatment with GP IIb/IIIa inhibitors is associated with a 27% reduction in 30-day mortality (P = .024). Ctrl indicates control group; trt, treatment group. (Modified with permission from Kong DF, Hasselblad V, Harrington RA, et al.[25])

[ ] GLYCOPROTEIN IIB/IIIA INHIBITION IN PERCUTANEOUS CORONARY INTERVENTION AND NON-ST-ELEVATION ACUTE CORONARY SYNDROME

The routine application of GP IIb/IIIa inhibitors as adjunctive therapy to elective and high-risk PCI has been modeled after an initial series of large, randomized, placebo-controlled trials: Evaluation of c7E3 for the Prevention of Ischemic Complications (EPIC),[26] Evaluation in Percutaneous Transluminal Coronary Angioplasty to Improve Long-term Outcome with Abciximab GP IIb/IIIa Blockade (EPILOG),[27] CAPTURE,[28] Integrilin to Minimize Platelet Aggregation and Coronary Thrombosis (IMPACT-II),[29] and Randomized Efficacy Study of Tirofiban for Outcomes and REstenosis (RESTORE).[30] Despite differences between the agents examined in these trials, they have consistently demonstrated reductions in early ischemic adverse events in addition to significant reductions in long-term morbidity and mortality. Furthermore, the addition of GP IIb/IIIa antagonists to coronary stenting is supported by the significant reduction in 30-day death, MI, or urgent revascularization observed in the Evaluation of IIb/IIIa Platelet Inhibitor for Stenting (EPISTENT) trial (5.3% in the stent-plus-abciximab group vs 10.8% in the stent-only group, P < .001).[31] A systematic overview of these trials has shown a highly significant reduction in the end point of death, nonfatal MI, or urgent revascularization at 48 to 96 hours (P < .001), 30 days (P < .001), and 6 months (P < .003).[25]

The more recent Enhanced Suppression of the Platelet IIb/IIIa Receptor with Integrilin Therapy (ESPRIT) trial not only confirmed that treatment with a GP IIb/IIIa inhibitor before stenting was the superior approach but also demonstrated improved outcomes among low-risk patients treated with more modern stenting techniques, thereby broadening the applicability of the therapy to nearly all patients undergoing PCI.[32] In the ESPRIT trial, the control arm was "rescue" or "bailout" GP IIb/IIIa inhibitor therapy. Among 2064 patients undergoing elective angioplasty with stenting, treatment with double-bolus eptifibatide was associated with a 37% relative reduction in the rate of the composite of death, MI, urgent revascularization, or "bailout" GP IIb/IIIa inhibitor therapy at 48 hours (P = .0015). The benefit of preprocedural eptifibatide administration was consistent across all components of the primary end point and was maintained at 30-day and 6-month follow-up.[32,33] At 1 year, the eptifibatide group showed continued benefit, with a significantly lower rate of death or MI (8.0% vs 12.4% with placebo, P = .001).[34]

A significant benefit of GP IIb/IIIa inhibition in PCI reflects a reduction in periprocedural MI, yet the long-term avoidance of adverse events cannot be attributed to the decrease in procedural ischemic complications alone. Although elevated cardiac enzymes clearly reflect myocardial injury and necrosis, the clinical significance of periprocedural myocardial necrosis has been debated. Depending on the clinical setting, up to 40% of patients develop periprocedural myocardial necrosis with elevation of creatine kinase myocardial band.[35] Although most of these events can be identified by angiography, a substantial number of "angiographically silent" events occur at the cellular level of myocardial perfusion. Despite epicardial vessel patency, disrupted microvascular function and inadequate myocardial perfusion often result from thromboembolic debris. New angiographic techniques, including the Thrombolysis in Myocardial Infarction (TIMI) myocardial blush score, and noninvasive diagnostic tests (eg, continuous ST-segment monitoring) have confirmed that epicardial TIMI grade 3 flow is an incomplete measure of reperfusion success and long-term outcome.[36] Studies evaluating balloon occlusion and filter devices to prevent distal embolization during high-risk PCI have been inconsistent and may depend on the extent of thrombus burden, lesion morphology, and clinical presentation (eg, acute MI vs elective PCI).[37,38] To date, these devices have not been systematically compared with GP IIb/IIIa inhibition, yet recent studies suggest that this latter therapy may be effective in improving myocardial perfusion and microvascular integrity.[39,40]

Despite the avoidance of early and late ischemic events, the inability of GP IIb/IIIa inhibition to influence restenosis appears more certain. By 6 months after initial PCI, restenosis accounts for the majority of repeat procedures, and clinical events accrue equally after 6 months independent of earlier GP IIb/IIIa inhibition, and the relative difference between groups diminishes.[41-43] Instead, greater uncertainty exists about the selection of a particular adjunctive GP IIb/IIIa inhibitor in PCI, and additional comparative studies are needed. In the only comparative trial of GP IIb/IIIa inhibition in PCI to date, the Do Tirofiban And ReoPro Give similar Efficacy outcomes? (TARGET) study showed a significant 26% reduction in the composite of death, MI, or urgent revascularization at 30 days with abciximab compared with tirofiban (6.01% vs 7.55%, $P = .038$).[44] Although this difference merits further exploration, one potential explanation is inadequate platelet inhibition with the tirofiban regimen used. Alternative dosing regimens that more effectively achieve platelet inhibition have been proposed and need to be evaluated,[45] and a randomized trial comparing revised tirofiban dosing with abciximab is forthcoming.

Other existing challenges to the use of intravenous GP IIb/IIIa inhibitors include recent trials suggesting the potential for equivalent outcomes with either novel antithrombin agents or pretreatment with high-dose thienopyridines in selected PCI patients with lower presenting clinical risk. (The Intracoronary Stenting and Antithrombotic Regimen-Rapid Early Action for Coronary Treatment [ISAR-REACT] trial is described below.) Results from the REPLACE-2 trial, comparing unfractionated heparin plus mandatory GP IIb/IIIa inhibition with bivalirudin plus provisional GP IIb/IIIa inhibitors in PCI, indicate that the latter treatment strategy may have similar efficacy yet results in less bleeding complications.[46] At 30 days, the occurrence of the composite end point did not differ between groups, but use of bivalirudin resulted in significantly less bleeding (4.2% vs 2.4%, $P < .001$). In higher risk populations, however, the recent ISAR REACT 2 trial has provided some insight for ACS patients who are treated with oral antiplatelet therapy alone. In this study, 2022 patients with NSTE ACS undergoing PCI were treated with 600 mg of clopidogrel and aspirin followed by randomization to treatment with either abciximab or placebo against the background of unfractionated heparin therapy. The primary endpoint was a clinical composite of death, MI, and ischemia-driven target vessel revascularization at 30 days postprocedure. Treatment with abciximab was associated with a significant reduction in both the primary endpoint (11.9% vs 8.9%, $P = .03$) in addition to a reduction in 30-day death or MI

(11.5% vs 8.6%, $P < .05$). This clinical benefit associated with abciximab was particularly apparent among patients with elevated troponin levels ($n = 1049$; 8.3% placebo versus 13.1% abciximab, $P = .02$ for death, MI, ischemic-driven urgent revascularization) compared with troponin-negative patients ($n = 973$; 4.6% vs 4.6%, $P = .98$). The occurrences of major and minor bleeding did not statistically vary between treatment groups. Thus, among higher risk NSTE ACS patients undergoing PCI who are treated with aspirin, clopidogrel (600 mg), and unfractionated heparin, the adjunctive use of abciximab is associated with a significant improvement in early clinical outcome.

【 】 "UPSTREAM" GLYCOPROTEIN IIB/IIIA INHIBITION AND EARLY INVASIVE TREATMENT STRATEGIES FOR NON-ST-ELEVATION ACUTE CORONARY SYNDROMES

Because many patients do not undergo PCI (the median time to PCI still approximates one day[47]) and most MIs do not occur in the periprocedural setting,[48] early administration of effective antithrombotic therapy for all high-risk patients with ACS and NSTE is essential prior to angiographic confirmation of coronary disease. Recently, large randomized trials have shown the efficacy of GP IIb/IIIa inhibition in broader populations of patients with ACS and NSTE to support practice guidelines recommending treatment in patients with high-risk features that include elevated biomarkers, ST-segment deviation, and those in whom an invasive strategy is planned.[49] Whether the mechanism of benefit with early GP IIb/IIIa inhibition is passivation of an unstable plaque, improved microvascular function, or greater epicardial patency, recent trials of early GP IIb/IIIa inhibition followed by PCI have fueled enthusiasm for this complementary approach.

In the Treat angina with Aggrastat and Determine Cost of Therapy with an Invasive or Conservative Strategy-Thrombolysis in Myocardial Infarction (TACTICS-TIMI 18) study, upfront administration of tirofiban coupled with an early invasive strategy resulted in lower rates of death and MI (4.7% with early invasive strategy vs 7.0% with conservative management at 30 days, $P = .02$).[47] The highest-risk patients (eg, troponin-positive, ST-segment depression) derived the greatest benefit from the early invasive strategy combined with GP IIb/IIIa inhibition. Similarly, all 410 high-risk patients with NSTE and ACS enrolled in the Intracoronary Stenting and Antithrombotic Regimen—Evaluation of Prolonged Antithrombotic Pretreatment ("Cooling-Off" Strategy) Before Intervention in Patients With Unstable Coronary Syndromes (ISAR-COOL) were randomized to early versus delayed intervention (median time to catheterization, 2.4 vs 86.0 hours) following treatment with aspirin, clopidogrel (600 mg loading dose), unfractionated heparin, and tirofiban.[50] At 30 days, an early invasive strategy following initial antithrombotic therapy was associated with a significant reduction in the occurrence of death or MI (11.6% vs 5.9%, $P = .04$), a difference largely attributable to the reduction is ischemic events prior to cardiac catheterization. An important limitation of both studies, however, is that all patients received tirofiban, precluding comparisons to early revascularization without GP IIb/IIIa inhibition. However, in a systematic overview of 6766 patients randomized to routine invasive vs conservative therapy, an invasive approach-in combination with use of GP IIb/IIIa antagonists and coronary stenting-was associated with significant and sustained reductions in death or MI at 30 days (RR, 0.61; 95% CI 0.45-0.84) and 1 year (RR 0.78; 95% CI 0.65-0.92).[51]

Although recent trials have associated an early invasive strategy with reductions in death and MI, analysis of GP IIb/IIIa inhibition in ACS trials suggests that the benefit of an invasive strategy is not strictly due to PCI alone. Though a more modest benefit than observed in PCI, early or "upstream" treatment with GP IIb/IIIa inhibitors before arrival in the catheterization laboratory may improve early outcomes for higher risk patients (eg, troponin-positive) irrespective of revascularization.[52] In an observational study from the National Registry of Myocardial Infarction-4 (NRMI-4) that included 60,770 patients with NSTE MI, the early use of GP IIb/IIIa inhibitors was associated with a highly significant reduction in in-hospital mortality (9.6% vs 3.3%, $P < .0001$), a clinical benefit that persisted even after excluding patients who underwent PCI (Figure 20-3). More recently however, a randomized trial comparing bivalirudin with standard therapies has demonstrated a similar clinical outcome. In the Acute Catheterization and Urgent Intervention Thrombotic Strategy (ACUITY) trial, 13,800 patients with moderate-high risk ACS were randomized to treatment with bivalirudin, bivalirudin and a GP IIb/IIIa inhibitor, or heparin (unfractionated or LMWH) and GP IIb/IIIa inhibition.[52a] Patients assigned to treatment with a GP IIb/IIIa inhibitor (with bivalirudin or heparin) underwent a second randomization to receive the GP IIb/IIIa inhibitor either at randomization or during PCI. The primary endpoint was the 30-day composite of all-cause death, myocardial infarction, ischemia-driven revascularization, and major bleeding. Comparing patients treated with bivalirudin and GP IIb/IIIa blockade versus heparin and GP IIb/IIIa inhibition, there were no significant differences in either ischemic or bleeding events. Similarly, 30-day ischemic events did not differ among patients treated with bivalirudin versus those receiving heparin and a GP IIb/IIIa inhibitor (7.3% heparin and GP IIb/IIIa inhibition vs 7.8% bivalirudin and GP IIb/IIIa inhi-

bition, $P = .011$ for noninferiority, $P = .32$ for superiority). However, major bleeding was significantly lower among patients treated with bivalirudin (5.7% vs 3.0%, $P < .0001$ for both noninferiority and superiority). In subgroup analysis, although there were no differences in net clinical outcome between bivalirudin and heparin/ GP IIb/IIIa inhibition relative to troponin positivity, early treatment with a thienopyridine prior to PCI was associated with a significant reduction in the primary endpoint among patients receiving bivalirudin. Thus, in moderate to high-risk NSTE ACS patients, treatment with bivalirudin may be an acceptable substitute for heparin and GP IIb/IIIa inhibition with similar efficacy and a significant reduction in bleeding events. These results will require further consideration against the background of recent trials examining alternative antithrombin agents and early treatment with intravenous GP IIb/IIIa antagonists. To further clarify the safety and efficacy of GP IIb/IIIa inhibition in the early management of high-risk patients, the ongoing EARLY ACS trial is a large, prospective, randomized study designed to verify the benefit of upfront treatment with eptifibatide for high-risk NSTE ACS patients.

[ ] GLYCOPROTEIN IIB/IIIA INHIBITION AND PERCUTANEOUS CORONARY INTERVENTION IN ST-ELEVATION MYOCARDIAL INFARCTION

Recent trials have established evidence supporting GP IIb/IIIa blockade as adjunctive therapy for primary PCI in acute ST-segment elevation MI. Addition of GP IIb/IIIa inhibition to PCI for ST-elevation MI has substantially lowered the incidence of recurrent ischemic events and improved early survival, ventricular function, and vessel patency.

Observations from early studies evaluating the use of GP IIb/IIIa inhibitors prior to primary PCI yielded TIMI grade 3 flow rates that exceeded previously reported rates of reperfusion with aspirin and heparin and were comparable to full-dose streptokinase.[53] Based on the clinical observation that abciximab exhibited intrinsic anticoagulant and clot-dissolving activity,[54,55] the GRAPE

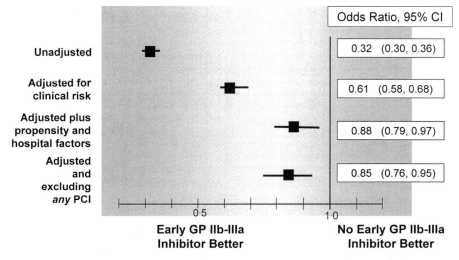

FIGURE 20-3. Odds ratios for in-hospital survival relative to early glycoprotein (GP) IIb/IIIa inhibitor use in the National Registry of Myocardial Infarction-4. PCI = percutaneous coronary intervention. *(Data from Peterson ED, Pollack CV, Roe MT, et al.[52])*

investigators showed that rates of TIMI grade 2/3 flow occurred in approximately 40% patients treated with abciximab prior to angioplasty.[56] More recently, nearly one third of patients randomized to abciximab alone in the TIMI 14 (32%) and Strategies for Patency Enhancement in the Emergency Department (SPEED) (27%) trials experienced grade TIMI 3 flow at 90 minutes.[57,58] Although treatment with GP IIb/IIIa inhibitors alone is not ideally suited to achieve early reperfusion, such observations reaffirm the potential of abciximab to restore infarct-artery patency prior to mechanical revascularization.

Aside from epicardial artery patency, pivotal trials demonstrating improved clinical outcomes with abciximab in unstable angina patients undergoing PCI also lead to studies extending the role of GP IIb/IIIa inhibitors in percutaneous revascularization for acute MI. Among the 893 patients in the EPIC trial[26] with evolving MI or unstable angina, abciximab was associated with an approximate 30% reduction in death, nonfatal MI, or recurrent ischemic complications at 30 days (7.0% vs 12.8%, 95% CI 0.5-1.1). For the 64 patients with MI undergoing primary or rescue angioplasty,[59] treatment with abciximab resulted in an 83% reduction in 30-day death, reinfarction, or urgent revascularization (26.1% vs 4.5%, $P = .06$). Similarly, in the ReoPro And Primary Percutaneous Transluminal Coronary Angioplasty Organization and Randomized Trial (RAPPORT) study, patients with acute infarction given abciximab in the catheterization laboratory before primary angioplasty experienced significant reductions in 30-day and 6-month death, reinfarction, or urgent revascularization (5.6% vs 11.2% at 30 days, $P = .03$).[60]

In the ISAR-2 trial,[41] 401 AMI patients within 48 hours of symptom onset for whom rescue or primary PCI was planned were randomized to abciximab bolus plus infusion or control (Table 20-2). Abciximab as an adjunct to coronary stenting improved 30-day clinical outcomes (5.0% vs 10.5%, $P = .038$) for the composite of death, reinfarction, or target lesion revascularization). At one year, although the absolute reduction in the composite end point was maintained with abciximab therapy, this early benefit no longer remained statistically significant, largely due to the accrual of restenotic events and the need for repeat revascularization.

More recently, the Abciximab Before Direct Angioplasty and Stenting in Myocardial Infarction Regarding Acute and Long-term Follow-up (ADMIRAL) study demonstrated that abciximab improved early and late TIMI 3 flow (post-PCI TIMI 3 flow, 95.1% for abciximab vs 86.7% for placebo, $P = .04$), was associated with higher left ventricular ejection fraction (57.0 + /−10.4% vs 53.9 + /−10.4%, $P < .05$), and more than halved the primary composite end point of death, recurrent MI, and urgent TVR at 30 days after enrollment (14.6% vs 6.0%, $P = .01$).[61] In the ADMIRAL trial, nearly one fourth of patients received early treatment with abciximab in the emergency department or even the ambulance (see Table 20-2). Consonant with prior studies showing improved epicardial TIMI flow with early abciximab, a significantly greater proportion of abciximab-treated patients had a patent infarct vessel (TIMI grade 2 or 3 flow) at baseline compared with those receiving placebo (25.8% vs 10.8%, $P = .006$). In contrast, initial TIMI 3 flow was present in 17.6% of patients receiving placebo in the ambulance compared with 6.8% of patients elsewhere (P = not significant).

In the Controlled Abciximab and Device Investigation to Lower Late Angioplasty Complications (CADILLAC) trial,[62] 2082 patients with acute ST-segment elevation MI were randomized to one of four treatment strategies: (1) balloon angioplasty alone, (2) balloon angioplasty plus abciximab, (3) stenting alone, or (4) stenting plus abciximab (see Table 20-2). Unlike the "upfront" treatment in the ADMIRAL trial, abciximab was administered only in the catheterization laboratory to patients in CADILLAC following the diagnostic angiogram. Among individual treatment groups, event-free survival was greatest in patients assigned to routine stenting (with or without abciximab), intermediate in patients assigned to percutaneous transluminal coronary angioplasty (PTCA) plus abciximab and lowest in those assigned to PTCA only (stent plus abciximab, 10.0%; stent alone, 10.9%; PTCA plus abciximab, 16.4%; PTCA only, 19.4%; $P = .0001$). In a combined analysis based on randomization to abciximab or no abciximab, although patients receiving abciximab tended to have higher baseline infarct-related artery TIMI 3 flow rates, treatment with abciximab was associated with significantly higher postprocedural flow rates and a significant reduction in the composite end point of death, recurrent MI, disabling stroke, and ischemic target vessel revascularization.[63] At 30 days, subacute thrombosis and length of hospital stay were also significantly decreased. By 6 months, however, restenosis was the predominant clinical event, and event-free survival rates converged, consistent with previous studies demonstrating the lack of influence by abciximab (or any GP IIb/IIIa inhibitor) on angiographic restenosis.[41,42] Thus, although the absolute benefit of abciximab therapy was maintained at 1 year, it remained no longer statistically significant.

In the most recent AMI trial evaluating the safety and efficacy of GP IIb/IIIa antagonists, the ACE study randomized 400 patients undergoing primary PCI with stenting to either abciximab or control therapy (see Table 20-2).[64] Crossover to abciximab occurred in 11% of patients assigned to the control group. At one month, abciximab treatment was associated with a significant reduction in the primary end point of death, MI, TVR, and stroke (4.5% vs 10.5%, $P = .023$). Early ST-segment resolution ($\geq$ 50% resolution at 30 minutes) was also achieved more commonly with abciximab (68% with stenting alone vs 85% with abciximab and stenting, $P < .001$). Although the occurrence of restenosis and TVR at 6 months was not significantly different between the treatment groups, patients randomized to abciximab therapy experienced sustained benefit with regard to the reduction in death and MI (5.5% vs 13.5% at 6 months, $P = .006$).

Considering the differences in trial design and study population, it is difficult to reconcile the somewhat divergent results regarding the relative impact of GP IIb/IIIa inhibition on mortality and ventricular function among the ADMIRAL, ACE, and CADILLAC trials. The apparently greater risk reduction of clinical events observed with abciximab in the ADMIRAL and ACE trials may be due to differences in patient selection, the stent used, the lack of abciximab crossover in ADMIRAL, differing end point definitions, or timing of abciximab administration. Collectively, however, trials evaluating GP IIb/IIIa inhibition as adjunctive therapy to primary angioplasty show benefits consistent with the abciximab versus no abciximab analysis of the CADILLAC results-reductions in early ischemic adverse events that are maintained but

TABLE 20-2

Selected Randomized Trials of Abciximab in Primary Percutaneous Coronary Intervention

STUDY	n	YEAR	ABCIXIMAB DOSE AND TIMING OF ADMINISTRATION	HEPARIN	STENT	THIENOPYRIDINE POST-PCI	PRIMARY END POINT
RAPPORT	483	1997	250 µg/kg bolus, 125 µg/kg/min infusion for 12 h, prior to diagnostic angiography	B to ACT > 300 s, I for 48 h	No	No	6-month D/reMI/TVR
ISAR-2	401	2000	250 µg/kg bolus, 10 µg/min infusion for 12 h, after diagnostic angiography	With abciximab: B 7500 U, control: B 15,000 U, I for 12 h	Yes	Yes	6-month angiographic late lumen loss
ADMIRAL	300	2002	250 µg/kg bolus, 125 µg/kg/min infusion for 12 h, prior to diagnostic angiography	B to ACT > 200 s, I for 24 h	Yes	Yes	30-day D/reMI/TVR
CADILLAC	2082	2002	250 µg/kg bolus, 125 µg/kg/min infusion for 12 h, after diagnostic angiography	With abciximab: B to ACT 200–300 s, no abciximab: B to ACT ≥ 350 s	Randomization to stent or PTCA	YES	6-month D/reMI/TVR disabling stroke

ACT = activated clotting time; B = bolus; I = infusion; D = death; PCI = Percutaneous coronary intervention; reMI = recurrent myocardial infarction; TVR = target vessel revascularization.

no longer statistically significant during longer term follow-up. In a recent systematic overview of four trials examining treatment with abciximab for primary PCI (ADMIRAL, CADILLAC, ISAR-2, and RAPPORT), treatment with abciximab significantly reduced the 30-day composite end point of death, reinfarction, or ischemic or urgent TVR (n = 3266; OR 0.54, 95% CI 0.40-0.72), with trends toward reduced 30-day death and death or reinfarction (Figure 20-4).[65] However, abciximab resulted in an increased likelihood of major bleeding (OR 1.74, 95% CI 1.11-2.72), although differences were not observed among more recent individual trials (ADMIRAL, CADILLAC) with more cautious heparin dosing. By 6 months, abciximab significantly reduced the occurrence of death, reinfarction, or any TVR (OR 0.80, 95% CI 0.67-0.97), and there were positive trends favoring a decrease in mortality alone and the composite of death or reinfarction (see Figure 20-4). Further, in another systematic overview of trials evaluating treatment with abciximab in ST-elevation myocardial infarction, treatment with GP IIb/IIIa inhibition was associated with significant reductions in 30-day death and recurrent infarction, but abciximab was not associated with benefit as adjunctive therapy to fibrinolysis.[65a]

【 】FACILITATED PERCUTANEOUS CORONARY INTERVENTION: COMBINATION FIBRINOLYSIS AND GLYCOPROTEIN IIB/IIIA INHIBITION

Facilitated PCI, or the strategy of planned early PCI after pharmacologic reperfusion therapy, is intended to combine the reperfusion benefits of fibrinolysis and primary angioplasty in the management of ST-elevation MI. On one hand, fibrinolysis can result in TIMI grade 3 flow as early as 60 minutes after administration. On the other hand, primary angioplasty achieves higher rates of normal epicardial artery blood flow but generally at later times. As a combined approach, facilitated PCI may provide the best outcomes based on TIMI flow and clinical events.

The rationale for facilitated PCI is derived from observations of the clinical benefit associated with a patent infarct artery prior to the performance of catheter-based revascularization. As described previously in the ADMIRAL trial, nearly one fourth of patients received early administration of abciximab in either the emergency room or the ambulance.[61] Baseline TIMI grade 3 flow was

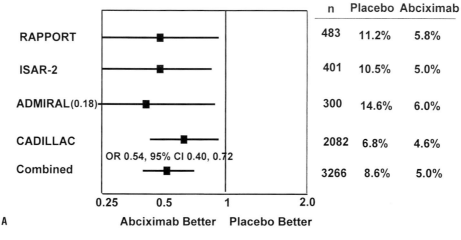

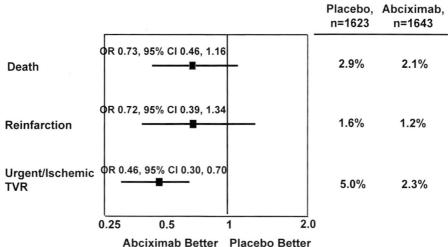

FIGURE 20-4. Odds ratios and 95% confidence intervals for 30-day risk of death, recurrent myocardial infarction, or urgent or ischemia-driven target vessel revascularization (**A**) and individual elements of composite end point (**B**) in trials evaluating the efficacy of abciximab in primary percutaneous coronary intervention. TVR = target vessel revascularization. *(Adapted with permission from Kandzari DE, Hasselblad V, Tcheng JE, et al.[65])*

significantly more common among patients receiving abciximab both immediately before and after revascularization, a finding consonant with prior studies showing a 25% to 35% rate of TIMI grade 3 flow with abciximab when given 60 to 90 minutes before angiography.[57,66] Although some of the marked benefit in the early-treatment group in ADMIRAL may be due to chance alone, resulting in an inexplicably high rate of adverse events in the placebo-treated patients, these data support ongoing trials of pharmacologic reperfusion before mechanical revascularization. These data are also consistent with the following:

1. A previous report from 2507 patients in the Primary Angioplasty in Myocardial Infarction (PAMI) trials, in which early and late mortality were strikingly reduced for patients with spontaneously recovery of TIMI 3 flow before the procedure, independent of the final TIMI flow grade (Figure 20-5).[67]

2. The randomized Primary Angioplasty Compatibility Trial (PACT) trial, in which early reperfusion with reduced dose alteplase resulted in greater early recovery of left ventricular function.[68]

3. A meta-analysis showing that mortality is reduced when thrombolytic therapy is started before arrival at the hospital rather than in the emergency room.[69]

The Global Use of Streptokinase and Tissue Plasminogen Activator for Occluded Arteries (GUSTO IV) SPEED investigators described the outcomes of 323 patients who underwent PCI approximately 1 hour after reperfusion therapy and compared them with a similar cohort who did not undergo early revascularization.[66] For the facilitated-therapy group, procedural success was 88%, and the 30-day composite end point of death, reinfarction, and urgent TVR occurred in 5.6% of patients (see Figure 20-5). Although these findings are more descriptive than comparative, they were encouraging, because earlier trials consistently showed lower immediate procedural success rates, higher mortality, and higher rates of reinfarction, bypass surgery, and bleeding than with a conservative approach. In contrast, the more recent ASSENT-4 PCI trial was halted prematurely following enrollment of 1667 patients based upon higher 30-day mortality among patients randomized to full-dose tPA-TNK and facilitated PCI compared with primary PCI alone (6.0% vs 3.8%, $P = .04$).[66a] By 90 days, the primary composite endpoint of death, heart failure, or cardiogenic shock was also significantly higher in the fibrinolytic PCI group (18.8% vs 13.7%, $P = .0055$), although the individual endpoints did not statistically vary. While a relatively shorter transit time may be one potential explanation for the absence of benefit with this strategy, still more trials are underway, including the FINESSE trial (abciximab/reteplase followed by early PCI).

[ ] GLYCOPROTEIN IIB/IIIA INHIBITOR DOSING AND MONITORING PLATELET INHIBITION IN PERCUTANEOUS CORONARY INTERVENTION

Despite the recent attention to the relationship between the pharmacodynamics of GP IIb/IIIa inhibition and clinical outcomes, the most effective intensity of platelet inhibition remains unknown. In the GOLD trial evaluating the intensity of platelet inhibition with GP IIb/IIIa therapy in patients undergoing PCI, less than 70% platelet inhibition after steady-state drug infusion was associated with a higher incidence of ischemic adverse events.[70]

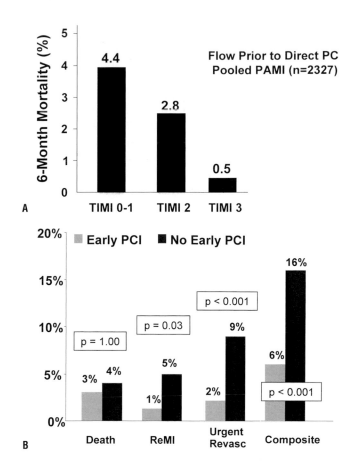

FIGURE 20-5. Influence of preprocedural TIMI infarct-related artery flow on 6-month mortality in the Primary Angioplasty in Myocardial Infarction trial (**A**). Thirty-day clinical outcomes for facilitated PCI in the GUSTO IV-SPEED trial (**B**). PCI = percutaneous coronary intervention; revasc = revascularization. *(From Herrmann HC, Moliterno DJ, Ohman EM, et al,[66] and Stone GW, Cox D, Garcia E, et al.[67])*

More adverse events likewise occurred among the approximate 25% of patients who did not achieve more than 95% inhibition within 10 minutes of administration.

Notably, the use of a calcium-chelating anticoagulant (such as citrate) in ex vivo platelet aggregation studies overestimates the in vivo inhibitory effects of GP IIb/IIIa inhibitors. This phenomenon confounded the identification of clinically optimal dosing regimins of eptifibatide and tirofiban. Doses of eptifibatide used in the IMPACT-II study[29] achieved 50% to 60% inhibition by standard platelet aggregometry. This finding led to higher dosing in the Platelet Glycoprotein IIb-IIIa in Unstable Angina: Receptor Suppression Using Integrilin Therapy (PURSUIT) and ESPRIT trials and may partly explain the larger clinical benefit observed in these studies compared with IMPACT-II.

Similarly, variable platelet inhibition may have contributed to the negative findings of the TARGET[44] and RESTORE[30] trials of tirofiban and the GUSTO-IV study of abciximab.[71] In the Comparison Of Measurements of Platelet Aggregation with Aggrastat, ReoPro, and Eptifibatide (COMPARE) trial, serial platelet aggregometry was performed in 73 patients randomized to receive either abciximab, eptifibatide, or tirofiban using doses established in contemporary ACS trials.[72] Platelet aggregation in the first 30 minutes after administration was reduced least with tirofiban (RESTORE dose regimen). The greatest variability in platelet aggregation was observed with abciximab during late infusion ($\geq$4 hours). In contrast, the most consistent inhibition of platelet aggregation occurred with the eptifibatide regimen (PURSUIT dose regimen). Although the RESTORE-tirofiban dosing regimen provided platelet inhibition comparable with that of eptifibatide and abciximab with extended infusion, it did not produce a similar degree of platelet inhibition during immediate PCI. Consistent platelet inhibition after several hours of continued infusion may account for the efficacy observed when PCI is delayed 4 to 48 hours after administration, as in the Platelet Receptor Inhibition for Ischemic Syndrome Management in Patients Limited by Unstable Signs and Symptoms (PRISM-PLUS) and TACTICS-TIMI 18 studies. Alternatively, recovery of platelet aggregability after several hours of abciximab therapy may in part explain the negative findings with abciximab in the GUSTO-IV trial, which discouraged early revascularization. Based on these findings, however, potent platelet inhibition at the time of intentional vessel injury likely determines benefit during PCI, whereas a more prolonged and consistent reduction in platelet aggregation may be required for ACS applications.

Further studies in ACS and PCI are required to determine how pharmacodynamic differences may influence the efficacy of GP IIb/IIIa antagonists. In addition, reasons for interpatient variability in response to GP IIb/IIIa inhibition need to be clarified. Potential contributing factors include individual cardiovascular risk profiles (eg, diabetes, age), resistance to adjunctive antiplatelet therapies (eg, aspirin), or inherited genetic polymorphisms regarding platelets. Moreover, there is a need for standardized, accurate methods of determining platelet inhibition, because current measures of platelet inhibition are imprecise.[73] Platelet aggregometry has been the accepted standard for determining the intensity of antiplatelet therapies, but this technique is limited by intra- and interindividual variation along with excessive time and cost to complete the assay. Moreover, this method does not specifically measure GP IIb/IIIa binding activity, but rather global platelet function. Newer assays such as the Ultegra Rapid Platelet Function assay may provide a more rapid and specific assessment of GP IIb/IIIa receptor occupancy. Because of the present variability in assays and lack of a uniform standard, routine platelet monitoring likely will be used to support clinical trial results, but routine clinical use is unlikely. Whether other measures of platelet function yield more consistent results than aggregometry is not well studied. Studies examining the effects of GP IIb/IIIa antagonists on inflammation (eg, inhibition of the $\alpha v \beta 3$ or Mac-1 integrin receptors) may instead provide more reliable and yet clinically relevant assessments of platelet activity.

【 】 BLEEDING AND THROMBOCYTOPENIA

Although further studies are needed to clarify the relationship between ischemic events and the level of platelet inhibition with GP IIb/IIIa blockade, the likelihood of bleeding complications correlates more directly with the level of impaired platelet activity. In the EPILOG study, a nonsignificantly lower bleeding rate was observed with abciximab and low-dose heparin versus standard heparin,[27] and bleeding may even be further reduced with throm-

bin inhibitors such as bivalirudin. Similarly, among trials examining GP IIb/IIIa antagonists in primary PCI, more attentive dosing of heparin likely accounts for the absence of differences in major bleeding. Further, unlike with fibrinolytic therapy, the risk of intracranial hemorrhage does not appear increased with intravenous GP IIb/IIIa inhibition.

All GP IIb/IIIa inhibitors are associated with some risk of thrombocytopenia, which occurs in 0.4% to 4% of patients. The precise mechanism and optimal treatment remain unknown, and treatment is usually limited to platelet transfusions. Thrombocytopenia is associated with not only a greater risk of hemorrhage but also a paradoxically greater likelihood of ischemic adverse events.[74] Pseudothrombocytopenia, or artifactual platelet clumping in vitro due to autologous antibodies, may occur in up to 1% of patients receiving abciximab but does not affect clinical outcome.[75]

Except for abciximab, readministration of GP IIb/IIIa antagonists remains uncertain, although adverse consequences do not appear common in routine clinical practice. In the ReoPro Readministration Study,[76] overall rates of thrombocytopenia with abciximab were similar to rates for first-time administration, yet there appeared to be a greater incidence of profound thrombocytopenia for those patients having human antichimeric antibodies or when the interval between doses was less than 30 days.[77] Despite the development of human antichimeric antibodies in a small number of patients after initial exposure to abciximab, neither hypersensitivity reactions nor neutralization of the abciximab effect was observed.

For most patients, the risk of thrombocytopenia does not preclude the use of a GP IIb/IIIa inhibitor. Instead, the uncertainty about which patients will develop thrombocytopenia and our inability to prevent it should reinforce the need for vigilant periprocedural monitoring of platelet counts. Advanced age and lower body weight are associated with a greater likelihood of thrombocytopenia, although no risk factor has been established with any certainty to preclude GP IIb/IIIa inhibitor administration. Importantly, the ReoPro Readministration study did not include patients who developed thrombocytopenia with initial therapy, such that potential risks from readministration to this particular subgroup are not well understood. Although it is customary among patients with abciximab-associated thrombocytopenia to avoid GP IIb/IIIa inhibition altogether or substitute a small-molecule inhibitor, there are few prospective data to support this practice.

ORAL ANTIPLATELET AGENTS: ASPIRIN AND THIENOPYRIDINES

Despite improved outcomes in high-risk patients with ACS, current standard therapies have limitations. Persistent reports of high clinical event rates among patients with ACS and NSTE following treatment have motivated the need for improved antiplatelet and anticoagulant therapy.[78,79]

Although aspirin remains a relatively weak antiplatelet agent, in a systematic overview of 60,000 high-risk patients with prior cardiovascular disease, aspirin therapy resulted in an approximate 25% relative reduction ($P <$ .00001) in subsequent vascular events, although the total event rate remained high despite aspirin therapy with a 15% incidence of recurrent MI, stroke, or vascular death.[80] In spite of numerous clinical trials involving more than 100,000 patients, the most effective aspirin dose has not been identified either in ACS or PCI. Nonetheless, a broad clinical consensus has developed, with recommendations for aspirin dosing between 75 mg and 325 mg per day in patients with coronary disease. Varied results from previous trials addressing aspirin dosing have underscored the uncertainty with regard to aspirin dosing in reducing secondary vascular events. In a recent observational analysis of aspirin dosing in the Clopidogrel in Unstable Angina to Prevent Recurrent Events (CURE) trial, the lowest rates of bleeding and ischemic events occurred among patients taking less than 100 mg/d of aspirin.[81] For patients receiving combined aspirin and clopidogrel (75 mg/d), adverse events were lowest among those patients taking less than 100 mg/d of aspirin compared with 100 to 200 mg/d and more than 200 mg/d; the benefit of combination therapy was largely due to the reduction in ischemic events compared with aspirin alone at doses more than 100 mg/d. Similarly, two recent systematic overviews of aspirin trials showed a greater benefit of lower doses of aspirin in reducing ischemic adverse events in ACS.[82,83] To date, no study evaluating variable aspirin dosing has been performed among patients undergoing PCI, yet the potential implications of aspirin dosing underscore the need for a large, randomized clinical trial.

More recent evaluations of orally administered antiplatelet agents not active through the cyclooxygenase pathway have been evaluated to prevent ischemic complications as alternatives to or in combination with aspirin. Ticlopidine, a thienopyridine that inhibits the ADP receptor on platelets, was shown in a series of clinical trials when combined with aspirin to significantly attenuate stent thrombosis compared with alternative antithrombotic regimens.[84-86] Clopidogrel is structurally similar to ticlopidine but is associated with a much lower rate of adverse events. Most notably, ticlopidine treatment carries troublesome rates of neutropenia, thrombocytopenia, and thrombotic thrombocytopenic purpura.[87] In contrast, these events have not been identified with clopidogrel in large clinical trials.

In the Clopidogrel versus Aspirin in Patients at Risk of Ischemic Events (CAPRIE) trial, the thienopyridine derivative clopidogrel significantly reduced the incidence of MI, stroke, or vascular death compared with aspirin (5.3% vs 5.8%; $P = .043$.[88] In addition, ACS patients treated with combined aspirin and clopidogrel in the CURE trial experienced significantly fewer ischemic events after a mean follow-up period of 9 months compared with patients assigned aspirin therapy alone (9.3% with clopidogrel and aspirin vs 11.5% with aspirin alone, $P = .00005$ for the primary composite end point of cardiovascular death, stroke, and MI).[89] Although the occurrence of major bleeding was significantly greater with combined therapy (3.6% with aspirin and clopidogrel vs 2.7% with aspirin alone, $P = .0003$), there was no excess in major bleeding in the clopidogrel group after the initial 30 days; this result suggested that most of the risk may have occurred in the setting of revascularization procedures. As a result, contemporary guidelines for the treatment of NSTE ACS emphasize prompt administration of aspirin and clopidogrel for patients in whom a noninvasive strategy is planned and for patients scheduled to undergo PCI.[49] However, consideration of potential bleeding risks among patients whose treatment outcomes are initially unknown

but who may undergo surgical revascularization has raised uncertainty regarding the role of combination therapy as initial therapy in NSTE ACS. In an observational study of 224 patients undergoing nonurgent bypass surgery and with background aspirin use, treatment with clopidogrel within 7 days of surgery was associated with significantly higher postoperative bleeding and a 10-fold greater likelihood to undergo repeat operation for bleeding complications (6.8% vs 0.6%, $P = .018$).[90]

Unlike surgical revascularization, however, treatment with clopidogrel in the periprocedural setting of catheter-based revascularization has been associated with significant early and long-term benefit. In the observational Percutaneous Coronary Intervention-Clopidogrel in Unstable Angina to Prevent Recurrent Events (PCI-CURE) trial, treatment with clopidogrel for a median of 6 days before PCI followed by long-term clopidogrel therapy was associated with a significant reduction in the rate of cardiovascular death, MI, or revascularization at 30 days (RR 0.70, $P = .03$).[91] In this study, use of GP IIb/IIIa inhibitors was infrequent, and the apparent benefit of early combined aspirin and clopidogrel has advanced the notion that IIb/IIIa inhibitors may not be warranted for patients receiving prolonged dual antiplatelet therapy with aspirin and clopidogrel.

The Clopidogrel for the Reduction of Events During Observation (CREDO) study randomized 2116 patients intended to undergo PCI to either pretreatment with 300 mg clopidogrel within 24 hours prior to PCI or alternatively 75 mg at the time of revascularization.[92] Patients randomized to the pretreatment arm also received combined aspirin and clopidogrel for 1 year following revascularization. Although a trend toward reduced 28-day ischemic adverse events favored pretreatment with clopidogrel (6.8% vs 8.3%, $P = .23$), long-term clopidogrel therapy was associated with a significant reduction in the 1-year occurrence of death, MI, and stroke compared with aspirin alone (8.5% vs 11.5%, $P = .02$) (Figure 20-6).

More recently, the potential efficacy of a higher loading dose of clopidogrel has been examined in patients undergoing PCI. Because administration of large loading doses of clopidogrel more

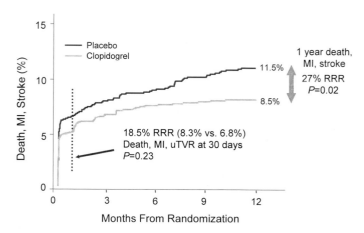

FIGURE 20-6. Occurrence of ischemic adverse events at 28 days and 1 year in the CREDO trial evaluating long-term treatment with clopidogrel following PCI. MI = myocardial infarction; RRR = relative risk reduction; uTVR = urgent target vessel revascularization. (*Data from Steinhubl SR, Berger PB, Mann III JT, et al, for the CREDO Investigators.*[92])

rapidly achieve inhibition of ADP-induced platelet aggregation,[93] the benefit of additional GP IIb/IIIa inhibition to a clopidogrel pretreatment strategy has been recently debated. The ISAR-REACT trial randomized 2159 patients scheduled for elective PCI to treatment with either abciximab or placebo.[94] All patients received a 600-mg dose of clopidogrel at least 2 hours prior to the procedure. At 30 days, the incidence of death, MI, and urgent TVR did not significantly differ between treatment groups (4.0% vs 4.0%, $P = .82$). Although the occurrence of major bleeding also did not differ, the development of profound thrombocytopenia was significantly more common with abciximab (1.0% vs 0, $P = .002$). Importantly, none of the patients enrolled in ISAR-REACT presented with high-risk ACS characteristics, and all patients underwent PCI. Instead, among higher risk NSTE ACS patients undergoing PCI who are treated with aspirin, clopidogrel (600 mg) and unfractionated heparin, the adjunctive use of abciximab was associated with a significant improvement in early clinical outcome in the ISAR-REACT 2 trial.[46a] Thus, outcomes appear less beneficial for NSTE ACS patients with high risk features (eg, recent MI or electrocardiographic ST-segment deviation > 0.1 mV) who are treated with oral antiplatelet therapy alone (and unfractionated heparin) and for those ACS patients who are not treated according to an early invasive strategy.

In the Antiplatelet Therapy for Reduction of Myocardial Damage During Angioplasty study (ARMYDA-2), 255 patients were randomized to a preprocedural loading dose of 300 mg or 600 mg of clopidogrel.[93a] Treatment with the higher loading does in this trial was associated with a significant reduction in the 30-day composite endpoint of death, myocardial infarction, or target vessel revascularization. In particular, a 600-mg clopidogrel loading dose resulted in an approximate 50% relative reduction in the occurrence of early myocardial infarction (odd ratio 0.48, 95% confidence interval 0.15 to 0.97, $P = .044$). As yet, however, there has been no large-scale randomized study powered to determine the clinical efficacy of the 300-mg loading dose compared with that of the 600-mg loading dose.

FUTURE DIRECTIONS: INTEGRATING ANTITHROMBOTIC THERAPIES AND REVASCULARIZATION

Despite remarkable achievements in the care of patients undergoing catheter-based revascularization, we remain ever more reliant on the results of clinical trials evaluations seeking to refine treatment strategies for patients relative to individual risk presentation, the availability of facilities for invasive procedures, and the timing of revascularization. Even with presently available therapies, ongoing trials are designed to tailor antiplatelet and anticoagulant treatment as adjunctive therapy in PCI and a variety of clinical presentations. Such trials may clarify the complementary—rather than exclusionary—benefits of presently available antiplatelet and antithrombin therapies to maintain efficacy (eg, reducing death and MI) while improving safety (eg, decreasing bleeding and thrombocytopenia). Aside from these clinical trials, translational research identifying the role of inflammation in thrombosis has further enhanced our understanding of the mechanism of benefit with current antiplatelet therapies.

Alone and combined with other pharmacologic and mechanical interventions, the application of antiplatelet therapies reflects considerable progress in the treatment of patients undergoing PCI. The limited efficacy of "standard" antithrombotic and anticoagulant therapy with aspirin and heparin alone should remind clinicians of the continued need to apply therapies with proven benefit. Even in spite of significant reductions in death or MI with contemporary antiplatelet therapies, many eligible patients still do not actually receive treatment with such agents. It is necessary to better understand the indications for GP IIb/IIIa antagonists relative to oral antiplatelet agents, novel antithrombin therapies, and even new devices and technologies (eg, distal protection, thrombectomy devices) as well as the reasons for the gap between health care achievements in clinical trials and contemporary "real world" practice.[95,96] This paradoxical quality of care emphasizes the continued need to encourage adherence to practice guidelines and participation in quality improvement initiatives. While unresolved issues mandate further clinical trials to refine the place of antithrombotic agents in a treatment algorithm for patients undergoing PCI relative to their clinical risk presentation, clinicians can apply the available evidence to select current therapies to achieve clinically meaningful benefit.

REFERENCES

1. Fuster V, Badimon L, Badimon JJ, Chesebro JH. The pathogenesis of coronary artery disease and the acute coronary syndrome. *N Engl J Med*. 1992;326:242–250, 310.
2. Lefkovits J, Plow EF, Topol EJ. Platelet glycoprotein IIb/IIIa receptors in cardiovascular medicine. *N Engl J Med*. 1995;332:1553.
3. Lefkovits J, Plow EF, Topol EJ. Platelet glycoprotein IIb/IIIa receptors in cardiovascular medicine. *N Engl J Med*. 1995;332:1553.
4. Phillips DR, Charo IF; Parisi LV, Fitzgerald LA. The platelet membrane glycoprotein IIb-IIIa complex. *Blood*. 1988;71:831.
5. Pytela R, Pierschbacher MD, Ginsberg MH, et al. Platelet membrane glycoprotein IIb/IIIa: member of a family of Arg-Gly-Asp specific adhesion receptors. *Science*. 1986;231:1559.
6. Coller BS, Peerschke EI, Scudder LE, Sullivan CA. A murine monoclonal antibody that completely blocks the binding of fibrinogen to platelets produces a thrombasthenic-like state in normal platelets and binds to glycoproteins IIb and/or IIIa. *J Clin Invest*. 1983;72:325.
7. Goldstein JA, Demetriou D, Grines CL, Pica M, Shoukfeh M, O'Neill WW. Multiple complex coronary plaques in patients with acute myocardial infarction. *N Engl J Med*. 2000;343:915.
8. Maehara A, Mintz GS, Bui AB, et al. Morphologic and angiographic features of coronary plaque rupture detected by intravascular ultrasound. *J Am Coll Cardiol*. 2002;40:902.
9. Heeschen C, Dimmeler S, Hamm CW, et al, for the CAPTURE Study Investigators. Soluble CD40 ligand in acute coronary syndromes. *N Engl J Med*. 2003;348:1104.
10. Varo N, de Lemos JA, Libby P, et al. Soluble CD40L: risk prediction after acute coronary syndromes. *Circulation*. 2003;108:1049.
11. Buffon A, Biasucci LM, Liuzzo G, D'Onofrio G, Crea F, Maseri A. Widespread coronary inflammation in unstable angina. *N Engl J Med*. 2002;347:5.
12. Kereiakes DJ. The fire that burns within: C-reactive protein. *Circulation*. 2003;107:373.
13. Blankenberg S, Luc G, Ducimetière P, et al, on behalf of the PRIME study group. Interleukin-18 and the risk of coronary heart disease in European men: the Prospective Epidemiological Study of Myocardial Infarction (PRIME). *Circulation*. 2003;108:2453–2459.
14. André P, Prasad KS, Denis CV, et al. CD40L stabilizes arterial thrombi by a beta3 integrin-dependent mechanism. *Nat Med*. 2002;8:247.
15. André P, Nannizzi-Alaimo L, Prasad SK, Phillips DR. Platelet-derived CD40L: the switch-hitting player of cardiovascular disease. *Circulation*. 2002;106:896.
16. Cipollone F, Ferri C, Desideri G, et al. Preprocedural level of soluble CD40L is predictive of enhanced inflammatory response and restenosis after coronary angioplasty. *Circulation*. 2003;108:2776.

17. Vivekananthan DP, Bhatt DL, Chew DP, et al. Clopidogrel pretreatment prior to percutaneous coronary intervention attenuates periprocedrual rise of C-reactive protein. *J Am Coll Cardiol.* 2003;41:24A.

18. Zidar FJ, Quinn MJ, Bhatt DL, et al. Clopidogrel pretreatment reduces platelet inflammatory marker expression in patients undergoing percutaneous coronary intervention. *J Am Coll Cardiol.* 2003;41:45A.

19. Serruys PW, de Jaegere P, Kiemeneij F, et al. A comparison of balloon expandable stent implantation with balloon angioplasty in patients with coronary artery disease. *N Engl J Med.* 1994;331:489.

20. Fischman DL, Leon MB, Baim DS, et al. A randomized comparison of coronary stent placement and balloon angioplasty in the treatment of coronary artery disease. *N Engl J Med.* 1994;331:496.

21. Serruys PW, van Hout B, Bonnier H, et al. Randomised comparison of implantation of heparin-coated stents with balloon angioplasty in selected patients with coronary artery disease (BENESTENT II). *Lancet.* 1998;352:673.

22. Adgey JAA. Overview of the results of clinical trials with glycoprotein IIb/IIIa inhibitors. *Am Heart J.* 1998;135(Suppl):S43.

23. Kong DF, Califf RM, Miller DP, et al. Clinical outcomes of therapeutic agents that block the platelet glycoprotein IIb/IIIa integrin in ischemic heart disease. *Circulation.* 1998;98:2829.

24. Karvouni E, Katritsis DG, Ioannidis JPA. Intravenous glycoprotein IIb/IIIa receptor antagonists reduce mortality after percutaneous coronary interventions. *J Am Coll Cardiol.* 2003;41:26.

25. Kong DF, Hasselblad V, Harrington RA, et al. Meta-analysis of survival with platelet glycoprotein IIb/IIIa antagonists for percutaneous coronary interventions. *Am J Cardiol.* 2003;92:651.

26. The EPIC Investigators. Use of a monoclonal antibody directed against the platelet glycoprotein IIb/IIIa receptor in high-risk coronary angioplasty. *N Engl J Med.* 1994;330:956.

27. The EPILOG Investigators. Platelet glycoprotein IIb/IIIa receptor blockade and low-dose heparin during percutaneous coronary revascularization. *N Engl J Med.* 1997;336:1689.

28. The CAPTURE Investigators. Randomised placebo-controlled trial of abciximab before and during coronary intervention in refractory unstable angina: the CAPTURE study. *Lancet.* 1997;349:1429.

29. The IMPACT-II Investigators. Randomised placebo-controlled trial of effect of eptifibatide on complications of percutaneous coronary intervention: IMPACT-II. *Lancet.* 1997;349:1422.

30. The RESTORE Study Group. Effects of platelet glycoprotein IIb/IIIa blockade with tirofiban on adverse cardiac events in patients with unstable angina or acute myocardial infarction undergoing coronary angioplasty. *Circulation.* 1997;96:1445.

31. The EPISTENT Investigators. Randomised placebo-controlled and balloon-angioplasty-controlled trial to assess safety of coronary stenting with use of platelet glycoprotein IIb/IIIa blockade. *Lancet.* 1998;352:87.

32. The ESPRIT Investigators. Novel dosing regimen of eptifibatide in planned coronary stent implantation (Enhanced Suppression of the Platelet IIb/IIIa Receptor with Integrilin Therapy): a randomised, placebo-controlled trial. *Lancet.* 2000;356:2037.

33. O'Shea JC, Hafley GE, Greenberg S, et al, for the ESPRIT Investigators. Platelet glycoprotein IIb/IIIa integrin blockade with eptifibatide in coronary stent intervention. The ESPRIT trial: a randomized controlled trial. *JAMA.* 2001;285:2468.

34. O'Shea JC, Buller CE, Cantor WJ, et al. Long-term efficacy of platelet glycoprotein IIb/IIIa integrin blockade with eptifibatide in coronary stent intervention. *JAMA.* 2002;287:618.

35. Califf RM, Abdelmeguid AE, Kuntz RE, et al. Myonecrosis after revascularization procedures. *J Am Coll Cardiol.* 1998;31:241.

36. Gibson CM, Cannon CP, Murphy SA, et al, for the TIMI Study Group. Relationship of the TIMI myocardial perfusion grades, flow grades, frame count, and percutaneous coronary intervention to long-term outcomes after thrombolytic administration in acute myocardial infarction. *Circulation.* 2002; 105:1909.

37. Baim DS, Wahr D, George B, et al, for the SAFER Investigators. Randomized trial of a distal embolic protection device during percutaneous intervention of saphenous vein aorto-coronary bypass grafts. *Circulation.* 2002;105:1285.

38. SoRelle R. Cardiovascular news. *Circulation.* 2004;109:e9017.

39. Wong GC, Morrow DA, Murphy S, et al, for the TACTICS-TIMI 18 Study Group. Elevations in troponin T and I are associated with abnormal tissue level perfusion: a TACTICS-TIMI 18 substudy. *Circulation.* 2002;106:202.

40. Gibson CM, Cohen DJ, Cohen EA, et al. Effect of eptifibatide on coronary flow reserve following coronary stent implantation (an ESPRIT substudy). Enhanced Suppression of the Platelet IIb/IIIa Receptor with Integrilin Therapy. *Am J Cardiol.* 2001;87:1293.

41. Neumann FJ, Kastrati A, Schmitt C, et al. Effect of glycoprotein IIb/IIIa receptor blockade with abciximab on clinical and angiographic restenosis rate after the placement of coronary stents following acute myocardial infarction. *J Am Coll Cardiol.* 2000;35:915.

42. The ERASER Investigators. Acute platelet inhibition with abciximab does not reduce in-stent restenosis. *Circulation.* 1999;100:799.

43. Gibson CM, Goel M, Cohen DJ, et al. Six-month angiographic and clinical follow-up of patients prospectively randomized to receive either tirofiban or placebo during angioplasty in the RESTORE trial. *J Am Coll Cardiol.* 1998;32:28.

44. Topol EJ, Moliterno DJ, Herrmann HC, et al. Comparison of two platelet glycoprotein IIb/IIIa inhibitors, tirofiban and abciximab, for the prevention of ischemic events with percutaneous coronary revascularization. *N Engl J Med.* 2001;344:1888.

45. Schneider DJ, Herrmann HC, Lakkis N, et al. Increased concentrations of tirofiban in blood and their correlation with inhibition of platelet aggregation after greater bolus doses of tirofiban. *Am J Cardiol.* 2003;91:334.

46. Lincoff AM, Bittl JA, Harrington RA, et al, for the REPLACE-2 Investigators. Bivalirudin and provisional glycoprotein IIb/IIIa blockade compared with heparin and planned glycoprotein IIb/IIIa blockade during percutaneous coronary intervention: REPLACE-2 randomized trial. *JAMA.* 2003;289:853.

46a. Kastrati A, Mehilli J, Neumann FJ, et al. for the Intracoronary Stenting and Antithrombotic Regimen: Rapid Early Action for Coronary Treatment 2 (ISAR-REACT 2) Trial Investigators. Abciximab in patients with acute coronary syndromes undergoing percutaneous coronary intervention after clopidogrel pretreatment: the ISAR-REACT 2 randomized trial. *JAMA* 2006;295: 1531–1538.

47. Cannon CP, Weintraub WS, Demopoulos L, et al. Comparison of invasive versus conservative strategy in patients with unstable coronary syndromes treated with the glycoprotein IIb/IIIa inhibitor tirofiban: the Treat Angina with Aggrastat and Determine the Cost of Therapy with an Invasive of Conservative Strategy (TACTICS-TIMI 18) Investigators. *N Engl J Med.* 2001;344:1879.

48. Mahaffey KW, Alexander JH, Roe MT, et al. Characterization of types of myocardial infarctions in two large acute coronary syndrome trials. *Circulation.* 2001;104:II-697.

49. Braunwald E, Antman EM, Beasley JW, et al. ACC/AHA guidelines for the management of patients with unstable angina and non-ST-segment elevation myocardial infarction. *J Am Coll Cardiol.* 2000;36:970.

50. Neumann FJ, Kastrati A, Pogatsa-Murray G, et al. Evaluation of prolonged antithrombotic pretreatment ("cooling-off" strategy) before intervention in patients with unstable coronary syndromes: a randomized controlled trial. *JAMA.* 2003;290(12):1593.

51. Bavry AA, Kumbhani DJ, Quiroz R, Ramchandano SR, Kenchaiah S, Antman EM. Invasive therapy along with glycoprotein IIb/IIIa inhibitors and intracoronary stents imporves survival in non-ST-segment elevation acute coronary syndromes: a meta-analysis and review of the literature. *Am J Cardiol.* 2004;93:830.

52. Peterson ED, Pollack CV, Roe MT, et al. Early use of glycoprotein IIb/IIIa inhibitors in non-ST-elevation acute myocardial infarction. *J Am Coll Cardiol.* 2003;42:45.

52a. Stone GW. Primary results of the Acute Catheterization and Urgent Intervention Thrombotic Strategy (ACUITY) trial. Presented at the 2006 American College of Cardiology Scientific Sessions, March 12, 2006, Atlanta, GA.

53. Chesebro JH, Knatterud G, Roberts R, et al. Thrombolysis in Myocardial Infarction (TIMI) Trial, phase I: a comparison between intravenous tissue plasminogen activator and intravenous streptokinase. *Circulation.* 1987;76:142.

54. Gold HK, Garabedian HD, Dinsmore RE, at al. Restoration of coronary flow in myocardial infarction by intravenous chimeric 7E3 antibody without exogenous plasminogen activators: observations in animals and humans. *Circulation.* 1997;95:1755.

55. Reverter JC, Beguin S, Kessels H, et al. Inhibition of platelet-medicated, tissue factor-induced thrombin generation by the mouse/human chimeric 7E3 antibody: potential implications for the effect of c7E3 Fab treatment on acute thrombosis and clinical restenosis. *J Clin Invest.* 1996;99:863.

56. van den Merkhof LFM, Zijlstra F, Olsson H, et al. Abciximab in the treatment of acute myocardial infarction eligible for primary percutaneous transluminal coronary angioplasty. *J Am Coll Cardiol.* 1999;33:1528.

57. Antman EM, Giugliano RP, Gibson CM, et al, for the TIMI-14 Investigators. Abciximab facilitate the rate and extent of thrombolysis. Results of the TIMI 14 trial. *Circulation.* 1999;99:2720.

58. Strategies for Patency Enhancement in the Emergency Department (SPEED) Group. Trial of Abciximab With and Without Low-Dose Reteplase for Acute Myocardial Infarction. *Circulation.* 2000;101:2788.

59. Lefkovits J, Ivanhoe RJ, Califf RM, et al, for the EPIC Investigators. Effects of platelet glycoprotein IIb/IIIa receptor blockade by a chimeric monoclonal antibody (abciximab) on acute and six-month outcomes after percutaneous transluminal coronary angioplasty for acute myocardial infarction. *Am J Cardiol.* 1996;77:1045.

60. Brener SJ, Barr LA, Burchenal JE et al. Randomized, placebo-controlled trial of platelet glycoprotein IIb/IIIa blockade with primary angioplasty for acute myocardial infarction. ReoPro and Primary PTCA Organization and Randomized Trial (RAPPORT) Investigators. *Circulation.* 1998;98:734.

61. Montalescot G, Barragan P, Wittenberg O, et al. for the ADMIRAL Investigators. Platelet glycoprotein IIb/IIIa inhibition with coronary stenting for acute myocardial infarction. *N Engl J Med.* 2001;344:1895.

62. Stone GW, Grines CL, Cox DA, et al. A prospective, randomized trial comparing primary balloon angioplasty with or without abciximab to primary stenting with or without abciximab in acute myocardial infarction-primary endpoint analysis from the CADILLAC Trial. *N Engl J Med.* 2002;346:957.

63. Tcheng JE, Kandzari DE, Grines CL, et al, for the CADILLAC Investigators. Abciximab treatment in primary angioplasty during acute myocardial infarction: final results of the CADILLAC trial. *Circulation.* 2003;108:1316.

64. Antoniucci D, Rodriguez A, Hempel A, et al. A randomized trial comparing primary infarct artery stenting with or without abciximab in acute myocardial infarction. *J Am Coll Cardiol.* 2003;42:1879.

65. Kandzari DE, Hasselblad V, Tcheng JE, et al. Improved clinical outcomes with abciximab therapy in acute myocardial infarction: a systematic overview of randomized clinical trials. *Am Heart J.* 2004;147:457.

65a. De Luca G, Suryapranata H, Stone GW, et al. Abciximab as adjunctive therapy to reperfusion in acute ST-segment elevation myocardial infarction: a meta-analysis of randomized trials. *JAMA* 2005;293:1759–1765.

66. Herrmann HC, Moliterno DJ, Ohman EM, et al. Facilitation of early percutaneous coronary intervention after reteplase with or without abciximab in acute myocardial infarction. Results from the SPEED (GUSTO-4 Pilot) Trial. *J Am Coll Cardiol.* 2000;36:1489.

66a. The ASSENT-4 PCI Investigators. Primary versus tenecteplase-facilitated percutaneous coronary intervention in patients with ST-segment elevation acute myocardial infarction (ASSENT-4 PCI): randomised trial. *Lancet* 2006;367:569–578.

67. Stone GW, Cox D, Garcia E, et al. Normal flow (TIMI-3) before mechanical reperfusion therapy is an independent determinant of survival on acute myocardial infarction. Analysis from the Primary Angioplasty in Myocardial Infarction Trials. *Circulation.* 2001;104:636.

68. Ross AM, Coyne KS, Reiner JS, et al. A randomized trial comparing primary angioplasty with a strategy of short-acting thrombolysis and immediate planned rescue angioplasty in acute myocardial infarction: the PACT trial. *J Am Coll Cardiol.* 1999;34:1954.

69. Morrison LJ, Verbeek PR, McDonald AC, et al. Mortality and prehospital thrombolysis for acute myocardial infarction: a meta-analysis. *JAMA.* 2000;283:2686.

70. Steinhubl SR, Talley JD, Braden GA, et al. Point-of-care measured platelet inhibition correlates with a reduced risk of an adverse cardiac event after percutaneous coronary intervention. Results of the GOLD (AU-Assessing Ultegra) Multicenter Study. *Circulation.* 2001;103:2572.

71. The GUSTO IV-ACS Investigators. Effect of glycoprotein IIb/IIIa receptor blocker abciximab on outcome in patients with acute coronary syndromes without early coronary revascularization: the GUSTO-IV ACS randomised trial. *Lancet.* 2001;357:1915.

72. Batchelor WB, Tolleson TR, Huang Y, et al. Randomized COMparison of Platelet Inhibition with Abciximab, TiRofiban and Eptifibatide during percutaneous coronary intervention in acute coronary syndromes: the COMPARE Trial. *Circulation.* 2002;106:1470.

73. Kereiakes DJ, Broderick TM, Roth EM, et al. Time course, magnitude, and consistency of platelet inhibition by abciximab, tirofiban, or eptifibatide in patients with unstable angina pectoris undergoing percutaneous coronary intervention. *Am J Cardiol.* 1999;84:391.

74. McClure MW, Berkowitz SD, Sparapani R, et al. Clinical significance of thrombocytopenia during a non-ST-elevation acute coronary syndrome: the Platelet glycoprotein IIb/IIIa in Unstable angina: Receptor Suppression Using Integrilin Therapy (PURSUIT) trial experience. *Circulation.* 2000;99:2892.

75. Sane DC, Damaraju LV, Topol EJ, et al. Occurrence and clinical significance of thrombocytopenia during abciximab therapy. *J Am Coll Cardiol.* 2000;36:75.

76. Tcheng JE, Kereiakes DJ, Lincoff AM, et al. Abciximab readministration: results of the ReoPro Readministration Study. *Circulation.* 2001;104:870.

77. Dery JP, Braden GA, Lincoff AM, et al, on behalf of the ReoPro Readministration Registry Investigators. Final results of the ReoPro Readministration Registry. *Am J Cardiol.* 2004;93:9744.

78. The TIMI IIIB Investigators. Effects of tissue plasminogen activator and a comparison of early invasive and conservative strategies in unstable angina and non-Q-wave myocardial infarction: results of the TIMI IIIB trial. *Circulation.* 1994;89:1545.

79. The Global Use of Strategies to Open Occluded Coronary Arteries (GUSTO) IIb Investigators. A comparison of recombinant hirudin with heparin for the treatment of acute coronary syndromes. *N Engl J Med.* 1996;335:775.

80. The Antiplatelet Trialists' Collaboration. Collaborative overview of randomised trials of antiplatelet therapy-I: prevention of death, myocardial infarction, and stroke by prolonged antiplatelet therapy in various categories of patients. *BMJ.* 1994;308:81.

81. Peters RJG, Mehta SR, Fox KAA, et al, for the CURE Trial Investigators. Effects of aspirin dose when used alone or in combination with clopidogrel in patients with acute coronary syndromes: observations from the Clopidogrel in Unstable angina to prevent Recurrent Events (CURE) Study. *Circulation.* 2003; 108:1682.

82. Antithrombotic Trialists' Collaboration. Collaborative meta-analysis of randomised trials of antiplatelet therapy for prevention of death, myocardial infarction, and stroke in high risk patients. *BMJ.* 2002;324:71.

83. Kong DF, Hasselblad V, Kandzari DE, Newby KL, Califf RM. Seeking the optimal aspirin dose in acute coronary syndromes. *Am J Cardiol.* 2002; 90:622.

84. Leon M, Baim D, Popma J, Gordon P, et al. A clinical trial comparing three antithrombotic-drug regimens after coronary-artery stenting. *N Engl J Med.* 1998;339:1665.

85. Schömig A, Neumann FJ, Kastrati A, et al. A randomized comparison of antiplatelet and anticoagulant therapy after the placement of coronary-artery stents. *N Engl J Med.* 1996;334:1084.

86. Berger PB, Bell MR, Hasdai D, Grill DE, Melby S, Holmes DR. Safety and efficacy of ticlopidine for only 2 weeks after successful intracoronary stent placement. *Circulation.* 1999;99:248.

87. Quinn MJ, Fitzgerald DJ. Cardiovascular drugs: ticlopidine and clopidogrel. *Circulation.* 1999;100:1667.

88. The CAPRIE Steering Committee. A randomised, blinded, trial of clopidogrel versus aspirin in patients at risk of ischaemic events (CAPRIE). *Lancet.* 1996;348:1329.

89. The CURE Study Investigators. Effects of clopidogrel in addition to aspirin in patients with acute coronary syndromes without ST-segment elevation. *N Engl J Med.* 2001;345:494.

90. Hongo RH, Ley J, Dick SE, Yee RR. The effect of clopidogrel in combination with aspirin when given before coronary artery bypass grafting. *J Am Coll Cardiol.* 2002;40:231.

91. Mehta SR, Yusuf S, Peters RJG, et al, for the CURE Investigators. Effects of pretreatment with clopidogrel and aspirin followed by long-term therapy in patients undergoing percutaneous coronary intervention: the PCI-CURE study. *Lancet.* 2001;358:526.

92. Steinhubl SR, Berger PB, Mann III JT, et al, for the CREDO Investigators. Early and sustained dual oral antiplatelet therapy following percutaneous coronary intervention: a randomized controlled trial. *JAMA.* 2002;288:2411.

93. Thebault JJ, Kieffer G, Cariou R. Single-dose pharmacodynamics of clopidogrel. *Semin Thromb Hemost.* 1999;25(suppl 2):3.

93a. Patti G, Colonna G, Pasceri V, Pepe LL, Montinaro A, Di Sciascio G. Randomized trial of high loading dose of clopidogrel for reduction of periprocedural myocardial infarction in patients undergoing coronary intervention: results from the ARMYDA-2 (Antiplatelet therapy for Reduction of Myocardial Damage during Angioplasty) Study. *Circulation* 2005;111:2099–2106.

94. Kastrati A, Mehilli J, Schühlen H, et al, for the Intracoronary Stenting and Antithrombotic Regimen-Rapid Early Action for Coronary Treatment (ISAR-REACT) Study Investigators. A clinical trial of abciximab in elective percutaneous coronary intervention after pretreatment with clopidogrel. *N Engl J Med.* 2004;350:232.

95. Roe MT, Ohman EM, Pollack CV, et al. Changing the model of care for patients with acute coronary syndromes-implementing practice guidelines and altering physician behavior. *Am Heart J.* 2003; 2003;146:605.

96. Peterson ED, Roe MT, Lytle BL, et al. The association between care and outcomes in patients with acute coronary syndrome: national results from CRUSADE. *J Am Coll Cardiol.* 2004;43:406A.

97. Kandzari DE, Califf RM. TARGET versus GUSTO-IV: appropriate use of glycoprotein IIb/IIIa inhibitors in acute coronary syndromes and percutaneous coronary intervention. *Curr Opin Cardiol.* 2002;17:332.

CHAPTER (21)

Thrombolytic Therapy

Abdul R. Halabi, MD, and James E. Tcheng, MD

THROMBOLYSIS IN ST-ELEVATION MYOCARDIAL INFARCTION

Thrombolytic therapy has revolutionized the care of patients with acute ST-elevation myocardial infarction (STEMI). In 1986, the Gruppo Italiano per lo Studio della Streptochinasi nell'Infarcto miocardico (GISSI) investigators established the life-saving potential of this novel approach.[1] In fact, the GISSI trial signaled the birth of the "thrombolytic era," marked by redefined treatment strategies coupled with improved clinical outcomes in STEMI. Recently, new generations of thrombolytic agents, adjunctive and combination pharmacologic strategies, and catheter-based interventions have further improved outcomes. Current indications for thrombolytic therapy go beyond the scope of cardiac disease and include a wide range of clinical conditions, such as acute pulmonary embolism, acute nonhemorrhagic stroke, acute peripheral vascular embolization, superior vena cava obstruction, deep venous thrombosis, and central venous catheter occlusions. In this chapter, we will summarize the early work that established the modern role of thrombolysis in acute STEMI, chronicle the ensuing search for better thrombolytic agents (including strategies for combining thrombolytic agents with antiplatelet and antithrombin therapies), and present the recent "merger" of pharmacologic and mechanical reperfusion.

【 】 EARLY WORK: A BRIEF HISTORICAL PERSPECTIVE

Cardiovascular disease is the most common cause of death in Western industrialized countries. In the United States in 2001,

cardiovascular disease accounted for more than 930,000, or approximately 38%, of all deaths.[2] In comparison, all cancers accounted for 554,000 deaths, or approximately 23% of the total number of deaths. The economic burden of cardiovascular disease is enormous, with the costs of cardiovascular disease in the United States in 2003 estimated at $351.8 billion. The only good news is that cardiovascular mortality rates have actually *decreased* over the past 50 years, largely because of improved preventive and therapeutic strategies. The application of thrombolytic therapies for the treatment of acute STEMI provided a major contribution to these reduced mortality rates.

Recognition that β-hemolytic streptococci possessed fibrinolytic properties provided the physiologic rationale for the development of thrombolytic agents (Table 21-1). Streptokinase was initially studied in the basic science laboratory for its clot-dissolving properties, even being applied to patients with myocardial infarction in the 1950s.[3] Another landmark advance was the identification of total coronary occlusion in the early hours of acute myocardial infarction as a potential mechanism leading to STEMI.[4] Streptokinase became the first thrombolytic agent to be prospectively studied in a large, multicenter, randomized clinical trial. The GISSI investigators randomized more than 11,000 STEMI patients to streptokinase or placebo. In-hospital mortality was strikingly reduced from 13% to 10.7% following streptokinase administration, thus establishing the role of fibrinolysis in the treatment of acute STEMI.[1]

Several large clinical trials subsequently redefined the role of streptokinase in acute STEMI. These included the Second International Study of Infarct Survival (ISIS-2) trial of more than 17,000 patients and the Global Utilization of Streptokinase and

---

A list of the clinical trials cited in Chapters 19 through 24 is presented in Appendix IV-1 at the end of Part IV.

TABLE 21-1

Pharmacological Characteristics of Thrombolytic Agents

	STREPTOKINASE	tPA (ALTEPLASE)	rPA (RETEPLASE)	TNK-tPA (TENECTEPLASE)	nPA (IANOTEPLASE)
Molecular Weight (kDa)	47	70	39	70	54
Dosage	1.5 million U Infusion over 30–60 minutes	15 mg bolus, then 0.75 mg/kg 30-min infusion (max 50 mg), then 0.5 mg/kg 60-min Infusion (max 35 mg)	double bolus 10 IU 30 minutes apart	single bolus 0.5 mg/kg	single bolus 120 IU/kg
Half-life (minutes)	20	4	15	17–25	25–45
Fibrin-specificity	−	++	+	+++	+
Antigenicity	+	−	−	−	−
90-min Coronary Patency	+	++	+++	++	+++
ICH risks	+	++	++	++	+++
Survival Benefit	++	+++	+++	+++	+++
Major RCTs	GISSI, ISIS-2, GUSTO-1	GUSTO-1, GUSTO-3	RAPID-1, RAPID-2, INJECT, GUSTO-3	TIMI-10B, ASSENT-1, ASSENT-2	In-TIME-1, In-TIME-2
Comments	first available thrombolytic; produces systemic fibrinolysis; may cause allergic reactions	gold-standard in thrombolytic therapy	double bolus administration	single bolus administration, dose-adjustment by weight to reduce bleeding	prolonged half-life, single bolus administration, but increased bleeding and ICH rates
FDA Approval	+	+	+	+	−

FDA = Food and Drug Administration; ICH = intracranial hemorrhage; RCT = randomized clinical trial.

Tissue Plasminogen Activator for Occluded Coronary Arteries (GUSTO) trial of 41,021 patients.[5,6] ISIS-2 yielded important findings, both confirming the 25% relative risk reduction of in-hospital mortality with streptokinase as well as identifying a synergistic beneficial effect when aspirin was administered in addition to streptokinase.[5] The GUSTO trial was the first large prospective trial comparing streptokinase with tissue plasminogen activator (tPA).[6] A significant 1% absolute risk reduction in 30-day mortality was noted when tPA was used instead of streptokinase (6.3% vs 7.4%). These early results generated significant enthusiasm among clini-

cians worldwide and clearly established thrombolytic therapy (and in particular, tPA) as a mainstay of initial acute STEMI care.

Unfortunately, several limitations to this success story became apparent.[7] First, approximately one third of STEMI patients did not "respond" to thrombolytic therapy and did not achieve optimal early coronary patency. Second, approximately 15% to 20% of thrombolysis patients experienced clinical reinfarction following initially successful reperfusion. Third, a non-negligible proportion of patients suffered from increased bleeding complications and devastating intracranial hemorrhage. These limitations stimulated

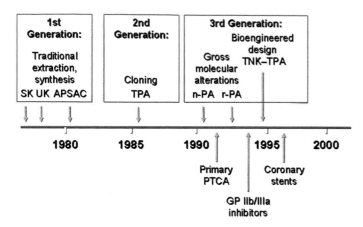

FIGURE 21-1. Evolution of pharmacologic reperfusion therapies. APSAC = acylated plasminogen-streptokinase activator complex; GP = glycoprotein; nPA = lanoteplase; PTCA = percutaneous transluminal coronary angioplasty; rPA = reteplase; SK = streptokinase; TNK-tPA = tenecteplase; tPA = tissue plasminogen activator.

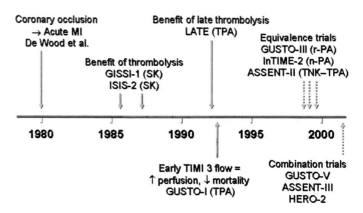

FIGURE 21-2. Selected major mortality trials in thrombolytic therapy. tPA = tissue plasminogen activator.

the development of new generations of thrombolytic agents and the development of combination strategies. The timelines of the evolution of thrombolytic therapies over the past two decades along with the conduct of major mortality trials are illustrated in Figures 21-1 and 21-2, respectively.

[ ] SEARCH FOR NEW AGENTS: NEW GENERATIONS OF THROMBOLYTIC AGENTS

Unlike streptokinase and other first-generation thrombolytic agents such as anistreplase and urokinase, second-generation agents (namely alteplase) were engineered to be fibrin-specific. Alteplase (tPA) is a product of recombinant DNA technology and has been extensively studied in a series of large, prospective trials. In a landmark trial, the GUSTO investigators compared the effects of four thrombolytic strategies in STEMI patients: (1) intravenous streptokinase and subcutaneous heparin, (2) intravenous streptokinase and intravenous heparin, (3) accelerated tPA and intravenous heparin, (4) and a combination of intravenous heparin, streptokinase, and intravenous heparin.[6] These four groups demonstrated the following 30-day mortality rates: 7.2%, 7.4%, 6.3%, and 7.0%, respectively. Thus, a statistically significant 1% absolute risk reduction (or a 14% RR reduction) was noted in the tPA group compared with the combined streptokinase groups. Hemorrhagic stroke occurred in 0.49%, 0.54%, 0.72%, and 0.94% in the four groups, respectively. Despite slightly increased risks of stroke with tPA therapy, the combined end point of death or disabling stroke was lower in the tPA group compared to the streptokinase groups (6.9% vs 7.8%, respectively). Importantly, a follow-up analysis from the GUSTO trial identified certain clinical predictors of non-hemorrhagic stroke in acute STEMI patients receiving thrombolytic therapies: older age, previous stroke, diabetes mellitus, prior angina, systemic hypertension, worse Killip class, coronary angiography or bypass surgery, and atrial arrhythmias.[8]

In an attempt to further improve clinical outcomes following thrombolysis, a third generation of fibrinolytic agents was developed and became available in the early 1990s. These agents are

derived from tPA and include rPA (reteplase), TNK-tPA (tenecteplase), and nPA (lanoteplase).

In comparison to tPA, rPA is mainly characterized by reduced fibrin specificity. The Reteplase versus Alteplase Infusion in Acute Myocardial Infarction (RAPID) trial, a dose-finding angiographic trial, compared early coronary patency rates after bolus administration of rPA versus standard-dose tPA in over 600 STEMI patients.[9] In this pilot trial, the double-bolus regimen of rPA given 30 minutes apart resulted in slightly more rapid and complete rates of reperfusion than tPA and was associated with slightly improved left ventricular function at discharge. The RAPID-II trial then compared rPA to a tPA accelerated 90-minute administration regimen.[10] At 90 minutes following thrombolysis, the rPA group achieved significantly higher coronary patency (83.4% vs 73.3%) and TIMI-3 flow rates (59.9% vs 45.2%). However, no differences were noted among treatment groups with regard to reocclusion of the infarct-related artery, left ventricular function, stroke, and 35-day mortality. Similarly, no differences in 35-day mortality and clinical outcomes were noted when streptokinase and rPA were compared in the International Joint Efficacy Comparison of Thrombolytics (INJECT) trial of 6010 STEMI patients.[11]

In an attempt to establish the superiority of rPA over tPA, the Global Use of Strategies to Open Occluded Coronary Arteries-3 (GUSTO-III) investigators compared the efficacy and safety of accelerated administration regimens of rPA versus tPA in over 15,000 patients.[12] However, the rPA and tPA groups demonstrated no differences in terms of rates of stroke (1.64% vs 1.79%, respectively) and 30-day mortality (7.47% vs 7.24%, respectively). It thus appeared that an improvement in early angiographic patency following rPA thrombolysis did not necessarily translate into a measurable mortality benefit. Moreover, follow-up data from GUSTO-III confirmed the lack of a survival difference between these two strategies at one-year following STEMI.[13] In summary, the potential benefits of rPA over tPA are related only to ease of administration rather than clinical outcomes.

TNK-tPA is another member of the third generation of thrombolytic agents. It provides two highly attractive characteristics: high fibrin specificity and a single bolus administration regimen. Several large trials have examined the effects of TNK-tPA in comparison to tPA in acute STEMI patients. The Thrombolysis in Myocardial Infarction-10B (TIMI-10B) study was the first large trial comparing the efficacy of a single TNK-tPA bolus to frontloaded 90-

minute tPA administration.[14] When the 40 mg TNK-tPA bolus dose was used, rates of 90-minute TIMI-3 flow and bleeding complications were similar in both arms. A second, larger randomized trial, Assessment of the Safety and Efficacy of a New Thrombolytic-2 (ASSENT-2), provided additional valuable information on the dosage and efficacy of TNK-tPA.[15] Approximately 17,000 patients were randomized to a weight-adjusted single dose of TNK-tPA or frontloaded tPA. This trial showed that TNK-tPA and tPA were equally effective; no differences were noted in 30-day mortality (6.18% vs 6.15%), stroke (1.78% vs 1.66%), intracranial hemorrhage (0.93% vs 0.94%), and overall bleeding (26.4% vs 28.9%) rates. TNK-tPA, in spite of the lack of additional clinical benefits over tPA, has nevertheless gained widespread support within the medical community because of ease of administration (single bolus) and its well-established equivalence to tPA.

Yet another derivative of tPA, nPA is another member of the third generation of thrombolytic agents. It provides fibrin specificity and a markedly longer half-life than tPA, thus allowing for a single bolus administration. Initial information on the dosing and safety profile of nPA was examined in the Intravenous nPA for Treatment of Infarcting Myocardium Early (InTIME) trial.[16] This angiographic study randomized 602 STEMI patients to either nPA or frontloaded 90-minute tPA administration. Initial results were encouraging and revealed slightly better coronary patency rates in the nPA group within 90 minutes of drug administration. Increased coronary patency with nPA appeared to be dose-dependent; the highest tested dose of nPA (120 IU/kg) was associated with greater 90-minute patency than tPA (83% vs 71%, respectively). The InTIME-II investigators examined clinical outcomes in a cohort of more than 15,000 patients randomized to high-dose nPA (120 IU/kg) versus frontloaded 90-minute tPA.[17] Mortality rates were similar between the nPA and tPA arms 30 days (6.75% vs 6.61%, respectively) and 6 months following STEMI. However, increased rates of hemorrhagic strokes (1.12% vs 0.64%, respectively) and minor bleeding (19.7% vs 14.8%, respectively) were associated with nPA administration. Despite ease of administration, these results have generated lasting concerns over increased risks of hemorrhagic stroke, and this has prevented approval of nPA and its use in clinical practice.

[ ] COMBINATION STRATEGIES

Platelet Glycoprotein IIb/IIIa Inhibitors

The glycoprotein IIb/IIIa inhibitors have substantially widened the therapeutic arsenal available to clinical cardiologists. Although this class of agents has demonstrated significant benefits in patients admitted with high-risk acute coronary syndromes (ACSs) and undergoing percutaneous coronary interventions (PCIs), conflicting evidence surrounding the magnitude of benefits in STEMI remains.[18] The theoretical ability of abciximab to facilitate the rate and extent of fibrinolysis in STEMI was first tested in the TIMI-14 trial.[19] This dose-finding and strategy-defining trial of 888 patients compared 90-minute coronary patency rates of several combinations and permutations of therapies. Tested strategies included tPA only, abciximab only, and a half-dose fibrinolytic agent (tPA or streptokinase) combined with abciximab. Ninety-minute TIMI-3 flow was indeed achieved in 57% of the tPA-only

group, 32% of the abciximab-only group, and 77% of the tPA-abciximab combination group. Major hemorrhage occurred in only 1% of the tPA-abciximab (with "very low dose" heparin) combination group. However, major hemorrhage rates were unacceptably elevated in the following groups: tPA-abciximab combination group using a higher heparin dose (7%), tPA-only group (6%), and streptokinase-abciximab combination group (10%). These results were consistent with those published by the Strategies for Patency Enhancement in the Emergency Department (SPEED) Group.[20] This latter angiographic study of 528 patients revealed enhanced early coronary patency rates with an rPA-abciximab combination strategy over rPA-only or abciximab-only strategies.

Unfortunately, the enthusiasm generated from these promising angiographic results using a combination therapy did not translate into a meaningful improvement in clinical outcomes. Both the GUSTO-V and ASSENT-3 investigators failed to demonstrate sustained clinical benefits from a combination strategy using a glycoprotein IIb/IIIa inhibitor and a fibrinolytic agent.[21,22] GUSTO-V was an ambitious, randomized, multicenter trial comparing the effects of rPA alone with a combination of half-dose rPA and abciximab in more than 16,000 STEMI patients.[21] Mortality rates were no different at 30 days. A slight reduction in secondary end points (ie, rates of reinfarction and need for acute PCI) was more than offset by increased hematologic side effects (ie, rates of severe bleeding, cerebral hemorrhage in elderly patients, and overall thrombocytopenia). Results from the ASSENT-3 trial reemphasized the GUSTO-5 conclusions.[22] More than 6000 STEMI patients were randomized to three strategies, including TNK-tPA in addition to one of these three drugs: unfractionated heparin (UFH), enoxaparin, or abciximab (with half-dose TNK-tPA). Again, 30-day mortality rates were no different among groups; only a composite end point of mortality, in-hospital reinfarction, and in-hospital refractory ischemia at 30 days was reduced (in both the enoxaparin and abciximab groups). Unfortunately, the incidence of major noncerebral bleeding was significantly higher in the abciximab group (4.3%) compared with the enoxaparin (3.0%) and UFH (2.2%) groups.

In summary, all recent attempts at "up front" combinations of a glycoprotein IIb/IIIa inhibitor and a thrombolytic agent have yielded mixed results. Clearly, the attenuation of platelet aggregation and reduction of proinflammatory endothelial interactions through glycoprotein IIb/IIIa inhibition translate into enhanced early coronary patency rates and lesser recurrence of ischemic events following STEMI. However, these benefits do not result in a significant reduction of mortality and appear to be associated with unacceptably increased rates of bleeding and thrombocytopenia in most patient subgroups. Although there is still an undeniable role for the concomitant administration of glycoprotein IIb/IIIa inhibitors in certain situations following thrombolysis, routine upstream administration in combination with thrombolysis cannot be recommended.

Antithrombin Therapies

Unfractionated Heparin. Ever since the first thrombolytic trials were conducted, the adjunctive role of antithrombin therapy has been recognized. Accordingly, UFH has been administered in conjunction with streptokinase, tPA, and the subsequent generations of thrombolytic agents in the respective clinical trials. Although the overall benefits of heparin are presently well-established, recent investigations have focused on clarifying the appropriate dosage. Several studies have indeed shown that a lower bolus dose and a lower weight-adjusted infusion dose are associated with a reduced incidence of intracranial hemorrhage.[23] In light of these findings, the recently updated 2004 AHA/ACC Guidelines stipulate in a class I recommendation that "unfractionated heparin should be given intravenously to patients undergoing reperfusion therapy with alteplase, reteplase, or tenecteplase with dosing as follows: bolus of 60 U/kg (maximum 4000 U) followed by an infusion of 12 U/kg (maximal 1000 U/kg) initially adjusted to maintain an activated partial thromboplastin time at 1.5–2.0 times control (approximately 50–70 seconds)."[24] Furthermore, in patients treated with non–fibrin-specific thrombolytic agents (streptokinase, anistreplase, urokinase), the guidelines strictly limit the indications for intravenous UFH administration to only those patients at "high risk for systemic emboli" (class I recommendation).

Low-Molecular-Weight Heparins. A high affinity for factor Xa inhibition, ease of administration, and lack of need for monitoring are valuable characteristics of low-molecular-weight heparin (LMWH) therapy in patients with acute coronary syndromes.[25,26] Several trials have now compared the administration of a LMWH to UFH in combination with thrombolysis for acute STEMI. The Heparin and Aspirin Reperfusion Therapy-II (HART-II) trial compared the efficacy and safety of enoxaparin versus heparin in combination with tPA in 400 STEMI patients.[27] Ninety-minute coronary patency rates were similar between both study groups, and there was a nonsignificant trend toward less coronary reocclusion within the first week in the enoxaparin group. Using TNK-tPA instead of tPA, the Enoxaparin and TNK-tPA with or without glycoprotein IIb/IIIa Inhibitor as Reperfusion Strategy in ST-elevation Myocardial Infarction (ENTIRE-TIMI-23) trial studied 483 STEMI patients randomized to either heparin or enoxaparin.[28] The results were in line with those from HART-2; the two regimens showed equivalence in terms of 60-minute coronary patency. A slight reduction in 30-day recurrent ischemic events was observed in the enoxaparin group in comparison to the heparin group.

Of all published trials examining the combination of various antithrombin strategies to thrombolytic therapy, the ASSENT-3 trial was the most comprehensive.[22] In ASSENT-3, more than 6000 patients were randomized to TNK-tPA with heparin, enoxaparin, or abciximab. Treatment with enoxaparin was associated with a significant reduction in the 30-day composite primary end point of mortality, in-hospital reinfarction, and recurrent ischemia compared with heparin. Furthermore, in comparison to the abciximab group, the enoxaparin group had a favorable safety profile and experienced significantly lower rates of major bleeding, need for transfusions, and thrombocytopenia. However, bleeding rates still showed a trend toward an increase in the enoxaparin group over the heparin group. Additional important observations were as follows: patients with significant renal dysfunction were excluded from ASSENT-3, and patients older than 75 experienced a higher incidence of major bleeding in the enoxaparin group.[29]

Despite encouraging efficacy results showing equivalence between LMWH and heparin, some unresolved safety concerns remain associated with the administration of a LMWH in combination with thrombolytic therapy. In turn, the administration of a LMWH in combination with a thrombolytic agent is therefore considered a class IIb indication for "patients aged less than 75 years, provided that significant renal dysfunction (serum creatinine >2.5 mg/dL in men and >2.0 mg/dL in women) is not present."[24]

Direct Thrombin Inhibitors. Direct and selective thrombin inhibition provides theoretical advantages over UFH in terms of ease of administration, predictability of anticoagulation, and bleeding risks. Two early trials using adjunctive hirudin versus heparin in combination with thrombolysis showed equivalent 30-day mortality and recurrent MI rates.[30,31] The Hirulog and Early Reperfusion or Occlusion-2 (HERO-2) trial compared bivalirudin (at the time known as Hirulog) with heparin in more than 17,000 STEMI patients initially treated with streptokinase.[32] This large randomized trial showed no improvement in 30-day mortality rates with bivalirudin over heparin with worrisome increases in rates of mild and moderate bleeding. These results thus suggest no role for bivalirudin as a routine substitute for UFH or a LMWH. Bivalirudin may therefore only be a "useful alternative to heparin to be used with streptokinase in patients with contraindications to indirect antithrombin therapy or known heparin-induced thrombocytopenia" (class 2a recommendation).[24]

Where Are We Today?

Thrombolytic therapy has clearly revolutionized STEMI care over the past two decades. A significant reduction in mortality and secondary cardiac outcomes has been documented with both streptokinase and tPA. The GUSTO trial showed an additional 1% absolute risk reduction in mortality favoring tPA over streptokinase,[6] with tPA considered as the "gold standard" in pharmacologic reperfusion therapy ever since. In addition to streptokinase and tPA, several second- and third-generation thrombolytic agents are presently available. Of these drugs, only rPA and TNK-tPA have been convincingly shown to provide equivalent efficacy and safety profiles to tPA while improving early coronary patency rates and simplifying dosage regimens.

The addition of combination therapies has so far focused on the administration of various antiplatelet and antithrombin agents, with the intention of facilitating thrombolysis and reducing the extent of injury. Aspirin remains a cornerstone of STEMI therapy as it was shown in the ISIS-2 trial to provide a survival benefit equivalent to that of streptokinase alone.[5] A relatively new and potent target of platelet inhibition has been the final common pathway of platelet aggregation through the administration of glycoprotein IIb/IIIa inhibitors. Although this class of medication has shown significant benefits in non-STEMI ACS patients, no clear survival benefit has been associated with their administration as adjunctive therapy to thrombolysis. The addition of intravenous heparin remains paramount to the efficacy of the fibrin-specific agents. However, a high degree of care with respect to dosing should be exercised to minimize the potential for untoward bleeding. More recently, the LMWH class has been investigated as an alternative to heparin due to ease of administration, predictability of anticoagulant effect, and specific antifactor Xa properties. Enoxaparin in particular has been shown to be a valid alternative to UFH following thrombolysis in patients younger than 75 years of age and without significant renal dysfunction.[29] Direct thrombin inhibitors have yielded only equivocal results, particularly with the use of bivalirudin. Concerns over safety bleeding end points have limited the widespread application of this agent in combination with thrombolytic agents.

The advances in pharmacologic reperfusion notwithstanding, several fundamental problems inherent to thrombolytic therapy persist. First, about one third of STEMI patients randomized to reperfusion therapy in large clinical trials do not achieve early patency and TIMI-3 flow in the infarct-related artery. The importance of this observation comes from the strong association between 90-minute TIMI-3 flow in the infarct-related artery and overall survival. Using the GUSTO patient population, Ross et al reported 30-day mortality rates of 4.6% and 8.0% for patients with initial TIMI-3 and TIMI-0-2 flow, respectively.[33] First, this association carries long-term prognostic value; the 2-year mortality rates are 7.9% and 15.7%, respectively. Second, even the best combination reperfusion regimens are associated with substantial reocclusion and early recurrent ischemia in approximately 15% to 20% of patients. Third, a limited number of STEMI patients have absolute contraindications to thrombolytic agents and are therefore not eligible for pharmacologic reperfusion. With these issues in mind, the role of mechanical reperfusion therapy is ever expanding. Advances in catheter-based reperfusion therapy have created a need to redefine interactions between pharmacologic and mechanical reperfusion. The role of the cardiac catheterization laboratory in rescue, delayed, and facilitated PCI will be discussed in a subsequent section.

THROMBOLYSIS IN UNSTABLE ANGINA

A reduction in intrinsic fibrinolytic activity has been reported in patients admitted with non-STEMI ACS. A number of investigations have thus explored the utility of thrombolytic therapy in this disease state. The TIMI-IIIB investigators evaluated the effects of tPA in 1473 patients with unstable angina or non-Q-wave myocardial infarction.[34] The combined primary end point of death, myocardial infarction, or failure of initial therapy at 6 weeks occurred in 54.2% of the placebo group and 55.5% of the tPA group. Paradoxically, rates of subsequent acute myocardial infarction were increased with tPA treatment along with intracranial hemorrhage (7.4% vs 4.9% for STEMI; 0.55% vs 0% for intracranial hemorrhage; tPA vs placebo, respectively). These findings were further supported by additional results from the ISIS-2[35] and GISSI[36] trials. Explanations for why thrombolytic treatment in ACS might be associated with increased event rates include plaque hemorrhage, inappropriate activation of the fibrinolytic cascade, and unwarranted bleeding complications. Consequently, fibrinolytic agents are absolutely contraindicated in the management of ACS patients (class 3 recommendation, 2002 ACC/AHA Guidelines Update for the Management of Patients with Unstable Angina and Non–ST-Segment Elevation Myocardial Infarction).[37]

THE CARDIAC CATHETERIZATION LABORATORY AND THROMBOLYTIC THERAPY

Over the past decade, primary PCI has emerged as the preferred option for reperfusion in STEMI. A meta-analysis by Keeley and colleagues of 7739 thrombolytic-eligible STEMI patients

demonstrated significant benefits in favor of mechanical reperfusion.[38] Primary PCI was superior to thrombolytic therapy at reducing mortality (7% vs 9%, respectively), nonfatal reinfarction (3% vs 7%, respectively), and stroke (1% vs 2%, respectively). Furthermore, the benefits attributed to primary PCI were sustained at long-term follow-up and were independent of thrombolytic agent, transfer delay (up to 3 hours), and on-site cardiac surgery availability at receiving hospitals (Figure 21-3). Nevertheless, thrombolytic therapy remains an essential strategy for STEMI care in view of the lack of availability of PCI because of geographic, logistic, and economic factors. Given the important association between prompt successful reperfusion and clinical outcomes on the one hand, and delays inherent to patients' transfer on the other hand, the role of thrombolytic therapy remains essential. Uncertainty and controversy persist about treatment strategies combining pharmacologic and mechanical reperfusion. The past few years have witnessed a rapid growth of data on the potential "merger" of these strategies. Issues concerning timing of drug administration (and potential benefits of prehospital fibrinolysis), failure of pharmacologic reperfusion (and the benefits and risks of rescue PCI), and potential benefits from early routine post-thrombolytic PCI (facilitated PCI) are particularly important and complex.

【 】 PREHOSPITAL THROMBOLYSIS AND RESCUE PERCUTANEOUS CORONARY INTERVENTION

Whether prehospital administration of a thrombolytic agent by experienced medical staff and the ensuing reduction of the time-to-reperfusion interval translate into improved clinical outcomes has generated significant debate. These questions were investigated by the Comparison of Angioplasty and Prehospital Thrombolysis in Acute Myocardial Infarction (CAPTIM) study group.[39] A total of 840 patients presenting within 6 hours of symptom onset were randomized to prehospital accelerated tPA or primary PCI. Although the median delay between symptom onset and treatment was significantly shorter in the accelerated thrombolysis group (190 vs 130 minutes), the combined primary end point of 30-day death, nonfatal reinfarction, and nonfatal disabling stroke was not different. In fact, there was a trend toward improved clinical outcomes with the use of primary PCI over accelerated prehospital thrombolysis. Furthermore, 26% of patients in the accelerated thrombolysis group underwent rescue PCI. Although these results demonstrate the feasibility of a prehospital thrombolysis protocol, they principally underline the importance of transferring STEMI patients to a PCI-capable hospital as the strategy of choice following thrombolysis.

【 】 FACILITATED PERCUTANEOUS CORONARY INTERVENTION

The role of a strategy of routine catheterization within hours of thrombolysis was examined by the Southwest German International Study in Acute Myocardial Infarction-III (SIAM-III) study.[40] The composite end point of death, reinfarction, ischemic events, and target lesion revascularization was significantly reduced in the group undergoing routine stenting within six hours of thrombolysis compared to the group undergoing catheterization at

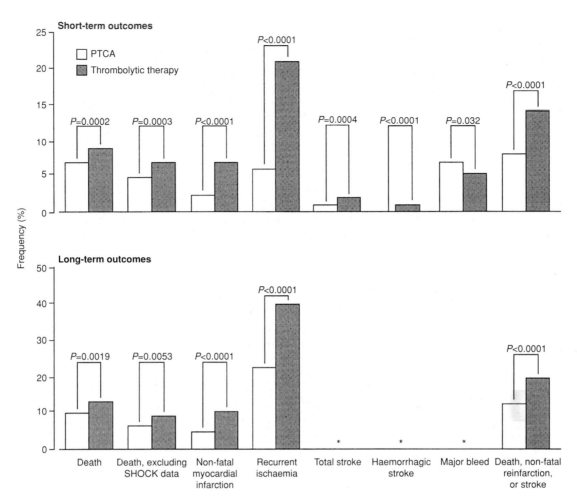

FIGURE 21-3. Short- and long-term clinical outcomes in patients with ST-elevation myocardial infarction treated with primary percutaneous transluminal coronary angioplasty (PTCA) or thrombolytic therapy. A meta-analysis of 23 trials showed that patients assigned to primary PTCA (clear bars) were less likely to die, have a nonfatal myocardial rein-farction, or experience the combined end point of death, nonfatal myocardial reinfarction, or stroke in comparison with patients initially treated with thrombolytic therapy (shaded bars). These outcomes were significantly decreased in the short-term (upper bars) and the long-term (lower bars). *(Reproduced with permission from Keeley, et al.[38])*

2 weeks. Although these results appear to favor a strategy of routine early catheterization following fibrinolytic therapy, the comparison is hardly applicable to the North American medical practice environment where "routine" angiography is usually performed well within 48 hours of presentation. Additional insights from the Primary Angioplasty After Transport of patients From General Community Hospitals to Catheterization Units With/Without Emergency Thrombolysis Infusion (PRAGUE) 1 and 2 trials provided a comparison between on-site thrombolysis, on-site thrombolysis followed by transfer to a PCI-capable center, and early transfer to a PCI-capable center without initial thrombolysis.[41,42]

Interestingly, the PRAGUE-1 trial showed that the most significant reduction in the 30-day composite end point of death, stroke, and reinfarction occurred in the group undergoing early transfer to a PCI-capable hospital without prior thrombolytic therapy.[41] Additionally, analysis of PRAGUE-2 patients who were transferred to PCI-capable hospitals and had presented 3 to 12 hours after symptom onset showed a significant reduction in mortality rates (6.0% vs 15.3%).[42] In comparison, patients transferred within 3 hours of symptom onset showed no mortality benefit

with early transfer to PCI compared to thrombolytic therapy (7.3% vs 7.4%). The Danish Multicenter Randomized Trial on Thrombolytic Therapy versus Acute Coronary Angioplasty in Acute Myocardial Infarction (DANAMI-2) is the largest experience so far to compare on-site thrombolysis to emergency transport for PCI.[43] A significant reduction in the combined 30-day end point of recurrent myocardial infarction, disabling stroke, and death was associated with PCI over thrombolysis (8.5% vs 14.2%). Overall, the DANAMI-2 results favor a strategy of early transfer to a PCI-capable institution whenever this is feasible. A recent meta-analysis by Keeley and colleagues confirmed these results and revealed a significant reduction of the combined end point of death, nonfatal reinfarction, and stroke in STEMI patients who were transferred for primary PCI over patients treated with on-site thrombolysis (Figure 21-4).[38]

The continual introduction of new agents, devices, strategies, catheter-based technologies, and vast amount of trials contribute to the ongoing confusion regarding the choice of optimal reperfusion strategy. The evidence is still accumulating, and the field should be considered highly dynamic. Consequently, the following

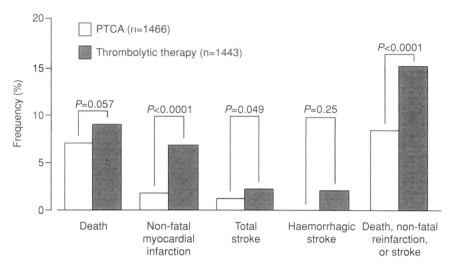

FIGURE 21-4. Meta-analysis of short-term clinical outcomes in patients with ST-elevation myocardial infarction treated with on-site thrombolysis versus transfer for primary percutaneous coronary intervention (PCI). Combined data from five trials comparing on-site thrombolysis (shaded bars) to emergent transfer for primary percutaneous transluminal coronary angioplasty (PTCA) (clear bars) reveal that, despite delays inherent to a transfer strategy, primary PCI was associated with significant reductions in nonfatal myocardial reinfarction, total stroke, and the combined end point of death, nonfatal reinfarction, or stroke in patients transferred to primary PTCA-capable institutions. *(Reproduced with permission from Keeley et al.[38])*

recommendations are derived from the recently updated 2004 AHA-ACC guidelines.[24] Patients with the following conditions are most likely to benefit from an invasive strategy: cardiogenic shock or Killip 3 class, estimated door-to-balloon time interval less than 90 minutes, contraindications to thrombolytic therapy, relatively late presentation (>3 hours after symptom onset), and doubtful STEMI diagnosis. Although a strategy of initial thrombolysis followed by PCI may still be intuitively appealing, current evidence does not suggest any benefits from the *routine* administration of thrombolytic agents prior to PCI if a skilled PCI laboratory and team are readily available. Two exceptions are important to note and warrant initial pharmacologic reperfusion: (1) patients presenting very early following symptom onset (<3 hours) to a non-PCI-capable institution with an anticipated delay for an invasive strategy, and (2) patients requiring a significantly prolonged transfer time (estimated door-to-balloon time interval >90 minutes). Under those specific circumstances, initial thrombolytic therapy should be strongly considered as the initial reperfusion modality.

REFERENCES

1. GISSI Investigators. Effectiveness of intravenous thrombolytic treatment in acute myocardial infarction. Gruppo Italiano per lo Studio della Streptochinasi nell'Infarto Miocardico (GISSI). *Lancet.* 1986;1:397.
2. Eyre H, Kahn R, Robertson RM and the ACS/ADA/AHA Collaborative Writing Committee. Preventing cancer, cardiovascular disease, and diabetes. A common agenda for the American Cancer Society, the American Diabetes Association, and the American Heart Association. *Circulation.* 2004;109:3244.
3. Fletcher AP, Alkjaersig N, Smyrniotis F, et al. The treatment of patients suffering from early myocardial infarction with massive and prolonged streptokinase therapy. *Trans Assoc Am Physicians.* 1958;71:287.
4. DeWood MA, Spores J, Notske R, et al. Prevalence of total coronary occlusion during the early hours of transmural myocardial infarction. *N Engl J Med.* 1980;303:897.
5. ISIS-2 Collaborative Group. Randomised trial of intravenous streptokinase, oral aspirin, both, or neither among 17,187 cases of suspected acute myocardial infarction: ISIS-2. *Lancet.* 1988;332:349.
6. GUSTO Investigators. An international randomized trial comparing four thrombolytic strategies for acute myocardial infarction. The GUSTO investigators. *N Engl J Med.* 1993;329:673.
7. Lincoff AM, Topol EJ. Illusion of reperfusion. Does anyone achieve optimal reperfusion during acute myocardial infarction? *Circulation.* 1993;88:1361.
8. Mahaffey KW, Granger CB, Sloan MA, et al. Risk factors for in-hospital non-hemorrhagic stroke in patients with acute myocardial infarction treated with thrombolysis: results from GUSTO-I. *Circulation.* 1998;97:757.
9. Smalling RW, Bode C, Kalbfleisch J, et al, and the RAPID Investigators. More rapid, complete, and stable coronary thrombolysis with bolus administration of reteplase compared with alteplase infusion in acute myocardial infarction. *Circulation.* 1995;91:2725.
10. Bode C, Smalling RW, Berg G, et al, for the RAPID II Investigators. Randomized comparison of coronary thrombolysis achieved with double-bolus reteplase (recombinant plasminogen activator) and front-loaded, accelerated alteplase (recombinant tissue plasminogen activator) in patients with acute myocardial infarction. *Circulation.* 1996;94:891.
11. INJECT Investigators. Randomised, double-blind comparison of reteplase double-bolus administration with streptokinase in acute myocardial infarction (INJECT): trial to investigate equivalence. *Lancet.* 1995;346:329.
12. GUSTO-III Investigators. A comparison of reteplase with alteplase for acute myocardial infarction. *N Engl J Med.* 1997;337:1118.
13. Topol EJ, Ohman EM, Armstrong PW, et al. Survival outcomes 1 year after reperfusion therapy with either alteplase or reteplase for acute myocardial infarction: results from the Global Utilization of Streptokinase and t-PA for Occluded Coronary Arteries (GUSTO) III Trial. *Circulation.* 2000; 102:1761.
14. Cannon CP, Gibson CM, McCabe CH, et al, for the Thromblysis in Myocardial Infarction (TIMI) 10B Investigators. TNK-Tissue plasminogen activator compared with front-loaded alteplase in acute myocardial infarction. Results of the TIMI 10B Trial. *Circulation.* 1998;98:2805.
15. ASSENT-2 Investigators. Single-bolus tenecteplase compared with front-loaded alteplase in acute myocardial infarction: the ASSENT-2 double-blind randomized trial. *Lancet.* 1999;354:716.
16. Heijer PD, Vermeer F, Ambrosioni E et al, on behalf of the InTIME Investigators. Evaluation of a weight-adjusted single-bolus plasminogen activator in patients with myocardial infarction: a double-blind, randomized angiographic trial of lanoteplase versus alteplase. *Circulation.* 1998;98:2117.

17. InTIME-II Investigators. Intravenous NPA for the treatment of infracting myocardium early. InTIME-II, a double-blind comparison of single-bolus lanoteplase vs accelerated alteplase for the treatment of patients with acute myocardial infarction. *Eur Heart J.* 2000;21:2005.

18. Bhatt DL, Topol EJ. Current role of platelet glycoprotein IIb/IIIa inhibitors in acute coronary syndromes. *JAMA.* 2000;284:1549.

19. Antman EM, Giugliano RP, Gibson CM, et al, for the TIMI 14 Investigators. Abciximab facilitates the rate and extent of thrombolysis. Results of the thrombolysis in myocardial infarction (TIMI) 14 Trial. *Circulation.* 1999;99:2720.

20. SPEED Group. Trial of abciximab with and without low-dose reteplase for acute myocardial infarction. *Circulation.* 2000;101:2788.

21. The GUSTO-V Investigators. Reperfusion therapy for acute myocardial infarction with fibrinolytic therapy or combination reduced fibrinolytic therapy and platelet glycoprotein IIb/IIIa inhibition: the GUSTO-V randomized trial. *Lancet.* 2001;357:1905.

22. ASSENT-3 Investigators. Efficacy and safety of tenecteplase in combination with enoxaparin, abciximab, or unfractionated heparin: the ASSENT-3 randomised trial in acute myocardial infarction. *Lancet.* 2001;358:605.

23. Giugliano RP, McCabe CH, Antman EM, et al, for the Thrombolysis in Myocardial Infarction (TIMI) Investigators. Lower-dose heparin with fibrinolysis is associated with lower rates of intracranial hemorrhage. *Am Heart J.* 2001;141:742.

24. ACC/AHA Guidelines for the Management of Patients with ST-Elevation Myocardial Infarction. *Circulation.* 2004;110:e82. Available at: http://www.acc.org/clinical/guidelines/stemi/index.pdf. Accessed September 28, 2004.

25. Cohen M, Demers C, Gurfinkel EP, et al. A comparison of low-molecular-weight heparin with unfractionated heparin for unstable coronary artery disease. Efficacy and Safety of Subcutaneous Enoxaparin in Non-Q-Wave Coronary Events Study Group. *N Engl J Med.* 1997;337:447.

26. Antman EM, McCabe CH, Gurfinkel EP, et al. Enoxaparin prevents death and cardiac ischemic events in unstable angina/non-Q-wave myocardial infarction. Results of the thrombolysis in myocardial infarction (TIMI) 11B trial. *Circulation.* 1999;100:1593.

27. Ross AM, Molhoek P, Lundergan C, et al, for the HART-II Investigators. Randomized comparison of enoxaparin, a low-molecular-weight heparin, with unfractionated heparin adjunctive to recombinant tissue plasminogen activator thrombolysis and aspirin: second trial of Heparin and Aspirin Reperfusion Therapy (HART-II). *Circulation.* 2001;104:648.

28. Antman EM, Louwerenburg HW, Baars HF, et al. Enoxaparin as adjunctive antithrombin therapy for ST-elevation myocardial infarction: results of the ENTIRE-Thrombolysis in Myocardial Infarction (TIMI) Trial. *Circulation.* 2002;105:1642.

29. Wallentin L, Goldstein P, Armstrong PW, et al. Efficacy and safety of tenecteplase in combination with the low-molecular-weight heparin enoxaparin or unfractionated heparin in the prehospital setting: the Assessment of the Safety and Efficacy of a New Thrombolytic Regimen (ASSENT)-3 PLUS randomized trial in acute myocardial infarction. *Circulation.* 2003;108:135.

30. GUSTO-2b Investigators. A comparison of recombinant hirudin with heparin for the treatment of acute coronary syndromes. *N Engl J Med.* 1996;335:775.

31. Antman EM. Hirudin in acute myocardial infarction. Thrombolysis and Thrombin Inhibition in Myocardial Infarction (TIMI) 9B trial. *Circulation.* 1996;94:911.

32. White H. and The Hirulog and Early Reperfusion or Occlusion (HERO)-2 Trial Investigators. Thrombin-specific anticoagulation with bivalirudin versus heparin in patients receiving fibrinolytic therapy for acute myocardial infarction: the HERO-2 randomised trial. *Lancet.* 2001;358:1855.

33. Ross AM, Coyne KS, Moreyra E, et al. Extended mortality benefit of early postinfarction reperfusion. GUSTO-I Angiographic Investigators. Global Utilization of Streptokinase and Tissue Plasminogen Activator for Occluded Coronary Arteries Trial. *Circulation.* 1998;97:1549.

34. TIMI-IIIB Investigators. Effects of tissue plasminogen activator and a comparison of early invasive and conservative strategies in unstable angina and non-q-wave myocardial infarction. Results of the TIMI-IIIB Trial. *Circulation.* 1994;89:1545.

35. Baigent C, Collins R, Appleby P, et al. ISIS-2: 10 year survival among patients with suspected acute myocardial infarction in randomised comparison of intravenous streptokinase, oral aspirin, both, or neither. The ISIS-2 (Second International Study of Infarct Survival) Collaborative Group. *BMJ.* 1998;316:1337.

36. Franzosi MG, Santoro E, De Vita C, et al. Ten-year follow-up of the first megatrial testing thrombolytic therapy in patients with acute myocardial infarction: results of the Gruppo Italiano per lo Studio della Sopravvivenza nell'Infarto-1 study. The GISSI Investigators. *Circulation.* 1998;98:2659.

37. ACC/AHA Guidelines Update for the Management of Patients with Unstable Angina and Non-ST-Segment Elevation Myocardial Infarction. *J Am Coll Cardiol.* 2002;40:366. Available at: http://www.acc.org/clinical/guidelines/unstable/update_index.htm. Accessed September 28, 2004.

38. Keeley EC, Boura JA, Grines CL. Primary angioplasty versus intravenous thrombolytic therapy for acute myocardial infarction: a quantitative review of 23 randomised trials. *Lancet.* 2003;361:13.

39. Bonnefoy E, Lapostolle F, Leizorovicz A, et al. Comparison of Angioplasty and Prehospital Thromboysis in Acute Myocardial Infarction study group. Primary angioplasty versus prehospital fibrinolysis in acute myocardial infarction: a randomised study. *Lancet.* 2002;360:825.

40. Scheller B, Hennen B, Hammer B, et al, for the SIAM III Study Group. Beneficial effects of immediate stenting after thrombolysis in acute myocardial infarction. *J Am Coll Cardiol.* 2003;42:634.

41. Widimsky P, Groch L, Zelizko M, et al. Multicentre randomized trial comparing transport to primary angioplasty vs immediate thrombolysis vs combined strategy for patients with acute myocardial infarction presenting to a community hospital without a catheterization laboratory. The PRAGUE study. *Eur Heart J.* 2000;21:823.

42. Widimsky P, Budesinsky T, Vorac D, et al, for the 'PRAGUE' Study Group Investigators. Long distance transport for primary angioplasty vs immediate thrombolysis in acute myocardial infarction. Final results of the randomized national multicentre trial–PRAGUE-2. *Eur Heart J.* 2003;24:94.

43. Andersen HR, Niesen TT, Rasmussen K, et al, for the DANAMI-2 Investigators. A comparison of coronary angioplasty with fibrinolytic therapy in acute myocardial infaction. *N Engl J Med.* 2003;349:733.

CHAPTER (22)

Radiographic Contrast Media

Abdallah G. Rebeiz, MD, and J. Kevin Harrison, MD

HISTORY OF CONTRAST AGENT DEVELOPMENT

Ever since Roentgen discovered x-rays in 1895,[1] efforts have been made to image internal body structures. The x-ray absorbance of a structure must be either greater or less than that of surrounding tissues for it to be imaged. Blood vessel walls and myocardium have similar x-ray absorbance to that of blood, making their imaging by conventional radiographic techniques virtually impossible without the use of an intravascular contrast agent. By virtue of their high absorbance of x-rays, contrast agents increase the radiographic density of a vascular structure's lumen. Initial efforts at imaging blood vessels focused on bromide-containing solutions,[2] but these were quickly abandoned because of toxicity. Researchers soon identified iodine as the element with optimal physical and biological properties for intravascular imaging. Since the first report of use of sodium iodide solution for arterial imaging in 1924,[3] there have been multiple breakthroughs and refinements in the manufacture of iodinated contrast agents. These have included the incorporation of iodine into organic molecules[4] and the synthesis of molecules with a higher iodine content, such as acetrizoic acid, a tri-iodinated aromatic molecule. Further modifications of this molecule led to the synthesis of diatrizoic acid (Hypaque, Renographin), which was the most commonly used intravascular contrast agent for more than two decades (Figure 22-1).[5]

Contrast agents in use before 1980 maintained their aqueous solubility by ionization in solution (ie, they were ionic agents). The cation associated with the iodinated molecules in ionic contrast solutions thus needed to be present in high concentrations in order to achieve adequate concentrations of the contrast agent

molecule for radiographic visualization. This precluded the use of simple cations (such as sodium) for intracoronary injection. Methylglucamine, or meglumine, is an organic cation with no electrophysiologic effects and was preferentially used in most commercially available contrast formulations. Because of the high viscosity of meglumine, a lower concentration of sodium was used in ionic contrast solutions, with a meglumine-to-sodium ratio of 6.6:1 to keep the sodium concentration in the isotonic range. One major drawback of ionic contrast agents is their high osmolality (up to five or six times that of plasma), which is associated with clinical side effects and complications, especially when large volumes of contrast media are used.[6]

Subsequently, attempts were made to synthesize contrast agents with lower osmolalities by replacing the ionizable group with a polar residue, hence maintaining aqueous solubility while halving the osmolality of the formulation. This led to the synthesis of the nonionic compounds iohexol (Omnipaque)[7] and iopamidol (Isovue).[8] Further efforts to decrease the osmolality of contrast formulations focused on the synthesis of ionic agents containing six iodine atoms per molecule, achieved by linking together two tri-iodinated aromatic molecules. The prototype of this class of dimeric contrast agents is ioxaglate (Hexabrix), which is an ionic compound (see Figure 22-1).[9] More recently, iodixanol (Visipaque), a nonionic dimer containing six iodine atoms per molecule, achieved iso-osmolality with blood (see Figure 22-1).

Table 22-1 lists all contrast agents currently available in the United States. It is important to note that the amount of iodine necessary for adequate imaging is many times the body's daily turnover of elemental iodine. Molecular weights of these agents range from 600 to 1700. Preservatives added to contrast agent formulations include ethylenediamine tetra-acetic acid (EDTA) and

A list of the clinical trials cited in Chapters 19 through 24 is presented in Appendix IV-1 at the end of Part IV.

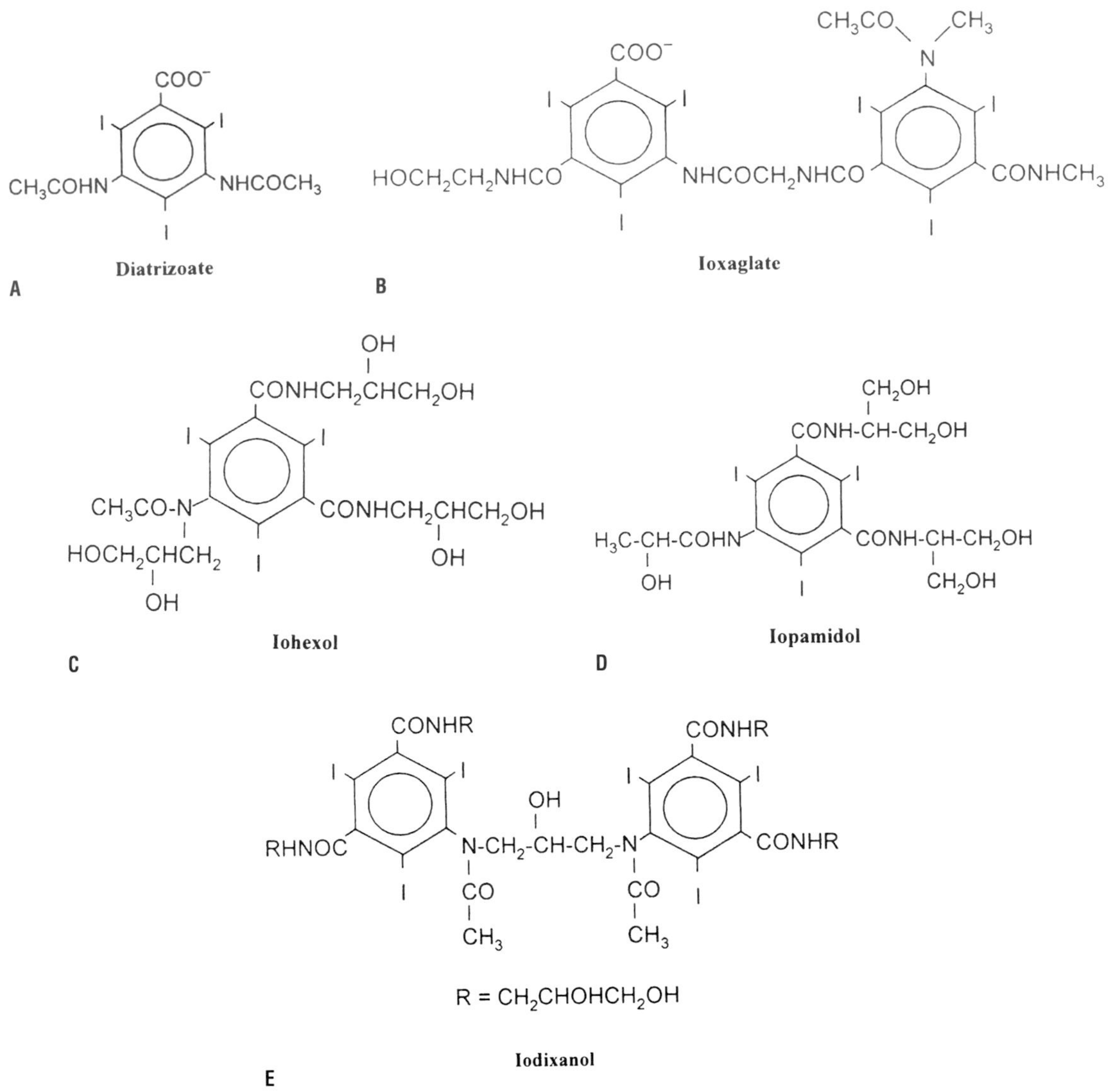

FIGURE 22-1. Schematic representation of the chemical structures of selected iodinated contrast molecules.

vary among different preparations. The calcium-binding properties of these agents led to a transient decrease in serum calcium concentration after contrast administration, but without significant systemic sequelae.[10] However, these calcium chelators play a role in some of the hemodynamic and electrophysiologic adverse reactions seen with intracoronary injection of radiographic contrast. Non-calcium-binding contrast media are associated with fewer hemodynamic alterations than calcium-binding agents.[11] The addition of calcium to contrast formulations reduces the negative inotropic effects caused by calcium-binding additives.[12] The risk of ventricular fibrillation associated with intracoronary contrast injection is also higher with the use of calcium-binding contrast media.[13]

Contrast agent molecules gain access to the entire extracellular fluid compartment promptly after intravascular administration.[14] They exhibit virtually no lipid solubility and minimal plasma protein binding. Given their size and low lipid solubility, contrast molecules do not cross cell membranes. They are filtered in renal glomeruli and are almost entirely excreted in the urine. The elimination half-life of contrast agents from the intravascular space is on the order of 30 minutes.[15]

CARDIOVASCULAR EFFECTS

[ ] HEMODYNAMIC EFFECTS

All contrast agents produce arteriolar vasodilation with a resultant decrease in systemic vascular resistance and a transient drop in arterial pressure shortly after administration.[9] Vasodilation occurs more commonly with high-osmolality agents,[16] high contrast agent volume use, and arterial (compared with venous) injection. Contrast agent administration also leads to an increase in intravascular volume, with agents of higher osmolarity having a greater effect. Ventricular filling pressures therefore rise following intravascular contrast media injection,[17] which is an important consideration in patients with depressed left ventricular function and preexisting elevation of diastolic filling pressures.

Intracoronary injections of contrast agents generally cause a mild decrease in left ventricular contractility, which is transient and of no clinical significance even in patients with moderate left ventricular dysfunction.[18] Lower osmolality agents appear to have

TABLE 22-1

Contrast Agents Approved in the United States

GENERIC NAME	TRADE NAME	IODINE (mg/mL)	OSMOLALITY (mOsm/Kg)
IONIC			
Diatrizoate	Renographin–76	370	1940
Diatrizoate	Hypaque–76	370	2016
Diatrizoate	Angiovist–370	370	2100
Ioxaglate	Hexabrix	320	580
NONIONIC			
Iohexol	Omnipaque	180	408
		240	520
		300	672
		350	844
Iopamidol	Isovue 300	300	616
	Isovue 370	370	796
Ioversol	Optiray 320	320	702
	Optiray 350	350	792
Ioxilan	Oxilan 350	350	695
Iodixanol	Visipaque 320	320	290

Adapted from Fischer HW. Catalog of intravascular contrast media. *Radiology.* 1986;159:561–563.

less of a negative inotropic effect than high-osmolality media.[19] The mechanism underlying the depressant effect of intracoronary contrast agents on myocardial contractile performance is probably multifactorial and related to calcium-binding properties,[20] osmolality of the solution, and transient ischemia.

Injection of contrast media into a coronary artery causes a transient decrease in coronary vascular resistance and an increase in coronary blood flow.[21] These changes do not appear to alter the angiographic assessment of epicardial artery size.[22]

[ ] ELECTROPHYSIOLOGIC EFFECTS

Contrast agents cause several electrophysiologic alterations when injected in coronary arteries. Intracoronary administration of contrast, especially of high osmolar ionic agents, causes transient sinus bradycardia for approximately 1 minute. This effect is also more pronounced after right coronary artery injections, presumably because this artery more commonly supplies the sinoatrial and atrioventricular nodes. The mechanism of this bradycardia involves vagal reflex activation in addition to direct effects on the sinoatrial node.[23] In addition, contrast agents cause QRS prolongation, axis shift, ST-segment depression, P-R prolongation, and QT prolongation on the surface electrocardiogram.[24] Many of these changes are markedly reduced with newer nonionic agents such as iodixanol.[25]

All contrast agents lower the heart's ventricular fibrillation threshold. The propensity for ventricular fibrillation is influenced by the quantity of intracoronary contrast injected, the duration of injection, and the properties of the contrast formulation used.[26] The combination of ischemia and intracoronary contrast reduces the ventricular fibrillation threshold even further.[26]

ADVERSE REACTIONS

[ ] ANAPHYLACTOID REACTIONS

Anaphylactic and anaphylactoid reactions are probably the most feared complication of radiographic contrast exposure. Typical symptoms include varying degrees of urticaria, bronchospasm, angioedema, vasodilation, and hypotension. Progression to cardiovascular collapse or total airway obstruction may occur. The exact mechanism of these reactions is unknown, but it does involve complement and kinin release and mast cell degranulation.[27] These reactions do not necessarily involve IgE release and can occur on first exposure to contrast agents.[28] The overall frequency of anaphylactoid reactions (including mild reactions) is approximately 5%, but the risk of severe reactions is on the order of 0.1%.[29] In patients with a history of immediate anaphylactoid reaction to iodinated contrast, the risk of a repeat reaction is about 15%.[29]

The management of mild or moderate anaphylactoid reactions is usually aimed at symptom alleviation, and includes fluid administration and H_1 and H_2 histamine receptor antagonists. The management of severe reactions may necessitate endotracheal intubation, fluid resuscitation and vasopressor support. It is therefore imperative for catheterization and angioplasty laboratories to be equipped with resuscitation carts.

The prevention of anaphylactoid complications is critical in patients with a history of prior contrast reactions. There are no placebo-controlled studies of prophylactic measures in this patient population. In a nonrandomized series of patients with prior anaphylactoid reactions, prophylaxis with prednisone and diphenhydramine was associated with a 10.8% rate of generalized reactions, but only 0.7% had transient hypotension. The addition of ephedrine to the prophylactic regimen reduced the incidence of reactions to 5%.[30] The use of sympathomimetic drugs such as ephedrine, however, is not safe in the patient with cardiac disease. In a randomized study of routine oral corticosteroid prophylaxis prior to intravenous ionic contrast administration in 6763 consecutive patients, methylprednisolone given as two doses, 12 hours and 2 hours prior to dye exposure, was associated with a significant reduction in all reactions compared to a 1-dose regimen (6.4% vs 9.4%, $P < .05$). The incidence of adverse reactions was comparable between the placebo group and the 1-dose regimen group.[31] Routine pretreatment with histamine receptor antagonists prior to contrast agent exposure has been shown to significantly reduce the incidence of nausea, angioedema, and urticaria.[32] A systematic strategy of diphenhydramine premedication (25 mg intravenous) for all patients undergoing cardiac catheterization or percutaneous intervention is recommended. For patients with a history of generalized reactions, 50 mg diphenhydramine, 300 mg cimetidine, and corticosteroid treatment (preferably 12 hours preprocedure) is often prescribed as a prophylactic regimen.

[ ] OTHER TOXIC EFFECTS

The most common adverse reactions to ionic contrast agents are nausea and vomiting, occurring in 10% to 20% of patients. These reactions have been virtually eliminated by the nonionic agents.[33] Contrast agents also cause erythrocyte deformation by osmolar extraction of intracellular water, which can result in capillary plugging due to decreased red blood cell conformation to the microcirculation. Ultrastructural changes in endothelial cells have also been reported following contrast injection, but their clinical significance is unknown.[34] Overall, large registry surveys show that the incidence of adverse reactions has been significantly reduced with the use of nonionic contrast media.[35] Randomized trials have also shown that the incidence of adverse reactions with nonionic low-osmolality agents is consistently lower than with ionic high-osmolarity agents.[36] Barrett et al reported the risk of moderate reactions to be 3-fold higher with ionic compared with nonionic agents in one study.[37]

NEPHROTOXICITY

Contrast nephropathy is a common cause of hospital-acquired renal failure and results in substantial morbidity, prolonged lengths of stay, higher hospitalization costs, and increased mortality.[38–40] Although the formal definition of contrast nephropathy varies among studies, the syndrome is most commonly defined as either a greater than 25% increase or a greater than 0.5 mg/dL absolute increase in the serum creatinine above baseline within 48 hours of contrast administration.[41] Depending on the definition used and the patient population studied, contrast nephropathy has been reported to occur in zero to two thirds of patients following contrast administration.[38,42–44] In a typical unselected population of patients undergoing coronary angiography and using a definition of an increase in serum creatinine of greater than 0.5 mg/dL over baseline, contrast nephropathy can be expected to occur in 2% to 10% of patients;[42,45] it ranges in severity from transient nonoliguric renal dysfunction to overt renal failure requiring dialysis. The risk of contrast nephropathy is low in patients with normal renal function, occurring in less than 2% of such patients.[38,39] In patients who develop contrast nephropathy, approximately 5% to 10% may require transient dialysis and about 1% will require long-term dialysis.[46]

The increase in serum creatinine concentration secondary to radiocontrast nephropathy usually peaks 3 to 5 days after contrast administration, with return to baseline levels in most cases by 7 to 10 days.[38] The single most important risk factor for the development of contrast nephropathy is baseline renal dysfunction. Other baseline characteristics and clinical conditions associated with increased risk of contrast-induced renal dysfunction include diabetes mellitus, congestive heart failure, volume depletion, and the concomitant administration of nephrotoxic drugs such as cyclosporine and nonsteroidal anti-inflammatory agents.[39,45] Given the age-related decline in renal function, the elderly have a 3-fold higher risk of contrast nephropathy compared with younger patients.[47] In patients with baseline serum creatinine concentra-

tions equal to or greater than 2.0 mg/dL, the risk of developing contrast nephropathy seems to increase with use of high volumes of contrast solution.[48] There does not seem to be a strong relation between volume of contrast administered and the incidence of contrast nephropathy in patients with normal baseline renal function.[45] Regardless of contrast volume used, the threat of contrast nephropathy does appear higher for patients receiving contrast for a second time within 72 hours of a first exposure.[49,50]

Although its pathogenesis remains unclear, contrast nephropathy is probably due to a combination of decreased renal medullary perfusion resulting in critical medullary ischemia and direct tubular toxicity.[51] Contrast administration causes a reduction in renal medullary blood flow and tissue oxygen content and an increase in red blood cell aggregability.[52] Several mechanisms for the contrast-induced alteration in medullary blood flow have been proposed, including alterations in the renin-angiotensin system, nitric oxide synthesis, adenosine metabolism, prostacyclin production, and endothelin synthesis.[46,53,54] In addition to impaired renal hemodynamics, contrast agents have a direct cytotoxic effect on renal tissue.[55] Iodinated contrast molecules have been shown to increase the production of oxygen free radicals in renal tissue, which in turn contributes to the vasoconstrictor response of the renal vasculature.[56] The mechanism of reactive oxygen species generation is not entirely clear but could result from direct contrast-mediated injury to the glomerular basement membrane and mesangium, with resultant polymorphonuclear chemotaxis and oxygen free radical release within the glomerulus. Another potential mechanism may be a direct generation of free radicals by the radiocontrast medium itself, with the iodine molecules on the benzoic acid moiety serving as a radical initiating species.[57]

Despite its predominantly transient nature, contrast nephropathy is a predictor of long-term adverse outcomes. In a case-control study, in-hospital mortality in 183 patients with radiocontrast nephropathy was 34% compared with 7% in control patients.[58] The degree of renal impairment appears to correlate with mortality as well. In one particular study, patients with an increase in serum creatinine of 0.5 to 0.9 mg/dL postcontrast exposure had an in-hospital mortality of 3.8% compared with 64% in those with a creatinine elevation greater than 3.0 mg/dL.[38] In patients undergoing percutaneous coronary intervention (PCI), the occurrence of contrast nephropathy also portends poor clinical outcomes. In a study of 1826 consecutive patients undergoing PCI, renal failure occurred in 14.5% of patients and dialysis-requiring renal failure occurred in 0.7%. In-hospital mortality was more than 30-fold greater in patients with diabetes who developed acute renal failure than in patients who did not (35.7 vs 1.1%, $P < .05$).[39] In another study of high-risk PCI patients with baseline serum creatinine concentrations greater than or equal to 1.8 mg/dL, there was a 37% incidence of contrast nephropathy. In-hospital mortality was significantly higher in patients who developed renal failure (14.9% vs 4.9%, $P = .001$). One-year mortality rates were 45.2% in patients who developed dialysis-dependent real failure, 35.4% in patients with milder degrees of contrast nephropathy, and 19.4% in patients who did not develop renal failure post-PCI.[59] Finally, in a study of 7586 patients undergoing coronary intervention, those with renal failure had a 5-year mortality rate of 44.6% compared with 14.5% in those who did not develop renal dysfunction following percutaneous revascularization.[45]

Several studies have compared the effect of different contrast agents on the risk of contrast nephropathy.[42,60–62] In 443 patients undergoing cardiac catheterization and randomized to iopamidol, a low-osmolality nonionic agent, or diatrizoate, a high-osmolality, ionic agent, Schwab and colleagues reported no significant difference in the incidence of nephropathy in both low-risk and high-risk patient cohorts.[60] In the larger Iohexol Cooperative Study, patients with baseline renal insufficiency experienced significantly lower rates of nephropathy with the nonionic agent iohexol compared with diatrizoate.[42] In a systematic overview of trials comparing high- and low-osmolality agents, low-osmolality contrast formulations were associated with a lower incidence of contrast nephropathy, particularly in patients with preexisting renal dysfunction.[63]

The Contrast Utilization in high-Risk PTCA (COURT) trial compared the low-osmolar, ionic agent ioxaglate with the iso-osmolar, nonionic, dimeric contrast iodixanol in 815 patients with acute coronary syndrome undergoing PCI; the patients had serum creatinine levels less than 2 mg/dL. No significant differences were observed in the incidence of contrast nephropathy between both arms.[61] In a recent study, patients with diabetes and baseline renal impairment undergoing coronary or aortofemoral angiography were randomized to receive either iodixanol or the low-osmolality, nonionic, monomeric contrast medium iohexol. The mean increase in serum creatinine concentration following contrast administration was significantly lower in the iodixanol group compared with the iohexol group ($P = .001$). Three percent of patients receiving iodixanol had a 0.5 mg/dL increase in serum creatinine from baseline compared with 26% of those receiving iohexol ($P = .002$).[62] The use of the iso-osmolar agent iodixanol is therefore recommended for patients undergoing PCI who are at increased risk of developing contrast related renal dysfunction.

Several prophylactic strategies for the prevention of contrast nephropathy have been investigated, including the use of diuretics,[64] calcium channel antagonists,[65] endothelin receptor antagonists,[66] dopamine,[67] and the selective dopamine-1 receptor agonist fenoldopam.[68] These interventions have not shown benefit to date. Hydration remains the essential prophylactic measure in high-risk patients;[64] isotonic 0.9% saline hydration is a superior regimen to half-isotonic saline, as shown in a large randomized trial of high-risk PCI patients.[69] N-acetylcysteine has also been shown to be beneficial in the prevention of contrast nephropathy and is recommended for patients with a baseline creatinine clearance less than 50 mL/min.[70]

CONTRAST MEDIA AND PERCUTANEOUS INTERVENTION: THROMBOEMBOLIC CONSIDERATIONS

Contrast media have been shown to interact with coagulation factors and platelets, which can influence the safety and clinical outcome of percutaneous revascularization procedures.[71] Ionic agents bind to thrombin's anion binding site and inhibit thrombin's ability to activate the platelet thrombin receptor. These agents prolong prothrombin time and inhibit platelet aggregation and degranulation.[72,73] Ionic agents exhibit greater inhibition of coagulation and platelet function compared with nonionic agents in vitro.[71,74]

Several studies have compared thrombotic complications of ionic and nonionic contrast agents in patients undergoing PCI, with varying results.[61,75–78]

In one of the earliest prospective randomized trials of ionic versus nonionic contrast use in PCI, Grines et al randomized 211 patients undergoing percutaneous transluminal coronary angioplasty (PTCA) for unstable coronary syndromes to ioxaglate (ionic medium) or iohexol (nonionic contrast agent).[75] Patients receiving ionic contrast were significantly less likely to experience a decrease in Thrombolysis In Myocardial Infarction (TIMI) flow during PCI compared with patients receiving nonionic contrast (8.1% vs 17.8%, $P = .04$). There were no differences in final percentage diameter stenosis and procedural success rates between groups. Patients in the nonionic contrast arm had a higher incidence of repeat catheterization and angioplasty during the index hospitalization than those in the ionic contrast arm.[75] In another study, 30 patients with unstable angina were also randomized at the time of PTCA to either ioxaglate or iohexol; all patients underwent coronary angioscopy before and after PTCA. After PTCA, 5 patients (33.3%) in the ioxaglate arm and 11 (73.6%) in the iohexol arm developed angioscopically visible new thrombus.[76] However, in another study comparing ioxaglate to iopamidol (nonionic contrast agent) in 210 patients undergoing PTCA for unstable angina, there were no differences between groups in the incidence of coronary dissection, thrombus formation, or abrupt vessel closure.[79]

In an analysis of patients enrolled in the Angioplasty Substudy of the Global Use of Strategies to Open Occluded Arteries in Acute Coronary Syndromes (GUSTO IIb) trial, the outcomes of patients undergoing primary angioplasty for acute ST-segment elevation myocardial infarction were compared based on whether they received ionic or nonionic contrast media. The choice of contrast was at the discretion of the individual investigators and was not randomized. The composite end point of death, reinfarction, or refractory ischemia occurred less frequently in the ionic contrast group compared with the nonionic contrast group during the index hospitalization (4.4% vs 11%, $P = .018$) and at 30 days (5.5% vs 11%, $P = .044$). These differences were no longer significant, however, after adjustment for imbalances in baseline characteristics between groups.[77]

The COURT trial was a large randomized study comparing iodixanol (nonionic) to ioxaglate (ionic) in 856 patients with unstable coronary syndromes undergoing PCI. Approximately one third of patients in each arm underwent stent placement. The primary end point of in-hospital (MACE) occurred significantly less frequently in the iodixanol group than in the ioxaglate group (5.4% vs 9.5%, $P = .027$). Angiographic success defined by a blinded core laboratory was more frequent in the iodixanol arm compared with the ioxaglate arm.[61] The Visipaque in percutaneous transluminal coronary angioplasty (VIP) trial also sought to compare iodixanol to ioxaglate in the PCI setting. In this trial, 1411 patients undergoing PCI for various indications (stable angina, unstable angina, silent ischemia) were randomized to iodixanol or ioxaglate. There was no difference in MACE between both groups at 2 days and at 1 month of follow-up.[78] However, in another large trial of patients undergoing coronary stent placement and randomly assigned to receive ioxaglate or one of several nonionic contrast media, ioxaglate was associated with a significant reduction in subacute stent thrombosis and in 12-month MACE (death or revascularization).[80] The stents used were early generation stents, however, and platelet glycoprotein IIb/IIIa inhibitors were only used in approximately 5% of patients.

With regards to peripheral vascular interventions, ioxaglate was compared to iobitridol (a nonionic low-osmolar contrast) in one randomized controlled trial that enrolled 189 patients undergoing renal artery angioplasty. There were no differences between both groups in the incidence of thromboembolic complications.[81]

It is evident that no unifying conclusion can be reached from the multitude of clinical trials that have compared ionic to non-ionic contrast agents with regards to thrombotic adverse events. It is critical to realize that thromboembolic complications in the setting of percutaneous intervention are influenced by a variety of factors, including adjunctive antithrombin and antiplatelet pharmacotherapy, procedural technique such as frequent flushing of guiding catheters, the specific devices used, and length and complexity of the procedure. One pivotal lesson to derive is the need to always avoid long "dwell times" of contrast-blood contact by frequently flushing catheters with heparinized saline, especially in long cases requiring use of different devices (brachytherapy, atherectomy, laser, etc), and to avoid "bloody" control syringes.

CONCLUSIONS

Intravascular contrast agents have been refined over the years to improve image quality and to reduce the frequency of adverse reactions. Nonionic agents have eliminated several untoward effects of intravascular contrast administration, and offer an excellent alternative to ionic agents. Recent trials in high-risk patients seem to favor the use of iodixanol in an attempt to reduce serious renal toxicity. Tailoring contrast choice based on contemporary evidence is recommended to optimize clinical outcomes in percutaneous intervention.

REFERENCES

1. Roentgen W. On a new kind of rays. *Erst Mitt Sitzber Phys Med Ges.* 1895;137.
2. Berberich J, Hirsch S. Die roentgenographische darstellun der arterien und venen am lebenden. *Muench Klin Wschr.* 1923;49:2226.
3. Brooks B. Intraarterial injection of sodium iodide. *JAMA.* 1924;82:1016.
4. Swick M. Intravenous urography by means of Uroselectan. *Am J Surg.* 1930;8:405.
5. Hoppe J, Larsen H, Coulston F. Observations on the toxicity of a new urographic contrast medium, sodium 3,5-diacetamido-2,4,6 triiodobenzoate (Hypaque sodium) and related compounds. *J Pharmacol Exp Ther.* 1956;116:394.
6. Almen T. Contrast agent design. *J Theor Biol.* 1969;24:216.
7. Lindgren E. Iohexol: a non-ionic contrast medium: pharmacology and toxicology. *Acta Radiol.* 1980;362(suppl).
8. McKinstry D, Rommel A, Sugarman A. Pharmacokinetics, metabolism, and excretion of iopamidol in healthy subjects. *Invest Radiol.* 1984;19:S171.
9. Hirshfeld JJ, Laskey W, Martin J, et al. Hemodynamic changes induced by cardiac angiography with ioxaglate: comparison with diatrizoate. *J Am Coll Cardiol.* 1983;2:954.
10. Berger R, Gomez L, Mallette L. Acute hypocalcemic effects of clinical contrast media injections. *Am J Roentgenol.* 1982;138:282.
11. Murdock D, Walsh J, Euler D, et al. Inotropic effects of ionic contrast media: the role of calcium-binding additives. *Cathet Cardiovasc Diagn.* 1984;10:455.
12. Hanley P, Holmes D, Julsrud P, et al. Use of conventional and newer and newer radiographic contrast agents in cardiac angiography. *Prog Cardiovasc Dis.* 1986;28:435.
13. Zukerman L, Friehling T, Wolf N, et al. Effect of calcium binding additives on ventricular fibrillation and repolarization changes during coronary angiography. *J Am Coll Cardiol.* 1987;10:1249.
14. Dean P, Kivissaari L, Kormano M. The diagnostic potential of contrast enhancement pharmacokinetics. *Invest Radiol.* 1978;13:533.
15. Aulie Michelet A. Effects of intravascular contrast media on blood-brain barrier. Comparison between iothalamate, iohexol, iopentol, and iodixanol. *Acta Radiol.* 1987;28:329.
16. Read R, Johnson J, Vick J, et al. Vascular effects of hypertonic solutions. *Circ Res.* 1960;8:538.
17. Higgins C, Gerber K, Mattrey R, et al. Evaluation of the hemodynamic effects of intravenous administration of ionic and nonionic contrast materials. *Radiology.* 1982;142:681.
18. Higgins C, Sovak M, Schmidt W, et al. Direct myocardial effects of intracoronary administration of new contrast materials with low. *Invest Radiol.* 1980;15:39.
19. Mancini G, Bloomquist J, Bhargava V, et al. Hemodynamic and electrocardiographic effects in man of a new nonionic contrast agent (iohexol): advantages over standard ionic agents. *Am J Cardiol.* 1983;51:1218.
20. Bourdillon P, Bettmann M, McCracken S, et al. Effects of a new nonionic and a conventional ionic contrast agent on coronary sinus ionized calcium and left ventricular hemodynamics in dogs. *J Am Coll Cardiol.* 1985; 6:845.
21. Kloster F, Griesen W, Green G, et al. Effects of coronary arteriography on myocardial blood flow. *Circulation.* 1972;46:438.
22. Hill J, Feldman R, Conti C, et al. Effects of selective injection of contrast media on coronary artery diameter. *Cathet Cardiovasc Diagn.* 1982;8:547.
23. Frink R, Merrick B, Lowe H. Mechanism of the bradycardia during coronary angiography. *Am J Cardiol.* 1975;35:17.
24. Hirshfeld JJ, Wieland J, Davis C, at el. Hemodynamic and elecrocardiographic effects of ioversol during cardiac angiography. *Invest Radiol.* 1989;24:138.
25. Hill J, Cohen M, Kou W, et al. Iodixanol, a new isosmotic nonionic contrast agent, compared with iohexol in cardiac angiography. *Am J Cardiol.* 1994;74:57.
26. Wolf G. Cardiovascular radiology. The fibrillatory propensities of contrast agents. *Invest Radiol.* 1980;15:S208.
27. Greenberger P, Patterson R. Adverse reactions to radiocontrast media. *Prog Cardiovasc Dis.* 1988;31:239.
28. Greenberger P. Contrast media reactions. *J Allergy Clin Immunol.* 1984;74:600.
29. Shehadi W. Contrast media adverse reactions: Occurence, recurrence, and distribution patterns. *Radiology.* 1982;143:11.
30. Greenberger P, Patterson R, Tapio C. Prophylaxis against repeated radiocontrast media reactions in 857 cases. Adverse experience with cimetidine and safety of beta-adrenergic antagonists. *Arch Intern Med.* 1985;145:2197.
31. Lasser E, Berry C, Talner L, al e. Pretreatment with corticosteroids to alleviate reactions to intravenous contrast material. *New Engl J Med.* 1987;317:845.
32. Ring J, Rothenberger K, Clauss W. Prevention of anaphylactoid reactions after radiographic contrast media infusion by combined histamine H1 and H2 receptor antagonists: results of a prospective controlled trial. *Int Arch Allergy Appl Immunol.* 1985;78:9.
33. Wisneski J, Gertz E, Dahlgren M, Muslin A. Comparison of low osmolality ionic (ioxaglate) versus nonionic (iopamidol) contrast media in cardiac angiography. *Am J Cardiol.* 1989;63:489.
34. Parvez Z, Khan T, Moncada R. Ultrastructural changes in rat aortic endothelium during contrast media infusion. *Invest Radiol.* 1985;20:407.
35. Katayama H, Yamaguchi K, Kozuka T, et al. Adverse reactions to ionic and nonionic contrast media. *Radiology.* 1990;175:621.
36. Barrett B, Parfrey P, Vavasour H, et al. A comparison of nonionic low-osmolality radiocontrast agents with ionic, high-osmolality agents during cardiac catheterization. *N Engl J Med.* 1992;326:425.
37. Steinberg E, Moore R, Powe N, et al. Safety and cost effectiveness of high-osmolality as compared with low-osmolality contrast material in patients undergoing cardiac catheterization. *N Engl J Med.* 1992;326:425.
38. Berns A. Nephrotoxicity of contrast media. *Kidney Int.* 1989;36:730.
39. McCullough P, Wolyn R, Rocher L, et al. Acute renal failure after coronary intervention: incidence, risk factors, and relationship to mortality. *Am J Med.* 1997;103:368.
40. Iakovou I, Dangas G, Lansky A, et al. Predictors of contrast induced nephropathy after percutaneous coronary intervention in patients with and without chronic renal failure. *J Am Coll Cardiol.* 2002;39:56A.
41. Brinker J. No CAN? *Cathet Cardiovasc Intervent.* 2001;52:417.
42. Rudnick M, Goldfarb S, Wexler L, et al. Nephrotoxicity of ionic and nonionic contrast media in 1196 patients: a randomized trial. The Iohexol Cooperative Study. *Kidney Int.* 1995;47:254.

43. Mason R, Arbeit L, Giron F. Renal dysfunction after arteriography. *JAMA*. 1985;253:1001.

44. Rich M, Crecelius C. Incidence, risk factors, and clinical course of acute renal insufficiency after cardiac catheterization in patients 70 years of age and older: a prospective study. *Arch Intern Med*. 1990;150:1237.

45. Rihal C, Textor S, Grill D, et al. Incidence and prognostic importance of acute renal failure after percutaneous coronary intervention. *Circulation*. 2002; 105:2259.

46. Deray G. Nephrotoxicity of contrast media. *Nephrol Dial Transpl*. 1999; 14:2602.

47. Batchelor W, Anstrom K, Muhlbaier L, et al. Contemporary outcome trends in the elderly undergoing percutaneous coronary interventions in 7,472 octogenarians. *J Am Coll Cardiol*. 2000;36:723.

48. Taliercio C, Vlietstra R, Fisher L, et al. Risks for renal dysfunction with cardiac angiography. *Ann Intern Med*. 1986;104:501.

49. Tublin M, Murphy M, Tessler F. Current concepts in contrast media-induced nephropathy. *Am J Roentgenol*. 1998;171.

50. Byrd L, Sherman R. Radiocontrast-induced acute renal failure: a clinical and pathophyciologic review. *Medicine*. 1979;58:270.

51. Brezis M, Rosen S. Hypoxia of the renal medulla–its implications for disease. *N Engl J Med*. 1995;332:647.

52. Barrett B. Contrast nephrotoxicity. *J Am Soc Nephrol*. 1994;5:125.

53. Pflueger A, Larson T, Nath K, et al. Role of adenosine in contrast media-induced acute renal failure in diabetes mellitus. *Mayo Clin Proc*. 2000;75:1275.

54. Margulies K, Hildebrand F, Heublein D, et al. Radiocontrast increases plasma and urinary endothelin. *J Am Soc Nephrol*. 1991;2:1041.

55. Tomasso C. Contrast-induced nephrotoxicity in patients undergoing cardiac catheterization. *Cathet Cardiovasc Intervent*. 1994;31:316.

56. Bakris G, Lass N, Gaber A, et al. Radiocontrast medium-induced declines in renal function: a role for oxygen free radicals. *Am J Physiol*. 1990;258:F115.

57. Janzen E. Spin trapping of oxygen radicals. *Methods Enzymol*. 1982;105:188.

58. Levy E, Viscoli C, Horwitz R. The effect of acute renal failure on mortality: a cohort analysis. *JAMA*. 1996;275:1489.

59. Gruberg L, Mintz G, Mehran R, et al. The prognostic implications of further renal function deterioration within 48 hours of interventional coronary procedures in patients with pre-existent chronic renal insufficiency. *J Am Coll Cardiol*. 2000;36:1542.

60. Schwab S, Hlatky M, Pieper K, et al. Contrast nephrotoxicity: a randomized controlled trial of a nonionic and an ionic radiographic contrast agent. *N Engl J Med*. 1989;320:149.

61. Davidson C, Laskey W, Hermiller J, et al. Randomized trial of contrast media utilization in high-risk PTCA: the COURT trial. *Circulation*. 2000; 10:2172.

62. Aspelin P, Aubry P, Fransson S, et al. Nephrotoxic effects in high-risk patients undergoing angiography. *N Engl J Med*. 2003;348:491.

63. Barrett B, Carlisle E. Meta-analysis of the relative nephrotoxicity of high- and low-osmolality iodinated contrast media. *Radiology*. 1993;188:171.

64. Solomon R, Werner C, Mann D, et al. Effects of saline, mannitol, and furosemide on acute decreases in renal function induced by radiocontrast agents. *N Engl J Med*. 1994;331:1416.

65. Neumayer H, Junge C, Kufner A, et al. Prevention of radiocontrast media induced nephrotoxicity by the calcium channel blocker nitrendipine: a prospective randomised trial. *Nephrol Dial Transplant*. 1989;4:1030.

66. Wang A, Holcslaw T, Bashore T, et al. Exacerbation of radiocontrast neprotoxicity by endothelial receptor antagonism. *Kidney Int*. 2000;57:1675.

67. Abizaid A, Clark C, Mintz G, et al. Effects of dopamine and aminophylline on contrast-induced acute renal failure after coronary angioplasty in patients with preexisting renal insufficiency. *Am J Cardiol*. 1999;83:260.

68. Stone G, Tumlin J, Madyoon H, et al. Design and rationale of CONTRAST–a prospective, randomized, placebo-controlled trial of fenoldopam mesylate for the prevention of radiocontrast nephropathy. *Rev Cardiovasc Med*. 2001;2(suppl 1):S31.

69. Mueller C, Buerkle G, Buettner H, et al. Prevention of contrast media-associated nephropathy: randomized comparison of 2 hydration regimens in 1620 patients undergoing coronary angioplasty. *Arch Intern Med*. 2002;162:329.

70. Tepel M, van der Giet M, Schwarzfeld C, et al. Prevention of radiographic-contrast-agent-induced reductions in renal function by acetylcysteine. *N Engl J Med*. 2000;343:180.

71. Dawson P, Hewitt P, Mackie J, et al. Contrast, coagulation, and fibrinolysis. *Invest Radiol*. 1986;21:248.

72. Rao A, Rao V, Willis J, et al. Inhibition of platelet function by contrast media: iopamidol and ioxaglate versis iothalamate. *Radiology*. 1985;156:311.

73. Chronos N, Goodall A, Wilson D, et al. Profound platelet degranulation is an important side effect of some types of contrast media used in interventional cardiology. *Circulation*. 1993;88:2035.

74. Stormorken H, Skalpe I, Testart M. Effect of various contrast media on coagulation, fibrinolysis, and platelet function: an in vitro and in vivo study. *Invest Radiol*. 1986;21:348.

75. Grines C, Schreiber T, Savas V, et al. A randomized trial of low osmolar ionic versus nonionic contrast media in patients with myocardial infarction or unstable angina undergoing percutaneous transluminal coronary angioplasty. *J Am Coll Cardiol*. 1996;27:1381.

76. Qureshi N, den Heijer P, Crijns H. Percutaneous soronary angioscopic comparison of thrombus formation during percutaneous coronary angioplasty with ionic and nonionic low osmolality contrast media in unstable angina. *Am J Cardiol*. 1997;80:700.

77. Batchelor W, Granger C, Kleiman N, et al. A comparison of ionic versus nonionic contrast medium during primary percutaneous transluminal coronary angioplasty for acute myocardial infarction. *Am J Cardiol*. 2000;85:692.

78. Bertrand M, Esplugas E, Piessens J, et al. Influence of a nonionic, iso-osmolar contrast medium (iodixanol) versus an ionic, low-osmolar contrast medium (ioxaglate) on major adverse cardiac events in patients undergoing percutaneous transluminal coronary angioplasty. *Circulation*. 2000;101:131.

79. Malekianpour M, Bonan R, Lesperance J, et al. Comparison of ionic and nonionic low osmolar contrast media in relation to thrombotic complications of angioplasty in patients with unstable angina. *Am Heart J*. 1998;135:1067.

80. Scheller B, Hennen B, Pohl A, et al. Acute and subacute stent occlusion: risk reduction by ionic contrast media. *Eur Heart J*. 2001;22:385.

81. Dieu V, Joffre F, Krause D, et al. A comparison of the efficacy and safety of ioxaglate and iobitridol in renal angioplasty. *Cardiovasc Intervent Radiol*. 2000;23:91.

CHAPTER (23)

Renal Complications of Contrast Media: Contrast-Induced Nephropathy

Peter A. McCullough, MD

HISTORICAL PERSPECTIVE

Radiocontrast was first described to cause nephrotoxicity in the 1960s.[1,2] Contrast-induced nephropathy (CIN) as a leading cause of acute renal failure (ARF) was reported with increasing frequency over the next 10 to 15 years, largely due to increasing use of radiocontrast studies in patients who were older, sicker, or had attendant comorbidities such as diabetes mellitus, renal failure, cardiac failure, and volume depletion.[3] CIN is currently described as the third most common cause of hospital-acquired renal failure, accounting for approximately 11% of cases.[4] The incidence of CIN reported in the literature has ranged between 1% and 45%, largely depending on the comorbidities of the study population and the parameters used to define CIN.[5] With more than a million radiocontrast procedures performed annually in the United States, the incidence of CIN is approximately 150,000 cases per year. At least 1% of these episodes require dialysis therapy (in half it will be permanent), with prolongation of hospital stay to an average of 17 days at an additional cost of approximately $32 million annually. For episodes that do not require dialysis, the average prolongation of the hospital stay is 2 days (at $500 per day; this translates into an added cost of $148 million annually).[6,7] The incidence and costs are higher in critically ill patients who have associated comorbidities such as hypotension, hypovolemia, diabetes, and congestive heart failure.

This chapter will first examine the important renal complications of contrast media. This will be followed by an evaluation of laboratory investigations that provide insights into the pathogenesis of this disorder. The last section deals with two important clinical issues: (1) the use of low-osmolality radiocontrast agents specifically to reduce the incidence of CIN, and (2) adjunctive methods currently used to prevent the development of CIN.

THE CARDIORENAL INTERSECTION

The obesity pandemic is a central driver of the dysmetabolic syndrome, hypertension, and diabetes. It is thus anticipated that there will soon occur a secondary epidemic of combined chronic kidney disease (CKD) and cardiovascular disease (CVD).[8] Among those with diabetes for 25 years or more, the prevalence of diabetic nephropathy in type 1 and type 2 diabetes is 57% and 48%, respectively. Approximately half of all cases of end-stage renal disease (ESRD) are due to diabetic nephropathy, with most of these cases driven by obesity related type 2 diabetes and hypertension.[9] With the graying of America, and cardiovascular care shifting toward the elderly, the imperative thus exists to understand the relationship between decreasing levels of renal function as a major adverse prognostic factor in cardiac patients. ARF after contrast exposure as the most proximal renal event is predictable and highlights an opportunity for the preventive measures outlined later in this chapter.

A list of the clinical trials cited in Chapters 19 through 24 is presented in Appendix IV-1 at the end of Part IV.

Freedom from death or MI

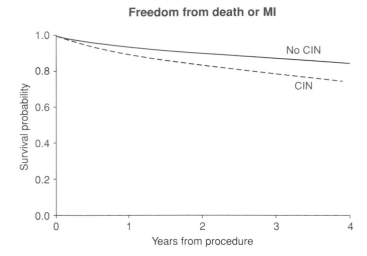

FIGURE 23-1. Adjusted, long-term outcomes in 7586 patients with and without acute renal failure after angioplasty, $P < .0001$. Contrast-induced nephropathy (CIN) is defined as a ≥0.5 mg/dL rise in Cr after percutaneous coronary intervention. MI = myocardial infarction. *(Reproduced with permission from Rihal CS, et al.[12])*

LINK BETWEEN SMALL INCREASES IN CREATININE AND POOR LONG-TERM OUTCOMES

The overall risk of CIN, defined as a transient rise in serum creatinine (Cr) more than 25% above the baseline, occurs in approximately 13% of patients without diabetes and in 20% of patients with diabetes undergoing procedures utilizing contrast.[10] Fortunately, rates of CIN leading to dialysis are quite low (0.5%–2.0%). However, the occurrence of CIN is associated with catastrophic outcomes, including a 36% in-hospital mortality rate and a 2-year survival of only 19%.[10] Transient rises in Cr are directly related to longer intensive care unit and hospital ward stays (3 and 4 additional days, respectively) after cardiac bypass surgery.[11] Recently, it has been shown that even transient elevations in Cr translate to differences in adjusted long-term outcomes after percutaneous coronary angioplasty (PCI) (Figure 23-1).[12,13] The leading explanation is that when renal function declines, the associated abnormal vascular pathobiology accelerates, and hence the progression of CVD events occurs more rapidly.

TABLE 23-1

Risk Factors for the Development of Contrast-induced Nephropathy

• eGFR ≤ 60 mL/min/1.73 m²	• Congestive heart failure
• Diabetes	• Preprocedural volume depletion
• Urine ACR >30	• Intraprocedural hypotension
• Hypertension	• Intra-aortic counterpulsation
• History of structural kidney disease or damage	• Cholesterol emboli syndrome
	• Use of large volume of contrast

ACR = urine albumin–serum creatinine ratio, eGFR = estimated glomerular filtration rate.
Reproduced with permission from McCullough PA, Sandberg KR.[6]

RISK FACTORS FOR CONTRAST-INDUCED NEPHROPATHY

Mild, transient decreases in the glomerular filtration rate occur after contrast administration in almost all patients.[14] There is a brief increase in renal blood flow followed by prolonged vasoconstriction within the kidneys after contrast exposure. The development of clinically significant ARF can be predicted based on the presence or absence of specific risk factors (Table 23-1). A multivariate analysis of prospective trials has shown that baseline renal impairment, diabetes mellitus, congestive heart failure, and higher doses of contrast media increase the risk of CIN.[15,16] Other risk factors include reduced effective arterial volume (eg, due to dehydration, nephrosis, or cirrhosis) or concurrent use of potentially nephrotoxic drugs such as nonsteroidal anti-inflammatory agents (NSAIDs) and aminoglycosides. Multiple myeloma has been suggested as a potential risk factor for CIN, but a large retrospective study failed to demonstrate an increased risk in these patients.[17] Of all these risk factors, preexisting renal impairment appears to be the single most important; patients with diabetes mellitus and renal impairment, however, have a substantially higher risk of CIN than patients with renal impairment alone.[18,19]

CLINICAL FEATURES OF CONTRAST-INDUCED NEPHROPATHY

CIN manifests usually as ARF and is typically nonoliguric. Nonoliguric ARF is generally more common in patients initially having a lower serum Cr prior to receiving contrast. In oliguric ARF, the time course of the oliguria and the rise in serum Cr depend on the preprocedure baseline serum Cr. Patients with normal renal function or mild renal functional impairment prior to receiving radiocontrast agents usually have oliguria lasting 2 to 5 days, with recovery to baseline renal function by day 7. Dialysis is infrequently required.[19,20] Some degree of residual renal impairment has been reported in as many as 30% of those affected by CIN.[19] Other comorbidities such as sustained hypotension, hypovolemia, atheroembolism, and the concurrent use of nephrotoxic medications can also contribute to CIN after coronary angiography and intervention. The occurrence of CIN usually prolongs the hospital stay.[21] Finally, mortality is increased in patients who develop CIN. In a retrospective study, Levy et al compared the outcomes of hospitalized patients with CIN to a control group of patients who did not develop CIN; controls were matched for age, baseline serum Cr, and type of diagnostic procedure. The mortality in the CIN group was 34% compared with 7% in the control group ($P <.001$, OR 5.5), even after controlling for baseline factors and in-hospital comorbidities.[22]

The antidiabetic agent metformin may lead to the development of lactic acidosis in the setting of CIN. This complication is rare and occurs only if the contrast administration results in significant renal failure and the patient continues to take metformin. In a recent review of this subject, no conclusive evidence was found to indicate that the use of contrast precipitated metformin-induced lactic acidosis in patients with serum Cr less than 1.5 mg/dL or 130 μmol/L at baseline. The complication was almost always observed in patients with non–insulin-dependent diabetes and decreased renal function before injection of contrast media. Thus, although there is no justification to discontinue metformin before the day of the contrast-requiring procedure, it is recommended that patients not take this drug for 48 hours or so after contrast administration and resume taking the drug only if there are no signs of nephrotoxicity. This is especially true for patients in high-risk subgroups, described above.[23]

DIAGNOSIS OF CONTRAST-INDUCED NEPHROPATHY

CIN usually develops within 24 to 72 hours following a radiocontrast study. This may rarely be accompanied with oliguria. One interesting feature of oliguric CIN is the presence of a low fractional excretion of sodium during the initial stages, despite the absence of clinical evidence of volume depletion.[24] Microscopic urinalysis demonstrates renal tubular epithelial cell casts or coarsely granular brown casts but may occasionally be negative. Even in the absence of a rise in serum Cr, radiocontrast agents may still alter the urinary sediment, showing epithelial cells, epithelial cell casts, granular or muddy brown coarsely granular casts, and occasional crystals. Hence routine urinalysis is not particularly specific and is not recommended after contrast procedures.[25,26] A persistent nephrogram 24 to 48 hours after the contrast study has been reported to be a sensitive indicator of the presence of renal failure (83% of patients with renal failure had a positive nephrogram) with high specificity (93% of patients without renal failure lacked the persistent nephrogram).[27] The persistent nephrogram has been related to an abnormal and persistent intrarenal vasoconstriction after contrast exposure.[27–29]

PATHOPHYSIOLOGY OF CONTRAST-INDUCED NEPHROPATHY

There are three core elements that are intertwined in the pathophysiology of CIN: (1) direct toxicity of iodinated contrast to nephrons, (2) "microshowers" of atheroemboli to the kidneys, and (3) contrast- and atheroemboli-induced intrarenal vasoconstriction.[28] Direct toxicity to nephrons with iodinated contrast has been demonstrated and appears to be related to the osmolality of the contrast.[29] Hence, low ionic or nonionic, and low-osmolar or iso-osmolar contrast agents have been shown to be less nephrotoxic in vitro. "Microshowers" of cholesterol emboli are thought to occur in up to 50% of percutaneous interventions in which a guiding catheter is passed through the aorta.[30] Most of these "showers" are clinically silent. However, in approximately 1% of high-risk cases, an acute cholesterol emboli syndrome can develop

manifested by ARF, mesenteric ischemia, decreased microcirculation to the extremities, and in some cases, embolic stroke. Because ARF occurs after coronary artery bypass surgery with nearly the same risk predictors as in patients undergoing contrast procedures, it is thought that atheroembolism may be a common pathogenic feature of both causes of renal failure.[30] Finally, intrarenal vasoconstriction as a pathologic vascular response to contrast media and (perhaps) to cholesterol emboli is a third mechanism leading to hypoxic/ischemic injury to the kidney.[31] Hypoxia triggers activation of the renal sympathetic nervous system and results in a reduction in renal blood flow, especially in the outer medulla (Figure 23-2).[31,32] It is important to note that animal studies do not demonstrate agreement regarding the direct vasoconstrictive and/or vasodilatory effects of contrast on the kidney.[33,34] In humans with vascular disease, endothelial dysfunction, and glomerular injury, it is believed that contrast and the multifactorial insult of renal hypoxia provokes a vasoconstrictive response and hence mediates in part an ischemic injury. The most important predictor of CIN is underlying renal dysfunction. The "remnant nephron" theory postulates that after sufficient chronic kidney damage has occurred and the estimated glomerular filtration rate (eGFR) is reduced to less than 60 mL/min/1.73 m^2, the remaining nephrons must pick up the remaining filtration load; they have increased oxygen demands and are thus more susceptible to ischemic and oxidative injury.

It is important to distinguish CIN from cholesterol emboli syndrome (CES) or atheroembolic renal disease. The incidence of CES following coronary angiography has been reported to be 1.4% in a recent study.[35] Scolari et al retrospectively reported that 15 of 16,223 vascular procedures were complicated with CES, an incidence of 0.09%.[36] In contrast, an autopsy study reported that the overall prevalence of CES was 25% to 30% of patients after cardiac catheterization.[37] Ramirez et al noted cholesterol emboli at autopsy in 30% of patients who died within 6 months of undergoing aortography and in 25.5% of patients who died within 6 months of undergoing coronary angiography. In contrast, the incidence of cholesterol embolism was 4.3% in age-matched controls who had not undergone a previous invasive vascular procedure. The cholesterol emboli in the control group may have resulted from spontaneous erosion of atheromatous plaques or from previous anticoagulant or thrombolytic therapy.[38]

In patients with CES occurring after angiographic and vascular surgical procedures, the interval from the inciting event to the onset of renal symptoms may vary greatly. Some patients have immediate clinical features, but in others the onset can be more insidious, with a delay of weeks or months between the precipitating event and clinical features. In 17 patients who developed atheroembolization after an arteriographic procedure, Frock et al found the mean interval between the inciting event and diagnosis of atheroembolic renal disease to be 5.3 weeks.[39] Contrast media–associated nephrotoxicity immediately follows the radiographic study. There is an increase in Cr level a few days after the procedure (usually within 72 hours); peak Cr level elevation occurs approximately 1 week after exposure and returns to baseline within 10 to 14 days.[40] Conversely, atheroembolic renal damage frequently has a delayed onset (days to weeks) and a protracted course; the outcome is often poor, resulting in progressive renal failure requiring dialysis. When fulminant disease develops

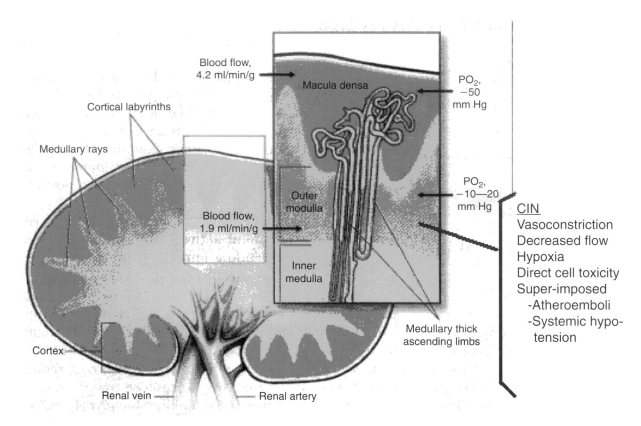

FIGURE 23-2. Pathophysiology of contrast-induced nephropathy involves acute ischemia to the outer medulla, the most vulnerable part of the kidney, due to direct cellular toxicity and sustained intrarenal vasoconstriction and reduction in renal blood flow. This process is worsened by multiple factors including hypoxia, anemia, and systemic hypoperfusion. CIN = contrast-induced nephropathy. *(Adapted from Brezis M, Rosen S.[32])*

rapidly after angiography, the concomitant cutaneous, neurological, and gastrointestinal complications usually accompany renal atheroembolic disease.[41–44]

RENAL PROTECTION FOR PATIENTS UNDERGOING CONTRAST PROCEDURES

Renal protection for CKD patients at risk (eGFR < 60 mL/min/1.73 m2) can be thought of in three separate spheres: (1) long-term cardiorenal protection, (2) removal of renal toxins, and (3) prevention measures carried out before contrast exposure. Long-term cardiorenal protection involves two important concepts. The first is blood pressure control in CKD to a target of approximately 125/75 mm Hg.[12] The second is to use an agent that blocks the renin-angiotensin system such as an angiotensin converting enzyme (ACE) inhibitor or an angiotensin-receptor blocker (ARB). Of note, both agents cause a chronic rise in Cr more than 25% above the baseline in approximately 10% of cardiovascular patients.[45] Even with an increase in Cr, the benefits of ACE inhibitor/ARB agents with respect to a reduction in new cases of ESRD, congestive heart failure (CHF), or cardiovascular death appear compelling.[46–52] It has been sufficiently shown that these benefits extend to nondiabetics and to African Americans with CKD.[51,52]

Removal of toxins largely refers to the discontinuation of NSAIDs, aminoglycosides, and cyclosporine. These agents all

complicate contrast procedures and increase the risk of CIN. Prevention measures taken prior to contrast exposure include hydration, approaches to reducing the direct cellular toxicity of the contrast, and measures to reduce the intrarenal vasoconstriction that occurs uniquely in CKD patients when exposed to iodinated contrast.[53]

PREDICTION OF CONTRAST-INDUCED NEPHROPATHY

Chronic kidney disease is defined through a range of eGFR values by the National Kidney Foundation Kidney Disease Outcomes Quality Initiative (KDOQI) as depicted in Figure 23-3.[54] Most studies of cardiovascular outcomes have associated the development of CIN, restenosis, recurrent myocardial infarction (MI), diastolic/systolic CHF, and cardiovascular death with an eGFR below 60 mL/min/1.73 m², which corresponds approximately to a serum Cr of more than 1.5 mg/dL in the general population.[55–58] Because Cr is a crude indicator of renal function and often underestimates renal dysfunction in women and the elderly, calculated measures of eGFR or Cr clearance (CrCl) by the Cockroft-Gault equation or by the Modification of Diet in Renal Disease (MDRD) equations (available on the Web, personal digital assistants, and with hand-held plastic estimators) are the preferred methods of estimating renal function. The four-variable MDRD

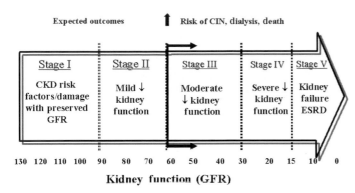

Expected outcomes   ↑ Risk of CIN, dialysis, death

Stage I	Stage II	Stage III	Stage IV	Stage V
CKD risk factors/damage with preserved GFR	Mild ↓ kidney function	Moderate ↓ kidney function	Severe ↓ kidney function	Kidney failure ESRD

130 120 110 100   90   80 70   60 50   40 30   20 15 10   0

Kidney function (GFR)

FIGURE 23-3. The classification of chronic kidney disease (CKD) according to the National Kidney Foundation Kidney Disease Outcomes Quality Initiative (KDOQI). Increased rates of adverse events are generally seen below an estimated glomerular filtration rate of 60 mL/min/1.73 m². CIN = contrast-induced nephropathy; ESRD = end-stage renal disease; GFR = glomerular filtration rate. *(Reproduced with permission from McCullough PA, Sandberg KR.[6])*

equation for CrCl is the preferred method since it does not rely on body weight.[54] This equation is given below (calculated values are multiplied by 0.742 for women and by 1.21 for African Americans):

$$186.3 \times (serum\ Cr - 1.154) \times (age - 0.203)$$

In addition, microalbuminuria (defined as random urine albumin/Cr ratio of 30–300 mg/g) at any level of eGFR is considered to represent CKD and has been thought to occur as the result of endothelial dysfunction in the glomeruli.[59] It is critical to understand that the risk of CIN is related in a curvilinear fashion to the eGFR, as shown in Figure 23-4.[6] Multivariate prediction scoring schemes have been developed and indicate that patients with multiple risk factors can have a very high, if not certain expectation for the development of CIN after contrast exposure during coronary

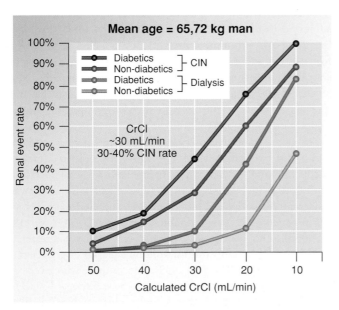

Mean age = 65,72 kg man

Diabetics / Non-diabetics — CIN
Diabetics / Non-diabetics — Dialysis

CrCl ~30 mL/min
30-40% CIN rate

Renal event rate (y-axis): 0%–100%
Calculated CrCl (mL/min) (x-axis): 50 40 30 20 10

FIGURE 23-4. Validated risk of radiocontrast nephropathy and dialysis after diagnostic angiography and ad hoc angioplasty by creatinine clearance (CrCl) and diabetes. This assumes a mean contrast dose of 250 mL and a mean age of 65 years. CIN = contrast-induced nephropathy. *(Reproduced with permission from McCullough PA, Sandberg KR.[6])*

angiography or PCI (Figure 23–5).[60] For example, a hypotensive, critically ill patient with heart failure, anemia, diabetes, and an eGFR < 60 mL/min/1.73 m² has an estimated 57.3% risk of CIN and a 12.6% risk of needing dialysis with a contrast procedure (derived from Figure 23-5).

PREVENTIVE STRATEGIES

For patients with significant CKD (ie, a baseline eGFR <60 mL/min/1.73 m² or other evidence of renal disease such as proteinuria), a CIN prevention strategy should be employed. In general, at an eGFR of 30 mL/min/1.73 m², the expected rate of CIN is 30% to 40% and the rates of ARF requiring dialysis is approximately 2% to 8% (see Figure 23-4).[6] These rates may be even higher and can be accurately predicted from multiple risk factors as shown in Figure 23-5 in the setting of the cardiac catheterization laboratory. There are four basic concepts in CIN prevention: (1) hydration; (2) choice and quantity of contrast; (3) pre-, intra-, and postprocedural end-organ protection with pharmacotherapy; and (4) postprocedural monitoring and expectant care.

Volume supplementation with intravenous (IV) normal saline or sodium bicarbonate solution, starting 3 to 12 hours prior to the procedure at a rate of 1 to 2 mL/kg/h, remains key.[3,61,62] Sodium bicarbonate was found to be superior to normal saline in a small trial in which there were too few outcomes to be definitive. Thus, confirmation of this finding will be needed to recommend bicarbonate as a routine IV hydration strategy.[62a] A simple IV rate to remember from clinical trials of hydration is 100 to 150 mL/h. In patients at risk, at least 300 to 500 mL of IV hydration should be received before contrast is administered. If there are any concerns regarding volume overload or heart failure, right-sided heart catheterization may be considered for management during and after the case. A urine output of 150 ml/h should be the target for hydration after the procedure. Importantly, if patients have a diuresis of more than a 150 ml/h, they should have replacement of extra losses with more IV fluid. In general, this strategy calls for hydration orders of 150 mL/h for at least 6 hours after the procedure. When adequate urine flow rates were achieved in a clinical trial setting, there was a 50% reduction in the rate of CIN observed.[62]

Using lower osmolality contrast agents and limiting the amount of contrast administered is associated with lower rates of CIN. This has now been confirmed in two large-scale, double-blind randomized controlled trials. In the Iohexol Cooperative Study, iohexol (Omnipaque) was found to be superior to high osmolality contrast (diatrizoate meglumine [Hypaque-76]) in patients with diabetes and baseline CKD.[19] In the recently completed Nephrotoxicity in High-Risk Patients Study of Iso-Osmolar and Low-Osmolar Non-Ionic Contrast Media Study (NEPHRIC), iodixanol (Visipaque), a nonionic, iso-osmolar contrast agent was proven to be superior to iohexol with lower rates of CIN observed.[63] Iodixanol has also been demonstrated to be less thrombogenic then other contrast agents in the Contrast Media Utilization in High-Risk Percutaneous Transluminal Coronary Angioplasty (COURT) Trial, with a 45% reduction in major adverse cardiac events compared to ioxaglate meglumine (Hexabrix). Iodixanol is thus the contrast agent of choice in patients at high renal risk undergoing intervention.[64]

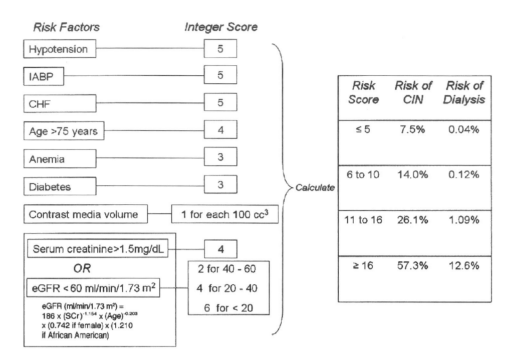

FIGURE 23-5. Risk prediction scheme for the development of contrast-induced nephropathy (CIN) and for serious renal failure requiring dialysis after coronary angiography or percutaneous coronary intervention. Anemia = baseline hematocrit value < 39% for men and < 36% for women; CHF = congestive heart failure functional class III/IV and/or history of pulmonary edema; eGFR = estimated glomerular filtration rate; hypotension = systolic blood pressure < 80 mm Hg for at least 1 hour requiring inotropic support with medications or intra-aortic balloon pump (IABP) within 24 hours periprocedurally. *(Reproduced with permission from Mehran R, Aymong ED, Nikolsky E, et al.[60])*

Although it is logically desirable to limit the amount of contrast to the smallest volume possible, there is disagreement as to whether there is a "safe" contrast limit.[65] This is mainly due to the fact that the lower the eGFR, the smaller the contrast needed to cause CIN. In general, it is desirable to limit contrast to less than 100 mL for any procedure.[10,53] If staged procedures are planned, it is desirable to have more than 10 days between the first and second contrast exposure if CIN has occurred on the first contrast exposure.[66]

There have been more than 40 randomized trials testing various strategies in the prevention of CIN. The majority have been small and underpowered and did not find the preventive strategy to be better than placebo. A few lessons have been learned from these trials:

1. Diuretics in the form of loop diuretics or mannitol can actually worsen CIN if there is inadequate volume replacement for the diuresis that follows.

2. Neither low-dose or "renal dose" dopamine nor fenoldopam provides renal protection, presumably because of counterbalancing forces of intrarenal vasodilatation via the dopamine-1 receptor versus the vasoconstrictive effects on the dopamine-2, alpha, and beta receptors.

3. Nephrotoxic agents, including NSAIDs, aminoglycosides, and cyclosporine should not be administered in the periprocedural period.

Although there are currently no approved agents for the prevention of CIN, studies of oral or IV N-acetylcysteine (NAC), a cytoprotective agent against oxidative injury, appear promising. A standard regimen widely followed is NAC 600 mg PO bid for a day before and the day of contrast study.[67] For emergency procedures involving radiocontrast, a 1-g oral dose 1 hour before and 4 hours after radiocontrast exposure may be given.[68] In one trial of NAC, patients with mild to moderate CKD undergoing PCI were randomized to receive NAC and IV hydration or IV hydration alone. An NAC infusion (150 mg/kg) was given intravenously before contrast exposure and was continued (50 mg/kg) over the following 4 hours. Thus, in a 70-kg patient, the cumulative NAC dose was 14,000 mg–a significantly higher dosage than that used in previous studies (~2400 mg). In the two groups, the contrast volumes were 238 mL and 222 mL, and CIN occurred in 5% and 21% of cases, respectively ($P = .045$).[69] In another study by Briguori et al, two different NAC dosages were compared (600 mg vs 1200 mg orally twice daily) before and after radiocontrast administration in patients with modest CKD who underwent coronary and/or peripheral procedures. The incidence of CIN was lower in patients receiving a double dose of NAC (3.5% vs 11%, $P = .038$). The benefit of double-dose NAC was greater in patients receiving a radiocontrast volume equal to or greater than 140 mL (5.4% vs 18.9%, $P = .039$) than in those who received a radiocontrast volume less than 140 mL (1.7% vs 3.6%, $P = 0.61$).[70] Thus, these results suggest that a higher dose of NAC is likely needed in CKD patients undergoing PCI, and they support the hypothesis of a dose-dependent protective effect of NAC. Further studies are needed to confirm these data and to test the effects of NAC using hard clinical end points.

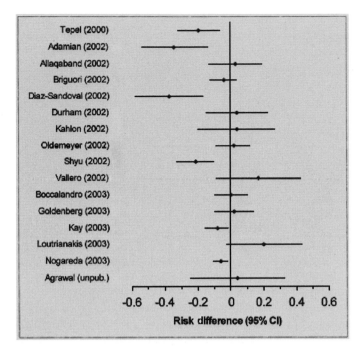

FIGURE 23-6. Odds ratio display of weighted risk differences of 16 controlled clinical trials of N-acetylcysteine in the prevention of contrast-induced nephropathy. (*Reproduced with permission from Kshirsagar AV, et al.*[71])

A recent meta-analysis of trials involving the use of NAC in prevention of CIN was undertaken to examine for (1) publication bias, (2) differences among the study results attributable to chance variation, and (3) current support of existing literature of a conclusion regarding the effectiveness of oral NAC in the reduction of the occurrence of radiocontrast-induced nephropathy.[71] This analysis found the results of oral NAC in the prevention of radiocontrast-induced nephropathy to be inconclusive. The analysis did not demonstrate an added benefit of oral NAC among all individuals with preexistent renal insufficiency (Figure 23-6). The authors concluded that, rather than the indiscriminate use of NAC, clinicians may better direct their efforts at proven interventions (IV saline, low-osmolality/iso-osmolality contrast media). The findings of this systematic review and others did not support the routine use of NAC for the prevention of radiocontrast-induced nephropathy.[71–72]

A trial of NAC in patients with acute MI undergoing primary angioplasty assigned 354 patients (eGFR~78mL/min,~15% diabetics) to one of three groups: 116 patients were assigned to a standard dose NAC (a 600-mg intravenous bolus before primary angioplasty and 600 mg orally twice daily for the 48 hours after angioplasty), 119 patients to a double dose of NAC (a 1200-mg intravenous bolus and 1200 mg orally twice daily for the 48 hours after intervention), and 119 patients to placebo. The rates of CIN (>25% rise in Cr from baseline) were 39 (33%) in controls, 17 (15%) for standard-dose NAC, and 10 (8%) for double-dose NAC, $P < .001$. Overall in-hospital mortality was 13 (11%) in the control group died, 5 (4%) in the standard-dose NAC group, and 3 (3%) in the high-dose NAC, $P = .02$. The rate for the composite end point of death, acute renal failure requiring temporary renal-replacement therapy, or the need for mechanical ventilation

was 21 (18%), 8 (7%) and 6 (5%) in the three groups, respectively ($P = .002$). Thus for high risk primary angioplasty candidates with $P = .02$ CKD, double-dose NAC may be a reasonable adjunctive strategy.

As indicated above, there have been many small trials of other strategies, including aminophylline, endothelin receptor antagonists, ascorbic acid, dopamine, fenoldopam, and a variety of other agents, all of which are either of neutral or equivocal benefit. There have been eight clinical trials involving the use of aminophylline or theophylline in the prevention of CIN; two studies did not show any protective effect, and six showed a positive preventive effect.[14,21,73–78] A recent meta-analysis of studies employing theophylline or aminophylline for prevention of CIN identified a statistically significant, favorable effect on the decline in kidney function. However, the authors note the translation of this effect to clinically meaningful benefit (reduced need for dialysis or in-hospital mortality) remains to be proven.[79] Because endogenous adenosine activates intrarenal adenosine receptors causing vasoconstriction, the adenosine antagonism provided by aminophylline may have a favorable effect on renal blood flow. Therefore, aminophylline is considered optional as a preventive strategy and certainly can be continued in pulmonary patients who are already taking the drug.

Prophylactic continuous hemofiltration has been proposed as an interventional strategy to prevent CIN in advanced CKD patients.[80] Hemofiltration works to (1) guarantee preprocedure hydration, (2) provide hemodynamic stability pre- and post procedure, and (3) provide a blood milieu lower in uremic toxins, thus allowing remnant nephrons to work more efficiently. A recent trial of hemofiltration before and after contrast exposure in patients with advanced CKD (mean Cr = 3.0 mg/dL) resulted in lower CIN rates compared to a control group (5% vs 50%, $P < .001$), as shown in Figure 23-7. Temporary hemodialysis was required in 25% of the control patients and in 3% of the patients in the hemofiltration group.[80] This trial needs replication. However, at the time of this writing, for patients with severe CKD, prophylactic hemofiltration as performed in the trial in an intensive care unit setting 4 to 6 hours before the coronary procedure and for 18 to 24 hours after the procedure is a reasonable option. The hemofiltration circuit requires a Y-shaped 12-Fr double-lumen catheter placed in a femoral vein. Blood is driven through the circuit at a rate of 100 mL/min. The flow of isotonic replacement fluid set at a rate of 1000 mL/h is exactly matched with the rate of ultrafiltrate production, so that no net fluid loss results. A heparin bolus of 5000 IU is required before hemofiltration and heparin is continued at a rate of 500 to 1000 IU/h through the inflow side of the circuit. In most centers, this process is managed by nephrologists and their dialysis staff.

It is important to realize that treatment before the procedure is critical and that preemptive dialysis after contrast exposure has not been shown to prevent CIN. Vogt et al evaluated prophylactic hemodialysis started soon after the administration of the contrast agent and continued for an average of 3 hours.[81] The rationale for the study was to remove the contrast agent efficiently by hemodialysis, thus reducing the concentration of contrast agent to which the kidneys would be exposed. However, this strategy did not show any beneficial effect as compared with saline hydration alone, and patients who were treated with hemodialysis were more likely to

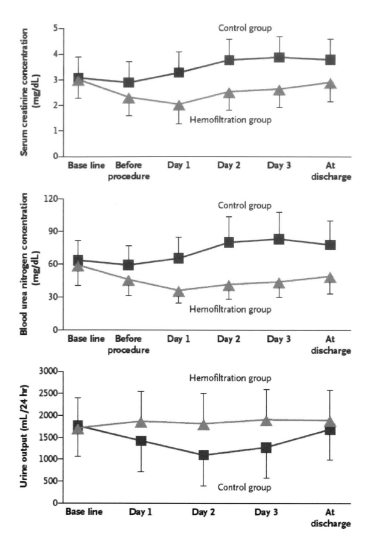

FIGURE 23-7. The lines represent changes in creatinine (Cr), blood urea nitrogen (BUN), and urine output in 114 patients randomized to prophylactic hemofiltration versus control. Changes from baseline in the Cr and BUN concentration were significant ($P < .01$) before the procedure and on days 1, 2, and 3 in the hemofiltration group and at day 2, day 3, and discharge in the control group; the difference between the two groups was significant beginning on day 1. Control urine output rates differed ($P < .01$) on day 2 and day 3 but not in the hemofiltration group; hemofiltration resulted in higher urine flow rates beyond day 2. (*Reproduced with permission from Marenzi G, Marana I, Lauri G, et al.[80]*)

have a decline in renal function and to require additional hemodialysis treatment.

A possible explanation for the difference in results with post-procedure hemodialysis compared with periprocedural continuous hemofiltration is that hemodialysis may induce hypovolemia and consequently may worsen renal ischemic injury, delay recovery of renal function, and result in a need for prolonged treatment. On the other hand, hemofiltration is associated with hemodynamic stability and safeguards against renal hypoperfusion by preserving the volume of circulating blood. This effect is particularly useful when coronary procedures are performed in patients with critical conditions such as MI or acute cardiovascular events such as pulmonary edema or severe left ventricular dysfunction. In addition to hemodynamic stability, hemofiltration provides controlled high-volume hydration and removal of contrast agent from the cir-

culation, with a resultant reduction in the kidneys' exposure to the agent.[82–86] It can also be speculated that in addition to high-volume controlled hydration, the removal of mediators of CIN toxicity by convective filtration and adsorption to the filter membrane may play a significant role.[87]

Once CIN has been recognized, there is no specific treatment, and management involves supportive treatment of ARF, including dialysis treatment as needed. Most operators believe that, given the seriousness of CIN as a complication, the relative safety of the strategies used, and the evolution of clinical trials shaping our practice, that the combination of hydration (saline or possibly sodium bicarbonate), iodixanol, and NAC is a reasonable three-pronged approach to minimize CIN and the risk of ARF requiring dialysis.

Postprocedural monitoring is an issue in the modern era of short stays and outpatient procedures. In general, high-risk patients in the hospital should have hydration started 3 to 13 hours before the procedure and continued at least 6 hours afterwards (Figure 23-8). A serum Cr should be measured 24 hours after the procedure. For outpatients, particularly those with eGFR less than 60 mL/h/1.73 m², either an overnight stay or discharge to home with 24 to 48–hour follow-up and Cr measurement is advised. It has been demonstrated that those individuals who develop severe CIN have a rise of Cr more than 0.5 mg/dL in the first 24 to 48 hours after the procedure.[88] Hence, for patients who have not had this degree of Cr elevation, and otherwise have had uneventful courses, discharge to home may be considered.

In summary, for CIN risk assessment and prevention, the action items as shown in Figure 23-8 are advised. It is important that CIN risks are discussed in the consent process. For patients with eGFR less than 30 mL/min/1.73 m², the possibility of dialysis should be mentioned. Lastly, in those with eGFR less than 20 mL/min/1.73 m², nephrology consultation is advised with possible planning for dialysis after the procedure.

CONCLUSION

Contrast-induced nephropathy is an important cause of ARF and death in critically ill patients. The presence of multiple risk factors can anticipate up to an approximately 50% probability of CIN in specific patients. Risk prediction and preventive measures are mandatory. Once ARF occurs, even with dialysis and expectant management, high-rates of in-hospital and long-term mortality can be expected.

Additional summary points include:

- Chronic kidney disease recognized by calculating the eGFR from the age, serum Cr, gender, race, and weight, and not from the serum Cr alone.

- Rates of contrast-induced nephropathy and other major adverse cardiac events increase with declines in eGFR below 60 mL/min/1.73 m².

- CIN prevention can be achieved with (1) hydration to a target urine output of more than 150 mL/h for the first 6 hours after the procedure, (2) use of iodixanol as the preferred contrast agent, (3) limiting contrast volume to less than 100 mL, (4) spacing out second contrast procedures more than 10 days from

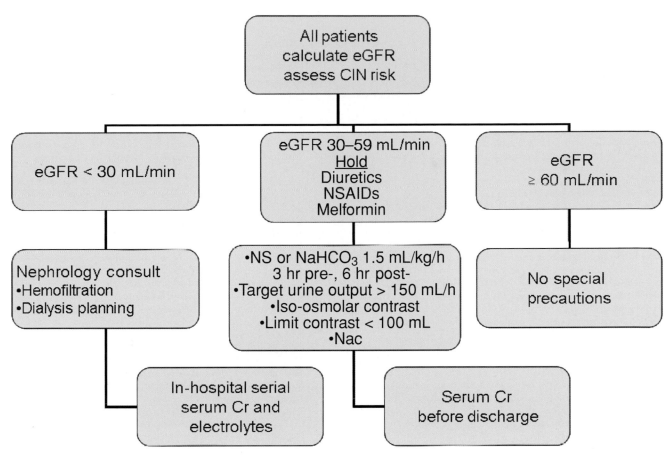

FIGURE 23-8. Suggested algorithm for patients undergoing coronary angiography and intervention. All patients should have the estimated glomerular filtration rate (eGFR) calculated and have an assessment for contrast-induced nephropathy (CIN) risk based on validated multivariate scoring schemes. NSAID = nonsteroidal anti-inflammatory agent; NS = normal saline; NaHCO₃ = sodium bicarbonate; NAC = N-acetylcysteine; Cr = creatinine.

each other, and (5) NAC 600 mg PO bid (2 doses prior and 2 doses after contrast exposure).

• For patients with advanced CKD, eGFR less than 15 to 20 mL/min/1.73 m^2 and serum Cr approximately 3.0 mg/dL, prophylactic periprocedural continuous hemofiltration may reduce the incidence of CIN.

REFERENCES

1. Cotton DB. Radiocontrast-induced renal failure. *Lancet.* 1979;2:1378.
2. Radiocontrast-induced renal failure. *Lancet.* 1979;2:835.
3. Solomon R, et al. Effects of saline, mannitol, and furosemide to prevent acute decreases in renal function induced by radiocontrast agents. *N Engl J Med.* 1994;331:1416.
4. Nash K, Hafeez A, Hou S. Hospital-acquired renal insufficiency. *Am J Kidney Dis.* 2002;39:930.
5. Taylor AJ, et al. PREPARED: Preparation for Angiography in Renal Dysfunction: a randomized trial of inpatient vs. outpatient hydration protocols for cardiac catheterization in mild-to-moderate renal dysfunction. *Chest.* 1998;114:1570.
6. McCullough PA, Sandberg KR. Epidemiology of contrast-induced nephropathy. *Rev Cardiovasc Med.* 2003;4(suppl 5):S3.
7. Gruberg L, Mehran R, Dangas G. Acute renal failure requiring dialysis after percutaneous coronary interventions. *Catheter Cardiovasc Interv.* 2001; 52:409.
8. Lewis CE, et al. Weight gain continues in the 1990s: 10-year trends in weight and overweight from the CARDIA study. Coronary Artery Risk Development in Young Adults. *Am J Epidemiol.* 2000;151:1172.
9. Bakris GL, et al. Preserving renal function in adults with hypertension and diabetes: a consensus approach. National Kidney Foundation Hypertension and Diabetes Executive Committees Working Group. *Am J Kidney Dis.* 2000; 36:646.
10. McCullough PA, et al. Acute renal failure after coronary intervention: incidence, risk factors, and relationship to mortality. *Am J Med.* 1997;103:368.
11. Mangano CM, et al. Renal dysfunction after myocardial revascularization: risk factors, adverse outcomes, and hospital resource utilization. The Multicenter Study of Perioperative Ischemia Research Group. *Ann Intern Med.* 1998;128:194.
12. Rihal CS, et al. Incidence and prognostic importance of acute renal failure after percutaneous coronary intervention. *Circulation.* 2002;105:2259.
13. McCullough PA. Cardiorenal risk: an important clinical intersection. *Rev Cardiovasc Med.* 2002;3:71.
14. Katholi RE, et al. Nephrotoxicity from contrast media: attenuation with theophylline. *Radiology.* 1995;195:17.
15. Barrett BJ. Contrast nephrotoxicity. *J Am Soc Nephrol.* 1994;5:125.
16. Morcos, SK. Prevention of contrast media nephrotoxicity-the story so far. *Clin Radiol.* 2004;59:381.
17. McCarthy CS, Becker JA. Multiple myeloma and contrast media. *Radiology.* 1992;183: 519.
18. Parfrey PS et al. Contrast material-induced renal failure in patients with diabetes mellitus, renal insufficiency, or both. A prospective controlled study. *N Engl J Med.* 1989;320:143.
19. Rudnick MR, et al. Nephrotoxicity of ionic and nonionic contrast media in 1196 patients: a randomized trial. The Iohexol Cooperative Study. *Kidney Int.* 1995;47:254.
20. Barrett BJ, et al. Contrast nephropathy in patients with impaired renal function: high versus low osmolar media. *Kidney Int.* 1992;41:1274.
21. Abizaid AS, et al. Effects of dopamine and aminophylline on contrast-induced acute renal failure after coronary angioplasty in patients with preexisting renal insufficiency. *Am J Cardiol.* 1999;83:260, A5.

22. Levy EM, Viscoli CM, Horwitz RI. The effect of acute renal failure on mortality. A cohort analysis. *JAMA*. 1996;275:1489.

23. Thomsen HS, Morcos SK. Contrast media and metformin: guidelines to diminish the risk of lactic acidosis in non-insulin-dependent diabetics after administration of contrast media. ESUR Contrast Media Safety Committee. *Eur Radiol*. 1999;9:738.

24. Fang LS, et al. Low fractional excretion of sodium with contrast media-induced acute renal failure. *Arch Intern Med*. 1980;140:531.

25. Tumlin J, McCullough CA, Adam A, Becker CR, Davidson C, Lameire N, Stacul F. CIN Consensus Working Panel. Pathophysiology & contrast-induced nephropathy. *Am J Cardiol*. 2006; in press.

26. Weinrauch LA, et al. Coronary angiography and acute renal failure in diabetic azotemic nephropathy. *Ann Intern Med*. 1977;86:56.

27. D'Elia JA, et al. Nephrotoxicity from angiographic contrast material. A prospective study. *Am J Med*. 1982;72:719.

28. Margulies K, Schirger J, Burnett J Jr. Radiocontrast-induced nephropathy: current status and future prospects. *Int Angiol*. 1992;11:20.

29. Andersen KJ, Christensen EI, Vik H. Effects of iodinated x-ray contrast media on renal epithelial cells in culture. *Invest Radiol*. 1994;29:955.

30. Keeley EC, Grines CL. Scraping of aortic debris by coronary guiding catheters: a prospective evaluation of 1,000 cases. *J Am Coll Cardiol*. 1998;32:1861.

31. Denton KM, Shweta A, Anderson WP. Preglomerular and postglomerular resistance responses to different levels of sympathetic activation by hypoxia. *J Am Soc Nephrol*. 2002;13:27.

32. Brezis M, Rosen S. Hypoxia of the renal medulla—its implications for disease. *N Engl J Med*. 1995;332:647.

33. Uder M, et al. Nonionic contrast media iohexol and iomeprol decrease renal arterial tone: comparative studies on human and porcine isolated vascular segments. *Invest Radiol*. 2002;37:440.

34. Rauch D, et al. Comparison of iodinated contrast media-induced renal vasoconstriction in human, rabbit, dog, and pig arteries. *Invest Radiol*. 1997; 32:315.

35. Fukumoto Y, et al. The incidence and risk factors of cholesterol embolization syndrome, a complication of cardiac catheterization: a prospective study. *J Am Coll Cardiol*. 2003;42:211.

36. Scolari F, et al. Cholesterol atheromatous embolism: an increasingly recognized cause of acute renal failure. *Nephrol Dial Transplant*. 1996;11:1607.

37. Rosansky SJ, Deschamps EG. Multiple cholesterol emboli syndrome after angiography. *Am J Med Sci*. 1984;288:45.

38. Ramirez G, et al. Cholesterol embolization: a complication of angiography. *Arch Intern Med*. 1978;138:1430.

39. Scolari F, et al. Cholesterol crystal embolism: a recognizable cause of renal disease. *Am J Kidney Dis*. 2000;36:1089.

40. Rudnick MR, et al. Nephrotoxic risks of renal angiography: contrast media-associated nephrotoxicity and atheroembolism—a critical review. *Am J Kidney Dis*. 1994;24:713.

41. Kassirer JP. Atheroembolic renal disease. *N Engl J Med*. 1969;280:812.

42. Fine MJ, Kapoor W, Falanga V. Cholesterol crystal embolization: a review of 221 cases in the English literature. *Angiology*. 1987;38:769.

43. Saleem S, Lakkis FG, Martinez-Maldonado M. Atheroembolic renal disease. *Semin Nephrol*. 1996;16:309.

44. Dahlberg, PJ, Frecentese DF, Cogbill TH. Cholesterol embolism: experience with 22 histologically proven cases. *Surgery*. 1989;105:737.

45. Pitt B, et al. Randomised trial of losartan versus captopril in patients over 65 with heart failure (Evaluation of Losartan in the Elderly Study, ELITE). *Lancet*. 1997;349:747.

46. Toto R. Angiotensin II subtype 1 receptor blockers and renal function. *Arch Intern Med*. 2001;161:1492.

47. Lewis EJ, et al. Renoprotective effect of the angiotensin-receptor antagonist irbesartan in patients with nephropathy due to type 2 diabetes. *N Engl J Med*. 2001;345:851.

48. Parving HH, et al. The effect of irbesartan on the development of diabetic nephropathy in patients with type 2 diabetes. *N Engl J Med*. 2001;345:870.

49. Dahlof B, et al. Cardiovascular morbidity and mortality in the Losartan Intervention For Endpoint reduction in hypertension study (LIFE): a randomised trial against atenolol. *Lancet*. 2002;359:995.

50. Brenner BM, et al. Effects of losartan on renal and cardiovascular outcomes in patients with type 2 diabetes and nephropathy. *N Engl J Med*. 2001;345:861.

51. Mann JF, et al. Renal insufficiency as a predictor of cardiovascular outcomes and the impact of ramipril: the HOPE randomized trial. *Ann Intern Med*. 2001;134:629.

52. Agodoa LY, et al. Effect of ramipril vs. amlodipine on renal outcomes in hypertensive nephrosclerosis: a randomized controlled trial. *JAMA*. 2001;285:2719.

53. McCullough PA, Manley HJ. Prediction and prevention of contrast nephropathy. *J Interv Cardiol*. 2001;14:547.

54. K/DOQI clinical practice guidelines for chronic kidney disease: evaluation, classification, and stratification. *Am J Kidney Dis*. 2002;39(2 suppl 1):S1.

55. McCullough PA, et al. Risks associated with renal dysfunction in patients in the coronary care unit. *J Am Coll Cardiol*. 2000;36:679.

56. Beattie JN, et al. Determinants of mortality after myocardial infarction in patients with advanced renal dysfunction. *Am J Kidney Dis*. 2001;37:1191.

57. Chertow GM, et al. Preoperative renal risk stratification. *Circulation*. 1997; 95:878.

58. Szczech LA, et al. Outcomes of patients with chronic renal insufficiency in the bypass angioplasty revascularization investigation. *Circulation*. 2002;105:2253.

59. Keane WF, Eknoyan G. Proteinuria, albuminuria, risk, assessment, detection, elimination (PARADE): a position paper of the National Kidney Foundation. *Am J Kidney Dis*. 1999;33:1004.

60. Mehran R, et al. A simple risk score for prediction of contrast-induced nephropathy after percutaneous coronary intervention: development and initial validation. *J Am Coll Cardiol*. 2004;44:1393.

61. Mueller C, et al. Prevention of contrast media-associated nephropathy: randomized comparison of 2 hydration regimens in 1620 patients undergoing coronary angioplasty. *Arch Intern Med*. 2002;162:329.

62. Stevens MA, et al. A prospective randomized trial of prevention measures in patients at high risk for contrast nephropathy: results of the P.R.I.N.C.E. Study. Prevention of Radiocontrast Induced Nephropathy Clinical Evaluation. *J Am Coll Cardiol*. 1999;33:403.

62a. Merten GJ, Burgess WP, Gray LV, Hollaman JH. Roush TS, Kowalchuk GJ, et al. Prevention of contrast-induced nephropathy with sodium bicarbonate: a randomized controlled trial. *JAMA*, 2004, May 19:291,2328.

63. Abassi ZA, et al. Urinary endothelin: a possible biological marker of renal damage. *Am J Hypertens*. 1993;6:1046.

64. Davidson CJ, et al. Randomized trial of contrast media utilization in high-risk PTCA: the COURT trial. *Circulation*. 2000;101: 2172.

65. Manske CL, et al. Contrast nephropathy in azotemic diabetic patients undergoing coronary angiography. *Am J Med*. 1990;89(5):615.

66. Stone GW, et al. Design and rationale of CONTRAST–a prospective, randomized, placebo-controlled trial of fenoldopam mesylate for the prevention of radiocontrast nephropathy. *Rev Cardiovasc Med*. 2001;2(suppl 1):S31.

67. Tepel M, et al. Prevention of radiographic-contrast-agent-induced reductions in renal function by acetylcysteine. *N Engl J Med*. 2000;343:180.

68. Ochoa A, et al. Abbreviated dosing of N-acetylcysteine prevents contrast-induced nephropathy after elective and urgent coronary angiography and intervention. *J Interv Cardiol*. 2004;17:159.

69. Baker CS, et al. A rapid protocol for the prevention of contrast-induced renal dysfunction: the RAPPID study. *J Am Coll Cardiol*. 2003;41:2114.

70. Briguori C, et al. Standard vs. double dose of N-acetylcysteine to prevent contrast agent associated nephrotoxicity. *Eur Heart J*. 2004;25:206.

71. Kshirsagar AV, et al. N-acetylcysteine for the prevention of radiocontrast induced nephropathy: a meta-analysis of prospective controlled trials. *J Am Soc Nephrol*. 2004;15:761.

72. Alonso A. et al. Prevention of radiocontrast nephropathy with N-acetylcysteine in patients with chronic kidney disease: a meta-analysis of randomized, controlled trials. *Am J Kidney Dis*. 2004;43:1.

72a. Marenzi G, et al. N-acetylcysteine and contrast-induced nephropathy in primary angioplasty. *N Engl J Med*. 2006; 354:2773.

73. Huber W, et al. Effect of theophylline on contrast material-nephropathy in patients with chronic renal insufficiency: controlled, randomized, double-blinded study. *Radiology*. 2002;223:772.

74. Kapoor A, et al. The role of theophylline in contrast-induced nephropathy: a case-control study. *Nephrol Dial Transplant*. 2002;17:1936.

75. Kolonko A, Wiecek A, Kokot F. The nonselective adenosine antagonist theophylline does prevent renal dysfunction induced by radiographic contrast agents. *J Nephrol*. 1998;11:151.

76. Erley CM, et al. Adenosine antagonist theophylline prevents the reduction of glomerular filtration rate after contrast media application. *Kidney Int*. 1994;45:1425.

77. Erley CM, et al. Prevention of radiocontrast-media-induced nephropathy in patients with pre-existing renal insufficiency by hydration in combination with the adenosine antagonist theophylline. *Nephrol Dial Transplant*. 1999;14:1146.

78. Huber W, et al. Effectiveness of theophylline prophylaxis of renal impairment after coronary angiography in patients with chronic renal insufficiency. *Am J Cardiol*. 2003;91:1157.

79. Ix JH, McCulloch CE, Chertow GM. Theophylline for the prevention of radiocontrast nephropathy: a meta-analysis. *Nephrol Dial Transplant.* 2004;19:2747.

80. Marenzi G, Marana I, Lauri G, Assanelli E, et al. The prevention of radiocontrast-agent-induced nephropathy by hemofiltration. *N Engl J Med.* 2003; 349:1333.

81. Vogt B, et al. Prophylactic hemodialysis after radiocontrast media in patients with renal insufficiency is potentially harmful. *Am J Med.* 2001;111:692.

82. Forni LG, Hilton PJ. Continuous hemofiltration in the treatment of acute renal failure. *N Engl J Med.* 1997;336:1303.

83. Marenzi G, et al. Circulatory response to fluid overload removal by extracorporeal ultrafiltration in refractory congestive heart failure. *J Am Coll Cardiol.* 2001;38:963.

84. Marenzi G, et al. Continuous veno-venous hemofiltration for the treatment of contrast-induced acute renal failure after percutaneous coronary interventions. *Catheter Cardiovasc Interv.* 2003;58:59.

85. Schindler R, et al. Removal of contrast media by different extracorporeal treatments. *Nephrol Dial Transplant.* 2001;16:1471.

86. Jungers P, et al. Incidence and risk factors of atherosclerotic cardiovascular accidents in predialysis chronic renal failure patients: a prospective study. *Nephrol Dial Transplant.* 1997;12:2597.

87. Marenzi G, Bartorelli AL. Recent advances in the prevention of radiocontrast-induced nephropathy. *Curr Opin Crit Care.* 2004;10:505.

88. Guitterez NV, Diaz A, Timmis GC, et al. Determinants of serum creatinine trajectory in acute contrast nephropathy. *J Interv Cardiol.* 2002;15:349.

CHAPTER (24)

Patient Sedation in the Cardiovascular Catheterization Laboratory

*Jon E. Gardner, RCIS, MBA, Laurie A. Vancamp, RN,
Tammey M. Wilkerson, RN, Annette A. Moore, RN,
and Georgann Bruski, RT(R)*

MODERATE SEDATION: ACHIEVING OPTIMAL COMFORT

Patients undergoing invasive procedures, such as coronary or peripheral vascular interventions, can be anxious about the hospital environment, outcomes of the procedures, and have generalized fears of the unknown. The multidisciplinary team of physician, nurse, and physician extender have the responsibility and obligation to assess the requirement for, explain, administer, and monitor sedative therapies given each patient.

The American Society of Anesthesiologists (ASA) identifies moderate sedation (formerly referred to as conscious sedation) as "a drug-induced depression of consciousness and sensorium during which patients continue to be able to respond purposefully to verbal commands either alone or accompanied by a light tactile stimulation."[1] No interventions are required to maintain a patent airway or cardiovascular function. Moderate sedation (with or without analgesia) includes the use of medications that, in the manner used, may be reasonably expected to potentially result in the loss of protective reflexes. Constant vigilance of the patient's

monitor is required to avoid loss of protective airway reflexes or the development of deeper levels of sedation and to ensure the safety of the patient undergoing a procedure requiring moderate sedation.

Reducing the patient's level of consciousness to a moderate level of sedation is intended to facilitate the successful performance of the therapeutic procedure.[9] The goals of moderate sedation are:

- Maintenance of airway by the patient.
- Independent maintenance of protective reflexes (swallow and gag).
- Sustained moderate sedation throughout the procedure (eg, as assessed by the Modified Ramsey Score).
- Minimal effects on vital signs and hemodynamics.
- Mild amnesia during the procedure.
- Acceptable degree of analgesia.
- Preserved response to physical and verbal commands.
- Cooperation during the procedure.
- Reduced (or eliminated) anxiety and fear.
- Recovery to preprocedural status safely and promptly.

See Staffing and Responsibilities section.
A list of the clinical trials cited in Chapters 19 through 24 is presented in Appendix IV-1 at the end of Part IV.

TABLE 24-1

American Society of Anesthesiologists Physical Status Classification

CLASS	DESCRIPTION
1	A healthy patient (eg, varicose veins in an otherwise healthy patient)
2	A patient with mild systemic disease that in no way interferes with normal activity (eg, controlled hypertension, controlled diabetes, or chronic bronchitis)
3	A patient with severe systemic disease that is not incapacitating (eg, insulin-dependent diabetes, angina, pulmonary insufficiency)
4	A patient with severe systemic disease that is a constant threat to life (eg, cardiac failure, major organ insufficiency)
5	A moribund patient who is not expected to survive for 24 hours with or without surgery (eg, intracranial hemorrhage in coma)

【 】 PATIENT SELECTION CRITERIA

Patients must be appropriately assessed and selected before receiving moderate sedation during invasive cardiovascular procedures. The ASA Physical Status Classification guidelines (Table 24-1) provide a useful approach for assessing and classifying patient risk related to sedative therapies. (Note that this may not be appropriate or applicable in the emergency situation.) The physician scheduling the procedure is responsible for assigning the patient an ASA classification. In the event an ASA classification cannot be determined, consultation with an anesthesiologist should be obtained.

【 】 INFORMED CONSENT

Current standards require that informed consent be obtained from the patient regarding the risks and alternatives associated with moderate sedation independent of the requirement for consent for the procedure proper. The consent should reflect that the risks and benefits of moderate sedation have been discussed with the patient prior to the procedure. The signed consent form then becomes part of the permanent medical record.[8,10]

【 】 STAFFING AND RESPONSIBILITIES

Throughout the entire procedure, a minimum of two persons must be involved in the care of patients undergoing moderate sedation: (1) the physician who performs the diagnostic, therapeutic, or surgical procedure, and (2) an individual whose responsibility is directed only to the patient: to administer medication, to monitor the patient, and to observe the patient's response to both the sedation and the procedure. Specific requirements and responsibilities are delineated in Table 24-2, and Figure 24-1 is a tool used at Duke University Hospital to document staff competencies related to the administration of moderate sedation. Finally, specific equipment required for the administration of moderate sedation is described in Table 24-3.[8,10]

【 】 DRUG DOSAGE GUIDELINES

Medications for the purpose of moderate sedation are not to be administered without the presence of the physician on the unit. A physician's order is required specifying route and dosage of medication. Dosages should be individually titrated for desired therapeutic effect. Table 24-4 includes a list of commonly used medications and dosages as a guide to the drug administration for moderate sedation. Note that this list includes commonly used medications but may not be all inclusive.[3,5]

Routes of administration of agents that induce moderate sedation include transmucosal, intramuscular, inhalation, topical, oral

TABLE 24-2

Personnel Involved With the Administration of Moderate Sedation

- Physicians are to be credentialed by the medical executive committee (or other governing body) to administer moderate sedation.

- Registered nurses are authorized to administer moderate sedation, assess, monitor and/or provide immediate postprocedure care to patients receiving moderate sedation. Specific competencies include airway management, use of medications and dosages, pulse oximetry, cardiac monitoring equipment, and arrhythmia recognition.

- Cardiac catheterization laboratory technicians, depending on local governance, are authorized to administer medications for moderate sedation and monitor or provide immediate postprocedure care to patients receiving moderate sedation. Specific competencies include airway management, use of medications and dosages, pulse oximetry, cardiac monitoring and equipment, and arrhythmia recognition.[a]

- Physician extenders (ie, CRNA, PA, NP), depending on local governance, are authorized to administer medications for moderate sedation, monitor, and provide immediate postprocedure care. Specific competencies include airway management, use of medications and dosages, pulse oximetry, cardiac monitoring and equipment, and arrhythmia recognition.[a]

- Initial competency must be established and maintained by re-evaluation annually. Successful completion of ACLS/PALS training is strongly recommended.

[a]Authorization for administration should be referred to specific institution and/or state regulations and guidelines.

ACLS = advanced cardiac life support; CRNA = Certified Registered Nurse Assistant; NP = nurse practitioner; PA = physician's assistant; PALS = pediatric advanced life support.

Competency Based Orientation
Moderate Sedation (MONITOR)

Name & Position: _____   Work Unit/Area:_____

1. When an item is successfully completed (independently and competently) in the clinical setting, the preceptor will initial and date in the *PRECEPTOR VALIDATION* column. Simulations and/or practice may be indicated in the *PRACTICED/REVIEWED* column.
2. The completed checklist will be given to the manager for inclusion in the employee's personnel file.

Preceptor Initials _____ Preceptor Name (PRINTED)_____
Preceptor Initials _____ Preceptor Name (PRINTED)_____

PERFORMANCE EXPECTATION	ASSESSMENT OF LEARNER OUTCOMES	PRECEPTOR VALIDATION (DATE/INITIALS)	PRACTICED / REVIEWED
Cares for the patient requiring Moderate Sedation	**Pre-procedure:** • Verifies consent for Moderate Sedation and procedure signed		
	• Gathers/verifies proximity of equipment: oxygen, suction, emergency airway management, BP cuff, pulse oximeter, code cart, and defibrillator		
	• Instructs patient/family on sedation and procedure		
	• Initiates flow sheet documentation		
	During Procedure: • Monitors BP, pulse, respiratory rate, oxygen saturation, and level of consciousness (using Modified Ramsey score) minimum of every 10 minutes and every 2 minutes X 3 following each dose of sedative medication		
	• Verbalizes expected & unexpected reactions of moderate sedation medications and their management		
	• Maintains flow sheet documentation including patient response to procedure and sedation		
	Post-procedure: • Monitors BP, pulse, respiratory rate, oxygen saturation, and level of consciousness (using Modified Ramsey score) minimum of every 15 minutes		
	• Maintains flow sheet documentation including patient response to procedure and sedation		
	• Instructs patient/family on discharge care		
	• Discontinues monitoring upon MD determination of patient's recovery		

FIGURE 24-1. Personnel competency assessment tool for the management of moderate sedation. BP = blood pressure.

or intravenous (IV) approaches.[2] In the cardiac catheterization laboratory, the route of moderate sedation is typically IV administration. The methods of administration of IV medications include single-dose injection, bolus technique, and drug combination therapy.[5,7] Frequently, drug combinations are used. Most commonly, benzodiazepines and opiates are combined to potentiate the effects of the individual agents and thus more effectively achieve the level of sedation and pain control required for moderate sedation.[4,6]

The benzodiazepines commonly used in the cardiac catheterization laboratory are midazolam and diazepam (Valium).[5,7] The actions and pharmacodynamic profiles of these drugs are predictable in reducing the level of anxiety, and these agents often induce a mild degree of amnesia. Additionally, the patient may achieve some skeletal muscle relaxation. The major potential adverse effect of benzodiazepines is depression of the respiratory system. It is vital that the nurse administering the drugs monitor the patient's respiratory rate and oxygen saturation. These drugs can also produce a slight decrease in cardiovascular function. Patients may experience a drop in blood pressure and cardiac output, and thus close monitoring of the blood pressure and heart rate is required.

TABLE 24-3

Essential Equipment for Moderate Sedation

- Intravenous access
- Emergency airway equipment (age-appropriate)
- Oxygen
- Noninvasive blood pressure monitor or manual blood pressure cuff
- Pulse oximeter
- Emergency code cart with defibrillator (age-appropriate)
- Reversing drugs such as naloxone (Narcan) and flumazenil (Romazicon)

The opiates produce a degree of anxiety relief, but the main use of narcotics during moderate sedation is to provide pain relief. The drugs commonly used in the cardiac catheterization laboratory are hydromorphone hydrochloride (Dilaudid), morphine sulfate, and fentanyl.[5,7] Opiates may depress respiration; inhibit the cough reflex; and produce bradycardia, nausea, and vomiting. It is therefore critical to monitor respiratory status, blood pressure, heart rate, level of sedation, and patient response when administering narcotics.

Antagonists, also known as reversal agents, act on the receptors in the central nervous system to reverse the pharmacologic effects of medications. Opiates and benzodiazepines both have antagonists to reverse their actions. Flumazenil (Romazicon) is the benzodiazepine antagonist and Naloxone (Narcan) is the opiate antagonist. Their lengths of action are relatively short, usually shorter than the length of opiate or benzodiazepine being reversed.[2,4] Additional doses may be required and should be repeated as needed.

For moderate sedation, the physician and nurse must be knowledgeable about the pharmacologic properties and therapeutic characteristics, including indications, contraindications, and other specific considerations. For percutaneous coronary interventions and stent deployment, the combination of drugs preferred at Duke University Hospital cardiovascular catheterization laboratory is hydromorphone (Dilaudid) with Versed. Starting doses of IV 0.5 mg of both Dilaudid and Versed are used. Appropriate dosing should be individualized to the response of the patient.[10]

[ ] STANDARDS FOR THE DELIVERY OF MODERATE SEDATION

The Joint Commission on Accreditation of Healthcare Organizations (JCAHO) clearly defines the standards and minimal requirements for administering and monitoring moderate sedation.[8] These standards establish a *uniform standard of care* for all patients. Moderate sedation guidelines may be more, but not less restrictive than hospital guidelines. The standards for sedation apply when patients receive moderate sedation, in any setting, for any purpose, and by any route. These are reproduced in Table 24-5.

[ ] CARE AND MONITORING OF PATIENTS RECEIVING MODERATE SEDATION

Specific recommendations for the preprocedural, intraprocedural, and postprocedural care and monitoring are listed below. Refer to JCAHO Consent Policy RI.2.40 (see Table 24–5).

Preprocedure Care and Monitoring

A baseline health evaluation includes a brief health history:

- Adverse experience with sedation/analgesia, regional and general anesthesia.
- Allergies and previous adverse drug reactions.
- Current medications.
- Disease, disorders, and abnormalities.
- Prior hospitalizations.
- Pertinent family history of disease or disorders.
- Review of systems.

A baseline physical examination includes:

- Height and weight.
- Vital signs.
- Baseline oxygen saturation.
- Airway assessment.
- Chest and cardiac examination.
- Level of consciousness.
- Laboratory and diagnostic testing relevant to the medical condition.
- Time and nature of the last oral intake.
- Baseline blood pressure, pulse and respiratory rates, oxygen saturation (on room air unless the patient arrives with oxygen) and level of consciousness, must be documented on the flow sheet.

Procedure Care and Monitoring

Immediately before the initiation of the procedure, a preprocedure assessment must be performed including the physician's verbal statement and written documentation that there has been no change from the baseline assessment.

The moderate sedation nurse must be able to monitor, document and respond appropriately to the patient's response to medications, including adverse drug reactions and, at a minimum, changes in the following:

- Vital signs.
- Degree of sedation (ie, Modified Ramsey Score).
- Presence or loss of a patent airway.
- Oxygen saturation.
- Pain level.
- Response to medication.

Blood pressure, pulse and respiratory rates, oxygen saturation, pain level and the degree of sedation must be assessed and

TABLE 24-4

Pharmacologic Agents Used for Moderate Sedation in the Cardiac Catheterization Suite

DRUGS	DOSE	MAX	ONSET (Min)	DURATION (Min)	CONSIDERATIONS
SEDATIVES					
Midazolam (Sedative, Amnesic)	0.5–1.0 mg	3.5 mg	3 min	15–30 min	This agent produces amnesia; patients may not be able to follow post procedure instructions. Slurred speech is a good end point for sedation. Use one third less if other central nervous system drugs, including narcotics, are in use.
Diazepam (Valium) (sedative, amnesic)	2.5–5.0 mg	30 mg	2–5 min	240 min	Pain on injection; phlebitis.
BENZODIAZEPINE ANTAGONIST					
Flumazenil (Romazicon)	0.2 mg	0.6–1.0 mg	1–3 min	45 min	Half life of the benzodiazepine may be longer than half life of flumazenil, resulting in residual sedation.
NARCOTIC					
Hydromorphone hydrochloride (Dilaudid) (Narcotic Analgesic)	0.5–1.0 mg	4 mg	10–15 min	120–240 min	Used to treat moderate to severe pain; Can cause serious reactions in patients who have taken MAO inhibitors within the previous 14 days.
Morphine sulfate (Narcotic analgesic)	2–4 mg	8–15 mg	1–2 min	240 min	Decreases the workload of the heart muscle by reducing myocardial wall tension and myocardial oxygen demand. Benefits patients with an acute MI as well as pulmonary edema and congestive heart failure.
Fentanyl (Sublimaze) (Narcotic Analgesic)	50–100 μg	Titrate in increments of μg to desired effect	1–2 min	30–60 min	Reduce dose when given with sedatives; useful as adjunct for sedative; beneficial for pain; airways monitor for respiratory depression.
NARCOTIC ANATAGONIST					
Naloxone (Narcan)	0.4–2.0 mg	Titrate patient's response	2–3 min	45–60 min	In patients with narcotic addictions, Narcan can cause severe withdrawal symptoms. Adverse reations include VF, VT, hypotension and pulmonary edema.

MAO = monoamine oxidase; MI = myocardial infarction; VF = ventricular fibrillation; VT = ventricular tachycardia.

documented on the flow sheet at least every 10 minutes during the procedure. Following an initial dose, and after each additional dose of IV sedative medication, these measurements should be recorded (every 2–3 minutes), depending on the drug selected, the route of administration, and the patient's clinical needs. Monitoring may need to be more frequent depending on the clinical needs of the patient and may also vary by organizational policy.

Postprocedure Care and Monitoring

On termination of sedation medication, patient monitoring must continue until the patient achieves his/her presedation level of consciousness and functionality.[8] Patients who receive moderate sedation must be monitored postprocedure. Recovery and discharge are based on one of two methods:

TABLE 24-5

2004 JCAHO Standards for the Administration of Moderate Sedation

Standard RI.2.40	Informed consent is obtained.
Rationale for RI.2.40	The goal of the informed consent process is to establish a mutual understanding between the patient and the physician or other licensed independent practitioner who provides the care, treatment, and services about the care, treatment, and services that the patient receives. This process allows each patient to fully participate in decisions about his or her care, treatment, and services.
Elements of Performance for RI.2.40	1. The hospital's policies describe the following: • Which procedures or care, treatment, and services require informed consent • The process used to obtain informed consent • How informed consent is to be documented in the record • When a surrogate decision maker, rather than the patient, may give informed consent • When procedures or care, treatment, and services normally requiring informed consent may be given without informed consent 2. Informed consent is obtained and documented in accordance with the hospital's policy 3. A complete informed consent process includes a discussion of the following elements: • The nature of the proposed care, treatment, services, medications, interventions, or procedures • Potential benefits, risks, or side effects, including potential problems related to recuperation • The likelihood of achieving care, treatment, and services goals • Reasonable alternatives to the proposed care, treatment, and service • The relevant risks, benefits, and side effects related to alternatives, including the possible results of not receiving care, treatment, and services • When indicated, any limitations on the confidentiality of information learned from or about the patient
Standard PC.2.120 **Elements of Performance for PC.2.120**	The hospital defines in writing the time frame(s) for conducting the initial assessment(s). 1. The hospital defines the time frames(s) for conducting the initial assessment(s). *The hospital specifies the following time frames for these assessments:* 2. A medical history and physical examination is completed within no more than 24 hours of inpatient admission 3. A nursing assessment is completed within no more than 24 hours of inpatient admission 4. A nutritional screening, when warranted by the patient's needs or condition, is completed within no more than 24 hours of inpatient admission 5. A functional status screening, when warranted by the patient's needs or condition, is completed within no more than 24 hours of inpatient admission *Some of these elements may have been completed ahead of time, but most meet the following criteria:* 6. The history and physical must have been completed within 30 days before the patient was admitted or readmitted 7. Updates to the patient's condition since the assessment(s) are recorded at the time of admission
Standard PC.13.20	Operative or other procedures and/or the administration of moderate or deep sedation or anesthesia are planned.
Rationale for PC.13.20	Because the response to procedures is not always predictable and sedation-to-anesthesia is a continuum, it is not always possible to predict how an individual patient will respond. Therefore, qualified individuals are trained in professional standards and techniques to manage patients in the case of a potentially harmful event.

TABLE 24-5

2004 JCAHO Standards for the Administration of Moderate Sedation *(continued)*

Elements of Performance for PC.13.20	1. Sufficient numbers of qualified staff are available to evaluate the patient, perform the procedure, monitor, and recover the patient. 2. Individuals administering moderate or deep sedation and anesthesia are qualified and have the appropriate credentials to manage patients at whatever level of sedation or anesthesia is achieved, either intentionally or unintentionally. 3. A registered nurse supervises perioperative nursing care. 4. Appropriate equipment to monitor the patient's physiologic status is available. 5. Appropriate equipment to administer intravenous fluids and drugs, including blood and blood components, is available as needed. 6. Resuscitation capabilities are available. *Before operative and other procedures or the administration of moderate or deep sedation or anesthesia:* 7. Patient acuity is assessed to plan for the appropriate level of postprocedure care. 8. Preprocedural education, treatments, and services are provided according to the plan for care, treatment, and services. 9. The site, procedure, and patient are accurately identified and clearly communicated, using active communication techniques, during a final verification process, such as "time out," prior to the start of any surgical or invasive procedure. 10. A presedation or preanesthesia assessment is conducted. 11. Before sedating or anesthetizing a patient, a licensed independent practitioner with appropriate clinical privileges plans or concurs with the planned anesthesia. 12. The patient is reevaluated immediately before moderate or deep sedation and before anesthesia induction.
Standard PC.13.30	Patients are monitored during the procedure and/or administration of moderate or deep sedation or anesthesia
Elements of Performance for PC.13.30	1. Appropriate methods are used to continuously monitor oxygenation, ventilation, and circulation during procedures that may affect the patient's physiological status. 2. The procedure and/or the administration of moderate or deep sedation or anesthesia for each patient are documented in the medical record.
Standard PC.13.40	Patients are monitored immediately after the procedure and/or administration of moderate or deep sedation or anesthesia.
Elements of Performance for PC.13.40	1. The patient's status is assessed on arrival in the recovery area. 2. Each patient's physiological status, mental status, and pain level are monitored. 3. Monitoring is at a level consistent with the potential effect of the procedure and/or sedation or anesthesia. 4. Patients are discharged from the recovery area and the hospital by a qualified licensed independent practitioner according to rigorously applied criteria approved by the clinical leaders. 5. Patients who have received anesthesia in the outpatient setting are discharged in the company of a responsible, designated adult.

- Recovery/discharge by a physician.
- Achievement of standardized monitoring, documentation, and continuing care requirements.

Prior to discharge, or transfer of care to an inpatient bed, the care nurse observes and documents any postprocedure complications, manages those events, and responds to the patient.

For the outpatient, absence of nausea and vomiting and ability to void is required prior to discharge. After the patient's vital signs and level of consciousness have returned to normal, the nurse provides verbal and written discharge instructions to the patient and a responsible designated adult accompanying the patient. The nurse has the patient verbalize the understanding of the instructions and then documents this on the flow sheet.

For the inpatient, the care nurse provides a verbal report to the nurse receiving the patient. The report includes preprocedure vital signs and level of consciousness, any problems encountered during or postprocedure, total drugs given, total IV fluid given, and status of IV administration. The nurse notes the time and name of person to whom the report is given and signs the flow sheet. All information is documented on the patient's permanent medical record.

Providing for patient safety and at the same time achieving an optimal comfort level is clearly the most important aspect of delivery of moderate sedation. Moderate sedation allows patients to recover and resume normal daily activities in a relatively short period.

Acknowledgment

Special mention and thanks to Cara A. Gardner, BA, Human Genetics, Duke University Medical Center, for her assistance in editing accompanying articles and chapters.

REFERENCES

1. American Society of Anesthesiologists Clinical Statement (2004). Continuum of Depth of Sedation: Definition of General Anesthesia and Levels of Sedation/Analgesia. Available at http://www.asahq.org/publicationsandservices/standards/20.pdf. Last accessed on July 7, 2006.
2. Trissel L, ed. *Pocket Guide to Injectable Drugs.* Bethesda, MD: American Society of Hospital Pharmacists; 2003.
3. Gahart BL, Nazareno AR. *Intravenous Medications: A Handbook for Nurses and Allied Health Professionals.* St. Louis: Mosby; 1998.
4. Pasero C. (1996) *Moderate Sedation/Analgesia for Adults.* City of Hope Pain Resource Center. Available at: http://www.cityofhope.org/prc/html/paserosedation.htm.
5. Yaniga L. Agents for the relief of pain and anxiety in the cath lab. *Cath Lab Dig.* 2004. Available at: http://www.hmpcommunications.com/CLD.
6. Lazear SE. *Moderate Sedation/Analgesia.* CME Resource. 2002. Available at: http://www.netce.com/course.asp?Course=1055.
7. Kern MJ ed. *The Interventional Cardiac Catheterization Handbook.* Philadelphia, Mosby; 2004.
8. Joint Commission Resource—2004 Hospital Standards, 3rd ed. Education, Program Workbook, 2003.
9. Webner C, Marzlin K. Conscious sedation. *ACVP CP Dig.* 2006; 49(2).
10. Duke Policy and Procedure. *Moderate Sedation.* Available at: http://www.hr.duke. edu.

APPENDIX IV-1

Clinical Trials Cited in Chapters 19 Through 24

ABBREVIATED NAME	COMPLETE NAME
ACE	Abciximab and Carbostent Evaluation
ACUITY	Acute Catheterization and Urgent Intervention Thrombotic StrategY
ADMIRAL	Abciximab Before Direct Angioplasty and Stenting in Myocardial Infarction Regarding Acute and Long-term Follow-up
ASSENT-2	Assessment of the Safety and Efficacy of a New Thrombolytic-2
BAT	Bivalirudin Angioplasty Trial
CACHET	Comparison of Abciximab Complications with Hirulog for Ischemic Events Trial
CADILLAC	Controlled Abciximab and Device Investigation to Lower Late Angioplasty Complications
CAPRIE	Clopidogrel versus Aspirin in Patients at Risk of Ischemic Events
CAPTIM	Comparison of Angioplasty and Prehospital Thrombolysis in Acute Myocardial Infarction
CAPTURE	Chimeric 7E3 Antiplatelet Therapy in Unstable Refractory Angina
COMPARE	Comparison Of Measurements of Platelet Aggregation with Aggrastat, ReoPro, and Eptifibatide
COURT	Contrast Utilization in high-Risk PTCA
CREDO	Clopidogrel for the Reduction of Events During Observation
CRUISE	Coronary Revascularization Using Integrilin and Single bolus Enoxaparin
CURE	Clopidogrel in Unstable Angina to Prevent Recurrent Events
DANAMI-2	Danish Multicenter Randomized Trial on Thrombolytic Therapy versus Acute Coronary Angioplasty in Acute Myocardial Infarction
EARLY ACS	Eptifibatide Administration Prior to Diagnostic Catheterization and Revascularization to Limit Myocardial Necrosis in Acute Coronary Syndromes
ENTIRE-TIMI-23	Enoxaparin and TNK-TPA with or without glycoprotein IIb/IIIa Inhibitor as Reperfusion Strategy in ST-elevation Myocardial Infarction
EPIC	Evaluation of c7E3 for the Prevention of Ischemic Complications
EPILOG	Evaluation in PTCA to Improve Long-term Outcome with Abciximab GP IIb/IIIa Blockade
ESSENCE	Efficacy Safety Subcutaneous Enoxaparin in Non-Q-Wave Coronary Events
EPISTENT	Evaluation of IIb/IIIa Platelet Inhibitor for Stenting
ESPRIT	Enhanced Suppression of the Platelet IIb/IIIa Receptor with Integrilin Therapy
FINESSE	Facilitated Intervention with Enhanced Reperfusion Speed to Stop Events

APPENDIX IV-1

Clinical Trials Cited in Chapters 19 Through 24 (continued)

GISSI	Gruppo Italiano per lo Studio della Streptochinasi nell' Infarcto miocardico
GOLD	Au-Assessing Ultegra Multicenter Study
GRAPE	Glycoprotein Receptor Antagonist Patency Evaluation
GUSTO-IIb	Global Use of Strategies to Open Occluded Arteries in Acute Coronary Syndromes
GUSTO-IV	Global Use of Streptokinase and Tissue Plasminogen Activator for Occluded Arteries
HART-II	Heparin and Aspirin Reperfusion Therapy-II
HERO-2	Hirulog and Early Reperfusion or Occlusion-2
IMPACT-II	Integrilin to Minimize Platelet Aggregation and Coronary Thrombosis
INJECT	International Joint Efficacy Comparison of Thrombolytics
InTIME	Treatment of Infarcting Myocardium Early
INTERACT	Integrilin and Enoxaparin Randomized assessment of Acute Coronary Syndrome Treatment
ISAR-REACT	Intracoronary Stenting and Antithrombotic Regimen-Rapid Early Action for Coronary Treatment
ISAR-COOL	Intracoronary Stenting and Antithrombotic Regimen-Evaluation of Prolonged Antithrombotic Pretreatment ("Cooling-Off" Strategy) Before Intervention in Patients With Unstable Coronary Syndromes
ISAR-2	Intracoronary Stenting and Antithrombotic Regimen
ISIS-2	Second International Study of Infarct Survival
KDOQI	National Kidney Foundation Kidney Disease Outcomes Quality Initiative
NICE	National Investigators Collaborating on Enoxaparin
PACT	Primary Angioplasty Compatibility Trial
PAMI	Primary Angioplasty in Myocardial Infarction
PCI-CURE	Percutaneous Coronary Intervention-Clopidogrel in Unstable Angina to Prevent Recurrent Events
PEPCI	Pharmacokinetics of Enoxaparin in PCI
PRAGUE	Primary Angioplasty After Transport of patients From General Community Hospitals to Catheterization Units With/Without Emergency Thrombolysis Infusion
PRISM	Platelet Receptor Inhibition in Ischemic Syndrome Management
PRISM-PLUS	Platelet Receptor Inhibition for Ischemic Syndrome Management in Patients Limited by Unstable Signs and Symptoms
PROTECT-TIMI 30	A Randomized Trial To Evaluate The Relative Protection Against Post-PCI Microvascular Dysfunction and Post-PCI Ischemia Among Antiplatelet and Antithrombotic Agents
PURSUIT	Platelet Glycoprotein IIb-IIIa in Unstable Angina: Receptor Suppression Using Integrilin Therapy
RAPID	Reteplase versus Alteplase Infusion in Acute Myocardial Infarction
RAPPORT	ReoPro And Primary Percutaneous Transluminal Coronary Angioplasty Organization and Randomized Trial
REPLACE	Randomized Evaluation in PCI Linking Angiomax to reduced Clinical Events
RESTORE	Randomized Efficacy Study of Tirofiban for Outcomes and REstenosis
SIAM-III	Southwest German International Study in Acute Myocardial Infarction-III
SPEED	Strategies for Patency Enhancement in the Emergency Department
STEEPLE	Safety and Efficacy of Enoxaparin in PCI Patients, an International Randomized Evaluation
SYNERGY	Superior Yield of the New strategy of Enoxaparin, Revascularization, and Glycoprotein IIb/IIIa Inhibitors
TACTICS-TIMI 18	Treat angina with Aggrastat and determine Cost of Therapy with an Invasive or Conservative Strategy-Thrombolysis in Myocardial Infarction
TIMI	Thrombolysis in Myocardial Infarction
TARGET	Do Tirofiban And ReoPro Give similar Efficacy outcomes?
VIP	Visipaque in PCTI

PART (5) Procedures

CHAPTER (25)

Diagnostic Procedures: Special Considerations

Spencer B. King III, MD

The interventional cardiologist must first and foremost be competent in performing, interpreting, and understanding the studies that define the coronary anatomy and function. Therefore, diagnostic high-quality coronary arteriography is not only a critical part of the armamentarium of the interventional cardiologist but is also important for all physicians performing coronary arteriograms. There are certain considerations for obtaining adequate coronary arteriograms and left ventricular function studies that are unique to the era of interventional cardiology. Prior to Gruentzig's seminal development, coronary arteriograms were largely used to discriminate patients with and without coronary artery disease and to select those who should be referred for coronary bypass surgery. Although these functions are still crucial, the demands of interventional cardiology place new requirements on understanding the principal diagnostic procedures that enable modern revascularization to be performed.

HISTORY OF CORONARY ANGIOGRAPHY

Prior to 1958, it was felt that any placement of catheters or injection of contrast media into the coronary arteries would be contraindicated as a life-threatening adventure. Mason Sones's development of coronary arteriography set the stage for the development of direct coronary bypass surgery and eventually coronary angioplasty.[1] Numerous others played a role in developing the currently applied techniques of coronary angioplasty, most notably Melvin Judkins.[2] The Seldinger approach from the femoral artery was used by the radiologist, and preformed catheters were shaped in the laboratory by literally bending them around plumbing pipes in

the laboratory and heating the catheters so that they would retain their shape. These shapes, designed by Judkins, withstood the test of time and remain the most commonly used devices today. Kurt Amplatz also designed catheters based partly on the designs of Castillo brachial catheters. Fred Schoonmaker and I worked on applying the Sones technique from the Seldinger femoral approach and finally settled on an existing multipurpose catheter as the best solution for a single catheter multipurpose technique.[3]

INDICATIONS FOR CORONARY ARTERIOGRAPHY

The American College of Cardiology/American Heart Association Task Force on Practice Guidelines published a report on the indications for coronary arteriography that identified the following indications:

- Patients with stable angina or asymptomatic individuals with high-risk criteria on noninvasive testing.

- Patients resuscitated from sudden cardiac death or having threatening ventricular arrhythmias.

- Patients with unstable coronary syndromes of all varieties, including acute myocardial infarction as a preamble to primary angioplasty and those who developed complications of acute infarction.

- Patients with ischemia at low levels of exercise following in the recovery phase of myocardial infarction.

- Patients with suspected or known coronary artery disease undergoing preoperative evaluation.

When the coronary anatomy is important for planning surgical procedures, such as in patients with valvular heart disease or in those with congestive heart failure in order to establish the correct etiology, coronary angiography is also recommended.[4]

To establish the need for coronary arteriography, results of the medical history, the electrocardiogram and various other indices of myocardial ischemia and coronary vascular abnormalities are needed. It is most critical to avoid errors in history taking. Without recognition of the many varieties of presentation of myocardial ischemia, the physician cannot proceed with the proper workup. Likewise, a superficial history identifying chest pain of any type is not a license to perform coronary arteriography. The judgment of a well-trained and knowledgeable physician skilled at taking an accurate history is of the utmost importance. Understanding the relationship of increased metabolic demands on fixed lesions and understanding the pathophysiology of acute coronary syndromes is required.

Once ischemic heart disease is suspected, stable patients should undergo electrocardiography and often stress testing, including electrocardiographic exercise stress testing and nuclear perfusion studies or stress echocardiography, or all of these diagnostic tests. Performance and interpretation of these procedures is beyond the scope of this chapter; however, interventional cardiologists should become skilled at interpreting these studies, not simply reading the reports. The location of ischemic defects and the extent of these defects, as well as the level of exercise performed, are important both prognostically and, when combined with the angiographic images, in determining the relative benefit of revascularization.

Finally, noninvasive diagnostic tests that examine the coronary arteries (eg, electron beam computed tomography and multislice computed tomography) often identify a need for coronary angiography. The detection of a large amount of calcium in the coronary arteries in young individuals heralds the presence of atherosclerosis but does not confirm obstructive disease. Multislice computed tomography is becoming increasingly accurate in identifying not only calcification in coronary arteries, but the course of vessels and in many cases the obstructive lesions themselves. This technology and perhaps magnetic resonance imaging in the future may supplant diagnostic coronary arteriography as the dominant strategy for investigating patients with coronary artery disease. That day, however, has not yet arrived and coronary arteriography remains the gold standard for selecting patients for coronary interventions and for planning the interventional approach.

EQUIPMENT

The catheters available for coronary arteriography are the Judkins shape, defined as the Judkins right, the Judkins left, the pigtail catheter for left ventriculography, the internal mammary artery catheter, and the shapes for intubating left and right coronary bypass grafts. The Amplatz shapes should also be available. The AL2 catheter is used predominantly for the left coronary artery and the AL1 catheter most commonly for difficult right coronary intubation. The multipurpose catheter is used by some operators as the dominant diagnostic catheter for coronary arteriography and left ventriculography, and there are specialty catheters for intubating difficult ostial positions, such as an anteriorly located right coronary ostium. Over the years, catheters used for coronary diagnostic arteriography have become smaller in diameter so that currently the most commonly used catheters are 6 French (Fr), with some operators utilizing 5-Fr and 4-Fr catheters. The advantage of 6-Fr diagnostic catheters over the 5-Fr and 4-Fr catheters is that

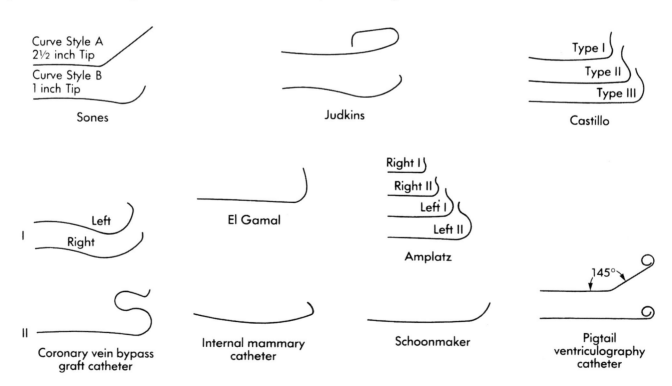

FIGURE 25-1. Commonly used catheter shapes for selective coronary arteriography and left ventriculography. *(Reproduced with permission from Kern MJ. Cardiac Catheterization Handbook. St Louis, MO: Mosby; 2003.)*

their shape retention and torque control is optimal. Devotees of the very small catheters point out that the femoral complications may be even less with these catheters than with the 6-Fr catheters, and adequate angiographic images can be obtained although sometimes various aids to injecting contrast media are used. Figure 25-1 illustrates the commonly used catheter shapes.

PROCEDURES

[ ] JUDKINS TECHNIQUE

Puncture of the femoral artery is the first critical step in performing coronary arteriography. The pulse should be palpated at the level of the inguinal ligament. If the right femoral artery is used, placing the index and middle finger of the left hand astride the pulsation can accurately identify the target for the Seldinger needle. The skin entry site is commonly the inguinal crease; however, the critical maneuver is to puncture the artery above the bifurcation of the femoral artery. The common femoral artery should be punctured, and the profunda or superficial femoral arteries should be avoided. Confirmation of the site of arterial puncture can be obtained by performing fluoroscopy of the needle tip.

The tip should enter the femoral artery in a position that is marked by the inner portion of the upper third of the femoral head when viewed in the anteroposterior projection. An effective technique for achieving this position is to palpate the inguinal ligament and then place the skin insertion site approximately one finger-breadth below the inguinal ligament, with the needle directed approximately 45 degrees from the vertical. Attempts should be made to puncture the anterior wall of the artery by advancing the bare needle until brisk backflow of blood is observed. For interventional cardiologists, the importance of obtaining the correct position for femoral puncture lies in the need to avoid bleeding complications in patients who undergo interventional procedures and are, therefore, anticoagulated. The correct puncture site above the bifurcation of the femoral artery is necessary for the utilization of the various closure devices that may be selected.

Using Judkins Catheters

After placing a properly sized femoral artery sheath, the left ventricular catheter, which is commonly the pigtail catheter, is selected and advanced over a 0.038-in guidewire. The guidewire is continued around the aortic arch, and the catheter is positioned above the aortic valve with the guidewire removed. Aspiration and flushing of the catheter should be performed to prevent introduction of air or embolic material. When crossing the normal aortic valve, gentle bending of the pigtail catheter on the aortic valve will usually cause it to prolapse into the left ventricle. Occasionally reinsertion of the guidewire may be required to stiffen the shaft of the catheter in order to facilitate crossing the valve. Rotation of the pigtail catheter in a clockwise and counterclockwise direction may also be helpful. Occasionally it may be necessary to use the guidewire as the lead in crossing the valve. Sometimes a straight guidewire is required after positioning the tip of the catheter so that it faces the orifices of a stenotic or sclerotic aortic valve.

Left ventriculography with a pigtail catheter is usually performed with the aid of a power injector. Judkins recommended that the loop on the catheter be rotated counterclockwise and withdrawn so as to position the loop near the entry of the open mitral valve. This facilitates good mixing of contrast material with blood flowing into the left ventricle so that adequate left ventriculography can be obtained with modest amounts of contrast media. This position often reduces the chance for ventricular ectopic beats, which are more common when injection is made into the left ventricular apex. Left ventriculography can be obtained in the right oblique and left oblique views, but the left oblique view is often unnecessary if right oblique ventriculography shows normal contractility. The finding of an occluded circumflex system should prompt the operator to perform left anterior oblique ventriculography in order to evaluate the motion of the posterolateral wall. Following left ventriculography, the catheter is flushed and pullback across the aortic valve is performed to identify any aortic valve gradient.

The left Judkins catheter selected for most patients should be the 4.0 device. This catheter is advanced over the guidewire into the aortic root. This maneuver is commonly performed in the left anterior oblique view in order to see the curve of the left Judkins catheter. If the tip does not engage the left coronary artery after removing the guidewire, the catheter can be advanced into the left aortic cusp, deflected slightly in the cusp, and then pulled back briskly to allow the tip to engage the ostium of the left coronary artery. In small aortic roots, a JL3.5 catheter may be preferred, and in very large aortic roots, it may be necessary to move to a JL5.0 catheter. Identification of these problems is easily made. If the secondary curve of the Judkins catheter remains in a vertical position in the aorta and the tip does not move up toward the ostium of the left coronary artery, then a small aortic root is present, requiring use of the smaller catheter. If, on the other hand, the secondary curve folds up on itself so the catheter tip comes to lie in the position it was in before insertion of the catheter, then the root is too large and a larger sized device may be required.

Right coronary cannulation with the Judkins catheter is usually accomplished with the catheter positioned above the left coronary cusp; then with clockwise rotation, the catheter can be swept across the anterior portion of the aortic root until it engages the right coronary artery. This maneuver causes the catheter tip to advance; therefore, simultaneous withdrawal of the catheter is usually required while rotating clockwise. An alternative maneuver, recommended by Judkins, is to place the catheter high in the aorta above the left coronary cusp and rotate clockwise, allowing the catheter tip to both sweep anteriorly along the aortic wall, as well as descend into the right coronary ostium.

[ ] OTHER CATHETER APPROACHES

The multipurpose catheter is used by some operators, including the author, as the principal catheter for coronary arteriography. This catheter is maneuvered in a manner similar to the Sones technique but performed from the femoral approach. The catheter can be maneuvered across the aortic valve in a similar manner as that used with the pigtail catheter. To avoid arrhythmias and intramyocardial injection, it is important to carefully position this catheter in the mid-left ventricular chamber. Usually a hand injection is performed with this technique, and by utilizing a 6-Fr catheter, adequate ventriculography can be obtained in a majority of cases.

Cannulation of the left coronary artery is performed by placing a catheter tip in the noncoronary cusp and advancing it until the catheter begins to buckle. Then, with clockwise rotation, the tip of the catheter is be flipped up into the left coronary cusp. Withdrawal of the catheter at the moment of that flip is usually required to maintain the correct position. If the tip does not enter the left coronary artery directly, then allowing the tip to fall into the left coronary cusp and subsequently advancing the catheter up the left coronary cusp with gentle counterclockwise rotation usually brings the tip up to the left coronary ostium.

Intubation of the right coronary artery is accomplished by positioning the patient in the left anterior oblique view and positioning the catheter initially above the left coronary ostium in a manner similar to that used for the Judkins catheter. The catheter is rotated clockwise and swept along the anterior portion of the aortic wall until it encounters the ostium in the right coronary artery. Although this maneuver was usually performed successfully with the original 8-Fr multipurpose catheters, the more flexible 6-Fr catheters often do not directly encounter the ostium in the right coronary artery. In that case, the 6-Fr catheter can be advanced into the right coronary cusp; gentle advancement will commonly cause the tip to migrate up and enter the right coronary ostium. If it enters deeply, then the catheter should be gently withdrawn until it lies in the ostium of that vessel.

The Amplatz curve catheters are sometimes required for entry into an ectopically placed left coronary ostium and some very large aortic roots. The Amplatz left coronary catheter is helpful in intubating high and anteriorly placed right coronary ostia. Other catheters, such as the hockey stick curve and the Amplatz right catheter, as well as the internal mammary catheter, can sometimes be helpful in intubating right coronary arteries. Of particular help in the anteriorly placed ostium of the right coronary artery is the out-of-plane right coronary catheter (Williams catheter).

The internal mammary artery catheter should be used to cannulate that vessel (Figure 25-2). The guidewire is used to advance the catheter around the aortic arch, and by placing the catheter at the top of the aortic arch and rotating it counterclockwise, the tip can be brought into the left subclavian artery. Sometimes the tip enters the left carotid artery; gentle withdrawal of the catheter will then cause it to slip into the left subclavian artery. Once the subclavian artery is entered, insertion of a guidewire distally in that vessel will facilitate easy passage of the catheter to the point of the internal mammary artery. The internal mammary arises caudally from the subclavian artery, and frequently some counterclockwise or clockwise rotation of the tip is required to enter that vessel. Vein graft cannulation is usually possible with the right Judkins catheter but other catheters may be helpful in that regard. The right coronary vein graft is commonly the most caudal position and rightward on the aorta. This is a graft that travels in an inferior direction, and the multipurpose catheter is usually ideal for entering that conduit. Left coronary vein grafts are usually arranged so that the lowest or most caudal is the anterior descending graft followed by diagonal grafts, and the most superior are the circumflex grafts. These grafts are commonly stacked one above the other, and entry is usually possible with right coronary or multipurpose catheters or left coronary bypass graft catheters. Occasionally the

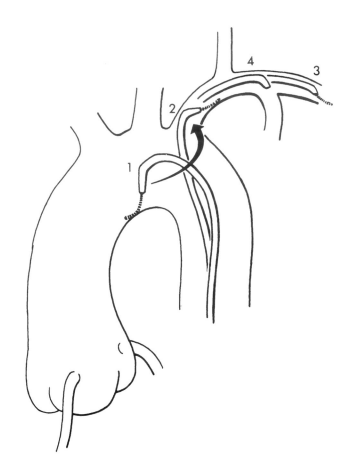

FIGURE 25-2. Technique for catheterizing the left internal mammary artery. A guidewire is used to enter the left subclavian artery and then removed in order to perform contrast injections to visualize the ostium of the vessel. *(Reproduced with permission from King SB, Douglas JS Jr. Coronary Arteriography and Angioplasty. New York, NY: McGraw-Hill; 1985.)*

ostia are distal in the ascending aorta and other devices, such as Amplatz curves, are required to contact those ostia.

Traversing tortuous iliac vessels, which are common in older patients with hypertension, can be problematic. The presence of peripheral vascular disease also complicates the process. If the needle has entered the femoral artery and the guidewire does not advance easily into the aorta, the operator should perform fluoroscopy of the femoral puncture area. If the guidewire has traversed in a lateral direction into the circumflex iliac vessel, it may be possible to pull it back and redirect into the femoral artery. If the wire passes partway into the iliac vessel but does not advance further, it is sometimes helpful to remove the guidewire and perform a contrast injection into the femoral artery through the needle.

Once an adequate entry into the femoral artery has been obtained, the sheath can be placed partway into the femoral artery and further, more vigorous injections used to visualize the course of the vessel and any obstructions that may be present. The use of the hydrophilic guidewires often facilitates crossing the tortuous iliac, although in many cases the best approach is to deflect the tip of the guidewire away from cul de sacs and obstructing plaque and toward the residual lumen. The use of the right Judkins diagnostic catheter has been helpful as a method of aiming the guidewire in the desired direction. Small contrast injections through the diagnostic catheter can be made to visualize the course of the iliac vessel. When tortuous segments are identified, it is usually helpful to place a long sheath, which will partially straighten the iliac system and allow easy entry into the aorta as well as facilitating catheter exchanges. Manipulation of the diagnostic catheter can be enhanced by placing the 0.038-in guidewire into the catheter to prevent kinking while torquing the catheter. If kinking of a diagnostic catheter occurs, the catheter should be rotated in the opposite direction while placing a guidewire back into the catheter before trying to remove it through the sheath.

[ ] ARM APPROACH

Some operators preferentially use the radial artery for coronary arteriography.[5] Most operators, however, resort to the use of radial or brachial approach when there is obstruction in the ileofemoral system. Radial artery catheterization was first reported in 1989, although brachial artery percutaneous catheterization has been performed by the Seldinger approach for many years. The radial approach has become the preferred method of some operators because it allows rapid ambulation at the end of the procedure. It is critical that the Allen test be performed before electing the radial approach to assure that there is adequate collateral circulation to the hand, because occlusion of the radial artery is not uncommon. Use of the radial artery enables very easy hemostasis, even in patients who have received anticoagulation therapy. The disadvantages of the radial approach are that large catheters are not very practical and use of the radial artery might compromise the future use of that vessel as an arterial conduit, should extensive arterial bypass grafting be needed in the future. When the radial artery approach is used, a short, 20-gauge needle is inserted and a 0.025-in guidewire is placed in the vessel. With the guidewire in place, a long sheath can be inserted through which heparin is usually administered during sheath insertion. Some operators administer 1% lidocaine and 200 µg of nitroglycerin into the sheath to prevent arterial spasm. A 6-Fr or smaller catheter is commonly used from the radial approach, and although the Sones catheters are seldom used today, the multipurpose catheter can be manipulated from the radial artery in a manner similar to Sones catheterization. Preformed catheters, such as the Judkins and Amplatz shapes, also are easily employed from the radial approach.

[ ] AVOIDING CONTRAST-INDUCED TOXICITY

All contrast media can induce nephropathy, and this is especially problematic in older patients with marginal creatinine clearance. No contrast agent is immune from this problem, and contrast agents are usually chosen for their relatively low osmolarity. The principal method for decreasing the likelihood of renal damage involves limiting the amount of contrast media used while maintaining good hydration and renal blood flow. Patients at risk of renal toxicity should be hydrated intravenously before the procedure, and liberal use of intravenous fluids throughout the procedure is also recommended. Diuretics, mannitol, and calcium channel blockers are not helpful in avoiding renal complications. N-acetylcysteine given prior to the procedure has been associated with reduced contrast-induced nephropathy. Fenoldopam, first thought to have a potent effect, was not helpful in a recently conducted randomized trial.

Limiting the volume of contrast media is an important goal for interventional cardiologists because many interventional procedures follow directly after diagnostic catheterization, thereby increasing the total volume of contrast media. If prior coronary arteriograms have been obtained, it may be possible to avoid repeating unnecessary views and if there has been no clinical change, it may also be possible to avoid ventriculography. In patients at very high risk for contrast-induced toxicity, left ventricular function may be assessed by other noninvasive means prior to the catheterization. Optimal views should be obtained first, and unnecessary additional views should be avoided, always bearing in mind that all segments of the coronary tree must be adequately visualized. One recently suggested approach is the method of rotating the x-ray tube or image tube gantry throughout an arc during coronary injection, thereby obtaining multiple views of the arteries with a single coronary injection.

[ ] SELECTING VIEWS

The optimal projections for viewing various segments of the coronary tree are illustrated in Figure 25-3. Modification of these views is necessary on an individual basis, based on the anatomy of the coronary circulation. In addition, the ostium of the left main coronary artery is often best seen in the straight posteroanterior view. The ostium of the right coronary artery will be best seen in a 45- to 60-degree left anterior oblique view with caudal angulation of the image intensifier. Visualization of the ostium of arteries and vein graft origins is critical when planning stent placement for ostial lesions. Modifications of the view should be made until the vessel is seen arising tangentially from the aorta with no overlap between the two vessels. The usual views for visualizing various segments of the coronary arterial tree are illustrated in Table 25-1.

[ ] AVOIDING PITFALLS IN OBTAINING ANGIOGRAPHIC VIEWS

Foreshortening

To estimate the length of arterial segments, especially the length of lesions, it is important to view the coronary artery segment in question *en face*. Views to assess the length of segments should be obtained where the segment achieves its maximum length, indicating that the x-ray beam is perpendicular to the artery segment in question.

Vessel Size

Estimation of vessel size usually is performed by comparison with the angiographic catheter tip. Larger angiographic catheters, such as 6-Fr and 7-Fr, provide easier calibration than smaller catheters. For the purpose of vessel size estimation, it is important to select views in which the catheter tip and the segment in question are in the same position relative to the x-ray tube and the image intensifier. Out-of-plane magnification errors will result if the catheter tip is materially closer to the image intensifier or the x-ray tube than the arterial segment to be calibrated. An example of such an error would be judging the size of the mid–anterior descending artery in

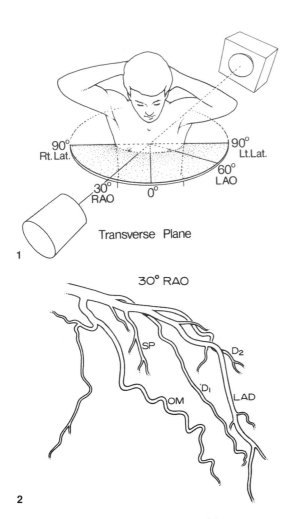

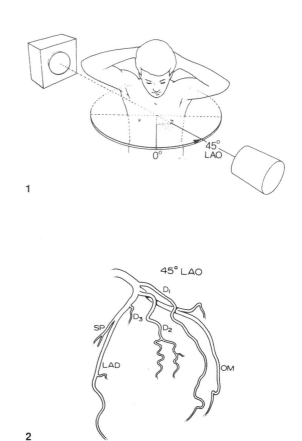

FIGURE 25-3A. Diagrammatic representation of the standard right anterior oblique (RAO) view of the left coronary arteriogram. The x-ray source is beneath the patient, the x-ray beam travels in a posterior-to-anterior direction, and the image intensifier is overhead. Most of the left coronary artery is well visualized in this projection, although there is considerable overlap of the mid-left anterior descending coronary artery and the diagonal branches. When the left main, circumflex, and diagonal branches have a leftward initial course, the long axis of these arterial segments is projected away from the image intensifier, preventing optimal visualization in this view. (D1, D2, D3 = first, second, third diagonal; OM = obtuse marginal; SP = septal perforator.) *(Reproduced from King SB III, Douglas JS Jr, Morris DC. New angiographic views for coronary arteriography. In: Hurst JW, ed. Update IV: The Heart. New York, NY: McGraw-Hill; 1981.)*

FIGURE 25-3B. Diagrammatic representation of the left anterior oblique (LAO) left coronary arteriogram. The image intensifier is above the patient in the LAO position, and the x-ray beam travels in a posterior-to-anterior direction. The value of this view depends in large part on the orientation of the long axis of the heart. When the heart is relatively horizontal, the left anterior descending (LAD) coronary artery and diagonal branches are seen end-on throughout much of their course. In this illustration, the heart is in an intermediate position, and there is moderate foreshortening of the LAD and diagonal branches in their proximal portions. The LAO projection is frequently inadequate to visualize the proximal LAD and its branches; the left main branch, which is directed toward the image tube and therefore foreshortened; and the proximal circumflex coronary artery, which may be obscured by overlapping vessels as in this illustration. The LAO projection is frequently used to visualize the proximal circumflex artery when there is not overlap, the distal LAD and its branches, the midcircumflex coronary artery in the atrioventricular groove, and the distal right coronary artery when it is filling via collaterals from the left coronary artery. (D1, D2, D3 = first, second, third diagonal; OM = obtuse marginal; SP = septal perforator.) *(Reproduced from King SB III, Douglas JS Jr, Morris DC. New angiographic views for coronary arteriography. In: Hurst JW, ed. Update IV: The Heart. New York, NY: McGraw-Hill; 1981.)*

the left anterior oblique cranial view. In this view, the anterior descending artery would be closer to the image intensifier, with the catheter tip lying in the aorta further away. This perspective would cause the image of the catheter to be magnified while decreasing magnification of the anterior descending artery, making it appear smaller than its actual size.

Cannulation of the right and left coronary ostia in the usual positions is ordinarily straightforward with any of the catheters described. The author favors either Judkins or multipurpose shapes. When the left main ostium is high in the sinus or above the sinus, the multipurpose catheter will not reach the ostium. When the aorta is dilated, larger Judkins catheters may be appropriate for the high left main ostium, but on some occasions an Amplatz II or

larger shape may be required. When the left main artery is very short or there are separate origins of the left anterior descending and circumflex arteries, selective entry into one or the other vessel is common. It is important to recognize the fact that one or the other vessel has not been cannulated. If the left circumflex artery is entered selectively with the left Judkins catheter, the operator should attempt to advance the catheter slightly, causing the tip to point more superiorly, thereby entering the anterior descending artery. In some cases it may be necessary to use a smaller left Judkins catheter for the anterior descending vessel. The Amplatz catheter will cannulate the circumflex artery selectively in these cases because it points caudally, but removal of Amplatz catheters can be problematic and may lead to dissection. These catheters should be handled very carefully to avoid complications. Operators should become competent in using Judkins, Amplatz, and multipurpose catheters so that all left coronary ostial locations can be cannulated.

The right coronary ostium is quite variable in location. It is sometimes located high on the right coronary cusp and may be positioned far anteriorly, causing intubation with the right Judkins catheter to be problematic. In cases involving such severe anterior locations, the use of the out-of-plane right coronary artery (Williams catheter) can be helpful.

Bifurcations

Bifurcations are best visualized from a perspective that affords no overlap of the arms of the bifurcation. This is critical in planning for the best interventional approach that will avoid plaque shifting and stenosis of side branches. Common views for left anterior descending diagonal bifurcations are the left anterior oblique cranial views and occasionally anteroposterior cranial views; for the circumflex marginal branches, the right anterior oblique caudal views; and for the right coronary artery posterior descending bifurcation, the shallow left anterior oblique cranial view.

The most common coronary anomaly is origin of the circumflex artery from the right coronary cusp. The vessel may arise from the right coronary artery itself or separately just anterior to the right coronary ostium. Commonly it arises in a caudal direction, and the multipurpose catheter is frequently helpful in selective cannulation of this vessel.

When the right coronary artery arises from the left coronary cusp, it is anterior to the left coronary ostium and sometimes can be cannulated with a left Judkins catheter or a long-tipped multipurpose catheter. The Amplatz II catheter is usually successful in engaging the ectopic origin of the right coronary artery from the left cusp.

[ ] USING DIAGNOSTIC CATHETERS TO BEGIN AN INTERVENTIONAL PROCEDURE

Occasionally it is very difficult to engage ectopic ostia cleanly with guide catheters despite successful insertion of the diagnostic catheter into the vessel. In these cases, the diagnostic catheters may be used to begin the interventional procedure by passing a long

TABLE 25-1

Optimal Angiographic Views for Specific Coronary Artery Segments

CORONARY SEGMENT	ORIGIN/BIFURCATION	COURSE/BODY
Left main	AP LAO cranial LAO caudal	AP LAO cranial
Proximal LAD	LAO cranial RAO caudal	LAO cranial RAO caudal
Mid-LAD	LAO cranial RAO cranial Lateral	
Distal LAD	AP RAO cranial Lateral	
Diagonal	LAO cranial RAO cranial	RAO cranial, caudal, or straight
Proximal circumflex	RAO caudal LAO caudal	LAO caudal
Intermediate	RAO caudal LAO caudal	RAO caudal Lateral
Obtuse marginal	RAO caudal LAO caudal RAO cranial (distal marginals)	RAO caudal
Proximal RCA	LAO Lateral	
Mid-RCA	LAO Lateral RAO	LAO Lateral RAO
Distal RCA	LAO cranial Lateral	LAO cranial Lateral
PDA	LAO cranial	RAO
Posterolateral	LAD cranial RAO cranial	RAO RAO cranial

AP = anteroposterior; LAD = left anterior descending artery; LAO = left anterior oblique; PDA = posterior descending artery (from RCA); RAO = right anterior oblique; RCA = right coronary artery.
ªHorizontal hearts.

exchange 0.014-in guidewire through the diagnostic catheter and well into the recipient artery. The diagnostic catheter is then removed, while keeping the 0.014-in guidewire deeply engaged into the recipient artery, and a guide catheter of the proper shape is inserted that contains a 0.038-in guidewire to stabilize passage around the aortic arch. This trick has avoided a lot of wasted time trying to engage extremely difficult ostial positions with less nimble guide catheters.

Before completing any angiographic evaluation of the coronary arteries, a careful review of the distribution of the arteries over the epicardial surface of the heart should be undertaken. If

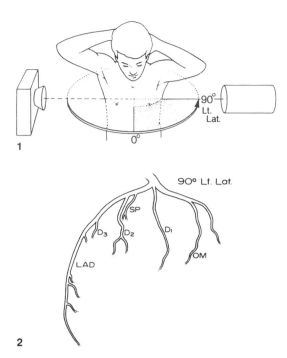

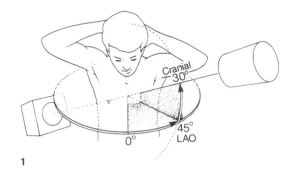

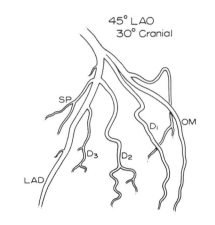

FIGURE 25-3C. Diagrammatic illustration of the 90-degree left lateral coronary arteriogram of the left coronary artery. The image intensifier is on the patient's left and the x-ray beam has a right-to-left direction in the horizontal plane. The lateral view of the left coronary artery is most useful for analyzing the proximal and mid-left anterior descending (LAD) coronary artery by avoiding overlap with the diagonal branches, which commonly take an inferior course from the LAD in this projection. The most proximal portion of the diagonal branches may not be well visualized, because the long axis of these segments may be in the direction of the x-ray beam. The leftward-directed left main coronary artery segment and the proximal circumflex artery are foreshortened in this view (compare with Figure 25-3B). (D1, D2, D3 = first, second, third diagonal; OM = obtuse marginal; SP = septal perforator.) *(Reproduced from King SB III, Douglas JS Jr, Morris DC. New angiographic views for coronary arteriography. In: Hurst JW, ed.* Update IV: The Heart. *New York, NY: McGraw-Hill; 1981.)*

FIGURE 25-3D. Diagrammatic illustration of the left coronary arteriogram in the 45-degree left anterior oblique (LAO) view with 30-degree cranial angulation. The image intensifier is on the patient's left and the direction of the x-ray beam is posterior to anterior. This is the most valuable view of the left coronary artery in most patients. Foreshortening of the left main and proximal left anterior descending (LAD) and diagonal branches, which occurs in the LAO view, is usually overcome by cranial angulation of the intensifier. The proximal left coronary artery segments are usually visualized at an angle almost perpendicular to their long axis. The ostium of the left main coronary artery, the proximal portion of the LAD, and the origin of the diagonal branches are usually well visualized without overlap (compare with Figure 25-3B). Some overlap may occur with branches of the proximal circumflex coronary artery, and this may be overcome by using a 60-degree LAO with 30-degree cranial angulation. The value of the LAO cranial view is considerably less when the proximal left coronary artery has a cephalad direction, in which case caudal angulation of the image intensifier is frequently helpful. (D1, D2, D3 = first, second, third diagonal; OM = obtuse marginal; SP = septal perforator.) *(Reproduced from King SB III, Douglas JS Jr, Morris DC. New angiographic views for coronary arteriography. In: Hurst JW, ed.* Update IV: The Heart. *New York, NY: McGraw-Hill; 1981.)*

segments of the heart are viewed that do not have a feeding artery, then it is likely that one of the arteries has not yet been visualized.

INTERPRETATION OF CORONARY ANGIOGRAMS

In interpreting coronary angiograms, it is important to be sure that all arteries are accounted for. Assessment of coronary artery disease should include lesion severity, lesion length, lesion character (ie, ulceration, thrombus, calcification), vessel size, ostial or bifurcation location, nature of the chronic total occlusions, and anatomic and functional significance of collateral filling. In addition, the angiographic assessment of coronary flow can be estimated. Figure 25-4 illustrates the difference in estimating the severity of stenoses expressed as diameter reduction and cross-sectional area reduction. Lesion severity is commonly judged in comparison to an adjacent "normal" segment. Ultrasound examination of arteries has been

convincing in showing that normal segments are frequently not normal and therefore the reference vessel size may not be accurate. Adaptive remodeling of the artery to accommodate plaque is also a feature that complicates assessment of lesion severity. However, utilization of the minimal diameter of the vessel compared with the "normal" reference segment remains a measure of clinical importance. Figure 25-5 shows the classic relationship of lesion severity to flow reduction as identified in the experiments of Gould. This cut point of 50% diameter stenosis has also been shown to correlate with reduction in maximal flow reserve measured by Doppler and pressure wire methods. Although on-line quantitative assessment is available in many laboratories, it is

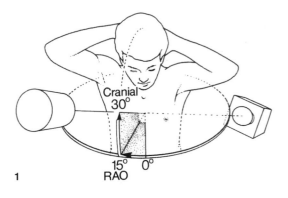

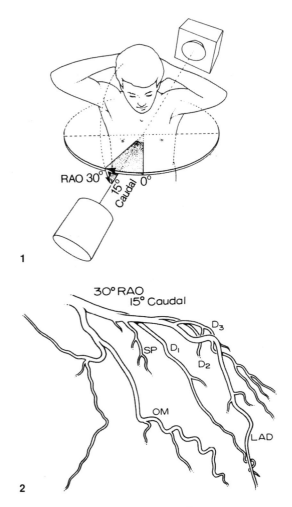

FIGURE 25-3E. Diagrammatic illustration of the left coronary arteriogram in the 30-degree right anterior oblique (RAO) view with 15-degree caudal angulation of the image intensifier. The image intensifier is positioned over the patient's liver and the direction of the x-ray beam is posterior to anterior. This view is helpful to unravel overlapping diagonal branches, to better visualize the proximal portion of the circumflex coronary artery, whose long axis was parallel to the x-ray beam in the routine RAO view, and to better visualize the mid–lateral anterior descending (LAD) artery, which overlaps diagonal branches in the standard RAO views. In this illustration, the mid-LAD is well visualized, as is a portion of the first diagonal, not well visualized in the RAO view. There is slight unfolding of the proximal circumflex artery as well. (D1, D2, D3 = first, second, third diagonal; OM = obtuse marginal; SP = septal perforator.) *(Reproduced from King SB III, Douglas JS Jr, Morris DC. New angiographic views for coronary arteriography. In: Hurst JW, ed. Update IV: The Heart. New York, NY: McGraw-Hill; 1981.)*

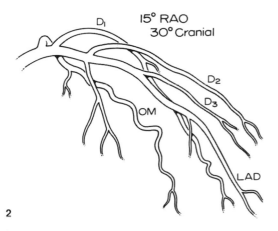

FIGURE 25-3F. Diagrammatic illustration of the left coronary arteriogram in the 15-degree right anterior oblique (RAO) view with 30-degree cranial angulation. This view is particularly helpful in analyzing the mid–left anterior descending (LAD) coronary artery and the origin of diagonal arteries and septal perforating arteries. Overlap with diagonal branches is usually avoided. The origin of the circumflex artery may be well seen, as in this illustration. (D1, D2, D3 = first, second, third diagonal; OM = obtuse marginal; SP = septal perforator.) *(Reproduced from King SB III, Douglas JS Jr, Morris DC. New angiographic views for coronary arteriography. In: Hurst JW, ed. Update IV: The Heart. New York, NY: McGraw-Hill; 1981.)*

approaches to the lesion. Ulcerations and irregularities within lesions may identify them as likely culprits in the acute coronary syndrome setting.

【 】 LESION LENGTH

Measurement of the length of the lesion should be accomplished using views in which foreshortening has been minimized. The most accurate measures of the lesion length are accomplished with guidewires having calibration marks or with balloon catheters utilizing the known distance between markers. Estimates of lesion length can be made from the diagnostic angiogram, however, by calibrating the guide catheter and then performing quantitative angiographic assessment of the lesion length. Although experienced interventionalists can often estimate lesion length from diagnostic angiograms within a reasonable margin of error, final assessment of lesion length should be obtained at the time of the interventional procedure.

seldom used in the decision-making process. However, to avoid significantly overestimating the severity of lesions, some form of quantitative angiography is helpful, if only to calibrate the operator's eye to replicate what would be found with quantitative angiography. A simple but accurate method is to utilize calipers to compare the minimal lumen diameter with the reference segment.

The composition of the lesion can help guide the interventional approach. The presence of dense calcification seen angiographically may lead to the use of intravascular ultrasound to determine whether rotary ablation should be applied prior to angioplasty. The presence of filling defects suggesting thrombus may appropriately lead to thrombus extraction or rheolytic thrombectomy

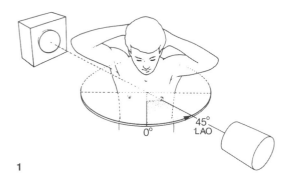

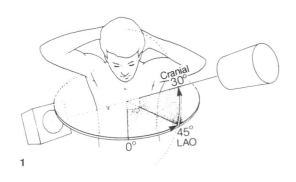

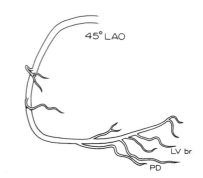

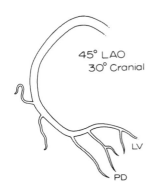

FIGURE 25-3G. Diagrammatic illustration of the right coronary artery in the 45-degree left anterior oblique (LAO) projection. The image intensifier is positioned on the patient's left and the x-ray beam travels in a posterior-to-anterior direction. This view is excellent for visualizing the proximal, mid, and distal right coronary artery in the atrioventricular groove, because the direction of the x-ray beam is perpendicular to these arterial segments. Ostial lesions of the right coronary artery are not well visualized if the proximal right coronary artery takes an anterior direction from the aorta and therefore travels in a direction parallel to the x-ray beam. This can usually be overcome by turning to a steeper LAO projection. The posterior descending (PD) and left ventricular (LV) branches of the right coronary artery, which pass down the posterior aspect of the heart toward the apex, may be severely foreshortened, because the long axis of these vessels is in the same direction as the x-ray beam. The proximal portion of the posterior descending branches can be visualized by cranial angulation of the overhead intensifier (see Figure 25-3H) or using a right anterior oblique view with cranial angulation. *(Reproduced from King SB III, Douglas JS Jr, Morris DC. New angiographic views for coronary arteriography. In: Hurst JW, ed. Update IV: The Heart. New York, NY: McGraw-Hill; 1981.)*

FIGURE 25-3H. Diagrammatic illustration of the right coronary artery in a 45-degree left anterior oblique (LAO) view with 30-degree cranial angulation. Cranial angulation of the image intensifier overcomes the problem of foreshortening of the posterior descending (PD) and left ventricular (LV) branches observed in Figure 25-3G. Lesions in the posterior descending or left ventricular branches can be well visualized. When the right coronary artery originates anteriorly from the aorta, the proximal portion of this vessel is frequently well seen in this projection. When the left anterior descending artery arises anomalously from the right sinus of Valsalva, this view is helpful, because the standard LAO view produces considerable foreshortening of the anomalous artery. *(Reproduced from King SB III, Douglas JS Jr, Morris DC. New angiographic views for coronary arteriography. In: Hurst JW, ed. Update IV: The Heart. New York, NY: McGraw-Hill; 1981.)*

【 】 CHRONIC TOTAL OCCLUSIONS

Total occlusions of coronary arteries that have been present for more than a few months may become extremely firm, and the success rate of crossing with the usual guidewires is diminished in these lesions compared with high-grade stenoses. Numerous features have been identified that predict the ability to cross chronic total occlusions, including whether there is a tapering into the occlusion or "a beak". This angiographic appearance sometimes signals the presence of small recanalized channels within a total occlusion and correlates with an increased success rate from interventions. Conversely, there is a lower chance of success in patients with total occlusions that are abruptly occluded. The least favorable appearance is the total occlusion that terminates in a side branch at the exit of the total occlusion; this scenario can cause wires to migrate into that side branch, minimizing the ability to cross the

【 】 BIFURCATION LESIONS

Bifurcation lesions should be examined in views in which there is no overlap between the two arms. Assessment should be made as to whether the lesion involves the parent vessel only or whether it compromises the ostium of the side branch. There should also be assessment of the projected need for angioplasty or stenting in a side branch rather than the main channel itself. Plaque shifting from the main vessel to the side branch should be estimated as part of the planning process for interventional procedures.

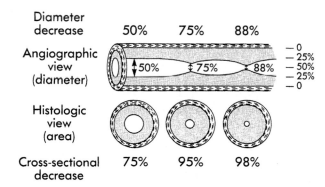

FIGURE 25-4. Diagrammatic representation of angiographic versus postmortem analysis of coronary artery stenosis. *(Reproduced with permission from Robert WC. Coronary heart disease: A review of abnormalities observed in the coronary arteries. Cardiovasc Med. 1977; 2:29.)*

total occlusion. Other characteristics that influence success include the curvature of the artery at the site of the total occlusion and beyond it and especially the length of the total occlusion. Visualization of collateral circulation from contralateral or ipsilateral injections can identify the length of the total occlusion and thereby influence the chance for success from interventional procedures. Such an assessment of total occlusions is very important in selecting patients for attempted intervention versus continued medical therapy or bypass surgery.

The observation of collateral circulation is critical in judging whether ischemic syndromes would likely be improved with restoration of flow. It is unusual to have no collateral filling into segments of viable myocardium in the chronic phase of coronary artery disease. Therefore the visualization of collateral vessels is not a signal that no revascularization is needed but is rather a sign that viable myocardium is possible in those zones. Examination of the left ventriculogram in combination with the collateral filling to discrete myocardial zones can help predict which patients will be benefited symptomatically from reperfusion therapy. In the future, magnetic resonance imaging will provide enormously improved data regarding functional recovery of revascularized arterial segments.

【 】 CORONARY FLOW JUDGED ANGIOGRAPHICALLY

Flow in the coronary arteries is judged primarily in the setting of acute infarction. The relative flow in coronary arteries has been classified according to the TIMI flow scale, as follows:

- TIMI 0 (no flow).
- TIMI 1 (opacification of the distal vessel without run off).
- TIMI 2 (reduced flow compared with nonobstructed arteries).

- TIMI 3 flow (flow in the affected artery that is equal to other unobstructed arteries).

This scale has been further refined to reflect the actual velocity of the flow in the coronary artery by judging the number of angiographic frames required for contrast media to traverse the coronary artery. The latter method[3] is obtained using 6-Fr catheters and filming at 30 frames per second. The number of frames from the appearance of the dye in the coronary artery to a distal predetermined landmark is then obtained.

Gibson has proposed a correction of this frame count called the *corrected TIMI frame count,* which uses the distal targets in the left anterior descending artery as the distal bifurcation, the distal target in the circumflex artery as the distal bifurcation of the terminal segments at the longest distance, and the right coronary artery as the first branch of the posterolateral artery. Because the anterior descending artery is longer than the other vessels, the normal TIMI frame count for the left anterior descending artery is 36; for the circumflex artery, 21; and for the right coronary artery, 22. The corrected TIMI frame count divides the anterior descending count by 1.7 to equate the three vessels. The force of injection into the coronary artery affects the TIMI frame count only marginally. An increase in the rate of injection of more than 1 mL/s by hand can decrease the frame count by 2 frames. These frame counts have been found to be of value in judging clinical response after reperfusion therapy in the setting of acute syndromes.

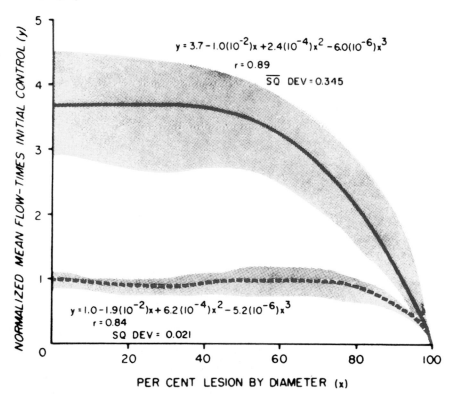

FIGURE 25-5. The relation of resting mean blood flow (dotted line) and hyperemic flows (solid line) to percentage of arterial diameter reduction. Flows are expressed as ratios to control resting mean values at the beginning of the experiment. The shaded area represents the range of values measured in individual dogs: r = correlation coefficient; SQ DEV = mean square of deviations. *(Reproduced from Gould KL, Lipscomb K, Hamilton GW. Physiologic basis for assessing critical coronary stenosis. Am J Cardiol. 1974;33:87.)*

The pattern of collateral circulation is important in planning interventional procedures. Because arteries that receive collateral blood flow may be partially protected during interventional procedures, there is an added margin of safety when approaching such lesions. Conversely, performing interventional procedures on arteries that supply collateral vessels to large segments of the myocardium puts those segments in jeopardy during the procedure, especially if occlusive dissection occurs at the time of the interventional procedure.

【 】 INTERPRETION OF THE LEFT VENTRICULOGRAM

The left ventriculogram provides important prognostic data. The formula of Sandler and Dodge, which utilizes the area length method, can be calculated; however, experienced operators frequently estimate the ejection fraction visually. Accurately assessed left ventricular function is a potent prognostic indicator of future clinical events, especially survival. Coronary artery disease commonly produces asynchronous myocardial contractility, with each segment identified as being either normal in contraction, hypokinetic, akinetic (no motion), or dyskinetic with paradoxical systolic expansion. These abnormalities, combined with the degree of thinning of the ventricular wall, have been used to predict recovery of segments following revascularization. Whereas akinetic and dyskinetic segments in areas of thinned left ventricular wall have traditionally been judged to have a low chance of recovery, more recent magnetic resonance assessment of viability have shown that even quite thin arterial segments can undergo significant recovery after revascularization. In the future, the degree of fibrosis and the degree of retained myocardial tissue will be much more important in assessing functional recoverability.

COMPLICATIONS OF CORONARY ARTERIOGRAPHY AND LEFT VENTRICULOGRAPHY

Insertion of catheters into the coronary arteries and left ventricle can result in serious complications. Fortunately these complications are unusual. Analysis of more than 200,000 patients indicates the incidence of death is less than 0.2%; myocardial infarction, less than 0.5%; stroke less than 0.7%; and serious ventricular arrhythmia, less than 0.5%. Major vascular complications at the catheterization access site, including thrombosis, bleeding requiring transfusion, or pseudoaneurysm, have been less than 1%.[4] Table 25-2 outlines complications of cardiac catheterization. The most potentially lethal condition leading to complications of diagnostic coronary arteriography is the presence of severe left main coronary artery stenosis, particularly ostial involvement. Placement of the diagnostic catheter into the coronary ostium, especially if it causes disruption of plaque, may lead to immediate hemodynamic instability and a downward spiral. All physicians performing angiography should be prepared to administer pressor agents immediately should blood pressure fall in the setting of left main artery stenosis. Increasing the filling pressure as

TABLE 25-2

Complications of Cardiac Catheterization

Major
  Cerebrovascular accident
  Death
  Myocardial infarction
  Ventricular tachycardia, fibrillation, or
    serious arrhythmia
Other
  Aortic or coronary dissection
  Cardiac perforation, tamponade
  Congestive heart failure
  Contrast reaction, anaphylaxis, nephrotoxicity
  Heart block, asystole
  Hemorrhage (local, retroperitoneal, pelvic)
  Infection
  Protamine reaction
  Supraventricular tachyarrhythmia, atrial fibrillation
  Thrombosis, embolus, air embolus
  Vascular injury, pseudoaneurysm
  Vasovagal reaction

quickly as possible is critical if one is to avoid the spiral of decreased coronary flow leading to decreased contractility, and to further decreases in arterial pressure. In centers equipped with interventional cardiology equipment, an early decision for urgent angioplasty and stenting as a bail-out technique for left main artery occlusion should always be added to the armamentarium. Lesser degrees of emergency can be dealt with using pressor agents, followed by balloon counterpulsation to stabilize the situation, and then definitive surgery; however, it is sometimes impossible to stabilize the patient quickly enough using these measures, and the emergency placement of left main artery stents has, in some cases, been lifesaving.

SUMMARY

Percutaneous coronary interventions can only be planned and executed based on accurate "intelligence" information supplied by the coronary arteriogram and left ventricular function measurements. Misleading information as a result of inadequate coronary angiography can lead to the wrong decision in the selection of appropriate candidates or in the performance of the interventional procedure. As interventional procedures become the focus of invasive cardiologists—with the placement of modern drug-eluting stents and performance of debulking techniques and intravascular ultrasound imaging assessment of coronary circulation—we must not forget the more "mundane" activity of coronary arteriography. The successful battle against coronary obstructive disease must start with the proper intelligence information that accurately predicts the outcome of our therapeutic endeavors.

REFERENCES

1. Sones FM Jr, Shirey EK. Cine coronary arteriography. *Modern Concepts Cardiovasc Dis.* 1962;31:735.
2. Judkins MP. Selective coronary arteriography: I. A percutaneous transfemoral technique. *Radiology.* 1967;89:815, 1967.
3. Schoonmaker FW, King SB III. Coronary arteriography by the single catheter percutaneous femoral technique: Experience with 6,800 cases. *Circulation.* 1974;50:735.
4. ACC/AHA Guidelines for Coronary Angiography: Executive summary and recommendations. *Circulation.* 1999;99:2345.
5. Kiemenei JF, Laarman G. Percutaneous transradial artery approach for coronary Palmaz-Schatz stent implantation. *Am Heart J.* 1994;129:167.

CHAPTER (26)

Diagnostic Procedures: Peripheral Angiography

Christopher J. White, MD, and Jose A. Silva, MD

THORACIC AORTOGRAPHY

Thoracic aortography is usually performed to confirm the diagnosis of pathologic entities such as aneurysms, aortic dissection, coarctation of the aorta, patent ductus arteriosus, vascular rings, or chest trauma, or to assess the origin of the aortic arch vessels. A classic indication for thoracic angiography is to identify the origin of the tear in an aortic dissection. However, in contemporary medicine, most of this pathology is initially viewed with cross-sectional imaging techniques with three-dimensional (3D) reconstruction, such as computed tomographic (CT) angiography, magnetic resonance (MR) angiography, and transesophageal echocardiography.

ASCENDING AORTOGRAPHY

【 】 GENERAL CONSIDERATIONS

Angiography of the ascending aorta, aortic arch vessels, and descending aorta is an integral element of the practice of an invasive and interventional cardiologist. The ascending aorta begins at the sinus of Valsalva and travels in an anterior-to-posterior direction (Figure 26-1). Indications for thoracic aortography were described earlier. Angiography is also indicated to determine the patency of aortocoronary bypass grafts, and to assess aortic valve competency (Figure 26-2). Arterial access may be obtained from either (right or left) upper extremity (radial, brachial, or axillary artery) or lower extremity (common femoral artery).

Imaging is performed on a large-format image intensifier (9 to 16 in). If the patient is able to breath-hold, digital subtraction angiography is desirable. Imaging is usually performed at 7.5 to 15 frames per second (fps).

A multiholed (4- to 6-Fr) angiographic catheter (pigtail, tennis racquet, etc) is advanced to the aortic root and positioned several centimeters above the aortic valve (Figure 26-3). This positioning is necessary because the catheter will "unwind" and descend into the aortic valve during the injection. To avoid having the angiographic catheter prolapse into the aortic valve, it must be positioned slightly higher than its estimated "final" position, which will occur during contrast flow. Contrast injection rates of 15 to 20 mL/s for 2 to 3 seconds at a maximum of 800 to 1200 pounds per square inch (psi), depending on catheter specifications, are often used. The amount of contrast delivered is dependent on the patient size and cardiac output. The ascending aortogram is often performed in a moderately steep, left anterior oblique (LAO) view of 30 to 60 degrees. In laboratories equipped with biplane equipment, the orthogonal right anterior oblique (RAO) may be obtained simultaneously.

【 】 AORTOCORONARY BYPASS GRAFTS

When performing angiography to assess aortocoronary bypass graft patency, it is important to stay on the cine pedal until the left internal mammary artery graft has filled via the subclavian artery (Figure 26-4). Saphenous vein grafts often may not readily fill if they are stenotic. To facilitate filling of the grafts, with an aortic injection, the operator should position the side holes of the pigtail catheter near the ostia of the grafts. The most common projection

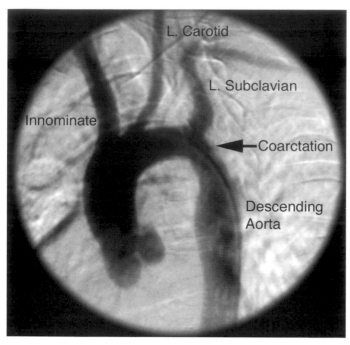

FIGURE 26-1. Ascending aorta, aortic arch, and descending aorta with coarctation (arrow). Note post-stenotic dilation of the descending aorta. Digital subtraction angiographic technique with pigtail catheter and 20 mL/s.

for this image is a left anterior oblique (LAO) view of 30 to 60 degrees. In catheterization laboratories that use biplane imaging, the orthogonal right anterior oblique (RAO) view is also obtained. The LAO projection is ideal for viewing the origin of the saphenous vein

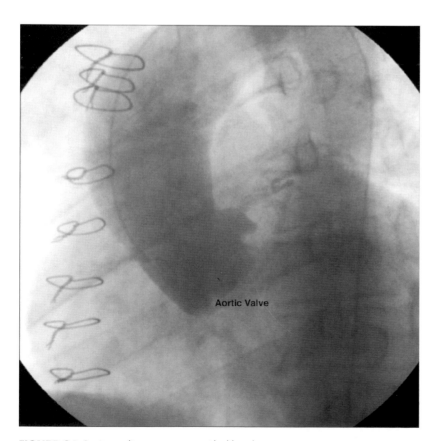

FIGURE 26-2. Ascending aortogram with dilated aortic root.

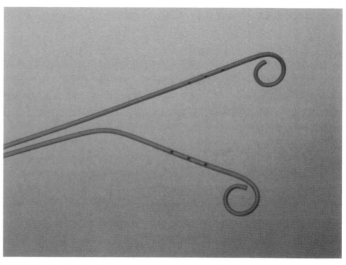

FIGURE 26-3. Multiholed straight and angled pigtail catheters.

graft to the right coronary artery. Occasionally the origin of the left-sided bypass grafts may be difficult to visualize and an RAO (15- to 45-degree) projection may be more desirable.

【 】 AORTIC DISSECTION OR ANEURYSM

When the indication for ascending aortography is dissection or aneurysm identification, it is important to fill the aorta from the aortic valve cusps to the aortic arch (see Figure 26-2). Placement of the pigtail catheter too high in the aorta may not allow contrast to fill the cusps. Placement of the catheter too low in the aorta may cause the catheter to prolapse into the ventricle or into the aortic valve, causing artifactual aortic insufficiency. Two-dimensional (2D) biplane aortography is not the imaging modality of choice to evaluate aortic aneurysm size or to determine the presence of dissection. This is better done with cross-sectional imaging techniques such as CT angiography, MR angiography, or transesophageal echocardiography. The value of contrast aortography is to visualize the origin and flow into the coronary arteries.

When planning to perform angiography in a patient with a suspected dissection of the ascending aorta, it is important to determine the blood pressure in each arm, which can help to determine involvement of the vessels of the aortic arch. Higher blood pressure in the right arm compared with the left arm may suggest that right arm arterial access is preferable to femoral access.

【 】 AORTIC VALVE COMPETENCY

When performing ascending aortography to assess the severity or presence of aortic insufficiency, either an LAO or RAO view is acceptable. The catheter must

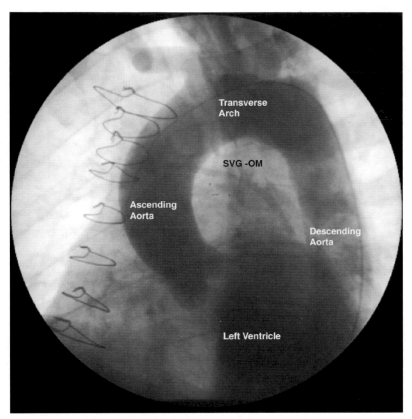

FIGURE 26-4. Severe aortic insufficiency.

remain above the valve during injection to avoid confounding the assessment of aortic insufficiency that occurs when the catheter prolapses into the valve. An injection rate that will fill the aortic cusps is required to adequately assess the aortic valve (see Figure 26-4).

AORTIC ARCH ANGIOGRAPHY

【 】 GENERAL CONSIDERATIONS

The transverse aortic arch begins as the ascending aorta crosses the main pulmonary artery and continues in a posterior direction, giving rise to the aortic arch vessels (innominate, left common carotid, and left subclavian arteries), and continues until the ligamentum arteriosus (remnant of the ductus arteriosus), as shown in Figure 26-5. The most common anatomic variation, the bovine arch, occurs in 10% of patients and is identified when the left common carotid artery arises from the innominate artery (Figure 26-6).[1]

Angiography of the aortic arch may be performed to assess the presence and severity of dissection or aneurysm, or as an overview image for supraclavicular and cervical vascular imaging. Arterial access may be obtained from the upper (radial, brachial, or axillary artery) or lower extremity (common femoral artery). Imaging is performed on a large-format image intensifier (9 to 16 in). The larger format permits a larger field of view, allowing more information to be obtained. A pigtail-type catheter is advanced to a position several centimeters proximal to the origin of the innominate artery to ensure adequate filling of this vessel. Contrast injection rates of 15 to 20 mL/s for 2 to 3 seconds are often used. The amount of contrast used is dependent on patient size and cardiac output. If the patient is able to breath-hold, digital subtraction angiography is desirable and will allow

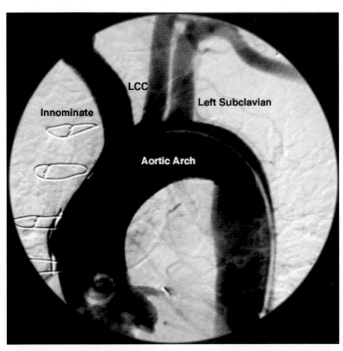

FIGURE 26-5. Normal aortogram (left anterior oblique 45-degree view). Digital subtraction technique. LCC = left common carotid artery.

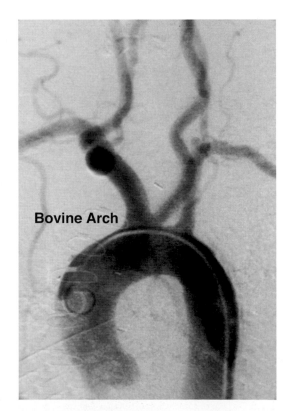

FIGURE 26-6. Bovine arch, digital subtraction technique (left anterior oblique 45-degree view).

less contrast to be used. Imaging is usually performed at 7.5 to 15 fps. The aortogram is often performed in a moderately steep, LAO view of 30 to 60 degrees. The optimal LAO angulation demonstrates the origin of the innominate, left common carotid, and left subclavian arteries.

【 】 AORTIC ARCH DISSECTION OR ANEURYSM

As in ascending aortography, when the indication for ascending aorta and arch angiography is to assess the presence and extent of dissection or aneurysm, it is important to fill the aorta from the aortic valve cusps to the aortic arch. Likewise, 2D biplane aortography is not the imaging modality of choice to evaluate aortic aneurysm size or to determine the presence of dissection involving the aortic arch. This is better done with cross-sectional imaging techniques such as CT angiography, MR angiography, or transesophageal echocardiography. As noted earlier, the value of contrast

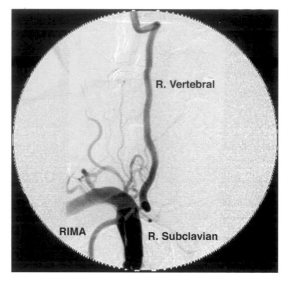

FIGURE 26-8. Right subclavian angiography filling right vertebral artery and right internal mammary artery (RIMA).

aortography is to visualize the origin and flow into the coronary arteries.

When planning to perform angiography in a patient with a suspected dissection of the ascending aorta, it is important to determine the blood pressure in each arm, which can help to determine involvement of the aortic arch vessels. Higher blood pressure in the right arm compared with the left arm may suggest that the dissection involves the left subclavian artery, but not the innominate artery, and that right arm arterial access is preferable.

【 】 IMAGING FOR SUPRACLAVICULAR AND CERVICAL ANGIOGRAPHY

When the indication for aortic arch angiography is to obtain an overview image prior to four-vessel (carotid and vertebral) selective angiography, it is important to use a large-field image intensifier (9 to 16 in) with subtraction techniques to remove the bony structures (Figure 26-7). Ideally the aortic arch is imaged with a 12-in (or larger) image intensifier in the LAO projection (30–60 degrees) to show the origin of the innominate, left common carotid, and left subclavian arteries.

It is important to identify the origins of the aortic arch vessels, and to view the subclavian arteries and their branches. Visualizing the origins and proximal segments of the vertebral arteries can be very helpful in planning further angiography (Figure 26-8). The operator can determine if one or the other vertebral artery is occluded or if one vertebral artery is dominant. Angiographic subclavian steal, the reversal of vertebral artery flow, in the presence of a subclavian or innominate stenosis can also be identified.

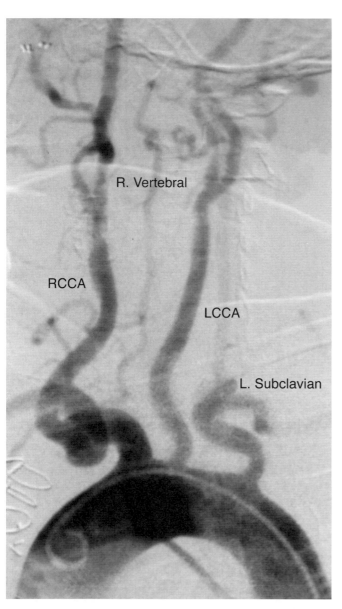

FIGURE 26-7. Digital subtraction technique (left anterior oblique 45-degree view). LCCA = left common carotid artery; RCCA = right common carotid artery.

DESCENDING AORTOGRAPHY

The descending aorta begins after the ligamentum arteriosus and extends to the diaphragm lying in the posterior portion of the

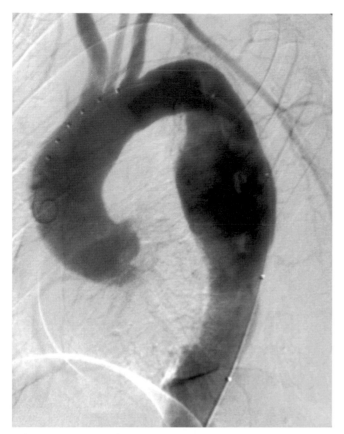

FIGURE 26-9. Descending aortic aneurysm.

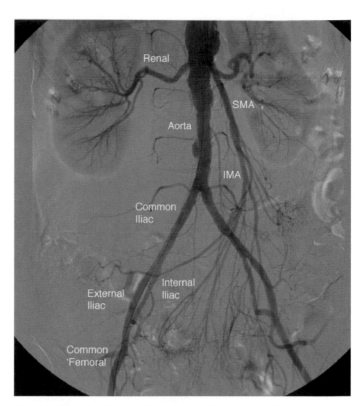

FIGURE 26-10. Abdominal aortogram. IMA = internal mesenteric artery; SMA = superior mesenteric artery.

chest. The descending aorta gives rise to nine pairs of intercostal arteries, which have clinical importance when assessing aortic dissections, or considering the risk of surgical repair.

Thoracic aortography is usually performed for the diagnosis of pathologic entities such as aneurysms, aortic dissection, coarctation of the aorta, patent ductus arteriosus, or vascular rings, as well as for the evaluation of vascular injuries such as blunt or penetrating chest trauma and stenoses in the origin of the great vessels (Figure 26-9). As with ascending aortography, arterial access may be obtained from the upper (radial, brachial, or axillary artery) or lower extremity (common femoral artery), and imaging is performed on a large-format image intensifier (9 to 16 in). A pigtail catheter is advanced to the ascending aorta. Contrast injection rates of 15 to 20 mL/s for 2 to 3 seconds are often used, and the amount of contrast used is dependent on patient size and cardiac output. As with other angiographic procedures, if the patient is able to breath-hold, digital subtraction angiography is desirable and will allow less contrast to be used. Imaging is usually performed at 7.5 to 15 fps. The descending aortogram is often imaged in the anteroposterior (AP) and lateral (LAT 90-degree) views.

ABDOMINAL AORTOGRAPHY

The abdominal aorta begins at the level of the diaphragm at the 12th thoracic vertebra (T12). At this level the aorta runs anterior to the spine and to the left of the inferior vena cava before it bifurcates into the common iliac arteries at the 4th lumbar vertebra (L4) (Figure 26-10). The normal diameter of the abdominal aorta ranges between 1.5 and 2.15 cm, and there is a slight increase in size with aging.[2] Three main branches originate on the ventral aspect of the abdominal aorta: The celiac trunk or celiac artery arises at the level of T12 to L1, the superior mesenteric artery (SMA) originates between L1 and L2, and the inferior mesenteric artery (IMA) takes off in a left anterolateral direction at the level of L3 to L4 (Figure 26-11). The renal arteries originate from the lateral aspect of the abdominal aorta at the level of L1 to L2, taking a lateral and posterior direction. In addition, four pairs of lumbar arteries arise in a posterolateral direction, below the main renal arteries.

Vascular access is usually obtained in the common femoral artery, although axillary, brachial, or radial access may also be used if the common femoral arteries are not accessible. A multiple-hole (4-Fr to 6-Fr) angiographic catheter (pigtail, tennis racquet, etc) is advanced to the level of the diaphragm. Contrast injection rates of 15 to 20 mL/s for 2 to 3 seconds at a maximum of 800 to 1200 psi, depending on catheter specifications, are often used. The amount of contrast delivered is dependent on patient size and cardiac output. The abdominal aortogram is usually imaged in the AP and lateral (LAT 90-degree) views. Two views should be obtained: The AP view allows good visualization of the renal arteries, and the lateral view enables adequate assessment of the origin of the celiac trunk and mesenteric arteries.

When imaging the renal arteries, care should be taken to rotate the image slightly in the LAO projection to optimize visualization of the ostium of the renal arteries. A common pitfall occurs when the superior mesenteric artery fills with contrast and obscures the origin of the left renal artery. Abdominal aortic aneurysms may not

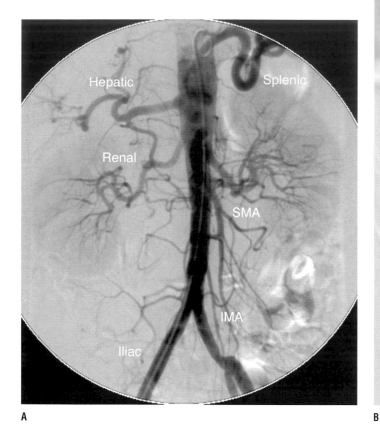

A

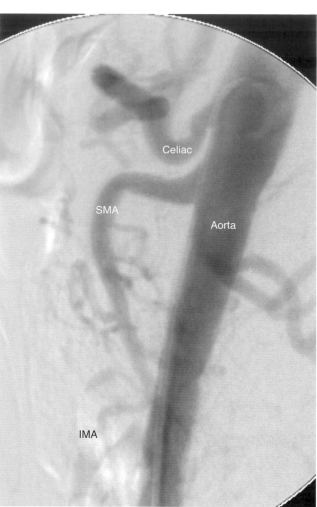

B

FIGURE 26-11. A. Anteroposterior abdominal aortogram. IMA = inferior mesenteric artery; SMA = superior mesenteric artery. **B.** Lateral abdominal aortogram.

be visualized with contrast angiography because the aneurysm sac may be filled with organized thrombus. If an abdominal aortic aneurysm is suspected, a cross-sectional imaging technique (ultrasound, CT, or MR) should be performed (Figure 26-12).

VISCERAL OR MESENTERIC ANGIOGRAPHY

【 】 GENERAL CONSIDERATIONS

The mesenteric circulation includes three arteries that originate from the ventral aspect of the abdominal aorta: the celiac artery, SMA, and IMA (see Figure 26-11). The celiac artery, which as previously noted arises at the level of diaphragm (T12 to L1), branches into the hepatic and splenic arteries. The SMA, originating at the level of L1 to L2, irrigates the lower half of the duodenum, ileum, cecum appendix, ascending colon, and proximal two thirds of the transverse colon. The IMA, arising at the level of L3 to L4, supplies blood to the distal third of the transverse colon, descending colon, sigmoid colon, rectum, and upper part of the anal canal.[3]

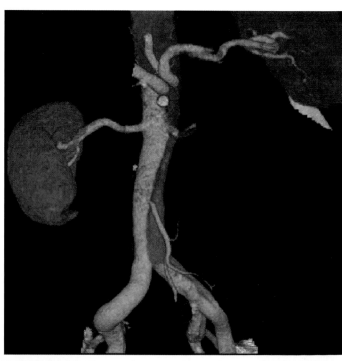

FIGURE 26-12. Computed tomographic angiogram of abdominal aortic dissection.

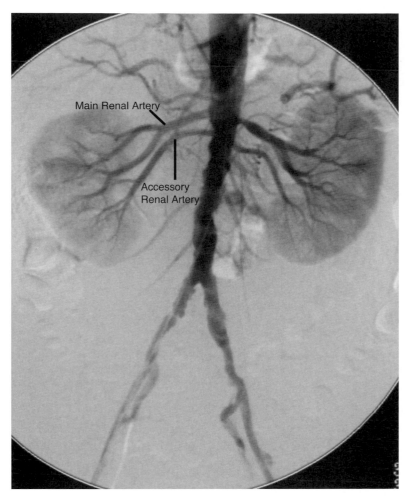

FIGURE 26-13. Abdominal aortogram. Bilateral renal accessory arteries are present.

The renal arteries arise from the lateral aspect of the abdominal aorta, usually between L1 and L2. They run in a lateral and posterior direction, and may take a caudal, horizontal, or cranial orientation although this last is less common (see Figure 26-11). In about 25% to 35% of the normal population, the lower part of the kidney may receive blood supply from an accessory renal artery, which may originate anywhere from the suprarenal aorta down to the iliac arteries (see Figure 26-13).

RENAL ANGIOGRAPHY

【 】 GENERAL CONSIDERATIONS

It is generally recommended that an abdominal aortogram be obtained prior to performing selective renal angiography. This enables the operator to locate the origins of the renal arteries, identify accessory renal arteries, and determine the presence of significant renal artery stenoses (Figure 26-13). After the abdominal aortogram has been obtained, selective renal angiography is indicated if the aortogram demonstrates a renal artery stenosis or if the operator wishes to obtain better images as well as measure pressure gradient across the stenosis. Selective renal angiography is also indicated if intrarenal vascular disease is suspected, as is the case in fibromuscular dysplasia, vasculitis, aneurysms, or radiation vasculopathy.

【 】 MESENTERIC ANGIOGRAPHY

Selective angiography of the mesenteric arteries remains the gold standard method to assess the anatomy of this segment of the vascular system. Before selective angiography is performed, an abdominal aortogram should be obtained in the AP and lateral projections. After the origin of the mesenteric vessels has been identified, selective angiography is carried out in the AP and lateral views using a diagnostic angiographic catheter [internal mammary, Judkins right coronary artery, or a shepherd crook-shaped diagnostic catheter (ie, Simmons or Sos catheter)]. Because the IMA often arises at a very acute caudal angle on the ventral portion of the abdominal aorta, a Simmons-1 catheter is often very useful to engage this vessel. When imaged from access in the upper extremity, a multipurpose-shaped catheter is ideal for engagement.

Using hand injections, selective angiography is performed in the lateral and AP views, which allows good visualization of the ostium, as well as the rest of the mesenteric vessels and their main branches. Selective engagement of the mesenteric arteries also allows measurement of a pressure gradient, as the majority of atherosclerotic stenoses in these vessels are located proximally. The classic teaching is that at least two or the three mesenteric arteries must be occluded to cause symptomatic ischemia.

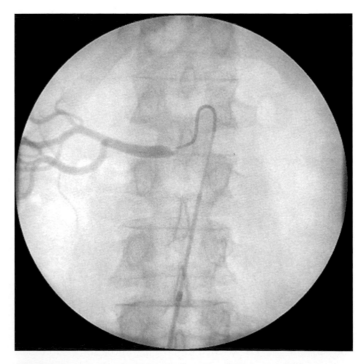

FIGURE 26-14. Shepherd crook–shaped catheter viewed from femoral approach in a patient with right renal artery ostial stenosis.

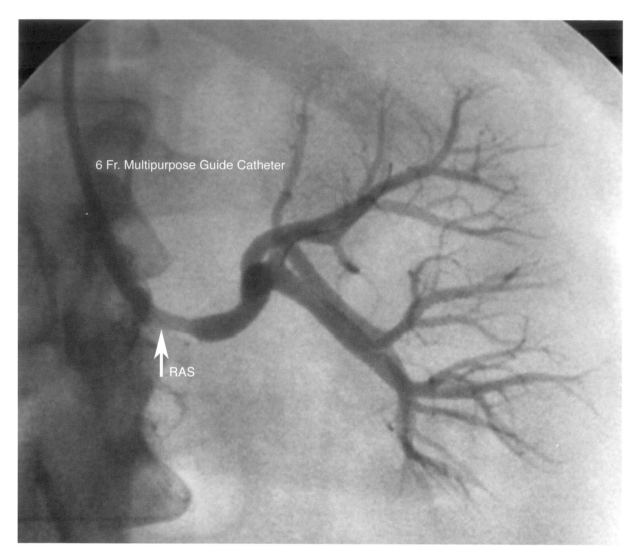

FIGURE 26-15. Renal angiogram from brachial approach in a patient with renal artery stenosis (RAS; arrow). Brachial artery access was obtained with a 6-Fr multipurpose guiding catheter.

【 】 RENAL TECHNIQUE

Several diagnostic catheters (4-Fr to 6-Fr) are available for selective engagement of the renal arteries from the femoral approach. We routinely use an internal mammary artery catheter; however, the Judkins right and shepherd crook–shaped catheters may also be useful (Figure 26-14). When imaging is obtained from an upper extremity access site, a multipurpose catheter is ideal for engagement (Figure 26-15). When placing catheters in a diseased aorta, care must be taken to avoid excessive trauma or manipulation, which may contribute to atheroembolism.

Selective renal angiography is performed at 15 to 30 fps with hand injections using a coronary manifold with pressure monitoring. A medium- (6- or 7-in) to large-format (9- or 12-in) image is preferred. It is desirable to be able to show the entire length of the renal artery from aorta to cortex during imaging. Usually a shallow LAO angulation (5–15 degrees) is preferred for imaging. If the aorta is tortuous, some caudal or cranial orientation (15–20 degrees) may occasionally be helpful for better visualization of ostial lesions.

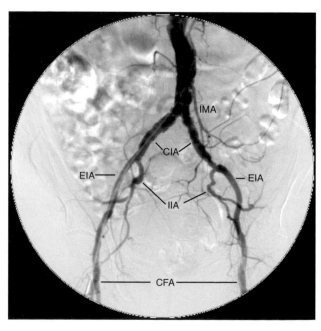

FIGURE 26-16. Lower extremity angiogram. CFA = common femoral artery; CIA = common iliac artery; EIA = external iliac artery; IIA = internal iliac artery; IMA = inferior mesenteric artery.

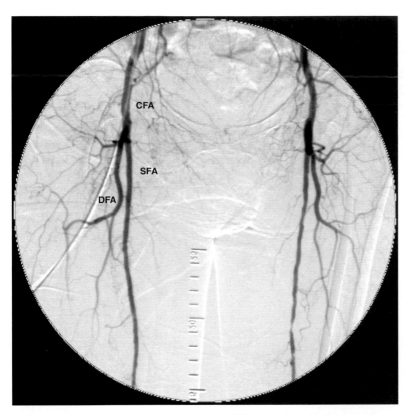

FIGURE 26-17. Lower extremity angiogram. CFA = common femoral artery; DFA = deep femoral artery; SFA = superficial femoral artery.

the anteromedial thigh, and in its distal portion runs deeper to cross the abductor or Hunter's canal, where it is now termed the popliteal artery (Figure 26-19). The popliteal artery crosses the knee and gives origin to small muscular branches, two sural branches, and three geniculate arteries (superior, medial, and inferior) at the knee.

Below the knee, at the level of the popliteus muscle, the popliteal artery bifurcates into the anterior tibial artery and continues as the tibioperoneal trunk (Figure 26-20). The anterior tibial artery runs laterally and anterior to the tibia toward the foot, and as it passes over the ankle onto the dorsum of the foot, it becomes the dorsalis pedis artery. The tibioperoneal trunk bifurcates into the posterior tibial and the peroneal artery. The posterior tibial artery courses posteromedially in the calf, whereas the peroneal runs near the fibula between the anterior tibial and posterior tibial arteries. The peroneal artery then rejoins the posterior tibial artery above the ankle via the posterior division, and the anterior tibial artery through the anterior division.

On the dorsum of the foot, the dorsalis pedis artery has lateral and medial tarsal branches. After the posterior tibial artery passes behind the medial malleolus, it divides into medial and lateral plantar arteries. The lateral plantar and distal dorsalis pedis arteries join to form the plantar arch.

LOWER EXTREMITY ANGIOGRAPHY

【 】 GENERAL CONSIDERATIONS

The abdominal aorta bifurcates into the common iliac arteries at the level of L4 to L5 (Figure 26-16). The common iliac artery bifurcates into the internal and external iliac arteries (IIAs) at the level of the lumbosacral junction. The external iliac artery emerges from the pelvis posterior to inguinal ligament. At the level of inguinal ligament, two small branches originate from the EIA, the inferior epigastric artery, which follows a medial direction, and the deep iliac circumflex, which takes a lateral and superior direction.

Once the EIA crosses the inguinal ligament, it is referred to as the common femoral artery (CFA); this artery runs over the femoral head (Figure 26-17). When it reaches the lower edge of the femoral head, the CFA divides into the superficial femoral artery (SFA) and profunda femoris or deep femoral artery (DFA; Figure 26-18). The DFA runs posteriorly and laterally along the internal aspect of the femur. A few centimeters after its origin, the DFA gives origin to two small branches, the lateral femoral circumflex and the medial femoral circumflex arteries, and subsequently to several small perforating arteries, which run laterally toward the femur. The SFA continues down

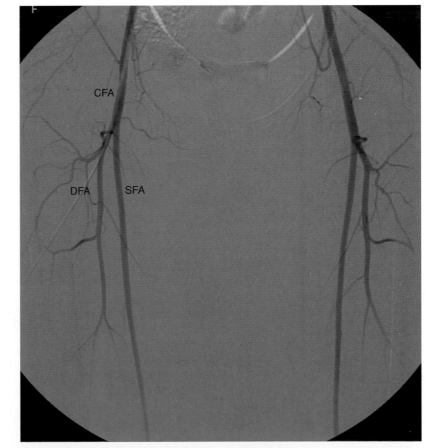

FIGURE 26-18. Bilateral lower extremity run-off angiography; anteroposterior view with digital subtraction technique. CFA = common femoral artery; DFA = deep femoral artery; SFA = superficial femoral artery.

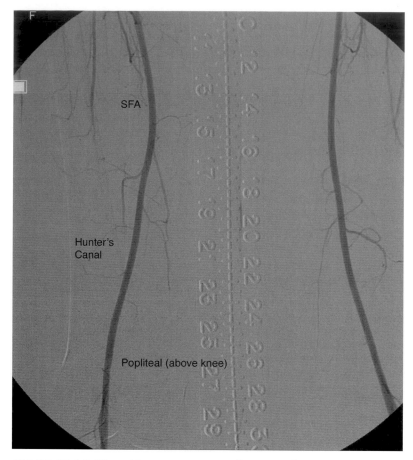

FIGURE 26-19. Bilateral lower extremity run-off angiography; anteroposterior view with digital subtraction technique. SFA = superficial femoral artery.

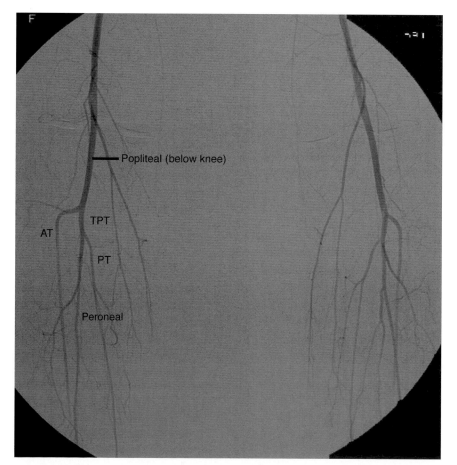

FIGURE 26-20. Bilateral lower extremity run-off angiography; anteroposterior view with digital subtraction technique. AT = anterior tibial; PT = posterior tibial; TPT = tibioperoneal trunk.

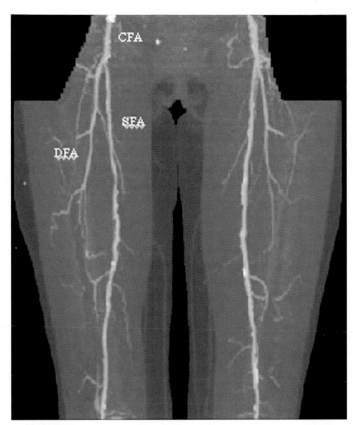

FIGURE 26-21. Computed tomographic angiography of lower extremity vessels. CFA = common femoral artery; DFA = deep femoral artery; SFA = superficial femoral artery.

【 】 LOWER EXTREMITY TECHNIQUE

Arteriography is still considered the gold standard for assessing patients with peripheral vascular disease, but noninvasive studies such as duplex ultrasound, CT angiography, or MR angiography are commonly used to detect the severity and the level of significant lower extremity vascular stenoses (Figure 26-21).

Vascular access is usually obtained in the CFA, preferably in the extremity that is least symptomatic. Brachial or radial artery access is preferred in patients with bilateral iliac artery occlusion. A 4-Fr to 6-Fr pigtail catheter is positioned above the renal arteries at L1 or L2. A stepping table with a large-format (15- or 16-in) image intensifier is used, and a single bolus of contrast material is injected at 8 to 12 mL/s for a total of 70 to 120 mL. Digital subtraction angiography (DSA) is performed to obtain images in a single AP run along the course of the contrast from the diaphragm to the feet. Follow-up selective imaging may be performed to clarify areas of concern.

An alternative is to use a moderate-sized (9- or 12-in) image intensifier with single leg dynamic run-off angiograms. Common femoral artery access is obtained with an arterial sheath (4-Fr to 6-Fr). An internal mammary catheter is advanced to the distal aorta over a guidewire. The tip of the mammary

catheter is placed at the ostium of the contralateral common iliac artery. A 0.035-in stiff-angled glide wire (Terumo, BSC, Watertown, MA) is then advanced carefully down to the common femoral artery. When the iliac bifurcation is at an acute angle, a shepherd crook–shaped catheter (Simmons-1 or -2) may be used to cannulate the contralateral common iliac artery. The internal mammary or Simmons catheter is then exchanged for an angiographic catheter (pigtail, tennis racquet, multipurpose, etc), which is placed securely in the common iliac artery. A test injection is performed, and the table is rapidly moved (panned) with the contrast bolus down the leg to the feet. Dynamic collimation is required to optimize vessel imaging. Angiography is performed by injecting 40 mL of contrast over 8 seconds. The drawback of this technique is that digital subtraction is not possible. The advantage is that the image intensifier may be angulated laterally to optimize viewing the bifurcation of the SFA and DFA. Following completion of the contralateral extremity, the angiographic catheter is withdrawn to the ipsilateral common iliac artery and the single leg dynamic run-off angiogram is repeated.

Selective angiograms at different angulations of a particular artery or segment are very useful when the nonselective angiogram shows stenoses of questionable significance or further anatomic clarification is needed. For instance, 20 degrees of caudal and 20 degrees of medial angulation is very useful to image the bifurcation of the IIA and EIA. To view the right IIA and EIA, we would use 20-degree caudal and 20-degree LAO angulation with the injection of contrast (10–15 mL) in the common iliac artery. A diagnostic catheter may be positioned at any level (iliac, femoral,

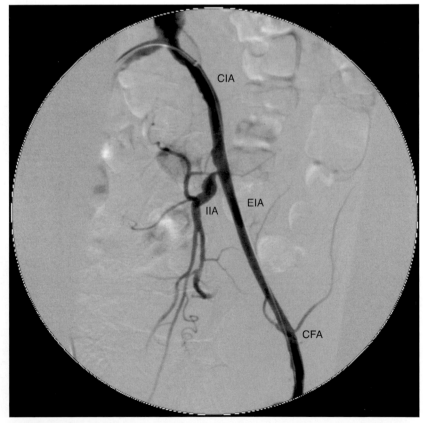

FIGURE 26-22. Twenty-degree oblique and 20-degree caudal view of internal iliac stenosis. CFA = common femoral artery; CIA = common iliac artery; EIA = external iliac artery; IIA = internal iliac artery.

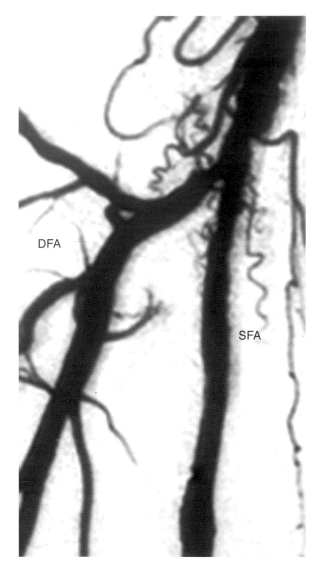

FIGURE 26-23. Separation of profunda and femoral artery with 30-degree oblique angulation. DFA = deep femoral artery; SFA = superficial femoral artery.

popliteal, or infrapopliteal) for a more detailed image of a particular arterial segment. These catheters should be as small as possible, usually 6-Fr or less in size, and always advanced over a guidewire to avoid trauma to the vessel.

Particular angiographic views are important to mention because they help to improve anatomical detail. In the AP view there is significant overlap of the origin of the EIA and the IIA, and ostial stenoses in either or both vessels may be missed. To "separate" these two segments, the contralateral 20-degree oblique angle with a 20-degree caudal view is very useful (Figure 26-22). Likewise, there is a great deal of overlapping between the ostia of the SFA and the DFA, which are frequently affected by atherosclerosis.[4] A view that separates the proximal segments of these two vessels is the ipsilateral 30-degree oblique (or steeper) view (Figure 26-23).

CORONARY SINUS ACCESS

Cannulation of the coronary sinus may be accomplished using either a superior or an inferior approach. For the superior approach, a central vein is cannulated (left brachial, cephalic, axillary, or subclavian veins or the right internal jugular vein). A J-tipped guidewire is advanced to the right atrium. A preformed "coronary sinus" long sheath or a catheter is advanced to the right ventricular inflow tract, then pulled back to the level of the tricuspid annulus at its inferior margin. The catheter is then pulled slowly back further with a counterclockwise rotation. This can be accomplished in either the LAO or RAO projection. In the LAO projection, counterclockwise rotation directs the sheath posteriorly toward the spine. Once the sheath (or catheter) appears to have crossed the midline of the spine without causing ventricular ectopy, it should then be slowly and gently advanced into the coronary sinus. In this position, the catheter appears to curve posteriorly. To confirm the correct position in the RAO view, the catheter takes off at an acute angle at the origin of the coronary sinus with the catheter pointing superiorly and rightward on the fluoroscopic screen.

Cannulation of the coronary sinus is sometimes complicated by variability in the anatomic location of the ostium. The coronary sinus ostium may be displaced inferiorly, superiorly, or posteriorly. Fortunately, there is usually a relationship with the tricuspid annulus, and the two structures are often located together.

The coronary sinus can also be cannulated using a transfemoral (inferior) venous approach. A multipurpose or cobra-shaped catheter is advanced across the tricuspid valve into the right ventricular inflow tract. The catheter is pulled down and back, such that its tip lies at the inferior margin of the tricuspid ring. At some point, the tip will dip into the coronary sinus ostium. In an LAO

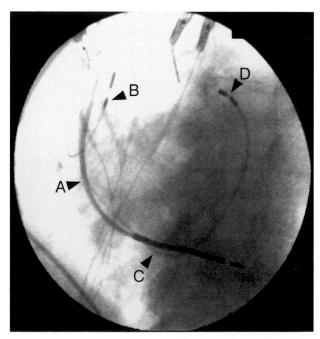

FIGURE 26-24. Cannulation of coronary sinus, left anterior oblique view. A indicates AICD lead; B, high right atrial pacing lead; C, origin of the coronary sinus; and D, distal coronary sinus lead.

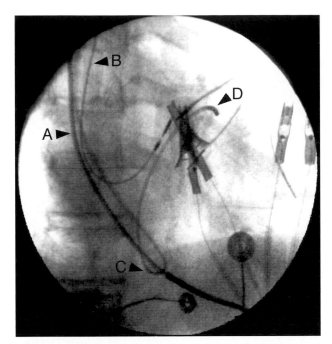

FIGURE 26-25. Coronary sinus, right anterior oblique view. A indicates AICD lead; B, high right atrial pacing lead; C, origin of the coronary sinus; and D, distal coronary sinus lead

view, the catheter will be pointing toward the spine with the shaft making an angle of approximately 110 degrees at the level of entry into the coronary sinus (Figure 26-24). In the RAO view, prior to cannulation, the tip of the catheter appears to be looped on itself, in an attempt to prolapse the catheter into the ostium of the coronary sinus (Figure 26-25). When the catheter has entered the coronary sinus, it will appear to have made a gentle U-turn at the level of the coronary sinus ostium, with the shaft directed first to the right of the screen, then making a 240-degree turn toward the left, and then back again, shooting to the right and the superior part of the screen.

Cannulation of the coronary sinus from the femoral approach may be somewhat easier compared with the superior approach because the catheter can be supported on the tricuspid valve and the floor of the coronary sinus. If it is necessary to cannulate the coronary sinus from above, then the femoral catheter may be left in place and used as a marker to direct further attempts from the superior approach. The coronary sinus may be a relatively large structure, and with the femoral approach, the operator tends to push the catheter against the roof of the coronary sinus (closer to the atria) whereas the superior approach tends to push the catheter toward the floor of the vein. It is feasible in most cases to place two catheters in the coronary sinus and still maneuver each independently. Therefore, if the femoral catheter is being used as a marker, it is not necessary to withdraw it immediately after successful cannulation from a superior approach. It can be kept through parts of the procedure and then removed only when the operator is confident that the superior catheter is quite stable in its position.

REFERENCES

1. Kadir S. Regional anatomy of the thoracic aorta. In: Kadir S, ed. Atlas of *Normal and Variant Angiographic Anatomy*. Philadelphia, PA: Saunders; 1991:19.
2. Horejs D, Gilbert PM, Burstein S, Vogelzang RL. Normal aortoiliac diameters by CT. *J Comput Assist Tomogr*. 1988;12:602.
3. Ulfacker R. Abdominal aorta and its branches. In: Ulfacker R, ed. *Atlas of Vascular Anatomy: An Angiographic Approach*. Philadelphia, PA: Lippincott, Williams and Wilkins; 1997:405.
4. Silva JA, White CJ, Ramee SR, et al. Percutaneous profundaplasty in the treatment of lower extremity ischemia: Results of long-term surveillance. *J Endovasc Ther*. 2001;8:75.

CHAPTER (27)

Adjunctive Diagnostic Techniques

William F. Fearon, MD, Mamoo Nakamura, MD, and Peter J. Fitzgerald, MD, PhD

Although coronary angiography remains the reference standard for diagnosing critical epicardial coronary artery disease, it has a number of limitations. Identifying functionally significant intermediate coronary narrowing, characterizing plaque morphology, detecting moderate diffuse intimal thickening, evaluating the results of percutaneous coronary intervention (PCI), and assessing the status of the microvasculature all remain challenging with coronary angiography alone.[1-6] Technologic advancements have made available several adjunctive diagnostic techniques that allow the interventional cardiologist to address the limitations of coronary angiography and more thoroughly assess the coronary circulation.

The goal of this chapter is to provide a review of adjunctive diagnostic procedures commonly used in the cardiac catheterization laboratory. The chapter focuses on intravascular ultrasound and the coronary pressure wire; however, other modalities, including the Doppler velocity wire and angiographic contrast flow and perfusion grading systems, are also discussed.

INTRAVASCULAR ULTRASOUND

【 】 HISTORICAL BACKGROUND

With its tomographic perspective and direct visualization of the vessel wall, intravascular ultrasound imaging (IVUS) provides valuable anatomic information regarding lesion morphology, the need for PCI, and the adequacy of PCI. IVUS was first introduced in the late 1980s as a mechanism for facilitating coronary atherectomy.[7-9] During the 1990s as imaging systems improved, facilitating interpretation, as the catheters became smaller and easier to use, and as appreciation regarding the importance of maximal stent expansion grew, IVUS became an indispensable adjunctive procedure in many catheterization laboratories.

【 】 IMAGING SYSTEMS AND PROCEDURE

IVUS systems consist of two major components: a catheter that is equipped with a miniaturized transducer and a console that processes electronic signals into cross-sectional images. Current IVUS catheters use the monorail design and are available in 2.5 to 3.5 French (Fr) (0.83–1.17 mm) sizes, allowing the use of a 6-Fr guiding catheter. IVUS images are generated using either mechanical or solid-state technology. A mechanical catheter is equipped with a flexible cable that rotates a single transducer mounted on the tip of the catheter. In the current commercially available system, the transducer is rotated at a speed of 1800 revolutions per minute (rpm) by a cable controlled by an external motor drive, yielding 30 images per second. The transducer operates within a protective transparent sheath that allows the transducer to move within the catheter without requiring motion of the catheter itself. Flushing the protective sheath with saline before use is necessary to remove air bubbles. The solid-state catheter consists of multiple transducer elements that are mounted on the catheter in an annular array and are activated sequentially to generate the image. In general, a mechanical probe offers better image quality, whereas a solid-state catheter is easier to set up and use.

Heparin and nitroglycerin should be administered prior to an IVUS procedure to prevent thrombus and vessel spasm. The IVUS catheter is advanced under fluoroscopic guidance over an

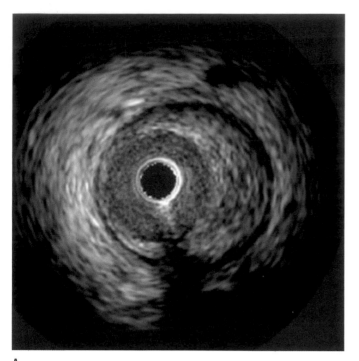

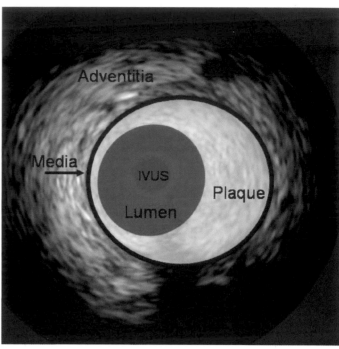

A

B

FIGURE 27-1. Common intravascular ultrasound (IVUS) measurements. **A.** A cross-sectional IVUS image of a diseased vessel. **B.** Key landmarks are identified. IVUS allows accurate measurement of vessel diameter and area, lumen diameter and area, and calculation of plaque area.

angioplasty guidewire until the transducer is beyond the region of interest. The catheter is retracted either by slow manual or automated pullback to the guiding catheter. The merit of an automated pullback is that it allows accurate determination of lesion length and it permits volumetric analyses. Several cross-sectional and longitudinal vessel measurements can be performed with IVUS, as outlined in Figures 27-1 and 27-2.

The safety of performing IVUS has been documented previously.[10,11] The most common complication is transient vascular spasm, which occurs at a rate of approximately 3%. Major complications such as coronary dissection and vessel closure are very rare, with an incidence of less than 0.5%. These severe complications occur mostly in patients who undergo PCI, rather than diagnostic IVUS alone.

【　】 PRACTICAL APPLICATIONS OF IVUS (TABLE 27-1)

Intermediate Lesions

Intermediate or ambiguous coronary lesions are frequently seen at specific locations such as bifurcations or vessel ostia, which are particularly difficult to image angiographically. In these cases, IVUS provides valuable information about the severity, morphology and anatomic location of the questionable lesion. Small population studies comparing IVUS parameters with stress myocardial perfusion or intracoronary physiologic measurements in intermediate lesions have found that the minimum lumen cross-sectional area (CSA) correlates with the presence of myocardial ischemia.[12,13] A minimum lumen CSA between 3.0 and 4.0 mm^2, depending on the study, has a sensitivity and specificity higher than 80% for predicting ischemia.[12–14]

Angiographic assessment of left main artery disease remains a frequent challenge. Although there are no absolute criteria regarding the IVUS definition of critical left main disease, a lumen CSA of less than 6 mm^2 and lumen CSA stenosis of more than 60% have been suggested.[15]

Preintervention

Aspects of a successful PCI include acute lumen gain, the avoidance of complications, and the prevention of restenosis. IVUS guidance during PCI may be an effective strategy for achieving these goals.

IVUS examination prior to intervention offers an assessment of lesion morphology and extent of atherosclerosis, as well as an evaluation of vessel size, all of which may facilitate safely maximizing acute lumen gain. Although the absolute benefit of routine IVUS use prior to PCI remains uncertain, the information obtained can be valuable for the appropriate selection of interventional devices. For instance, in hard-type lesions with dense fibrous or calcified plaque based on IVUS evaluation, larger acute lumen gain may be effectively achieved using rotational atherectomy or cutting balloon angioplasty rather than using plain balloon angioplasty or direct stenting.[16,17] By providing accurate measurements of vessel dimensions, IVUS can also help in the selection of the appropriate atherectomy burr size, leading to optimal lumen gain and minimizing complications. Furthermore, in bifurcation lesions, in which IVUS reveals excessive plaque burden at the main branch immediately distal to the side branch takeoff, plaque debulking may help prevent side branch occlusion by plaque shift.

Using IVUS to determine the remodeling pattern of a culprit lesion may predict the risk of restenosis after PCI. Previous studies examining the impact of the remodeling pattern on subsequent

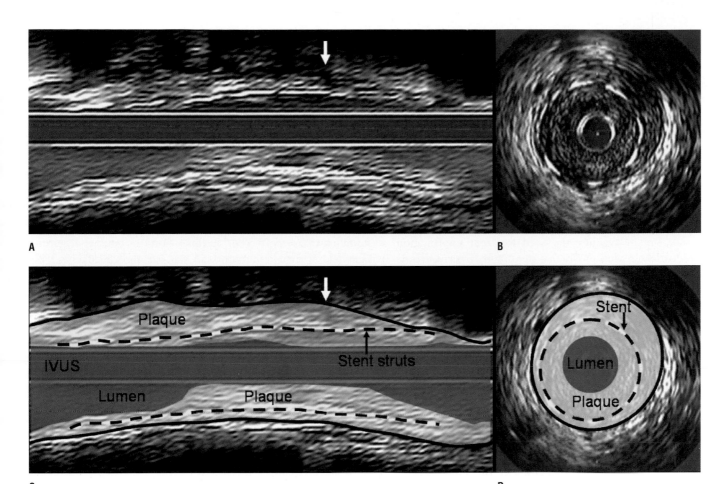

FIGURE 27-2. Volumetric intravascular ultrasound (IVUS) analysis. **A.** A longitudinal reconstruction of multiple cross-sectional IVUS images in a previously stented vessel. **B.** Cross-sectional image at the site corresponding to the white arrow in A. **C, D.** The same longitudinal and cross-sectional image as in A and B, with key landmarks noted. Using this technique, volumetric measurements such as vessel, lumen, and plaque volume can be determined.

restenosis suggest that outward remodeling is a risk factor for restenosis after balloon angioplasty.[18,19] The impact of outward remodeling on in-stent restenosis after bare-metal stenting remains controversial.

Finally, IVUS evaluation of vessel size at both the site of the lesion and the reference vessel facilitates the precise selection of device size and may prevent unnecessary excessive vascular injury caused by an oversized device. In the era of drug-eluting stents, determination of vessel size and lesion length appears to be critical. Recent drug-eluting stent trials suggest that minimizing vessel injury and completely covering the diseased segment may further reduce restenosis rates.[20]

TABLE 27-1

Indications for Intravascular Ultrasound Examination

Preintervention assessment of ambiguous lesion morphology
Preintervention assessment of lesion length
Preintervention assessment of bifurcation, ostial, or left main stenoses
Postintervention assessment of stent deployment

Postangioplasty

Cumulative observations from previous IVUS studies have suggested that the final residual plaque burden and lumen area or diameter are predictors of restenosis after conventional balloon angioplasty alone.[21,22] The Clinical Outcomes with Ultrasound Trial (CLOUT) examined the efficacy of IVUS guidance on treatment outcome in patients undergoing angioplasty. IVUS-guided balloon sizing was performed after successful angiographically guided balloon angioplasty. In this trial, 73% of lesions received additional balloon angioplasty using a larger diameter balloon catheter.[23] After IVUS-guided percutaneous transluminal coronary angioplasty (PTCA), the nominal balloon-to-artery ratio increased from 1.12 to 1.30, resulting in an increase of the IVUS lumen area from 3.16 to 4.52 mm^2 without an increase in dissection or ischemic complications. Several subsequent small studies confirm these findings, showing improved short- and long-term outcomes with IVUS guidance.[24,25]

IVUS is useful for evaluating vessel wall injury after angioplasty. Fracture or dissection of plaque after angioplasty is frequently observed by IVUS and regarded as a principal mechanism for lumen enlargement. For example, in the Guidance by Ultrasound Imaging for Decision Endpoints (GUIDE) trial, larger acute lumen gain after balloon angioplasty was associated with the presence of plaque dissection rather than the absence of any tearing in the vessel wall.[26] This observation was further confirmed in small studies examining the impact of deep vessel wall fracture on subsequent lumen change after either conventional balloon angioplasty or cutting balloon angioplasty.[27,28] Although the presence of dissection or tearing can favorably impact the acute lumen gain, extensive dissection may also compromise the lumen area and become a potential risk factor for acute vessel occlusion, in the absence of coronary stenting.

At the present time when coronary stent implantation is a dominant, albeit more expensive, strategy in PCI, several investigators have studied the role of IVUS in determining an optimal angioplasty result and in avoiding the need for stent implantation. IVUS-guided PTCA with provisional stenting may decrease medical costs while obtaining equivalent outcomes compared with an elective bare-metal stenting strategy.[29,30] A percent lumen area stenosis of less than 30% to 35% and a minimum lumen area of 6 mm^2 or less without flow-limiting dissection defines an optimal angioplasty result based on IVUS evaluation.[31]

Post-Stenting

Since the introduction of the bare-metal stent, IVUS has played an essential role in the development of an optimal strategy for stent deployment. In general, criteria for optimal stent deployment have focused on the achievement of complete apposition of the stent struts to the vessel wall, a large enough minimum stent area with complete expansion of the stent, and complete coverage of the diseased segment, as well as any dissection.[32,33] Early in the clinical experience with stent implantation, IVUS studies demonstrated an unexpectedly high incidence of inadequate stent deployment, despite an optimal angiographic result.[34,35]

Incomplete stent expansion is generally defined as less than 70% expansion of a portion of the stent compared with the distal and proximal reference lumen dimensions; it frequently occurs in lesions with hard plaque, such as dense fibrocalcific or fully calcified plaque. Incomplete stent apposition refers to the situation when more than one stent strut is clearly separated from the vessel wall, with evidence of blood speckles behind the stent at a site without side branch involvement.[36] Immediately after stent implantation, incomplete apposition may result from incomplete stent expansion or inadequate stent size selection. Incomplete apposition that develops late after stent deployment (late stent incomplete apposition) is often related to the use of specific interventional devices, such as directional coronary atherectomy, brachytherapy or drug-eluting stents.[37–40] Several recent retrospective studies suggest that incomplete stent deployment is a strong risk factor for subacute thrombosis.[41,42] Fortunately, the current rate of this complication is reasonably low with higher pressure stent deployment, improvement of stent design, and application of antiplatelet therapy. Therefore, routine use of IVUS for the purpose of reducing stent thrombosis may be impractical, particularly from the standpoint of cost-effectiveness, and thus should be reserved for high-risk cases such as patients with complex lesions, small vessels, or left main artery disease.

In current practice, optimal stent deployment is probably more critical for the reduction of in-stent restenosis, particularly in the context of bare-metal stenting. Because late lumen loss after stent implantation depends on the degree of intrastent neointimal hyperplasia, the final minimum stent CSA immediately after stenting is regarded as the most powerful IVUS predictor for in-stent restenosis.[43,44] Over the past few years, several multicenter trials have investigated whether IVUS-guided bare-metal stenting improves stent CSA and clinical outcome compared with an angiography-guided procedure. The Can Routine Ultrasound Influence Stent Expansion (CRUISE) trial found that IVUS-guided stenting achieved a significantly larger angiographic minimum lumen diameter (2.9 ± 0.4 mm vs 2.7 ± 0.5 mm) as well as minimum stent CSA (7.78 ± 1.72 mm^2 vs 7.06 ± 2.13 mm^2), which translated into a 44% relative reduction in the need for target vessel revascularization (8.5% vs 15.3%).[4] In this cohort, the optimal diagnostic threshold of stent minimum CSA was 6.5 mm^2, predicting 94% freedom from repeat revascularization at 9 months.[45] A similar trend in the increase of minimum stent CSA was observed after the acute procedure and at 6-month follow-up in the IVUS-guided stenting group of the Restenosis after IVUS-guided Stenting (RESIST) trial, although the rate of in-stent restenosis was not statistically different compared with the angiography-guided group (6.3% relative restenosis reduction in the IVUS-guided group).[46] The Optimization with ICUS to Reduce Stent Restenosis (OPTICUS) trial, however, showed no difference in angiographic and long-term clinical results between the groups of IVUS-guided and angiography-guided stenting, probably due to equivalent acute gain in the angiography and IVUS-guided groups.[47] Finally, the Angiography Versus Intravascular Ultrasound-Directed Stent Placement (AVID) study identified specific lesion subsets that may receive particular benefit from IVUS-guided bare-metal stenting for better long-term outcome. These included angiographic vessel size less than 3.25 mm, severe original angiographic percent diameter stenosis greater than 70%, and saphenous vein graft target vessels.[48]

At this point, there is no strict consensus regarding optimal IVUS procedural end points for bare-metal stenting. In general, complete apposition of the stent struts to the vessel wall and achievement of a minimum stent CSA comparable to the lumen area in the reference segments have been used in the IVUS-guided studies.

In addition, a minimum stent CSA of greater than 6.5 to 7 mm^2 may be required to minimize the risk of in-stent restenosis for the major epicardial coronary artery segment, although this threshold will vary with vessel size. In a single-center real-world experience that included 1248 lesions treated with IVUS-guided bare-metal stenting, patients who ultimately developed restenosis had significantly smaller minimum stent CSA after the initial procedure (6.5 ± 2.1 mm^2 vs 8.0 ± 2.6 mm^2). Multivariate analysis found that total stent length and IVUS minimum stent CSA were the most powerful predictors of in-stent restenosis; the risk of restenosis decreased 19% for every 1 mm^2 increase in minimum stent CSA.[49]

In addition to evaluating stent expansion and apposition, IVUS can also be useful for detecting edge dissection, which is often angiographically obscure.[50,51] For example, one single-center retrospective study examining 124 lesions with nonocclusive residual dissections after angioplasty (n = 43) or stent implantation (n = 81) found that an IVUS-derived percent area stenosis at the site of the dissection that was greater than 60% was a predictor for acute or subacute major adverse cardiac events (Table 27-2).

TABLE 27-2

IVUS Criteria for Optimal Bare-metal Stent Deployment

Complete stent expansion (> 90% of the average reference area)
Complete stent apposition
Minimum stent CSA > 7 mm^2
Absence of edge dissection

CSA = coronary artery stenosis; IVUS = Intravascular, ultrasound imaging.

Drug-Eluting Stents

Current results of European and US clinical trials evaluating drug-eluting stents strongly support the potential of this new device as the most effective approach to preventing restenosis.[52–54] Because neointimal hyperplasia, a main cause of in-stent restenosis, is better visualized with IVUS than angiography, IVUS has played a major role in evaluating the effects of various drugs on neointimal proliferation.[55–57]

IVUS can also be useful for optimizing drug-eluting stent deployment. For instance, despite the dramatic reduction of restenosis inside the stented segment, the pivotal US multicenter trial with sirolimus-eluting stenting (Sirolimus-Eluting Stents versus Standard Stents in Patients with Stenosis in a Native Coronary Artery: SIRIUS trial) found that the greatest degree of restenosis occurred in the coronary segment just proximal to the proximal stent edge.[58] Although the exact mechanism is unclear, stent edge injury or residual peri-stent disease have been implicated. In fact, preliminary results from the SIRIUS trial indicate that higher pressure deployment, particularly in smaller sized vessels, may be associated with this phenomenon. From the analysis of 126 serial IVUS cases, including 74 sirolimus-eluting stent cases and 52 bare-metal stent cases, the minimum stent CSA immediately after stenting was a stronger predictor of outcome in the sirolimus-eluting stent group than in the bare-metal stenting group; moreover, the optimal threshold of minimum stent CSA in the sirolimus-eluting stent group was significantly smaller than in the bare-metal stent group (5.0 mm^2 vs 6.5 mm^2).[59] On the other hand, underexpansion of the drug-eluting stent may increase the risk of stent thrombosis.

Complete stent apposition to the vessel wall is important for proper drug delivery to the vessel wall. IVUS evaluation of strut apposition after stent deployment may be valuable for determining the need for additional balloon dilation to maximize the effect of this device. Several reports describing IVUS follow-up of drug-eluting stents have revealed the late development of incomplete apposition, characterized by the vessel wall moving away from the stent struts.[55,60] Although the exact clinical impact of late incomplete apposition is still not clear, to date, late thrombotic events have not been reported related to this problem. For these reasons, at least until greater experience is obtained, IVUS may have an important role in ensuring appropriate drug-eluting stent deployment.

DOPPLER VELOCITY WIRE

HISTORICAL BACKGROUND

Estimating coronary flow by measuring velocity using Doppler technology was first introduced in the early 1990s.[61] Initially, the Doppler transducer was mounted on a catheter, but as technology advanced the transducer was miniaturized and it is now available mounted on a standard 0.014-in coronary guidewire.

DERIVATION OF CORONARY FLOW RESERVE

The main utility of the Doppler velocity wire is to estimate the coronary flow reserve (CFR), by measuring the coronary velocity reserve (CVR). CFR, first introduced by Gould and colleagues, is defined as the ratio of the maximal coronary flow to resting flow.[62] With a Doppler wire, coronary flow can be estimated by measuring the velocity of blood flow and by multiplying the velocity by the vessel area. In general, it is assumed that as long as the velocity is measured in the same spot at rest and at peak hyperemia and as long as nitroglycerin is administered before the resting measurements, the vessel area remains constant and CFR is equal to CVR, defined as simply the average peak velocity at maximal hyperemia divided by the average peak velocity at rest.

CFR provides information regarding the status of both the epicardial coronary artery, or large vessel, and the coronary microvasculature. Therefore, patients with microvascular dysfunction, such as diabetics, or those with left ventricular hypertrophy, may have an abnormal CFR despite a normal epicardial artery. This can be a limitation when measuring CFR to determine the physiologic significance of an intermediate epicardial stenosis.[63]

CFR is also limited by its dependence on resting hemodynamics and by the fact that there is no absolute normal value. For example, tachycardia can increase resting flow and thereby lower CFR. An increase in mean arterial pressure can have a similar effect. In the normal setting, CFR should be greater than 3; however, it can be as high as 6 or 7.

In an attempt to address these limitations, an index called relative CFR (rCFR) was introduced.[64] rCFR is defined as the CFR of the target vessel divided by the CFR of a normal adjacent vessel. This index is not applicable in patients with disease involving three vessels, and it assumes that microvascular pathology is evenly distributed throughout the myocardium, which may not be the case in some situations (eg, myocardial infarction). rCFR has an absolute normal value of 1.0 and should be epicardial specific. Studies suggest that rCFR (or relative coronary velocity reserve; rCVR) predicts ischemia-producing lesions better than CVR.[65,66]

INDICATIONS FOR USING THE DOPPLER VELOCITY WIRE

The main indication for using the Doppler velocity wire is to measure CVR to help determine the significance of an epicardial artery stenosis. Despite the previously outlined limitations, several studies have demonstrated a correlation between CVR and noninvasive tests for ischemia in patients with intermediate coronary lesions.[67] In general, CVR less than 2.0 is considered abnormal and indicative of myocardial ischemia. The value of measuring CVR to determine if a PCI result is optimal has also been extensively studied.[68–70]

Another application of Doppler velocity measurements is in the setting of acute myocardial infarction. For example, the finding of systolic flow reversal or a short diastolic deceleration time, or both, on Doppler velocity recordings is indicative of severe microvascular damage and portends a worse outcome.[71,72]

Lastly, Doppler velocity measurements have been made distal to a balloon occlusion of the epicardial artery in an attempt to assess for the presence of collateral circulation. In one study, the presence and degree of both antegrade and retrograde Doppler-derived flow at balloon occlusion, compared with antegrade flow after PCI was used to define a collateral flow index.[73] The development of ischemia at the time of balloon occlusion was found to be related to the degree of collateral circulation based on the Doppler velocity measurements.

[ ] EQUIPMENT AND TECHNIQUE

The Doppler velocity wire (Volcano Therapeutics) is a standard 0.014-in angioplasty guidewire with a piezoelectric ultrasound transducer integrated into the tip of the wire. The wire is connected to a real-time spectrum analyzer, a videocassette recorder, and a video page printer via an interface connector at its distal end. After administration of heparin and nitroglycerin, the wire is introduced into the coronary artery using standard angioplasty equipment. The tip of the wire should be positioned at least 5 to 10 artery-diameter lengths beyond the stenosis in question. Attempts should be made to position the wire in the middle of the vessel to maximize the velocity signal. Obtaining an accurate and reliable Doppler signal can be challenging, particularly in tortuous vessels. The wire should not be moved between the resting and hyperemic measurements. Hyperemia can be induced with intracoronary or intravenous adenosine or papaverine, as described in more detail in the later section on fractional flow reserve. If necessary, PCI can be performed using this wire simply by disconnecting the distal end from the interface connector.

CORONARY PRESSURE WIRE

[ ] HISTORICAL BACKGROUND

The significance of intracoronary pressure gradients and their reflection of the severity of underlying coronary artery disease have been appreciated for many years.[74] However, it was not until the advent of miniaturized pressure sensors that allowed a wire-based approach to measuring coronary pressure and not until the development and validation of the fractional flow reserve (FFR) index by Pijls and De Bruyne that intracoronary pressure measurements have become a routine procedure in many catheterization laboratories.[75,76]

[ ] DERIVATION OF FRACTIONAL FLOW RESERVE

Currently, the main indication for assessing intracoronary pressure is to determine the FFR to guide the operator's decision about performing PCI on a stenosis of unclear physiologic significance. FFR is defined as the fraction of maximal blood flow perfusing the myocardium in the presence of stenosis compared with the maximal blood flow that would reach the myocardium in the theoretical absence of the stenosis. Because the measurement is made at maximal vasodilation, resistance is minimized and flow becomes proportional to pressure. In a normal epicardial artery there is little pressure decrement along the vessel and distal pressure is roughly equal to proximal pressure. Therefore, in a diseased vessel, one can estimate the distal flow or pressure in the theoretical absence of the disease by measuring the proximal pressure. FFR then can be calculated easily in a diseased vessel by dividing the distal pressure, measured with a coronary pressure wire, by the proximal pressure, measured with the guiding catheter during peak hyperemia[75] (Figure 27-3).

Compared with other techniques for determining the functional significance of a coronary narrowing, measuring FFR has several inherent advantages. It has an absolute normal value of 1.0 and a narrow range of normal values extending from 0.94 to 1.0.[77] Because the measurements are made at maximal vasodilation, the effects of resting hemodynamics are eliminated, making FFR an extremely reproducible index, independent of blood pressure and heart rate.[78] Compared with measuring CFR to evaluate intermediate coronary lesions, FFR is advantageous because it is epicardial artery–specific and independent of the microcirculation (Figure 27-4). As described in more detail below, FFR has a narrow cutoff range for identifying ischemia-producing lesions. Numerous studies have shown that an FFR less than 0.75 correlates strongly with the presence of ischemia on a variety of noninvasive stress tests.

[ ] INDICATIONS FOR MEASURING FRACTIONAL FLOW RESERVE (TABLE 27-3)

The primary indication for measuring FFR is to determine the physiologic significance of an intermediate coronary lesion. As more and more patients present to the catheterization laboratory without a prior noninvasive assessment for myocardial ischemia and as awareness of the limitations of angiography alone to identify functionally important moderate lesions has grown, the role of a relatively simple method, such as measuring FFR, for interrogating this challenging subset has expanded. Pijls and colleagues performed

---

TABLE 27-3

Indications for Measuring Fractional Flow Reserve

Functional assessment of intermediate coronary lesions
Determination of culprit stenosis in multivessel disease
Distinguishing focal coronary disease from diffuse disease
Guiding treatment of serial stenoses
Assessment of collateral circulation

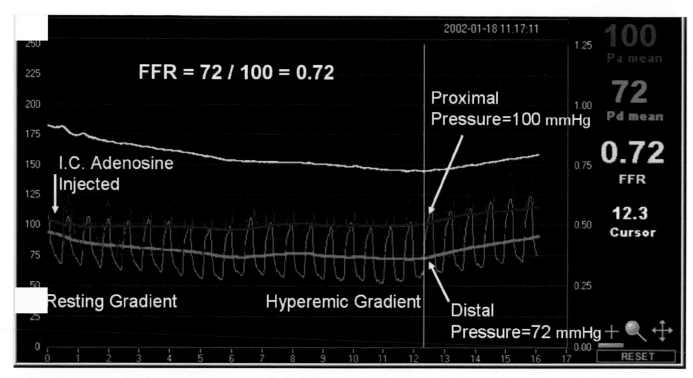

FIGURE 27-3. Example of fractional flow reserve determination. The upper tracing represents the mean and phasic pressure recorded from the guiding catheter and the lower tracing represents the mean and phasic pressure recorded from the pressure wire in a patient with a moderate, but physiologically significant, stenosis of the left anterior descending artery. The nearly horizontal line above the two tracings represents the continuous fractional flow reserve calculation, and the vertical line marks the peak gradient.

a landmark trial comparing FFR with three noninvasive stress tests.[1] They showed that an FFR less than 0.75 is 100% specific for predicting myocardial ischemia; the sensitivity was 88% and the predictive accuracy was 93%. Other studies have confirmed the high specificity of an FFR less than 0.75 and further suggest a "gray zone" between 0.75 and 0.80, where a minority of patients will have inducible ischemia on noninvasive stress test.[79–82] If the FFR is greater than 0.80, it is extremely unlikely that inducible ischemia is present.

To determine the safety of employing FFR to guides the operator's decision to defer PCI, Bech and colleagues measured FFR in 325 patients with chest pain, no prior stress test, and intermediate coronary lesions who had been referred for PCI.[83] One hundred and forty-four of these patients had an FFR less than 0.75, underwent PCI as planned, and formed a reference group. One hundred and eighty-one had an FFR of 0.75 or greater and were randomized to deferral of PCI (n = 91) or performance of PCI (n = 90) with bare-metal stents. The deferral group had a greater freedom from major adverse cardiac events at 2 years, although not statistically significant, compared with the performance group, 89% versus 83%, respectively. The reference group had a significantly worse event-free survival compared with the deferral group (78% vs 89%, P = 0.03), presumably because they had more significant coronary artery disease. This trial clearly showed that it is safe to defer PCI in stable patients with an intermediate lesion and an FFR of 0.75 or greater.

Besides assessing intermediate coronary lesions in patients with single vessel coronary artery disease, FFR is useful for determining culprit stenoses in patients with multivessel coronary artery disease. The use of FFR in this setting has become particularly relevant as

our appreciation of the limitations of nuclear perfusion imaging in patients with multivessel disease has grown.[84–86] Furthermore, the spatial resolution of FFR in patients with multiple lesions in a single vessel is superior to noninvasive stress imaging studies. The noninvasive test may identify an ischemic myocardial region, but measuring FFR and doing a pullback of the pressure wire allows localization of the ischemia-producing region of a coronary artery.

Two recent studies evaluating the cost-effectiveness of measuring FFR to assess intermediate coronary lesions should further expand the use of this technology.[87,88] In the first study, a decision model was created comparing the long-term costs and benefits of three strategies for treating patients with an intermediate coronary lesion and no prior functional study: (1) deferring the decision for PCI to obtain a nuclear stress imaging study (NUC strategy); (2) measuring FFR at the time of angiography to help guide the decision for PCI (FFR strategy); and (3) stenting all intermediate lesions (STENT strategy). The FFR strategy saved $1795 per patient compared with the NUC strategy and $3830 compared with the STENT strategy. Quality-adjusted life expectancy was similar among the three strategies.

In the second study, 70 patients presenting with an acute coronary syndrome, who were found to have an intermediate culprit stenosis, were randomized to deferral of PCI so that a nuclear perfusion study could be performed or randomized to measurement of FFR at the time of the initial catheterization. The patients who had nuclear perfusion imaging then returned to the catheterization laboratory for PCI if the noninvasive test revealed ischemia; otherwise they were treated medically. Patients randomized to measurement of FFR underwent PCI immediately if the FFR was less than 0.75; otherwise they were treated medically. The group of patients

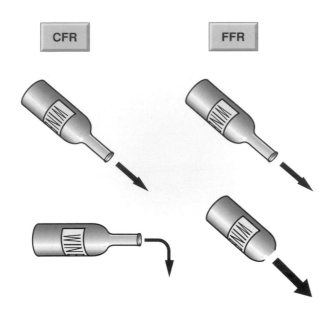

FIGURE 27-4. Analogy comparing fractional flow reserve (FFR) with coronary flow reserve (CFR). Imagine that a wine bottle represents the epicardial coronary artery and the bottle neck represents an epicardial stenosis. Assume that one's ability to tilt and pour the wine represents the ability of the microvasculature to maximally dilate. Using this analogy, CFR is defined as the amount of wine poured with the bottle fully tilted (maximally vasodilated) and in the presence of the bottle neck (epicardial stenosis), compared with the amount of wine poured with the bottle on its side (at rest) and in the presence of the bottle neck. FFR on the other hand is the amount of wine poured with the bottle fully tilted in the presence of the bottle neck compared with the amount of wine poured again with the bottle fully tilted, but in the theoretical absence of the bottle neck. From this analogy, one can see how CFR interrogates both the microvasculature and the epicardial stenosis. The impact of resting hemodynamics on the calculation of CFR is also apparent. FFR on the other hand is independent of resting hemodynamics because both measurements are made at maximal vasodilatation. FFR also interrogates the status of the epicardial artery, only, and is "independent" of the microvasculature.

randomized to measurement of FFR had a significantly shorter hospital stay (11 vs 49 hours, $P < .001$) and lower hospital costs ($1329 vs $2113, $P < .05$). There were no significant differences in procedure time, radiation exposure, or adverse cardiac events at 1-year follow-up.

A final indication for determining FFR is to optimize PCI. In a study evaluating 58 patients who had undergone angioplasty alone, it was shown that the combination of an excellent angiographic outcome (residual percent diameter stenosis of 35% or less) and an excellent functional result (FFR of 0.90 or more, measured 15 minutes after angioplasty), which occurred in 26 patients, resulted in a significantly better event-free survival rate at 2-year follow-up (88% compared with 59% in the 32 patients with suboptimal angiographic or functional results).[89]

A number of studies have compared FFR after stenting with intravascular ultrasound criteria for determining optimal stent deployment and have found a significant correlation between the two techniques.[90–92] However, the strongest evidence supporting a role for measuring FFR after PCI comes from a registry in which 750 patients who had FFR measured after bare-metal stenting

were followed for 6 months to determine the relationship between the post-procedure FFR and clinical outcomes.[5] Multivariate analysis showed that FFR was the strongest predictor of major adverse cardiac events. In the 36% of patients with a final FFR of more than 0.95, the 6-month adverse event rate (after bare-metal stenting) was 4.9%, and in the 32% with a final FFR between 0.90 and 0.95, the event rate was 6.2%. In comparison, if the final FFR was less than 0.90, the event rate was 20.3%, and in the 6% of patients with a final FFR of less than 0.80, the event rate was 29.5%. Of note, angiographic results were not at all predictive of adverse events.

One should be cautious when measuring FFR in certain patient subgroups. For example, in the setting of acute myocardial infarction, microvascular stunning may result in diminished hyperemic flow across a moderate stenosis, a lower pressure gradient, and a higher FFR. Once the stunning has resolved, allowing greater peak flow to the myocardium, the same stenosis may produce a larger gradient and a lower FFR. De Bruyne and colleagues demonstrated that if one waits at least 6 days after a myocardial infarction, then an FFR cutoff value of 0.75 still correlates well with noninvasive testing for myocardial ischemia.[93] Another limitation of FFR includes significant left ventricular hypertrophy. Because the hypertrophic myocardium can outgrow the blood supply, the fraction of normal flow required to prevent myocardial ischemia may be higher. In other words, a higher cutoff value for FFR may be appropriate, although this has not been well studied.[94]

【 】 EQUIPMENT AND TECHNIQUE

The coronary pressure wire is a standard 0.014-in angioplasty guidewire with a high-fidelity pressure transducer mounted 3 cm from the tip of the wire, at the junction of the radiopaque and radiolucent segments. Currently there are two manufacturers of the pressure wire (Radi Medical Systems and Volcano Therapeutics) each of which have their own consoles, which analyze and display the pressure recordings.

To measure FFR it is first necessary to connect the pressure console to the catheterization laboratory pressure monitoring system and to calibrate the guiding catheter and pressure wire. After administering intravenous heparin and intracoronary nitroglycerin, the pressure wire should be advanced out of the guiding catheter so that the pressure transducer is positioned at the ostium of the coronary artery. At this location, both the pressure wire and the guiding catheter should display identical pressures. If this is not the case, the pressure wire can be equalized to the guiding catheter. The pressure wire is then advanced to the distal part of the vessel and a vasodilating agent such as adenosine or papaverine is administered. The FFR of the vessel is the lowest value achieved by dividing the simultaneously measured mean distal pressure by the mean proximal pressure.

Achieving maximal hyperemia is critical in order to accurately measure FFR. If hyperemia is submaximal, the gradient across the stenosis in question will be underestimated and FFR will be overestimated. The reference standard agent for achieving peak vasodilatation is intravenous adenosine. It is administered through a central vein with an onset and offset within minutes. Its main side effect is chest pain (not due to ischemia), which is generally well tolerated if the patient is forewarned. Because the hyperemia lasts as long as the infusion continues, intravenous adenosine is advantageous in that it allows more careful determination of the peak gradient. In addition, it affords the operator the ability to slowly pull back the pressure wire proximally in order to identify the area of stenosis. This can be particularly useful if there is diffuse disease or multiple lesions in the vessel.

In the United States, intracoronary adenosine is often used to measure FFR because it is less expensive and easier to administer. Its major drawback is its short peak effect, which is roughly 5 to 10 seconds. In addition, because it is given via the coronary artery, the potential exists for incomplete administration down the coronary artery and partial injection or reflux into the aorta. Recently, it has been shown that higher doses than previously used are necessary to achieve peak hyperemia, and some patients do not respond to intracoronary adenosine.[95,96] If there is any doubt regarding adequate hyperemia, it is important to use either intravenous adenosine or intracoronary papaverine.

Using intracoronary papaverine to measure FFR is advantageous because its peak effect is longer lasting than intracoronary adenosine, roughly 45 seconds, which makes more accurate determination of FFR possible and which allows time to perform a slow pullback of the pressure sensor. In addition, papaverine is inexpensive and easy to prepare and administer. Its major drawback is its potential arrhythmogenic effect. In an older series, the incidence of a serious arrhythmia (ventricular tachycardia or torsades de pointes) was approximately 1%.[97] Fortunately, these arrhythmias were usually self-limited. Papaverine can precipitate in ionic contrast medium, which may induce the arrhythmia (Table 27-4).

If the FFR is abnormal and PCI is necessary, the operator can disconnect the pressure wire from the interface coupler and a balloon catheter or stent can be advanced over the pressure wire in the usual fashion. During balloon inflation the pressure wire can be reconnected and the coronary wedge pressure, a reflection of collateral flow, can be recorded.[98] After completing the PCI, the pressure wire can be reconnected and FFR remeasured. Finally, it is important after measuring FFR, whether or not PCI has been performed, to reposition the pressure sensor at the ostium of the guiding catheter before removing the wire completely to ensure that equal pressures are recorded from the guiding catheter and the pressure wire (ie, that no "drift" in either pressure recording system has occurred).

In summary, FFR is advantageous compared with other invasive indexes for determining myocardial ischemia because it is easy to determine and very reproducible; it has an absolute normal value of 1.0; it is specific for the epicardial artery and independent of the microvasculature; it accounts for collateral flow; it is not affected by resting hemodynamics; and it has unmatched spatial resolution (ie, the pressure pullback curve allows localization of critical stenoses).

ANGIOGRAPHIC FLOW GRADING SCORES

Several grading systems, based on the speed and quality of the flow of intracoronary contrast dye material, have been proposed to assess coronary and myocardial perfusion. The first of these techniques to be introduced was the Thrombolysis in Myocardial Infarction (TIMI) flow grade, which was originally developed to assess reperfusion after administration of fibrinolytics in the setting of acute myocardial infarction. The grades are defined as follows:

- Grade 0 signifies complete absence of flow beyond the area of occlusion.
- Grade 1 signifies penetration without perfusion; contrast passes beyond the obstruction but does not opacify the distal vessel.
- Grade 2 is defined as complete filling of the vessel, but at a slower rate than an adjacent artery.
- Grade 3 means normal filling of the coronary artery.[99]

Numerous studies have shown that patients with TIMI grade 3 flow in the setting of an acute myocardial infarction have better survival compared with patients who have slower flow.[100,101] The TIMI flow grade is the easiest to measure and has been the best studied; however, it is the most qualitative and it provides little information regarding the status of the coronary microcirculation.

More recently, Gibson and others introduced the more quantitative TIMI frame count.[102] It is based on the ability to count the number of angiographic frames necessary for contrast dye to reach specific coronary arterial landmarks. The specific landmarks used are the mustache of the left anterior descending coronary artery and the first branch off of the continuation of the right coronary artery after the origin of the posterior descending artery. In the circumflex system, one counts the number of frames necessary for contrast dye to reach the last branch of the longest obtuse marginal artery beyond the culprit lesion. Validation studies showed that the right coronary and circumflex arteries had similar frame counts, but the frame count for the left anterior descending artery was on average 1.7 times greater. To allow for comparisons between the different vessels, the corrected TIMI frame count for the left anterior descending artery is defined as the number of frames divided by 1.7.[102]

These investigators have found that in patients treated with fibrinolytic therapy for acute myocardial infarction, the corrected TIMI frame count at 90 minutes after reperfusion

TABLE 27-4

Characteristics of Common Hyperemic Agents

	IV ADENOSINE	IC ADENOSINE	PAPAVERINE
Dose	140 μg/kg/min	≥ 30 μg	≥ 10 mg
Peak effect	Indefinite	Seconds	30–60
Pullback possible	Yes	No	Yes
Side effects	Chest pain, Bronchospasm	Transient bradycardia	Rare ventricular tachycardia

IC = ionic contrast; IV = intravenous.

therapy was strongly predictive of in-hospital mortality; moreover, in patients with TIMI grade 3 flow, the corrected TIMI frame count further stratified patients at risk for in-hospital mortality. These findings applied to 1-month survival as well.[103]

Both the TIMI flow grade and frame counting provide information regarding the status of the epicardial coronary artery. Recently, the importance of the coronary microcirculation in determining outcomes has gained greater attention, particularly in the setting of acute myocardial infarction.[104] In an attempt to measure microvascular function, the TIMI investigators introduced the TIMI myocardial perfusion grading system. Grade 0 is defined as no apparent tissue-level perfusion in the distribution of the culprit artery, based on the lack of contrast "blush" in the myocardium.

- Grade 1 indicates the presence of microvascular blush without clearance (ie, the blush remains present on the next injection).

- Grade 2 is defined as blush that clears slowly.

- Grade 3 is defined as blush that clears normally during washout.[105]

In a study of 762 patients with acute myocardial infarction treated with fibrinolytic therapy, the TIMI myocardial perfusion grade predicted 30-day mortality. Patients with grade 3 had the lowest mortality (2%); those with grade 2 had an intermediate mortality (4.4%); and those with grade 0 or 1 had the highest mortality (6%). Even among patients with TIMI grade 3 flow, the myocardial perfusion grade further stratified patients for risk of mortality.[105]

REFERENCES

1. Pijls NH, De Bruyne B, Peels K, et al. Measurement of fractional flow reserve to assess the functional severity of coronary-artery stenoses. *N Engl J Med.* 1996;334:1703.

2. Metz JA, Yock PG, Fitzgerald PJ. Intravascular ultrasound: Basic interpretation. *Cardiol Clin.* 1997;15:1.

3. Fearon WF, Nakamura M, Lee DP, et al. Simultaneous assessment of fractional and coronary flow reserves in cardiac transplant recipients: Physiologic Investigation for Transplant Arteriopathy (PITA Study). *Circulation.* 2003;108:1605.

4. Fitzgerald PJ, Oshima A, Hayase M, et al. Final results of the Can Routine Ultrasound Influence Stent Expansion (CRUISE) study. *Circulation.* 2000;102:523.

5. Pijls NH, Klauss V, Siebert U, et al. Coronary pressure measurement after stenting predicts adverse events at follow-up: A multicenter registry. *Circulation.* 2002;105:2950.

6. Pijls NH, Bech GJ, el Gamal MI, et al. Quantification of recruitable coronary collateral blood flow in conscious humans and its potential to predict future ischemic events. *J Am Coll Cardiol.* 1995;25:1522.

7. Yock PG, Linker DT, Angelsen BA. Two-dimensional intravascular ultrasound: Technical development and initial clinical experience. *J Am Soc Echocardiogr.* 1989;2:296.

8. Yock PG, Linker DT. Intravascular ultrasound. Looking below the surface of vascular disease. *Circulation.* 1990;81:1715.

9. Yock PG, Fitzgerald P, White N, et al. Intravascular ultrasound as a guiding modality for mechanical atherectomy and laser ablation. *Echocardiography.* 1990;7:425.

10. Hausmann D, Erbel R, Alibelli-Chemarin MJ, et al. The safety of intracoronary ultrasound. A multicenter survey of 2207 examinations. *Circulation.* 1995;91:623.

11. Batkoff BW, Linker DT. Safety of intracoronary ultrasound: Data from a Multicenter European Registry. *Cathet Cardiovasc Diagn.* 1996;38:238.

12. Abizaid A, Mintz GS, Pichard AD, et al. Clinical, intravascular ultrasound, and quantitative angiographic determinants of the coronary flow reserve before and after percutaneous transluminal coronary angioplasty. *Am J Cardiol.* 1998;82:423.

13. Takagi A, Tsurumi Y, Ishii Y, et al. Clinical potential of intravascular ultrasound for physiological assessment of coronary stenosis: Relationship between quantitative ultrasound tomography and pressure-derived fractional flow reserve. *Circulation.* 1999;100:250.

14. Nishioka T, Amanullah AM, Luo H, et al. Clinical validation of intravascular ultrasound imaging for assessment of coronary stenosis severity: Comparison with stress myocardial perfusion imaging. *J Am Coll Cardiol.* 1999;33:1870.

15. De Franco AC, Safian RD, Ziada KM, et al. Intravascular ultrasound. In: Safian RD, Feed MS, eds. *The Manual of Interventional Cardiology,* 3rd ed. Royal Oak, MI: Physicians' Press; 2001:693.

16. Mintz GS, Potkin BN, Keren G, et al. Intravascular ultrasound evaluation of the effect of rotational atherectomy in obstructive atherosclerotic coronary artery disease. *Circulation.* 1992;86:1383.

17. Kovach JA, Mintz GS, Pichard AD, et al. Sequential intravascular ultrasound characterization of the mechanisms of rotational atherectomy and adjunct balloon angioplasty. *J Am Coll Cardiol.* 1993;22:1024.

18. Dangas G, Mintz GS, Mehran R, et al. Stent implantation neutralizes the impact of preintervention arterial remodeling on subsequent target lesion revascularization. *Am J Cardiol.* 2000;86:452.

19. Okura H, Morino Y, Oshima A, et al. Preintervention arterial remodeling affects clinical outcome following stenting: An intravascular ultrasound study. *J Am Coll Cardiol.* 2001;37:1031.

20. Holmes DR Jr, Leon MB, Moses JW, et al. Analysis of 1-year clinical outcomes in the SIRIUS trial: A randomized trial of a sirolimus-eluting stent versus a standard stent in patients at high risk for coronary restenosis. *Circulation.* 2004;109:634.

21. Investigators TGT. IVUS-determined predictors of restenosis in PTCA and DCA: An interim report from the GUIDE Trial, Phase II. *Circulation.* 1994;90:I-23.

22. Mintz GS, Popma JJ, Pichard AD, et al. Intravascular ultrasound predictors of restenosis after percutaneous transcatheter coronary revascularization. *J Am Coll Cardiol.* 1996;27:1678.

23. Stone GW, Hodgson JM, St Goar FG, et al. Improved procedural results of coronary angioplasty with intravascular ultrasound-guided balloon sizing: The CLOUT Pilot Trial. Clinical Outcomes With Ultrasound Trial (CLOUT) Investigators. *Circulation.* 1997;95:2044.

24. Haase KK, Athanasiadis A, Mahrholdt H, et al. Acute and one year follow-up results after vessel size adapted PTCA using intracoronary ultrasound. *Eur Heart J.* 1998;19:263.

25. Schroeder S, Baumbach A, Haase KK, et al. Reduction of restenosis by vessel size adapted percutaneous transluminal coronary angioplasty using intravascular ultrasound. *Am J Cardiol.* 1999;83:875.

26. Fitzgerald PJ, Yock PG. Mechanisms and outcomes of angioplasty and atherectomy assessed by intravascular ultrasound imaging. *J Clin Ultrasound.* 1993;21:579.

27. Okura H, Shimodozono S, Hayase M, et al. Impact of deep vessel wall injury and vessel stretching on subsequent arterial remodeling after balloon angioplasty: A serial intravascular ultrasound study. *Am Heart J.* 2002;144:323.

28. Nakamura M, Yock PG, Kataoka T, et al. Impact of deep vessel wall injury on acute response and remodeling of coronary artery segments after cutting balloon angioplasty. *Am J Cardiol.* 2003;91:6.

29. Narins CR, Holmes DR Jr, Topol EJ. A call for provisional stenting: The balloon is back! *Circulation.* 1998;97:1298.

30. Schiele F, Meneveau N, Gilard M, et al. Intravascular ultrasound-guided balloon angioplasty compared with stent: Immediate and 6-month results of the multicenter, randomized Balloon Equivalent to Stent Study (BEST). *Circulation.* 2003;107:545.

31. Abizaid A, Pichard AD, Mintz GS, et al. Acute and long-term results of an intravascular ultrasound-guided percutaneous transluminal coronary angioplasty/provisional stent implantation strategy. *Am J Cardiol.* 1999;84:1298.

32. Colombo A, Hall P, Nakamura S, et al. Intracoronary stenting without anticoagulation accomplished with intravascular ultrasound guidance. *Circulation.* 1995;91:1676.

33. de Jaegere P, Mudra H, Figulla H, et al. Intravascular ultrasound-guided optimized stent deployment. Immediate and 6 months clinical and angiographic results from the Multicenter Ultrasound Stenting in Coronaries Study (MUSIC Study). *Eur Heart J.* 1998;19:1214.

34. Goldberg SL, Colombo A, Nakamura S, et al. Benefit of intracoronary ultrasound in the deployment of Palmaz-Schatz stents. *J Am Coll Cardiol.* 1994;24:996.

35. Nakamura S, Colombo A, Gaglione A, et al. Intracoronary ultrasound observations during stent implantation. *Circulation.* 1994;89:2026.

36. Honda Y, Grube E, de La Fuente LM, et al. Novel drug-delivery stent: Intravascular ultrasound observations from the first human experience with the QP2-eluting polymer stent system. *Circulation.* 2001;104:380.

37. Shah VM, Mintz GS, Apple S, Weissman NJ. Background incidence of late malapposition after bare-metal stent implantation. *Circulation*. 2002;106:1753.

38. Nakamura M, Kataoka T, Honda Y, et al. Late incomplete stent apposition and focal vessel expansion after bare metal stenting. *Am J Cardiol*. 2003;92:1217.

39. Kozuma K, Costa MA, Sabate M, et al. Late stent malapposition occurring after intracoronary beta-irradiation detected by intravascular ultrasound. *J Invasive Cardiol*. 1999;11:651.

40. Lemos PA, Saia F, Ligthart JM, et al. Coronary restenosis after sirolimus-eluting stent implantation: Morphological description and mechanistic analysis from a consecutive series of cases. *Circulation*. 2003;108:257.

41. Uren NG, Schwarzacher SP, Metz JA, et al. Predictors and outcomes of stent thrombosis: An intravascular ultrasound registry. *Eur Heart J*. 2002;23:124.

42. Cheneau E, Leborgne L, Mintz GS, et al. Predictors of subacute stent thrombosis: Results of a systematic intravascular ultrasound study. *Circulation*. 2003;108:43.

43. Hoffmann R, Mintz GS, Mehran R, et al. Intravascular ultrasound predictors of angiographic restenosis in lesions treated with Palmaz-Schatz stents. *J Am Coll Cardiol*. 1998;31:43.

44. Kasaoka S, Tobis JM, Akiyama T, et al. Angiographic and intravascular ultrasound predictors of in-stent restenosis. *J Am Coll Cardiol*. 1998;32:1630.

45. Morino Y, Honda Y, Okura H, et al. An optimal diagnostic threshold for minimal stent area to predict target lesion revascularization following stent implantation in native coronary lesions. *Am J Cardiol*. 2001;88:301.

46. Schiele F, Meneveau N, Vuillemenot A, et al. Impact of intravascular ultrasound guidance in stent deployment on 6-month restenosis rate: A multicenter, randomized study comparing two strategies-with and without intravascular ultrasound guidance. RESIST Study Group. REStenosis after Ivus guided STenting. *J Am Coll Cardiol*. 1998;32:320.

47. Mudra H, di Mario C, de Jaegere P, et al. Randomized comparison of coronary stent implantation under ultrasound or angiographic guidance to reduce stent restenosis (OPTICUS Study). *Circulation*. 2001;104:1343.

48. Russo RJ, Attubato MJ, Davidson CJ, et al. Angiography versus intravascular ultrasound-directed stent placement: final results from AVID. *Circulation*. 1999;100(suppl I):I-234.

49. Kasaoka S, Tobis JM, Akiyama T, et al. Angiographic and intravascular ultrasound predictors of in-stent restenosis. *J Am Coll Cardiol*. 1998;32:1630.

50. Ziada KM, Tuzcu EM, De Franco AC, et al. Intravascular ultrasound assessment of the prevalence and causes of angiographic "haziness" following high-pressure coronary stenting. *Am J Cardiol*. 1997;80:116.

51. Schuhlen H, Hadamitzky M, Walter H, et al. Major benefit from antiplatelet therapy for patients at high risk for adverse cardiac events after coronary Palmaz-Schatz stent placement: Analysis of a prospective risk stratification protocol in the Intracoronary Stenting and Antithrombotic Regimen (ISAR) trial. *Circulation*. 1997;95:2015.

52. Morice MC, Serruys PW, Sousa JE, et al. A randomized comparison of a sirolimus-eluting stent with a standard stent for coronary revascularization. *N Engl J Med*. 2002;346:1773.

53. Colombo A, Drzewiecki J, Banning A, et al. Randomized study to assess the effectiveness of slow- and moderate-release polymer-based paclitaxel-eluting stents for coronary artery lesions. *Circulation*. 2003;108:788.

54. Schofer J, Schluter M, Gershlick AH, et al. Sirolimus-eluting stents for treatment of patients with long atherosclerotic lesions in small coronary arteries: Double-blind, randomised controlled trial (E-SIRIUS). *Lancet*. 2003;362:1093.

55. Serruys PW, Degertekin M, Tanabe K, et al. Intravascular ultrasound findings in the multicenter, randomized, double-blind RAVEL (RAndomized study with the sirolimus-eluting VElocity balloon-expandable stent in the treatment of patients with de novo native coronary artery Lesions) trial. *Circulation*. 2002;106:798.

56. Tanabe K, Serruys PW, Degertekin M, et al. Chronic arterial responses to polymer-controlled paclitaxel-eluting stents. Comparison with bare metal stents by serial intravascular ultrasound analyses: Data From the randomized TAXUS-II trial. *Circulation*. 2004;109:196.

57. Degertekin M, Lemos PA, Lee CH, et al. Intravascular ultrasound evaluation after sirolimus eluting stent implantation for de novo and in-stent restenosis lesions. *Eur Heart J*. 2004;25:32.

58. Moses JW, Leon MB, Popma JJ, et al. Sirolimus-eluting stents versus standard stents in patients with stenosis in a native coronary artery. *N Engl J Med*. 2003;349:1315.

59. Sonoda S, Morino Y, Ako J, et al. Impact of final stent dimensions on long-term results following sirolimus-eluting stent implantation: Serial intravascular ultrasound analysis from the SIRIUS trial. *J Am Coll Cardiol*. 2004;43:1959.

60. Degertekin M, Serruys PW, Tanabe K, et al. Long-term follow-up of incomplete stent apposition in patients who received sirolimus-eluting stent for de novo coronary lesions: An intravascular ultrasound analysis. *Circulation*. 2003;108:2747.

61. Doucette JW, Corl PD, Payne HM, et al. Validation of a Doppler guide wire for intravascular measurement of coronary artery flow velocity. *Circulation*. 1992;85:1899.

62. Gould KL, Lipscomb K, Hamilton GW. Physiologic basis for assessing critical coronary stenosis. Instantaneous flow response and regional distribution during coronary hyperemia as measures of coronary flow reserve. *Am J Cardiol*. 1974;33:87.

63. Kern MJ. Coronary physiology revisited: Practical insights from the cardiac catheterization laboratory. *Circulation*. 2000;101:1344.

64. Gould KL, Kirkeeide RL, Buchi M. Coronary flow reserve as a physiologic measure of stenosis severity. *J Am Coll Cardiol*. 1990;15:459.

65. Baumgart D, Haude M, Goerge G, et al. Improved assessment of coronary stenosis severity using the relative flow velocity reserve. *Circulation*. 1998;98:40.

66. Voudris V, Avramides D, Koutelou M, et al. Relative coronary flow velocity reserve improves correlation with stress myocardial perfusion imaging in assessment of coronary artery stenoses. *Chest*. 2003;124:1266.

67. Kern MJ, de Bruyne B, Pijls NH. From research to clinical practice: Current role of intracoronary physiologically based decision making in the cardiac catheterization laboratory. *J Am Coll Cardiol*. 1997;30:613.

68. Serruys PW, di Mario C, Piek J, et al. Prognostic value of intracoronary flow velocity and diameter stenosis in assessing the short- and long-term outcomes of coronary balloon angioplasty: The DEBATE Study (Doppler Endpoints Balloon Angioplasty Trial Europe). *Circulation*. 1997;96:3369.

69. Serruys PW, de Bruyne B, Carlier S, et al. Randomized comparison of primary stenting and provisional balloon angioplasty guided by flow velocity measurement. Doppler Endpoints Balloon Angioplasty Trial Europe (DEBATE) II Study Group. *Circulation*. 2000;102:2930.

70. Albertal M, Voskuil M, Piek JJ, et al. Coronary flow velocity reserve after percutaneous interventions is predictive of periprocedural outcome. *Circulation*. 2002;105:1573.

71. Yamamoto K, Ito H, Iwakura K, et al. Two different coronary blood flow velocity patterns in thrombolysis in myocardial infarction flow grade 2 in acute myocardial infarction: Insight into mechanisms of microvascular dysfunction. *J Am Coll Cardiol*. 2002;40:1755.

72. Yamamuro A, Akasaka T, Tamita K, et al. Coronary flow velocity pattern immediately after percutaneous coronary intervention as a predictor of complications and in-hospital survival after acute myocardial infarction. *Circulation*. 2002;106:3051.

73. Seiler C, Fleisch M, Garachemani A, Meier B. Coronary collateral quantitation in patients with coronary artery disease using intravascular flow velocity or pressure measurements. *J Am Coll Cardiol*. 1998;32:1272.

74. Peterson RJ, King SB 3rd, Fajman WA, et al. Relation of coronary artery stenosis and pressure gradient to exercise-induced ischemia before and after coronary angioplasty. *J Am Coll Cardiol*. 1987;10:253.

75. Pijls NH, van Son JA, Kirkeeide RL, et al. Experimental basis of determining maximum coronary, myocardial, and collateral blood flow by pressure measurements for assessing functional stenosis severity before and after percutaneous transluminal coronary angioplasty. *Circulation*. 1993;87:1354.

76. De Bruyne B, Bartunek J, Sys SU, Heyndrickx GR. Relation between myocardial fractional flow reserve calculated from coronary pressure measurements and exercise-induced myocardial ischemia. *Circulation*. 1995;92:39.

77. De Bruyne B, Hersbach F, Pijls NH, et al. Abnormal epicardial coronary resistance in patients with diffuse atherosclerosis but "Normal" coronary angiography. *Circulation*. 2001;104:2401.

78. de Bruyne B, Bartunek J, Sys SU, et al. Simultaneous coronary pressure and flow velocity measurements in humans. Feasibility, reproducibility, and hemodynamic dependence of coronary flow velocity reserve, hyperemic flow versus pressure slope index, and fractional flow reserve. *Circulation*. 1996;94:1842.

79. Chamuleau SA, Meuwissen M, van Eck-Smit BL, et al. Fractional flow reserve, absolute and relative coronary blood flow velocity reserve in relation to the results of technetium-99m sestamibi single-photon emission computed tomography in patients with two-vessel coronary artery disease. *J Am Coll Cardiol*. 2001;37:1316.

80. Fearon WF, Takagi A, Jeremias A, et al. Use of fractional myocardial flow reserve to assess the functional significance of intermediate coronary stenoses. *Am J Cardiol*. 2000;86:1013, A10.

81. Fearon WF, Yeung AC. Evaluating intermediate coronary lesions in the cardiac catheterization laboratory. *Rev Cardiovasc Med*. 2003;4:1.

82. Bartunek J, Marwick TH, Rodrigues ACT, et al. Dobutamine-induced wall motion abnormalities: Correlation with fractional flow reserve and quantitative coronary angiography. *J Am Coll Cardiol.* 1996;27:1429.

83. Bech GJ, De Bruyne B, Pijls NH, et al. Fractional flow reserve to determine the appropriateness of angioplasty in moderate coronary stenosis: a randomized trial. *Circulation.* 2001;103:2928.

84. Lima RS, Watson DD, Goode AR, et al. Incremental value of combined perfusion and function over perfusion alone by gated SPECT myocardial perfusion imaging for detection of severe three-vessel coronary artery disease. *J Am Coll Cardiol.* 2003;42:64.

85. Chamuleau SA, Meuwissen M, Koch KT, et al. Usefulness of fractional flow reserve for risk stratification of patients with multivessel coronary artery disease and an intermediate stenosis. *Am J Cardiol.* 2002;89:377.

86. Aarnoudse WH, Botman KJ, Pijls NH. False-negative myocardial scintigraphy in balanced three-vessel disease, revealed by coronary pressure measurement. *Int J Cardiovasc Intervent.* 2003;5:67.

87. Fearon WF, Yeung AC, Lee DP, et al. Cost-effectiveness of measuring fractional flow reserve to guide coronary interventions. *Am Heart J.* 2003;145:882.

88. Leesar MA, Abdul-Baki T, Akkus NI, et al. Use of fractional flow reserve versus stress perfusion scintigraphy after unstable angina. Effect on duration of hospitalization, cost, procedural characteristics, and clinical outcome. *J Am Coll Cardiol.* 2003;41:1115.

89. Bech GJ, Pijls NH, De Bruyne B, et al. Usefulness of fractional flow reserve to predict clinical outcome after balloon angioplasty. *Circulation.* 1999;99:883.

90. Hanekamp CE, Koolen JJ, Pijls NH, et al. Comparison of quantitative coronary angiography, intravascular ultrasound, and coronary pressure measurement to assess optimum stent deployment. *Circulation.* 1999;99:1015.

91. Fearon WF, Luna J, Samady H, et al. Fractional flow reserve compared with intravascular ultrasound guidance for optimizing stent deployment. *Circulation.* 2001;104:1917.

92. Katritsis DG, Ioannidis JP, Korovesis S, et al. Comparison of myocardial fractional flow reserve and intravascular ultrasound for the assessment of slotted-tube stents. *Catheter Cardiovasc Interv.* 2001;52:322.

93. De Bruyne B, Pijls NH, Bartunek J, et al. Fractional flow reserve in patients with prior myocardial infarction. *Circulation.* 2001;104:157.

94. Pijls NH, Kern MJ, Yock PG, De Bruyne B. Practice and potential pitfalls of coronary pressure measurement. *Catheter Cardiovasc Interv.* 2000;49:1.

95. Jeremias A, Whitbourn RJ, Filardo SD, et al. Adequacy of intracoronary versus intravenous adenosine-induced maximal coronary hyperemia for fractional flow reserve measurements. *Am Heart J.* 2000;140:651.

96. De Bruyne B, Pijls NH, Barbato E, et al. Intracoronary and intravenous adenosine 5'-triphosphate, adenosine, papaverine, and contrast medium to assess fractional flow reserve in humans. *Circulation.* 2003;107:1877.

97. Talman CL, Winniford MD, Rossen JD, et al. Polymorphous ventricular tachycardia: A side effect of intracoronary papaverine. *J Am Coll Cardiol.* 1990;15:275.

98. Pijls NH, Bech GJ, el Gamal MI, et al. Quantification of recruitable coronary collateral blood flow in conscious humans and its potential to predict future ischemic events. *J Am Coll Cardiol.* 1995;25:1522.

99. Sheehan FH, Braunwald E, Canner P, et al. The effect of intravenous thrombolytic therapy on left ventricular function: A report on tissue-type plasminogen activator and streptokinase from the Thrombolysis in Myocardial Infarction (TIMI Phase I) trial. *Circulation.* 1987;75:817.

100. Lenderink T, Simoons ML, Van Es GA, et al. Benefit of thrombolytic therapy is sustained throughout five years and is related to TIMI perfusion grade 3 but not grade 2 flow at discharge. The European Cooperative Study Group. *Circulation.* 1995;92:1110.

101. Gersh BJ. Current issues in reperfusion therapy. *Am J Cardiol.* 1998;82:3P.

102. Gibson CM, Cannon CP, Daley WL, et al. TIMI frame count: A quantitative method of assessing coronary artery flow. *Circulation.* 1996;93:879.

103. Gibson CM, Murphy SA, Rizzo MJ, et al. Relationship between TIMI frame count and clinical outcomes after thrombolytic administration. Thrombolysis In Myocardial Infarction (TIMI) Study Group. *Circulation.* 1999;99:1945.

104. Roe MT, Ohman EM, Maas AC, et al. Shifting the open-artery hypothesis downstream: The quest for optimal reperfusion. *J Am Coll Cardiol.* 2001;37:9.

105. Gibson CM, Cannon CP, Murphy SA, et al. Relationship of TIMI myocardial perfusion grade to mortality after administration of thrombolytic drugs. *Circulation.* 2000;101:125.

CHAPTER (28)

Coronary Guidewire Manipulation

J. Dawn Abbott, MD, and David O. Williams, MD

In percutaneous coronary intervention (PCI), appropriate selection and manipulation of equipment is critical to successful outcomes and low complication rates. The guidewire is the first piece of interventional equipment to contact the lesion to be treated. Proper intraluminal advancement of the guidewire through the lesion and into the distal vessel allows the coronary guidewire to serve as the backbone for the safe delivery of diagnostic and therapeutic devices while maintaining secure access to the vessel lumen. Although the current standard 0.014-in wires are suitable for the majority of interventions, operator familiarity and facility with guidewire placement are still paramount. The advent of specialty guidewires, such as those designed for chronic total occlusions, have furthered our ability to treat successfully more complex lesions but require an understanding of the possible complications that can result from their use. Given the wide variety of guidewires that are available for use, knowledge of their design, materials and structure aids the operator in understanding unique differences in performance and ultimately in proper selection for an individual patient or lesion.

In this chapter, we review specific characteristics of coronary guidewires, including their construction and clinical features. To optimize guidewire selection we have developed a general classification scheme based on wire performance features. We discuss techniques for guidewire manipulation in selected subsets of coronary lesions with the caveat that minimal comparative literature is available. As with other aspects of interventional cardiology, there are multiple guidewires that can be used for each lesion and operator selection may change with experience or as technologic advances are made.

HISTORY OF THE GUIDEWIRE

More than 25 five years has passed since the introduction of a catheter system allowing an independently movable, flexible-tipped guidewire for coronary intervention. Unlike the initial balloon catheters with fixed-wire systems, the two component balloon and independent, steerable guidewire systems greatly enhanced coronary artery and lesion accessibility.[1-3] The guidewires were designed to allow the tip to be shaped or curved so that the wire could be purposefully directed into the desired artery and across the target lesion using rotation and advancement. The independent catheter-guidewire system also brought increased safety with the ability to exchange devices without recrossing the coronary lesion.[4,5]

The first available guidewire, 1979 to 1982, for the removable guidewire system was a 0.018-in standard wire (Cook Group Inc). This wire had a safety wire, a precursor to the shaping ribbon, in the tip that allowed it to be shaped but resulted in a stiff tip. The next wire to be developed (ACS) was a standard wire that replaced the safety wire with a metal ribbon, which made the tip more flexible while retaining the ability for shaping. Further advances allowed construction of a floppy wire, which lacked a shaping ribbon and had greater flexibility and safety but sacrificed some directional control. Thus the objective was to develop wires that combined flexible and safe tips while maintaining shapability and torsional control.[6] Currently, because no guidewire meets all needs or preferences, several manufacturers offer a "line" of coronary guidewires, many with subtle variations, to allow artery- or lesion-specific guidewire selection.

GUIDEWIRE DESIGN AND CONSTRUCTION

Knowledge of the underlying construction of the guidewire provides an understanding of the expected performance features, including steerability and trackability. *Steerability* relates to the ability to direct the wire to a desired location within an artery or lesion, and *trackability* is the ability of a wire to follow the course of an artery during advancement with minimal resistance or buckling. Multiple characteristics, including flexibility, radiopacity, torquability and kink resistance, and the frictional resistance of the guidewire within the system it is used, all contribute to the fundamental properties that result in maneuverability of guidewires (Figure 28-1). *Torquability* is a term that describes the relationship between rotational movement of the proximal wire (the site where the operator grasps the wire) and the tip rotation. Torquability that is 1:1 means that for every degree of rotation by the operator, a similar rotation will occur at the tip.

Coronary guidewires are composed of three main components: a central core that tapers distally, a flexible tip, and a lubricious coating (Figure 28-2). These components all influence the ability of a wire to reach and cross a lesion and also to support the delivery of balloon catheters or other devices to the lesion. For example, the core provides the support for device advancement but is also integrally related to trackability, steerability, and torque transmission.

Core

The core may be constructed as a single continuous unit or have more than one segment. As the core extends distally, the diameter tapers, and the degree of tapering and the location of tapering vary. These variations in core diameter, length, and degree of tapering affect performance. Cores that extend to the distal wire tip provide

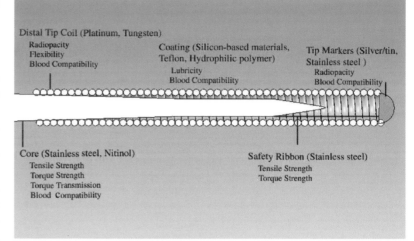

FIGURE 28-2. Coronary guidewires are composed of three main components: a central core, a flexible tip, and a lubricious coating (see text for details).

extra support and torque transmission but are stiff. Cores that do not extend to the distal tip and that gradually taper are more flexible and retain more trackability than wire cores that abruptly end.[7] For this reason, wires that have a single core construction have the smoothest transition into the flexible preshaped tip and provide a high degree of steerability and trackability. The core strength also varies with the core material and diameter, and as stiffness increases, flexibility may be compromised but vessel straightening and device delivery improve. The core wire is commonly composed of stainless steel or alternative alloys such as nitinol. The nitinol core increases wire trackability, including the ability to traverse acute artery angulations without wire prolapse. Nitinol wires, therefore, might be more capable of entering a retroflexed circumflex takeoff than a stainless steel core wire. The limitation of a nitinol core wire is that it tends to store, rather than transmit, torque. Wires, therefore, with single nitinol cores may result in the wire "winding up."

Tip

The tip of the wire may be composed of a coil or spring that provides a flexible leading tip that enhances safety and steerability. The ability to shape the tip into a retainable and variably shaped curve is accomplished by a shaping ribbon. This is a thin metallic strip that runs parallel to the longitudinal axis of the wire and allows the tip to retain a curved shape or **J** configuration that provides directionality to the guidewire. The degree to which the tip retains its shape during use relates to the properties of the shaping ribbon, such as material selection and thickness, the material of the distal tapered core, and, additionally, to the coatings, which are discussed below. Wires with straight tips and shaping ribbons can be shaped to more acute angles, or sequential bends can be placed to negotiate unusual or severe (>90 degree) instances of vessel tortuosity. Wires that have preshaped tips are also available. Some preshaped wires retain the shaping ribbon; in others it is lacking, which results in less ability to alter the tip shape.

The wire tip also varies in stiffness. Highly flexible tips are termed *floppy* or *soft,* and these wires are particularly safe and atraumatic in that the likelihood of subintimal dissection or vessel perforation is very low. Commonly such wires include a core of

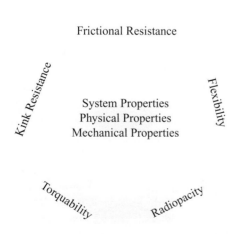

FIGURE 28-1. Guidewire performance. Multiple characteristics contribute to the fundamental properties that result in the steerability and maneuverability of a guidewire.

moderate flexibility and support and are accordingly used as "workhorse wires." Because of enhanced tip flexibility, they can prolapse or form a large J configuration when advanced. Such a configuration is an advantage if it occurs after the wire crosses the lesion to be treated in that the wire can readily and safely be advanced into the distal artery without the need for steering. This configuration is also preferred for crossing stents within the vessel, because the tip cannot slide between a stent strut and the vessel.

Other potential features of the wire tip that may be manipulated include the distal diameter and tip load. Guidewire tips can have a tapered coil from the shaft of 0.014-in down to 0.009-in. Some lines of wires also are designed with incremental tip loads, or grams of force at the wire tip. The tip load, in this case, is the amount of force required to deflect the tip into a predetermined configuration based on the manufacturer's measurement methods. These wires with reduced profile or increased tip load, discussed below, are designed to improve crossing subtotally or totally occluded arteries. Caution must be exercised with these wires to avoid coronary dissection or perforation.

The distal coil tip is constructed of a platinum or tungsten alloy, or an alternative radiopaque material. Radiopacity is critical for monitoring fine wire manipulation and advancement. The standard wire has a radiopaque tip of 2 to 3 cm in length, and although the entire wire is visible with fluoroscopy, the entire length of the wire may be difficult to follow. Problems with the wire, such as kinks or the development of loops, particularly outside the guiding catheter and within the aorta, may be difficult to detect. These situations, however, are usually recognized by accompanying clues such as loss of 1:1 torque, pushability, guide stability, or the ability to deliver devices. The benefit of a short radiopaque tip is that it can be advanced past the target lesion so as not to influence the identification of devices or evaluation of the targeted lesion. The radiopaque segment may also interfere with the ability to perform quantitative coronary angiography. Certain wires have longer radiopaque tips of 11 to 40 cm. This "high-radiopacity" feature is found on more aggressive wires in which more force may be applied to wire advancement and intense monitoring of the entire length of the wire in the coronary and guiding sheath is needed for safety. Outside the safety issue, the longer radiopaque tip does not offer additional benefits.

Coating

The third component of the coronary wire is the lubricious coating, which can be silicone, Teflon, polytetrafluoroethylene (PTFE), or a hydrophilic polymer. The coating decreases the friction within the device lumen and across lesions and improves wire and device tracking in tortuous vessels. The hydrophilic wires are well suited for severe stenoses and total occlusions, but they may create vessel dissections or perforations if not manipulated cautiously. As with other aspects of wire construction, each feature may improve one or more clinical aspects of the wire but at the expense of another.

GENERAL GUIDEWIRE FEATURES

The majority of current coronary wires are 0.014-in diameter for compatibility with low-profile coronary balloon and stent systems. Specialty wires, discussed later, may be designed with larger diameters and therefore require special delivery microcatheters. Wires come in two general lengths. Standard-length guidewires are 175 to 190 cm, and exchange-length wires are 270 to 400 cm. The choice of wire length depends largely on the balloon catheter system chosen by the operator: single operator or rapid exchange (RX) versus over the wire (OTW). Details of these techniques are discussed in the next section. Importantly, most but not all standard-length guidewires can be extended with compatible extension wires if conversion to an OTW technique is required. Additional features on some wires include marker bands on the proximal body of the wire that can reduce fluoroscopy time. These bands allow passage of the wire through the guide or balloon to the appropriate distance without fluoroscopy, ensuring that the wire has not exited from the guide catheter. Wires can also be designed with radiopaque markers at the distal tip that are a known distance apart, allowing for more precise estimation of lesion length. These wires are termed *marker wires*.

GUIDEWIRE TECHNIQUES FOR SPECIFIC CATHETER SYSTEMS

【 】 OVER-THE-WIRE SYSTEMS

In an OTW system the wire traverses the entire length of the balloon catheter lumen, which is generally 135 to 150 cm. Standard coronary balloon and stent catheters are designed for 0.014-in wires. Often the tolerances of the balloon catheter lumens and the guidewires overlap such that there is little clearance between lumen and wire. There are two approaches to using an OTW system. In the more common approach the operator first places the guidewire through the balloon lumen and then the guidewire-loaded device is advanced into the guiding catheter to the coronary ostium. The guidewire is manipulated through the vessel across the target lesion and with the wire fixed in place the balloon can be advanced across the lesion for dilation. The advantage of this technique is that the balloon catheter can be advanced over the wire into the coronary artery for more precise guidewire manipulation. Additionally, if the operator requires a different guidewire, the balloon catheter can be left in place to maintain access. For example, OTW balloon catheters are of special value when attempting recanalization of total occlusions. The greatest challenge for successfully treating total occlusions is to cross the lesion with a guidewire, and accordingly, an assortment of different guidewires is often necessary in these cases. The OTW catheter can be positioned directly proximal to the total occlusion and facilitate guidewire exchanges.

Either a standard-length wire (175 to 190 cm) or an exchange-length wire (300 cm) can be used to cross the lesion with the OTW system. If a standard wire successfully crosses the target lesion, the wire can usually be extended with an extension wire to remove the balloon catheter or the balloon can be advanced distal to the lesion and the wire can be exchanged through the balloon for an exchange-length wire prior to balloon withdrawal.

In an alternative technique, the operator advances a guidewire alone into the guiding catheter and across the target lesion. In this so-called bare-wire technique, the balloon or stent is then advanced over the wire into the lesion. This approach allows better visualization in smaller diameter guiding catheters, but given the low profile of current OTW balloons the advantage of this approach is minimized. Although passage and removal of OTW balloon catheters over standard-length wires has been reported, it is preferable to use an RX catheter in these situations.[8,9]

【 】 RAPID EXCHANGE SYSTEMS

The RX system is commonly referred to as a single-operator exchange system. The coronary balloon and stent catheters are labeled *RX* (for rapid exchange) or *monorail* and are compatible with 0.014-in wires. The catheters were modified from the OTW type and the distal portion is similar, with the guidewire traversing through the balloon lumen. The "OTW" segment, however, is short and the remainder of the wire tracks outside the catheter adjacent to the body of the dilation catheter. The RX system is ideal for the single operator and can reduce fluoroscopy time. A standard-length guidewire can be used for all RX intracoronary catheters. Initially, the bare-wire technique is used to cross the lesion; then, the balloon catheter is loaded on the distal end of the guidewire. The catheter is advanced until the wire exits the catheter lumen, and the wire is then fixed in place as the remainder of the catheter is advanced across the lesion. Although the RX catheters have less pushability and trackability and cannot act as a device for exchanging wires, the current balloon catheters are low profile, easy to deliver, and can be used in most cases.

When using an RX system the operator must be prepared change to an OTW system when necessary. In certain situations (eg, inability to cross a lesion with a wire or balloon or an unanticipated nondilatable lesion), the wire may need to be exchanged for a specialty wire such as an extra support wire or rotational atherectomy wire. If balloon inflations have been performed, and in particular if a dissection in the vessel is present, maintenance of distal wire position is essential. Normally these situations pose no problem as the majority or standard-length wires can be extended to exchange length with extension wires, and a microcatheter or OTW balloon catheter can be used to secure position during the wire exchange.

If a 0.014-in wire has no compatible extension wire, alternative mechanisms for balloon removal and wire exchange are possible. If the lesion was crossed with a standard-length wire delivered through an OTW balloon, then the best method for wire exchange is to advance the balloon across the lesion and place an exchange-length or extension compatible wire for removal of the balloon. If the balloon will not advance and the wire is already across the lesion, exchange will be difficult without losing wire position. The hydroglide method can be attempted in this case.[9] This method uses hydrostatic pressure applied to the central lumen of the balloon catheter with a saline-filled syringe or inflation device. Loss of wire position is the main drawback of this approach. Because this situation can lead to loss of vessel access, it should be avoided, which requires knowledge of the extendibility of standard-length wires.

【 】 MULTI-EXCHANGE PLATFORM

Another approach to conversion of a standard wire to an exchange-length wire is to use a Zipper Multi-Exchange (MX) platform (Metronic Inc). The catheter is designed with a **Z** component that temporarily separates a portion of the guidewire; then, as the catheter is advanced, the separation closes and the wire is fed into the catheter lumen. The MX platform may have more trackability than RX systems and allows catheters of different lengths to be exchanged during the procedure without using an exchange-length guidewire.

GUIDEWIRE SELECTION

There may be many appropriate guidewire choices for each coronary intervention. Categorizing the guidewires into groups according to their general performance features and becoming familiar with a few wires from each group is a sound initial approach. Subsequently, each operator may find subtle differences among the guidewires in each group and develop a personal preference for a specific guidewire. Most operators will choose an "all-purpose" guidewire for the majority of cases and then have preferred wires for circumstances in which "extra support" is needed or for specific lesion subsets, such as distal tortuous lesions. A guidewire classification grouping according to the general performance features is provided in Table 28-1.

【 】 SPECIALTY WIRES FOR TOTAL OCCLUSIONS

Many wires have been developed to cross severely narrowed or totally occluded coronary stenosis. Most can be classified into a generic category (eg, hydrophilic coating/nitinol core) but others are more unique. This section reviews examples of these types of wires.

Glidewire Gold

The Glidewire Gold (SCIMED/Boston Scientific Corporation) wires are hydrophilic coated and are well suited for chronic total occlusions because of their larger core diameters of 0.016-in and 0.018-in. They are constructed with a superelastic alloy core and a radiopaque gold tip that provides optimum visibility. The tip is preformed and available with angles of 45 and 70 degrees for vessels of varying tortuosity. They are 180-cm wires and are available in nonstandard diameters; accordingly, they will not fit within standard balloon or stent catheters. The length and size features require that the wire be placed through a special delivery catheter such as a Tracker or Transit catheter that can subsequently be exchanged for a standard 0.014-in wire once the lesion is crossed. The benefit of the larger diameter is that it has increased steerability and support. In addition, with the superelastic core, these wires would tend to store torque were they not provided in a larger core wire diameter. These wires may be successful in crossing a total occlusion when all other wires have failed. Once advanced into a lesion, the wire has the ability to finds its own way forward. On the other hand, precise tip control is difficult, and subintimal wire entry or distal perforation may occur.

Several other hydrophilic wires that may or may not have a nitinol core can be included in this category. Typically these wires are 0.014 in and are not as stiff as the Glidewire Gold but have similar

TABLE 28-1

Guidewire Classification

GENERAL PERFORMANCE FEATURES	DESIRED USE	EXAMPLES

All purpose
  Soft floppy tip
  Light to moderate support core wire
	Simple to complex lesions	CholCE Floppy (SCIMED)
		ATW (Cordis)
		Hi-Torque Balance Middle Weight (Guidant)
		Hi-Torque Floppy II (Guidant)
		Stabilizer BP (Cordis)

Extra-support High to extra-high support core wire	Vessel straightening	CholCE Extra Support (SCIMED) Stabilizer Plus or XS (Cordis) Hi-Torque Iron Man (Guidant)
Stiff tipped/tapered tip Added pushability	Severe stenoses Total occlusions	CholCE Intermediate (SCIMED) WIZDOM Soft (Cordis) Hi-Torque Cross-It XT Series (Guidant) SHINOBI (Cordis) Hi-Torque Floppy Intermediate (Guidant)
Hydrophilic-coated polymer cover	Total occlusions Severe tortuosity	Hi-Torque WISPER (Guidant) CholCE PT or PT Graphix (SCIMED)
Firm tip and core (without polymer cover)	Chronic total occlusions Uncrossable lesions	Asahi MiracleBros line (Biomedicon) CholCE Standard (SCIMED) SHINOBI Plus (Cordis)

lubricious coatings. Examples include the Whisper wire, Choice PT wire, and the Crosswire.

Magnum Wire

The Magnum wire is an unusual wire in that, in addition to a Teflon-coated solid-steel shaft with diameters of 0.014 to 0.021 in, it has a shapeable distal segment with a large olive-shaped tip (0.7–1.0 mm). The shaft provides steerability, and the stability facilitates passage of the balloon catheter. The flexible portion of the wire requires catheter backup support for optimal pushability. The olive tip is designed for blunt dissection and avoidance of creating subintimal flaps as it is pushed, supported by the delivery catheter over the occlusion. The original Magnum wire (0.021 in) requires at least a 7 French guiding catheter and a special balloon or delivery catheter, whereas the 0.014-in version can be used with standard equipment.

The technique for using the Magnum wire in chronic total occlusions is to direct the wire to the occlusion, supported by a balloon or delivery catheter, and use the olive tip to push across the lesion. The wire can be advanced independently or, as a single unit in conjunction with the balloon catheter, across the lesion providing there is adequate guide support. The wire has a J curve, so it can be withdrawn and steered into the lesion in different orientations. Some operators have inflated the balloon in the stump of the occlusion to enhance the backup when forcing the Magnum wire through the occlusion. Once free in the distal lumen, the balloon catheter can be advanced over the wire into the channel created by the olive tip. The magnum wire results in a 10% to 20% improvement in success rates over conventional wires for crossing chronic

total occlusions.[10,11] The wire has also been used safely for routine PCI of nonoccluded vessels.[12–14]

Asahi MiracleBros Line

The Asahi MiracleBros line of 0.014-in wires is also designed for highly stenosed or occluded vessels. The wires have a single continuous core construction with a jointless spring coil for tracking and silicone, fluororesin, and hydrophilic coatings to reduce friction and highly radiopaque 11-cm tip. The wires are manufactured according to a tip load, or the weight of force required to deflect the tip, with 3 g, 4.5 g, 6 g, and 12 g available (ie, MiracleBros 3 has a tip load of 3 g). The flexibility of the wire is reduced and support increased as the tip weight increases. The progression in tip load translates in to greater retention of tip shape, responsiveness, and ability to push the wire in a desired direction. The wire with the most support and penetration ability for chronic total occlusions is the Asahi Confianza. The wire has a 20-cm radiopaque segment, a tip load of 9 g, and is distally tapered to 0.009 in. Use of these wires is based on a strategy of crossing total occlusions that differs from the conventional approach, in which emphasis is placed on detecting the original lumen and slipping through that segment of the total occlusion. The Asahi concept features blunt but highly direct dissection. This technique is more complex and technically demanding but may achieve success when others fail.

Other stiff-tipped wires, such as the Cross-it line of wires, may be more steerable than the "glide" type wires and are well suited for total occlusions. These wires have a unique tapered 0.010-in tip and are available with three levels of tip stiffness (Cross-it 100, 200, and 300).

GUIDEWIRE MANIPULATION TECHNIQUES

【 】 UNIVERSAL TECHNIQUES

The "workhorse" wires are flexible-tipped 0.014-in wires. These are often the initial wires of choice as they offer adequate support, excellent steerability, and are atraumatic. Some vessels and lesions, however, are particularly challenging and require alternative wires and techniques. The operator should be familiar with alternative wires and have a logical stepwise approach planned to accomplish a complicated intervention. In addition to wire choice, appropriate selection of additional equipment, such as a guiding catheter with sufficient backup, is needed. Common lesion subsets are discussed here.

【 】 TORTUOUS VESSELS AND DISTAL LESIONS

Severely angulated or tortuous vessels and distal lesions may be technically difficult to access. Even proximal lesions may pose a challenge if the origin of the left anterior descending artery, or more commonly the left circumflex, arises from the left main coronary artery at an extreme angle. Although the tip of the flexible guidewire can be shaped to accommodate increased angulation, the guidewire will often prolapse into the alternative artery or branch rather than advance into the target branch. Stiffer-tipped wires may prolapse less in angulations of less than 90 degrees, but even these wires will have poor tip steerability. Distal lesions in tortuous arteries may represent the greatest challenge for access because as the wire traverses curved segments, steerability is lost.

For these reasons, additional support and ability for wire exchange is offered by an OTW approach. A low-profile OTW balloon can be advanced near the guidewire tip to decrease wire prolapse and to make wire removal and reshaping easier. The OTW system also increases the torque responsiveness and decreases frictional drag of the wire. On occasion, even low-profile OTW balloons cannot be advanced without compromising guide or wire position. Alternatively placing a second wire adjacent to the initial wire, the "buddy wire" technique, may augment access. A third option advocated by many operators is the use of a more flexible system in these cases. Microcatheters, such as perfusion or Tracker catheters, have been used successfully in these difficult cases.[15–17] Delivery of devices such as balloons and stents may also be difficult in tortuous arteries or distal lesions. Vessel straightening and increased support can be achieved by exchanging the initial wire for an extra-support wire. Dual wires, or a buddy wire, can also be used in tortuous vessels to keep the balloon tips free.

【 】 CHRONIC TOTAL OCCLUSIONS

Approximately 10% of percutaneous coronary interventions are for chronic total occlusions.[18] The success rate for these lesions is lower than for other lesion subsets and ranges from 40% to 80% in various studies.[19–24] As noted earlier, the most common reason for failure in a chronic total occlusion is inability to cross the lesion with a guidewire.[25] Careful evaluation of the preintervention angiogram should help determine the appropriate course of the occluded vessel segment. If an angiogram was obtained prior to vessel occlusion, it should be reviewed to gain information regarding the vessel course and characteristics. Careful advancement toward the distal reconstituted vessel can be aided by visualization of the vessel supplying collateral circulation, which may require simultaneous contralateral artery injection.[26,27] Recanalization of chronic total occlusions requires the availability of a broader range of coronary wires. An OTW technique is preferred because advancement of the balloon catheter proximal to the site of occlusion allows more "pushability" for a given wire stiffness and exchange to progressively more aggressive wires as needed. Figure 28-3 illustrates a chronic total occlusion of the left anterior descending artery that was treated using contralateral coronary injections and the Asahi Confianza wire (Biomedicon Systems).

Hydrophilic wires have been used successfully in lesions previously attempted with conventional wires. In several series, lesions previously uncrossable with conventional wires were crossed with clinical success in 39% to 79% of attempts.[28,29] Coronary perforations were higher than previously reported at approximately 2%. In a larger series of 106 patients with chronic total occlusions and previous failed PCI, a hydrophilic wire was employed; 42% of these attempts were successful. In a multivariate regression analysis, TIMI flow grade and occlusion age were independent predictors of success. In five cases, pericardial contrast staining due to vessel perforation occurred.[30]

Whether to use a hydrophilic wire as the initial wire in patients with chronic total occlusions is debatable, but in one small randomized study of 88 patients, this strategy resulted in a lower number of guidewires being used, a trend toward shorter procedural and fluoroscopy times, and decreased use of contrast media compared with a strategy of using one or two 0.014-in soft- or intermediate-tip guidewires.[31] Since that time, many nonhydrophilic wires suitable for chronic total occlusions have been developed, such as the Cross-it and Asahi MiracleBros series. These wires may offer the same success rate in crossing chronic total occlusions as the hydrophilic wires, with more directability and less risk for dissection or perforation.

【 】 STENTS

Advancing the guidewire through new or previously placed stents must be done cautiously. Even in situations of in-stent restenosis, the guidewire may exit through the stent struts, which will prohibit delivery of balloons and other devices and may even lead to stent avulsion.[32] One manipulation technique that may decrease the chances of the wire advancing through stent struts is to place a large J curve on the wire in an attempt to loop or prolapse the wire through the stent. If the wire passes through the stent but there is difficulty delivering another stent through the initial one, an option is to use a specialty wire such as the "Wiggle" wire (Guidant, Inc). This is a 0.014–in wire manufactured with a distal core that has multiple undulations or bends, a shapeable flexible tip, and a low friction coating. The "wiggle" portion of the tip begins 6 cm and extends 12 cm from the distal radiopaque tip and has a span of 3 mm that is designed to reduce the incidence of the stent delivery system becoming entrapped against a stent strut. This wire should be placed "bare" or backloaded through an OTW balloon catheter, because the "wiggle" portion will not pass through the catheter lumen.

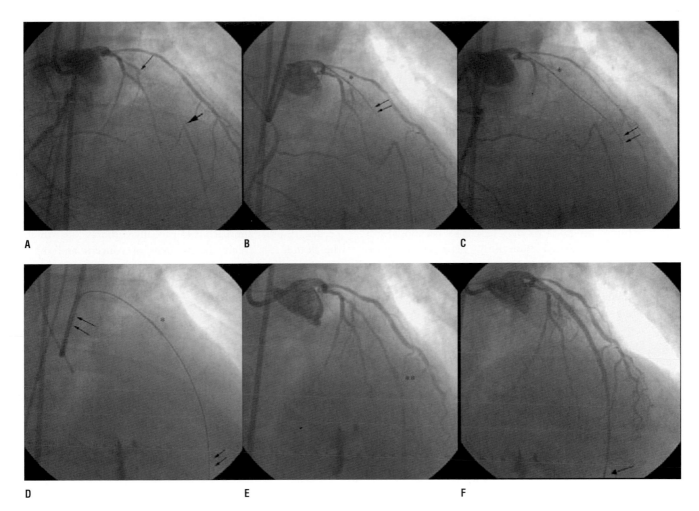

FIGURE 28-3. Procedural cineangiograms from a percutaneous coronary intervention in a 45-year-old man with chronic stable angina and a chronic total occlusion of the left anterior descending (LAD) coronary artery. **A.** Simultaneous injections of the left coronary artery (8-Fr guide) and right coronary artery (5-Fr diagnostic) allow visualization of the length of the LAD occlusion. The *small arrow* shows antegrade filling from the left and the *large arrow*, retrograde filling from the right. **B.** *Double arrows* show the tip of the Asahi Confianza wire extending partially through the occlusion through an over-the-wire (OTW) balloon (*). **C.** The guidewire is shown exiting the LAD and passing into the diagonal artery, demonstrated by contralateral injection. **D.** The Confianza wire was redirected into the distal LAD successfully. Note the long radiopaque segment of the wire (*double arrows*). **E.** The wire was exchanged to a floppy wire using the OTW balloon so that the LAD could be better visualized. A dissection was seen by angiography (**) that was confirmed by intravascular ultrasound. **F.** Several drug-eluting stents were delivered over a floppy guidewire (tip in distal LAD, *arrow*).

【 】 BIFURCATION LESIONS AND SIDE BRANCH ACCESS

Dual coronary guidewires are often needed for bifurcation lesions. If provisional stenting will be used for the side branch, then the side branch wire should be removed before stenting the main artery to avoid wire entrapment.[33] Some operators, however, believe this cautionary step is not necessary and that leaving the side branch wire in place improves side branch patency during stent placement. Dual wires can be used for bifurcation lesions during balloon dilation. The wire should be retracted during stent placement and then readvanced across the stent struts into the side branch for postdilation with simultaneous or "kissing" inflations of the main and side branch.

A complication that may occur with dual wires in bifurcation lesions or with the use of a buddy wire is wire "braiding." This occurs when the two wires become entwined and cannot be manipulated independently. This phenomenon occurs mostly with RX systems and must be recognized to avoid inadvertent removal of both wires.

WIRE COMPLICATIONS

Recognition and management of guidewire-related complications are critical to patient safety and successful procedural outcomes.

【 】 CORONARY VASOSPASM AND PSEUDOSTENOSIS

Coronary vasospasm occurs in less than 5% of interventions and is mostly at the target lesion or the distal vessel.[34] The incidence is similar among devices with the exception of intracoronary ultrasound and rotational atherectomy, in which varying degrees of spasm can occur in up to a third of cases. Vessel closure secondary to spasm is uncommon, less than 2%, even with this device.[35] Guidewire-induced vasospasm is uncommon and the presentation is not uniform. Rare instances of diffuse coronary vasospasm solely due to guidewire insertion and responsive to nitrates have been described.[36] Additionally, wire-induced spasm may accompany angioplasty, making the recognition of the vasospasm more difficult.[37] Multiple sites of spasm remote from the target lesion may occur, due to wire or equipment manipulation.[38] Most vasospasm is responsive to intracoronary vasodilators such as nitroglycerin (100–200 μg), but some patients may require higher doses or a continuous intravenous infusion. The calcium channel blockers verapamil (100 μg/min up to 1.0–1.5 mg) and diltiazem (0.5–2.5 mg over 1 minute, up to 5–10 mg) have also been used.[39,40] Vasospasm distal to the dilated lesion during percutaneous transluminal coronary angioplasty (PTCA) may be refractory to vasodilators if the guidewire is contributing to the spasm; in that case, guidewire removal is necessary.[41]

Distinguishing newly acquired coronary narrowing due to vasospasm from coronary dissection is important. Removal of the guidewire, a potential therapy for wire-induced spasm, may be detrimental if a dissection, thrombus, or other mechanical complication is not recognized. Intravascular ultrasound may be helpful in this situation to rule out a dissection prior to wire removal. Recognition of this phenomenon of guidewire-induced vasospasm is important so that it does not interfere with selection of appropriate balloon and stent sizes or result in unnecessary interventions for "pseudolesions."

Another well-described cause of coronary narrowing attributable to a guidewire is pseudostenosis. Tortuous vessels, including the right coronary, left circumflex, and internal mammary arteries, are prone to these artifacts. Pseudostenosis results from the creation of pleats or kinks in the artery due to artificial straightening induced by passage of the straight section of the guidewire through a tortuous or redundant arterial segment.[42–49] In addition, stiffer guidewires, which are often used for the purpose of improved device delivery in more complicated cases such as calcified or tortuous vessels, are more likely to cause these false lesions. The lesions often appear as a linear defect and may be difficult to distinguish from a dissection, thrombus, or vasospasm. Pseudostenosis usually resolves once the guidewire is removed; however, it can also result in erroneous hemodynamic measurements or assessment of stenosis severity.[50]

Prior to complete removal of the wire, a few approaches can be taken to evaluate for a true lesion. If a stiff or extra-support wire is being used, it can be exchanged for a floppy wire to see if less vessel straightening resolves the lesion. Relief of pseudostenosis may occur with a transit catheter or OTW balloon catheter.[51] The catheter can be placed distal to the lesion in question and the wire removed. This technique is particularly useful if the catheter has been used during the procedure so that an additional wire is not needed. Another approach is to partially withdraw the wire so that the flexible tip enters the segment of concern and the pseudostenosis disappears as the segment assumes its normal tortuous configuration (Figure 28-4). Such an approach is not suitable for clarifying multiple lesions.[52] If the etiology is still unclear intravascular ultrasound imaging can be helpful.[53]

【 】 WIRE PERFORATIONS

Coronary perforations are a rare complication of PCI; one study found they occurred in 0.3% of patients in 12,658 cases, more with debulking devices (1%) than with balloon angioplasty and stent techniques (0.2%).[54] Importantly, this study observed that 51% of the coronary perforations were guidewire related. The majority of guidewire perforations result from distal migration and buckling of the wire during exchanges and delivery of devices. In this situation, the wire is advanced through progressively smaller arterial branches until it exceeds the lumen diameter and penetrates the thin wall of the distal branch. Perforations can also occur when attempting to cross a chronic total occlusion. Guidewires that have a distal hydrophilic polymer coating are more prone to cause perforations because of both wire and lesion characteristics. Operator experience is also a factor. In fact, reports of perforation often follow the release to market of new wires.[55] As with other coronary perforations, wire perforations can be classified as type I

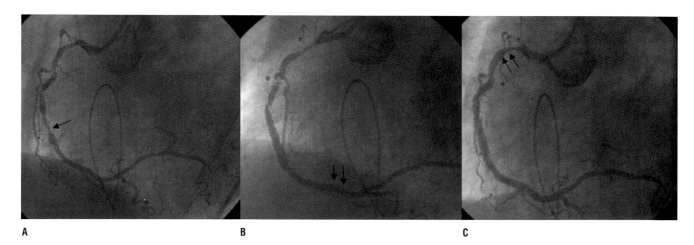

A   B   C

FIGURE 28-4. Procedural cineangiograms of a right coronary intervention. **A.** Diagnostic angiography shows a tortuous right coronary artery with a culprit lesion mid vessel (*arrow*). **B.** After the stent was delivered over an extra-support wire (radiopaque floppy tip, *double arrows*) two lesions were noted proximally (*). **C.** The diagnosis of pseudolesions was made by progressively withdrawing the guidewire until its floppy segment rested equally on either side of the suspect lesion(s).

through III, and risk of tamponade increases with higher classification. Importantly, wire perforations may not be readily apparent during the PCI procedure. Patients with undetected perforations may present with features of cardiac tamponade, notably hypotension, several hours after completion of what was judged to be an uncomplicated intervention. A high index of suspicion is essential for the prompt diagnosis and management of these patients.

Initial treatment of perforation should consist of reversal of anticoagulation and, if needed, prolonged balloon inflation, up to 15 minutes, which in the case of a distal or chronic total occlusion perforation should not result in significant ischemia.[56] Wire-induced perforations typically cannot be treated with a covered stent. An OTW balloon should be used if time allows so that the wire can be removed, but if a RX balloon is in place, the wire can be withdrawn into the distal balloon lumen. Further management is individualized, but if a significant pericardial effusion or tamponade is present pericardiocentesis should be performed.

For perforations that persist despite prolonged inflations, particularly when immediate reversal of anticoagulation is not possible (eg, with administration of a glycoprotein (GP) IIb/IIIa inhibitor), several unique treatment strategies have been reported. In two cases, a small dose (100–300 IU) of thrombin was injected via the lumen of a balloon catheter during prolonged low-pressure balloon inflation, just proximal to the wire perforation site.[57] The thrombin can be prepared at a concentration of 50 to 100 IU/mL, with a delivery of 2 to 5 mL and a 10- to 20-minute balloon inflation following the thrombin injection to prevent retrograde effects of the activated thrombin. In one case report, 2-mm pieces of gel foam soaked in contrast were injected into the distal vessel via a transit catheter, with successful sealing of the perforation.[58] Microcoil embolization, distal delivery of polyvinyl alcohol, or the patient's organized thrombus have also been used successfully to treat wire perforations.[59–61]

[ ] WIRE FRACTURES, EMBOLI, AND RETAINED FRAGMENTS

Guidewire entrapment or embolization is a rare complication of PCI that may be related to operator technique or less commonly to manufacturing flaws or wire component failure.[62] Tip entrapment may occur when the wire is advanced into a small side branch or distal vessel due to resultant vessel vasospasm or with excessive rotation in total occlusions. Initially, an attempt to release the wire should include administration of intracoronary nitroglycerin with gentle retraction. Another technique that can be used is to advance a low-profile balloon over the wire close to the wire tip, and then retract the wire into the balloon catheter. After removal of the wire, angiography should be performed to exclude vessel perforation. Attempts to remove an entrapped wire may lead to fracture and unwinding of the distal tip coil or wire embolization. Another situation that can lead to wire entrapment is the use of a wire to maintain side branch patency during stenting. The wire, therefore, should be retracted from the side branch before placement of the stent. A wire may also become inadvertently trapped behind a stent if a loop in the nonradiopaque segment goes unrecognized. We had this experience once during treatment of a bifurcation lesion, and the stent-entrapped wire fractured during attempted removal. Fracture of a coronary guidewire during thrombectomy of an occluded coronary bypass graft with the X-Sizer catheter has also been reported as a result of entrapment with a coronary stent.[63] Guidewire transection can also occur during rotational atherectomy if the wire prolapses or kinks in the path of the rotating burr.[64]

The optimal strategy for retrieval of wire fragments and the consequences of retained fragments are unclear because the largest series reported outcomes in only eight patients.[65] Four of five extraction procedures were successful, including retrieval of a wire segment totally contained within a distal coronary artery. Retrieval of wires with segments extending into the coronary guide or aorta has been achieved with bioptomes, or compression of the wire in the guiding catheter by inflation of a balloon within the guide and simultaneous withdrawal of the balloon and catheter.[66] Guidewire segments retained totally within the coronary circulation can be removed with improvised or commercially available snares that can be looped around the wire fragment.[67] Some retained fragments may be benign, particularly if within the coronary or in total occlusions. At late follow-up in the observations of Hartzler and colleagues,[65] up to 5 years, five patients with retained wire segments had no sequelae attributable to the PTCA component debris.

SUMMARY

The guidewire is one of the most critical instruments in coronary interventions. This chapter has reviewed the construction and fundamental physical properties of guidewires, general manipulation techniques, and potential guidewire complications. As coronary anatomy becomes more challenging, understanding of the advantages and limitations of available guidewires can complement operator experience for successful outcomes.

ACKNOWLEDGMENTS

The authors would like to thank Ed McNamara and John Schreiner for sharing their guidewire expertise and Arlene Grant for her technical assistance.

REFERENCES

1. Dervan JP, Baim DS, Cherniles J, et al. Transluminal angioplasty of occluded coronary arteries: Use of a movable guide wire system. *Circulation.* 1983;68:776.
2. Simpson JB, Baim DS, Robert EW, et al. A new catheter system for coronary angioplasty. *Am J Cardiol.* 1982;49:1216.
3. Levin DC, Ganz P, Friedman P, et al. Percutaneous transluminal coronary angioplasty with an over-the-wire system. *Radiology.* 1985;155:323.
4. Dervan JP, McKay RG, Baim DS. The use of an exchange guide wire in coronary angioplasty. *Cathet Cardiovasc Diagn.* 1985;11:207.
5. Kaltenbach M, Vallbracht C, Kober G. The long wire technique for coronary angioplasty. *Cathet Cardiovasc Diagn.* 1986;12:337.
6. McAuley BJ, Oesterle S, Simpson JB. Advances in guidewire technology. *Am J Cardiol.* 1984;53:15.
7. McDermott EA. Coronary angioplasty guidewire technology. *Z Kardiol.* 1987;6:29.
8. Ahmad T, Webb JG, Carere RG, et al. Guide wire extension may not be essential to pass an over-the-wire balloon catheter. *Cathet Cardiovasc Diagn.* 1995;36:59.
9. Nanto S, Ohara T, Shimonagata T, et al. A technique for changing a PTCA balloon catheter over a regular-length guidewire. *Cathet Cardiovasc Diagn.* 1994;32:274.

10. Pande AK, Meier B, Urban P, et al. Magnum/Magnarail versus conventional systems for recanalization of chronic total coronary occlusions: A randomized comparison. *Am Heart J.* 1992;123:1182.

11. Allemann Y, Kaufmann UP, Meyer BJ, et al. Magnum wire for percutaneous coronary balloon angioplasty in 800 total chronic occlusions. *Am J Cardiol.* 1997;80:634.

12. Jaup T, Allemann Y, Urban P, et al. The Magnum wire for percutaneous coronary balloon angioplasty in 723 patients. *J Invasive Cardiol.* 1995;7:259.

13. Gunnes P, Meyer BJ, Kessler B, et al. Magnum wire for angioplasty of total and non-total coronary lesions. *Int J Cardiol.* 1997;60:1.

14. Nukta ED, Meier B, Urban P, et al. Magnum system for routine coronary angioplasty: A randomized study. *Cathet Cardiovasc Diagn.* 1992;25:272.

15. Hibbard MD, Holmes DR Jr. The Tracker catheter: A new vascular access system. *Cathet Cardiovasc Diagn.* 1992;27:309.

16. Tatineni S, Kern MJ, Aguirre F, et al. The usefulness of a tracking catheter in complex coronary angioplasty. [see comment]. *Cathet Cardiovasc Diagn.* 1992;27:75.

17. Pimentel CX, Schreiter SW, Gurbel PA. The use of the Tracker catheter as a guidewire support device in angioplasty of angulated and tortuous circumflex coronary arteries. *J Invasive Cardiol.* 1995;7:66.

18. Detre K, Holubkov R, Kelsey S, et al. Percutaneous transluminal coronary angioplasty in 1985–1986 and 1977–1981. The National Heart, Lung, and Blood Institute Registry. *N Engl J Med.* 1998;318:265.

19. Bell MR, Berger PB, Bresnahan JF, et al. Initial and long-term outcome of 354 patients after coronary balloon angioplasty of total coronary artery occlusions. [see comment]. *Circulation.* 1992;85:1003.

20. Melchior JP, Meier B, Urban P, et al. Percutaneous transluminal coronary angioplasty for chronic total coronary arterial occlusion. *Am J Cardiol.* 1987;59:535.

21. Ivanhoe RJ, Weintraub WS, Douglas JS Jr, et al. Percutaneous transluminal coronary angioplasty of chronic total occlusions. Primary success, restenosis, and long-term clinical follow-up. [see comment]. *Circulation.* 1992;85:106.

22. Finci L, Meier B, Favre J, et al. Long-term results of successful and failed angioplasty for chronic total coronary arterial occlusion. *Am J Cardiol.* 1990;66:660.

23. Serruys PW, Umans V, Heyndrickx GR, et al. Elective PTCA of totally occluded coronary arteries not associated with acute myocardial infarction; short-term and long-term results. *Eur Heart J.* 1985;6:2.

24. Kinoshita I, Katoh O, Nariyama J, et al. Coronary angioplasty of chronic total occlusions with bridging collateral vessels: Immediate and follow-up outcome from a large single-center experience. *J Am Coll Cardiol.* 1995;26:409.

25. Tan K, Sulke N, Taub N, et al. Clinical and lesion morphologic determinants of coronary angioplasty success and complications: Current experience. *J Am Coll Cardiol.* 1995;25:855.

26. Grollier G, Commeau P, Foucault JP, et al. Angioplasty of chronic totally occluded coronary arteries: Usefulness of retrograde opacification of the distal part of the occluded vessel via the contralateral coronary artery. *Am Heart J.* 1987;114:1324.

27. Sherman CT, Sheehan D, Simpson JB. Simultaneous cannulation: A technique for percutaneous transluminal coronary angioplasty of chronic total occlusions. *Cathet Cardiovasc Diagn.* 1987;13:333.

28. Gray DF, Sivananthan UM, Verma SP, et al. Balloon angioplasty of totally and subtotally occluded coronary arteries: Results using the Hydrophillic Terumo Radifocus Guidewire M (glidewire). [see comment]. *Cathet Cardiovasc Diagn.* 1993;30:293.

29. Corcos T, Favereau X, Guerin Y, et al. Recanalization of chronic coronary occlusions using a new hydrophilic guidewire. [see comment]. *Cathet Cardiovasc Diagn.* 1998;44:83.

30. Kahler J, Koster R, Brockhoff C, et al. Initial experience with a hydrophilic-coated guidewire for recanalization of chronic coronary occlusions. *Cathet Cardiovasc Interv.* 2000;49:45.

31. Lefevre T, Louvard Y, Loubeyre C, et al. A randomized study comparing two guidewire strategies for angioplasty of chronic total coronary occlusion. *Am J Cardiol.* 2000;85:1144.

32. Jain D, Kurowski V, Katus HA, et al. A unique pitfall in percutaneous coronary angioplasty of in-stent restenosis: Guidewire passage out of the stent. [see comment]. *Cathet Cardiovasc Interv.* 2001;53:229.

33. Thew ST, Klein LW. Report of an undeployed stent causing the unraveling of a coronary artery guidewire being used for sidebranch protection. *J Invasive Cardiol.* 2002;14:106.

34. Fischell TA, Derby G, Tse TM, et al. Coronary artery vasoconstriction routinely occurs after percutaneous transluminal coronary angioplasty. A quantitative arteriographic analysis. *Circulation.* 1988;78:1323.

35. Warth DC, Leon MB, O'Neill W, et al. Rotational atherectomy multicenter registry: Acute results, complications and 6-month angiographic follow-up in 709 patients. *J Am Coll Cardiol.* 1994;24:641.

36. Moukarbel GV, Dakik HA. Diffuse coronary artery spasm induced by guidewire insertion. *J Invasive Cardiol.* 2003;15:353, 2003.

37. Zanchetta M, Pedon L, Rigatelli G, et al. Pseudo-lesion of internal mammary artery graft and left anterior descending artery during percutaneous transluminal angioplasty—a case report. *Angiology.* 2004;55:459.

38. Douard H, Broustet JP. Unusual multiple spasm during coronary angioplasty. *Heart.* 2001;86:558.

39. McIvor ME, Undemir C, Lawson J, et al. Clinical effects and utility of intracoronary diltiazem. *Cathet Cardiovasc Diagn.* 1995;35:287.

40. Babbitt DG, Perry JM, Forman MB. Intracoronary verapamil for reversal of refractory coronary vasospasm during percutaneous transluminal coronary angioplasty. *J Am Coll Cardiol.* 1988;12:1377.

41. Takahashi M, Ikeda U, Sekiguchi H, et al. Guide wire-induced coronary artery spasm during percutaneous transluminal coronary angioplasty. A case report. *Angiology.* 1996;47:305.

42. Lau KW, Ding ZP, Gao W, et al. Pseudo-dissection in percutaneous transluminal coronary angioplasty. *J Invasive Cardiol.* 1994;6:296.

43. Tenaglia AN, Tcheng JE, Phillips HR 3rd, et al. Creation of pseudo narrowing during coronary angioplasty. *Am J Cardiol.* 1991;67:658.

44. Shea PJ. Mechanical right coronary artery shortening and vessel wall invagination: A fourth cause of iatrogenic coronary obstruction during coronary angioplasty. A case report and review of the literature. *Cathet Cardiovasc Diagn.* 1992;26:136.

45. Hays JT, Stein B, Raizner AE. The crumpled coronary: An enigma of arteriographic pseudopathology and its potential for misinterpretation. *Cathet Cardiovasc Diagn.* 1994;31:293.

46. Blankenship JC. Right coronary artery pseudo-transection due to mechanical straightening during coronary angioplasty. *Cathet Cardiovasc Diagn.* 1995;36:43.

47. Deligonul U, Tatineni S, Johnson R, et al. Accordion right coronary artery: An unusual complication of PTCA guidewire entrapment. *Cathet Cardiovasc Diagn.* 1991;23:111.

48. Grewe K, Presti CF, Perez JA. Torsion of an internal mammary graft during percutaneous transluminal angioplasty: A case report. *Cathet Cardiovasc Diagn.* 1990;19:195.

49. Rauh RA, Ninneman RW, Joseph D, et al. Accordion effect in tortuous right coronary arteries during percutaneous transluminal coronary angioplasty. *Cathet Cardiovasc Diagn.* 1991;23:107.

50. Escaned J, Flores A, Garcia P, et al. Guidewire-induced coronary pseudostenosis as a source of error during physiological guidance of stent deployment. *Cathet Cardiovasc Interv.* 2000;51:91.

51. Fortuin FD, Sweeney JP, Lee RW. Relief of pseudostenosis using the transit exchange catheter. *Cathet Cardiovasc Interv.* 2004;63:457.

52. Chalet Y, Chevalier B, el Hadad S, et al. "Pseudo-narrowing" during right coronary angioplasty: How to diagnose correctly without withdrawing the guidewire. *Cathet Cardiovasc Diagn.* 1994;31:37.

53. Alfonso F, Delgado A, Magalhaes D, et al. Value of intravascular ultrasound in the assessment of coronary pseudostenosis during coronary interventions. *Cathet Cardiovasc Interv.* 1999;46:327.

54. Witzke CF, Martin-Herrero F, Clarke SC, et al. The changing pattern of coronary perforation during percutaneous coronary intervention in the new device era. [see comment]. *J Invasive Cardiol.* 2004;16:257.

55. Wong CM, Kwong Mak GY, Chung DT. Distal coronary artery perforation resulting from the use of hydrophilic coated guidewire in tortuous vessels. *Cathet Cardiovasc Diagn.* 1998;44:93.

56. Flynn MS, Aguirre FV, Donohue TJ, et al. Conservative management of guidewire coronary artery perforation with pericardial effusion during angioplasty for acute inferior myocardial infarction. *Cathet Cardiovasc Diagn.* 1993;29:285.

57. Fischell TA, Korban EH, Lauer MA. Successful treatment of distal coronary guidewire-induced perforation with balloon catheter delivery of intracoronary thrombin. *Cathet Cardiovasc Interv.* 2003;58:370.

58. Dixon SR, Webster MW, Ormiston JA, et al. Gelfoam embolization of a distal coronary artery guidewire perforation. *Cathet Cardiovasc Interv.* 2000;49:214.

59. Gaxiola E, Browne KF. Coronary artery perforation repair using microcoil embolization. *Cathet Cardiovasc Diagn.* 1998;43:474.

60. Yoo BS, Yoon J, Lee SH, et al. Guidewire-induced coronary artery perforation treated with transcatheter injection of polyvinyl alcohol form. *Cathet Cardiovasc Interv.* 2001;52:231.

61. Cordero H, Gupta N, Underwood PL, et al. Intracoronary autologous blood to seal a coronary perforation. *Herz.* 2001;26:157.

62. Ceschinski H, Henkes H, Weinert HC, et al. Torquability of microcatheter guidewires: The resulting torsional moment. *Bio Medical Materials & Engineering.* 2000;10:31.

63. Cafri C, Rosenstein G, Ilia R. Fracture of a coronary guidewire during graft thrombectomy with the X-sizer device. *J Invasive Cardiol.* 2004;16:263.

64. Foster-Smith K, Garratt KN, Holmes DR, Jr. Guidewire transection during rotational coronary atherectomy due to guide catheter dislodgement and wire kinking. *Cathet Cardiovasc Diagn.* 1995;35:224.

65. Hartzler GO, Rutherford BD, McConahay DR. Retained percutaneous transluminal coronary angioplasty equipment components and their management. *Am J Cardiol.* 1987;60:1260.

66. Patel T, Shah S, Pandya R, et al. Broken guidewire fragment: A simplified retrieval technique. *Cathet Cardiovasc Interv.* 2000;51:483.

67. Mikolich JR, Hanson MW. Transcatheter retrieval of intracoronary detached angioplasty guidewire segment. *Cathet Cardiovasc Diagn.* 1988;15:44.

CHAPTER (29)

Coronary Balloon Angioplasty

Ziyad Ghazzal, MD

Percutaneous coronary balloon angioplasty was first described by Andreas Gruentzig. In 1976, he reported the successful application in canine coronary experiments. Dr Gruentzig designed and assembled balloon dilation catheters in his own kitchen. He performed the first coronary angioplasty in a conscious patient in September 1977 in Zurich. The dilation catheter consisted of a balloon attached to a long shaft and a short wire attached to its tip. Soon after, balloon catheters were designed with a central guidewire lumen. Despite the major advances in the technology, the basic equipment used in today's percutaneous coronary interventions still includes a guide catheter, guidewire, balloon catheter, and contrast agent. This chapter addresses the basic elements of a percutaneous coronary balloon intervention procedure.

GUIDE CATHETERS

Guiding catheters have several important characteristics: shape, size, inner diameter, stiffness, torquability, and pushability. The outer diameter of a guide catheter can be as small as 4 French (3-Fr = 1 mm). However, most guide catheters used in the United States are 6- to 8-Fr in diameter. Large catheters allow for better dye visualization and, in general, provide better backup, but they tend to be somewhat stiffer. There is no definitive proof that smaller catheters cause fewer groin complications.

Selection of a guide catheter takes into consideration the shape and orientation of the vessel to be cannulated as well as the shape and width of the aorta.

【 】 LEFT CORONARY ARTERY

Several guiding catheter configurations are suitable for engaging the left main coronary artery. The commonly used Judkins curve is available in different sizes. The most popular is the "four curve," which refers to the distance in centimeters between the primary and secondary curves of the catheter. The smaller 3.5-cm curve is used in patients with smaller ascending aortas, and larger curves are used with larger aortas. In general, the left anterior descending (LAD) artery originates from the left main coronary artery in an anterior and superior direction. A left Judkins catheter can be made coaxial with the LAD if it is advanced so that the secondary curve is pushed down in the ascending aorta, allowing the tip of the catheter to point superiorly. A gentle counterclockwise rotation will allow the tip to point anteriorly in the direction of the LAD.

In case of a short or absent left main artery, a shorter curve will help the Judkins catheter point in the direction of the LAD, while a longer curve will help the catheter stay more coaxial with the circumflex artery. In addition, because the circumflex artery takes off posteriorly and inferiorly from the left main artery, gentle withdrawal of the Judkins catheter will bring the secondary curve higher in the aorta, allowing the tip to point inferiorly and in the direction of the artery. However, the backup support in this situation would likely be suboptimal, because the secondary curve of the catheter will not be pushing against the back wall of the aorta.

A short (3.5-cm) Judkins curve is suitable to engage a left main artery with a superior takeoff, whereas a 4.5-cm curve is appropriate for a left main artery with an inferior takeoff. Other guiding catheters suitable for the left main system include the Amplatz and the "extra backup."

The Amplatz catheter provides very good support when engaging the left coronary system because its secondary curve sits securely in the root of the aorta. It is important to remember that the Amplatz catheter needs to be pushed down and rotated before it is disengaged from the left main coronary artery. This will prevent the tip of the catheter from plunging and possibly traumatizing the left main artery.

The extra backup catheter has a very wide secondary curve, which allows a strong guide support as it sits tightly against the contralateral aortic wall. Extra backup catheters tend to provide superior coaxial support. Therefore, care should be taken when withdrawing a winged balloon back into the guiding catheter as the tip of the guider may be pulled in deep into the ostium of the artery.

【 】 RIGHT CORONARY ARTERY

Most right coronary arteries are easily engaged with a right Judkins catheter with its regular 4F curve. A small aorta may require a smaller curve, whereas a dilated aorta may require a larger curve.

Some situations, however, may be more challenging. When the orientation of the ostium of the right coronary artery is very anterior, a misalignment exists between the Judkins catheter tip and the ostium of the artery. Gentle clockwise rotation allows the catheter tip to become more coaxial with the artery. Care should be taken not to allow the catheter tip to engage the artery too deeply.

When the proximal right coronary artery takes a superior orientation (shepherd crook shape), the backup provided by the Judkins catheter can be suboptimal. Catheters that have the capability of providing better support or those that can point more superiorly include the Amplatz, hockey stick, left coronary bypass, Arani, and internal mammary catheters.

If the orientation of the origin of the right coronary artery is very inferior, an "inferior takeoff" Judkins or "short right curve" catheters can prove adequate. If the orientation is markedly inferior but otherwise straight, a multipurpose catheter can be tried.

【 】 SAPHENOUS VEIN BYPASS GRAFTS

A right coronary artery bypass graft can be best engaged with a multipurpose guiding catheter, which usually sits within the graft in a coaxial manner and provides adequate support. The left saphenous vein bypass graft is usually accessed with a regular left coronary bypass guiding catheter. However, the Amplatz catheter may provide a better backup. Other guiding catheters include the hockey stick and the right Judkins guider.

【 】 INTERNAL MAMMARY ARTERY

The internal mammary catheter is shaped similarly to a Judkins right catheter, however, the primary curve is very sharp. It can be used for cannulation of both left and right internal mammary arteries. The catheter comes in the conventional 100-cm length as well as a 90-cm length. The 10-cm shorter length in the guiding catheter allows additional working length for the interventional devices. This can help in reaching more distal lesions in the native circulation past the mammary artery.

On rare occasions, cannulation of the internal mammary catheter can prove difficult from the femoral approach. An alternative approach is to cannulate the artery from the brachial or radial access site. This is not necessarily easier, depending on where the mammary artery originates from the subclavian artery.

【 】 CORONARY ARTERY ANOMALIES

Coronary artery anomalies occur in approximately 2% of the population. The choice of the guiding catheter does not follow any general rule, but rather depends on the specific variation in the anatomy. The most common coronary artery anomaly is origin of the circumflex artery from the right cusp or sharing of a common ostium with the right coronary artery. The multipurpose catheter usually sits well in the ostium of the anomalous coronary artery that points inferiorly and then courses posteriorly toward the atrioventricular groove.

GUIDEWIRES

Despite the rapid advancement in interventional technology, the guidewire remains an important gadget without which a coronary intervention cannot be performed. All currently approved catheter devices are designed to track over a guidewire. If a lesion cannot be crossed with a guidewire, a coronary intervention cannot be completed. The only exception is a balloon-on-the-wire catheter (see "Balloon Catheters," later).

Most coronary or vein graft lesions can be crossed without much difficulty. However, certain complex anatomic situations can be challenging. These include acutely tortuous vessel, severely angulated lesions, bifurcations, and chronic total occlusions. Accordingly, an angioplasty guidewire must fulfill several important characteristics.

【 】 TIP FLEXIBILITY AND WIRE SHAPING

The distal 2 to 3 cm of a guidewire is radiopaque and ranges in stiffness from the very floppy to the very stiff. Most guidewires have a flexible or floppy tip and are suitable to negotiate the majority of coronary lesions. A wire with a stiff distal tip is used to attempt crossing chronic total occlusions.

Shaping of the wire tip is tailored to the vessel and lesion. Most lesions can be crossed with a wire that has a 45-degree bend in the distal 2 to 3 mm of the wire tip. Crossing of lesions in bifurcating branches is best achieved with the wire tip shaped so that the radius of the bend approximates the diameter of the parent vessel. This allows the tip to reach the branch vessel.

The wire tip can be shaped in a number of ways to suit the different anatomic situations. A common shape is a double curve consisting of primary and secondary curves. In crossing a lesion in a branch, the secondary curve can be formed so as to have the distance to the wire tip approximate the diameter of the parent vessel. After the wire enters the branch vessel with the help of the secondary curve, the smaller primary curve will help negotiate the lesion in the branch.

【 】 TRANSITION POINT

It is helpful to understand how wires on the market today compare. One difference may be the transition zone of the wire between the shaft of the wire and the softer distal tip. In negotiating a branch that takes off at a very acute angle, a wire with a stiff transition will have the tendency to "buckle" or prolapse into the parent vessel. To compensate, the operator may reshape the wire by increasing the angle on the bend and lengthening the arm. Once the wire engages the branch, there may be difficulty in crossing a particular lesion because of the excessive bend on the wire.

【 】 SHAFT SUPPORT AND DEVICE DELIVERY

One important characteristic of a guidewire is shaft stiffness. Although a stiff shaft can provide better support for device delivery, it generally lacks the torque control that a softer wire offers. In the case of a very tortuous artery, softer wires tend to conform better to the vessel curvatures. A stiff guidewire that spans a tortuous segment of an artery creates an angiographic appearance referred to as "pseudolesions," which can be mistakenly interpreted as a coronary dissection. Instead, it is an indication of vessel straightening by the guidewire, resulting in the creation of kinks along the course of the tortuous vessel. When this condition is suspected, the operator may pull the wire back, keeping the soft tip across the "lesions" and allowing the vessel to relax. If the kinks are reduced and the angiographic appearance is improved, the diagnosis of "pseudolesions" can be made.

BALLOON CATHETERS

Despite the wide use of stents, balloon catheters remain an integral element of the procedure. Balloons are used to predilate lesions before stent deployment or to perform stand-alone balloon angioplasty. However, the most important role for balloon catheters in the current era is stent deployment, because most stents chosen in clinical practice are balloon expandable.

【 】 BALLOON CATHETER SYSTEMS

Fixed-Wire System

In this system, the wire is attached to the balloon tip. Historically, such balloons had the best crossing profile. Today, although they are much less popular and almost abandoned, fixed-wire catheters may still be used in distal arteries and bifurcating lesions.

Over-the-Wire System

In this system, the balloon catheter has a central lumen permitting free guidewire movement. The over-the-wire system is helpful when crossing difficult anatomy such as a chronic total occlusion, where balloon support is helpful and wire exchange is anticipated. Another advantage of this system is the option of keeping the wire across the lesion after balloon inflation so that the lesion can be examined angiographically without sacrificing wire access.

Rapid Exchange System

The rapid exchange system is preferred by most single operators. The lesion is crossed with a standard-length guidewire. The wire is then fixed with one hand while the balloon catheter is advanced with the other (the wire exits a few centimeters from the distal end of the balloon catheter rather than its proximal end). Balloon pushability may not be as good as with a full-length over-the-wire system. However, the main disadvantage is that the wire cannot be pulled out for reshaping and cannot be exchanged for another wire without taking the entire system out.

Cutting Balloon

The cutting balloon is the newest addition to the balloon catheter technology. It consists of an over-the-wire balloon catheter with 3 or 4 microtomes—sharp metal blades mounted longitudinally on the surface of the balloon. The balloon is inflated slowly, allowing the blades to "cut" into the lesion before actual balloon dilation. It is felt that these controlled microsurgical incisions may limit overall vessel wall injury, therefore reducing the balloon dissection rate and possibly also the elastic recoil. The cutting balloon has gained popularity for angioplasty of in-stent restenosis. In these situations, it has the advantage of preventing "watermelon seeding" of the balloon and may result in better balloon dilatation.[1] The balloon comes in 6-, 10-, and 15-mm lengths. It is important to keep in mind that the device is stiff and has a high crossing profile. Some anatomic situations, such as lesions in very tortuous segments, may be out of reach with the cutting balloon.

Perfusion Balloon

The perfusion balloon catheter has small holes in the shaft proximal and distal to the balloon that allow blood to perfuse the distal artery while the balloon is inflated. Although the catheter is still available commercially, it is rarely used because of the availability of stents for treatment of coronary dissections. Rather, it can be used as a temporizing method in coronary perforations.

【 】 BALLOON MATERIALS

The first balloon catheter used by Andreas Gruentzig was made of polyvinylchloride, a low compliance material. Since then significant advances have been reached, addressing important issues such as crossing profile, trackability, pushability, conformability, strength, and balloon compliance.

Most balloon catheters available on the market today are derived from one of four families of balloon materials: polyolefin, nylon, polyester, and urethane. It is the type of balloon material derived from these categories of plastic that will largely determine the characteristics that differentiate dilatation catheters.

An example of the polyester category is a balloon made of polyethylene terephthalate (PET). This material is classified among the highest in tensile strength and is typically noncompliant and highly durable but has the tendency to "wing" after deflation. The nylons (polyamide) are classified as semicompliant, but the compliance is also partly dependent on the manufacturing process. The polyolefin family of plastic material is a low-strength polymer that is considered highly compliant. Examples include the polyethylene

(PE) and the polyolefin copolymer (POC). These can stretch to higher diameters with higher pressures.

PERCUTANEOUS BALLOON ANGIOPLASTY IN THE DRUG-ELUTING STENT ERA

Since Andreas Gruentzig performed the first coronary balloon angioplasty on a living human in September of 1977, a balloon remains a fundamental tool in almost any revascularization procedure. This is true even in the event of primary stenting, because most stents are balloon expandable. It is also true when adjunctive methods, such as rotational atherectomy or laser, are used because these rarely consist of stand-alone devices. A balloon is used to predilate a lesion or postdilate a stent.

Stents have significantly reduced the problem of acute closure or threatened vessel closure. Drug-eluting stents, in particular, have dramatically improved the problem of restenosis. However, in some situations, percutaneous coronary revascularizations still rely on "poor old balloon angioplasty (POBA)." Examples include:

- The use of a plain balloon or a cutting balloon in a bifurcating ostial lesion.

- Treatment of in-stent restenosis.

- Small vessel lesions.

- Distal lesions in which severe proximal tortuosities, especially with calcifications, prohibit the advancement of a stent.

- Poorly dilatable lesions in which placing a stent is felt to be inadvisable because of the risk of poor stent expansion.

- Some bifurcating lesions, when a balloon result is adequate and a stent is avoided to prevent jailing of the side branch.

- Treatment of lesions at the anastomosis of the left internal mammary artery (LIMA) or more distally in the native artery. In such instances, advancing a stent in a tortuous LIMA may be difficult. Moreover, data suggest that the long-term result with stenting is not favorable over ballooning in LIMA anastomosis lesions.

- Rare situations in which prolonged antiplatelet therapy is contraindicated, such as in the presence of severe thrombocytopenia, the potential for active bleeding, or the anticipation of certain types of non-elective surgeries postangioplasty.

These examples, as well as other situations, lead to the performance of percutaneous coronary angioplasty without placing a stent in approximately 10% to 15% of cases. On the other hand, drug-eluting stents, which are very commonly used in the United States, are used much less often in most parts of the world because of economic concerns. With that in mind, the interventionalist needs to be familiar with what to expect from a balloon result both in the short and long term.

【 】 MECHANISM OF BALLOON ANGIOPLASTY AND PROCEDURAL RISK

Balloon angioplasty stretches the arterial wall. However, arterial stretching as well as plaque compression plays a very limited role in enlarging the lumen. The most important mechanism by which a balloon expands the lumen in a stenotic artery is by causing fissuring of the atherosclerotic plaque. If the fissures are severe, they can be apparent on a coronary angiogram as intimal tears or dissections. These can be hemodynamically significant and can cause acute vessel closure, which used to be the most important cause of morbidity and mortality in the present era.

Several studies have addressed the predictors of acute closure in the balloon era. These include diffuse disease, bulky eccentric atherosclerotic plaques, heavy calcification, extremely angulated segments, ostial lesions, bifurcation lesions, and the presence of thrombus. Accordingly, the well-known American College of Cardiology/American Heart Association classification emerged, which helped stratify procedural risk with balloon angioplasty according to lesion characteristics, and was later modified so that it becomes applicable to the a more recent era of percutaneous coronary interventions[2] (Table 29-1).

TABLE 29-1

Lesion Classification System

ANATOMIC RISK GROUPS,[a] 2000, PCI STENT ERA

Low Risk
Discrete (length < 10 mm)
Concentric
Readily accessible
Nonangulated segment (< 45 degrees)
Smooth contour
Little or no calcification
Less than totally occlusive
Not ostial in location
No major side branch involvement
Absence of thrombus

Moderate Risk
Tubular (length 10–20 mm)
Eccentric
Moderate tortuosity of proximal segment
Moderately angulated segment (> 45, < 90 degrees)
Irregular contour
Moderate or heavy calcification
Total occlusions < 3 mo old
Ostial in location
Bifurcation lesions requiring double guidewires
Some thrombus present

High Risk
Diffuse (length > 20 mm)
Excessive tortuosity of proximal segment
Extremely angulated segments (> 90 degrees)
Total occlusions > 3 mo old or bridging collaterals, or both
Inability to protect major side branches
Degenerated vein grafts with friable lesions

PCI = percutaneous coronary interventions.
[a]This classification of lesion risk is cited from the ACC-National Cardiovascular Data Registry
Catheterization Laboratory Module version 2.0 (15). This classification scheme is also cited in the ACC Clinical Data Standards.[22]

[ ] BALLOON ANGIOPLASTY AND CLINICAL OUTCOME

Patients enrolled in the 1985–1986 National Heart, Lung, and Blood Institute (NHLBI) registry were compared with those in the 1997–1998 Dynamic Registry.[3] In the NHLBI registry, balloon angioplasty was the primary device in 100% of patients, whereas stents were used in 70% of patients in the Dynamic Registry. In the balloon-only era, procedural success was considerably lower (81.8% vs 92.0%; $P < .001$) and the composite rate of in-hospital death, myocardial infarction, and emergency coronary bypass surgery was significantly higher (7.9% vs 4.9%; $P < .001$). The 1-year rate for coronary artery bypass grafting was lower in the Dynamic Registry (6.9% vs 12.6%; $P < .001$).

When stents became available in the mid-1990s, there was still an interest in trying to achieve an adequate balloon result without resorting to a stent in order to avoid the then-growing concern of cost and acute stent thrombosis. However, a retrospective analysis from the 1985–1986 NHLBI registry failed to show any advantage of a "stent-like result" on the long-term risk of death or myocardial infarction.[4]

[ ] SPECIAL LESION SUBSETS

Ostial Lesions and Bifurcating Lesions

The current era of stent and new technology has considerably limited the use of balloon angioplasty in aorto-ostial lesions. This stems from the fact that aorto-ostial lesions in locations such as the right coronary artery posed a big challenge for the balloon technology. In one study from the present era involving 53 patients who underwent percutaneous transluminal angioplasty of a right coronary artery ostial stenosis, a procedure success rate of only 79% was reported.[5] Five patients required emergency coronary artery bypass grafting because of abrupt closure. One-year follow-up revealed clinical recurrence of angina in 20 patients (48%) and restenosis in 16 (38%). A nonrandomized study that compared different strategies, including balloon angioplasty in right coronary artery ostial lesions, reported that stenting provided the best short- and long-term outcomes.[6]

For ostial lesions located at bifurcation points, such as the ostium of the left anterior descending (LAD) or circumflex arteries, stenting poses a particular challenge. Possibilities of an untoward outcome in such situations include a proximal stent edge tear that could propagate into the left main artery, plaque shift into the adjacent large vessel, and complete or partial jailing of the bifurcating artery. The latter problem tends to occur when the stent is precisely positioned so as to cover the ostium of the branching vessel completely. A stent that is positioned slightly more distally will miss the ostium.

These problems can at times be circumvented by avoiding use of a stent altogether. For example, one way to approach an ostial LAD would be to debulk the lesion with rotational atherectomy prior to balloon angioplasty. Use of a stent would follow only if a suboptimal result was obtained post–balloon angioplasty. Another approach would be to use cutting balloon angioplasty with provisional stenting. No randomized trials have been performed to test these different strategies. In a retrospective study from the current

era of percutaneous coronary interventions, we compared the outcome in patients with ostial lesions versus proximal nonostial lesions.[7] The procedure was completed without resorting to a stent in 30 of 223 patients (13%) with ostial lesions and 239 of 2261 patients (11%) with nonostial lesions. Procedural success was similar for ostial and nonostial percutaneous coronary interventions (96% vs 95%). The 1-year event-free survival rate was lower in patients who underwent ostial interventions (69% vs 80%, $P = .0019$), largely due to a greater need for repeat interventions (19% vs 10%, $P < .0001$). It seems, therefore, that even with the availability of stents, ostial lesions remain somewhat of a challenge.

Ostial lesions have been excluded from the landmark randomized trials of drug-eluting stents. The efficacy of such stents in challenging anatomic subsets is being studied from large postmarket registry data.

Long Lesions

A long lesion with diffuse disease is one of the most powerful predictors of a reduced procedural success rate and an increased risk of hemodynamically important dissections with balloon angioplasty.[8–10] The ADVANCE study investigated the clinical benefit of additional stenting after optimal balloon angioplasty in lesions between 20 and 50 mm in length.[11] Of the 437 patients enrolled in the study, optimal balloon angioplasty was achieved in only two thirds of the patients. In the remaining 149 patients (34%), stenting was necessary because of either flow-limiting dissections or angiographic failure with inability to attain a diameter stenosis of less than 50%. This group was also associated with an increased risk of periprocedural infarctions. The remaining 288 patients in whom optimal balloon angioplasty was achieved (diameter stenosis < 30% without significant dissection) were randomized to balloon angioplasty alone versus additional stenting, which resulted in a superior early minimal lumen diameter and led to reduced angiographic restenosis (27% vs 42%, $P = .022$). Freedom from major adverse cardiac events at 9 months was similar in both groups (77%).

Stents have dramatically reduced the chance of dissections in long lesions and helped restore flow in hemodynamically important dissection caused by balloon angioplasty. However, bare-metal stents are associated with the risk of increased restenosis with longer stented segments.[12,13] Colombo and colleagues advocated a strategy of spot stenting for long lesions whereby stents are placed only in the segments of a lesion in which the luminal result after balloon angioplasty does not meet prespecified intravascular ultrasound criteria.[14] This approach led to lower rates of angiographic restenosis and follow-up major adverse events compared with traditional stenting. Drug-eluting stents seem to have a clear advantage in long lesions[15,16] and appear for now to be the treatment of choice, when economically feasible.

Small Vessel Disease

In general, percutaneous revascularization of small coronary vessels carries a lower chance of success and a relatively higher risk compared with revascularization of large vessels, specifically when located in proximal coronary segments.[17] Consequently, a distinction must be made between a small vessel supplying a small amount of myocardium and a proximal lesion in a small artery that supplies a large amount of myocardium, either because it travels a considerable length or it supplies important collaterals. In the first case, where the amount of myocardium in jeopardy is small, the benefit from an angioplasty may not outweigh the risks and medical therapy is most often the first choice. The second case, in which a large amount of myocardium is at risk, presents a challenging problem for the interventionalist. When performing percutaneous revascularization to a small vessel, especially in association with diffuse disease, options are limited because the risk associated with the use of debulking techniques such as rotational atherectomy or laser in such vessels is increased.

Deployment of stents is fraught with the risk of underexpansion and the possibility of subacute thrombosis. In the early stent era, the French multicenter registry reported a subacute stent thrombosis rate of 10% in vessels with diameters less than 2.5 mm.[18] Comparison of balloon angioplasty of small coronary vessels with bare-metal stenting can be derived from subanalysis of randomized trials such as BENESTENT, which showed that decreasing vessel size was associated with an increasing risk of cardiac events for both the stent and balloon angioplasty groups.[19] A small retrospective study of percutaneous treatment of coronary vessels with diameters less than 3.0 mm showed that elective stent implantation in small vessels with complex lesions does not improve early and late outcomes.[20] Alternatives to conventional short balloon dilations include gradual and prolonged balloon angioplasty (GPBA) and cutting balloon angioplasty. These three methods of balloon dilation were tested in a randomized study of 263 patients with reference vessel diameter of less than 3.0 mm.[21] The rationale was derived from previous studies that had shown that GPBA caused less arterial trauma with fewer major dissections and larger arterial lumina.[22,23] GPBA and cutting balloon angioplasty resulted in more favorable angiographic and clinical outcomes compared with POBA, resulting in a lower restenosis and target lesion revascularization rates.

Saphenous Vein Grafts

One of the main limitations of coronary artery bypass surgery is the lifespan of the saphenous vein graft. At 10 years postsurgery, more than half of these bypasses are severely diseased or completely closed. Since the early days of percutaneous transluminal revascularization, balloon angioplasty of saphenous vein grafts was viewed as a logical approach in selected cases compared with the less-attractive alternative of repeat bypass surgery.[24–26] However, the procedure was associated with more significant risks than balloon angioplasty of native coronary vessels. The short-term risks included distal embolization, no-reflow phenomenon, and myocardial infarction, and in the long term, there was a significant occurrence of late cardiac events and a restenosis rate that can exceed 50%. It became clear that balloon angioplasty treatment of saphenous vein grafts was a suboptimal solution that carried significant limitations.

With the advent of stents, the Saphenous Vein De Novo (SAVED) randomized trial compared the safety and efficacy of the Palmaz-Schatz stent with balloon angioplasty in 220 venous bypasses.[27] There was no significant improvement in angiographic restenosis, which was the primary end point of the study. However, stenting was associated with more favorable procedural outcomes, a larger gain in luminal diameter, and a reduction in major cardiac events. This advantage, seen with stenting, led to the widespread use of stents in saphenous vein grafts.

The reduction of restenosis has yet to be demonstrated with drug-eluting stents. What must be kept in mind is that the long-term failure of saphenous vein grafts postintervention correlates not only with restenosis, but also with the natural course that these bypasses follow in the years following surgery.[28,29]

Balloon Angioplasty Through a LIMA Bypass

The challenge posed by performing percutaneous angioplasty to a native artery via an internal mammary artery bypass is primarily correlated with the tortuosities of the conduit.[30] Severe bends may be prohibitive and bear the increased risk of acute closure of the bypass during angioplasty. Moderate tortuosities may allow advancement of a low-profile balloon without permitting advancement of a stent, therefore limiting the chance of a bailout for acute vessel closure during angioplasty. Relatively straight internal mammary conduits are usually approachable with stents. A good balloon result at the anastomosis with the native vessel does not necessarily need to be followed by stenting.

A recent retrospective analysis[31] of 50 patients who underwent percutaneous revascularization of the LAD artery via a LIMA bypass (16 patients) or at the anastomosis site (34 patients), reported a success rate of 88%. The main reasons for failure were lack of adequate guide catheter support and excessive tortuosities of the LIMA. Thirty-four of the successfully treated patients were restudied with angiography. Restenosis was documented in 14 patients (41%). Restenosis rate was significantly higher if stenting was performed (65% vs 18%; $P = .005$). In particular, lesions at the anastomosis did better with balloon angioplasty compared to stenting (restenosis rate 14% vs 80%; $P = .001$).

Other studies have also reported good short- and long-term outcomes with balloon angioplasty.[30,32]

Balloon Angioplasty in Multivessel Disease

Several randomized trials have compared balloon angioplasty with bypass surgery in patients with multivessel disease.[33–35] The derived conclusions were similar: angioplasty in general causes less discomfort to patients and allows for a faster recovery and return to work, while it is associated with a much higher chance of requiring additional revascularization procedures in the follow-up period. Bypass surgery usually offers a more complete revascularization and is associated with less recurrent angina and need for antianginal treatment. The randomized trials found no significant difference in the long-term survival and incidence of myocardial infarction.

The bearing of the balloon angioplasty versus coronary bypass trials is diminishing with time. The evolving technology has resulted in newer modalities of treatment, including the widespread use of the drug-eluting stents and the availability of the IIb/IIIa platelet receptor blockers. The approach to secondary prevention has become more aggressive. Bypass surgery is frequently performed without the use of the heart-lung machine, and new approaches such as the minimally invasive bypass operation are gaining experience. Therefore, a comparison of the most modern percutaneous revascularization technology and pharmacotherapy with the latest approaches in bypass surgery for multivessel disease will be more relevant to our practice.

【 】 RESTENOSIS FOLLOWING CORONARY BALLOON ANGIOPLASTY

The most important limitation of balloon angioplasty second to acute vessel closure is the problem of restenosis. Coronary arteries dilated with a balloon are prone to elastic recoil and acute lumen loss, a process that predisposes to restenosis and is eliminated by coronary stenting. A more important mechanism of restenosis following balloon angioplasty is the development of intimal hyperplasia.

Longitudinal plaque fissures that commonly occur with balloon angioplasty expose the subendothelial and medial components to the circulating blood. Platelets deposit and aggregate at the site of balloon injury and release thromboxane A_2, a very powerful platelet aggregator and vasoconstrictor. Platelets also release platelet-derived growth factor, transforming growth factor-β_1, and insulin-like growth factor 1.[36] Inflammatory cells also release a wide variety of mitogens. Thrombin, which is the most potent known platelet activator, plays a key role following balloon injury and endothelial denudation. Thrombin activity and thrombin receptor expression are upregulated.[37–40] All the growth factors and mitogens in turn will stimulate cell migration and proliferation. Vascular smooth muscle cells will migrate from the media to the intima and deposit extracellular connective tissue matrix proteins. This results in what is referred to as *intimal hyperplasia*. It is the magnitude of this neointimal proliferation and hyperplasia, as well as the degree of geometric remodeling of the vessel, that will determine which lesions will progress to clinically important restenosis following balloon angioplasty.

The most popular angiographic definition of restenosis is a renarrowing of the lumen to 50% or greater in diameter stenosis. When using this definition, restenosis following balloon angioplasty has been estimated to occur at a rate of 30% to 50%. More important than the angiographic appearance of the lesion in follow-up is the clinical relevance of the restenotic process in terms of the emergence of symptoms, documentation of ischemia by noninvasive testing, and long-term events (myocardial infarction, death, and target lesion revascularization).

Restenosis following coronary balloon angioplasty usually occurs within the first few months, most commonly between 6 and 12 weeks. It is very unusual for restenosis to present as an acute myocardial infarction. Rather, the recurrence of a lesion treated with angioplasty is often exposed by the reappearance of symptoms or by functional testing. If a lesion treated with balloon angioplasty does not recur within the first few months, the chance of restenosis thereafter is dramatically reduced to less than 3%.

The risk factors that could potentially play a role in restenosis are many and range from clinical, angiographic, morphologic, and procedural variables to biologic and geometric variables. The mechanism of restenosis following balloon angioplasty is so complex that to this date many of these factors remain poorly defined or totally unknown. It is likely that a confluence of factors has a synergetic effect in causing restenosis. Previous studies that have attempted to identify the importance of clinical variables have found some that correlated with restenosis, such as unstable angina, insulin-dependent diabetes, chronic hemodialysis, hyperlipidemia, hypertension, and prior restenosis. Angiographic variables that seem to increase the risk of restenosis following balloon angioplasty include long lesions, ostial and bifurcating lesions,

small vessels with diffuse disease, total occlusions, and degenerate saphenous vein grafts. The predictive power of many of these variables is poor and derived from small studies. The one factor that is probably the most accepted is that a large lumen postangioplasty favors a lower restenosis rate. This may be explained by the fact that for the same degree of intimal hyperplasia, a larger residual lumen will less likely cause significant renarrowing. The theory of "bigger is better" is probably unrelated to the type of device used in a percutaneous coronary revascularization.

Over the past two decades, numerous studies have been conducted in an effort to find a pharmacologic solution to restenosis following balloon angioplasty. These studies tested agents that could alter one or more of the multiple pathways that are believed to play a role in the restenotic process. Although many animal studies showed promising results, human studies have been largely disappointing. Probucol, an agent with antioxidant and lipid-lowering properties, and AGI-1067, a metabolically stable modification of probucol, may reduce restenosis if administered a few weeks prior to balloon angioplasty.[41] Probucol is not available for use in the United States. Cilostazol, an antiplatelet agent and an inhibitor of intracellular phosphodiesterase activity, has been shown to reduce restenosis following balloon angioplasty.[42] But in the more important randomized Cilostazol for Restenosis (CREST) study,[43,44] cilostazol was shown to reduce restenosis when used as adjunct therapy with bare-metal stenting.

【 】 ADJUNCTIVE PERCUTANEOUS DEVICES

Prior to coronary stenting, several devices emerged that achieve percutaneous arterial revascularization mainly through tissue ablation (rotational atherectomy, excimer laser), tissue excision (directional atherectomy), or controlled plaque fissuring (cutting balloon angioplasty). These newer devices have been used as standalone therapy but more commonly are used as an adjunct to balloon angioplasty. The hope in developing these techniques was to improve the success rate of percutaneous coronary revascularization and to lower restenosis. Several randomized trials have compared each device with balloon angioplasty. A recent meta-analysis by Bittl[45] and colleagues showed no clear advantage for the routine use of these devices.

CONTRAST AGENTS

The first quarter of the 20th century marked the recognition of iodine as the element with the appropriate characteristics for intravascular imaging. Iodine has since remained the element of choice in contrast agent preparations.

Several contrast agents suitable for coronary angiography are currently marketed in the United States (Table 29-2). Similarities and differences between agents can best be appreciated by comparing a few of the important chemical and pharmacologic characteristics: iodine concentration, osmolality, viscosity, and the presence or absence of an ionic salt. In turn, these characteristics can influence some of the immediate effects that these agents have on the cardiovascular and noncardiovascular systems.

TABLE 29-2

Pharmacologic and Chemical Properties of Several Commercially Available Contrast Agents

	IODINE-CONTAINING MOLECULE	IONIC RATIO	CATIONS	OSMOLALITY (mOsm/kg)	VISCOSITY
Angiovist	Diatrizoate	1.5	Methylglucamine, sodium	2076	8.4
Hexabrix	Ioxaglate	3	Methylglucamine, sodium	600	7.5
Hypaque	Diatrizoate	1.5	Methylglucamine, sodium	1690	9.0
Isovue	Iopimadol	3	None	796	9.4
Omnipaque	Iohexol	3	None	844	10.4
Renografin	Diatrizoate	1.5	Methylglucamine, sodium	1940	8.4
Visipaque	Iodixanol	6	None	290	11.8

【 】 IONIC SALT

All currently available contrast agents have in common a tri-iodinated benzene ring. To preserve the solubility condition in aqueous solutions, the benzene ring relies on an ionizing functional group in its molecular structure. This ionizing functional group (anion) must be associated with an ionic salt (cation). Ionic salts that are most commonly used are sodium and methylglucamine (meglumine).

If the ionizable functional group is replaced by a nonionizing functional group that would preserve aqueous solubility (eg, the carboxyl group is replaced by a sugar), the need of an associated cation would not be required. Such agents are termed "nonionic" and have only one osmotically active particle (see later discussion).

【 】 IODINE RATIO

This is the ratio of the number of iodine atoms in a molecule to the osmotically active particles that the molecule produces in solution. The osmotically active particles are the anions and the cations. For example, a contrast agent with a basic structure of a tri-iodinated benzene ring contains three iodine atoms, an anion, and a cation. The iodine ratio in this situation is 1.5 (three iodine atoms and two osmotically active particles). An iodine ratio of 3 is obtained by linking two tri-iodinated benzene rings and converting one of the carboxyl groups to an amide. Such an ionic agent would contain six iodine atoms, an anion, and a cation (iodine ratio of 3). If in this same situation the ionizable functional group is replaced by a nonionizing functional group, the iodine ratio would be 6 (six iodine atoms and one osmotically active particle).

The higher the iodine ratio, the better the radiopacity of the contrast agent. A higher ratio can be achieved either by increasing the iodine content or by reducing the osmotically active particles.

【 】 OSMOLALITY

This term refers to the number of active particles in solution and is, therefore, related to the iodine ratio. A solution can be hypertonic, isotonic, or hypotonic. The osmolality of a contrast agent can be reduced by replacing the ionizable functional group with a nonionizing functional group. Compared with nonionic agents, ionic agents are significantly hyperosmolar because they dissociate into separate ions in solution.

【 】 VISCOSITY

This term refers to the friction of the contrast agent's molecular component in blood. Solutions that are very viscous are more difficult to inject during angiography. Higher iodine concentration offers better radiopacity at the expense of increasing the contrast agent's viscosity. Viscosity also depends on the size of the molecular component of the contrast agent. Viscosity can be significantly decreased by warming the contrast agent to body temperature.

【 】 SIDE EFFECTS

Ionic and high-osmolar contrast agents are more likely to cause electrophysiologic disturbances such as bradyarrhythmias, prolongation of the QT and QRS intervals, ST-segment depression and T-wave inversion.[46,47] They can also be responsible for causing hemodynamic alterations, including transient reduction in left ventricular contractility and systolic blood pressure. Some of the untoward effects are felt to be related in part to the calcium-chelating properties of these agents. Nonionic and low-osmolar contrast agents, on the other hand, cause fewer side effects.

The issue of increased thrombogenicity with nonionic agents has been the focus of much debate. It appears, however, that nonionic contrast agents do not add a significant risk of thromboembolism when used in percutaneous interventions. Despite the fact that low-osmolar contrast agents are considerably more expensive than the high-osmolar agents, their use in high-risk patients is totally justified.

REFERENCES

1. Albiero R, Silber S, Di Mario C, et al. Cutting balloon versus conventional balloon angioplasty for the treatment of in-stent restenosis: Results of the restenosis cutting balloon evaluation trial (RESCUT) *J Am Coll Cardiol*. 2004;43:943.
2. Smith SC, Dove JT, Jacobs AK, et al. ACC/AHA Guidelines for percutaneous coronary intervention (revision of the 1993 PTCA Guidelines). *J Am Coll Cardiol*. 2001;37:2239.
3. Williams DO, Holubkov R, Yeh W, et al. Percutaneous coronary intervention in the current era compared with 1985–1986. The NHLBI Registries. *Circulation*. 2000;102:2945.

4. Holmes DR Jr, Kip KE, Yeh W, et al. Long-term analysis of conventional coronary balloon angioplasty and an initial "stent-like" result. The NHLBI PTCA Registry. *J Am Coll Cardiol.* 1998;32:590.

5. Topol EJ, Ellis SG, Fishman J, et al. Multicenter study of percutaneous transluminal angioplasty for right coronary artery ostial stenosis. *J Am Coll Cardiol.* 1987;9:1214.

6. Jain SP, Liu MW, Dean LS, et al. Comparison of balloon angioplasty versus debulking devices versus stenting in right coronary ostial lesions. *Am J Cardiol.* 1997;79:1334.

7. Mavromatis K, Ghazzal Z, Veledar E, et al. Comparison of outcomes of percutaneous coronary intervention of ostial versus nonostial narrowing of the major epicardial coronary arteries. *Am J Cardiol.* 2004;94:583.

8. Meier B, Gruentzig B, Hollman J, et al. Does length or eccentricity of coronary stenoses influence the outcome of transluminal dilatation? *Circulation.* 1983;67:497.

9. Ellis SG, Roubin GS, King SB III, et al. Importance of stenosis morphology in the estimation of restenosis risk after elective percutaneous transluminal coronary angioplasty. *Am J Cardiol.* 1989;63:30.

10. Tenaglia A, Zidar J, Jackman J, et al. Treatment of long coronary artery narrowings with long angioplasty balloon catheters. *Am J Cardiol.* 1993;71:1274–1277.

11. Serruys PW, Foley DP, Suttorp MJ, et al. A randomized comparison of the value of additional stenting after optimal balloon angioplasty for long coronary lesions: Final results of the additional value of NIR stents for treatment of long coronary lesions (ADVANCE) study. *J Am Coll Cardiol.* 2002;39:393.

12. Bauters C, Hubert E, Prat A, et al. Predictors of restenosis after coronary stent implantation. *J Am Coll Cardiol.* 1998;31:1291.

13. Kastrati A, Elezi S, Dirschinger J, et al. Influence of lesion length on restenosis after coronary stent placement. *Am J Cardiol.* 1999;83:1617.

14. Colombo A, De Gregorio J, Moussa I, et al. Intravascular ultrasound-guided percutaneous transluminal coronary angioplasty with provisional spot stenting for treatment of long coronary lesions. *J Am Coll Cardiol.* 2001;38:1427.

15. Moses JW, Leon MB, Popma JJ, et al. Sirolimus-eluting stents versus standard stents in patients with stenosis in a native coronary artery. *N Engl J Med.* 2003;349:1315.

16. Degertekin M, Arampatzis CA, Lemos PA, et al. Very long sirolimus-eluting stent implantation for de novo coronary lesions. *Am J Cardiol.* 2004;93:826.

17. Schunkert H, Harrell L, Palacios IF. Implications of small reference vessel diameter in patients undergoing percutaneous coronary revascularization. *J Am Coll Cardiol.* 1999;34:40.

18. Karrillon GJ, Morice MC, Benveniste E, et al. Intracoronary stent implantation without ultrasound guidance and with replacement of conventional anticoagulation by antiplatelet therapy. 30-day clinical outcome of the French Multicenter Registry. *Circulation.* 1996;94:1519.

19. Keane D, Azar AJ, de Jaegere P, et al. Clinical and angiographic outcome of elective stent implantation in small coronary vessels: An analysis of the BENESTENT trial. *Semin Interv Cardiol.* 1996;1:255.

20. Briguori C, Nishida T, Adamian M, et al. Coronary stenting versus balloon angioplasty in small coronary artery with complex lesions. *Cathet Cardiovasc Interv.* 2000;50:390.

21. Umeda H, Iwase M, Kanda H, et al. Promising efficacy of primary gradual and prolonged balloon angioplasty in small coronary arteries: A randomized comparison with cutting balloon angioplasty and conventional balloon angioplasty. *Am Heart J.* 2004;147:E4.

22. Ohman EM, Marquis JF, Ricci DR, et al. A randomized comparison of the effects of gradual prolonged versus standard primary balloon inflation on early and late outcome. Results of a multicenter clinical trial. Perfusion Balloon Catheter Study Group. *Circulation.* 1994;89:1118.

23. Miketic S, Carlsson J, Tebbe U. Influence of gradually increased slow balloon inflation on restenosis after coronary angioplasty. *Am Heart J.* 1998;135:709.

24. Douglas JS Jr, Gruentzig AR, King SB III, et al. Percutaneous transluminal coronary angioplasty in patients with prior coronary bypass surgery. *J Am Coll Cardiol.* 1983;2:745.

25. Dorros G, Johnson WD, Tector AJ, et al. Percutaneous transluminal coronary angioplasty in patients with prior coronary artery bypass grafting. *J Thorac Cardiovasc Surg.* 1984;87:17.

26. Platko WP, Hollman J, Whitlow PL, Franco I. Percutaneous transluminal angioplasty of saphenous vein graft stenosis: Long-term follow-up. *J Am Coll Cardiol.* 1989;14:1645.

27. Savage MP, Douglas JS Jr, Fischman DL, et al. Stent placement compared with balloon angioplasty for obstructed coronary bypass grafts. Saphenous Vein De Novo Trial Investigators. *N Engl J Med.* 1997;337:740.

28. Lawrie GM, Lie JT, Morris GC Jr, Beazley HL. Vein graft patency and intimal proliferation after aortocoronary bypass: Early and long-term angiopathologic correlations. *Am J Cardiol.* 1976;38:856.

29. Hamby RI, Aintablian A, Handler M, et al. Aortocoronary saphenous vein bypass grafts: Long-term patency, morphology and blood flow in patients with patent grafts early after surgery. *Circulation.* 1979;60:901.

30. Hearne SE, Davidson CJ, Zidar JP, et al. Internal mammary artery graft angioplasty: Acute and long-term outcome. *Cathet Cardiovasc Diagn.* 1998;44:153; discussion 157.

31. Kockeritz U, Reynen K, Knaut M, Strasser RH. Results of angioplasty (with or without stent) at the site of a narrowed coronary anastomosis of the left internal mammary artery graft or via the internal mammary artery. *Am J Cardiol.* 2004;93:1531.

32. Gruberg L, Dangas G, Mehran R, et al. Percutaneous revascularization of the internal mammary artery graft: Short- and long-term outcomes *J Am Coll Cardiol.* 2000;35:944.

33. King SB, Lembo NJ, Weintraub WS, et al. A randomized trial comparing coronary angioplasty with coronary bypass surgery. Emory Angioplasty versus Surgery Trial (EAST). *N Engl J Med.* 1994;331:1044.

34. Comparison of coronary bypass surgery with angioplasty in patients with multivessel disease. The Bypass Angioplasty Revascularization Investigation (BARI) Investigators [published erratum appears in *N Engl J Med* 1997;336:147]. *N Engl J Med.* 1996;335:217.

35. Hamm CW, Reimers J, Ischinger T, et al. A randomized study of coronary angioplasty compared with bypass surgery in patients with symptomatic multivessel coronary disease. German Angioplasty Bypass Surgery Investigation (GABI). *N Engl J Med.* 1994;331:1037.

36. Ruggeri ZM. New insights into the mechanisms of platelet adhesion and aggregation. *Semin Hematol.* 1994;31,229.

37. Patterson C, Stouffer GA, madamanchi N, Runge MS. New tricks for old dogs: Nonthrombotic effects of thrombin in vessel wall biology. *Circ Res.* 2001;88:987.

38. McNamara CA, Sarembock IJ, Bachhuber BG, et al. Thrombin and vascular smooth muscle cell proliferation: Implications for atherosclerosis and restenosis. *Semin Thromb Hemost.* 1996;22:139.

39. Marmur JD, Merlini PA, Sharma SK, et al. Thrombin generation in human coronary arteries after percutaneous transluminal balloon angioplasty. *J Am Coll Cardiol.* 1994;24:1484.

40. Wilcox JN, Rodriguez J, Subramanian R, et al. Characterization of thrombin receptor expression during vascular lesion formation. *Circ Res.* 1994;75:1029.

41. Tardif JC, Gregoire J, Schwartz L, et al. Canadian Antioxidant Restenosis Trial (CART-1) Investigators. Effects of AGI-1067 and probucol after percutaneous coronary interventions. *Circulation.* 2003;107:552.

42. Tsuchikane E, Fukuhara A, Kobayashi T, et al. Impact of cilostazol on restenosis after percutaneous coronary balloon angioplasty. *Circulation.* 1999;100:21.

43. Weintraub WS, Foster J, Culler SD, et al. Cilostazol for RESTenosis trial. Methods for the economic and quality of life supplement to the cilostazol for RESTenosis (CREST) trial. *J Invasive Cardiol.* 2004;16:257.

44. Douglas JS, Weintraub WS, Holmes D. Rationale and design of the randomized, multicenter, cilostazol for RESTenosis (CREST) trial. *Clin Cardiol.* 2003;26:451.

45. Bittl JA, Chew DP, Topol EJ, et al. Meta-analysis of randomized trials of percutaneous transluminal coronary angioplasty versus atherectomy, cutting ballon atherotomy, or laser angioplasty. *J Amer Coll Card.* 2004;43:936.

46. Brinker J. What every cardiologist should know about intravascular contrast. *Rev Cardiovasc Med.* 2003;4(suppl 5):S19.

47. Matthai WH Jr, Hirshfeld JW Jr. Choice of contrast agents for cardiac angiography: Review and recommendations based on clinically important distinctions. *Cathet Cardiovasc Diagn.* 1991;22:278.

Note Added in Proof:

As this book is going to press in late 2006, issues have arisen that deserve some comment. Stenting has become the default strategy for interventional cardiology procedures. And in the past few years, drug-eluting stenting has been almost universally adopted in the United States. Whereas none of the clinical trials have individually suggested increased complication rates, none have proved a decrease in death or myocardial infraction.

Two recent meta-analyses conducted by investigators in Switzerland showed, in one case, a trend toward increased total mortality in the patients receiving drug-eluting stenting compared to those receiving metal stents. In the other, the events of death and myocardial infarction were excessive in the drug-eluting stent groups. Although noncardiac death seems to have driven much of this difference, these reports heighten the concern expressed by many cardiologists who have observed late stent thrombosis, especially after discontinuation of thienopyridine and aspirin therapy. That issue was highlighted by the report of the Basket Late Trial at the American College of Cardiology Scientific Sessions in 2006. In that study, patients were given aspirin and clopidogrel for six months after which only aspirin was continued. During the subsequent year, there was excess death and myocardial infarction suggesting late stent thrombosis in the drug-eluting stent group. The two meta-analyses reported at the European Society of Cardiology meeting in September of 2006 only heightened this concern. Pathologic evidence reported by Virmani showed that patients who had died secondary to late stent thrombosis had impaired endothelialization over the drug-eluting stents.[1]

Whereas the evidence for increased risk of late thrombosis in drug-eluting stents is far from definitive, the extensive utilization of these stents in more complex cases and the documented association of discontinuation of double antiplatelet therapy and late stent thrombosis have created concern about the total duration of these antithrombotic measures. Some would argue that the clear reduction in need for repeat intervention outweighs the small risk of late stent thrombosis. Others would say that any decrease in safety would offset the benefit of avoiding repeat interventions. As pointed out in Chapter 30, the almost universal shift to drug-eluting stents has resulted in avoidance of approximately five repeat interventions per 100 patients treated. Examination of registries which do not mandate angiographic follow up continue to suggest a re-intervention rate with bare metal stents below 10% within the first year.[2]

From the perspective of the physician recommending stenting, it is clear that judgment should be exercised, weighing the relative risk of restenosis for the individual patient and lesion being treated against the necessity and risk for long-term antithrombotic therapy. Patients facing a need for discontinuation of antiplatelet therapy who have a relatively low risk of restenosis may benefit greater from bare metal stents. On the other hand, patients with lesions with a high risk of restenosis without contraindications to double antiplatelet therapy will be best served by drug-eluting stenting. Obviously there will be many shades of gray.

For the future, improved technology will certainly evolve. Returning to less effective technology is seldom a solution, and at present there are many approaches to reducing the risk of late stent thrombosis including polymeric codings that may be antithrombotic, methods of drug release from polymers that are biodegradable and therefore will not exist after a period of time, and methods of drug release that will not require a polymer at all. The issue of the drugs being utilized is also of interest. Will drugs that inhibit endothelialization to a major degree pose a long-term risk necessitating permanent antiplatelet therapy in some patients?

Patients who have had drug-eluting stents implanted should realize the absolute risk posed by these devices in the late follow-up is very small and there is significant heterogeneity in that risk depending on patient factors and lesion factors. The overall outcomes in the drug-eluting stent era with improved adjunctive and preventive therapy as reflected in the ARTS II registry are impressive. The duration of antiplatelet therapy at the present time should depend on informed physician judgment as to the relative benefits of such therapy balanced against bleeding risk for the patient. It is anticipated that in the future stent technology will evolve to the point that late stent thrombosis will no longer be an issue in interventional cardiology.

Spencer B. King III, September 2006

---

[1] Jones M, Finn AV, Farb A, et al. Pathology of drug-eluting stents in humans: delayed healing and late thrombotic risk. J Am Coll Cardiol 48:193–202, 2006.

[2] Yock CA, Isbill JM, King SB. Bare metal stent outcomes in an unselected patient population. Clin Cardiol 29:352–356, 2006.

CHAPTER (30)

Coronary Stenting

Spencer B. King, III, MD, and Alan C. Yeung, MD

Balloon angioplasty opened the era of interventional cardiology, however, next to the steerable guidewires, the development of coronary stenting was the most important breakthrough since the birth of this new specialty. The first coronary stents were implanted by Sigwart in Lausanne and Puel in Toulouse in 1986.[1] These were self-expanding stents made of a stainless steel. The following year, coil stents were implanted in the United States at Emory University[2,3] and the first slotted tube stent was implanted in Sao Paulo, Brazil. These stents were initially used to scaffold the artery and prevent the early recoil and reclosure of the vessel leading to the need for emergency bypass surgery. The evaluation of stents for reduction in restenosis would proceed over the next several years, and it was not until 1994 that elective use of stents was approved by the Food and Drug Administration (FDA).[4] Additional improvement in stenting outcomes came with the understanding that complete expansion of stents with good apposition to the wall required high-pressure balloon inflations. Intravascular ultrasound played a pivotal role in showing that stents were commonly underexpanded, and this led to early restenosis and thrombotic complications.[5]

In the first few years of stenting, it was considered necessary to use warfarin anticoagulation, which produced a prolonged hospitalization and a high incidence of thrombotic and bleeding complications. A randomized trial of stent placement comparing warfarin anticoagulation with a combination of aspirin and ticlopidine (Intracoronary Stenting and Antithrombotic Regimen [ISAR]) showed a significantly decreased incidence of bleeding and improved efficacy of the strategy using double antiplatelet therapy.[6] This was confirmed by the Stent Anticoagulation Regimen Study (STARS), again showing that a lower stent thrombosis rate was associated with the simpler strategy of aspirin and ticlopidine. The duration of therapy for these strategies was 30 days; however, a sub-

sequent report suggested that 14 days of ticlopidine might be adequate for prophylaxis against stent thrombosis.[7] More recently with performance of the Clopidogrel Aspirin Stent Interventional Cooperative Study (CLASSICS), ticlopidine has largely been abandoned in the United States in favor of clopidogrel based on equal efficacy and fewer complications of neutropenia, thrombocytopenia, or early discontinuation of the drug because of rashes or gastrointestinal disturbances.[8]

BARE-METAL STENTS

【 】 USE OF STENTING TO PREVENTING ACUTE VASCULAR CLOSURE

Before the introduction of stenting, dissections and incomplete dilation of coronary arteries commonly resulted in acute closure necessitating bypass surgery. The major reduction in this complication has been the principal contribution of stenting. In the years between 1980 and 1987, the need for urgent bypass surgery following balloon angioplasty was approximately 5% to 6%. After full introduction of stenting in the years 1996 through 1999, that rate had dropped to 1.2%, and currently it is far below 1%.[9]

Trials were carried out testing the routine use of coronary stenting versus balloon angioplasty with stenting only used for complications and inadequate results. The Optimal Angioplasty Versus Primary Stenting (OPUS-1) trial showed that routine stenting resulted in a significantly lower incidence of death, myocardial infarction, and target vessel revascularization than occurred in the provisional stenting group (6.1% vs 14.9%; *P* = .003).[10] It was also necessary to place stents in 37% of the provisional stenting group. Other studies involving careful assessment of angioplasty results with intravascular ultrasound and pressure wires have shown that when balloon angioplasty is completely successful in opening the artery without any residual obstruction or pressure gradient, then the results are comparable to stenting. Nonetheless, stenting has become the dominant strategy in interventional cardiology for well over 90% of lesions.

A meta-analysis of 29 trials of routine stenting versus balloon angioplasty with provisional stenting for inadequate results did not show a difference in the major outcomes of death, myocardial infarction, or the need for coronary bypass surgery. Nonetheless, routine stenting resulted in a reduction in the need for repeat interventions, with an odds ratio of 0.59. Translated into an absolute reduction, this meant that 5 patients per 100 treated would avoid reintervention when routine stenting strategy was used.[11] These data were particularly convincing for native coronary arteries ranging from 3 to 4 mm in diameter, stenotic saphenous vein grafts, total occlusions, and restenotic lesions following balloon angioplasty in the setting of acute myocardial infarction. The data have been somewhat less convincing in small coronary arteries and those with long diffuse disease, ostial disease, and side branch lesions and bifurcation situations.

[ ] TRIALS THAT SUPPORT THE USE OF STENTING OVER BALLOON ANGIOPLASTY

Some of the pivotal trials that have resulted in stenting becoming the dominant therapy in interventional cardiology are important to review. The Stent Restenosis Study (STRESS)[4] showed a reduction in restenosis from 42.1% to 31.6% with stenting. The Belgian Netherlands Stent (BENESTENT) study from Europe produced a reduction from 32% to 22% with stenting and BENESTENT-2, utilizing the same Palmaz-Schatz stent but with heparin coating, resulted in a reduction in restenosis from 31% to 16%. Each of these trials was performed in native arteries with de novo lesions. Arteries with restenosis after balloon angioplasty were investigated in the Restenosis Stent Trial (REST),[12] which showed that restenosis was reduced from 32% with balloon angioplasty to 18% with stenting. Vein grafts with stenotic lesions were investigated in the Saphenous Vein De Novo (SAVED) trial.[13] The investigators found reduction in restenosis from 47% to 36%, which was not significant; however, clinical events were significantly reduced. Finally, chronic total occlusion was investigated in the Total Occlusion Study of Canada (TOSCA) trial, which showed reduction in restenosis from 70% to 55% with stenting and, more importantly, a very significant reduction in follow-up total occlusion in the group that underwent stenting. These studies were carried out using the initial Palmaz-Schatz stent, which used a slotted tube design.

[ ] COMPARISON OF PALMAZ–SCHATZ STENT WITH NEW DESIGNS

When newly designed stents became available, the FDA mandated that they be tested against the Palmaz-Schatz stent. Four trials of these second-generation stents were carried out, testing the Multi-link, Paragon, Nirstent, and Radius stents against the Palmaz-Schatz stent. Follow-up angiography demonstrated no significant difference in restenosis rates with these new designs. Nonetheless, improvements in stent technology have resulted in lower profile stents and safer delivery systems. In recent years improvement in stent design has not required head-to-head comparison with previous designs, because the FDA has streamlined the process for stent development.

[ ] OTHER IMPROVEMENTS IN MATERIALS

Most stents were manufactured using standard 316L stainless steel because this was a widely approved material in medical applications. Other materials, such as cobalt chromium stents, have been approved, leading to development of thinner and stronger stent struts. Stents have also been coated with heparin and other materials to try to decrease thrombogenicity. The architecture of stents continues to evolve with a balance being solved between open cells enabling access to side branches and adequate coverage to ensure proper scaffolding of the stented arterial segment (Figure 30-1).

[ ] STENTING AS AN ALTERNATIVE TO BYPASS SURGERY

Previous trials comparing balloon angioplasty with bypass surgery in patients with multivessel coronary artery disease demonstrated comparable clinical outcomes in selected patients with the exception of those with diabetes mellitus, who benefited disproportionately from the surgical approach. Since the development of coronary stenting, reevaluation of stenting versus angioplasty has been performed in three trials: the Arterial Revascularization Therapy Study (ARTS),[14] the Stent or Surgery (SOS) trial,[15] and the ERACI trial.[16] The ARTS trial showed comparable survival without stroke or myocardial infarction at 3 years of 87.2% for percutaneous coronary intervention (PCI) and 88.4% for surgery. The need for repeat revascularization was 26.7% at 3 years, a dramatic reduction from that seen in previous balloon angioplasty trials. The SOS trial randomized 998 patients with multivessel disease to stenting or surgery and showed a 2-year mortality rate of 5% in the stent group and 2% in the surgery group. The ERACI trial of 230 patients showed no difference in survival at followup (96.4% for PCI vs 95% for surgery).

There is no doubt that stenting has improved the need for repeat revascularization in these patients with multivessel disease and has made PCI more competitive with surgery for some selected patients. It is yet unclear whether stenting will provide comparable long-term survival to bypass surgery in patients with diabetes. A meta-analysis of 13 interventional trials, dominated by balloon angioplasty trials, showed a mortality advantage for surgery, which was not apparent at 1 or 3 years but became evident at 5 years.[17] A summary of the results of some of these trials is listed in Figure 30-2. The stent versus surgery trials have included too few diabetic patients for too short a follow-up period to make any claims to comparability with surgery for this group.

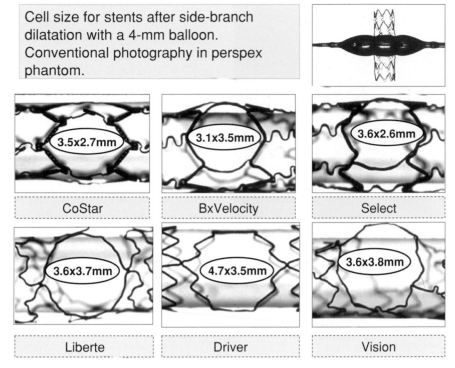

Cell size for stents after side-branch dilatation with a 4-mm balloon. Conventional photography in perspex phantom.

CoStar	BxVelocity	Select
3.5x2.7mm	3.1x3.5mm	3.6x2.6mm

Liberte	Driver	Vision
3.6x3.7mm	4.7x3.5mm	3.6x3.8mm

FIGURE 30-1. The appearance of several different stent design following the expansion of a 4 mm balloon through the cells is illustrated. The ability to expand the cells is sometimes helpful for side branch access. *(Courtesy of Dr. John Ormiston.)*

【 】 STENTING IN SMALL VESSELS

Several trials of second-generation stents have been carried out in vessels smaller than those studied in the pivotal stent versus balloon angioplasty trials. Because restenosis is inversely related to vessel size, studies have been carried out in vessels smaller than 3 mm that compare stenting with balloon angioplasty, with use of stenting only for complications or inadequate results. Eleven of these studies were combined in a meta-analysis.[18] Stents studied

were the Nir, Multilink, Hepacoat B, Jostent, Biodivysio, and Tenax. Baseline features included reference vessel diameter of 2.35, length of 9.9 mm, and final minimum lumen diameter in the balloon group of 1.96 and in the stent group of 2.26. Cross-over from balloon to stenting occurred in 19% of the patients, and stents could not be delivered in 2% of the stent group.

Only three of these trials showed a significant reduction in restenosis; however, the aggregate restenosis rate was 34.2% in the balloon angioplasty group and 25.8% in the stent groups. Late loss as expected was greater in the stent group (0.76 mm) compared with the balloon angioplasty group (0.54 mm). These results translated into improved clinical outcomes due to a reduction in the need for new revascularization procedures. Routine stenting resulted in less target vessel revascularization (12.5% for stenting vs 17% for balloon angioplasty). Thus, 4.5 patients per 100 avoided a repeat procedure by being enrolled in the routine stenting arm. This difference may be slightly exaggerated because of the requirement for routine angiographic follow up in these patients. Although small vessels undergo restenosis more frequently than larger vessels, the clinical manifestation of this might be less because of the smaller area of myocardium supplied by the vessel.

Historical CABG vs PCI Trials

Trial	No stents used / Stents used	Superior Treatment Modality			
	Clinical Parameters			Angiographic Endpoints	Cost Assessment
	Mortality & MI	Angina Relief	Repeat Revascularization		
GABI	PCI	PCI	CABG	No difference	n/a
EAST	No difference	CABG	CABG	CABG	PCI
RITA	No difference	CABG	CABG	n/a	n/a
ERACI	No difference	CABG	CABG	n/a	PCI
CABRI	No difference	CABG	CABG	n/a	n/a
BARI	No difference	n/a	CABG	n/a	n/a
MASS-2	CABG (MI)	n/a	CABG	n/a	No difference
AWESOME	No difference	No difference	CABG	n/a	n/a
ERACI-2	PCI	n/a	CABG	CABG	No difference
SoS	CABG (Mortality)	CABG	CABG	n/a	n/a
ARTS	No difference	n/a	CABG	n/a	PCI

FIGURE 30-2. Eleven of the coronary artery by pass grating (CABG) vs percutaneous coronary intervention (PCI) trials are summarized. All of the stent trials use bare-metal stents. n/a = not applicable.

DRUG–ELUTING STENTS

Coronary stents eliminate two of the components of restenosis—namely, early vascular recoil and late constrictive remodeling—but they accentuate neointimal proliferation compared with balloon

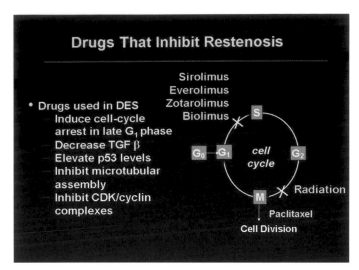

FIGURE 30-3. Effect on cell cycle of sirolimus and paclitaxel and other agents under investigation for use in drug-eluting stents.

angioplasty alone. The understanding of this accentuated tissue growth within the stent led to the development of local delivery methods for controlling that process.

Drug-eluting stents have now rapidly been developed, and two platforms have been approved for clinical use. They are the sirolimus-eluting stent of Johnson & Johnson/Cordis and the paclitaxel stent of Boston Scientific. Other agents with antiproliferative or antineoplastic properties are being tested. Sirolimus is an immunosuppressive macrolide antifungal agent that acts to block the G1S phase of cellular replication, and paclitaxel is an antimicrotubular agent that has its effect at the G0/G1 and G1/M phases of the cell cycle. Both of these agents interrupt the cell cycle and act to block smooth muscle proliferation and migration, resulting in decrease in neointimal formation (Figure 30-3). The pivotal trials resulting in approval of these two stents were the SIRIUS and TAXUS trials.

The SIRIUS trial, which randomized 1058 patients with lesions ranging from 15 to 30 mm assigned to treatment with BX Velocity stent coated with the polymer containing sirolimus or the BX Velocity stent without coating or drug. Restenosis within the stent was reduced from 35% to 3.2%, and when the stent edges were included, the reduction in restenosis was from 37% to 9%, ($P >$. 001). In this trial with a mandated angiographic follow up at 9 months, the target lesion revascularization was reduced from 17% with the bare-metal stent to 4% with the drug-eluting stent.

The paclitaxel-eluting stent was investigated in several trials. The pivotal trial, TAXUS 4, randomized 1314 patients to use of a bare-metal stent versus a paclitaxel-impregnated polymer-coated stent. The restenosis rate for patients receiving the bare-metal stent was 26.6% compared with 7.9% in the group receiving the TAXUS stent. The rapamycin- and paclitaxel-eluting stents have been effective for a broad range of vessel sizes, lesion lengths, and clinical conditions.

Interestingly, in the SIRIUS trial, the restenosis rate for bare-metal versus sirolimus-eluting stents was reduced from 30.2% to 1.9% in 3.3-mm vessels, from 36.5% to 6.3% in 2.8-mm vessels, and from 42.9% to 18.6% in 2.3-mm vessels. Similar data were reported from the TAXUS 4 trial, which showed reductions in vessels greater than 3 mm from 15.2% to 6.8%, in vessels from 2.5

to 3 mm from 27.8% to 6.7%, and in vessels smaller than 2.5 mm from 38.5% to 10.2%.[19] Therefore, although small vessels continue to have higher restenosis rates with bare-metal and drug-eluting stents, the absolute impact on reduction of restenosis is clearly substantial in small vessels. The REALITY trial compared to the two stents available in the United States. Among 1353 patients, there was no significant difference in stent restenosis: 7% for CYPHER and 8.3% for TAXUS. Major adverse cardiac events were also not different: 9.2% for CYPHER and 10.6% for TAXUS.[19a]

The restenosis risk with drug-eluting stents has been associated in part with injury at the end of the stent placement. Predilation with balloons prior to stenting may account for some of this effect. The PIXEL trial, in which stents were placed without predilation, showed a particularly low restenosis rate at the edges of the stent in the group without predilation.

【 】 WHAT IS THE VALUE OF DRUG-ELUTING STENTS OVER EXISTING BARE-METAL STENTS?

To examine this question, we should understand the contemporary results with use of bare-metal stents as a baseline for appreciating the added benefit of drug-eluting stents. The comparative trials of drug-eluting stents versus bare-metal stents were carried out to establish safety and efficacy of the new product in order to gain FDA approval. The study design and end points were agreed on by the sponsor and the FDA. The primary end point of these trials was the occurrence of restenosis, defined by the amount of narrowing within the stent exceeding 50% at follow up and the relative loss of lumen diameter between the immediate post-stenting angiogram and the follow-up angiogram at 6 to 9 months. The rationale for using late loss and restenosis rates as the end points was based on the fact that these generate a variable number that can demonstrate a significant difference with a relatively small sample size, thereby reducing the cost and time required to perform the trials. Following patients with real clinical end points would require larger sample sizes.

In addition to the angiographic end points, however, the clinical events are also recorded. Major adverse cardiac events (MACE) are defined as death, myocardial infarction, and revascularization of the target vessel. Examination of the SIRIUS trial late results shows that the difference in "clinical events" is entirely determined by late target vessel revascularization (3.9% vs 16.6%). There was no difference in mortality or death in the hospital or out of the hospital. Because MACE ranges from the hard clinical end point of death to redilation, we should examine how well MACE reflects the impact of drug-eluting stents in the practice of interventional cardiology.

MACE is confounded by the mandated angiographic follow up. Clinical events of repeat intervention are counted after the protocol angiogram is obtained, whether or not the patient has symptoms or even documented ischemia; thus, the overall incidence of MACE may be inflated compared with that of patients not enrolled in clinical trials. It is estimated that as many as 50% of reinterventions in bare-metal stent groups may be performed in the absence of a clinical indication. The Kaplan-Meier curves of

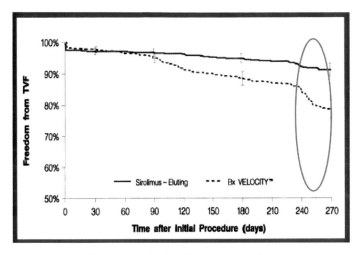

FIGURE 30-4. SIRIUS trial: Kaplan-Meier curves of freedom from target vessel failure. "Ocular-stenotic" effect at nine months angiographic follow-up.

freedom from target vessel failure from the SIRIUS trial illustrate this point (Figure 30-4). At the time of the follow-up angiogram, there is a bolus of patients undergoing repeat interventional procedures. This scenario is greater in the control group, probably because neointimal proliferation is greater in this group and even if a patient has not been symptomatic, repeat intervention may be tempting. It should be understood that with bare-metal stenting, the narrowing seen at 6 to 9 months is usually greater than would be seen at 3 years due to retraction and volume loss of the neointimal tissue.[20]

Results from the ARTS II registry are encouraging. Patients similar to those in ARTS were registered. One year major coronary and cerebrovascular events were equal to the CABG group from ARTS and significantly improved compared to the stent group from ARTS.[20a]

Balancing the reduction in revascularization is the concern about late stent thrombosis. The BASKET registry showed a threefold higher thrombosis rate with DES compared to bare metal stents.

[ ] IS RESTENOSIS A RISK FACTOR FOR FUTURE DEATH?

Several trials have failed to show that the occurrence of restenosis is a factor leading to increased mortality. The largest study of this subject compared patients who developed restenosis following balloon angioplasty with those who remained free from restenosis on follow-up angiograms.[21] After 6 years' follow up, no difference was noted between patients who underwent restenosis and those who did not. Therefore, restenosis is not a fatal event.

[ ] WHAT IMPACT WILL DRUG–ELUTING STENTS HAVE ON SURVIVAL, MYOCARDIAL INFARCTION, AND REVASCULARIZATION?

The RESEARCH registry, conducted in Rotterdam, was a consecutive case registry of patients treated with sirolimus-eluting stents and followed for 1 year. Data from this registry were compared with results collected from a consecutive series of patients the year before drug-eluting stents became available. There was no difference in mortality between these two consecutive series from the same institution (pre-drug-eluting stent, 4.1% vs post–sirolimus-eluting stent, 3.7%; P = .69).[22] The same registry examined the 6-month reintervention rate in the two cohorts. Reintervention in the sirolimus-eluting group was 2.7% at 6 months and in the presirolimus stent group, 7.1%. This translates to 4.4 reinterventions avoided per 100 patients routinely treated with drug-eluting stents. At 1 year, the difference had widened to more than 6 procedures avoided per 100 patients treated.[23]

A large clinical registry, the *Goodroe Data Warehouse*, was used to examine outcomes in patients treated with bare-metal stents prior to the availability of drug-eluting stents. Patients, who were entered from 23 hospitals (n = 14,025 patients), were followed for the occurrence of reintervention and classified as to whether reintervention was performed in the target vessel, at the target site, and whether other lesions were also treated. At 1 year follow up, 20% of patients had undergone diagnostic catheterization, 11.5% had undergone PCI, and 1.5%, bypass surgery. Intervention involved the target vessel in 9.7% of patients; however, that reintervention was attributed to the target segment in only 5.7%.[24] Revascularization of segments that were not initially treated will not be altered by the use of drug-eluting stents. There is no doubt, however, that drug-eluting stents will reduce the target segment reintervention rate. The e-cypher registry, from Europe, reported remarkably low target lesion revascularization rate of 1% at 6 months with use of drug-eluting stents. This registry also reported an exceptionally low non–Q-wave myocardial infarction rate of 0.62%, far below any other reported series. It is important to note, however, that such volunteer registries may reflect some underreporting of events.

A carefully performed registry, sponsored by the National Heart Lung and Blood Institute (NHLBI), is the NHLBI Dynamic Registry. This series registers consecutive cases from 13 tertiary referral centers to obtain a snapshot of interventional cardiology practice. The Dynamic registry is the outgrowth of the original NHLBI registry in the late 1970s and the registry performed in 1985 and 1986. The current Dynamic registry has now undergone four waves of collection. The third wave of data, collected in 2000 and 2001, was the last to represent practice just before the advent of drug-eluting stents. This wave-3 registry was examined to develop a benchmark for reintervention rates for patients not enrolled in clinical trials.[25] The total repeat PCI reintervention rate was 13.1% at 1 year, and the target vessel revascularization rate represented 77% of that group; however, target segment revascularization was performed in only 61.7% of the total. Reintervention on the target segment by percutaneous means was 7.9%. In addition, 2.34% of patients underwent coronary bypass surgery, which was almost always performed on multiple segments, usually including the original target segment. Therefore, the potentially reducible 1-year target segment revascularization rate in this unselected consecutive series lies between 7.9% and 9.4%. Within these average reintervention rates, some subgroups (eg, patients with vessels smaller than 3 mm in diameter or longer than 12 mm in length, and those with diabetes or multivessel disease) had higher reintervention rates.

[ ] WHICH SUBSETS OF PATIENTS ARE MOST SUITABLE FOR TREATMENT WITH DRUG-ELUTING STENTS?

Because the greatest impact of drug-eluting stents will be reflected by the absolute reduction of repeat procedures, rather than the relative reduction, the greatest benefit will be seen in those patients and lesions most likely to require reintervention. These are well known to be long lesions, relatively smaller vessels, and chronic total occlusions, as well as patients with diabetes or multiple risk factors.

Some lesions for which restenosis rates are high remain problematic for drug-eluting stents; these include bifurcation lesions and lesions involving the ostium of the left anterior descending coronary artery (LAD). Colombo reported relatively high restenosis rates when using T-stenting in bifurcation lesions. This has led to numerous recommendations for coping with these problems. Stenting the main vessel and using a balloon to open the side branch is successful in many cases of bifurcation lesions in which the side branch patency appears adequate. In other situations (eg, those in which side branch arteries do not remain open with balloon dilation or in which the lesion encroaches significantly far into the side branch), stenting with the so-called crush technique may be necessary. It is not necessary to crush the side branch stent extensively within the parent vessel; however, the opening of the side branch should be covered when this technique is employed. This technique can be facilitated by placing an uninflated balloon in the main channel while placing the side branch stent at the ostium of the side branch, and then inflating the balloon to ensure that the second stent can be delivered in the main channel. This technique enables a very minimal crush of the side branch stent. Most operators recommend "kissing" balloon dilation within the bifurcation stent when this technique is used.

Another lesion with a very high restenosis rate is the ostium of the LAD. A recent matched series of 43 patients who underwent bare-metal stenting of the LAD ostium was compared with an equal number treated with drug-eluting stents. The need for target lesion revascularization at 9 months was 7% in patients receiving drug-eluting stents compared with 25.6% for bare-metal stents. Thus, a lesion in this location is a clear indication for use of drug-eluting stents.[26]

Restenosis of chronic total occlusions was significantly improved with stenting; however, both restenosis and recurrent total occlusions have been dramatically reduced with drug-eluting stents.

[ ] WHICH LESIONS CAN BE ADEQUATELY TREATED WITH BARE-METAL STENTS?

As previously mentioned, very low reintervention rates are associated with vessels having large diameters or short lesions; therefore, bare-metal stents may be entirely appropriate in these cases. Vein grafts have not been studied extensively and, because preexisting, degenerating vein grafts commonly develop new lesions elsewhere in the vein graft, use of a drug-eluting stent may not solve this problem completely.

Treatment of acute myocardial infarction is aimed primarily at rapidly reestablishing flow, thereby interrupting the infarction. Reduction of restenosis is clearly a secondary goal in this subset

of patients and, again, bare-metal stents may be entirely appropriate here. Examination of the results of the Controlled Abciximab and Device Investigation to Lower Late Angioplasty Complications (CADILLAC) trial showed a reintervention rate of 7% in nondiabetic patients who were treated with primary angioplasty. It is likely that patients with acute myocardial infarction who undergo stenting outside the setting of a clinical trial might have even lower reintervention rates. There may be several reasons why reintervention is unlikely following primary angioplasty for acute myocardial infarction. Because varying degrees of myocardial loss have been experienced, a decreased demand for blood flow may exist in the zone supplied by that vessel. An analysis of the RESEARCH registry to identify outcomes for patients who underwent primary angioplasty for acute myocardial infarction found no significant difference in 1-year mortality.

In-stent restenosis has been inadequately treated with balloon angioplasty, repeat stenting, rotary ablation, and cutting balloon angioplasty. Endovascular brachytherapy was approved for the treatment of in-stent restenosis and has been widely applied. There is interest in evaluating whether drug-eluting stents inserted within previously placed stents can offer successful therapy for in-stent restenosis, as well. The Intracoronary Stenting and Antithrombotic Regimen (ISAR) DESIRE study, presented at the European Society of Cardiology in 2004, evaluated approximately 300 patients with in-stent restenosis treated either with Cypher or Taxus stents. The repeat restenosis rate was 14% with Cypher stents and 22% with Taxus stents. Target vessel revascularization was 8% with Cypher and 19% with Taxus, and late loss was 0.45 mm with Cypher and 0.66 with Taxus. It is unclear whether these results will be comparable to those that could be obtained with intravascular brachytherapy. Trials are currently underway testing both the Taxus stent (TAXUS V-ISAR) and the Cypher stent (SISR) for in-stent restenosis versus endovascular brachytherapy using beta sources.

ISSUES AND CONSIDERATIONS

Two important considerations related to the use of drug-eluting stents are now being evaluated:

1. How will the change in therapy associated with use of these stents affect long-term outcomes of patients?, and

2. Will the availability of these stents change the selection process for revascularization therapy?

A meta-analysis of the second-generation stent trials provides another benchmark for long-term clinical events. The four trials comparing second-generation stents with the Palmaz-Schatz stent underwent FDA-mandated 5-year follow up to identify clinical events. Analysis of the pooled data from this follow up showed that clinical events related to the originally treated lesion, classified as restenosis events, occurred in approximately 20% of the patients.[27] Most of these events occurred within the first year and were indeed related to restenosis. Very few of these events occurred after the first year. The clinical events that were not related to the initially treated lesion, however, occurred in 38% of the patients. There were almost twice as many events unrelated to the original lesion treated, and these would not have been altered by the use of drug-eluting stents. This observation highlights the importance of long-term preventive therapy to alter the progression of disease if major impact on clinical events is to be achieved.

Although it is tempting to use an assumed marked decrease in restenosis risk to broaden the indications for PCI, one should remember the limited impact of these devices. The reduction in restenosis has not been associated with a reduction in mortality, and any change in therapy that increases the risk of complications could negatively alter the outcome for those patients. Thus, it is premature to conclude that the availability of drug-eluting stents will materially change the selection process for patients previously selected for medical therapy or for surgery. Certainly in the years to come, there will be expansion of the use of drug-eluting stents and, through clinical observations as well as controlled randomized trials, the safe and effective application of these stents will be discovered. Trials currently underway and those yet to be proposed will shed light on the relative value of medical and surgical therapy compared with stenting.

At the time of this writing, the COURAGE and the Bypass Angioplasty Revascularization Investigation 2D (BARI 2D) trials have completed enrollment and are now in the follow-up phases. Both of these trials examine revascularization versus continued medical therapy in patients who are asymptomatic or whose symptoms can be adequately controlled with medical means. COURAGE includes a broad segment of patients; however, approximately 30% have diabetes mellitus, a subset of great interest for stenting. BARI 2D is limited entirely to diabetic patients with multivessel disease who are randomized either to medical therapy or revascularization with stenting or surgery. Approximately 40% of the BARI 2D PCI patients will have received drug-eluting stents.

Four additional trials are designed to compare the use of drug-eluting stents with coronary bypass surgery. The FREEDOM trial is an NHLBI-sponsored study enrolling patients with diabetes mellitus and multivessel disease to PCI using drug-eluting stents or to coronary artery bypass surgery. This trial will run for 5 years, with the primary end point being death, Q-wave myocardial infarction, and stroke. Another trial, largely taking place in Europe, is the SYNTEX trial which uses the paclitaxel-eluting stent and includes diabetic and nondiabetic patients randomized between stenting and bypass surgery. A third trial is in the planning phase and is being organized by the Veterans Administration to test a high-risk group of patients with diabetes mellitus randomized to PCI with drug-eluting stents or coronary bypass surgery. A trial in the United Kingdom, CARDIA is also evaluating revascularization modes in diabetic patients. These trials will provide an opportunity to understand the additional impact of drug-eluting stents in the overall clinical outcome of patients with multivessel disease.

CONCLUSION

Major advances in stenting have occurred over the past 15 years, and stents have become the primary method for performing PCI. The development of drug-eluting stents has been an important breakthrough in the reduction of neointimal proliferation and resulting clinical necessity for repeat intervention. Whereas the great contribution of stenting was to nearly eliminate the need for emergency bypass surgery and markedly decrease interventional complications, the promise of drug-eluting stents is to further reduce late restenosis by varying degrees, depending on the type of lesion being treated. Both stenting and drug-eluting stents have been important contributions to interventional cardiology; however, stenting per se certainly is the most important development since Gruentzig's launch of percutaneous intervention 30 years ago.

REFERENCES

1. Sigwart U, Puel J, Mirkovitch V, et al. Intravascular stents to prevent occlusion and restenosis after transluminal angioplasty. *N Engl J Med*. 1987;316:701.
2. Roubin GS, King SB III, Douglas JS Jr, et al. Intracoronary stenting during percutaneous transluminal coronary angioplasty. *Circulation*. 1990;81(suppl IV):IV-92.
3. Hearn JA, King SB III, Douglas JS Jr, et al. Clinical and angiographic outcomes after coronary artery stenting for acute or threatened closure after percutaneous transluminal coronary angioplasty: Initial results with a balloon-expandable, stainless steel design. *Circulation*. 1993;88:2086.
4. Fischman DL, Leon MB, Baim DS, et al. A randomized comparison of coronary-stent placement and balloon angioplasty in treatment of coronary artery disease. *N Engl J Med*. 1994;331:496.
5. Colombo A, Hall P, Nakamura S, et al. Intracoronary stenting without anticoagulation accomplished with intravascular ultrasound guidance. *Circulation*. 1995;91:1676.
6. Schoemig A, Newmann FJ, Kastrati A, et al. A randomized comparison of antiplatelet and anticoagulant therapy after the placement of coronary artery stents. *N Engl J Med*. 1996;334:1084.
7. Berger PB, Bell MR, Hasdai D, et al. Safety and efficacy of ticlopidine for only 2 weeks after successful intracoronary stent placement. *Circulation*. 1999;99:248.
8. Bertrand ME, Rupprecht H-J, Urban P, Gershlick AH, for the CLASSICS Investigators. Double blind study of the safety of clopidogrel with and without a loading dose in combination with aspirin compared with ticlopidine in combination with aspirin after coronary stenting. The Clopidogrel Aspirin Stent International Cooperative Study (CLASSICS). *Circulation*. 2000;102:624.
9. Douglas JS Jr, Ghazzal ZMB, Morris DC, et al. Twenty years of angioplasty at Emory University. *Circulation*. 2000;102(suppl II):II-753.
10. Weaver WD. Late breaking trials in interventional cardiology: Optimal angioplasty versus primary stenting (OPUS). *J Am Coll Cardiol*. 1999;34:1.
11. Brophy JM, Belisle P, Lawrence J. Evidence for use of coronary stents. *Ann Intern Med*. 2003;138:777.
12. Erbel R, Hsude M, Hopp H, et al. Coronary-artery stenting compared with balloon angioplasty for restenosis after initial balloon angioplasty. *N Engl J Med*. 1998;339:1672.
13. Savage MP, Douglas JS Jr, Fischman DL, et al. Stent placement compared with balloon angioplasty for obstructed coronary bypass grafts. Saphenous Vein De Novo Trial Investigators. *N Engl J Med*. 1997;337:740.
14. Serruys PW, Unger F, Sosa JE, et al for the Arterial Revascularization Therapies Study Group. Comparison of coronary artery bypass surgery and stenting for the treatment of multivessel disease. *N Engl J Med*. 2001;334:1117.
15. Stables RH and the SOS Investigators. Coronary artery bypass surgery versus percutaneous coronary intervention with stent implantation in patients with multivessel coronary artery disease (the Stent or Surgery Trial). *Lancet*. 2002;360:965.
16. Rodriguez A, Rodriguez AM, Navia J. Coronary stenting vs. coronary bypass surgery in patients with multiple vessel disease and significant LAD stenosis: Results from the ERACI II study. *Heart*. 2003;89:184.
17. Hoffman SN, TenBrook JA, Wolf M, et al. A meta-analysis of randomized controlled trials comparing coronary artery bypass graft with percutaneous transluminal coronary angioplasty: One to eight year outcomes. *J Am Coll Cardiol*. 2003;41:1293.
18. Moreno R, Fernandez C, Alfonso F, et al. Coronary stenting vs. balloon angioplasty in small vessels. *J Am Coll Cardiol*. 2004;43:1964.
19. Stone C, Ellis SG, Cox DA, et al. A polymer based paclitaxel eluting stent in patients with coronary artery disease. *N Engl J Med*. 2004;350:221.
19a. Morice M-C. Presented at American College of Cardiology. Scientific Session. March 2005.
20. Kimura T, Yokoi H, Nakagawa Y. Three year followup after implantation of metallic coronary artery stents. *N Engl J Med*. 1996;334:561.

20ᵃ. Serruys PW. Presented at the American College of Cardiology Scientific Session. March 2005.

21. Weintraub W, Ghazzal ZM, Douglas JS Jr, et al. Long-term clinical follow-up in patients with angiographic restudy after successful angioplasty. *Circulation.* 1993;87:831.

22. Serruys PW. Presented at the European Society of Cardiology meeting, August 2003; Vienna, Austria.

23. Lemos P, Serruys P, van Damburg R, et al. Unrestricted utilization of sirolimus-eluting stents compared with conventional bare metal stent implantation in the "real world". The rapamycin-eluting stent evaluated at Rotterdam Cardiology Hospital (RESEARCH) Registry. *Circulation.* 2004;109:190.

24. Yock CA, Conte-Matos AP, King SB III. Bare metal stent outcomes in an unselected patient population: The opportunity for drug-eluting stents. *Cardiology.* (in press).

25. King SB III, Selzer F, Detre K. Reintervention in the pre-drug-eluting stent era: One-year target segment revascularization in the NHLBI Dynamic Registry [abstract]. *Circulation.* 2004;117:III-689.

26. Tsagalou E, Stancovic G, Iakovou I, et al. Early outcome of treatment of ostial de novo left anterior descending coronary artery lesions with drug eluting stents. *J Am Coll Cardiol.* 2006;97:187.

27. Cutlip DE, Chambra A, Baim D, et al. Beyond restenosis—five-year clinical outcomes from second generation coronary stent trials. *Circulation.* 2004; 110:1226.

CHAPTER (31)

Rotational Atherectomy: Concepts and Practice

Mark Reisman, MD, and Lou Vadlamani, MD

The advent of drug-eluting stents has ushered in an exciting new era in the management of coronary artery disease. Restenosis, the bane of interventional cardiology, is almost a nonissue. Complex lesions now are amenable to percutaneous therapy, if the stents can be delivered to the lesions.

The goal of lesion preparation in these patients is to facilitate stent delivery, reduce plaque shift, and allow optimal stent expansion. Balloon angioplasty is usually adequate for lesion preparation to facilitate stent delivery. Often we encounter bifurcating lesions or lesions that are calcific or fibrocalcific and inelastic, resisting expansion with a balloon and making it very difficult to effectively deliver and deploy a stent. Aggressive high-pressure inflations of these lesions can increase the risk of adverse events such as vessel dissection or perforation.[1,2]

Plaque ablation with rotational atherectomy (RA) is an excellent alternative for these lesions. Its capacity to preferentially ablate diseased and calcified plaque, while sparing healthy tissue, makes RA a unique device to facilitate stent delivery in vessels with such lesions (Figure 31-1).

BACKGROUND AND HISTORY

The Rotablator system was developed by David C. Auth, PhD, PE (Boston Scientific Corporation, Redmond WA) over a period of 13 years. After years of experimentation and animal studies, on January 6, 1988, Fourrier and colleagues[3] performed the first procedure in a human coronary artery. At the same time, Zacca and colleagues performed the procedure in the peripheral vasculature in humans.[4] Since then, RA has become a major part of the interventional cardiologist's arsenal.

【 】 COMPONENTS

The components of the RA system include the console, burr, drive shaft, and turbine. Figure 31-2 shows the Rotablator system.

Console

This is a reusable part of the system which controls the rotational speed of the drive shaft and burr.

Burr

The Rotablator system consists of a nickel-plated brass burr, which is elliptical in shape. It is coated with diamond chips that are between 20 and 30 μ in size, of which only 5 μ protrude from the nickel plating, forming the abrasive surface that is responsible for the cutting or ablation (Figure 31-3). The burr is bonded to a drive shaft.

Drive Shaft

The drive shaft is flexible, housed in a 4.3–French (Fr) Teflon sheath, and connected to a turbine. Potential injury to the arterial wall (by the spinning drive shaft) is prevented by the Teflon sheath, which also acts as a conduit, delivering flush at 7 mL/min to 13 mL/min when activated.

Turbine

The turbine is driven by compressed air or nitrogen and rotates the shaft and burr at speeds of 150,000 to 200,000 revolutions per minute (rpm). The turbine is activated by a foot pedal and controlled by the console.

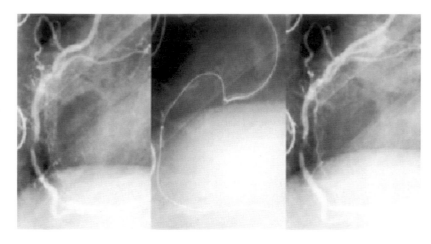

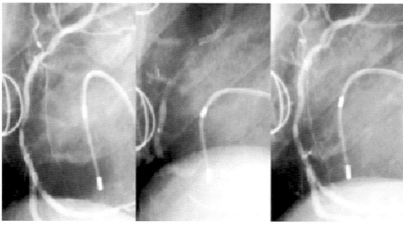

FIGURE 31-1. Example of a lesion in which stent delivery was facilitated by RA.

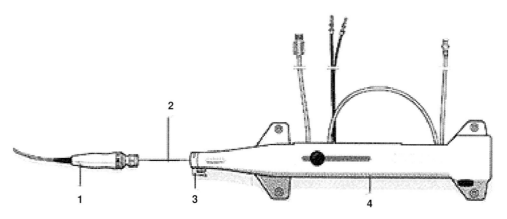

FIGURE 31-2. Components of the RotaLink Advancer system: (1) RotaLink catheter; (2) driveshaft connection; (3) connector latch; (4) Rotablator advancer; (5) burr control knob; (6) saline infusion port; (7) fiber-optic tachometer; (8) advancer hose to compressed gas (turbine) connector.

Mechanism

Depressing the foot pedal (Figure 31-4) initiates rotation of the burr and activates a locking system that prevents the coaxial guidewire from spinning along with the burr. A fiber-optic light probe (tachometer) monitors the rotational speed and displays it on the console.

[ ]   BURRS AND GUIDEWIRES

Burrs

Burrs for use in the coronary arteries are available in 1.25, 1.5, 1.75, 2.0, 2.15, 2.25, 2.38, and 2.5 mm sizes. Current recommendations are to use an 8-Fr sheath for the 1.25, 1.5, 1.75, 2.0, and 2.15 mm burrs, a 9-Fr sheath for the 2.25 and 2.38 mm burrs, and a 10-Fr sheath for the 2.5 mm burr. The inner diameter of the guide catheter must be 0.004-in greater than the burr size to provide adequate clearance for device advancement and withdrawal.

Guidewires

Four types of guidewires are currently available. The original, type C, is a 0.009-in stainless steel wire with a 3.7-cm flexible 0.017-in diameter platinum radiopaque tip. The clearance between the inner lumen of the burr and the guidewire is 0.001 in. The type A wire is similar to the type C except that the inner core extends to the distal end of the guidewire and the platinum radiopaque tip is 2.7 cm in length. Extending the stainless steel to the distal tip adds further stiffness, and the shorter segment of platinum is beneficial in vessels with limited distal beds.

The more commonly used wires, the RotaWires, come in floppy and extra support versions (Figure 31-5). These wires are transitional wires with 0.014-in radiopaque platinum tips. The distal platinum tip of the guidewire is larger and, therefore, not designed for burr advancement and should be placed beyond the lesion. Details of each wire follow.

- RotaWire Floppy (Figure 31-5C)
  - Diameter of the distal 44 cm tapers from 0.009 to 0.007 to 0.005 in.
  - 2.2-cm long platinum tip.
  - Soft tip.
  - 0.014-in diameter tip.
  - 325-cm length.
  - Long, tapered shaft.
  - Shaft maximizes flexibility.
  - Reduces vessel straightening in situations of unfavorable guidewire bias (discussed in more detail later).
- RotaWire Extra Support (Figure 31-5A)
  - Diameter of the distal 5 cm tapers from 0.009 to 0.005 in.
  - 2.8-cm long platinum tip.
  - Soft tip.
  - 0.014-in diameter tip.
  - 325-cm length.
  - Short, tapered shaft increases vessel straightening.
  - Shaft helps create favorable guidewire bias.
  - Added support aids in steering the Rotablator burr into lesions.

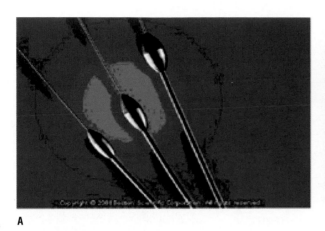 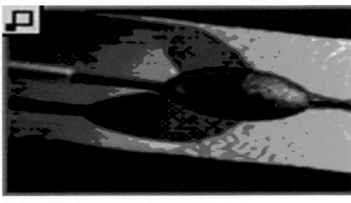

A **B**

FIGURE 31-3. Nickel-plated brass burr coated with diamond chips. *(Copyright © 2001 Boston Scientific Corporation.)*

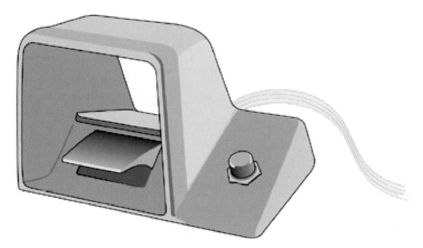

FIGURE 31-4. Dynaglide foot pedal.

- RotaWire Floppy Gold (Figure 31-5B)
  - Similar to RotaWire Floppy guidewire, but provides these additional features:
  - Gold-coated distal tip provides excellent radiopacity.
  - Increased visibility aids in anticipating the path of the Rotablator burr.
  - Long, tapered shaft maximizes flexibility and minimizes unfavorable guidewire bias.

BASIC PRINCIPLES AND CHARACTERISTICS

The Rotablator system is analogous to a low-powered rotary sander. The two principles that govern the operation and effectiveness of the Rotablator system are *differential cutting* and *orthogonal displacement of friction*.

【 】 DIFFERENTIAL CUTTING

Differential cutting is the ability to selectively ablate one material while preserving the integrity of the other, based on differences in the composition and texture of the substrate. This is analogous to taking a knife and scraping it across the skin versus the fingernail. The elasticity of the skin deflects the cutting surface whereas the inelastic properties of the nail activate the cutting ability of the knife and generated microparticulate debris. Shaving is also another very good example of differential cutting. Whiskers are relatively inelastic when compared with skin, and a razor will preferentially cut these while sparing the skin. The atherectomy burr acts much in the same way on the vascular tree, selectively cutting and ablating inelastic tissue and sparing healthy, elastic tissue. Calcium, fibrous tissue, fatty deposits, and intimal hyperplasia (restenotic tissue) increase the inelastic properties of vascular tissue, making it susceptible to ablation by the cutting edges of the atherectomy burr.

【 】 ORTHOGONAL DISPLACEMENT OF FRICTION

Orthogonal displacement of friction is essential in allowing easy passage of the burr through diseased and tortuous vascular segments. The sliding motion and high rotational speeds virtually eliminate the longitudinal friction vector, allowing for unhindered advancement and withdrawal of the burr. This principle also comes into play when a corkscrew is removed from a bottle. The twisting motion reduces the friction on the surfaces and facilitates easy removal of the corkscrew. The faster it is turned, the easier it is to remove it.

These two basic principles allow for the burr to effectively ablate diseased and atherosclerotic tissue, without harming normal tissue. This was confirmed with early animal studies using cholesterol-fed New Zealand white rabbits. After treatment, the minimum lumen diameter (MLD) was reduced from $81 \pm 9\%$ to $38 \pm 22\%$ ($P <$ .001, paired t-test).[5] Histologic specimens showed effective intimal plaque removal, with minimal medial injury and no medial or intimal dissections. Similar results were shown by Ahn et al, in cadaveric human coronary arteries.[6]

THERAPEUTIC AND SIDE EFFECTS

As mentioned earlier, based on the principles of differential cutting, high-speed RA effectively ablates calcified, inelastic atherosclerotic tissue while sparing healthy, elastic tissue. The ultimate

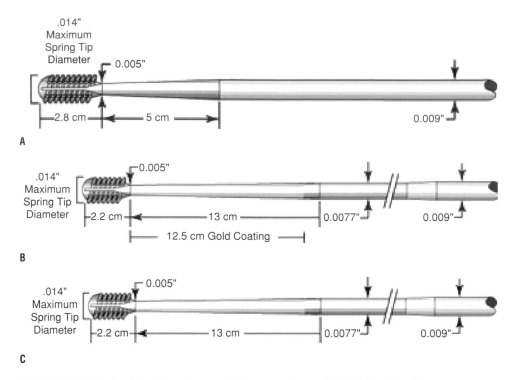

FIGURE 31-5. A. RotaWire Extra Support. **B.** Rotawire Floppy Gold. **C.** RotaWire Floppy.

goal in treatment of atherosclerotic disease is to effectively enlarge the lumen and facilitate stent placement. RA effectively leads to lumen enlargement, reducing cross-sectional atherosclerotic plaque area (by selective intimal plaque removal). There is also minimal trauma to normal "healthy" tissue. Data from human and animal studies confirm these findings.[3,7–9]

Quantitative coronary angiography has been used to evaluate the efficiency of RA in debulking lesions. Early studies using quantitative coronary angiography in 109 patients showed that a predictable MLD can be achieved across the range of burr sizes. Expressing MLD as a burr ratio (MLD/burr size), the Rotablator achieved immediate results of 0.72 ± 0.19 of the burr selected (ie, a 2.0-mm burr predicted a MLD of approximately 1.4 mm). Mintz and colleagues confirmed this using intravascular ultrasound (IVUS).[10,11] They found that this ratio ranged from 0.93 to 1.45 ($1.19 \pm .19$). There was minimal injury to the media and adventitia of adjacent tissue. Measured 24 hours later, the burr ratio increased to 0.84 ± 0.15. This change 24 hours later was confirmed by analyzing 186 patients who were studied before, immediately after, and 24 hours later. Comparing the post-procedure ratio to that at 24 hours, it appeared that 17% of those studied had lost more than 0.05 mm, 10% were within $\pm$ 0.05 mm, and 73% had gained more than 0.05 mm.[12,13]

It is possible that once the vessel is "unbound" there is restoration of vasomotor function with some late vasodilation. Another possibility is that eccentric guidewire orientation can result in preferential ablation of the plaque, causing greater cross-sectional ablation area than the burr size.

The high-speed rotations of RA are effective in increasing lumen diameter through plaque ablation. They also have some untoward effects. These include microcavitations, thermal effects, hematologic effects, and embolization of microparticulate debris.

【 】 MICROCAVITATIONS

Microcavitations are essentially gas bubbles dissolved in blood. The critical speed for this to occur is 14.7 m/s. A 2.0-mm burr operating at 160,000 rpm would rotate at a speed of 16.7 m/s, and would establish the appropriate conditions necessary to produce microcavitations. Zotz and colleagues studied in vivo and in vitro production of microcavitations.[14] Transthoracic and transesophageal echocardiograms were obtained before and after treatment from nine patients undergoing RA. None of the patients had a decrease in regional ejection fraction during or after the procedure. During activation of the burr, transient enhancement of contrast occurred in the area of the myocardium subtended by the artery and disappeared immediately after the burr rotation was stopped. It was unlikely that debris were responsible for this finding, because the opacification was transient and occurred prior to burr advancement. Therefore, it appears that high-speed RA may result in the formation of microcavitations that are relatively large, but collapse quickly without any clinical significance.

【 】 THERMAL EFFECTS

Thermal injury can lead to smooth muscle proliferation, increasing restenosis rates, as well as cause red blood cell aggregation and platelet activation.[15–17] In vitro and in vivo studies have been conducted to assess the extent of thermal injury caused by RA.[18] Using 122-mm cylinders derived from bovine femurs with a 0.35-mm core lumen to allow passage of the Rotablator guidewire, four thermal probes were placed at 3-mm intervals. Temperature changes were noted as the burr engaged the segment of the bone. With continuous saline infusion at body temperature, 2.0-mm burrs were activated and advanced through the model and simultaneous data on revolutions per minute and temperature were noted. Two burr advancement methods were used: (1) a continuous advancement through the entire segment, or (2) an intermittent or oscillating technique that consisted of a 2-second engagement followed by a 2-second withdrawal (to establish antegrade flow). Both techniques were tested using an aggressive ablation involving excessive decelerations (14,000–18,000 rpm) or a gentle advancement technique that limited decelerations to 4000 to 6000 rpm. The gentler technique, limiting decelerations, produced lower temperature elevations than the more aggressive method. The intermittent or oscillating technique was also more efficient at reducing the temperature changes when compared with the continuous method.[19]

In summary, to minimize thermal injury, it is prudent to minimize decelerations, while using an intermittent (pecking) movement to reduce temperature changes and minimize thermal injury during high-speed RA.

HEMATOLOGIC IMPACT

The high rotational speed of the burr establishes a shear field and affects both erythrocytes and platelets. A study using eight samples of porcine blood exposed to a spinning burr demonstrated evidence of platelet aggregation as measured by optical microscopy.[19] The number of aggregates was affected by the speed of the burr. Larger platelet aggregates (> 60 μm diameter) were seen in all eight samples at 180,000 rpm, and in only one of eight samples at 140,000 rpm. These findings support the importance of lowering the burr speed to minimize the hematologic impact of RA.

MICROPARTICULATE DEBRIS

The effect of microparticulate debris produced by RA was a major concern in early studies. In experimental studies to assess the in vivo effects of such debris, human particulate debris was injected into the left circumflex artery of three dogs. Myocardial blood flow was analyzed using radiolabeled microspheres. In two dogs, there was no detectable change in myocardial blood flow. The third dog was subjected to larger blouses of heavily calcified debris, which reduced blood flow between 50% and 100%. However, the amount injected was approximately 10 to 30 times the volume produced during coronary interventions.[20]

The effects of debris embolization were investigated in humans using positron emission tomography as well as other imaging modalities. These studies showed no evidence of long-term perfusion defects or wall motion abnormalities.[21,22] Pavlides and colleagues showed that balloon angioplasty was associated with significantly more wall motion abnormalities when compared with RA.[23] In contrast to these studies, Huggins and colleagues found transient wall motion impairment with RA, likely related to myocardial stunning.[24]

These observations establish the basic foundation for understanding the mechanism of RA. The untoward effects can be preempted by taking certain precautions. Heat generation and thermal injury can be minimized by advancing the device gently and intermittently and by avoiding significant decelerations. Platelet aggregation and other hematologic affects can be controlled by lowering the rotational speeds. Although it is difficult to prevent embolization of the microparticulate debris, no significant long-term sequelae appear to be associated with this finding.

PERFORMING THE ROTATIONAL ATHERECTOMY PROCEDURE

PREPROCEDURAL EVALUATION

Patient Selection and Evaluation

As is requisite for any other procedure (cardiac or otherwise), a complete history and physical examination are essential prior to RA. Information about the patient's medical regimen, allergies, and past medical history should be obtained. The patient's clinical status-stable versus unstable angina-should be noted. Patients with acute myocardial infarction (MI) and postinfarction angina may have a high thrombus burden and are not suitable for treatment with RA. The status of the myocardium subtended by the vessel should be evaluated, along with overall left ventricular function.

Lesion Morphology and Evaluation

In an elective setting, it would certainly be worthwhile to thoroughly assess vessel and lesion characteristics. Patency of remaining vessels and patterns of collateral flow should also be noted. Because RA has been associated with transient left ventricular dysfunction, the status of the remaining vessels is extremely important. Retrospective analysis of a multicenter registry shows a higher complication rate when treating a vessel in the left coronary system with an occluded right coronary artery (RCA).[25]

Although most lesions are suitable for RA, the procedure has often been "niched" for lesions with significant calcification in a diffuse pattern that are not usually amenable to balloon dilation. Lesions with thrombus, extensive dissection, and those in saphenous vein grafts should, however, be excluded. The choice of guide catheter (based on vessel takeoff, need for support, etc), guidewire, and burr size should be determined at the start of the procedure.

PREPROCEDURAL MANAGEMENT

The preinterventional management of patients undergoing RA is similar to that of patients undergoing other interventional procedures. Premedication with aspirin, 325 mg, is essential. Patients should be adequately hydrated for prevention of contrast nephropathy as well as maintenance of blood pressure if vasodilators are required during the procedure.

Adjunctive Mechanical Therapy

Temporary pacemakers are used when treating vessels associated with a high frequency of bradyarrhythmias and complete heart block. These vessels include RCA and the dominant left circumflex artery. Occasionally heart block is seen when ostial lesions of the left anterior descending (LAD) coronary artery are treated or with large burrs (≥ 2.25 mm). The mechanism of bradyarrhythmia is unclear. One theory suggests that it may be secondary to microparticulate emboli in the conductive tissue. Release of intracellular material, including adenosine, may also play a role (for this reason, some operators advocate the use of theophylline preprocedurally). Therefore, prior to heparinization, in high-risk patients, it is worthwhile to prophylactically place a transvenous pacemaker.

Because diastolic blood pressure and, therefore, coronary blood flow are reduced with pacing, therefore, when a pacemaker is placed prophylactically, longer runs are advisable. Patients undergoing for RA of the RCA, left circumflex, or LAD may also benefit from placement of an intra-aortic balloon pump, particularly if there is existing left ventricular dysfunction.

【 】 PROCEDURAL CONSIDERATIONS AND TECHNIQUE

Guide Catheter Selection

Appropriate guide catheter selection is essential for RA procedures. In most interventional procedures, the primary function of the guiding catheter is to provide a conduit to deliver the device to the lesion. In RA procedures, however, the guide catheter determines the ease of advancement of the burr and the trajectory of the guidewire that orients the burr and affects the direction of the ablation plane.

Guide catheter shape should be selected to ensure appropriate coaxial alignment. Coaxial alignment will reduce the tension or pull required on the guidewire when advancing the burr. Significant support or deep intubation is not required, because activation of the burr provides orthogonal displacement of friction, which reduces drag to ease the passage of the burr through the vessel (see later discussion of burr advancement techniques). Therefore, it is important to ensure that the guide is coaxial, in order to orient the guidewire centrally, avoiding guidewire bias (discussed below). An example is the use of an Amplatz guide catheter shape for an ostial left circumflex lesion. Amplatz guides can be manipulated to "telescope" into the circumflex artery, resulting in a centrally positioned guidewire. A Judkins guide catheter, however, would not generally direct toward the left circumflex artery and would cause the burr to cut primarily the inner curve of the ostial lesion.

The concept of an "active" guide catheter can be applied during RA. When treating eccentric lesions, the guide catheter can be manipulated to permit the guidewire to orient closer to the lesion, so that the advancing burr can achieve optimal engagement or "purchase" on the lesion. This concept has been referred to as *directional* rotational atherectomy.

The internal diameter of the guiding catheter should be at least 0.004 in larger than the burr. Selection of the guide catheter should take into account the possibility of using larger burrs during the procedure. In lesions such as those involving the ostial RCA, rotation of the guide catheter may be necessary, but this should be limited to cases in which the alignment is coaxial with the lesion. Therefore, oversizing the guide catheter may be helpful even when larger burrs are not being used. Firm tips are also recommended, because softer tips can "fish-mouth" and hinder advancement of larger burrs.

Guidewire Selection and Placement

Guidewire Selection. Several of the guidewires available for RA were described earlier. The RotaWire Extra Support is our workhorse wire. Prior to placement, the distal tip is gently curved by compressing the tip between the thumb and the forefinger. A "ribboning" technique can stretch the platinum spring and should be performed carefully. The bare guidewire is then inserted into an introducer sheath (this helps to minimize blood loss and prevents kinking), advanced to the ostium of the vessel, and then gently manipulated across the lesion. Of note, it helps to remove the guidewire from the packaging loop and maintain it straight on the table. This technique can help to increase the torque performance of the guidewire.

The platinum tip must be distal to the lesion, because the burr cannot track over this larger segment. The tip should not be placed in a minor branch; in general, the branch should be large enough so that contrast media can be demonstrated flowing past the tip. Occasionally, in cases where the vessel has limited length beyond the lesion, guidewires with the shorter distal tip can be beneficial. Every attempt should be made to keep the guidewire from prolapsing or coiling, because any rotation during burr activation can result in fracture or trapping of the tip in the vessel wall.

In the event a lesion cannot be crossed by a RotaWire, a conventional guidewire can be placed across the lesion, and exchanged for a RotaWire using a transfer catheter or a balloon. Using the floppy wire can be beneficial in tortuous or rigid vessels.

Guidewire Placement. In RA, the guidewire plays a vital role in establishing the cutting vector of the device; therefore, the position is crucial to the outcome of the procedure. The goal is to set the optimal ablation vector for treatment of a lesion while minimizing side load forces at segments proximal and distal to the lesion site. When the guidewire has greater rigidity than the vessel, pseudolesions occur and the vessel is deformed from the native architecture. On the other hand, when the vessel is more rigid than the guidewire, the guidewire yields to the configuration of the artery and places tension on the wall at points of contact, making burr advancement more difficult and affecting ablation efficiency. Often, in vessels with significant tortuosity beyond the lesion, the distal vector forces may change the orientation of the guidewire at the lesion, producing preferential cutting toward one wall. The guidewire should also be retracted to a more proximal position if pseudolesions are prominent distally. Deformity of the artery due to placement of the guidewire proximal to the lesion will affect the vector of the burr as it approaches the lesion and will often limit the burr sizes that can be used. These proximal pseudolesions may result in ablation of normal tissue if the strain on the wall by the guidewire is excessive.

From the preceding discussion, it is evident that the position of the guidewire in the artery is a major determinant of optimal RA. Divergence from the central axis of the vessel is referred to as *guidewire bias*. Guidewire bias is unfavorable, because it may orient the burr out of the central plane and result in radial or tangential cutting. Guidewire bias can, however, be beneficial if it orients the burr into the lesion.

Burr Selection and Placement

Early RA strategies incorporated a two-burr approach, with the burr-to-artery ratio of the first burr being approximately 0.5 to 0.6, and the second approximately 0.75 to 0.8. However, current literature has led most operators to use a single burr with a burr-to-artery ratio of 0.6 to 0.7 in conjunction with percutaneous transluminal coronary angioplasty (PTCA) or (usually) stenting (see later discussion). A burr-to-artery ratio of less than 0.5 is usually reserved for total occlusions, lesions on bends, or long lesions (> 30 mm).

Therefore, in the modern era in which most if not all lesions are stented, moderate debulking to improve vessel characteristics and allow for stent delivery and deployment using a single burr with a burr-to-artery ratio of 0.6 to 0.7 is usually appropriate.[26-29]

The appropriately sized burr should be selected, tested outside the body, and then advanced and placed just proximal to the lesion: the so-called *platform segment*. In this position, the burr should be able to rotate unimpeded, because if the burr is activated while in contact with the vessel wall, the risk of injury is significantly increased. If the operator experiences difficulty advancing the burr, it may be helpful to place further tension on the guidewire. However, excessive tension, especially in tortuous vessels, can cause the guidewire to become taut, resulting in excessive force being directed against the vessel wall.

In cases where extra tension is required to advance the burr, it is prudent to relieve the tension before activating the device. To do this, the operator should first relieve the drive shaft tension, then activate the device by depressing the brake defeat button with the wireclip in place, and minimally advance and withdraw the guidewire to confirm that there is "play" or the lowest possible tension in the system. After the burr has been advanced to the platform segment, just proximal to the lesion, the lie of the guidewire should be reassessed and adjusted if necessary.

The operator can confirm appropriate positioning by ensuring that there is free flow of contrast around the burr. By gently retracting the drive shaft, all forward tension on the burr should be removed prior to activation. The operator should "jiggle" the advancer knob to ensure that no resistance is felt. The presence of tension on the drive shaft can cause the device to jump forward, increasing the risk of dissection. Once the operator is certain that the tension on the burr has been released, the burr is activated in the platform segment, and the platform speed is adjusted based on the burr size. Current recommendations are 160,000 rpm for burrs that are 2 mm or larger and 180,000 rpm for burrs less than 2 mm.

Ablation Methods

As mentioned earlier, good ablation technique is essential to minimize some of the untoward side effects of RA. Ablation of the lesion should be performed using a "pecking" technique. Burr advancement should be gentle. Monitoring the decelerations and avoiding excessive decelerations (eg, a drop of > 5000 in rpm) helps to avoid aggressive burr advancement. Intermittent contrast injections should be performed to evaluate the progress of the burr and identify any problems with burr orientation or burr-to-artery relationship. If contrast fails to penetrate past the burr, gentle retraction of the burr is required to reestablish antegrade flow and allow for clearance of the microparticulate debris.

Although the optimal duration of each run is based on several factors, including lesion characteristics and hemodynamic stability, the usual duration is 15 to 30 seconds, with an interval of 30 seconds to 2 minutes between each run (depending on patient response). If electrocardiographic changes, hypotension, chest pain, or bradycardia develop, the time interval between each run should be increased to allow the patient's readings to return to baseline. The burr can be removed when there is no tactile resistance or when a drop in revolutions per minute is noted during burr advancement.

Repeat angiographic images and reevaluation of the lesion should be obtained to select the next course of action. A final "polishing" run should be associated with no drop in revolutions per minute and no perception of mechanical resistance as the burr crosses the treated segment.

Complications

The major clinical complication rates for RA are similar to those reported for balloon angioplasty and include death in 0.9% of patients, Q-wave MI in 1.3%, and emergency bypass surgery in 1.9%, even in the context of higher risk lesions. There is, however, a trend toward a higher rate of non–Q-wave MI (6%), defined as a creatine kinase, myocardial bound (CK-MB) level elevated to more than twice the normal value.[30] Most of these complications can be avoided by using proper procedural technique and pharmacotherapy.

【 】 INTRAPROCEDURAL PHARMACOTHERAPY

Adjunctive pharmacology for patients undergoing RA is similar to that for patients undergoing balloon angioplasty. All patients should be pretreated with 325 mg of aspirin. If heparin is the only anticoagulant used, the ACT should be >300 seconds; with the addition of GPIIb/IIIa, an ACT of 250 seconds is acceptable. Bivalirudin has also shown to be effective for this purpose.[31] It is worthwhile to note that use of glycoprotein IIb/IIIa inhibitors has been shown to reduce post-procedural elevation of cardiac enzymes by almost 50%, which may translate to a reduction in long-term adverse events.[32,33] Glycoprotein IIb/IIIa use has also been shown to attenuate the transient wall motion abnormality sometimes associated with RA,[34] and in vitro studies have shown that abciximab can reduce platelet activation caused by a high-speed burr.[35] Although there is significant benefit in using these agents, care is needed when lesions are at high risk for perforation, because the level of anticoagulation could have catastrophic effects.

Vasospasm can sometimes complicate RA; therefore, it is important to have vasodilating agents such as nitroglycerine (100–200 μg) available during the procedure. Some operators prefer to use a cocktail of nitroglycerine, verapamil, and heparin in a flush solution for continuous infusion, and some data support this approach.[36] Intracoronary adenosine administration has also shown to reduce the rates of no-reflow.[37] Rotaglide lubricant is also usually added to the flush solution to reduce friction between the drive coil and guidewire. Vasopressors should also be readily available; dopamine, epinephrine, and phenylephrine are the usual agents.

【 】 POST-PROCEDURAL MANAGEMENT

Management of patients after RA is similar to that of patients undergoing other coronary interventional procedures.

CLINICAL TRIALS

Since the advent of RA, several major clinical trials have been undertaken to evaluate therapy with RA as standalone or adjunctive therapy with other tools for percutaneous coronary intervention.

The following paragraphs discuss several of these important trials in depth.

[ ] MULTICENTER REGISTRY

The earliest multicenter investigation of RA started in 1988. The study included patients whose lesions were deemed suboptimal for standard balloon angioplasty and patients who were previously treated with balloon angioplasty who presented with restenosis or had not achieved adequate results. Patients with acute MI were excluded as were patients with postinfarction angina, because the presence of thrombus is an inadequate substrate for the device. Patients with saphenous vein graft lesions were also excluded, as were those with lesions greater than 25 mm and those with left ventricular ejection fractions less than 35%.

This multicenter registry, which included 2953 procedures involving 3717 lesions, was a benchmark study that led to other clinical trials. The mean age of the patients was 63 ± 11 years (SD), and 71.4% of the enrollees were men. Slightly less than 50% of the patients had previous MI or unstable angina. A majority of the patients had stable angina and multivessel disease. The lesions were distributed with predominance in the LAD, as follows: LAD, 47%; RCA, 30%; left circumflex, 19%; and protected left main coronary artery, 3%. When assessed by lesion morphology, most lesions were classified as American Heart Association/American College of Cardiology (AHA/ACC) type B (A = 17%, B = 66%, C = 17%).

The procedural success rate was 85% with the Rotablator system alone, and increased to 95% with adjunctive balloon angioplasty. Major clinical complications included Q-wave MI (1.2% of patients), coronary artery bypass grafting (2.5%), and death (1.0%). Other complications included creatine kinase elevation (non–Q-wave MI) in 6.1% of patients, and angiographic complications, including perforation (0.7%), dissection (13.7%), and abrupt vessel closure (1.1%).[38]

Quantitative coronary angiography was performed on 92 patients who underwent both 24-hour and 6-month follow-up. MLD decreased from 1.72 ± 0.32 mm at 24-hours post-procedure to 1.45 ± 0.48 mm at 6 months.

Based on the data from this multicenter registry, the Food and Drug Administration granted approval for the Rotablator system for use by interventional cardiologists who had attended and participated in a training course conducted by Boston Scientific Corporation, Northwest Technologies, Inc (formerly Heart Technology Inc).

[ ] OBSERVATIONAL DATA

Several investigators have presented findings based on single-center experience with RA procedures (Tables 31-1 through 31-3). Table 31-1 lists the initial studies and their procedural success rates, while Tables 31-2 and 31-3 show the in-hospital and angiographic complications. It is interesting to note the wide range of success and complications with the device. This is likely secondary to the heterogeneity in the technique of the initial investigators. The improvement in the later studies and in more complex lesion subsets is a testimony to the evolution of the technique and greater comfort with the device.

[ ] ROTATIONAL ATHERECTOMY VERSUS OTHER MODES OF PERCUTANEOUS REVASCULARIZATION

ERBAC (Excimer Laser, Rotational Atherectomy, and Balloon Angioplasty Comparison)

The purpose of this study was to test whether coronary revascularization with ablation of either excimer laser or RA can improve the initial angiographic and clinical outcomes compared with dilation (balloon angioplasty) alone. At a single center, a total of 685 patients with symptomatic coronary disease warranting elective percutaneous revascularization for a complex lesion were randomly assigned to balloon angioplasty (n = 222), excimer laser angioplasty (n = 232), or RA (n = 231). Patients enrolled in this study had lesions that were rated as AHA/ACC types B2 and C. The primary end point was procedural success (diameter stenosis < 50%; absence of death, Q-wave MI, or coronary artery bypass surgery). The patients who underwent RA had a higher rate of procedural success than those who underwent excimer laser angioplasty or conventional balloon angioplasty (89% vs 77% and 80%; P =.0019), and no difference was observed in major in-hospital complications (3.2% vs 4.3% and 3.1%; P = .71). At the 6-month follow-up, while the incidence of target lesion revascularization was higher for RA (42.4%) and laser (46.0%) than for balloon angioplasty (31.9%), the differences in angiographic restenosis rates failed to achieve significance (P = .13).[39]

COBRA (Comparison of Balloon Angioplasty vs Rotational Atherectomy)

This multicenter, prospective, randomized trial compared short- and long-term effects of PTCA and rotablation in patients with angiographically predefined complex coronary artery lesions. Seven sites enrolled 502 patients with predefined complex coronary artery lesions and assigned them to receive either PTCA (n = 250) or rotablation (n = 252). Primary end points were procedural success, 6-month restenosis rates in the treated segments, and major cardiac events during follow-up. Procedural success was achieved in 78% (PTCA), and 85% (rotablation) (P = .038) of cases. Crossover from PTCA to rotablation was 4% and 10% vice versa (P = .019). There was no difference between PTCA and rotablation with respect to procedure-related complications such as Q-wave infarctions (2.4% each), emergency bypass surgery (1.2% vs 2.4%), and death (1.6% vs 0.4%). However, more stents were required after PTCA (14.9% vs 6.4%; P < .002), predominantly for bailout or unsatisfactory results. Including bail-out stents as an end point, the procedural success rates were 73% for angioplasty and 84% for rotablation (P = .006). At 6 months, symptomatic outcome, target vessel reinterventions, and restenosis rates (PTCA 51% vs rotablation 49%; P = .33) were not different.[40] This study showed that complex coronary artery lesions could be treated with a high level of success and low complication rates either by PTCA with adjunctive stenting or by rotablation alone.

TABLE 31-1

Procedural Success Rates in Initial Studies of Rotational Atherectomy

AUTHOR	NO.	TYPE OF LESION	PROCEDURAL SUCCESS (%)	ADJUNCTIVE BALLOON (%)	RESIDUAL STENOSIS (%)	RESTENOSIS (%)	TLR (%)
Kiesz et al	111	B = 18.5%; C = 81.5%	98	All	18	28	23
Kini et al	574	A = 10%; B1= 12%; B2 = 54%; C = 26%	98	All	14	—	—
	254	A = 12%; B1= 13%; B2 = 44%; C = 31%	95	All	21	—	—
	172	A = 13%; B1 = 8%; B2 = 42%; C = 37%	94	All	24	—	—
Braden et al	100	B2, C = 75%	99	All	26	28	—
Levin et al	178	A = 3%; B1 = 26%; B2 = 46%; C = 25%	94	93	19	—	14
Brown et al	525	A = 6%; B1 =24%; B2 = 57%; C = 14%	88	88	26	—	26
DART	222	A or B1	99	—	—	—	—
ERBAC	231	A = 1%; B1 = 20%; B2 = 65%; C = 14%	89	93	33	57	42
Reisman et al	200	A = 8%; B = 75%; C = 17%	96	—	—	—	—
	2953	A = 17%; B = 66%; C = 17%	95	—	—	—	—
MacIsaac et al	2161	Calcified = 50%; noncalcified = 50%	94.5	74	22	—	—
Sterzer et al	656	A = 11%; B1 = 14%; B2 = 29%; C = 46%	96.5	65	—	—	—
Ellis et al	316	A = 24%; B = 70%; C = 6%	89.8	82	27	—	—
Warth et al	709	A = 27%; B = 59%; C = 14%	94.7	44	—	38	—
Borrione et al	166	Complex = 63%	95	All	18	—	—
Guerin et al	61	B2 = 100%	93.4	All	—	39	—
Gilmore et al	108	—	91.7	—	—	—	—
Stertzer et al	42	A = 7.5%; B/C = 92.5%	94	77	—	—	38
Safian et al	104	A = 20%; B = 76%; C = 4%	95.2	77	30	51	36

DART = Dilation versus Ablation Revascularization Trial Targeting Restenosis; ERBAC = Excimer Laser, Rotational Atherectomy, and Balloon Angioplasty Comparison; TLR = target lesion revascularization.

TABLE 31-2

In-Hospital Complication Rates Reported in Initial Rotational Atherectomy Studies

AUTHOR	NO.	DEATH (%)	CABG (%)	Q MI (%)	NON–Q-WAVE MI (%)
Kiesz et al	111	None	None	None	4.5
Kini et al	574	0.2	0.2	0.7	—
	254	0.8	0.8	1.2	—
	172	1.7	1.7	2.3	—
Levin et al	178	1.1	2.2	2.8	0.6
Brown et al	525	0.8	0.4	1.1	5.2
ERBAC	231	0.9	0.9	1.3	2.2
MacIsaac et al	2161	0.8	2.0	0.7	8.8
Sterzer et al	656	0.5	1.4	3.4	—
Ellis et al	316	0.3	0.9	2.9	5.7
Reisman et al	200	3.0	2.5	0.5	6.0
	2953	1.0	2.5	1.2	6.1
Warth et al	709	0.8	1.7	0.9	3.8
Borrione et al	166	1.8	None	0.6	8.4
Guerin et al	61	None	1.6	1.6	6.6
Gilmore et al	108	0.9	2.8	0.9	2.8
Safian et al	104	1.0	1.9	4.8	2.9
Stertzer et al	302	None	1.0	2.6	—

CABG = coronary artery bypass grafting; ERBAC = Excimer Laser, Rotational Atherectomy, and Balloon Angioplasty Comparison; MI = myocardial infarction.

TABLE 31-3

Angiographic Complications Reported in Initial Rotational Atherectomy Studies

AUTHOR	NO.	ABRUPT CLOSURE (%)	SLOW FLOW OR NO REFLOW (%)	PERFORATION (%)	DISSECTION (%)	SIDE-BRANCH OCCLUSION (%)	SPASM (%)
Kini et al	574	1.1	2.0	1.0	4.0	5.0	5.0
	254	2.3	4.0	0.7	4.0	5.0	5.0
	172	4.0	9.0	0.6	5.0	4.0	7.0
Levin et al	178	—	—	1.7	—	—	—
Brown et al	525	1.0	1.0	1.0	15.0	1.0	2.0
MacIsaac et al	2161	3.6	—	0.7	13.0	—	—
Sterzer et al	710	2.7	1.8	0.6	10.4	1.7	5.3
Ellis et al	316	5.5	7.6	1.5	—	—	—
Reisman et al	200	3.4	—	0.4	11.6	—	—
	2953	4.1	—	0.6	11.0	—	—
Warth et al	709	3.1	1.2	0.5	10.5	0.1	1.6
Borrione et al	166	1.8	—	0.6	—	—	—
Safian et al	104	11.2	6.1	None	—	1.8	—

TABLE 31-4

Summary of Major Rotational Atherectomy Trials

STUDY	AIM AND NO. OF CASES	PRIMARY END POINT	RESULT
ERBAC	Comparison between device Rotablator (n = 231) POBA (n = 222) ELCA (n = 232)	Procedure success	Procedural success: 89% vs 80% vs 77% TLR: 42% vs 32% vs 46%
STRATAS	Comparison between strategy Aggressive (B/A = 0.7–0.9; n = 250) Conservative (B/A = 0.6–0.8; n = 250)	MACE at 6 mo MLD at 6 mo	Death: 2.5% vs 5.1% MI: 2.5% vs 1.0% TLR: 35% vs 27%
DART	Comparison between device Rotablator (n = 250) POBA (n = 220)	Composite procedural success without major complications	MACE: 1.3% vs 0% Slow flow/No reflow: 8.0% vs 0.5% Major dissection: 8% vs 16% Bailout stenting: 6% vs 14%
CARAT	Comparison between strategy Aggressive (B/A > 0.7; n = 104) Conservative (B/A < 0.7; n = 118)	Procedural success and TLR at 6 mo Final diameter stenosis	Angiographic complication: 16% vs 8% TLR: 21% vs 22%

B/A = burr-to-artery ratio; CARAT = Coronary Angioplasty and Rotablator Trial; DART = Dilation versus Ablation Revascularization Trial Targeting Restenosis; ELCA = Excimer Laser Coronary Angioplasty [registry]; ERBAC = Excimer Laser, Rotational Atherectomy, and Balloon Angioplasty Comparison; MACE = main adverse coronary event; MI = myocardial infarction; MLD = minimum lumen diameter; POBA = plain old balloon angioplasty; STRATAS = Study to Determine Rotablator and Transluminal Angioplasty; TLR = target lesion revascularization.

[ ] "AGGRESSIVE" VERSUS "ROUTINE" ROTATIONAL ATHERECTOMY

STRATAS (Study to Determine Rotablator and Transluminal Angioplasty Strategy)

In this study, patients being considered for elective RA were randomized to either an "aggressive" strategy (n = 249; maximum burr/artery > 0.70 alone, or with adjunctive balloon inflation ≤ 1 atm) or a "routine" strategy (n = 248; maximum burr/artery ≤ 0.70, and routine balloon inflation ≥ 4 atm). Patient age was 62 ± 11 years. Fifty-nine percent of patients assigned to the routine group and 60% of those receiving aggressive RA had class III to IV angina. Fifteen percent of routine and 16% of aggressive strategy patients received treatment for a restenotic lesion; lesion length was 13.6 versus 13.7 mm. Reference vessel diameter was 2.64 mm. Maximum burr size (1.8 vs 2.1 mm), burr/artery ratio (0.71 vs 0.82), and number of burrs used (1.9 vs 2.7) were greater for those receiving the aggressive strategy ($P < .0001$). Final MLD and residual stenosis were 1.97 mm and 26% for routine strategy patients versus 1.95 mm and 27% for aggressive strategy patients. Clinical success was 93.5% for the routine strategy and 93.9% for the aggressive strategy. CK-MB was greater in the patients receiving aggressive RA (> 5 times normal in 7% of the routine vs 11% of the aggressive group). CK-MB elevation was associated with a decrease in revolutions per minute of more than 5000 from baseline for a cumulative time more than 5 seconds ($P = .002$).

At 6 months, 22% of the patients receiving routine RA versus 31% of those receiving aggressive RA had target lesion revascularization. Angiographic follow-up (77%) showed MLD of 1.26 mm in the routine group versus 1.16 mm in the aggressive group, and the loss index was 0.54 versus 0.62. Binary restenosis was 52% for the routine strategy versus 58% for the aggressive strategy. Multivariable analysis showed that left anterior descending location (odds ratio 1.67, $P = .02$) and operator-reported excessive speed decrease greater than 5000 rpm (odds ratio 1.74; $P = .01$) were significantly associated with restenosis. Thus, the aggressive RA strategy offers no advantage over more routine burr sizing plus routine angioplasty. Operator technique reflected by a decrease in revolutions per minute of more than 5000 from baseline is associated with CK-MB elevation and restenosis.[41] Therefore, "aggressive" debulking is not indicated when using RA; this is more true now, in the era of drug-eluting stents.

CARAT (Coronary Angioplasty and Rotablator Atherectomy Trial)

The purpose of this study was to compare the immediate and late results after rotablation of two treatment strategies: (1) a lesion-debulking strategy, in which large burrs (burr/artery ratio > 0.7) were used to achieve maximal debulking, or (2) a lesion modification strategy, in which small burrs (burr/artery ratio ≤ 0.7) were used to modify lesion compliance. Two hundred twenty-two patients at six centers were prospectively enrolled in this study and randomly assigned to receive treatment with large (n = 104 patients with 118 lesions) or small (n = 118 patients with 136 lesions) burrs. The primary end point was final diameter stenosis at the end of the procedure, and secondary end points included in-hospital angiographic and clinical complications, and target lesion revascularization at 6 months. Baseline demographic and angiographic characteristics were similar for the two groups.

There were no differences in procedural success, the extent of immediate lumen enlargement, in-hospital ischemic complications, or late target vessel revascularization. However, patients randomized to the large burr group were more likely than those in the small burr group to experience serious angiographic complications (5.1% vs 12.7%; $P < .05$) immediately after atherectomy. This study suggests that a routine lesion modification strategy employing small burrs (burr/artery ratio ≤ 0.7) achieves similar immediate lumen enlargement and late target vessel revascularization compared with a more aggressive debulking strategy (burr/artery ratio > 0.7), but with fewer angiographic complications.[42]

The preceding studies conclusively showed that "aggressive" atherectomy provides no benefit (and may even be harmful) when compared with "routine" atherectomy. Thus, most operators today use a burr-to-artery ratio of less than 0.7 (usually with burr sizes between 1.5 and 1.75 mm) for lesion modification.

[ ] ROTATIONAL ATHERECTOMY AND STENTING

EDRES (Effects of Debulking on Restenosis)

This prospective randomized trial compared RA with stenting to use of stenting alone. The goal was to evaluate immediate angiographic results and long-term restenosis rates. One hundred and fifty patients were enrolled at a single center. The study showed that while RA before stenting did not improve final stent diameter at the end of the procedure, it did reduce binary restenosis at 6 months (27% vs 34%; $P = .05$).[43]

SPORT (Stenting Post-Rotational Atherectomy)

This large multicenter trial enrolled 735 patients who were randomized to receive either balloon angioplasty (n = 375) or RA (n = 360) prior to stenting. The mean burr-to-artery ratio was 0.7(0.1. The RA group had a higher procedural and clinical success rate with no differences in in-hospital major cardiac events. This strategy also led to a higher post-treatment MLD; however, there was no difference in the incidence of angiographic restenosis or target lesion revascularization at the 6-month follow-up. This study[43a] showed that while there was a modest improvement in immediate results with RA before stenting, the long-term angiographic outcomes were no different. In contrast, Kobayashi and colleagues showed that "aggressive" debulking with RA prior to stent placement led to a lower restenosis rate.[44] However, as previously mentioned, "aggressive" debulking increases the risk of complications and in the era of drug-eluting stents is unnecessary.

[ ] ROTATIONAL ATHERECTOMY FOR SMALL ARTERIES

DART (Dilation vs Ablation Revascularization Trial targeting restenosis)

This multicenter, randomized, blinded end point trial compared RA with balloon angioplasty in the prevention of restenosis of obstructed small coronary arteries (< 3 cm). A total of 446 patients with myocardial ischemia associated with an angiographic stenosis in a native coronary artery 2 to 3 mm in diameter and 20 mm or less in length without severe calcification were randomly assigned to receive RA (n = 227) or balloon angioplasty (n = 219). The primary end point was target vessel failure at 12 months (defined as the composite of death, Q-wave MI, and clinically driven repeat revascularization of the target vessel). The mean reference vessel diameter was 2.46 ± 0.40 mm, the mean lesion length was 9.97 ± 5.59 mm, and the prevalence of diabetes mellitus was 32%. Acute procedural success (91.6% for RA, 94.1% for balloon angioplasty; $P = .36$) and target vessel failure at 12 months were not significantly different (30.5% vs 31.2%; $P = .98$). At 8 months, there were no significant differences in MLD (1.28 ± 0.63 mm vs 1.19 ± 0.54 mm; $P = .26$), percent diameter stenosis (28% ± 12% vs 29% ± 15%; $P = .59$), binary restenosis rate (50.5% vs 50.5%; $P = 1.0$), or late loss index (0.57 vs 0.62; $P = .7$). No Q-wave MIs occurred in either arm of the study, and non–Q-wave MIs (defined as CK level more than 2 times normal with an elevated CK-MB isoenzyme level) occurred in 2.2% and 1.4% of the patients in the RA and balloon angioplasty groups, respectively ($P = .72$). It is clear that while RA is safe in the treatment of obstructed small arteries, lower rates of target vessel failure were not achieved with RA when compared with balloon angioplasty.[45] Table 31-4 summarizes these major trials.

[ ] ROTATIONAL ATHERECTOMY FOR SPECIFIC LESIONS

Calcified Lesions

Treating calcified lesions can be a challenging endeavor. It is often difficult to successfully deliver and deploy a stent to the diseased segment. RA has proven to be particularly useful in this lesion subset. Complication and procedural success rates have been shown to be equivalent, and RA has been shown to be quite effective.[46,47] Hoffmann and colleagues found that debulking using RA, prior to stent placement in large calcified lesions in large arteries, is associated with infrequent complications, the largest acute angiographic results, and the most favorable late clinical event rates.[48]

Complex Lesions

As previously mentioned, the ERBAC and COBRA trials enrolled patients with type B2 and C lesions. Although initial results and procedural success were better with RA, long-term angiographic restenosis rates were comparable to those obtained with balloon angioplasty. Complication rates were found to be similar in both the balloon angioplasty and RA subsets.

Chronic Total Occlusions

Success with chronic total occlusions has been limited. Stenting has been shown to be better than angioplasty alone,[49] and with the advent of drug-eluting stents, success rates may increase substantially. A multicenter registry involving 145 lesions showed a success rate of 91% with an in-hospital death rate of 1.4% and non-Q-wave MI rates of 4.3%. In the 49% of patients who had angiographic follow-up, the restenosis rate was 62.5%.[50] The BAROCCO (Balloon Angioplasty vs Rotational Angioplasty in Chronic Coronary Occlusions) study showed that in chronic coronary occlusions of tapered morphology, RA is not superior to conventional angioplasty. In procedures involving stump-like occlusions, the primary success rate is higher with the RA technique.[51] However, these lesions are sometimes fibrotic and calcified, making them resistant to stent delivery and deployment. In these cases, RA may play role in debulking and "preparing" the lesions for stenting.

Ostial Lesions

Restenosis rates and procedural success are limited with these types of lesions. Several nonrandomized studied have shown that RA may improve procedural and clinical success rates.[52–55] Popma and colleagues reported on the largest series. They found a success rate of 97%, with 27% dissection and 2.8% spasm rates, respectively. Urgent or emergent coronary artery bypass grafting was required in 1.9% of patients, and the restenosis rate was reported at 32%.[52] No clinical trials have evaluated drug-eluting stents as an adjunct to RA in this setting. Extrapolating from existing data, it would seem that this would offer a useful alternative, particularly in ostial LAD or left circumflex lesions, where plaque shift could have significant adverse consequences.

Bifurcation Lesions

Walton and colleagues revaluated the angiograms of 418 patients with 320 side branches to determine the rate, predictors, and outcome of side-branch occlusion after RA.[56] Vessels were scored as either perfused (thrombolysis in MI 2 or 3 flow) or occluded (thrombolysis in MI 0 or 1 flow) before and after the procedure. A detailed quantitative angiographic analysis was performed on a total of 108 side branches, including all cases of branch occlusion. Clinical outcomes were determined in all cases involving side-branch loss. There were 24 occlusions in 21 patients after the procedure, giving a rate of branch loss of 7.5%. Follow-up angiography of 24 hours or longer was available for 13 of the occluded branches and 12 were found to be patent. In the 21 patients with branch occlusion, 6 patients sustained an MI (of which 5 were non–Q-wave), 2 underwent coronary artery bypass grafting, and 2 died.

Lesion-associated side branches are frequently present in the types of vessels to undergo high-speed RA. These branches remained patent 92.5% of the time, with occlusion occurring infrequently and usually being transient. When occlusion did occur, there was a 29% incidence of MI. Although no large-scale randomized studies have evaluated the utility of RA in bifurcating lesions, several retrospective analyses have shown a high procedural success rate with RA, with a decreased incidence of side-branch occlusion. It is possible that adequately debulking the lesions prior to stenting prevents plaque shift, and therefore may salvage the side branch.[56] Figure 31-6 shows a bifurcating lesion in which RA prior to stent delivery "spared" the diagonal vessel.

Angulated Lesions

Chevalier and colleagues reported a higher rate of complications (death, 2.7 % vs 0.3%; total ischemic events, 5.4% vs 1.3%) and lower procedural success rates (86% vs 94%) in angulated lesions (defined as > 45 degrees).[56a] When approaching angulated lesions, it is important to use a floppy wire, and to pick a guide catheter that will centralize wire placement and avoid wire bias, while using a stepped burr approach (burr-to-artery ratio of 0.5–0.6).

Tortuous Vessels

Although no large-scale trials have assessed the most efficient way to deal with lesions in tortuous vessels, it is helpful to use a floppy wire to avoid pseudolesions, and low speed with a stepped burr approach.

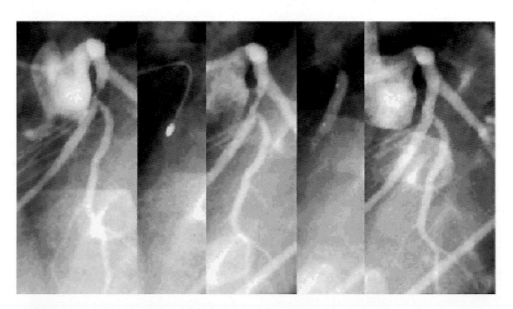

FIGURE 31-6. Bifurcating lesion. RA before stent delivery spared the diagonal.

Lesions Resistant to Balloon Dilation

The clinical and angiographic outcome of patients undergoing rotational coronary atherectomy after unsuccessful balloon angioplasty was evaluated using quantitative angiography by Brogan and colleagues. They found that RA may be effective in selected patients when standard balloon angioplasty is unsuccessful.[57] Sievert and colleagues reported a high success rate (almost 90%) using RA in the treatment of high-grade coronary stenoses and occlusions that could not be crossed with a balloon catheter.[58] Rosenblum and colleagues reported a series of 41 lesions; in 26, balloon expansion was inadequate within the lesion, and in 15, balloon delivery was unsuccessful. RA was technically successful in 40 of 41 (97.6%) of the lesions attempted. Follow-up of 24 patients (mean time = 9 ± 5 mo) showed a restenosis rate similar to that of balloon angioplasty.[59] Thus, it would seem that RA is an excellent alternative for patients with lesions in which balloon angioplasty is unsuccessful, either because the balloon cannot be delivered or because the lesion is resistant to balloon dilation as a result of inelasticity.

In-Stent Restenosis

Improvements in drug-eluting stents may soon eliminate the problem of in-stent restenosis resulting from neointimal proliferation. In current practice, however, interventional cardiologists have had limited long-term success in treating these lesions, particularly if the restenosis is diffuse in nature. IVUS and angiographic studies have shown that RA of in-stent restenosis appears to increase lumen gain by effective plaque removal.[60] Adjunctive angioplasty results in additional lumen gain by further stent expansion. Two large-scale trials, ROSTER and ARTIST, evaluated the use of RA in these types of lesions.

ROSTER. Rotational Atherectomy vs Balloon Angioplasty for Diffuse In-Stent Restenosis. This single-center, randomized trial compared RA with balloon angioplasty (both with IVUS guidance) in the treatment of diffuse in-stent restenosis in 200 patients. In the RA group (n = 100), rotablation was performed using a burr-to-artery ratio greater than 0.7 followed by adjunctive balloon dilation at low pressure (4–6 atm). In the angioplasty group (n = 100), high-pressure (> 12 atm) balloon dilation was performed using an optimal size balloon. The primary end point was target lesion revascularization at 9 months, and secondary end points included clinical events at 1 year and angiographic restenosis in a substudy of the last 75 patients enrolled.

The investigators found that procedural and angiographic success rates were similar. However, a higher rate of repeat stenting occurred in the angioplasty group (31% vs 10%; $P < .001$). Although the angiographic acute luminal gain was similar between the two groups, IVUS analysis revealed a lower residual intimal hyperplasia area after RA versus angioplasty (2.1 ± 0.9 mm² vs 3.3 ± 1.8 mm²; $P = .005$). At a mean follow-up of 12 ± 2 months, there were two deaths, three MIs, and three coronary artery bypass graft procedures in each group. The incidence of target lesion revascularization was 32% in the RA group and 45% in the angioplasty group ($P = .042$), with a similar trend noted in the angiographic substudy. Thus, this trial showed that for diffuse in-stent restenosis, both RA and angioplasty are safe and effective, but

RA resulted in less residual intimal hyperplasia, lower repeat stent use, and decreased target lesion revascularization.[61]

ARTIST (European Angioplasty vs Rotational Atherectomy for Treatment of Diffuse In-Stent Restenosis Trial). The primary goal of this study was to compare RA followed by balloon angioplasty with balloon angioplasty alone in patients with diffuse in-stent restenosis. This was a multicenter, randomized, prospective European trial involving 298 patients with in-stent restenosis greater than 70% (mean lesion length, 14 ± 8 mm) in stents, implanted in coronary arteries for 3 months or longer. In the angioplasty group, angioplasty was performed at the discretion of the local investigator, and RA was performed by using a stepped-burr approach followed by adjunctive PTCA with low (≤ 6 atm) inflation pressure. IVUS during the intervention and at follow-up was used in a substudy involving 86 patients (45 PTCA, 41 RA).

Angiography demonstrated no difference in the short-term outcome, with equivalent procedural success rates defined as remaining stenosis less than 30% (89% PTCA, 88% RA). However, the results showed that, in the long term, PTCA was a significantly better strategy than RA. Mean net gain in MLD was 0.67 mm and 0.45 mm for PTCA and RA, respectively ($P = .0019$). Mean gain in diameter stenosis was 25% and 17% ($P = .002$), resulting in restenosis (≥ 50%) rates of 51% for PTCA and 65% for RA ($P = .039$). By IVUS, the major difference was the missing stent overexpansion during PTCA after RA. Six-month event-free survival was significantly higher after PTCA (91.3%) compared with RA (79.6%; $P = .0052$). This study showed that angioplasty produced a significantly better long-term outcome than RA for the treatment of diffuse in-stent restenosis.[62] Dauerman and colleagues reported a trend toward decreased target lesion revascularization with RA as opposed to PTCA; however, this finding did not reach statistical significance (28% vs 46%; $P = .18$).[63]

It is interesting to note the contradictory results of these large trials. It is possible that routine use of IVUS in the ROSTER study, which led to the exclusion of one third of the patients (due to underdeployment of the stent), may have played a role in selecting a subgroup of patients who would benefit from RA. It is also possible that operator experience may have played a significant role in the findings.

CONCLUSION

Interventional cardiology has evolved considerably since the advent of RA. RA continues to have a unique role in treatment of arteries or lesions in which stent delivery is difficult or unfeasible. Rigid calcific or fibrocalcific lesions can be made more elastic after pretreatment with RA, facilitating stent delivery. With appropriate guide catheter, guidewire, and burr selection (burr-to-artery ratio < 0.7) and proper ablation techniques, complication rates can be significantly minimized. Aggressive burr advancement, indicated by decelerations greater than 5000 rpm, should be avoided and run times should be limited to 15 to 30 seconds with 30-second to 2-minute intervals (depending on artery and patient response) between runs. Today, drug-eluting stents have made interventions for previously unapproachable lesions relatively routine. RA can play a pivotal role in ensuring stent delivery in subset of these lesions.

REFERENCES

1. Reimers B, Von Birgelen C, van der Giessen WJ, et al. A word of caution on optimizing stent deployment in calcified lesions: Acute coronary rupture with tamponade. *Am Heart J.* 1996;131:192.
2. Goldberg SL, Colombo A, Nakamura S, et al. Benefit of intracoronary ultrasound in the deployment of Palmaz-Schatz stents. *J Am Coll Cardiol.* 1994;24:996.
3. Fourrier JL, Bertrand ME, Auth DC, et al. Percutaneous coronary rotational angioplasty in humans: Preliminary report. *J Am Coll Cardiol.* 1989;14:1278.
4. Zacca NM, Raizner AE, Noon GP, et al. Treatment of symptomatic peripheral atherosclerotic disease with a rotational atherectomy device. *Am J Cardiol.* 1989;63:77.
5. Hansen DD, Auth DC, Vracko R, et al. Rotational atherectomy in atherosclerotic rabbit iliac arteries. *Am Heart J.* 1988;115(1 Pt 1):160.
6. Ahn SS, Auth D, Marcus DR, Moore WS. Removal of focal atheromatous lesions by angioscopically guided high-speed rotary atherectomy. Preliminary experimental observations. *J Vasc Surg.* 1988;7:292.
7. Mintz GS, Potkin BN, Keren G, et al. Intravascular ultrasound evaluation of the effect of rotational atherectomy in obstructive atherosclerotic coronary artery disease. *Circulation.* 1992;86:1383.
8. Kovach JA, Mintz GS, Pichard AD, et al. Sequential intravascular ultrasound characterization of the mechanisms of rotational atherectomy and adjunct balloon angioplasty. *J Am Coll Cardiol.* 1993;22:1024.
9. Cowley M, Buchbinder M, Warth D, et al. Effect of coronary rotational atherectomy abrasion on vessel segments adjacent to treated lesions [abstract]. *J Am Coll Cardiol.* 1992;19:333A.
10. Mintz GS, Potkin BN, Keren G, et al. Intravascular ultrasound evaluation of the effect of rotational atherectomy in obstructive atherosclerotic coronary artery disease. *Circulation.* 1992;86:1383.
11. Mintz GS, Potkin BN, Keren G, et al. Cross-sectional and three dimensional intravascular ultrasound analysis of coronary artery geometry after rotational atherectomy [abstract]. *Circulation.* 1994;90:I-203.
12. Reisman M, Buchbinder M, Harms V, et al. Quantitative angiography of coronary artery dimensions 24 hours after rotational atherectomy. *Am J Cardiol.* 1998;81:1427.
13. Reisman M, Burchbinder M, Bass T, et al. Improvement in coronary dimensions at early 24-hour follow-up after coronary rotational ablation: Implications for restenosis [abstract]. *Circulation.* 1992;86:I-332.
14. Zotz RJ, Erbel R, Philipp A, et al. High-speed rotational angioplasty-induced echo contrast in vivo and in vitro optical analysis. *Cathet Cardiovasc Diagn.* 1992;26:98.
15. Yamashita K, Satake S, Ohira H, Ohtomo K. Radiofrequency thermal balloon coronary angioplasty: A new device for successful percutaneous transluminal coronary angioplasty. *J Am Coll Cardiol.* 1994;23:336.
16. Snabre P, Baumler H, Mills P. Aggregation of human red blood cells after moderate heat treatment. *Biorheology.* 1985;22:185.
17. Gader AM, al-Mashhadani SA, al-Harthy SS. Direct activation of platelets by heat is the possible trigger of the coagulopathy of heat stroke. *Br J Haematol.* 1990;74:86.
18. Hong MK, Tjurmin A, Haudenschild CC, et al. Historical finding in tirectional atherectomy specimens after rotational atherectomy in calcified coronary arteries [abstract]. *Circulation.* 1994;90:I-213.
19. Resiman M, DeVore LJ, Ferguson M, et al. Analysis of heat generation during high-speed rotational ablation: Technical implication [abstract]. *J Am Coll Cardiol.* 1996;27:292A.
20. Prevosti LG, Cook JA, Unger EF, et l. Particulate debris from rotational atherectomy: Size distribution and physiologic effects [abstract]. *Circulation.* 1988;78:II-83.
21. Friedman HZ, Elliot MA, Gottlieb GJ, et al. Mechanical rotary atherectomy: The effects of microparticle embolization on myocardial blood flow and function. *J Int Cardiol.* 1989;2:77.
22. Sherman CT, Brunken R, Chan A, et al. Myocardial perfusion and segmental wall motion after rotational atherectomy [abstract]. *Circulation.* 1992;86: I-652.
23. Pavlides GS, Hauser AM, Grines CL, et al. Clinical, hemodynamic, electrocardiographic and mechanical events during non-occlusive coronary atherectomy and comparison with balloon angioplasty. *Am J Cardiol.* 1992;70:841.
24. Huggins GS, Williams MJA, Yang J, et al. Transient wall motion abnormalities following rotational atherrectomy are reflective of myocardial stunning more than myocardial infarction [abstract]. *J Am Coll Cardiol.* 1995;25:96A.
25. Reisman M, Buchbinder M, Warth D, et al. Comparison of patients with either < 70% diameter narrowing or > or = 70% narrowing of the right coronary artery when performing rotational atherectomy on > or = 1 narrowing in the left coronary arteries. *Am J Cardiol.* 1997;79:305.
26. Kaplan BM, Safian RD, Mojares JJ, et al. Optimal burr and adjunctive balloon sizing reduces the need for target artery revascularization after coronary mechanical rotational atherectomy. *Am J Cardiol.* 1996;78:1224.
27. Stertzer SH, Pomerantsev EV, Fitzgerald PJ. Effects of technique modification on immediate results of high speed rotational atherectomy in 710 procedures on 656 patients. *Cathet Cardiovasc Diagn.* 1995;36:304.
28. Kobayashi Y, De Gregorio J, Kobayashi N, et al. Lower restenosis rate with stenting following aggressive versus less aggressive rotational atherectomy. *Cathet Cardiovasc Interv.* 1999;46:406.
29. Braden G, et al. Restenosis following minimally traumatic rotational atherectomy: The acute and long-term results of the Rotablator and Restenosis (R&R) study. *J Am Coll Cardiol.* 1998;31(suppl):378A.
30. Warth DC, Leon MB, O'Neill W. Rotational atherectomy multicenter registry: Acute results, complications and 6-month angiographic follow-up in 709 patients. *J Am Coll Cardiol.* 1994;24:641.
31. Lincoff AM, Bittl JA, Harrington RA, et al. Bivalirudin and provisional glycoprotein IIb/IIIa blockade compared with heparin and planned glycoprotein IIb/IIIa blockade during percutaneous coronary intervention: REPLACE-2 randomized trial. *JAMA.* 2003;289:853. Erratum in: *JAMA.* 2003;289:1638.
32. Kini A, Reich D, Marmur JD, et al. Reduction in periprocedural enzyme elevation by abciximab after rotational atherectomy of type B2 lesions: Results of the Rota ReoPro randomized trial. *Am Heart J.* 2001;142:965.
33. Kereiakes DJ. Preferential benefit of platelet glycoprotein IIb/IIIa receptor blockade: Specific considerations by device and disease state. *Am J Cardiol.* 1998;81:49E.
34. Koch KC, vom Dahl J, Kleinhans E. Influence of a platelet GPIIb/IIIa receptor antagonist on myocardial hypoperfusion during rotational atherectomy as assessed by myocardial Tc-99m sestamibi scintigraphy. *J Am Coll Cardiol.* 1999;33:998.
35. Williams MS, Coller BS, Vaananen HJ. Activation of platelets in platelet-rich plasma by rotablation is speed-dependent and can be inhibited by abciximab (c7E3 Fab; ReoPro). *Circulation.* 1998;98:742.
36. Cohen BM, Weber VJ, Blum RR, et al. Cocktail attenuation of rotational ablation flow effects (CARAFE) study: Pilot. *Cathet Cardiovasc Diagn.* 1996;(suppl 3):69.
37. Hanna GP, Yhip P, Fujise K, et al. Intracoronary adenosine administered during rotational atherectomy of complex lesions in native coronary arteries reduces the incidence of no-reflow phenomenon. *Cathet Cardiovasc Interv.* 1999;48:275.
38. MacIsaac A, Whitlow P, Cowley M, Buchbinder M. Angiographic predictors of outcome of coronary rotational atherectomy from the completed multicenter registry. *J Am Coll Cardiol.* 1994;23:353A.
39. Reifart N, Vandormael M, Krajcar M, et al. Randomized comparison of angioplasty of complex coronary lesions at a single center. Excimer Laser, Rotational Atherectomy, and Balloon Angioplasty Comparison (ERBAC) Study. *Circulation.* 1997;96:91.
40. Dill T, Dietz U, Hamm CW, et al. A randomized comparison of balloon angioplasty versus rotational atherectomy in complex coronary lesions (COBRA study). *Eur Heart J.* 2000;21:1759.
41. Whitlow PL, Bass TA, Kipperman RM, et al. Results of the study to determine rotablator and transluminal angioplasty strategy (STRATAS). *Am J Cardiol.* 2001;87:699.
42. Safian RD, Feldman T, Muller DW, et al. Coronary angioplasty and Rotablator atherectomy trial (CARAT): Immediate and late results of a prospective multicenter randomized trial. *Cathet Cardiovasc Interv.* 2001;53:213.
43. Braden G, Kutcher M, Ranking K, et al. The Effects of Debulking on Restenosis: EDRES trial. *Circulation.* 1998;98(suppl I):709.
43a. Buchbinder M, Fortuna R, Sharma SK. Debulking prior to stenting improves acute outcomes: early results from SPORT trial. *J Am Coll Cardiol.* 2000;35:8A.
44. Kobayashi Y, De Gregorio J, Kobayashi N, et al. Lower restenosis rate with stenting following aggressive versus less aggressive rotational atherectomy. *Cathet Cardiovasc Interv.* 1999;46:406.
45. Mauri L, Reisman M, Buchbinder M, et al. Comparison of rotational atherectomy with conventional balloon angioplasty in the prevention of restenosis of small coronary arteries: Results of the Dilatation vs Ablation Revascularization Trial Targeting Restenosis (DART). *Am Heart J.* 2003;145:847.

46. MacIsaac AI, Bass TA, Buchbinder M, et al. High speed rotational atherectomy: Outcome in calcified and noncalcified coronary artery lesions. *J Am Coll Cardiol.* 1995;26:731.

47. Altman D, Popma J, Kent K, et al. Rotational atherectomy effectively treats calcified lesions. *J Am Coll Cardiol.* 1993;21:443A.

48. Hoffmann R, Mintz GS, Kent KM, et al. Comparative early and nine-month results of rotational atherectomy, stents, and the combination of both for calcified lesions in large coronary arteries. *Am J Cardiol.* 1998;81:552.

49. Rahel BM, Suttorp MJ, Laarman GJ, et al. Primary stenting of occluded native coronary arteries: Final results of the Primary Stenting of Occluded Native Coronary Arteries (PRISON) study. *Am Heart J.* 2004;147:e22.

50. Omoigui N, Booth J, Reisman M, et al. Rotational atherectomy in chronic total occlusions. *J Am Coll Cardiol.* 1995;25:97A.

51. Danchin N, Cassagnes J, Juilliere Y, et al. Balloon angioplasty versus rotational angioplasty in chronic coronary occlusions (the BAROCCO study). *Am J Cardiol.* 1995;75:330.

52. Popma JJ, Brogan WC 3rd, Pichard AD, et al. Rotational coronary atherectomy of ostial stenoses. *Am J Cardiol.* 1993;71:436.

53. Koller PT, Freed M, Grines CL, O'Neill WW. Success, complications, and restenosis following rotational and transluminal extraction atherectomy of ostial stenoses. *Cathet Cardiovasc Diagn.* 1994;31:255.

54. Zimarino M, Corcos T, Favereau X, et al. Rotational coronary atherectomy with adjunctive balloon angioplasty for the treatment of ostial lesions. *Cathet Cardiovasc Diagn.* 1994;33:22.

55. Sabri MN, Cowley MJ, DiSciascio G, et al. Immediate results of interventional devices for coronary ostial narrowing with angina pectoris. *Am J Cardiol.* 1994;73:122.

56. Walton AS, Pomerantsev EV, Oesterle SN, et al. Outcome of narrowing related side branches after high-speed rotational atherectomy. *Am J Cardiol.* 1996;77:370.

56a. Chevalier B. Techniques of coronary atherectomy. *Sang Thrombose Vaisseaux.* 1992;4:513.

57. Brogan WC 3rd, Popma JJ, Pichard AD, et al. Rotational coronary atherectomy after unsuccessful coronary balloon angioplasty. *Am J Cardiol.* 1993;71:794.

58. Sievert H, Tonndorf S, Utech A, Schulze R. High frequency rotational angioplasty (rotablation) after unsuccessful balloon dilatation. *Z Kardiol.* 1993;82:411.

59. Rosenblum J, Stertzer SH, Shaw RE, et al. Rotational ablation of balloon angioplasty failures. *J Invasive Cardiol.* 1992;4:312.

60. Radke PW, Klues HG, Haager PK, et al. Mechanisms of acute lumen gain and recurrent restenosis after rotational atherectomy of diffuse in-stent restenosis: A quantitative angiographic and intravascular ultrasound study. *J Am Coll Cardiol.* 1999;34:33.

61. Sharma SK, Kini A, Mehran R, et al. Randomized trial of Rotational Atherectomy Versus Balloon Angioplasty for Diffuse In-stent Restenosis (ROSTER). *Am Heart J.* 2004;147:16.

62. Vom Dahl J, Silber S, Niccoli SE, et al. Angioplasty vs. rotational atherectomy for treatment of diffuse in-stent restenosis: Clinical and angiographic results from a randomized multicenter trial (ARTIST study). *J Am Coll Cardiol.* 2000;35(suppl A):7A.

63. Dauerman HL, Baim DS, Sparano AM, et al. Balloon angioplasty versus debulking for treatment of diffuse in-stent restenosis. *J Am Coll Cardiol.* 1998;31:455A.

CHAPTER (32)

Brachytherapy

Pramod Kuchulakanti, MD, and Ron Waksman, MD

Vascular brachytherapy, using beta and gamma emitters, revolutionized the treatment of percutaneous coronary interventions, particularly in-stent restenosis (ISR). Vascular brachytherapy following angioplasty for the prevention of restenosis was introduced in 1992 by several investigators who performed a series of preclinical studies and consistently demonstrated profound reduction of neointima formation following balloon injury. The results of these preclinical trials were encouraging and facilitated the initiation of the feasibility clinical trials first in the peripheral arteries, later in coronary arteries through pivotal trials, and then onto commercialization of the technology for clinical use in Europe in 1999.

In November 2000, the Food and Drug Administration approved vascular brachytherapy for ISR. Since then, brachytherapy has become an established modality of treatment for ISR, while expanding indications include ISR in saphenous vein grafts, lower extremities, renal arteries, and de novo lesions in coronary and femoropopliteal vessels. With the advent of DES for the treatment of ISR, brachytherapy may be of historic interest, but every interventionalist still should learn about this modality of treatment.

RADIATION BIOLOGY AND MECHANISM

Radiation inhibits smooth muscle cell proliferation and intimal hyperplasia in the irradiated atherosclerotic arteries by intervening in the cell cycle to cause cell death to radiosensitive cells, especially those undergoing mitosis following vascular injury. Cells in the M and G2 phases are the most sensitive to radiation, G1 are sensitive only in the early G1 phase, and cells in G0 are radio-resistant. Radiation affects tissue damage either directly, by absorbing into the target molecules such as DNA, RNA, or enzymes, or indirectly, by interacting with these molecules via formation of highly reactive

hydroxyl free radicals. Another mechanism is by inducing programmed cell death, also called *apoptosis*.

The potential mechanisms by which radiation may reduce restenosis is by inhibiting the first wave of cell proliferation in the adventitia and the media, and by inducing favorable remodeling.[1] Additional mechanisms include suppression of macrophages and adventitial myofibroblasts.[2,3] Cells can repair radiation damage; therefore, subtherapeutic doses may only delay the restenosis, because the surviving cells will continue to divide and eventually occupy the lumen wall. Dose optimization is thus important to achieve adequate results. Late effects of vascular brachytherapy may be seen 5 to 10 years after treatment and include late thrombosis, fibrosis, thinning of the media, aneurysm formation, and late restenosis.

RADIATION PHYSICS, DOSIMETRY, AND DELIVERY SYSTEMS

Among several isotopes developed for the use in vascular brachytherapy, only three have seen widespread use in clinical application; namely, the gamma emitter iridium 192 (^{192}Ir) and the beta emitters strontium 90 (^{90}Sr)/yttrium 90 (^{90}Y) and phosphorus 32 (^{32}P). Requirements for an ideal radioisotope in vascular brachytherapy include dose distribution of a few millimeters from the source with minimal dose gradient, low dose levels to the surrounding tissues, treatment time of less than 10 minutes, and a sufficient half-life for multiple applications when used in a catheter-based system. Gamma- and beta-emitting radionuclides currently investigated and used in the clinical trials for vascular brachytherapy are presented in Table 32-1. The main platforms that deliver radiation are catheter-based systems such as line source wires, radioactive seeds, radioactive gas- and liquid-filled balloons, or stents utilizing beta or gamma emitters. The latter are no longer

TABLE 32-1

Radionuclides for Vascular Brachytherapy

EMISSION	ISOTOPE	HALF-LIFE	ENERGY (MeV)		ACTIVITY (mCi)	RADIATION SYSTEM
			MAXIMUM	AVERAGE		
Gamma	^{192}Ir	74 d	0.67	0.18	500	Checkmate (Cordis)
Beta	^{90}Sr/$^{-90}$Y	29 y	2.28	0.93	50	BetaCath (Novoste)
	^{90}Y	64 h	2.28	0.93	50	
	^{32}P	14 d	1.71	0.69	40	Galileo (Guidant), RDX (RadianceMedical)
	^{186}Re	90 h	1.08	0.38	300	Liquid-filled balloon
	^{133}Xe	5.2 d	0.35^a	0.10^a	300	Gas-filled balloon
Beta and gamma	^{188}Re	17 h	2.12^a	0.77^a	100	Liquid-filled balloon
	^{106}Rh	130 d	3.54^a	1.42^a	30	—
	^{188}W/$^{-188}$Re	69 d	2.12^a	0.77^a	50	—

^{a}Beta energy, only.

used because they created the problem of narrowing at the ends of the stent the so-called *candy-wrapper effect.*

Source selection depends on the source energy half-life, available activity, penetration and dose distribution, radiation exposure to the patient and the operator, shielding requirement, availability, and cost. Isotope selection and dosimetry for intracoronary brachytherapy are derived from the anatomy of the vessel and the treated lesion, the target tissue (intima, media, or adventitia), the diameter and curvature of the vessel, the eccentricity and composition of the plaque, lesion length, amount of calcium, and the

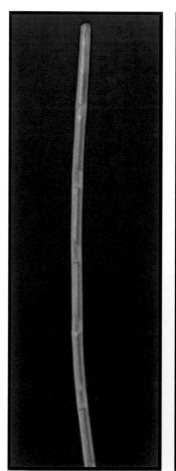
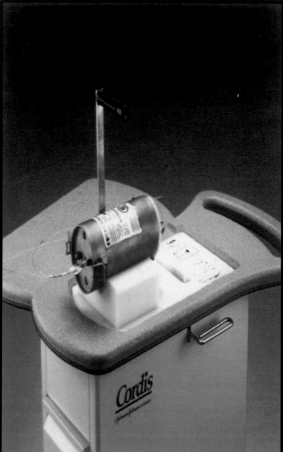
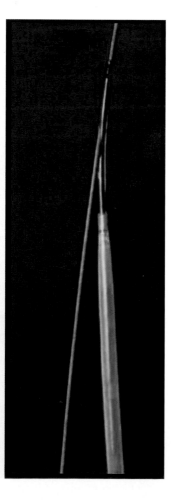

FIGURE 32-1. Cordis CheckMate system.

presence or absence of a stent in the treated segment. Dosimetry issues considered include the choice of isotope, beta- versus gamma-emitting radioisotopes, centering versus noncentering devices, administration of high- versus low-dose rates of radiation, centering versus noncentering of the source in the vessel wall, and the need for stepping. Intravascular ultrasound (IVUS) can assist in treatment planning and dosing because it determines the actual lumen size and the distances from the source to the lumen and the adventitia. Nevertheless, fixed radial prescription points seem to be easier and more practical without compromising the outcome.

^{192}Ir is administered by the CheckMate system (Cordis Corporation, Miami, FL), which requires manual loading of the radioactive seeds (Figure 32-1). The AngioRad system (Vascular Therapies, Norwalk, CT) uses a flexible, 30-mm ^{192}Ir wire source. The Galileo system (Guidant Corporation, Irvine, CA) administers ^{32}P with automated stepping technology and a centering balloon (Figure 32-2). The RDX system (Radiance Medical, San Diego, CA) also administers ^{32}P; however, the isotope is incorporated directly into the balloon material of the percutaneous transluminal coronary angiography (PTCA)-type catheter. ^{90}Sr/Y is administered by BetaCath system (Novoste Corporation, Norcross, GA), which employs a hydraulic technique to deliver the radioactive seeds (Figure 32-3). Rhenium 188 (^{188}Re) is obtained from the Tungsten 188 (^{188}W)/^{188}Re radionuclide generator as a solution that is injected into the coronary dilation balloon and can be applied at the target by inflating the balloon.

BRACHYTHERAPY IN ANIMAL MODELS

In a porcine stent model of restenosis, Schwartz and colleagues applied external radiation therapy (400–800 cGy) with an orthovoltage x-ray unit to the coronary vessels following stent placement and showed accentuated development of neointimal hyperplasia.[4] In later studies, higher doses of 21 Gy to the entire heart showed inhibition of the neointima formation with the same model. The degree of injury and lack of precise delivery to moving epicardial arteries are potential explanations for these findings. Higher volumes of radiation, even though helpful, may result in late fibrosis to the whole heart, and are therefore less attractive compared with the endovascular approaches.

Several groups using catheter-based systems have obtained consistent evidence for the efficacy and safety of radiation using both beta and gamma emitters. Studies separately conducted by Waksman and colleagues at Emory University,[5,6] Wiedermann and colleagues at Columbia University,[7,8] and Raizner and colleagues at Baylor University[9] have shown marked reduction with ^{192}Ir neointimal hyperplasia following balloon injury in the short term (2–4 weeks) as assessed by histomorphometric studies in the porcine restenosis model. In two of the studies, the reduction in the neointimal hyperplasia in the irradiated arteries was shown at 6 months.[5,8] Waksman and colleagues demonstrated complete reendothelialization by electron microscopy at 2 weeks in balloon-injured and irradiated arteries (dose of 14 Gy).[5] However, incomplete reendothelialization was seen after stent implantation with similar doses. Wiedermann and colleagues[10] studied endothelial function after irradiation and reported normal vasodilatory response to acetylcholine at 4 weeks. It was realized that there was no evidence of malignant or premalignant transformation, excess fibrosis, or aneurysm formation in any of the arteries.

Verin and colleagues[11] delivered intra-arterial radiation through ^{90}Y and a centering balloon catheter in atherosclerotic rabbit iliac and carotid arteries using 6, 12, and 18 Gy and demonstrated reduction in neointimal cells in all treated groups. At 6 weeks, however, the reduction in neointima was maintained only in the rabbits that received 18 Gy. Waksman and colleagues[12] demonstrated reduction in neointima in a dose-dependent manner (7–56 Gy) with ^{90}Sr/Y in porcine coronary arteries. A consistent effect of reduction of neointima was seen with doses above 21 Gy, without an increase in adverse effects. Raizner showed a similar effect of reduction of neointima formation, postballoon and stent injury with another pure beta emitter, ^{32}P, using doses of 32 Gy. In summary, both beta and gamma emitters appear to be equally effective in stented arteries, particularly when radiation is delivered before stent implantation.

Radioactive stents have been produced by cyclotron activation, ion implantation, and proton bombardment for beta, gamma, and combination isotopes. The earliest experiments of radioactive stents were conducted by Fischell and colleagues.[13] Hehrlein and colleagues[14,15] conducted studies on rabbit iliac arteries and demonstrated reduction of neointima compared with control

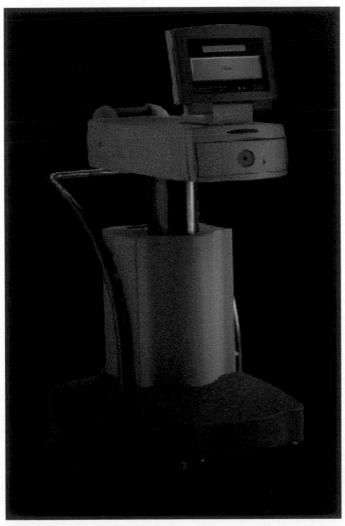

FIGURE 32-2. Guidant Galileo system source delivery unit.

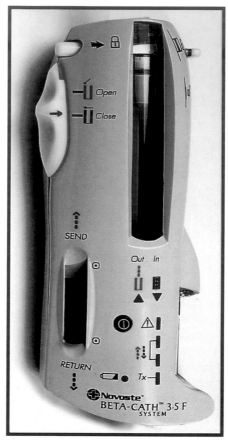
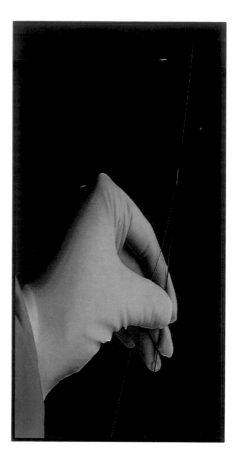
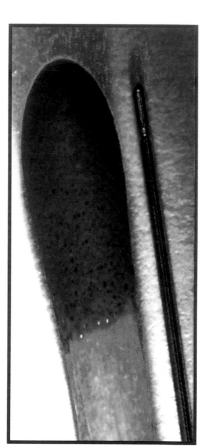

FIGURE 32-3. Novoste BetaCath system.

stents placed in the contralateral arteries. In this and another study preformed by this group, this reduction was better in the high-dose groups. Laird and Carter and their colleagues[16,17] in two different studies on pig iliac and coronary arteries, used pure beta-emitting (^{32}P) Strecker and Palmaz-Schatz stents, respectively, and demonstrated significant reductions of neointima at 4 weeks; however, at 6-month follow-up, inferior results were observed compared with controls. Radioactive stents, which were implanted in an atherosclerotic pig model, failed to show superiority over control nonradioactive stents with any of the treated doses at 6 months.[17]

Waksman,[18] Weinberger,[19] Robinson,[20] Makkar,[21] Kim,[22] and their colleagues used liquid isotope-filled balloons to irradiate porcine coronaries. The emitters used for this technology were xenon 133 (^{133}Xe), ^{188}Re (14Gy), and holmium 166 (^{166}Ho) (at 9 and 18 Gy). These preclinical studies showed reduction in neointimal tissue as assessed by IVUS and histomorphometry. The concept of the radioisotope-filled balloons is attractive because it has the advantages of centering and ease of use; however, a potential leakage hazard is of great concern.

LONG-TERM ANIMAL STUDIES

Long-term animal studies using beta and gamma emitter sources were disappointing. Wiedermann reported that at 6 months, arteries subjected to gamma radiation had less neointima formation compared with control. Waksman in 6-month studies utilizing ^{32}P

in a balloon-injury model had similar findings. However, with beta emitters (^{32}P and ^{90}Sr/Y) in a stented porcine coronary artery model, radiation was associated with increased mortality, thrombosis, and neointima formation compared with control. Similarly, 6-month studies with radioactive stents demonstrated an excess of neointima formation in the radioactive stents compared with control. Although few of the observations in long-term animal studies are reproduced in humans, results that carry over include the late thrombosis phenomenon, delayed restenosis, and inferior results using stent and radiation versus balloon and radiation. The discrepancy between the long-term animal results and the human results at 3- to 5-year follow-up can be explained by the differences in the species, normal porcine coronary artery versus atherosclerotic human coronary artery, and the age of the animals (younger animals subjected late radiation effects).

CLINICAL TRIALS

Both gamma and beta radiation were studied for the treatment of ISR, but only beta sources were studied for the treatment of de novo lesions. The only gamma isotope that was used in clinical trials is ^{192}Ir. Detailed discussion of these trials is beyond the scope of this chapter, but a brief summary of the landmark clinical trials conducted to date with gamma and beta emitters is presented. Summaries of these trials are displayed in Tables 32-2 through 32-4.

TABLE 32-2

Clinical Trials for In-Stent Restenosis Using Catheter-Based Systems With Gamma Radiation

STUDY NAME	DESIGN	RADIATION SYSTEM	DOSE (Gy)	RESULTS AND STATUS
SCRIPPS	Single-center, double-blind, randomized study in 55 patients with restenosis	Hand-delivered 0.030-in nylon ribbon with seeds (Best Medical) into noncentered, closed end lumen, 4.5-Fr catheter (Navius)	≥ 8 to < 30 to media by IVUS	Completed; showed reduction of restenosis in irradiated group maintained at 3 y
SCRIPPS II	Single-center, randomized study of 100 patients with diffuse ISR	Hand-delivered 0.030-in nylon ribbon with ^{192}Ir seeds into noncentered, closed end lumen, 4.0-Fr catheter (Cordis)	≥ 8 to < 30 to media by IVUS	Completed; demonstrated safety and efficacy of radiation in complex lesions, including SVGs
SCRIPPS III	Registry of 500 patients with ISR receiving 6 mo of clopidogrel with no stent and 12 mo of clopidogrel with stenting	Hand-delivered 0.030-in nylon ribbon with ^{192}Ir seeds into noncentered, closed end lumen, 4.0-Fr catheter (Cordis)	14 at 2 mm distance from source	Completed; underscored value of avoidance of additional stenting and need for prolonged antiplatelet therapy for preventing late thrombosis
SCRIPPS IV	Double-blind, randomized trial in 358 patients comparing 14 Gy vs 17 Gy at 2 mm from source	Hand-delivered 0.030-in nylon ribbon with ^{192}Ir seeds into noncentered, closed end lumen, 4.0-Fr catheter (Cordis)	14 and 17 Gy at 2 mm from source	Completed; modest but significant 36% decrease in restenosis at 8 mo, 41% decrease in MACE in 17 Gy group
WRIST	Single-center, double-blind, randomized trial in 130 patients with ISR (100 natives, 30 vein grafts)	Hand-delivered 0.030-in nylon ribbon with ^{192}Ir seeds (Best Medical) into noncentered, closed end lumen, 5.0-Fr catheter (Medtronic)	15 at 2.0 mm for vessels 3–4 mm; 18 for vessels > 4 mm	Completed; showed reduction in restenosis (67%) and revascularization (63%); at 2 y, reduction in TLR and TVR < 40%
SVG-WRIST	Multicenter, double-blind, randomized study in 120 patients with ISR	Hand-delivered 0.030-in nylon ribbon with seeds (Best Medical) into noncentered, closed end lumen, 5.0-Fr catheter (Medtronic)	15 at 2.4 mm for vessels ≥ 4.0 mm	Completed; showed reduction in restenosis (21% vs 44% placebo) at 6 mo; TLR and MACE reduced by 70% and 49%, respectively, compared with placebo group at 1y
Long WRIST	Two-center, double-blind, randomized trial in 120 patients with ISR lesions (36–80 mm)	Hand-delivered 0.030-in nylon ribbon with seeds (Best Medical) into noncentered, closed end lumen, 5.0 Fr catheter (Medtronic)	15 at 2.0 mm for vessels 3–4 mm	Completed; 6-mo restenosis rates lower in irradiated group (45%) versus control arm (73%)
Long WRIST High Dose	Single-center registry in 120 patients with ISR lesions (36–80 mm); 60 patients received 1 mo and 60 patients received 6 mo of clopidogrel therapy	Hand-delivered 0.030-in nylon ribbon with seeds (Best medical) into noncentered, closed end lumen, 5.0 Fr catheter (Medtronic)	18 at 2.0 mm for vessels 3–4 mm	Completed; restenosis was low (38%) and 1-y MACE 18%; late thrombosis was 9% in those who received clopidogrel for 6 mo

(continued)

TABLE 32-2 (continued)

Clinical Trials for In-Stent Restenosis Using Catheter-Based Systems With Gamma Radiation

STUDY NAME	DESIGN	RADIATION SYSTEM	DOSE (GY)	RESULTS AND STATUS
WRIST Plus	Registry of 120 patients with ISR receiving 6 mo of clopidogrel, 75 mg qd	Hand-delivered 0.030-in nylon ribbon with ^{192}Ir seeds into noncentered, closed end lumen, 4.0-Fr catheter (Cordis)	14 at 2 mm distance from source	Completed; late thrombosis was 4.2%; MACE, 36%; and TLR, 35% at 6 mo
WRIST 12	Registry of 120 patients with ISR receiving 12 mo of clopidogrel and 15 mo of angiographic study	Hand-delivered 0.030-in nylon ribbon with ^{192}Ir seeds into noncentered, closed end lumen, 4.0-Fr catheter (Cordis)	14 at 2 mm distance from source	Completed; late thrombosis was 3.3%; MACE, 21%; and TLR, 20% at 15 mo follow-up
EDGE WRIST	Registry of 120 patients with ISR having a longer treatment margin	Hand-delivered 0.030-in nylon ribbon with ^{192}Ir seeds into closed end lumen, 4.0-Fr catheter (Cordis)	14 at 2 mm from source	Ongoing
WRIST 21	Registry of patients with diffuse in-stent restenosis	Hand-delivered 0.030-in nylon ribbon with ^{192}Ir seeds into closed end lumen, 4.0-Fr catheter (Cordis)	21 at 2 mm from source	Ongoing
GAMMA-1	Multicenter, randomized double-blind study in 252 patients with ISR	Hand-delivered 0.030-in nylon ribbon with seeds (Best Medical) into noncentered, closed end lumen, 4.0-Fr catheter (Cordis)	$\geq$ 8 to < 30 to media by IVUS	Completed; patients with radiation therapy have significant reduction of restenosis (21.6% vs 50.5%) and clinical TLR at 9 mo
GAMMA-2	Multicenter registry in 125 patients with ISR	Hand-delivered 0.030-in nylon ribbon with seeds (Best Medical) into noncentered, closed end lumen, 4.0-Fr catheter (Cordis)	14 at 2 mm from source	Completed; similar to GAMMA-1; MACE was reduced by 36% and TLR was reduced by 48% compared with placebo group
GAMMA-5	Multicenter registry in 600 patients receiving 12 mo of therapy with clopidogrel for new stent and 6 mo for nonstent	Hand-delivered 0.030-in nylon ribbon with seeds (Best Medical) into noncentered, closed end lumen, 4.0-Fr catheter (Cordis)	14 at 2 mm from source	Ongoing
ARTISTIC I	Multicenter, double-blind, randomized trial of 115 patients with ISR	30-mm ^{192}Ir wire source	12, 15, and 18 at 2 mm	At 3 y, MACE is 22.8% in irradiated group compared with 24.1% in placebo group
ARTISTIC II	Multicenter study of 236 patients	30-mm ^{192}Ir wire source	18 at 2 mm	At 9 mo, irradiated patients had acute procedural success rate of 86.9% compared with 92.3% in placebo group

TABLE 32-2 (continued)

Clinical Trials for In-Stent Restenosis Using Catheter-Based Systems With Gamma Radiation

STUDY NAME	DESIGN	RADIATION SYSTEM	DOSE (GY)	RESULTS AND STATUS
CURE	Registry of 120 patients with ISR who were not considered good candidates for coronary artery bypass grafting or medical therapy	Hand-delivered 0.030-in nylon ribbon with ^{192}Ir seeds into closed end lumen, 4.0-Fr catheter (Cordis)	14 at 2 mm from source	Enrollment extended; clinical follow-up available for initial 120 patients; 31% TVR and 33% MACE at 6 mo
GRANITE	European registry of 96 patients with ISR	Hand-delivered ^{192}Ir seeds (Best Industries, VA) into closed end lumen, 3.7-Fr cather (Cordis, Waterloo, Belgium)	14 at 2 mm from source	32% repeat restenosis at 6 mo; 38.4% MACE and 58% event-free survival at 1-y follow up

ARTISTIC = AngioRAd Technology for In-Stent restenosis Trial in native Coronaries; CURE = Columbia University Restenosis limination; GRANITE = Gamma Radiation to Atheromatous Neointima using Intracoronary Therapy in Europe; ISR = in-stent restenosis; IVUS = intravascular ultrasound; MACE = major adverse coronary event; SCRIPPS = Scripps Coronary Radiation to Inhibit Proliferation Post = Stenting; SVG = saphenous vein graft; TLR = target lesion revascularization; TVR = target vessel revascularization; WRIST = Washington Radiation for In-Stent restenosis Trial.

[ ] CLINICAL TRIALS OF GAMMA RADIATION

The first study of intracoronary radiation in human coronary arteries was conducted in 1994 by Condado and colleagues. In this study, 21 patients (22 lesions; two thirds being de novo lesions) were treated with ^{192}Ir after routine balloon angioplasty. Serial quantitative coronary angioplasty detected a binary restenosis rate of 28.6% at 6 months,[23] which remained the same at 5 years. Angiographic complications included four aneurysms (two procedure related and two occurring within 3 months). At 3 and 5 years, all aneurysms except one remained unchanged and no other angiographic complications were observed.[24]

Gamma Radiation for In-Stent Restenosis

The efficacy of ^{192}Ir in reducing clinical and angiographic restenosis in patients with in-stent restenosis (Figures 32-4 through 32-8) was confirmed by several studies, including two single-center trials, SCRIPPS and WRIST; and multicenter trials, GAMMA-1 and -2, and ARTISTIC.

SCRIPPS Trials. SCRIPPS (Scripps Coronary Radiation to Inhibit Proliferation Post-Stenting) was the first randomized trial to evaluate the safety and efficacy of intracoronary gamma radiation as adjunctive therapy to stents. Fifty-five patients were randomized to either ^{192}Ir therapy (n = 26) or to placebo (n = 29). The angiographic follow-up at 6.8 months and 3 years showed significantly lower restenosis rates in the ^{192}Ir group (17% and 33%, respectively) compared with placebo (54% and 63%). A subgroup analysis of the 35 patients enrolled due to ISR showed a 70% reduction in the recurrence rate in the irradiated group compared with the placebo group.[25,26] There were no evident clinical complications resulting from the radiation treatment, and clinical benefits were

maintained at 5 years with a significant reduction in the need for target lesion revascularization (TLR).[27]

SCRIPPS II for ISR in diffuse lesions (30–80 mm), SCRIPPS III with prolonged antiplatelet therapy (6–12 months of clopidogrel), and SCRIPPS IV to evaluate higher doses (17 Gy versus 14 Gy) followed the original SCRIPPS study and have shown, respectively, that radiation is effective for diffuse lesions, that prolonged platelet therapy reduces late thrombosis and additional stenting is to be avoided, and that optimization of radiation dose improves the outcomes further in diffuse lesions.

WRIST Series. Original WRIST (Washington Radiation for In-Stent restenosis Trial) was the first study that evaluated the effectiveness of radiation therapy in patients with ISR. In this study, 130 patients (100 with native coronaries and 30 with saphenous vein grafts [SVGs]), with ISR lesions (up to 47 mm in length) were randomized to receive either ^{192}Ir or placebo. At 6 months the radiation group showed a reduction in restenosis (19% vs 58% in placebo) and 79% and 63% reduction in the need for revascularization and major adverse cardiac events (MACE), respectively, compared with the placebo group.[28] This study showed that intracoronary gamma radiation, as adjunct therapy to intervention for the treatment of ISR, is feasible, safe, and effective. Extended follow-up of these patients showed durable beneficial effect of radiation at 1 year, 3 years,[29] and 5 years[30] in MACE rates compared with placebo. MACE rates were significantly lower at 5 years follow-up, albeit at the expense of repeat revascularization procedures, suggesting that radiation may delay, in part, the biologic processes and that a late catch-up phenomena or late thrombosis will reduce the long-term benefit of radiation.

Other landmark trials in this series were SVG-WRIST, which evaluated the effect of radiation therapy in patients with diffuse ISR lesions in saphenous vein grafts[31]; Long WRIST in patients

TABLE 32-3

Clinical Trials for In-Sent Restenosis Using Catheter-Based Systems With Beta Radiation

STUDY NAME	DESIGN	RADIATION SYSTEM	ISOTOPE AND DOSE	RESULTS AND STATUS
Beta WRIST	Registry of 50 patients with ISR	Schneider system ^{90}Y source, centering balloon, and afterloader	^{90}Y, 20.6 at 1 mm from balloon surface	Completed; restenosis rate of 22% at 6 mo; MACE 46% at 2 y; results similar to those of gamma WRIST group
START	Multicenter, rendomized, double-blind design for 476 ISR lesions (20 mm)	BetaCath system, 30-mm source train	^{90}Sr/Y, 18–20 Gy at 2 mm	Completed; showed reduction in TLR, TVR, and MACE (35%) in irradiated group; no late thrombosis
START 40/20	Registry of 207 patients with ISR	BetaCath system, 40 mm source train	^{90}Sr/Y, 18–20 Gy at 2 mm	Reduction in restenosis of 44%; MACE, 26%; and repeat revascularization
INHIBIT	Multicenter, doubleblind, randomized trial of 332 patients with ISR	Automatic afterloader (Nucletron) 0.018-in, 27-mm fixed wire via helical centering balloon	^{32}P, 20 Gy at 1 mm into vessel wall	Completed; demonstrated 50% reduction in restenosis (analysis segment) and 55% in MACE
Galileo INHIBIT	International, multicenter registry of 120 patients with ISR	Automatic afterloader (Guidant Galileo system) via helical centering balloon	^{32}P, 20 Gy at 1mm into vessel wall	Reduction in TLR-MACE by 49% and reduction in in-stent and in-lesion restenosis of 74% and 27%, respectively
BRITE	Feasibility study in patients with ISR lesions < 25 mm	Radiance system, with deployable ^{32}P balloon	^{32}P, 20 Gy at 1.0 mm from balloon	Enrollment completed; demonstrated safety at 30 d and lower restenosis rates at 6 mo
BRITE-II	Randomized study of 429 patients	RDX system (hot balloon), ^{32}P balloon	^{32}P, 20 Gy at 1.0 mm from balloon	ISR of 10.9% and geographic miss of 8.5% at 9 mo
4R	Registry of 50 patients in South Korea with ISR	Liquid-filled balloon 36 mm in length following rotational atherectomy	^{188}Re, 15 Gy at 1 mm into vessel wall	Angiographic restenosis rate was 10.4% at 6 mo
CURE	Open-label registry of 60 patients	Liquid injected into perfusion balloon	^{188}Re, 20 Gy to balloon surface	TLR-free survival was 75% in first 37 patients at 12 mo
RENO	Registry of 1098 patients in Europe and Middle East	Novoste BetaCath system	^{90}Sr/Y source train, 14–18 Gy at 2 mm from centerline of source axis	6-mo follow-up MACE rate was 18.7%

BRITE = Beta Radiation to prevent In-sTent rEstenosis; CURE = Columbia University Restenosis Elimination; INHIBIT = Intimal Hyperplasia Inhibition with Beta In-stent Trial; ISR = in-stent restenosis; MACE = major adverse cardiac event; START = STents and Radiation Therapy; TLR = target lesion revascularization; WRIST = Washington Radiation for In-Stent restenosis Trial.

TABLE 32-4

Clinical Trials for Using Catheter-Based System With Beta Radiation in De Novo Lesions

STUDY NAME	DESIGN	RADIATION SYSTEM	ISOTOPE AND DOSE	RESULTS AND STATUS
Geneva	Open-label registry of 15 patients post-PTCA	Mechanical loading of fixed wire via segmented, centered balloon	^{90}Y, 18 Gy to balloon surface	Demonstrated feasibility and safety in de novo lesions; high restenosis rate (40%)
BERT	Open-label registry of 23 patients post-PTCA	Hydraulic hand delivery of seed train in noncentered 5-Fr catheter	^{90}Sr/Y, 12, 14, or 16 Gy at 2 mm from source	Restenosis rate of 15%, late loss of 10%, and loss index of 5%
BRIE	Registry of 149 patients	BetaCath System	^{90}Sr/Y, 14–18 Gy at 2 mm from centerline of source axis	TVR with PTCA, 22% and 31% at 6-mo and 1-y follow-up, respectively
Beta-Cath	Multicenter, prospective, randomized, double-blind study of 1455 patients post-PTCA and provisional stenting	BetaCath System	^{90}Sr/Y, 14–18 Gy at 2 mm from centerline of source axis	240-day TVF rate was 14.2% with 31% restenosis rate
Dose-Finding Study Group	Prospective, randomized, multicenter dose-finding study	Automatic afterloader of fixed wire via centered balloon	^{90}Y 9 (n = 45), 12 (n = 45), 15 (n = 46), or 18 (n = 45) Gy at 1 mm depth	Significant dose-dependent benefit at 6-mo follows-up.
PREVENT	Multicenter, prospective, randomized, sham controlled study of 105 patients post-PTCA or stenting	Automatic afterloader	^{32}P, 16, 20, or 24 Gy to 1 mm into artery wall	22.4% restenosis rate at 6 mo with MACE of 16% at 1 y
CURE	Open-label registry of 60 patients	Liquid injected into perfusion balloon	^{188}Re, 20 Gy to balloon surface	TLR-free survival was 75% in first 37 patients at 12 mo
SVG BRITE	Feasibility study of 24 patients	RDX system using hot balloon	^{32}P, 20 Gy at 1 mm from balloon surface	8% TVR and 13% restenosis rates at 1 y
ECRIS	Single-center, randomized trial of 225 patients	Liquid-filled balloon catheter	^{188}Re, 22.5 Gy at 0.5 mm	TVR (6.3%) and late loss significantly lower at 6-mo follow-up
BRIDGE	Multicenter, randomized trial of 112 patients	Galileo system	^{32}P, 20 Gy at 1 mm from balloon surface	Higher TVR and MACE (20.4% and 25.9%) compared with control (12.1% and 17.2%)

BERT = Beta Energy Restenosis Trial; BRIE = Beta Radiation in Europe; BRIDGE = Beta-Radiation Investigation with Direct Stenting and Galileo; BRITE = Beta Radiation to prevent In-sTent rEstenosis; CURE = Columbia University Restenosis Elimination; ECRIS = EndoCoronary-Rhenium-Irradiation-Study; MACE = major adverse coronary event; PTCA = percutaneous transluminal coronary angioplasty; SVG = Saphenous rein graft; TLR = target lesion revascularization; TVF = target vessel failure; TVR = target vessel revascularization.

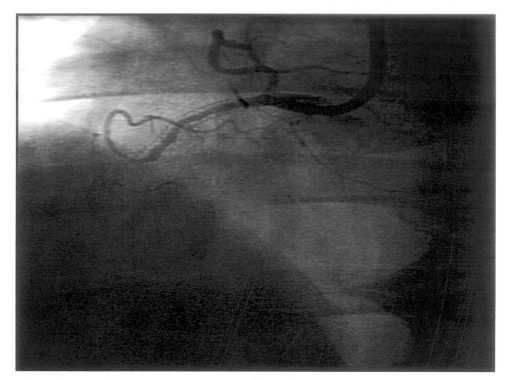

FIGURE 32-4. Total occlusion in-stent restenosis of the right coronary artery.

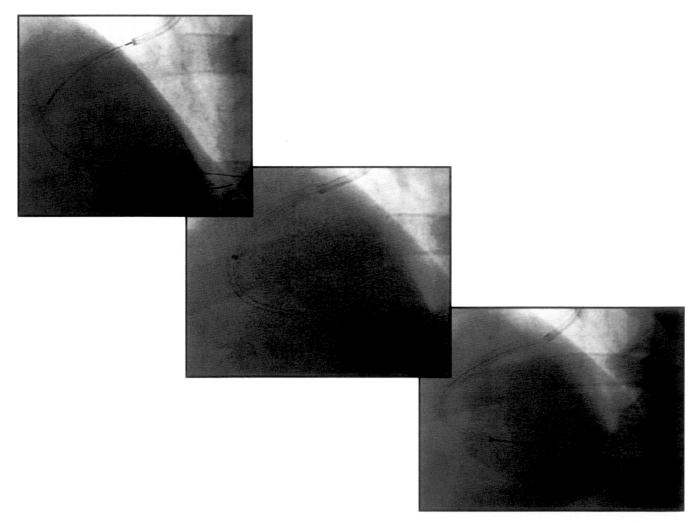

FIGURE 32-5. Novoste 40-mm radiation source train: Stepping × 3.

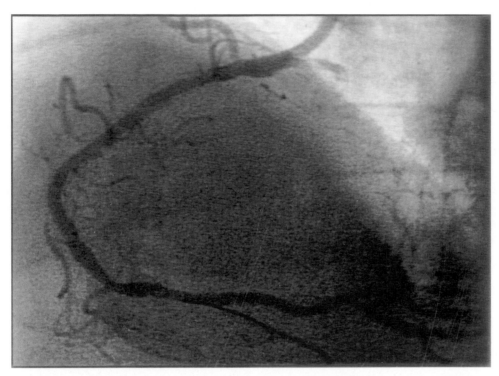

FIGURE 32-6. Final angiographic result postradiation.

with diffuse ISR in native coronary arteries (lesion length 36–80 mm)[32]; Long WRIST High Dose, which tested the efficacy of an 18-Gy dose of radiation; and WRIST Plus and WRIST 12, which tested the efficacy of prolonged clopidogrel therapy (up to 6 months and 12 months, respectively) to reduce the incidence of late thrombosis. WRIST 21 is an ongoing trial evaluating the optimization of dosimetry (with 21 Gy) in diffuse ISR lesions.

These trials have demonstrated superiority of radiation therapy in the treatment of ISR in vein graft disease (SVG-WRIST) and diffuse lesions (Long WRIST). The Long WRIST High Dose registry showed that a 3-Gy increase in the dose, from 15 to 18 Gy, provided additional reduction in MACE rates.[33] The strategy of prolonged antiplatelet therapy for 6 months in WRIST Plus reduced thrombosis rates from 9.6% to 2.5%-levels comparable to nonirradiated controls.[34] WRIST 12 has demonstrated further reduction in MACE and TLR with 12 months of clopidogrel therapy.[35] Based on these observations, it has become standard practice to provide at least 12 months of clopidogrel therapy for patients undergoing radiation therapy for ISR. High-dose radiation studies such as Long WRIST High Dose (18 Gy) and WRIST 21 (21 Gy) indicate that dose optimization will further reduce MACE rates and should be considered generally and particularly for the treatment of diffuse ISR.

GAMMA Trials.

GAMMA-1 was a multicenter, randomized trial of 252 patients with ISR treated with 8 to 30 Gy, hand-delivered using IVUS-guided dosimetry. This trial showed significant reductions in the in-stent (21.6%) and in-lesion (32.4%) restenosis rates compared with 50.5% and 55.3% in the control group at 6-month angiographic follow-up. The greatest benefit was obtained in patients with long lesions or diabetes, or both. Although TLR rates were lower in GAMMA-1, the rates of death and acute myocardial infarction were higher in the irradiated group compared with control. These complications were related in part to the late thrombosis phenomenon, which was more frequent in patients treated with radiation therapy than with placebo (5.3% vs 0.8%). All patients in the ^{192}Ir group who presented with late thrombosis had new stents placed within the in-stent target lesion at the time of the procedure.[36] This trial demonstrated the efficacy of intracoronary gamma radiation for the prevention of ISR recurrence, and increased awareness regarding the correlation between late thrombosis and an increased risk of MI.

GAMMA-2, a registry of 125 patients including complex lesions such as calcific lesions requiring rotablation, used a fixed dose of 14 Gy at 2 mm

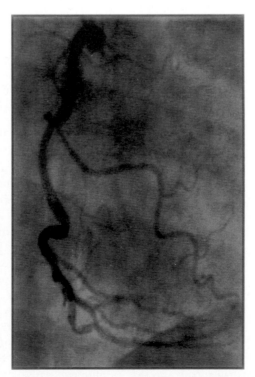

FIGURE 32-7. Six-month follow-up angiography.

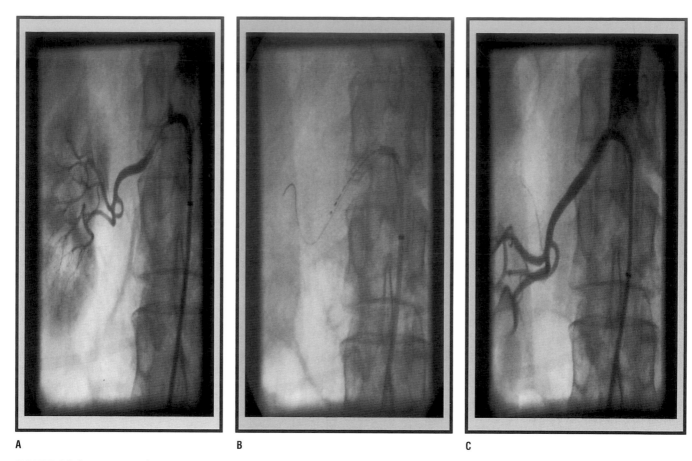

A **B** **C**

FIGURE 32-8. In-stent renal artery stenosis. **A.** In-stent restenosis in 20% renal stents. **B.** Ribbon with ^{192}Ir seeds prior to percutaneous transluminal angiography. **C.** Angiographic follow-up at 6 months.

from the center of the source and showed a reduction of 52% and 40% in in-stent and in-lesion restenosis, respectively, and a reduction of 48% and 36% in TLR rates and MACE rates, respectively.[37]

ARTISTIC I and II. ARTISTIC (AngioRad Radiation Technology for In-Stent restenosis Trial In native Coronaries) examined the usage of the AngioRad system in 115 patients (radiation = 57; placebo = 58) with ISR in native coronary arteries. At 3 years, the cumulative MACE rate was 24.1% in placebo patients and 22.8% in the AngioRad group.[38] ARTISTIC II used the same system in 236 patients and tested the efficacy as measured by a composite clinical end point at 9 months after radiation. These results were compared with the historical control group of 104 patients from the ARTISTIC I and WRIST studies. The Kaplan-Meier estimate of freedom from target vessel failure (TVF) for the placebo group was 52% whereas in the irradiated group it was 85.5%.[39]

【 】 CLINICAL TRIALS OF BETA RADIATION

Large-scale clinical studies testing the effectiveness of beta radiation for de novo, restenotic, and ISR lesions (Tables 32-3 and 32-4) have paralleled the encouraging results of gamma radiation.

Beta Radiation for In-Stent Restenosis

Beta WRIST. Beta WRIST showed that beta radiation is effective in the treatment of ISR in 50 patients. These patients demon-

strated a 58% reduction in the rate of TLR and a 53% reduction in target vessel revascularization (TVR) at 6 months compared with the historical control group of WRIST.[40] The clinical benefit was maintained at 2-year follow-up with a reduction in TLR (42 % vs 66%), TVR (46% vs 72%), and MACE (46 % vs 72%) compared with placebo. This study showed that the efficacy of beta and gamma emitters for the treatment of ISR appeared similar at longer-term follow-up.

START and START 40/20. In the START (STents And Radiation Therapy) trial, 476 patients were randomized to either placebo or an active radiation train 30 mm in length using the BetaCath system.[41] Late thrombosis as a complication of brachytherapy was first recognized during this trial and antiplatelet therapy was prolonged to at least 90 days. Angiographic restenosis rates at 8 months were 24% in the irradiated segments versus 46% in the placebo group. The rates of TLR, TVR, and MACE were 13%, 16%, and 18% in the irradiated group and 22%, 24%, and 26% in the control group, respectively.

During multiple studies of radiation, including START, the medical community became aware of the mismatch between the interventional injury length and radiation length-the so-called *geographic miss* phenomenon—with the potential to compromise clinical outcome.[42] START 40/20 was a 207-patient registry that mirrored START and ensured an adequate irradiation margin with 10 mm of radiation therapy applied proximal and distal to the injury zone (additional 5 mm each end). Compared with the control arm of START, patients in START 40/20 had a reduction of 44% in restenosis in the analysis segment, 50% reduction in TLR, 34% reduction in TVR, and 26% reduction in MACE. This registry demonstrated no deleterious effects of adding 10 mm of length to the source train, but there was a lack of a relationship between geographic miss and clinical or angiographic outcomes for ISR.

INHIBIT and Galileo INHIBIT.

INHIBIT (Intimal Hyperplasia Inhibition with Beta In-stent Trial) examined the efficacy of the Galileo system for the treatment of ISR in 332 patients.[43] At 9 months, treatment with ^{32}P reduced binary restenosis by 67% and 50% in the stented and analysis segments, respectively. There were no differences in the edge effect rates between the active and control-treated groups.

At 9 months, ^{32}P significantly reduced rates of TLR and MACE. Tandem positioning to cover diffuse lesions greater than 22 mm with ^{32}P was safe and effective. Galileo INHIBIT was an international, multicenter registry of 120 patients with ISR in which ^{32}P was delivered at a dose of 20 Gy to a depth of 1 mm into the vessel wall. There was a reduction in the primary clinical end point, defined as MACE-TLR, by 49%, reduction in angiographic end point of binary restenosis by 74% in the stented segment, and by 27% in the analysis segment.[44] The thrombosis rate was low, 1.5%, and similar to the control group, 1.2%.

Balloon Catheter-based Beta Radiation Trials for In-Stent Restenosis

BRITE, BRITE-II, 4R, and CURE.

BRITE (Beta Radiation to prevent In-sTent rEstenosis) was a feasibility study in 27 patients to test the Radiance system with a prescribed dose mean of 19.8 ± 0.4 Gy. Seventy percent of the dose was administered when the balloon was inflated. At 6 months, TVR (3.7%), MACE (3.7%), and angiographic binary restenosis rates (7.7%) were the lowest reported to date in any vascular brachytherapy series.[45] The BRITE II study evaluated the efficacy of beta radiation using the RDX system in 429 patients randomized to either radiation (n = 321) or placebo (n = 108). The RDX system demonstrated safety characterized by high technical success rates (> 95%), low periprocedural complications (< 1%), and low 30-day MACE (< 1%). The most prevalent location of restenosis was within the radiated vessel outside the injured zone despite lower rates of geographic miss (8.5%).[46] The RDX system demonstrated a very low ISR rate (10. 9% vs 46.1%) and proved to optimize the results when compared with historical studies.

4R, a South Korean registry evaluated beta-radiation therapy with ^{188}Re-filled balloons following rotational atherectomy for diffuse ISR in 50 patients. Radiation was delivered successfully with a dose of 15 Gy to a depth of 1 mm into the vessel wall. The mean irradiation time was 201.8 ± 61.7 seconds. No adverse events occurred during the follow-up period. The 6-month binary angiographic restenosis rate was 10.4%. Two potential limitations of this technology included reduced dosing at the balloon margins (edge effect) and the risks of balloon rupture with radiation spill. In the event of balloon rupture using ^{188}Re, concomitant administration of potassium perchlorate may mitigate thyroid uptake.[47]

The CURE (Columbia University Restenosis Elimination) study evaluated liquid ^{188}Re injected into a perfusion balloon. Of the 60 patients, half were treated with balloon alone and the other half were stented (with subsequent ^{188}Re therapy). The delivered dose was 20 Gy to the balloon surface, with a dwell time of 6.9 ± 2.2 minutes. At 12 months follow-up in the first 37 patients, the rate of TLR-free survival was 75%.[48]

RENO and BRIE.

Other studies assessing the efficacy of beta radiation are currently underway. RENO (Registry Novoste) is a registry of 1098 consecutive patients using the Novoste BetaCath system. Six-month follow-up data show nonocclusive restenosis in 18.8% of patients, total occlusion in 5.7%, and a MACE rate of 18.7% (1.9% deaths from any cause, 2.6% from acute myocardial infarction, 13.3% from TVR by percutaneous coronary interventions and 3.3% from TVR by coronary artery bypass grafting).[49] The BRIE (Beta Radiation in Europe) study is evaluating the safety and efficacy of the BetaCath system in patients with up to two discrete (treatable with a 20-mm balloon) lesions in different vessels. In the initial 149 patients, 6-month and 1-year rates of TVR with PTCA were 22% and 31%, respectively.[50]

Beta Radiation for De Novo Lesions

Several clinical studies were undertaken to test the effectiveness of beta radiation for de novo lesions concurrent with the trials of ISR. Important early studies included the Geneva trial[51]; the dose-finding study BERT,[52] which used ^{90}Y; and PREVENT,[53] which used ^{32}P.

BERT.

Beta Energy Restenosis Trial (BERT) was a feasibility study of 23 patients using the Novoste system with prescribed doses of 12, 14, or 16 Gy and treatment times less than 3.5 minutes.[52] No complications or adverse events were noticed at 30 days and at 9 months follow-up. Three patients underwent repeat revascularization to the target lesion. The Canadian arm of this study included 30 patients, and at 6 months follow-up, the angiographic restenosis rate was 10% with negative late loss and late loss index.[54] The European arm of BERT (BERT 1.5) was conducted at the Thoraxcenter in Rotterdam, The Netherlands, and involved an additional 30 patients who were treated successfully with balloon angioplasty. Angiographic restenosis in this cohort was higher than reported in the US and Canadian trials. Overall, the restenosis rate based on 64 of the 80 patients in the BERT series is 17%, and the late loss and late loss indexes are below 5%. Over 50% of the patients had larger minimal lumen diameter at follow-up compared with control, and a substudy involving IVUS demonstrated vessel remodeling at the irradiated site.[55]

PREVENT.

Proliferation Reduction with Vascular Energy Trial (PREVENT) was a randomized study of 105 patients with de novo (70%) or restenotic (30%) lesions using three different doses of beta radiation (16, 20, or 24 Gy to a depth of 1 mm in the artery wall) with ^{32}P. Angiographic restenosis at 6 months was 8.2% (target site) and 22.4% (target site plus adjacent segments) compared with 39.1% and 50.0% in the control group, respectively.[53] The incidence of MACE (death, myocardial infarction, and TLR) at 1 year was less in the radiation group although not statistically significant. Myocardial infarction due to thrombotic events after discharge occurred in seven patients who received radiotherapy and in none of the patients in the control group.

Dose-Finding Study Group. In this study, 183 patients were randomized; 181 received beta radiation (9–18 Gy) with ^{90}Y at a tissue depth of 1 mm. Stenting after radiation was required in 47% of the patients because of residual stenosis or major dissection. At 6-month angiographic follow-up, a significant dose-dependent benefit was evident. Thrombosis or late occlusion of the target vessel occurred in 3.3% of patients who were treated with only balloon angioplasty and in 14.3% of patients who received new stents. This study demonstrated a marked reduction in restenosis in non-stented arteries after administration of 18 Gy of beta radiation, especially in patients who underwent plain balloon angioplasty, suggesting that beta radiation therapy should be evaluated as an adjunct to PTCA.[56]

Beta-Cath. In this large randomized study, 1455 patients with suboptimal results after balloon angioplasty were treated with a stent and then assigned to ^{90}Sr/Y or placebo treatment.[57] In patients treated with balloon angioplasty alone, those receiving radiation treatment (n = 264) tended to have lower TVF (14.2%) compared with placebo (20.4%, n = 240). In the 452 patients treated with extended antiplatelet therapy who received a new stent, there were no differences in the 240-day TVF rate. Comparison of placebo and radiation treatment from pooled PTCA and stent groups (antiplatelet therapy ≥ 60 days) showed similar 8-month TLR and TVF-MACE.

An interesting point in this study was the low TVF in the irradiated balloon-only group. This was attributed to a reduction in angiographic restenosis within the initial lesion site in these patients (21.4% vs 34.3% in the placebo group), although the restenosis rates were similar in the analysis segment (treated segment plus the radiation margins). The loss of benefit at the treatment margins is attributable to geographic miss owing to the relatively short treatment length in the study. This was the first study to identify the higher-than-expected rate of late stent thrombosis when radiation was used with new stent implantation.

SVG BRITE. This study examined the RDX system using a ^{32}P emitter at a dose of 20 Gy at 1 mm from the balloon surface in saphenous vein grafts (SVG) of 49 patients; 24 of whom were treated for de novo lesions. New stents were implanted in most patients with de novo lesions. The outcome of the patients with de novo lesions was encouraging, with only 8% demonstrating TVR at 12-month follow-up, and 13% angiographic restenosis rates from the entire analysis segment (allowing for edge effect). These data warrant further investigation of this promising application, especially as the efficacy of potential alternatives, such as drug-eluting stents, has not yet been investigated in SVG lesions.[58]

ECRIS. EndoCoronary-Rhenium-Irradiation-Study (ECRIS) was a randomized trial in which 225 patients (71% de novo lesions) were randomly assigned to receive 22.5 Gy of beta irradiation to a depth of 0.5-mm using a ^{188}Re-filled balloon catheter (n = 113) or no additional intervention (n = 112). Clinical and procedural data did not differ between the groups except that there was a higher rate of stenting in the control group (63%) compared with the ^{188}Re group (45%). At 6-month follow-up, late loss was significantly lower in the irradiated group compared with the control group, both of the target lesion (0.11 ± 0.54 vs 0.69 ± 0.81 mm) and of the total segment (0.22 ± 0.67 vs 0.70 ± 0.82 mm). This was also evident in the subgroup of patients with de novo lesions

and independent from stenting. Binary restenosis rates and TVR were significantly lower after ^{188}Re brachytherapy compared with the control group.[59]

BRIDGE. The Beta-Radiation Investigation with Direct Stenting and Galileo (BRIDGE) study was a multicenter, randomized, controlled trial of 112 patients that evaluated the acute and long-term efficacy of intravascular brachytherapy with ^{32}P (20 Gy to a depth of 1 mm in the coronary wall) immediately following direct stenting in de novo lesions. TVR and MACE rates at 1 year in the irradiated group (20.4% and 25.9%, respectively) were higher than rates in the control group (12.1% and 17.2%, respectively).[60]

Clinical Trials with Radioactive Stents

In contrast to brachytherapy using removable sources, radioactive stents (permanent implants) have beta-emitting atoms (^{32}P) on the stent surface and emit beta particles that are absorbed by neointimal tissue to a depth of 1 to 2 mm into the vessel wall over longer periods of time. The first clinical trials included IRIS, the Milan dose-finding study, and the Vienna experience. In the IRIS (Isostent for Restenosis Intervention Study) pilot trials, ^{32}P radioactive Palmaz-Schatz stents were developed with varying radioactivities and were implanted with a high rate of technical success but limited by an angiographic restenosis rate (stent and edges) of 40% at 6-month follow-up.[61] The Milan dose-finding study showed that activities greater than 3 µCi (^{32}P stents 0.75–12 µCi) profoundly inhibited intimal hyperplasia; however, restenosis still occurred in more than 40% of lesions at the stent edges (ie, the "candy wrapper" effect).[62,63] These findings were replicated in the Vienna study using high-activity (6–21 µCi) stents.[64] An effort to circumvent edge restenosis by so-called *hot and cold end stents* failed to prevent edge effect, with an angiographic restenosis rate of 33% in 56 implanted stents.[65] In summary, although radioactive stents effectively inhibit intrastent neointimal hyperplasia, the problem of edge restenosis has not been solved with either less aggressive stent implantation or modification of the stent ends. Currently there is no indication for their clinical use.

【 】 BETA VERSUS GAMMA BRACHYTHERAPY

Although contemporaneous clinical trials to date have demonstrated comparable clinical efficacy for beta and gamma brachytherapy,[66] beta systems have several inherent advantages-such as reduced radiation exposure to operators and catheterization laboratory personnel, less shielding requirements, and easier handling of sources-that have led to more widespread acceptance of this technology. Potential limitations of beta sources in larger vessels (eg, vein grafts, peripheral arteries, and renal access grafts) may be offset by the use of sources with higher activity, centering mechanisms, and appropriately longer dwell times.

BRACHYTHERAPY: OTHER APPLICATIONS

Other than coronary and vein grafts, brachytherapy has been studied in the peripheral arterial system, including superficial femoral artery, popliteal artery, renal arteries, and hemodialysis vascular access dysfunction.

[ ] PERIPHERAL ARTERIAL SYSTEM

In the peripheral system, restenosis following percutaneous transluminal angioplasty (PTA) is mainly seen in small- and medium-sized peripheral arteries such as the saphenous femoral-popliteal arteries (SFAs) and renal arteries. Restenosis may also affect bypass grafts (anastomosis) and arteriovenous dialysis grafts, or occur following the placement of transjugular intrahepatic portosystemic shunts (TIPS).

Radiation Systems for the Peripheral Vascular System

Several radiation systems for peripheral endovascular brachytherapy have been suggested and are currently under development. A brief description of these systems follows.

External beam radiation is a viable option, but unfortunately, attempts to treat SFA lesions and arteriovenous dialysis grafts with external radiation failed to reduce the restenosis rate. Unacceptable recurrences of restenosis at the edges of the stent resulting from dose fall-off the so-called *edge effect*-precludes the usage radioactive stents. A new approach involving the use of radioactive nitinol self-expanding stents utilizing gamma emitters is currently under investigation as a potential therapy for primary SFA lesions. An example of SFA brachytherapy is shown in Figure 32-9.

Among catheter-based systems, the MicroSelectron HDR (Nucletron-Odelft, the Netherlands) system (Figure 32-10) uses a computerized, high-dose rate afterloader system that delivers a 3-mm, stepping, 10-Ci activity of ^{192}Ir into a centered, closed end lumen, segmented balloon radiation catheter. The Peripheral Brachytherapy Centering Catheter (PARIS catheter) (Guidant, Santa Clara, CA) is a 7-Fr double-lumen catheter with multiple centering balloons near its distal tip that enable the catheter to be centered in the lumen of large peripheral vessels during inflation. Another catheter-based system uses an ^{192}Ir radioactive wire that is delivered manually or by hand into a closed end lumen catheter. The activity of the source is limited to 500 mCi, and it is only practical for use in short lesions of small vessels (diameters < 4.0 mm) that require a dwell time of 20 minutes. Similar to this gamma system, a catheter-based system utilizing high-activity beta sources may eventually be an option for intermediate-sized vessels.

The Radiance balloon system is particularly attractive for peripheral applications because it is associated with apposition of a solid beta ^{32}P source attached to the inner balloon surface. Use of the system is limited to lesions less than 33 mm in length requiring one step, but it can accommodate longer lesions with manual stepping. To date, there is no clinical data to support the use of this technology in peripheral arteries. Another approach is the use of low x-ray energy delivered intraluminally via a catheter. The emitter would be between 5 and 7 mm in length and 1.25 and 2.0 mm

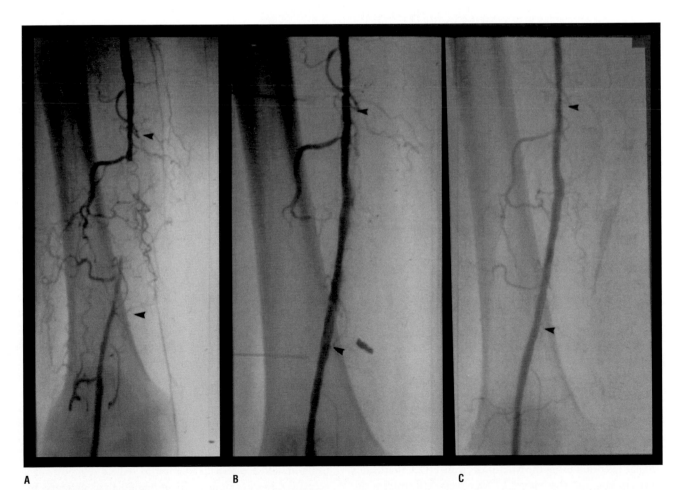

A   **B**   **C**

FIGURE 32-9. Brachytherapy of saphenous femoral-popliteal artery. **A.** Prior to percutaneous transluminal angiography (PTA). **B.** Following PTA. **C.** At 12-month follow-up.

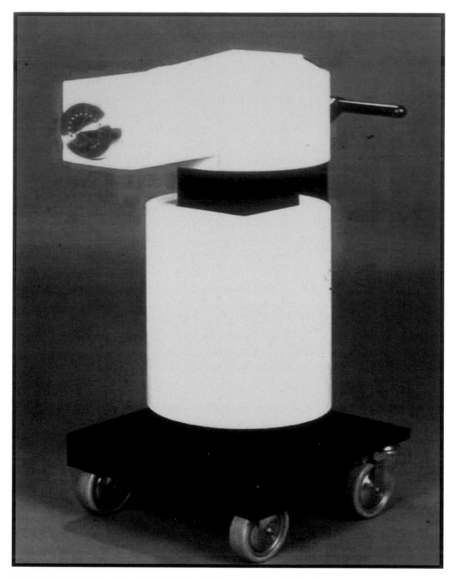

FIGURE 32-10. Nucletron-Odelft MicroSelectron HDR afterloader system.

within the treated segment was reported. Late total occlusion developed in 7% of patients after 37 months.

In the Vienna trial, 113 patients with de novo or recurrent femoropopliteal lesions were randomized PTA plus brachytherapy (n = 57) versus angioplasty alone (n = 56). The primary end point of cumulative patency rates at 12-month follow-up were higher in the group that received PTA plus brachytherapy (63.6%) compared with angioplasty alone (35.3%).[68] The group from Vienna continued to investigate a series of patients with a higher dose of 18 Gy to improve the outcome of the radiation group. In another series of studies, the effectiveness of radiation as adjunct therapy with primary stenting of the SFA was evaluated in 33 patients. In this series, the recurrence rate at 6 months was 30%; however, this finding was attributed to a high rate of late thrombosis (nearly 10%) following thrombolysis. Only 12% of patients had ISR. Late thrombosis was reduced significantly once prolonged antiplatelet therapy was administered, as shown in the Vienna 5 trial, in which 90 patients were randomized to stent plus radiation versus stent alone for the treatment of SFA lesions.

Preliminary analysis of the PARIS trial, which includes 203 patients, reported that restenosis was not different at follow-up between the radiated and control groups (28.6% vs 27.5%, respectively). In this trial, a 14-Gy dose was administered using the MicroSelectron HDR afterloader following PTA to SFA stenosis.[69] These data have shown the safety of high-dose radiation to treat femoropopliteal disease, but failed to show improvement in restenosis or functional symptoms when compared with balloon angioplasty treatment.

in diameter and could be administered distally to the lesion and pulled back to cover the entire lesion length. Miniaturizing the emitter is a technical challenge, and no preclinical data are as yet available to support this theory. The CORONA system, a modification of the BetaCath system, is used to accommodate beta systems with the $^{90}Sr/Y$ emitter in the peripheral system. With this system, a balloon filled with CO_2 allows centering and prevents dose attenuation. A clinical study of SFA for ISR lesions, entitled MOBILE, has been initiated.

Clinical Trials Involving Peripheral Arteries

Liermann and Schopohl (Frankfurt, Germany) were the first to perform vascular brachytherapy for the prevention of restenosis in the peripheral arteries. Known as the Frankfurt Experience, this pilot study was conducted in 30 patients with ISR in their SFAs.[67] The patients underwent atherectomy and PTA followed by endovascular radiation using the MicroSelectron-HDR afterloader and a noncentering catheter with ^{192}Ir. No adverse effects from the radiation treatment were reported up to 7 years later. The 5-year patency rate of the target vessel was 82%, and only 11% stenosis

Arteriovenous Dialysis Studies

An initial study was conducted at Emory University in 1994 to treat patients who had failed to respond to PTA of arteriovenous dialysis grafts. This study, which used the MicroSelectron HDR afterloader, reported 40% patency rate at 44 weeks[70]; however, the long-term results of the study were similar to stand-alone PTA without radiation. Similar disappointing results were reported by Nori and colleagues (personal communication) from a pilot study using external radiation doses of 12 and 18 Gy for arteriovenous dialysis shunts in 10 patients. At 6 months the TLR was 40%, but at 18 months all grafts failed and required intervention. Cohen and colleagues (personal communication) randomized 31 patients to PTA or stent placement alone followed by external radiation, prescribing 14 Gy in two 7-Gy fractions. They reported restenosis rates of 45% versus 67% in the irradiated and control groups, respectively at 6 months. New studies are currently underway using low-dose external radiation to reduce restenosis of vascular access for arteriovenous grafts of hemodialysis patients, and other studies are using a centering device to deliver an accurate homogenous dose of radiation following PTA.

Recently a new study was initiated at Scripps using endovascular radiation therapy for the prevention of restenosis following TIPS for patients with portal hypertension. Overall, the restenosis rate due to intimal hyperplasia of TIPS at 6 months has been reported to be as high as 70%. Complete thrombosis as early as 2 weeks after the procedure has also been reported.[71] However, in the long term, brachytherapy may be the best means of preventing occlusion for these patients.

LIMITATIONS TO BRACHYTHERAPY

Although clinical trials using vascular brachytherapy for both coronary and peripheral applications have demonstrated positive results in reducing restenosis rates, these trials have also identified two major complications related to the technology: late thrombosis and edge stenosis.

Late thrombosis probably results from the delay in healing associated with radiation. It has been estimated that late thrombosis can be remedied through the prolonged administration of antiplatelet therapy following intervention.

The main explanation for the edge effect is a combination of low dose at the edges of the radiation source and an injury created by the device for intervention that is not covered by the radiation source. Wider margins of radiation treatment to the intervening segment significantly reduce the edge effect.

DRUG-ELUTING STENTS AND BRACHYTHERAPY

Evidence is favorable for the efficacy of drug-eluting stents to reduce restenosis in de novo lesions, and experience is growing with other lesions. With these expanding indications, there will certainly be failures of drug-eluting stents. At present there are no data on how to treat these cases, but brachytherapy may be a potential method. Vascular brachytherapy is definitely a step ahead in the treatment of ISR and vein graft disease, and further simplification of the procedures for administering brachytherapy will help interventional cardiologists to explore additional uses of this therapy.

REFERENCES

1. Waksman R, Rodriquez JC, Robinson KA, et al. Effect of intravascular irradiation on cell proliferation, apoptosis and vascular remodeling after balloon overstretch injury of porcine coronary arteries. *Circulation.* 1997;96:1944.
2. Rubin P, Williams JP, Riggs PN, et al. Cellular and molecular mechanisms of radiation inhibition of restenosis. Part I: Role of the macrophage and platelet-derived growth factor. *Int J Radiat Oncol Biol Phys.* 1998;40:929.
3. Wang H, Griendling KK, Scott NA, et al. Intravascular radiation inhibits cell proliferation and vascular remodeling after angioplasty by increasing the expression pf p21 in adventitial myofibroblasts. *Circulation.* 1999;100:I-700.
4. Schwartz RS, Koval TM, Edwards WD, et al. Effect of external beam irradiation on neointimal hyperplasia after experimental coronary artery injury. *J Am Coll of Cardiol.* 1992;19:1106.
5. Waksman R, Robinson KA, Crocker IR, et al. Endovascular low-dose irradiation inhibits neointima formation after coronary artery balloon injury in swine. A possible role for radiation therapy in restenosis prevention. *Circulation.* 1995;91:1533.
6. Waksman R, Robinson KA, Crocker IR, et al. Intracoronary radiation before stent implantation inhibits neointima formation in stented porcine coronary arteries. *Circulation.* 1995;92:1383.

7. Wiedermann JG, Marboe C, Amols H, et al. Intracoronary irradiation markedly reduces restenosis after balloon angioplasty in a porcine model. *J Am Coll Cardiol.* 1994;23:1491.
8. Wiedermann JG, Marboe C. Amols H, et al. Intracoronary irradiation markedly reduces neointimal proliferation after balloon angioplasty in swine: Persistent benefit at 6-months follow-up. *J Am Coll Cardiol.* 1995;25:1451.
9. Mazur W, Ali MN, Khan MM, et al. High dose rate intracoronary radiation for inhibition of neointimal formation in the stented and balloon injured porcine models of restenosis: Angiographic, morphometric and histopathological analyses. *Int J Radiot Oncol Biol Phys.* 1996;36:777.
10. Wiedermann JG, Leavy JA, Amols H, et al. Effects of high dose intracoronary irradiation on vasomotor function and smooth muscle histopathology. *Am J Physiol.* 1994;267(*Heart Circ Physiol.* 36):H125.
11. Verin V, Popowski Y, Urban P, et al. Intra-arterial beta irradiation prevents neointimal hyperplasia in a hypercholesterolemic rabbit restenosis model. *Circulation.* 1995;92:2284.
12. Waksman R, Robinson KA, Crocker IR, et al. Intracoronary low-dose beta-irradiation inhibits neointima formation after coronary artery balloon injury in the swine restenosis model. *Circulation.* 1995;92:3025.
13. Fischell TA, Kharma BK, Fischell DR, et al. Low dose beta particle emission from stent wire results in complete localized inhibition of smooth muscle cell proliferation. *Circulation.* 1994;90:2956.
14. Hehrlein C, Kniser S, Kollum M, et al. Effects of very low dose endovascular irradiation via an activated guidewire on neointima formation after stent implantation. *Circulation.* 1995;92:I-69.
15. Hehrlein C, Gollan C, Donges K, et al. Low dose radioactive endovascular stent prevent smooth muscle cell proliferation and neointimal hyperplasia in rabbits. *Circulation.* 1995;92:1570.
16. Laird JR, Carter AJ, Kufs WM, et al. Inhibition of neointimal proliferation with low-dose irradiation from a beta-particle-emitting stent. *Circulation.* 1996;93:529.
17. Carter AJ, Laird JR, Bailey LR, et al. Effects of endovascular radiation from a beta-particle-emitting stent in a porcine coronary restenosis model. A dose-response study. *Circulation.* 1996;94:2364.
18. Waksman R, Chan RC, Vodovotz Y, et al. Radioactive 133-xenon gas-filled angioplasty balloon: A novel intracoronary radiation system to prevent restenosis. *J Am Coll Cardiol.* 1998;31:356A.
19. Weinberger J. Solution-applied beta emitting radioisotope (SABER) system. In Waksman R, Serruys P, eds: *Handbook of Vascular Brachytherapy*, 1st ed. London, England: Martin Dunitz Ltd; 1998.
20. Robinson KA, Pipes DW, Bibber RV, et al. Dose response evaluation in balloon injured pig coronary arteries of a beta emitting 186Re liquid filled balloon catheter system for endovascular brachytherapy. Paper presented at: Advances in Cardiovascular Radiation Therapy II; March 8–10, 1998; Washington, DC.
21. Makkar R, Whiting J, Li A, Cordero H, et al. A beta emitting liquid isotope filled balloon markedly inhibits restenosis in stented porcine coronary arteries. *J Am Coll Cardiol.* 1998;31:350A.
22. Kim HS, Cho YS, Kim JS, et al. Effect of transcatheter endovascular holmium-166 irradiation on neointimal formation after balloon injury in porcine coronary artery. *J Am Coll Cardiol.* 1998;31:277A.
23. Condado JA, Waksman R, Gurdiel O, et al. Long-term angiographic and clinical outcome after percutaneous transluminal coronary angioplasty and intracoronary radiation therapy in humans. *Circulation.* 1997;96:727.
24. Condado JA, Waksman R, Saucedo JF, et al. Five-year clinical and angiographic follow-up after intracoronary iridium-192 radiation therapy. *Cardiovasc Radiat Med.* 2002;3:74.
25. Teirstein PS, Massullo V, Jani S, et al. Catheter-based radiotherapy to inhibit restenosis after coronary stenting. *N Engl J Med.* 1997;336:1697.
26. Teirstein PS, Massullo V, Jani S, et al. Two-year follow-up after catheter-based radiotherapy to inhibit coronary restenosis *Circulation.* 1999;99:243.
27. Grise MA, Massullo V, Jani S, et al. Five-year clinical follow-up after intracoronary radiation: Results of a randomized clinical trial. *Circulation.* 2002;105:2737.
28. Waksman R, White RL, Chan RC, et al. Intracoronary radiation therapy for patients with in-stent restenosis: 6-month follow-up of a randomized clinical study. *Circulation.* 1998;98:17.
29. Ajani AE, Waksman R, Sharma AK, et al. Three-year follow-up after intracoronary gamma radiation therapy for in-stent restenosis. Original WRIST. Washington Radiation for In-Stent Restenosis Trial. *Cardiovasc Radiat Med.* 2001; 2:200.
30. Waksman R, Ajani AE, White RL, et al. Five-year follow-up after intracoronary gamma radiation therapy for in-stent restenosis. *Circulation.* 2004;109:340.
31. Waksman R, Ajani AE, White RL, et al. Intravascular gamma radiation for in-stent restenosis in saphenous-vein bypass grafts. *N Engl J Med.* 2002;346:1194.

32. Waksman R, Cheneau E, Ajani AE, et al. Intracoronary radiation therapy improves the clinical and angiographic outcomes of diffuse in-stent restenotic lesions: Results of the Washington Radiation for In-Stent Restenosis Trial for Long lesions (Long WRIST) studies. *Circulation.* 2003;107:1744.

33. Javed MH, Mintz GS, Waksman R, et al. Serial intravascular ultrasound assessment of the efficacy of intracoronary γ radiation therapy for preventing recurrence of very long, diffuse, in-stent restenosis lesions. *Circulation.* 2000;104:856.

34. Waksman R, Ajani AE, White RL, et al. Prolonged antiplatelet therapy to prevent late thrombosis after intracoronary gamma-radiation in patients with in-stent restenosis: Washington Radiation for In-Stent restenosis Trial plus 6 months of clopidogrel (WRIST PLUS). *Circulation.* 2001;103:2332.

35. Waksman R, Ajani AE, Pinnow E, et al. Twelve versus six months of clopidogrel to reduce major cardiac events in patients undergoing γ-radiation therapy for in-stent restenosis. Washington Radiation for In-Stent restenosis Trial (WRIST) 12 Versus WRIST PLUS. *Circulation.* 2002;106:776.

36. Leon MB, Teirstein PS, Moses JW, et al. Localized intracoronary gamma-radiation therapy to inhibit the recurrence of restenosis after stenting. *N Engl J Med.* 2001;344:250.

37. Kim HS, Ajani AE, Waksman R. Vascular brachytherapy for in-stent restenosis. *J Interv Cardiol.* 2000;13:417.

38. Waksman R, Bhargava B, Chan RC, et al. Intracoronary radiation with gamma wire inhibits recurrent in-stent restenosis. *Cardiovasc Radiat Med.* 2001;2:63.

39. Kereikas DJ, Waksman R, Mehra A, et al. Multi-center experience with a novel Ir-192 vascular brachytherapy device for in-stent restenosis: Final results of the AngioRad™ T radiation therapy for in-stent restenosis intracoronaries II (ARTISTIC II) trial. *J Am Coll Cardiol.* 2003;41:49A.

40. Waksman R, White RL, Chan RC, et al. Intracoronary beta radiation therapy inhibits recurrence of in-stent restenosis. *Circulation.* 2000;101:1895.

41. Popma J. Late clinical and angiographic outcomes after use of ^{90}Sr/^{90}Y beta radiation for the treatment of in-stent restenosis: Results from the ^{90}Sr treatment of angiographic restenosis (START) trial. *J Am Coll Cardiol.* 2000;36:311.

42. Kim HS, Waksman R, Cottin Y, et al. Edge stenosis and geographical miss following intracoronary gamma radiation therapy for in-stent restenosis. *J Am Coll Cardiol.* 2001;15:1026.

43. Waksman R, Raizner AE, Yeung AC, et al. Use of localized intracoronary beta radiation in treatment of in-stent restenosis: The INHIBIT randomized controlled trial. *Lancet.* 2002;359:551.

44. Waksman R on behalf of the Galileo INHIBIT and INHIBIT investigators. Manual stepping of 32P β-emitter for diffuse in-stent restenosis lesions, tandem versus single position. Clinical and angiographic outcome from a multi-center randomized study. Paper presented at the annual meeting of the American Heart Association; 2001.

45. Waksman R, Buchbinder M, Reisman M, et al. Balloon-based radiation therapy for treatment of in-stent restenosis in human coronary arteries: Results from the BRITE I study. *Cathet Cardiovasc Interv.* 2002;57:286.

46. Waksman R on behalf of the BRITE II investigators. Balloon based radiation for coronary in-stent restenosis: 9 months results from the BRITE II study. Paper presented at the annual meeting of the American College of Cardiology; 2003.

47. Park S-W, Kong M-K, Moon DH, et al. Treatment of diffuse in-stent restenosis with rotational atherectomy followed by radiation therapy with a rhenium-188-mercaptoacetyltriglycine-filled balloon. *J Am Coll Cardiol.* 2001;38:631.

48. Weinberger J, Giedd KN, Simon AD, et al. Radioactive beta-emitting solution filled balloon treatment prevents porcine coronary restenosis. *Cardiovasc Radiat Med.* 1999;1:252.

49. Urban P, Serruys P, Baumgart D, et al. A multicentre European registry of intraluminal coronary beta brachytherapy. *Eur Heart J.* 2003;24:604.

50. Sianos G, Kay P, Costa MA, et al. Geographical miss during catheter-based intracoronary beta-radiation: Incidence and implications in the BRIE study. *J Am Coll Cardiol.* 2000;38:415.

51. Verin V, Urban P, Popowski Y, et al. Feasibility of intracoronary beta-irradiation to reduce restenosis after balloon angioplasty. A clinical pilot study. *Circulation.* 1997;95:1138.

52. King SB III, Williams DO, Chougule P, et al. Endovascular beta-radiation to reduce restenosis after coronary balloon angioplasty. Results of the beta energy restenosis trial (BERT). *Circulation.* 1998;97:2025.

53. Raizner AE, Osterle SN, Waksman R, et al. Inhibition of restenosis with β-emitting radiotherapy report of the proliferation reduction with vascular energy trial (PREVENT). *Circulation.* 2000;102:951.

54. Bonan R, Arsenault A, Tardif JC, et al. Beta energy restenosis trials, Canadian arm. *Circulation.* 1997;96:I-219.

55. Gijzel AL, Wardeh AJ, van der Giessen WJ, et al. β-Energy to prevent restnosis: The Rotterdam contribution to the BERT 1.5 trial-1 yr. follow up [abstract]. *Eur Heart J.* 1999;370:1945.

56. Verin V, Popowski Y, deBruyne B, et al. Endoluminal beta-radiation therapy for the prevention of coronary restenosis after balloon angioplasty. *N Engl J Med.* 2001;344:243.

57. Results from late-breaking clinical trails sessions at ACC 2001. *J Am Coll Cardiol.* 2001;38:595.

58. Stone GW, Mehran R, Midei M, et al. Usefulness of beta radiation for de novo and in-stent restenotic lesions in saphenous vein grafts. *J Am Coll Cardiol.* 2003;92:312.

59. Höher M, Wöhrle J, Wohlfrom M, et al. Intracoronary beta-irradiation with a rhenium-188-filled balloon catheter: A randomized trial in patients with de novo and restenotic lesions. *Circulation.* 2003;7:3022.

60. Serruys PW, Wijns W, Sianos G, et al. Direct stenting versus direct stenting followed by centered beta-radiation with IVUS-guided dosimetry and long-term antiplatelet treatment; results of a randomized trial: Beta-Radiation Investigation with Direct Stenting and Galileo in Europe (BRIDGE). *J Am Coll Cardiol.* 2004;44:528.

61. Moses J. IRIS trials low activity 32P stent. Presented at: Advances in Cardiovascular Radiation therapy III; Washington, DC; 1999;387–388 [abstract].

62. Albeiro R, Adamian M, Kobayashi N, et al. Short- and intermediate-term results of (32)P radioactive beta emitting stent implantation in patients with coronary artery disease: The Milan Dose-Response Study. *Circulation.* 2000; 101:18.

63. Albeiro R, Nishida T, Adamian M, et al. Edge restenosis after implantation of high activity (32)P radioactive beta-emitting stents. *Circulation.* 2000; 101:2454.

64. Wexberg P, Siostrzonek P, Kirisits C, et al. High activity radioactive BX-stents for reduction of restenosis after coronary interventions: The Vienna P-32 dose response study. *Circulation.* 1999;100:I-156.

65. Wardeh A, Wijns W, Albiero R, et al. Angiographic follow-up after 32-P beta emitting radioactive "cold ends" Isostent implantation. Results from Aalst, Milan and Rotterdam [abstract]. *Circulation.* 2000;102:II-442.

66. Shirai K, Lansky AJ, Mintz, GS et al. Comparison of the angiographic outcomes after beta versus gamma vascular brachytherapy for treatment of in-stent restenosis. *Am J Cardiol.* 2003;92:1409.

67. Liermann DD, Bottcher HD, Kollath J, et al. Prophylactic endovascular radiotherapy to prevent intimal hyperplasia after stent implantation in femoropopliteal arteries. *Cardiovasc Intervent Radiol.* 1994;17:12.

68. Minar E, Pokrajac B, Maca T, et al. Endovascular Brachytherapy for prophylaxis of restenosis after femoropopliteal angioplasty: Results of a prospective randomized study. *Circulation.* 2000;102:2694.

69. Waksman R, Laird JR, Jurkovitz CT, et al. Intravascular radiation therapy after balloon angioplasty of narrowed femoropopliteal arteries to prevent restenosis: Results of the PARIS feasibility clinical trial. *J Vasc Interv Radiol.* 2001; 12:915.

70. Waksman R, Crocker IA, Kikeri D, et al. Long term results of endovascular radiation therapy for prevention of restenosis in the peripheral vascular system. *Circulation.* 1996;94:1745.

71. Raat H, Stockx L, Ranschaert E, et al. Percutaneous hydrodynamic thrombectomy of acute thrombosis in transjugular intrahepatic portosystemic shunt (TIPS): A feasibility study in five patients. *Cardiovasc Intervent Radiol.* 1997;20:180.

CHAPTER (33)

Basic Wire-Handling Strategies for Chronic Total Occlusions

Osamu Katoh, MD

When treating chronic total occlusions (CTOs) of the coronary arteries, the most important question remains how to get the wire across the occlusion. The lack of a revolutionary new device for use in CTOs means that the treatment strategy depends on the experience, expertise, and instincts of the operator.

The purpose of this chapter is to set out, as specifically as possible, basic wire-handling strategies for CTOs. Wire-handling is everything when performing percutaneous coronary interventions for CTOs, but to obtain the best handling from a wire, it is necessary to evaluate the lesion before intervention to identify the most suitable approach and the best treatment strategy. All CTO procedures require endless delicacy and patience, which is what differentiates them from procedures involving other lesions, even if the simplest available strategy is often the best treatment option. Today, individual lesion characteristics no longer have much direct influence on the success or failure of interventional procedures in other lesions. This cannot be said of CTOs, however, where the greater range of factors in play means that the specific characteristics of each lesion can have a direct bearing on procedural success.

Another key difference is that the operator cannot expect anything near a 100% success rate with CTOs and should always be prepared for the unexpected. The best way to increase the chances of success is to adapt the treatment strategy to the conditions with which one is faced.

LESION STRUCTURE: PATHOLOGIC AND IMAGING FINDINGS

Pathologic studies and intravascular ultrasound (IVUS) findings provide helpful information both in wiring a CTO and in optimal dilation after successful recanalization. In the pathologic studies, neovascular channels with diameters of 100 to 200 μ are frequently found, especially (85%) in CTOs that have been present for more than 1 year. The neovascular channels developing in preexisting plaque often connect with vasa vasorum in the adventitia, whereas those in an older thrombus communicate with the distal lumen (recanalization channels). A tapered CTO, as seen angiographically, represents a lesion with the later channels; therefore, there is a route that a guidewire can follow in this kind of CTO. However, in an older CTO especially one with no stump, a guidewire easily reaches to subintima through the neovascular channels connecting to vasa vasorum. Moreover, there are other pathologic findings that might restrict wire movement inside a CTO.

CTOs consist of relatively soft tissues composed of scattered fibrous tissue, lipid core, and neovascular system, and hard tissues composed of dense fibrous tissue and calcium. The dense fibrous tissue forms fibrous bundles, not only cross-sectionally but also longitudinally, which partition soft tissues (Figure 33-1). These partitions can restrict wire movement. When a guidewire is unable to pass through the partition from one soft tissue to another, it tends to slip into the soft tissue. This could be one of the major reasons why guidewires pass so easily into the subintima, creating a subintimal space. In evaluating the structure of CTOs, components such as calcification, dense fibrous tissue, and proximal fibrous cap, as well as vessel shrinkage, influence wire movement.

Recent IVUS findings indicate that subintimal space created by a guidewire is a strong factor in the failure to recanalize CTOs. Figure 33-2 illustrates a typical example of subintimal space, as visualized by IVUS. Once the subintimal space is created by the guidewire, the wire tends to slip into the space and extend it along the circumference, as seen in panels E and F of Figure 33-2.

This chapter is based on a presentation given at CCT, Kobe, Japan, 2004.

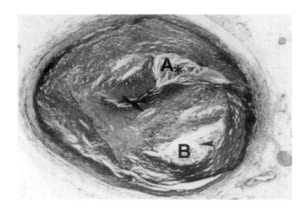

FIGURE 33-1. In this slice, two sections are visible, consisting of relatively scattered fibrous tissue (labeled *A* and *B*), with intervening bundles. Although a guidewire tends to pass though relatively soft tissue such as that in *A* or *B*, it is difficult for the guidewire to penetrate the fibrous bundle.

Difficulty is encountered when the guidewire in the subintimal space, extended in circumference, reaches beyond the distal true lumen. It is well known that the most difficult point in wiring a CTO comes when the operator seeks to penetrate tissue into the distal true lumen at the distal end of a CTO. IVUS findings indicate that a thick fibrous membrane rarely exists at the distal end of a CTO, in contrast to the proximal end. Thus, the major cause of difficulty in penetrating into the distal true lumen is considered to be the false lumen made around the distal true lumen by a guidewire, as shown in Figure 33-3.

PREPARATION

【 】 GETTING THE BEST HANDLING FROM THE WIRE

It is important to use an over-the-wire balloon catheter or wire delivery catheter (Transit, Interpass, or the Multifunction Probing Catheter) that allows the wire to move freely inside the CTO. Maneuverability of the wire may be complicated by natural tortuosity in the shape of the access artery (brachial of femoral), or by tortuosity, or proximal to the lesion.

Another cause of poor guidewire maneuverability is bifurcation of the right coronary artery forward from the right Valsalva sinus, so that the artery slants toward the atrioventricular sulcus at a very sharp angle, or branching of the left main trunk from the aortic posterior wall. To address these situations, when the lesion is distal and there is no proximal lesion, a 5 French (Fr) or 6-Fr guiding catheter can be inserted deep into the coronary artery to prevent any dangerous bending at the ostium (Figure 33-4). When the lesion is proximal, or when for some reason the guide catheter cannot be inserted deep into the coronary artery, a support wire can be used in parallel (Figure 33-5). The support wire is inserted into the side branch that bifurcates immediately before the occluded portion, and the guide catheter is then brought properly into line.

For stable wire-handling, the guide catheter needs to be stable as well. A problem can arise with a Judkins right (JR) catheter in the right coronary artery, or a Judkins left (JL) catheter in the left coronary artery, when the guide catheter does not advance deep into the

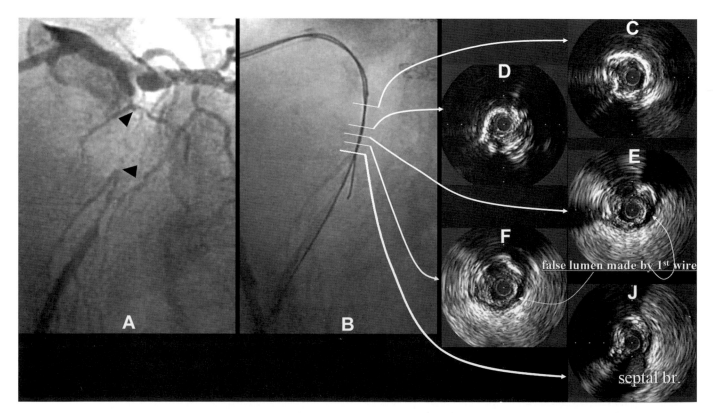

FIGURE 33-2. A typical example of subintimal space created by guidewire handling. After successful wiring (**B**), subintimal space was observed on intravascular ultrasound (**E** and **F**). The major cause of the failed wire attempt was shown, by IVUS, to be calcification inside the occlusion.

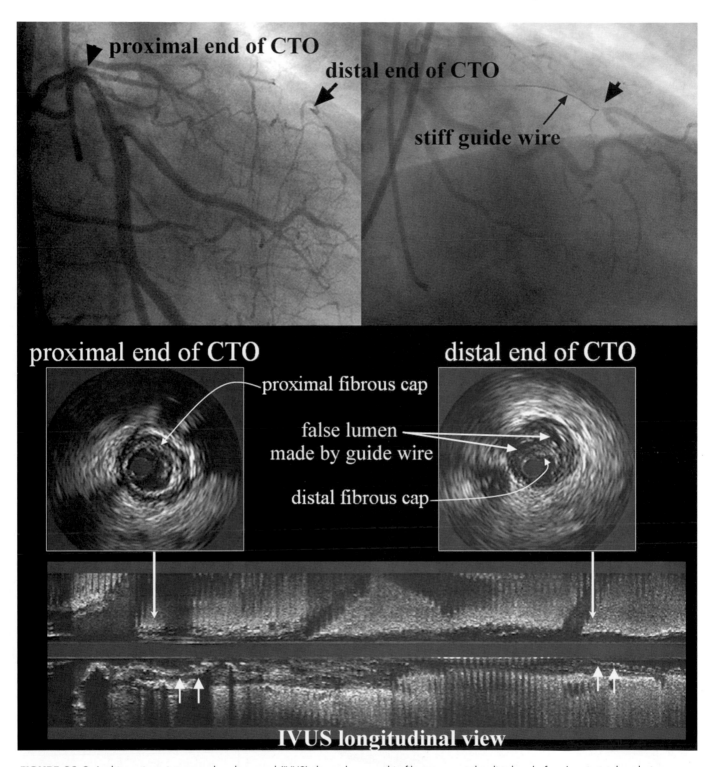

FIGURE 33-3. In this patient, intravascular ultrasound (IVUS) showed a very thin fibrous cap at the distal end of a chronic total occlusion (CTO) compared with a thick fibrous cap at the proximal end. Despite the thin distal cap, it was difficult to advance into the distal true lumen because of the intimal dissection made along the circumference of the distal true lumen by a guidewire.

artery. This situation makes the guide catheter unstable, allowing it to fall down the Valsalva sinus while the wire is being maneuvered. In this situation, a change of the guide catheter as soon as possible is advised. When an operator receives backup force from the guide catheter acting against the balloon catheter, he or she would usually torque the JR catheter in a clockwise direction and at the same time change the shape of the catheter inside the Valsalva sinus to secure it, but this strategy is not effective to secure the position of the guide

catheter in CTO wire-handling. It is better to exchange the guide catheter or dilate a balloon (3.0–4.0 mm) proximal to the CTO, leaving the balloon catheter in the artery for backup (Figure 33-6).

One factor that affects maneuverability of the guidewire is bending or tortuosity in the vessel proximal to the CTO lesion. One potential solution is to stretch and straighten the bends in the vessel; this can be done simply by inserting a balloon catheter into the vessel, which usually stretches it sufficiently to improve maneuverability of

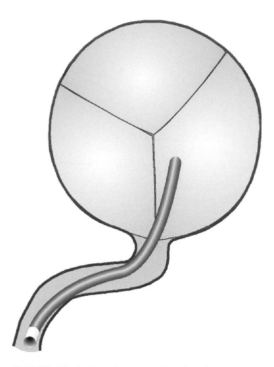

FIGURE 33-4. Straightening a bend at the ostium by deep engagement of a small-caliber guide catheter.

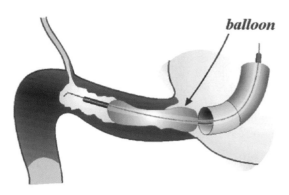

FIGURE 33-6. Fixing the balloon catheter position during wire-handling.

the wire. In some cases, however, this maneuver can cause the balloon catheter to be bent, and the wire lumen to be crushed, with the result that wire maneuverability is considerably diminished. If this happens, (1) exchange the balloon catheter for a Transit catheter, (2) use a wire with a hydrophilic coating, or (3) use a support wire in parallel to try to force the vessel to stretch and straighten (Figure 33-7). In all of these scenarios, correct identification of the conditions beforehand, under fluoroscopy, is extremely important.

【 】 CORRECT INTERPRETION OF THE LESION

Interpreting the lesion enables the physician to choose the optimal treatment modality and gain an insight into potential problems before starting the procedure; it is an essential part of strategy design for interventions involving CTOs. Although it may seem obvious, even interventional cardiologists with plenty of experience of normal lesions should recognize the differences inherent in interpretation of CTOs.

Duration of Occlusion

It is often difficult to identify exactly how long a vessel has been occluded, but even in the absence of a detailed history of myocardial infarction, the physician can gain an understanding of occlusion duration by obtaining a detailed medical history from the patient. Some CTOs that present with bridging collaterals, and appear to be quite old, turn out to be relatively young. Careful evaluation is essential, as in these lesions, a stiff wire may easily and suddenly push through the occlusion and create a false lumen. Because occlusion duration has an important impact on wire selection and wire-handling technique, finding out as much as possible about the patient's history is a great advantage.

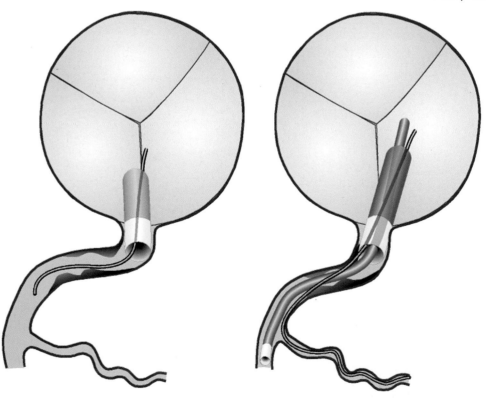

FIGURE 33-5. Insertion of a support wire into the side-branch proximal to a chronic total occlusion (CTO) to serve as a parallel wire. This approach can improve guidewire maneuverability, which would otherwise be difficult because of the bend at the ostium (*left*). Subsequent placement of a support catheter (balloon or Transit) in the coronary artery can improve coaxiality of the guide catheter with the vessel. This technique is not effective in proximal ostial CTOs.

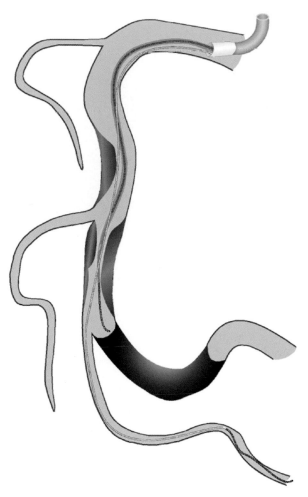

FIGURE 33-7. Straightening the vessel with a parallel wire.

Location of Lesions and Vessel Shape

The location of the coronary artery ostium, the direction of bifurcations, and the shape of the vessel all influence the choice of guide catheter. When a lesion is located at the entry to the CTO or proximal to it, the guide catheter can cause ischemia or coronary artery dissection; therefore, all the available angiographic information must be carefully analyzed when choosing the correct guide catheter and identifying the best way to maneuver it. This is especially important in the right coronary artery; although the actual approach will depend on individual circumstances, the operator may want to predilate ostial or proximal lesions and implant a stent. This approach often results in improved wire-handling and can also reduce and prevent complications (Figure 33-8).

Lesion Morphology

It is well known that lesion morphology, (ie, whether or not there is a dimple inside the occlusion) affects the success rate of interventions for CTOs, and care must be taken not to overlook dimples when viewing the angiographic images. For this reason, the operator should look at the images frame by frame and from a number of angles (Figure 33-9), while at the same time looking to see if there are any potential recanalization channels or existing lumina inside the CTO. Pursuing such paths through the CTO will not rule out the creation of a false lumen, but these paths can often suggest a passageway for the wire. Bends in the vessel inside the CTO are also sometimes missed. In addition, because calcification configuration is often a good indicator of vessel shape, it can sometimes be useful to delay infusion of the contrast medium for two to three heartbeats during fluoroscopy to obtain a better image of the calcification. When the proximal and distal portions of the

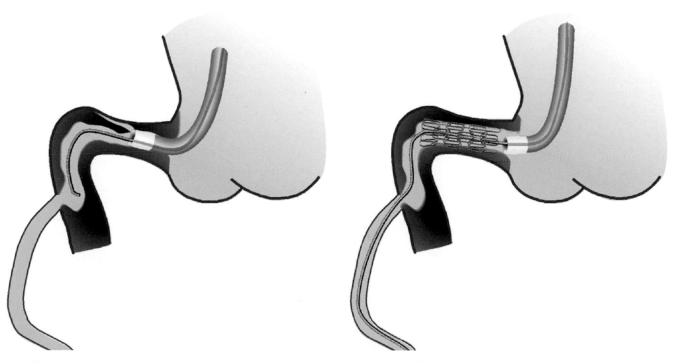

FIGURE 33-8. Ostial CTO lesions demand strong backup, and the risk of ostial dissection is high. Operators should be aware of this, proceed carefully, and be ready to act quickly if required.

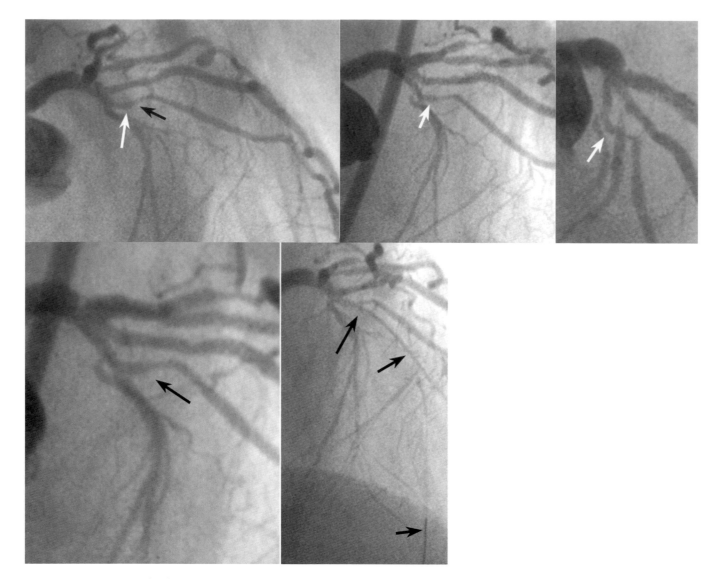

FIGURE 33-9. An example of a chronic total occlusion (CTO) in the proximal left anterior descending (LAD) coronary artery, just behind the bifurcation of the LAD and the diagonal branch. The duration of the occlusion was not clear, but the medical history suggested it had been present for several years. The CTO ostium in the LAD is not clearly visible on angiogram in the panel at upper left. The *white arrow* shows what appears to be the ostium, but the *black arrow* turned out to be the true dimple. The dimple was only detectable from the AP cranial view, and even then only after frame-by-frame analysis. [This] would normally tend to be overlooked.

occlusion seem to slip out of alignment with each heartbeat, it is a sign of tortuosity inside the CTO.

In addition to looking closely at morphology in the proximal part of the CTO, it is important to observe the situation at the distal end. For this purpose, obtaining a clear image of the distal vasculature supplied by collateral flow is crucial. This step is also important in gauging lesion length. An operator can sometimes mistake a short CTO for a long one, setting the penetration point he or she is aiming for as the true lumen too far down the CTO, and failing to realize that a false lumen is being created. The presence of a tapering distal portion and chronic buildup of jagged hard plaque around the true lumen can make it extremely difficult for the wire to penetrate the CTO (Figure 33-10). There must be only a single penetration point at the distal end of the CTO, because once a false lumen is created any-

where in the vicinity of the fibrous cap, the true lumen is easily collapsed and becomes very difficult to locate. Thus, identifying the shape of the end of the occlusion provides valuable information for determining how to maneuver the wire.

Collateral Flow

Monitoring collateral flow when maneuvering the wire is also a very important part of the strategy for recanalizing CTOs. It is relatively straightforward to identify the vessels supplying and receiving collateral blood flow, as well as the main collateral channels, but the operator must be on the lookout for pitfalls. For instance, if one of the supply channels is an atrial branch or a conus artery branch bifurcating from the proximal right coronary artery, the catheter tip may advance down one of these branches. In this case, collateral flow will not show up on the coronary angiogram (CAG). It is not uncommon, when CTOs involve the lateral anterior descending (LAD) coronary arteries, for a separated conus branch to be the supply channel for collateral flow, and operators often miss, on CAG, the collateral flow coming from the separated conus.

Knowledge of whether the vessel bifurcates toward the distal end of the CTO, as well as the angle of bifurcation and whether or not stenosis or plaque is present at the bifurcation ostium, are all extremely important.

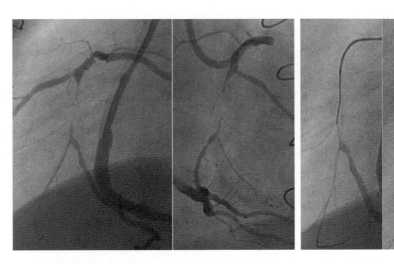

FIGURE 33-10. In this case, crossing the wire through the lesion was difficult because of the tapering distal end of the chronic total occlusion (CTO). This vessel had been occluded for more than 10 years, and hard tissue (fibrous cap) was present at the distal lumen. It was difficult to penetrate even the proximal portion of the CTO, probably because of a problem with the course of the wire up to the proximal end.

【　】 CONTRALATERAL INJECTION

Contralateral injection is an indispensable part of the strategy in percutaneous coronary interventions for CTOs. It is no exaggeration, in fact, to say that all expertise as to how to maneuver the CTO wire comes from the use of this technique. Contralateral injection not only tells the operator how to move the wire forward, but continually provides information, during the procedure and while the wire is moving, about the distal course of the true lumen and any bifurcations.

Following are several points to be aware of when using contralateral injection.

1. Interference between the guide and CAG catheters. This happens quite frequently, and the operator may find that it is very difficult or impossible to engage the guide catheter or the CAG catheter. Using the left radial artery approach for the CAG catheter is one way to avoid this problem. If it is still difficult to obtain a stable CAG catheter position, it may be easier to place a guidewire in the CAG catheter.

2. Ischemia. The operator must use care to prevent the catheter from finding its way deeper into the vessel and causing ischemia. If the CAG catheter continues to become wedged, passing a guidewire along the CAG catheter and forcing it back is a good method of freeing it from the wedge.

3. Amount of contrast medium. A large amount of contrast medium tends to be used during contralateral injection, but the quantity depends on how the procedure is performed. "Superselective" angiography (usually with the Transit catheter) is a good method to be used to minimize the amount of contrast medium used. The parallel wire technique, described later in this chapter, is another way of economizing on the amount of contrast medium used.

【　】 IMAGING VIEW

Even experienced operators should remember that they can become so involved during a procedure that they forget to look at the vessel from multiple directions. Although a three-dimensional (3D) image of the relative positions is provided, it is sometimes useful, during angiography, to rotate an intensifier (rotational angiography). Similarly, use of a biplane imaging system helps to cut down on the amount of contrast medium required.

BASIC WIRE TECHNIQUE

【　】 WIRE CHARACTERISTICS: WHICH ONE TO CHOOSE?

Types of Wires

Wires designed for treating CTOs are largely divided into two groups, polymer-coated wires and coil wires.

Polymer-coated wires have a hydrophilic coating, which means they attract very little resistance when they come into contact with the tissue in the lumen, and move quite easy through soft tissue. These wires offer good maneuverability in tortuous vessels. However, the operator must use care, because they can easily find their way down false lumina, and may not respond as well to the operator's attempts to make them to follow a precise, predetermined path through hard plaque.

Coil wires tend to encounter more resistance inside the lumen than polymer-coated wires, but because these wires have been developed to have good torquability, even inside a hard, tight CTO, they respond well to the most precise commands.

The operator can usually learn the feel of the guidewire tip, but the following cautions should be noted. The harder the wire tip, the higher the torquability of the wire; and the less resistance at the tip that is felt by the operator, the easier it is to find oneself in a false lumen. Also bear in mind that, because the tip of the coil wire attracts a lot of resistance, it is more difficult for it to end up in or select very small channels.

Recently the field of interventional cardiology has seen the introduction of tapered wires (Asahi Confianza 0.014-0.009 in; Guidant Cross-it 0.014–0.010 in). Notwithstanding the fact that these wires tend to slip into or select very narrow channels more easily than normal coil wires, the tapered wires are useful for making the penetration point in the fibrous cap. With the Confianza and the Cross-it XT300–400 wires, however, the hard tip means that these wires have a tendency to end up in false lumina just after tight bends, and it is hard to feel the resistance if they do so. Bear in mind, also, that the tapered wires can easily cause perforations in the vessel wall.

Wire Selection

When attempting recanalization of CTOs, wire selection must be tailored to the specific characteristics of the lesion and exchanged for more suitable wires during the procedure if circumstances demand it. There is no one wire that fits all eventualities.

When the occlusion has been present for 6 months or less, an intermediate wire is usually the first choice. The Asahi Miracle 3 g, with its superior torquability, may sometimes be a good choice for such occlusions. For a relatively hard, tapered CTO that has been present for 6 months to a year, Miracle 3 g is still a good choice.

If a recanalization or some other type of channel is present and the operator spots a light bend in the channel, a polymer-coated wire such as the Choice or Whisper wire is probably a good option. However, the polymer-coated wire should be exchanged for a coil wire if there is any indication that the wire has started along a false lumen.

When dealing with a convex-type lesion with no dimpling, a hard wire, such as the Miracle 12 g, or a tapered wire, such as the Confianza or the Cross-it XT300–400), is a good choice. In opt-

ing for a less-hard wire, the operator may run the risk of creating a false lumen, especially in CTOs of long duration with a side branch. Keep in mind that the stiffness of the wire tip depends on the position of the support catheter tip. In longer CTOs, however, especially if the course of the lumen is not obvious, the operator should try to avoid making a false lumen by judging from the feel of the resistance at the wire tip. It is usually better, after the initial breakthrough into the CTO, to switch to a Miracle 4.5 g or smaller or, on a case-by-case basis, to an intermediate wire.

If, because of tortuosity or tight bends, resistance is strong and handling difficult, the best strategy may be to switch to a polymer-coated wire when trying to locate a channel through relatively soft CTO tissue. Once the distal fibrous cap has been penetrated, the operator can then return to a hard (Miracle 6 g or 12 g) or tapered wire; this approach can help to minimize the risk of creating false lumina. Again, however, once the wire passes along a false lumen in the distal fibrous cap, it may be necessary to use the parallel wire technique or IVUS guidance (described later in the chapter) to find another channel with a stiff or tapered wire.

【 】 WIRE TIP SHAPES

Conventional CTO wires are available with four different tip shapes, as shown in Figure 33-11A–D. The most common, or basic shape has a 2- to 3-mm, 45-degree curve, as shown in part A of the figure. When selecting a branch with the wire and then

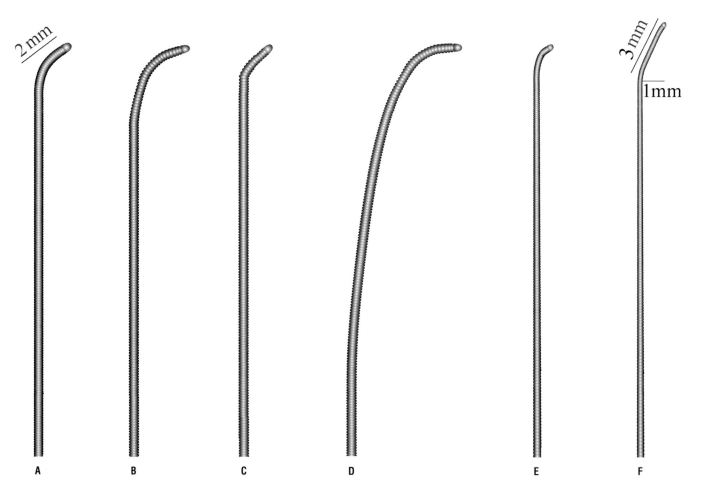

FIGURE 33-11. Types of wire tips: Conventional (**A–D**) and newer, tapered wires (**E, F**).

planning to cross it forward to the CTO, an operator can use a wire of the type shown in part D. The wire type shown in B, with its large curve, is effective when a large false lumen has been created and the operator needs to retract the wire and locate the true lumen. One thing to bear in mind, however, is that tips with large curves have a tendency to find their way through the intima. Because these tips can make existing false lumina even larger, an operator should try to use a tip with as small a curve as possible. With a wire of the type shown in part C, the core wire can become bent as the wire is bent, meaning this wire can quickly wear out inside highly resistant, hard CTOs.

The newer, tapered wires have quite different properties from their conventional counterparts. Their tip shapes are also designed for different uses than those of normal wires. When trying to advance the wire through a hard proximal fibrous cap, the slightly curved tip of the type shown in Figure 33-13E is probably best, but only if the operator is sure the wire is coaxial with the direction of the CTO. The tiny curve of the type shown in part F of the figure was, until recently, too difficult technically to incorporate into wire manufacture. The enhanced sensitivity for wire-tip control that this small curve offers is of great use when an operator is creating a new channel or looking for an existing one. The fact that tapered wires have enabled the development of these small curve-type wires is one of their key contributions.

【 】 TECHNIQUES OF WIRE-HANDLING

Maneuvering the Wire

The two fundamental elements of wire handling are rotating and "pushing" (feeding the wire forward). Because it is also important to feel the resistance at the wire tip when maneuvering the wire, it is recommended that the left hand be used to feed the wire back and forward, and the right hand to rotate the wire. There are two things to be careful of: (1) wire rotation should be minimized to avoid missing the point one is aiming at when making the penetration, and (2) the operator must ensure that the wire rotation does not enlarge the channels too much.

Another technique is to advance the wire, little by little, toward the target without rotating it at all. This method has the advantage over the rotational approach of minimizing the size of any channels that are created with the wire. However, as the wire is deflected by hard tissue, it can easily end up only going through softer tissue.

Either method has advantages and disadvantages, and the key is differentiating which method best suits one's specific needs. To summarize, when advancing the wire along the vessel, the operator should continually check for resistance at the tip, but when attempting to penetrate the fibrous tip, the tip should be pushed in the desired direction.

When trying to decide on the correct path inside a CTO, a route that meets very little resistance usually is the correct one, if the proximal portion of the CTO is tapered. When the CTO ends abruptly, however, the wire sometimes meets very little or no resistance even while moving down that wrong path. The only way to determine whether the wire tip is in the subintima is to withdraw the wire 1 to 2 mm. If the tip is in the subintima, the operator will feel an unusual and unmistakable sense of it being stuck. A good rule of thumb is as follows: If any kind of crunching sensation is felt from the hard tissue at the wire tip, the operator can be pretty certain that the tip is in the intima. The next step, in this case, is to bring the wire back and look for a new channel down which to continue.

Getting the Wire to Go Where Intended

Penetrating the Proximal Fibrous Cap. Consider the following common scenarios involving a CTO of several years' duration with no dimpling at the proximal end: (1) an operator is unable to insert a normal CTO wire into the lesion, or (2) the wire slips and the operator cannot get a fix on the point he or she wants to pierce, or (3) the operator does not know the ideal spot for the penetration point. For the first two scenarios, a Miracle 12 g or a Confianza wire should be used. When the wire and vessel cannot be made coaxial, adjusting the size and angle of the curve may often solve the problem (see Figure 33-11D). There are certain times (ie, CTOs of the ostial LAD) when it is useful to insert the guide catheter very deep. If the wire continues to slip down a side branch immediately before the ostium of CTO, use of a balloon to block the side branch sometimes is helpful (Figure 33-12). In a proximal CTO, IVUS can often be invaluable in locating the correct entry

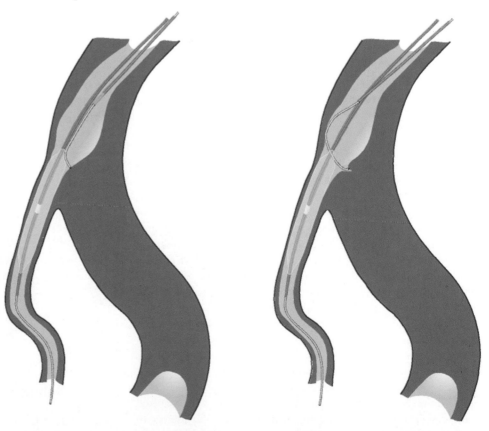

FIGURE 33-12. Balloon dilation to preventing the wire from slipping into a side branch.

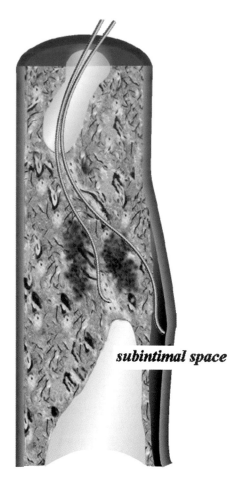

FIGURE 33-13. This tortuous channel inside a chronic total occlusion developed as a resulting of lack of coaxiality of proximal and the distal true lumina and the distribution of hard tissue inside the lesion.

point for perforation when an operator is unsure of where to aim the guide catheter.

Advancing the Wire to the Distal End of the CTO. There is no easy way to master the technique of advancing the wire to the distal end of a CTO; it really is a process of trial and error and learning from one's mistakes. The presence of a portion of surviving lumen inside the CTO, or a recanalization channel, can serve as a guide. And, as previously noted, calcification can also provide a guide to vessel course. Whether the path is signposted or not, sensitivity to resistance at the tip of the wire is crucial. Furthermore, even if the vessel is completely straight, the operator should proceed with caution because there is no guarantee that the channel being navigated will be as straight (Figure 33-13). If the wire tip repeatedly creates a false lumen, one is unlikely to achieve a better result with the same or an identical wire. Although exchanging wires in this situation can be difficult, it is an indispensable part of basic wire-handling technique for CTOs.

In many cases, to avoid making the false lumen even bigger, it is a good idea, once a route has been opened into a new channel using a stiff wire, to switch to a softer wire such as the Miracle 3 g. If it is still difficult to locate another channel, the operator may find that changing to a tapered wire with a small curved tip helps. Bear in mind, however, that using the parallel wire technique with a tapered wire (described later) is a key component of a successful strategy in this type of case (Figure 33-14). As previously noted, positioning the

wire at the outer part of the curve at the bend can often cause the tip to enter the subintima.

If the development of a false lumen is not connected with a bend in the vessel, it is often the case that the path of the wire has been obstructed by hard tissue, causing the wire to pass instead into the subintima. The best course of action in this case is to pull back proximal to the point where the false lumen was created and switch to a stiff wire (Miracle 6 g or higher) or a stiff tapered wire. A Confianza wire is normally the best choice, because the resistance at the wire tip offers the operator a good feel for the best pathway. The curve at the tip should also be kept as small as possible, except when the false lumen has already been enlarged. When making a new channel, the operator should, as a matter of course, be certain of its position relative to existing channels.

Changing Wires Inside the CTO. As previously mentioned, there are times when an operator will need to change wires during the procedure. The following discussion briefly summarizes three available methods for exchanging wires.

Bare wire exchange. This technique, which involves simply removing the first wire and inserting a new one in the same channel, is easier to accomplish if the CTO is relatively hard and not peppered with numerous false lumina. Disadvantages are that it adds to the overall procedural time, uses more contrast medium, and is technically challenging. The operator must be especially careful to avoid creating false lumina in a CTO with a bend; it is better to try a different technique before too much damage is provoked.

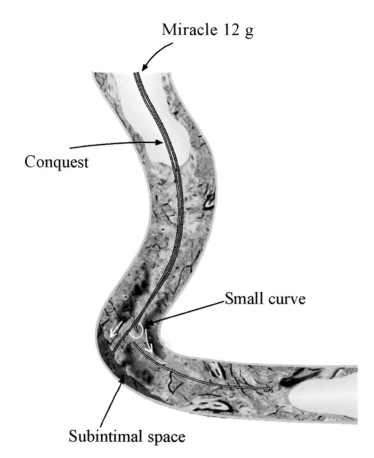

FIGURE 33-14. A Conquest wire can help locate a channel, but the operator must use the parallel wire technique.

Catheter-based wire exchange. If a 1.5-mm over-the-wire balloon catheter can be inserted inside the CTO, the operator will be able to exchange wires while keeping the tip of the balloon catheter inside the CTO. This method carries a risk of causing a dissection inside the CTO as the balloon catheter is inserted.

Parallel wire method. The parallel wire method is increasingly used for exchanging wires; the two other methods described above are, in fact, rarely used today. As shown in Figure 33-15, this method essentially involves feeding the second wire along the same path as the first wire, in parallel, using the first wire as the guide or marker to make the whole process fairly straightforward. The trick is to advance the tip of the second wire alongside the shaft of the first wire, so that it looks as though one is on top of the other from the various angiographic views. It is a good idea to bring the support catheter for the balloon catheter up to a point just proximal to the lesion.

Penetrating the Distal Fibrous Cap. Before considering how to penetrate the distal fibrous cap with the wire, it is necessary to first advance the wire tip to the point one wishes to target. A usable channel is often present, and if the wire is not in this channel and the operator is trying to reach the distal true lumen at the distal fibrous cap, the chances of success are low even with the use of various stiff wires. Again, if the wire is not in the correct channel, the operator should pull back and try to find the the correct pathway before making the false lumen any larger.

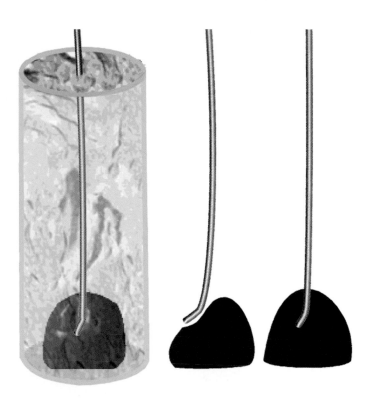

FIGURE 33-16. Wire tip position in the distal fibrous cap (3D view).

The end of the CTO is a dome-like 3D shape that does not show up clearly on two-dimensional (2D) images such as those provided by fluoroscopy. The operator must use particular care once the wire touches the distal fibrous cap at the optimal perforation point, because in the 2D view, the wire can look as if it is already in the distal true lumen (Figure 33-16). In this case, experience may not be enough to prevent mistakes, and extreme vigilance on the part of the operator is essential.

Most important of all, if the wire has been deflected by the fibrous cap, the operator must bring the wire tip back and attempt to locate a new channel that will provide a different route to the distal cap. If this attempt fails, the operator should pull back to avoid making the false lumen even larger, and should switch to a stiff or tapered wire.

In practice, most operators will find that the successful penetration of the distal fibrous cap remains far from easy. There are at least two possible reasons for this: (1) The wire has already strayed into the subintima at the distal end, and it is hard to penetrate through to the distal true lumen because the tissue there is thicker; or (2) maneuverability at the distal end of the CTO is poor, and the distal fibrous cap moves as the wire tip does, so that the operator cannot pin down a spot to make the penetration point (Figure 33-17). For scenario 1, all that can be done is to pull back and change the access route; for scenario 2, the operator should use a wire with a sharp stiff tip and keep rotation to a minimum to position it securely at the perforation point using the parallel wire technique described below.

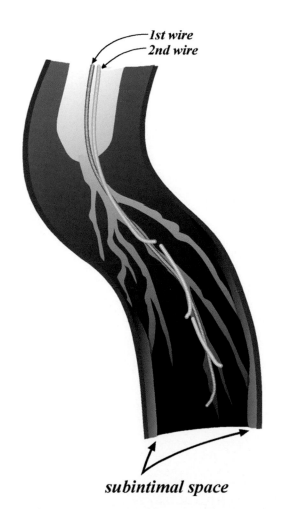

subintimal space

FIGURE 33-15. Wire exchange using the parallel wire technique.

PARALLEL WIRE TECHNIQUE

The parallel wire technique requires the insertion of a second wire into the CTO while the first wire is still in place. I believe that this

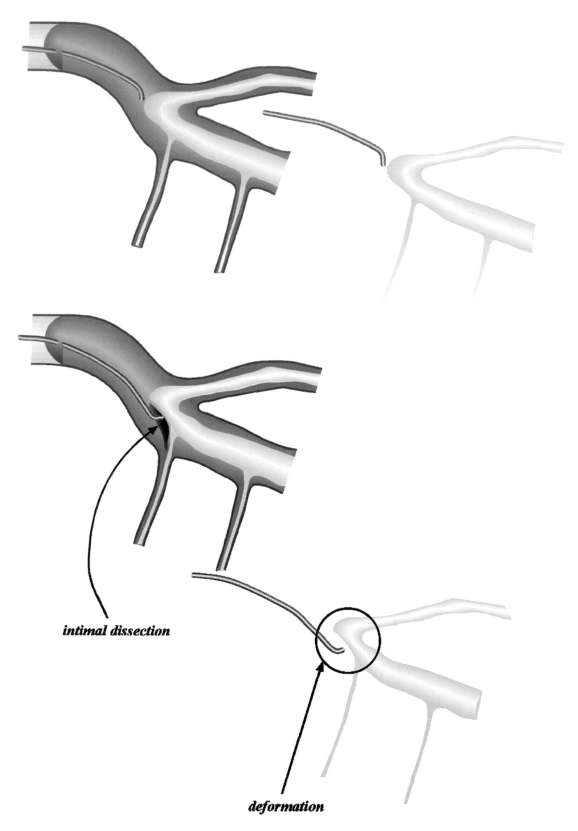

intimal dissection

deformation

FIGURE 33-17. The distal fibrous cap can be distorted or moved by the approaching wire.

technique will become the principal wire-handling technique for CTOs. It has the advantage over the other techniques in use until now of being applicable to all CTOs, irrespective of individual lesion characteristics.

【 】 BASIC CONSIDERATIONS

Five conditions, described below, must be observed for successful execution of the parallel wire technique.

Preconditions

One absolute condition is that the distal end of the CTO in the distal true lumen must be clearly visible on CAG from the collateral flow. To ensure the efficacy of the parallel wire technique, the operator must be absolutely sure that he or she can see, under fluoroscopy, the relative positions of the distal true lumen and first wire, using the full range of available angiographic views (Figure 33-18).

Importance of a Support Catheter

When inserting the second wire, the operator must use a 1.5-mm over-the-wire balloon, a Transit catheter, or even an Interpass catheter, and not simply a bare wire. This requirement is necessary to avoid twisting of the wire and, even more importantly, to maintain maneuverability of the second wire. As such, it is a key factor in the simplification and successful execution of this technique.

Wire-Handling in Theory

As the second wire is fed inside the CTO, the operator must ensure that the second wire closely follows the course of the first, "hugging" it as it advances. It is vital to use every available fluoroscopic view to confirm that the two wires occupy the same channel inside the CTO. With experience this will become easier, requiring the need for fewer views, and the use of less contrast medium.

Wire-Handling in Practice

Preferably, the second wire will be stiffer than the first, with superior torque transfer, because during these procedures the wires can become twisted. Furthermore, stiffer wires are less likely to become twisted in the first place. Most commonly the second wire is a Miracle 12 g or Confianza wire. When the second wire is stiffer and has better torque (and therefore better maneuverability) than the first, the first wire can be used more efficiently as a marker, reducing the risk of making new false lumina or of perforating the vessel.

Timing

Most operators will find that their success in advancing the first wire to the distal true lumen on the first attempt depends on the tissue inside the CTO. If the first attempt does not prove successful, the operator should try again, cautiously, because of the risk of creating a false lumen. It follows that an operator should always switch to the parallel wire technique before risking the creation of a large false lumen.

The preceding conditions represent the fundamental requisites of this technique. Neglecting any of these points will make wire-handling extremely difficult and more likely to result in failure.

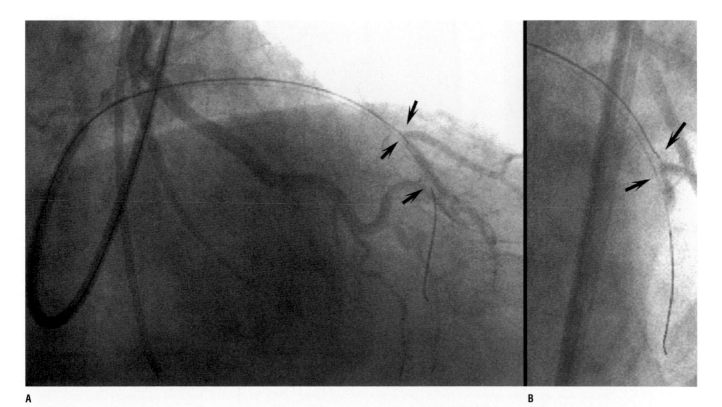

A   **B**

FIGURE 33-18. The ability to visualize the distal circulation via collateral flow is essential in the execution of the parallel-wire technique.

【 】 PERFECTING THE PARALLEL WIRE TECHNIQUE

This is not the most straightforward of techniques, and mastering it entails something of a learning curve. Lesions that have some degree of tortuosity offer particularly good practice opportunities. Similarly, when a wire passes relatively easily through a CTO, the operator can attempt, before dilating the balloon, to cross a stiff wire through using the parallel technique. With practice, the operator should be able to feed the wire across nearly 100% of the time.

【 】 APPLYING THE PARALLEL WIRE TECHNIQUE

The list that follows provides examples of specific situations in which the parallel wire technique can be expected to be of use in the clinical setting of an intervention for a CTO.

1. Exchanging wires (see earlier discussion).
2. Finding or creating a new channel inside the CTO. The difficulty in this instance is knowing in which direction to go. This factor is largely dependent on operator instinct, because there are no visual markers to show the correct direction or the exact spot at which to rotate the wire. Operators usually find that once they have made a channel, the wire tip tends naturally to slip away into the same channel (Figure 33-19). One advantage of the parallel wire technique is that the first wire acts as a marker, giving the operator a 3D view and making it easier to compensate for this jumping effect. Another merit of the technique is that the operator can use the first wire as an anchor, enabling him or her to guard against any slipping of the second wire while it is being rotated.
3. Navigating a bend inside the CTO. If an operator realizes that the first wire has entered the subintima at a bend, the wire can be left where it is, helping to straighten the bend, and the operator can use it as a marker to maneuver the second wire around the smaller, inner side of the bend.
4. Negotiating the tissue inside the CTO. Often, when an operator tries to push the wire through a new point, the existence of a false lumen means that the tissue shifts or "escapes" from the stiff wire tip, and actual penetration is difficult. If the operator switches quickly to the parallel wire technique, he or she can make use of the first wire by leaving it in the false lumen, where it can help steady or pin down the tissue, thus making it easier to find a route through the lesion.

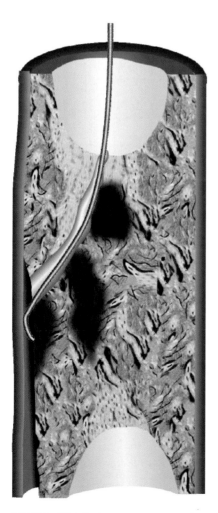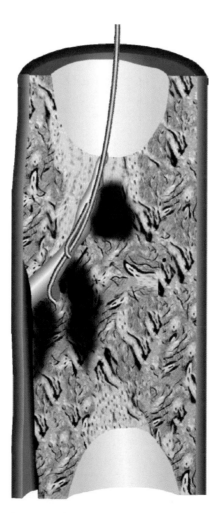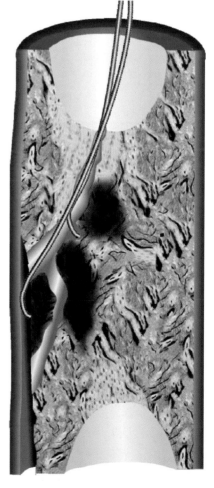

FIGURE 33-19. Once a wire enters the subintimal space (*left*), a new channel cannot easily be created. The wire repeatedly slips back into the space and changing its direction is very difficult (*center*). A new channel can be created relatively easily, however, using the parallel wire technique (*right*).

SPECIAL WIRE TECHNIQUES

[ ] SIDE-BRANCH TECHNIQUE

If, at the distal portion of the CTO, there is more than a 30° angle between the direction in which the wire is proceeding and the true lumen, it is often quite easy to create a false lumen around the true lumen. In such situations, if a side-branch forks out from the distal portion of the CTO, the operator should try, from the beginning, to feed the wire into the side branch through its ostium. This is actually the ideal scenario for utilizing the side-branch technique. The operator first passes the wire into the side branch, restoring blood flow in the parent artery by dilating a 1.5-mm balloon at the side branch ostium. Then, after changing to a softer wire, he or she pulls back from the side branch and returns to the parent artery. When the wire penetrates too far down the side-branch ostium, even if blood flow has been restored by balloon dilation, it is often impossible to maneuver the wire out of the side branch and into the parent artery. For this reason, operators must be very careful in directing the wire. If the wire advances just slightly past the side-branch ostium, and if the side branch is relatively large, use of a 1.25-mm Rotablator burr at the ostium to ablate the obstruction can facilitate advancement of the wire through to the main trunk. A word of caution: Because Rotablator use carries a high risk of vessel perforation, it should only be attempted when the operator is confident that it can be performed safely. In most situations, the parallel wire technique should be used to advance the wire into the true lumen in the parent vessel.

[ ] RETROGRADE APPROACH

This technique is possible when the lesion can be approached from the opposite (downstream) direction (eg, in the presence of large collateral channels without serious tortuosity; this is often the case with a septal branch or some channel connecting with the atrial branch, or an approach from a graft). One wire is advanced up to the distal fibrous cap of the CTO, to be used as a marker when piercing the distal cap with a second wire that is advanced from the proximal direction in the conventional way.

THE ROLE OF INTRAVASCULAR ULTRASOUND IN WIRE TECHNIQUE

It is sometimes difficult to obtain a clear idea from CAG about the entry to the proximal edge of a CTO. CTOs are especially difficult to assess in the ostial LAD, when the LAD is totally occluded immediately after the bifurcation of a large diagonal branch or septal branch; in the right coronary artery, when the occlusion occurs just after the bifurcation of the right ventricular branch; or in the left circumflex artery immediately after the obtuse marginal branch. In these situations, the operator can often confirm the location of the occlusion by inserting an IVUS catheter into a side branch. IVUS will be of no use, however, when the catheter cannot be advanced very far into the side branch, or when heavy calcification is present on the vessel wall at the CTO ostium or side branch.

IVUS can be used initially to check the CTO ostium and to visualize the transducer position from which the operator can get a good look at the CTO ostium using CAG. The transducer position can then be used to check the position of the CTO ostium. Although it may be possible to confirm the position of the CTO ostium from longitudinal positions, it is often difficult to see this clearly from the axial view. This is not usually a problem if one uses CAG.

Yet another use for IVUS occurs when the wire has reentered the true lumen from a false lumen and the operator wants to see where the wire entered or exactly where the false lumen was made (and, in particular, whether the wire went through the subintima). Advanced application of IVUS for CTO wiring is illustrated in Figure 33-20. When a CTO is not successfully wired with angiographic guidance, the operator can use IVUS as an alternative guidance method. In unsuccessful CTO cases, operators often lose sight of the collateral flow on CAG and cannot continue the procedure. However, it is usually possible to observe the distal true lumen via IVUS, by leaving an IVUS catheter in the false lumen after the collateral flow has disappeared on the angiographic view. If the distal true lumen can be imaged using IVUS, the operator can continue wire-handling with simultaneous IVUS guidance. Similarly, if the wire is in a side branch, it is very important, when feeding the wire to the parent vessel, to establish the location of any plaque buildup at the bifurcation of the side branch and parent vessel. IVUS is the best way to obtain this information.

CONCLUSION

It is important to bear in mind, while developing one's wire-handling skills for CTOs, that acquiring the ability to attempt these lesions is a gradual process. To put it another way, the chances are rather remote that an operator will suddenly be able to successfully recanalize a CTO of several years' duration if that operator has performed the procedure in fewer than 100 patients. Of course, the low initial success rate will dissuade some operators from attempting to treat CTOs altogether, and the high incidence of complications is another disincentive.

In this chapter, I have not addressed strategies to reduce and prevent complications associated with CTOs. These lesions are different from other lesions in the sense that there is a very little risk of dangerous coronary occlusion; but, conversely, there are other complications peculiar to CTOs. A thorough grounding in normal interventional procedures is a good starting point for coming to grips with these CTO-specific complications.

As an operator's experience with CTOs expands to include more indications, it should first be possible to achieve a success rate of 90% for CTOs that have been present for 3 months or less. For CTOs of longer duration, the operator should expect gradually to work up from tapered occlusions to abruptly closing CTOs, from CTOs with no tight bends to moderately tortuous ones, from CTOs less than 20 mm in length to longer CTOs, and from occlusions of up to 1 year's duration to those that have been present for much longer. A solid grasp of how to "read" the lesions and a thorough understanding of the pitfalls and important

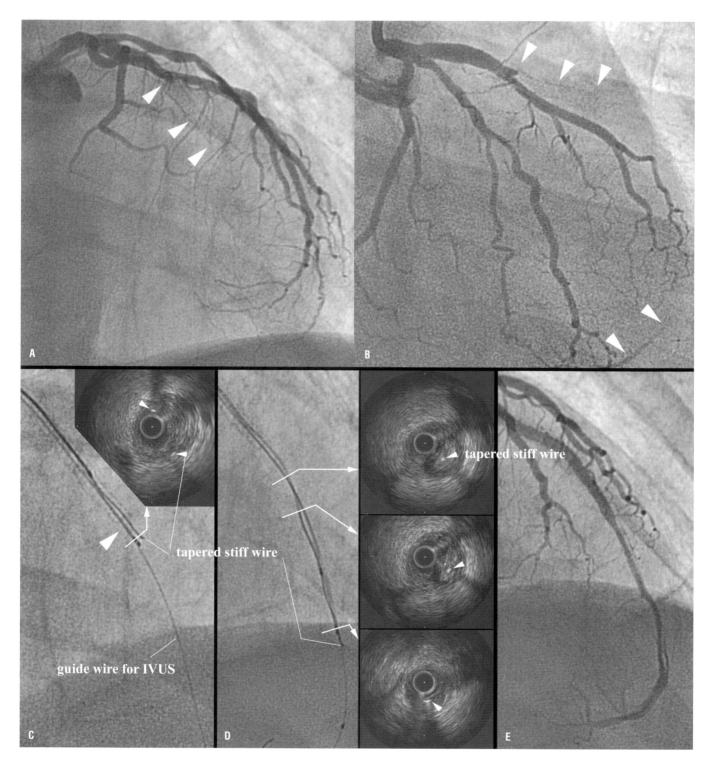

FIGURE 33-20. An example of a stent occlusion of 1 year's duration in the middle of the left anterior descending (LAD) artery. **(A)** Recanalization of this occlusion was attempted twice, causing the distal true lumen to collapse. It was subsequently occupied by a thrombus after the procedures. In this situation, to locate the distal true lumen with a guidewire is extremely difficult, because the target cannot be seen on angiogram (ie, the distal LAD was filled by collateral, as shown in panel **B**). The first wire was fed into the false lumen all the way [after] the stent. Next, the false channel was dilated with a 1.5-mm balloon to enable insertion of the intravascular ultrasound (IVUS) catheter into the channel. While observing the distal true lumen occupied by a thrombus just distal to the stent, penetration into the distal true lumen was attempted with a Confianza wire **(C)**. The wire was manipulated under IVUS guidance, as shown in panel **D**. After dilation of the true lumen, the false lumen was collapsed and good blood flow was restored **(E)**.

details are crucially important before an operator attempts to intervene in patients with CTOs.

Finally, I have, in this chapter, concentrated entirely on wire-handling and not on the handling of the other devices used in interventions for CTOs. It goes without saying that good CTO technique requires that the operator possess a greater degree of skill and ability than is required for normal interventions, in backing up the guide catheter, crossing the balloons, implanting stents, and using rotational and directional coronary atherectomy. All would-be operators would do well to bear this in mind.

CHAPTER (34)

Percutaneous Intervention in Chronic Total Coronary Occlusions

John S. Douglas, Jr, MD

Treatment of chronic total occlusions (CTOs) of the coronary arteries represents, in many respects, one of the last great challenges in percutaneous coronary intervention (PCI). CTOs account for a disparate proportion of denials of PCI and result in referral to coronary bypass graft surgery (CABG) or continued medical therapy. However, successful treatment of CTOs has been demonstrated to improve anginal symptoms, reduce the need for subsequent CABG, and in some studies, improve longevity. The aim of this chapter is to provide the reader with as clear a statement as possible of the contemporary treatment of CTOs, realizing that the techniques, equipment, and indications are still evolving.

EVOLUTION OF THERAPY FOR CHRONIC TOTAL OCCLUSIONS

One of the earliest reported series of successful percutaneous recanalization of total coronary occlusions was from Emory University in 1982 and described treatment of patients who, while waiting PCI, progressed to total occlusion.[1] Subsequently, following development of an over-the-wire balloon catheter and stiffer guidewires in the mid-1980s, it became possible to successfully recanalize carefully selected true CTOs.

Between 1990 and 1992, series of patients who had undergone attempted PCI of CTO lesions were reported from the Mid-America Heart Institute, Emory University, and the Mayo Clinic. In these studies, involving 1739 patients, angiographic success was reported in 66% to 72%, emergency CABG in 1% to 3%, myocardial infarction (MI) in 1% to 4%, and in-hospital death in 1% to 2%.[2–4] Although the restenosis rate following these balloon-alone cases averaged 40%, with reocclusion in 15%, each of these series reported a reduction in the need for subsequent CABG in patients with successful CTO recanalization (CABG was reduced from approximately 40% to 15%; $P < .04$). In 2001, a 20-year experience with more than 2000 CTOs was reported from the Mid-America Heart Institute, 93% of which utilized balloon-alone treatment. This report showed improving success rates over time with rates of major adverse cardiac events (MACE) similar to non-CTOs and a distinct 10-year survival advantage for successful CTO treatment compared with failed CTO treatment (73.5% vs 65.1%; $P = .001$).[5] More than 1000 patients were enrolled in eight clinical trials of balloon angioplasty versus bare-metal stenting in CTOs, and these studies showed that stenting was associated with about a 50% reduction in reocclusion (from approximately 20% to 10%), restenosis (about 60% to 30%), and target vessel revascularization (approximately 40% to 20%).[6–13] A multicenter registry of 29 Italian centers in 1999 to 2000 reported contemporary CTO therapy (90% of patients received bare-metal stents) in 419 consecutive patients. Technical success was reported in 77.2% and in-hospital MACE in 5.1% (death, 0.3%; Q-wave MI, 0.36%; non-Q-wave MI, 4.3%; perforation, 2.1%).[14] Multivariate analysis identified CTO length greater than 15 mm, moderate to severe calcification, duration of occlusion greater than 180 days, and multivessel disease as significant predictors of PCI failure. At 12 months, patients with successful CTO therapy had a lower incidence of cardiac death or MI (1.0% vs 7.2%; $P = .005$), experienced a reduced need for CABG (2.4% vs 16%; $P < .0001$), and were more frequently free of angina (89% vs 75%; $P = .008$).

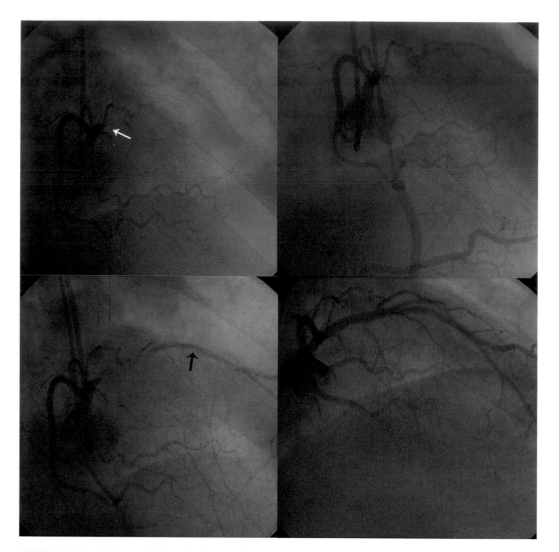

FIGURE 34-1. A 69-year-old [psychologist] with a 2-year history of stable angina underwent a positron emission tomography scan that revealed a very large anterior ischemic defect estimated to involve 35% of the left ventricle. The electrocardiogram at rest and the ventriculogram were normal. Coronary angiography revealed a chronic total occlusion (CTO) of the left anterior descending (LAD) coronary artery at its ostium (*upper left; right anterior oblique, cranial view, white arrow* indicates site of occlusion). The LAD at the occlusion was moderately calcified. Bilateral coronary artery injections revealed the length of the CTO to be about 15 mm and the length of the diseased segment to be approximately 25 mm (*upper right; same view*). Prior surgical repair of a pectus excavatum deformity was a complicating feature. It was possible to cross the CTO with the radiofrequency energy and optical coherence reflectometry guidance of the Safe-Cross guidewire (IntraLuminal Therapeutics, Carlsbad, CA). A safe intraluminal distal position of the guidewire was confirmed by contrast injection in the right coronary artery (*lower left panel; black arrow* indicates distal tip of guidewire). The proximal LAD was dilated and a 3.0-by-33 mm Cypher stent was deployed and, using ultrasound guidance, expanded to more than 4 mm, resulting in a superb angiographic result (*lower right*). Currently available studies (see references 17, 18, 20 and 21) indicate a very low recurrence rate can be expected with this approach.

In the past 5 years, CTO therapy has been substantially improved by the development of more effective techniques for successfully passing a guidewire across the CTO into the true lumen of the distal vessel. These include stiffer wires with greater torque control, hydrophilic coatings, a blunt dissection strategy with the Front Runner (Lumend, Redwood City, CA), and use of the Safe-Cross guidewire (IntraLuminal Therapeutics, CA), which incorporates radiofrequency energy with guidance via optical coherence reflectometry[15,16] (Figure 34-1). Of equal or greater importance, long-term results of PCI for CTO lesions have been enhanced by the advent of drug-eluting stents to retard restenosis. Although randomized, controlled trials of drug-eluting stents versus bare-metal stents in CTOs have not been conducted, observational studies strongly suggest safety and efficacy of drug-eluting stents in CTOs, and these stents have become standard therapy in CTO therapy in most centers.

Studies supporting routine use of drug-eluting stents in CTOs include the Research Registry (target lesion revascularization [TLR] in 4% of 56 consecutive patients at 1 year)[17]; the multicenter Asian Registry,[18] in which restenosis at 6 months occurred in only 3.4% of patients and MACE in 4.5%; and a report by Werner and colleagues of 48 CTOs treated with paclitaxel-eluting stents that had better outcomes than a bare-metal historical control group with respect to angiographic restenosis at 5 months (8.3% vs 51%; $P < .001$), reocclusion (2.1% vs 23%; $P < .001$), and MACE at 1 year (12% vs 48%; $P < .001$).[19] In a larger experience, 158 CTO patients treated with sirolimus-eluting stents were compared with 290 noncontemporaneous patients with bare-metal stents; outcomes at 6 months for patients receiving Cypher stents were better with respect to restenosis (11% vs 34%; $P = .005$), TLR (7.5% vs 23%; $P < .001$), and MACE (17% vs 31%. $P = .005$).[20] Among 360 CTO patients followed for 6 months in the e-Cypher Registry, TLR and MACE were low (1.4% and 3.3%, respectively).[21] Similarly, in a prospective nonrandomized study of 308 patients (128 treated with Cypher and 180 with Taxus) with 358 CTOs in five high-volume Asian centers, MACE at 30 days was zero and restenosis was low for both stents (1.5% and 1.7%; $P = NS$), as was MACE (2.3% vs 2.2%; $P = NS$).[22] The reduction in restenosis with drug-eluting stents compared with bare-metal stents (from ~30% to ~10%) and in TLR (from ~20% to ~5%) represents a very substantial improvement in outcomes and has fueled interest in new approaches to CTO therapy, resulting in formation of an American CTO Club along the lines of the Japanese CTO Club. The Japanese CTO Club, which was formed over a decade ago, has pioneered new stiff guidewire strategies, such as the parallel wire technique, "seesaw" wiring, and ultrasound-guided CTO recanalization (see Chapter 33 and below), with improved success rates from about 70% to well over 80%.

PATIENT AND LESION CHARACTERISTICS

A CTO is usually defined angiographically as a complete coronary obstruction with no luminal continuity, and Thrombolysis in Myocardial Infarction (TIMI) 0 or 1 flow, in a patient whose clinical history or prior angiography indicates that the occlusion is not a recent event. CTOs are present in about one quarter of patients with angiographically documented coronary disease yet accounted for only 15% of PCIs in the 1997–1998 National Heart, Lung, and Blood Index Dynamic Registry.[23] The perception that CTOs were poor targets for PCI resulted in CTOs being the most common reason for excluding patients from randomized studies of PCI and CABG.

The majority of patients undergoing CTO interventions have chronic stable or chronic progressive angina. Accompanying heart failure symptoms are not a contraindication to PCI, because left ventricular function may be improved by opening the CTO.[24] Both duration of symptoms and lesion complexity influence the success of PCI in CTO lesions, the more recent, simpler lesions faring better. Heavy calcification, long length, very old occlusions, rich collateral network, blunt occlusion, and side branches arising at the site of occlusion have traditionally predicted PCI failure. Recent experiences by Japanese colleagues suggest that bridging collaterals, formerly the best predictor of PCI failure, may be associated with a success rate of about 75% compared with over 80% when absent.[25] Katsuragawa and colleagues correlated histologic findings with CTO success, noting that tapered CTOs frequently had recanalized channels up to 200 μm in diameter that were not visualized angiographically.[26] It is difficult to see by angiography a lumen smaller than 300 μm. The presence of these recanalized microchannels explains why successful guidewire passage is more likely in tapered occlusions and indicates why a 0.009-in or 0.010-in guidewire is sometimes successful when a 0.014-in wire is not. Stated differently, angiographic CTOs and especially tapered CTOs are frequently not complete occlusions when examined histologically.

Other pertinent histologic findings include atherosclerotic plaque, fibrous tissue, calcification, and organized or partially organized thrombi. The presence of dense fibrocalcific tissue correlates with age of occlusion and reduced PCI success. Very fibrotic plaque probably accounts for many PCI failures, causing even stiff wires to deviate along the path of least resistance into softer subintimal tissue, producing dissection. Even when the guidewire can be successfully passed through a CTO, difficulty may be encountered in passing even the lowest profile balloon, or the lesion may be undilatable; in either case, laser or rotablator may be required and, of course, superb guide catheter support is essential (Figure 34-2). In my experience with very difficult CTOs, the Safe-Cross radiofrequency-assisted wire has been successful in about a half of otherwise unsuccessful cases. The presence of a partially organized thrombus is the rationale for prolonged local thrombolytic therapy to improve PCI success in otherwise unsuccessful cases.

EQUIPMENT

[ ] GUIDE CATHETER

The principal requirement is a catheter that will safely provide robust support to advance balloons and stents once the lesion is crossed with a guidewire. For this reason, many experienced operators prefer 8 French guide catheters, EBU types for the left coronary artery and Amplatz-shaped catheters for the right coronary artery. Less supportive catheters may be required to satisfy anatomic constraints.

[ ] GUIDEWIRES

Inability to cross a CTO with a guidewire is the most common failure mode, and recent improved success is largely related to improved guidewires. A host of guidewires is available with varying stiffness, tapered tips, and lubricious coatings. "Simple" stiffened wires include High Torque Intermediate and Standard guidewires with 2- to 4-g tip stiffness (Guidant) and the line of Miracle wires with 3- to 12-g tip stiffness (Asahi), popularized by Japanese colleagues. These are discussed in detail in Chapter 33. Tapered wires include the 0.010 in-tipped Cross-it line with 2- to 6-g tip stiffness (Guidant) and the 0.009-in tipped Confianza, 9-g tip stiffness, and Confianza Pro, 12-g tip stiffness (Asahi). Hydrophilic-coated guidewires listed by increasing tip stiffness include the Whisper wire, 1-g tip stiffness (Guidant); Choice PT and PT Graphix, 2- to 4-g tip stiffness (Boston Scientific); Pilot 50, 100 and 150, with 2- to 4-g tip stiffness (Guidant); and Shinobi and Shinobi Plus, 2- to 4-g tip stiffness (Johnson & Johnson).

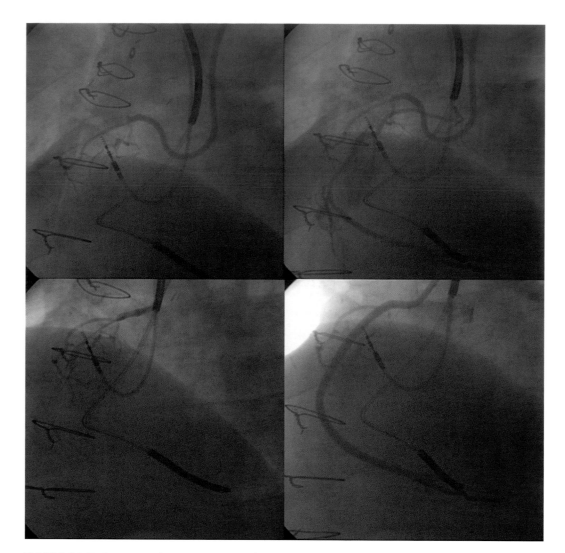

FIGURE 34-2. Five years after coronary artery bypass graft surgery, a 50-year-old man developed recurrent angina and experienced a cardiac arrest followed by successful resuscitation. Recanalization of a chronic total occlusion (CTO) of the right coronary artery (RCA) was attempted. The RCA was known to have been occluded for at least 3 years. The CTO (*upper right;* left anterior oblique view) had several unfavorable features, including lengthy occlusion, lack of tapering, calcification, side branches arising from the site, bridging collaterals, and an occlusion length of more than 15 mm (as demonstrated in the *upper right* panel). Use of multiple coronary guidewires was required (Safe-Cross, Confianza, and Pilot 50) to traverse the CTO. The occlusion could be crossed with a 1.5-mm diameter balloon, but was not dilatable until treated with a 1.5-mm Rotablator burr, shown approaching the lesion (*lower left*). Subsequently the vessel was dilated and stented with 3.0-mm diameter Taxus stents, providing an excellent angiographic and clinical result (*lower right*).

【 】 SPECIAL DEVICES FOR CROSSING CTOs

Use of the laser wire and the olive-tipped Magnum wire have failed to gain acceptance, and blunt microdissection with the Frontrunner (Lumend) catheter appears to me to be less effective than other options for coronary CTOs. The recently introduced Safe-Cross system (IntraLuminal Therapeutics) combines a forward-looking fiber-optic system, which emits and detects reflected near-infrared light and is reported to recognize vessel walls, with ablative radiofrequency energy to facilitate safe passage of the wire across the CTO into the distal lumen. There have been no randomized trials testing this system, but anecdotal published reports suggest that success can be expected in over half of patients who failed conventional

wire attempts, and this has been my experience in a limited number of about 35 cases.[16,17,27] Success was highest in straight vessels such as the left anterior descending coronary artery and lowest in the right coronary artery, which is unfortunately the most frequent target of CTO interventions. Importantly, the Safe-Cross wire has proved to be safe if the operator ensures that the wire is in the distal lumen before advancing balloon catheters over it.

【 】 ULTRASOUND

The Japanese pioneered use of intravascular ultrasound during interventions for CTO, and the reader is referred to Chapter 33 for discussion of this important adjunct to PCI.

STEP-BY–STEP INTERVENTION

【 】 INDICATIONS

Patients with CTOs who are selected for PCI generally have bothersome anginal symptoms or objective evidence of ischemic viable myocardium, a reasonable chance for PCI success, and do not have compelling indications for CABG or major contraindications to PCI. In most patients, the goal is relief from angina pectoris, but relief from silent ischemia may improve exercise tolerance and symptoms of heart failure. In addition, recanalization of a CTO may set the stage for safe PCI of contralateral coronary artery stenoses. Selection of patients for CTO PCI requires a classical risk-benefit analysis, balancing probability of success or complication against the potential gain. Factors that must be considered include duration and length of occlusion, tapered versus blunt shape of CTO, presence of bridging collaterals, calcification, vessel tortuosity, side branch origin from site of occlusion, amount of ischemic myocardium, clarity of distal vessel visualization, potential jeopardy to contralateral collaterals, and presence of renal insufficiency limiting use of contrast media. The difficulty of the CTO should also be commensurate with the experience level of the operator.

【 】 SELECTION OF ADJUNCTIVE THERAPY

Because of the small but increased risk of coronary perforation, most experienced CTO operators use a modest dose of unfractionated heparin to achieve an activated clotting time (ACT) of 200 to 250 and do not use glycoprotein IIb/IIIa receptor inhibitors or Angiomax, because it cannot be easily reversed. Antiplatelet therapy with aspirin and clopidogrel is usually administered routinely. Once the lesion is successfully crossed and the threat of guidewire perforation is reduced, additional antithrombotic therapy may be administered.

【 】 GUIDEWIRE MANIPULATION

An appropriate guide catheter is selected and multiple angiographic views of the CTO are recorded in an attempt to visualize the lesion free of overlap and foreshortening. Use of biplane angiography is favored by many operators to minimize the need for contrast media. Because clear visualization of the distal vessel is essential throughout the procedure, contralateral coronary artery injections are frequently necessary. In some cases, subselective injection in a contralateral vessel may reduce contrast usage. An example is use of a support catheter placed subselectively in a right ventricular branch of the right coronary artery to visualize the distal portion of an occluded left anterior descending artery.

A guidewire is selected and advanced through a support catheter or low-profile 1.5- or 2.0-mm over-the-wire balloon catheter. If the target lesion is distally located or a tortuous segment must be traversed, a soft, floppy guidewire should be used to deliver the support catheter to a position just proximal to the CTO. Selection of the least aggressive guidewire that the operator believes has a reasonable possibility for success and incremental increases in wire stiffness are preferences of many operators, but some very experienced Japanese operators elect immediate or early use of the Confianza wires. If the CTO is tapered, some operators prefer to start with a hydrophilic wire, taking advantage of unvisualized microchannels, but hydrophilic wires frequently find their way into subintimal spaces, resulting in dissection. Hydrophilic wires frequently shorten the case "one way or the other." Japanese operators have shown that when a guidewire passes subintimally, creating a false channel, leaving the wire in position and using a second or even third wire may be successful in reaching the distal true lumen (see Chapter 33). This has been termed the *parallel wire technique.*

Once the guidewire reaches the true distal lumen, the CTO can be crossed with a small balloon, or laser if necessary, predilated, and stented. If there is uncertainty about the location of the wire advanced distally, the operator should resist the urge to follow with a balloon or other device. When an operator is relying on collaterals from the target vessel to visualize the distal vessel, it is not uncommon for changes in collateral flow to occur during the procedure due to vessel dissection, necessitating contralateral femoral puncture to achieve contralateral coronary injections. Many operators therefore prefer to use the more reliable contralateral injections from the outset.

It is wise to define limits with respect to procedural time, fluoroscopy time, contrast media dose, and other parameters, before initiating the procedure. Operator experience determines choice of guidewires, balloons, guide catheters, and other equipment. In the era of drug-eluting stents, stenting is usually from "healthy to healthy." In some cases, a second attempt may be warranted after the vessel is allowed to heal for 6 weeks. Use of the Safe-Cross system resulted in success in about 50% of failed cases in my own experience and that of my colleagues. In prolonged cases, the operator should be aware of the importance of altering the views used to minimize radiation dose to the skin (see discussion of complications, later). Japanese operators have used ultrasound to assist in determining the true lumen when wire passage is difficult (see Chapter 33). Some operators have reported that a local infusion of a thrombolytic agent may lead to success when conventional guidewires have failed, but bleeding is a potential complication.[28]

TIPS AND PITFALLS

1. Use contralateral injections to demonstrate the distal true lumen.
2. Biplane fluoroscopy is preferred.
3. Avoid injecting through a balloon or support catheter to confirm proper distal position (if the catheter tip is subintimal, dissection will occur; contralateral injections are safer).
4. Never inflate a balloon catheter in an unconfirmed distal site.
5. Consider laser for uncrossable lesions and rotablator for undilatable CTOs that can be crossed with guidewire.
6. Use hydrophilic wires cautiously.
7. Use multiple views to confirm distal guidewire position.
8. Do not attempt a longstanding, difficult CTO without powerful guide catheter support.

COMPLICATIONS

The most common "complication" of PCI in patients with CTO lesions is failure to cross the lesion with a steerable guidewire, and this accounted for 81% of failures in a recently reported series.[14] Because of the need for excellent guide catheter support, guide catheter trauma is more common, but frequently less significant than with non-CTO PCI. Use of Amplatz guide catheters in the right coronary artery is especially liable to cause proximal coronary dissection. Because of subintimal guidewire passage and other vessel trauma, side-branch occlusion is common, as is loss of collaterals, and the latter may be more significant when PCI of CTO lesions is unsuccessful. Distal embolization is difficult to recognize, but may account for the no-reflow phenomenon following otherwise successful CTO PCI. Mid or distal coronary dissection may result in reestablishing flow to only a portion of the distal coronary artery. Penetration through the vessel wall with a guidewire is usually of no consequence unless IIb/IIIa platelet receptor inhibitors have been administered or unless the wire is followed by a balloon or other device. Among 420 consecutive CTO attempts between 1995 and 1999 at the Mid-America Heart Institute, four guidewire-induced perforations occurred (1%), two of which involved cardiac tamponade requiring urgent percardiocentesis.[5] Of 376 patients treated from 1999 to 2000 in a multicenter registry, eight patients (2.1%) experienced perforation, none with clinical sequelae. There was one death (0.25%), one Q-wave MI (0.26%), 16 non-Q-wave MIs (4.3%), two urgent CABGs (one retrograde left main dissection and one thrombosis of non-CTO stent; 0.53%), and two urgent repeat PCIs, for a total MACE rate of 5.1%.[14]

Because of the need for multiple contrast injections, contrast media usage in PCI of CTO lesions exceeds that of most non-CTO interventions and this is especially problematic in patients with impaired renal function. In these cases, optimal patient preparation in terms of hydration, N-acetylcysteine, and sodium bicarbonate administration, and use of the smallest amount of iodixanol possible is recommended.[29,30]

Radiation associated with prolonged fluoroscopy during CI for CTO can lead to skin injury. Approximately 60 minutes of fluoroscopy results in about 200 rems, which exceeds the radiation exposure received in 10,000 chest x-rays. Changing the position of the imaging system should be carried out during prolonged procedures to avoid skin injury.

CONCLUSION

Improved guidewire technology, including the Safe-Cross system and the stiffer Miracle wires, has resulted in substantially higher rates of CTO recanalization in recent years. Coupled with the advent of antiproliferative drug-eluting stents, these strategies have enhanced significantly the ability to achieve long-term patency in CTO interventions with improved symptomatic palliation, reduced need for CABG, and the prospect of improved longevity.

REFERENCES

1. Savage R, Hollman J, Gruentzig AR, et al. Can percutaneous transluminal coronary angioplasty be performed in patients with total occlusion? *Circulation.* 1982;66(suppl II):II-330. (Presented at the 55th Scientific Sessions of the American Heart Association, November 18, 1982).
2. Stone GW, Rutherford BD, McConahay DR, et al. Procedural outcome of angioplasty for total coronary artery occlusion: An analysis of 971 lesions in 905 patients. *J Am Coll Cardiol.* 1990;15:849.
3. Ivanhoe RJ, Weintraub WS, Douglas JS, et al. Percutaneous transluminal coronary angioplasty of chronic total occlusions. Primary success, restenosis, and long-term clinical follow-up. *Circulation.* 1990;85:106.
4. Bell MR, Berger PB, Bresnahan JF, et al. Initial and long-term outcomes of 354 patients after coronary balloon angioplasty of total coronary artery occlusions. *Circulation.* 1992;85:1003.
5. Suero JA, Marso SP, Jones PG, et al. Procedural outcomes and long-term survival among patients undergoing percutaneous coronary intervention of a chronic total occlusion in native coronary arteries: A 20-year experience. *J Am Coll Cardiol.* 2001;38:409.
6. Sirnes PA, Golf S, Myreng Y, et al. Stenting in Chronic Coronary Occlusion (SICCO): A randomized, controlled trial of adding stent implantation after successful angioplasty. *J Am Coll Cardiol.* 1996;28:1444.
7. Rubartelli P, Niccoli L, Verna E, et al. Stent implantation versus balloon angioplasty in chronic coronary occlusions: Results from the GISSOC trial. *J Am Coll Cardiol.* 1998;32:90.
8. Mori M, Kurogane H, Hayashi T, et al. Comparison of results of intracoronary implantation of the Palmaz-Schatz stent with conventional balloon angioplasty in chronic total coronary arterial occlusion. *Am J Cardiol.* 1996;78:985.
9. Hoher M, Wohrle J, Grebe OC, et al. A randomized trial of elective stenting after balloon recanalization of chronic total occlusions. *J Am Coll Cardiol.* 1999;34:722.
10. Buller CE, Dzavik V, Carere RG, et al. Primary stenting versus balloon angioplasty in occluded coronary arteries: The Total Occlusion Study of Canada (TOSCA). *Circulation.* 1999;100:236.
11. Lotan C, Rozenman Y, Hendler A, et al. Stents in total occlusion for restenosis prevention. *Eur Heart J.* 2000;21:1960.
12. Rahel MB, Suttorp MJ, Laarmen GJ, et al. Primary stenting of occluded native coronary arteries: Final results of Primary Stenting of Occluded Native Coronary Arteries (PRISON) study. *Am Heart J.* 2004;147:e22.
13. Sievert H, Rohde S, Utech A, et al. Stent or angioplasty after recanalization of chronic coronary occlusions? *Am J Cardiol.* 1999;84:386.
14. Olivari Z, Rubartelli P, Piscione F, et al; TOAST-GISE Investigators. Immediate results and one-year clinical outcome after percutaneous coronary interventions in chronic total occlusions: Data from a multicenter, prospective, observational study (TOAST-GISE). *J Am Coll Cardiol.* 2003;41:1672.
15. Whitbourn RJ, Vincotta M, Mossop P, et al. IntraLuminal blunt microdissection for angioplasty of chronic total occlusions. *Cathet Cardiovasc Interv.* 2003;58:194.
16. Baim DS, Braden G, Heuser R, et al. Utility of the Safe-Cross-guided radiofrequency total occlusion crossing system in chronic total occlusions. *Am J Cardiol.* 2004;94:853.
17. Hoye A, Tanabe K, Lemos P, et al. Significant reduction in restenosis after use of sirolimus-eluting stents in the treatment of chronic total occlusions. *J Am Coll Cardiol.* 2004;43:1954.
18. Nakamura S, Selvan TS, Bae JH, et al. Impact of sirolimus-eluting stents on the outcome of patients with chronic total occlusions: Multicenter registry in Asia. *J Am Coll Cardiol.* 2004;43:35A.
19. Werner GS, Krack A, Schwarz G, et al. Prevention of lesion recurrence in chronic total coronary occlusions by paclitaxel-eluting stents. *J Am Coll Cardiol.* 2004;44:2301.
20. Ge L, Iakovow I, Sangiori GM, et al. Immediate and mid-term outcomes of sirolimus-eluting stent implantation for chronic total occlusion lesions. *J Am Coll Cardiol.* 2005;45(suppl A):47A.
21. Lotan C, Gershlick A, Guagliumi G, et al. Treatment of chronic total occlusion with sirolimus-eluting stent. *J Am Coll Cardiol.* 2005;45(suppl A):47A.
22. Nakamura S, Muthasamy TS, Bae JH, et al. Comparison of efficacy and safety between sirolimus-eluting stent (Cypher) and paclitaxel-eluting stent (TAXUS) on the outcome of patients with chronic total occlusions: Multicenter Registry of Asia. *J Am Coll Cardiol.* 2005;45(suppl A):48A.
23. Suzuki T, Hosokawa H, Yokya K, et al. Time-dependent morphologic characteristics in angiographic chronic total coronary occlusions. *Am J Cardiol.* 2001;88:167.
24. Dzavik V, Carere RG, Mancini GBJ, et al. Predictors of improvement in left ventricular function after percutaneous revascularization of occluded coronary arteries. *Am Heart J.* 2001;142:301.

25. Kinoshita I, Katoh O, Nariyama J, et al. Coronary angioplasty of chronic total occlusions with bridging collateral vessels: Immediate and follow-up outcome from a large single-center experience. *J Am Coll Cardiol.* 1995;26:409.

26. Katsuragawa M, Fujiwara H, Miyamae M, et al. Histologic studies in percutaneous transluminal coronary angioplasty for chronic total occlusion: Comparison of tapering and abrupt types of occlusion and short and long occluded segments. *J Am Coll Cardiol.* 1993;21:604.

27. Wong P, Tse KK, Chan W. Recanalization of chronic total occlusion after conventional guidewire failure: Guided by optimal coherent reflectometry and facilitated by radiofrequency energy ablation. *J Invas Cardiol.* 2004;16:54.

28. Zidar FJ, Kaplan BM, O'Neill WW, et al. Prospective, randomized trial of prolonged intracoronary urokinase infusion for chronic total occlusions in native coronary arteries. *J Am Coll Cardiol.* 1996;27:1406.

29. Merten GJ, Burgess WP, Gray LV, et al. Prevention of contrast-induced nephropathy with sodium bicarbonate. A randomized controlled trial. *JAMA.* 2004;291:2328.

30. Aspelin P, Aubry P, Fransson SG, et al. Nephrotoxic effects in high-risk patients undergoing angiography. *N Engl J Med.* 2003;348:491.

CHAPTER (35)

Directional Coronary Atherectomy

Tomoaki Hinohara, MD, and Yasushi Asakura, MD

HISTORICAL OVERVIEW

The concept of atherectomy was introduced by JB Simpson in the mid-1980s; at the time, the major limitations of balloon angioplasty were acute failure resulting from dissection or elastic recoil and a high incidence of restenosis. Based on information obtained from surgical endarterectomy experiences involving diffusely diseased arteries with atherosclerosis, it was hypothesized that removal of atheromatous plaque would improve both acute and long-term outcomes following percutaneous coronary interventions (PCI). *Atherectomy* was defined as removal of atheromatous plaque using a transcatheter technique.

The initial success in testing this approach in patients with peripheral vascular disease led to development and testing of a coronary catheter. Subsequently, it was demonstrated that atheromatous plaque could be excised safely using the catheter technology. Simpson's directional coronary atherectomy (DCA) catheter (Devices for Vascular Intervention, Inc, Redwood City, Calif) was then approved by the Food and Drug Administration (FDA) in August 1990.

The initial experiences with DCA produced favorable clinical outcomes; the angiographic appearance of treated lesions was much wider and smoother, with less dissection, compared with percutaneous transluminal coronary angioplasty (PTCA). Furthermore, it appeared that the incidence of restenosis was respectable, and possibly lower than PTCA. By the early 1990s, DCA had become a widely applied procedure, accounting for close to 5% of overall PCI procedures. DCA was considered to be a technically difficult procedure, however, and it required experienced skills of the operator to obtain an optimal DCA result.

In the mid-1990s, as a consequence of improved stent technology, the simplicity of stenting, and the use of antiplatelet agents rather than anticoagulation to prevent acute in-stent thrombosis, DCA became a niche procedure for ostial lesions, bifurcation lesions, or eccentric lesions with a large plaque burden. Restenosis was shown to be related to the existing plaque burden even after stenting; thus, debulking prior to stenting was an attractive approach to further reduce restenosis in the stent era. However, subsequent multicenter randomized trials failed to demonstrate any benefits of debulking prior to stenting to reduce restenosis. Most recently, the introduction of drug-eluting stents (DES) has changed the approach for various complex lesions with PCI. The role of DCA in the DES era has significantly diminished; unless DCA or DCA with DES is shown to be more effective than DES alone, DCA may become a procedure of the past, except for a few exceptional, selected cases.

A new atherectomy catheter (SilverHawk, FoxHollow Technologies, Redwood City, Calif) was recently introduced. Its method of plaque excision, which differs significantly from previous atherectomy methods, enables this new catheter to treat long, diffuse lesions effectively, particularly in vessels of the lower extremities. Experience with this method is limited in the coronary artery. Further improvements of devices are necessary to apply this technology for treatment of coronary artery disease.

PIVOTAL TRIALS

Several pivotal trials were carried out to evaluate the safety and efficacy of DCA. These studies not only examined the concept of debulking and scientifically evaluated its efficacy, but also guided the evolution of procedural techniques to achieve "optimal" atherectomy outcomes.

In response to initial favorable results, CAVEAT (Coronary Angioplasty versus Excisional Atherectomy Trial) was carried out to evaluate the efficacy of DCA versus PTCA in reducing the restenosis rate.[1] CAVEAT was a historical landmark for device trials, because it was the first multicenter randomized trial to evaluate the performance of new interventional devices compared with PTCA. Although DCA was associated with lower restenosis (DCA 50% vs PTCA 57%; $P = .06$), the overall restenosis rate was considered to be too high. There were no overall clinical benefits compared with PTCA, and DCA was associated with some increased risk of early complications (11% vs 5%; $P < .001$) and slightly higher incidence of death or myocardial infarction (MI) at 6 months (DCA 8.6% vs PTCA 4.6%; $P = .007$). The potential explanation for a failure to reduce restenosis with DCA was that the angiographic result of DCA was suboptimal for atherectomy, with a high residual post-procedural stenosis. The suboptimal DCA outcome was considered to be the result of rapidly evolving procedural techniques without standardization, and the use of first-generation devices with features that were more limited than devices of subsequent generations.

Based on OARS (Optimal Atherectomy Restenosis Study), which showed improved outcomes of DCA with the use of appropriate technique to achieve optimal atherectomy,[2] a second multicenter randomized trial, BOAT (Balloon versus Optimal Atherectomy Trial), was subsequently carried out.[3] Immediate post-procedural angiographic residual stenosis was lower with DCA than with PTCA (DCA 15% vs PTCA 28%; $P < .0001$), and this was associated with a lower angiographic restenosis rate (DCA 31% vs PTCA 40%; $P = .016$). Despite these angiographic benefits, the target lesion revascularization rate was the same (DCA 15% vs PTCA 18%; $P = .23$) and there were no clinical benefits with DCA over PTCA. It was noted, however, that the incidence of non–Q-wave MI was higher in the DCA arm (DCA 16% vs PTCA 6%; $P < .0001$). In this trial, the increased incidence of MI was not associated with clinical adverse events; however, other studies have demonstrated adverse long-term clinical outcomes associated with creatine kinase (CK) and myocardial bound (CK-MB) elevation following PCI.

Post-procedural MLD visualized by angiography as well as post-procedural residual plaque burden by intravascular ultrasound (IVUS) are significant predictors of restenosis; thus, one of the goals of DCA was to achieve an optimal result with more effective debulking to reduce the plaque burden. With IVUS-guided DCA, the ABACUS (Adjunctive Balloon Angioplasty vs. Coronary Atherectomy Study) trial demonstrated that optimal atherectomy to minimize residual plaque burden could be achieved safely (residual plaque area: adjunctive PTCA group 42.6% vs DCA alone 45.6%; $P < .001$), with a respectable overall restenosis rate of 21.6%.[4] START (STent versus directional coronary Atherectomy Randomized Trial), a single-center, randomized trial, demonstrated that the restenosis rate following optimal DCA was lower than stenting (DCA 15.8% vs stenting, 32.8%; $P = .032$).[5]

Because plaque burden shown by IVUS was one of the predictors for restenosis following stenting, debulking to reduce plaque burden prior to stenting might have a potential effect on reducing restenosis.[6,7] To test this hypothesis, two large, randomized trials, AMIGO (Atherectomy before Multilink stent Improves lumen Gain and clinical Outcomes Study)[8] and DESIRE (DEbulking and Stenting In Restenosis Elimination)[9] were carried out. Although entry criteria and end points for both trials were similar, the use of IVUS-guided DCA was required to achieve optimal DCA prior to stenting in DESIRE. In AMIGO, the 8-month angiographic restenosis rates were similar (for stenting following DCA, 26.7% vs. stenting alone, 22.1%; $P = .2$). Despite more aggressive debulking with IVUS-guided DCA in DESIRE, the overall restenosis rates were also similar between the two groups. In-stent restenosis was slightly lower with debulking prior to stenting (for stent with DCA, 10.4% vs stent alone, 15.1%; $P = .16$); however, in-segment restenosis was the same (15.3% vs 16.1%; $P = NS$). These studies have concluded that there were no significant clinical benefits to debulking with DCA prior to stenting. Potential benefits of debulking as standalone therapy or prior to stenting for selected lesions such as bifurcation or ostial lesions, have been suggested, and this application of DCA needs to be further tested. At present, there is no information available regarding the effect of debulking prior to DES. In addition, with DES there is a potential risk of aneurysm formation by preventing the healing process of any deep-wall cuts occurring with DCA.

A peripheral version of the directional atherectomy device was approved by the FDA in 1987 for the treatment of peripheral vascular disease (PVD). No large observational studies or randomized studies were performed to evaluate the efficacy of atherectomy in superficial femoral or iliac arteries, and clinical follow-up, other than small observational series, was limited. Because of the limited lesion length that could be treated with this device, due to the relatively short window length, peripheral atherectomy was used infrequently and production of this device was subsequently discontinued. More recently, the SilverHawk longitudinal atherectomy device, manufactured by FoxHollow, has been approved by the FDA. This device was introduced to treat long, diffusely diseased or occluded segments of the superficial femoral artery, popliteal, and distal vessels. Preliminary results suggest favorable initial acute results and intermediate long-term patency. Further studies are necessary to evaluate the efficacy of this new technology.

DIRECTIONAL CORONARY ATHERECTOMY PROCEDURE

【 】 CASE SELECTION

Lesions Suitable for DCA

Randomized studies have not identified specific lesions that are better treated with DCA, as a standalone or an adjunctive treatment, than with any other devices; however, there are still some potential benefits of debulking for specific lesions. The following are potential applications of DCA when the suitable lesion is in a noncalcified, nontortuous vessel greater than 2.5 mm in size.

DCA has been an effective method to treat ostial lesions, particularly in the left anterior descending (LAD) ostial location, with a high success rate and low risk of complication. The potential advantage of standalone DCA or DCA prior to stenting for this location is to prevent plaque shifting toward the circumflex artery. DCA can be effectively applied as well to those circumflex ostial lesions that have a shallow takeoff from the LAD; those with steep angulation may not be good candidates because of the potential risk of deep wall cuts and fewer potential clinical benefits with a relatively low risk of significant plaque shifting. Debulking of left main ostial and right coronary artery (RCA) ostial lesions may enhance complete stent expansion where often restenosis occurs due to inadequate expansion of the stent.

Similar to ostial lesions, DCA may be used for bifurcation lesions. DCA can be used for the main artery only or side branch ostial lesions only, or both to prevent elastic recoil or plaque shifting. DCA can be used as a standalone procedure, particularly for ostial side branch lesions, or with stenting.

The other potential application for DCA is in-stent restenosis. The efficacy of DCA for this application has not been demonstrated in studies, but it is technically feasible. Lesions that may be considered for DCA are those with diffuse in-stent restenosis despite a fully expanded stent. Restenosis associated with inadequately expanded stents or stents with angles should be avoided because the risk of cutting into a stent strut is increased and, in the worst case scenario, the device cutter may become trapped in a strut.

Lesions to Be Avoided

Because of the profile and stiffness of the device, diffusely diseased vessels, calcified vessels, or tortuous vessels should be avoided. Small vessels (< 2.5 mm) and angulated lesions should be avoided because of the risk of perforation. DCA is not effective for calcified lesions because of the high incidence of failure to cross with the device as well as a failure to effectively excise calcified tissue. Lesions with significant thrombus are considered to be a contraindication due to the potential risk of distal embolization.

【 】 DCA CATHETER

The DCA device consists of several functional components: (1) the nosecone, for device tracking and tissue collection; (2) the housing with window and cutter, for tissue excision; (3) the balloon, which supports the device against the vessel wall during cutting; (4) the shaft, and (5) the motor drive unit, for cutter rotation. Since being approved by the FDA in 1990, there have been continuous improvements of the device, and the most current version is fourth generation.

The first-generation device (Simpson Coronary Atherocath) demonstrated the efficacy of DCA for plaque removal; however, that device was not user-friendly and the procedure itself was too demanding, technically, for most interventionists. The second-generation device improved the nosecone housing transition, thus improving trackability of the catheter. The third-generation device (GTO) had significantly improved torqueability, which allowed

operators to orient the device precisely, thus enabling them to excise plaque accurately and aggressively. The first three generations of these devices required a 10 French (Fr) guiding catheter. Despite such stepwise improvements in the device, DCA continued to be a complex and technically demanding procedure, and only a few interventionists could perform optimal atherectomy.

In the most current device, the FlexiCut, (Guidant, Santa Clara, Calif), major structural and design changes have been incorporated to make the device more user-friendly without decreasing the efficacy of tissue removal. The device was downsized to a 6-Fr platform to accommodate the use of an 8-Fr guiding catheter. To improve the deliverability of the device, specifically to help with the exit of the device from the guide, the housing length was shortened without changing the length of the window. These changes were made without the loss of debulking effectiveness. In fact, this new device may be more effective than previous devices for tissue removal. This was accomplished because of the introduction of a wider window opening (127 degrees) and a larger supporting balloon.

【 】 TECHNIQUE

Guiding Catheter Selection

An 8-Fr, large-lumen guiding catheter is required to accommodate the device size. For DCA, coaxial alignment of the guiding catheter and artery is more important than for other, lower profile, devices. For left coronary arteries, a broad curved guide such as the XB or C-curve guide is recommended. These broad curved guides rather than the Judkins left 4 (JL4) type guides will support the device exit without deforming the guide shape. For right coronary arteries, a Judkins right (JR) guide is most appropriate. For a right saphenous vein graft (SVG), a right graft catheter or a multipurpose (MP) guiding catheter, is best fitted for the procedure; and for a left SVG, left graft catheters.

Guidewire Selection

With the FlexiCut, a moderate support wire is adequate to give enough support for device deliverability. In difficult cases with less guide alignment and support, an extra support wire is helpful.

Device Selection

For earlier-generation devices, 5-Fr, 6-Fr, 7-Fr, and 7-Fr with large balloon devices were available; the FlexiCut is provided in three sizes: the same housing size (6-Fr) with a small, medium, or large supportive balloon. The recommendation for device size is as follows: a small-sized balloon for 2.5- to 2.9-mm vessels, a medium-sized balloon for 3.0- to 3.4-mm vessels, and a large-sized balloon for vessels of 3.5 mm or larger. If necessary, to remove more plaque, vessels less than 3.5 mm can be treated with a large balloon device, using caution.

Device Placement

When advancing the device, gentle rotation with constant forward pressure will often overcome any resistance that is encountered. Unless the lesion is calcified or composed of a hard fibrous plaque, predilation is not necessary. Once the device is advanced into the

TABLE 35-1

Relationship of Window Orientation on Fluoroscopic View, Location of Diagonal Artery, and Window Rotation

	WINDOW ORIENTATION BY FLUOROSCOPIC VIEW (RAO)	WINDOW ORIENTATION RELATIVE TO DIAGONAL ARTERY	WINDOW ROTATION FROM POINT A
A	Upward	90 degrees CW from DA	—
B	Toward II	Opposite from DA	90 degrees CW
C	Downward	90 degrees CCW from DA	180 degrees
D	Away from II	Toward DA	90 degrees CCW

CW = clockwise; CCW = counter-clockwise; DA = diagonal artery; II = image intensifier; RAO = right anterior oblique.

target vessel, the device (window) needs to be precisely placed to avoid deep cuts in normal arterial segments. For longitudinal device placement, the use of side branches as markers and the use of fluoroscopic views with minimal foreshortening of the vessel provides the most accurate information. For long lesions, multiple longitudinal device placements are necessary to cover the entire length of the diseased segment. Because many lesions contain eccentric plaques, device window orientation is critical to ensure adequate removal of plaque without causing deep cuts or perforation. Although operators may have some general idea of eccentricity from angiographic information, IVUS is an essential tool to determine plaque distribution.

IVUS-guided Atherectomy

IVUS information is important to determine vessel size; plaque composition, particularly the presence of calcification; plaque distribution, to assist with device orientation; and the end point of the procedure.

Evaluation of Lesions. IVUS provides important information for appropriate case selection. Vessel size greater than 2.5 mm by IVUS is required for DCA, and vessels with significant negative remodeling should be excluded. An absence of calcium in the vessel or lesion is the most desirable situation for DCA. The presence of deep wall calcification is not contraindicated, because the plaque over the calcification can be excised. However, plaque with superficial calcification cannot be excised with the current device; therefore, the presence of superficial calcium greater than 180 degrees should be considered a contraindication for DCA. The presence of low echogenicity in plaque may be associated with post-procedural no or slow flow possibly due to multiple microembolism.

【 】 DETERMINATION OF PLAQUE DISTRIBUTION AND DEVICE ORIENTATION

Plaque distribution can be accurately determined by using information obtained about side branches, test cuts, guidewire location, guiding catheter side holes, and the relative position of the IVUS catheter in the vessel. All of these methods use the same concepts: establishment of the relationship between fluoroscopic reference points and IVUS reference points to guide the device window orientation.

Firstly, the plaque distribution is determined with the IVUS image relative to an IVUS reference point (eg, side branch). Secondly, the relationship between the IVUS reference point and the fluoroscopic reference point is determined. Lastly, based on this information, the plaque distribution on the fluoroscopic view is determined.

The combined use of these methods will increase accuracy in determining the plaque orientation. Precise orientation of the window allows the operator to perform aggressive DCA using a larger balloon device or higher balloon inflation pressure for more efficient removal of tissue without an increased risk of perforation.

Use of Side Branches

Use of side branches as an index to determine plaque distribution is useful, particularly for lesions in the LAD using the circumflex artery, diagonal, septal, and right ventricular branches. Suppose the epicardial segment is at 12 o'clock, the diagonal originates from the 9 o'clock position, the septal from 4 o'clock, the circumflex from 8 o'clock, and the right ventricular branch from 12 o'clock. Among these, the relationship to the diagonal artery is the most consistent and reliable whereas the other branches tend to have more variation. When the LAD is observed from the right anterior oblique (RAO) 30-degree or caudal views, the proximal LAD and diagonal artery tend to completely overlap, indicating the diagonal originates opposite from the location of the image intensifier in the fluoroscopic view. The relationship between window orientation in the RAO view and location of the diagonal artery is summarized in Table 35-1. Similar concepts can be applied to other side branches, using either complete overlap views or perpendicular views on fluoroscopy.

Test Cuts

Following the initial determination of plaque distribution with IVUS, index cuts are made to further define the relationship between window orientation and plaque distribution. A few cuts with 20 psi in the same orientation will create a trough in the plaque. A trough location in IVUS images following the cuts will supply further detailed information regarding catheter rotation. If, for example, more plaque is present 45 degrees counter-clockwise from the index cuts, then the device needs to be rotated an additional 45 degrees counter-clockwise from the original fluoroscopic reference point. Appropriate fluoroscopic views may be selected

TABLE 35-2

Relationship of Plaque Distribution Relative to Side Holes, Window Orientation on Fluoroscopic View, and Window Rotation

	PLAQUE LOCATION RELATIVE TO SIDE HOLE	LAO FLUOROSCOPIC VIEW[a] WINDOW ORIENTATION	WINDOW ROTATION FROM POINT A
A	Same as SH	Complete profile (left side of screen)	—
B	90 degrees CW	Away from II	90 degrees CW
C	Opposite to SH	Complete profile (right side of screen)	180 degrees
D	90 degrees CCW	Toward II	90 degrees CCW

CW = clockwise; CCW = counter-clockwise; II = image intensifier; LAO = left anterior oblique; SH = side hole.
[a]In most cases, LAO of 30–60 degrees will provide complete profile of the side hole.

during index cuts; it is helpful to use fluoroscopic views with the window in complete profile.

Use of the Guidewire

When the guidewire is well separated from the crystal of the IVUS catheter (mostly proximal to the lesion), the relationship between fluoroscopic orientation and IVUS orientation can be determined. It is important to select a fluoroscopic view that provides the maximum separation of the wire from the IVUS crystal. When the plaque or a side branch is located 90 degrees clockwise from the wire position on IVUS, the window opening toward the wire location on fluoroscopy needs to be rotated 90 degrees clockwise.

Use of the Guiding Catheter Side Hole

This approach is particularly useful for the treatment of proximal or mid-RCA lesions. The side holes of JR4 guiding catheters (Cordis Brite Tip) located in the internal curvature are useful to determine the reference point for vessel orientation. The relationship between plaque distribution relative to the side hole and window orientation under fluoroscopy is summarized in Table 35-2.

Relationship Between Vessel Wall and IVUS Catheter Location

This approach is often useful, particularly in the RCA. With the curvature of the vessel, the IVUS catheter tends to bias toward the outside curvature of the vessel wall. It is important to select a view (often the LAO view in the RCA) with the catheter in close contact with the edge of the vessel proximal or distal to the lesion. When the plaque is located 90 degrees clockwise from the contact point of the IVUS crystal to the vessel wall, then the window needs to be rotated 90 degrees clockwise from a contact point to aim toward the plaque.

Plaque Excision

Once a catheter is appropriately positioned, the supporting balloon is inflated with each cut. The balloon inflation allows the window to engage into the vessel wall. Advancement of the rotating cutter excises the plaque that is invaginated into the window; the excised tissue is then collected into the nosecone. Low-pressure balloon inflations (10–20 psi) is recommended for the first series of cuts; then, gradually, the balloon pressure can be increased to a maximum of 60 to 80 psi. Slow advancement of the cutter is important to create a smoother cutting edge. Multiple cuts (20–40 or more, if necessary) are usually required to remove an adequate amount of tissue.

The operator must pay attention to both window orientation and longitudinal positioning based on IVUS information and fluoroscopy. The ideal views for window orientation and device positioning may differ, and multiple x-ray views may be necessary for precise placement of the device. Most often deep wall cuts occur when cuts are made in normal vessel segments.

End Points

Previous studies have suggested that adequate plaque excision is necessary to reduce restenosis following DCA. A post-procedure plaque area of less than 40% to 50%, as measured by IVUS, is considered optimal atherectomy. When angiographic appearance alone is used to determine the end point, it is necessary to achieve close to or 0% residual stenosis without the appearance of overtreatment. In general, however, angiographic appearance alone does not correlate well with IVUS-measured residual plaque area; thus, IVUS-guided DCA is strongly recommended to achieve and evaluate optimal atherectomy results (Figure 35-1).

【 】 TIPS AND PITFALLS

Optimal Atherectomy

Long-term outcome and restenosis are generally related to residual plaque mass; thus, the lower the residual plaque, the lower the restenosis. Optimal atherectomy is considered to be achieved when there is no angiographic residual stenosis and a plaque area of less than 50%, as measured by IVUS. There is no shortcut to achieving an optimal atherectomy result. Use of IVUS is essential both before and after atherectomy. Preprocedure IVUS provides not only lesion characteristics but also information regarding plaque distribution. Operators need to be familiar with interpretation of IVUS images and understand the relationship between IVUS images, fluoroscopic images, and device orientation, as previously described. Multiple device insertions, with a larger balloon device,

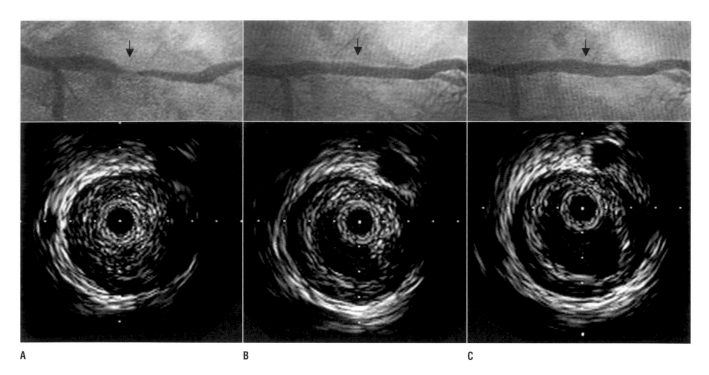

FIGURE 35-1. Optimal directional coronary atherectomy of a left anterior descending artery (LAD). **A.** Preintervention; the proximal LAD lesion appeared eccentric in the angiogram (*top*). However, the corresponding intravascular ultrasound (IVUS) image showed a fairly concentric, fibrofatty plaque (*bottom*). **B.** Post-procedure; angiography shows substantial improvement, but IVUS reveals a residual plaque burden of more than 70%. Minimum lumen area is 6.38 mm². **C.** Further angiographic improvement after additional cuts were made. Minimum lumen area by IVUS was 10.27 mm² with a residual plaque burden of less than 50%. Total tissue weight removed was 33.7 mg.

if appropriate, are often necessary. Precise device placement (window orientation and longitudinal positioning) allows aggressive debulking (frequent cuts and the use of higher balloon pressures) without increasing the risk of perforation. The final end point should be assessed by both angiography and IVUS.

Avoidance of Complications

Complications that are specifically related to DCA include dissection and nose cone injury, perforations, and wire fracture.

Dissection and Nosecone Injury. Case selection and appropriate technique are essential to avoid these complications. Diffuse disease, calcification, and tortuosity proximal to the lesion should all be avoided, because aggressive manipulation of the large, stiff device may cause significant dissection or nosecone injury. The nosecone may cause vessel wall damage beyond the lesion if a moderate degree of disease already exists. These dissections and nosecone injuries can be avoided with appropriate case selection. When the device is pulled back to the guiding catheter, the guiding catheter often tends to move deeply into the artery. Attention therefore needs to be paid at the guiding catheter tip when the device is pulled back.

Perforations. Perforation is the most devastating complication of DCA. Moderate to severe angulation at the lesion is associated with an increased risk of perforation; thus, these lesions are considered to be a contraindication to DCA. Vessels with significant negative remodeling, as indicated by IVUS, also should be avoided. Administration of intracoronary nitroglycerin prior to

device insertion is important to prevent device- or excision-related coronary spasm that may cause significant deep wall cuts. Most perforations occur when inappropriate DCA technique is used. Perforation is usually associated with deep wall cuts in a normal segment of vessel wall that does not contain atherosclerotic plaque. Accurate longitudinal positioning of the device and IVUS-guided precise window orientation, as previously described, is essential to avoid this complication.

Wire Fracture. During activation of the motor drive unit, the wire may rotate due to friction of the wire and cutter drive cable. If the wire tip becomes buried in a small branch, the wire may become fixed. Rotation of the fixed trapped tip may cause the wire to fracture. This complication is preventable with careful placement of the wire in the main vessel and by holding the wire while the motor drive unit is activated.

Management of Perforations

When a perforation occurs, its severity should be assessed quickly. If the perforation is small (localized, self-contained, or caused by a pinhole), the leakage can be sealed completely with prolonged balloon dilation, with or without the administration of protamine. With significant perforations (wide mouth, free communication to the pericardial space, tamponade), the leakage must first be quickly controlled with balloon inflations. A PTFE-covered stent of the appropriate length to cover the entire section should then be deployed to seal the perforation. It is important to note that covered stents require high-pressure deployment. If complete hemostasis is achieved with a covered stent, adequate antiplatelet agents

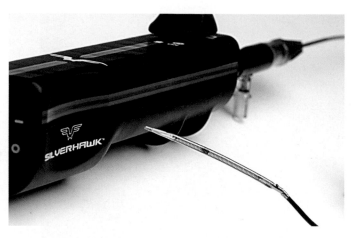

FIGURE 35-2. New atherectomy device: SilverHawk peripheral catheter. *Image courtesy of FoxHollow Technologies, Redwood City, Calif.*

(aspirin and clopidogrel) then need to be administered in a manner similar to that used in stent patients following the procedure. When bivalirudin is used, its action can be reversed with the administration of fresh frozen plasma. Administration of platelets will reverse the antiplatelet effect of abciximab but not eptifibatide.

SILVERHAWK ATHERECTOMY CATHETER

A new longitudinal atherectomy catheter, the SilverHawk, was approved by the FDA in 2005 for the treatment of peripheral vascular disease. However, at present, this device has not been approved for the treatment of coronary artery disease. These devices are designed to overcome some of the limitations of DCA.

The SilverHawk device consists of a nosecone, housing, cutter, shaft, and multifunctional motor drive unit (Figure 35-2). This system is operated over-the-wire with a monorail system. When the cutter is activated, the base of the housing actively bends to push the housing against the vessel wall. A rotation cutter is then shifted 0.013-in outside through the window. By advancing the entire catheter with the cutter exposed over the wire, tissue is excised and rolls into the nosecone. With deactivation of the cutter, the cutter lowers into the housing and the excised tissue is parted off. Usually multiple cuts are made, but much fewer than in the DCA procedure.

Table 35-3 compares features of the new device with the DCA catheter. The SilverHawk device has several potential advantages over the DCA catheter. There is no supporting balloon and the cutter is mechanically forced toward the vessel wall with active angulation of the catheter; therefore, there is no balloon dilation effect and luminal improvement is solely achieved by debulking. Because the catheter is advanced during cutting action, there is virtually no limitation to the treatable lesion length; thus, the procedure is suited for the treatment of long, diffusely diseased segments. The solid housing section is short; thus, the catheter deliverability is excellent and less maneuvering is required. The procedure is relatively simple and fast, with a specifically designed multifunction motor drive unit, and can be easily performed by a single operator.

For peripheral artery application, three sizes are available: 5.5-Fr for 2.0- to 2.5-mm vessel size; 6.5-Fr for 2.5- to 3.5-mm vessels; and 7.5-Fr for 3.5- to 6-mm vessels. For coronary artery application (Europe only), two sizes are available: 5.5-Fr for 2.0- to 3.0-mm vessels and 6.5-Fr for 3.0- to 4.0-mm vessels.

TABLE 35-3

Comparison of the FlexiCut, DCA Device and the SilverHawk Atherectomy Device

	FLEXICUT	SILVERHAWK
Housing length	11 mm	5 mm
Cutter	Inside housing	Exposed "outside" housing
Housing support	Balloon inflation	Active angulation of housing-shaft transition
Tissue excision	Excision of tissue invaginated into housing through window	Advance of catheter with exposed rotating cutter
Treated lesion length	Window length	Any length
Excised tissue thickness	Depends on thickness of tissue invaginated into housing	Constant
Dilatation effect	Significant with balloon dilation	None other than initial Dotter effect
Orientation of device	Directional	Directional
Tissue collection	Nosecone	Nosecone
Tissue packing in the nosecone	Passive	Active packing by tamper
Motor drive unit	Activates cutter rotation	Multifunctional: Cutter exposure, cutter rotation, activate angulation of catheter, tamper advancement

DCA = directional coronary atherectomy.

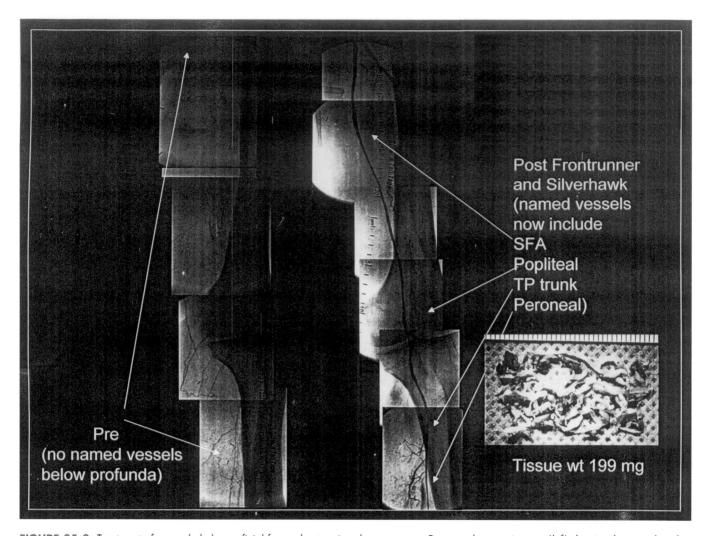

FIGURE 35-3. Treatment of an occluded superficial femoral artery in a long segment. Preprocedure angiogram (*left*) showing long total occlusion of superficial femoral artery (SFA) and popliteal artery and diffuse distal vessel disease with minimal collateral vessels. Patient suffered from ischemic leg with threatening necrosis of toes. Post-procedure angiogram (*right*) shows totally occluded vessels that were recanalized using a FrontRunner (LuMend, Redwood City, Calif) total occlusion device and then treated with a SilverHawk atherectomy catheter. Tissue retrieved totaled 199 mg.[DF14] (TP = tibia peroneal trunk.)

Indications for atherectomy with this device in peripheral vessels are lesions in the common femoral, superficial femoral, and popliteal arteries, as well as the distal vessels (peroneal, anterior tibial, posterior tibial) for critical limb ischemia.[10] Lesions of any length can be treated. This procedure is particularly attractive and suited for diffusely diseased segments, because current approaches with stents have a high incidence of restenosis (Figure 35-3). The device is also used to treat in-stent restenosis. This procedure has also been applied with clinical success in the treatment of diffuse, occlusive, small distal vessels for limb salvage.

REFERENCES

1. Topol EJ, Leya F, Pinkerton CA, et al, for the CAVEAT Study Group. A comparison of directional atherectomy with coronary angioplasty in patients with coronary artery disease. *N Eng J Med.* 1993;329:221.
2. Simonton CA, Leon MB, Baim DS, et al. 'Optimal' directional coronary atherectomy. Final results of the optimal atherectomy restenosis study (OARS). *Circulation.* 1998;97:332.
3. Baim DS, Cutlip EC, Sharma SK, et al. Final results of the balloon vs. optimal atherectomy trial (BOAT). *Circulation.* 1998;97:322.
4. Suzuki T, Hosokawa H, Katoh O, et al. Effects of adjunctive balloon angioplasty after intravascular ultrasound-guided optimal directional coronary atherectomy. The result of adjunctive balloon angioplasty after coronary atherectomy study (ABACAS). *J Am Coll Cardiol.* 1999;34:1028.
5. Tsuchikane E, Sumitsuji S, Awata N, et al. Final results of the stent versus directional coronary atherectomy randomized trial (START). *J Am Coll Cardiol.* 1999;34:1050.
6. Moussa I, Moses J, Di Mario C, et al. Stenting after optimal lesion debulking (SOLD) registry. *Circulation.* 1998;98:1604.
7. Prati F, Di Mario C, Moussa I, et al. In-stent neointimal proliferation correlates with the amount of residual plaque burden outside the stent. An intravascular ultrasound study. *Circulation.* 1999;99:1011.
8. Stankovic G, Colombo A, Bersin R, et al. Comparison of directional atherectomy and stenting versus stenting alone for the treatment of de novo and restenotic coronary artery narrowing. *Am J Cardiol.* 2004;15:953.
9. Aizawa T, Tamai H, Asakura Y, et al. Clinical and angiographic results of the debulking and stenting in restenosis elimination (DESIRE) trial. *Circulation.* 2001;104:2954.
10. Kandzari DE, Kiesz RS, Allie D, et al. Procedural and clinical outcomes with catheter-based plaque excision in critical limb ischemia. *J Endovasc Ther* 2006; 13:12.

CHAPTER (36)

Distal Embolic Protection Devices

Donald S. Baim, MD

Distal embolization of atherosclerotic debris was not initially felt to be a problem during catheter-based intervention, but recent data suggest that it is a common occurrence and the root cause of many procedural complications.[1] The first conclusive demonstration of this was in diseased saphenous vein grafts, where post-procedural cardiac enzyme elevation (17% of cases) and the "no-reflow" phenomenon (8% of cases) are common complications[2,3] that reflect impaired myocardial perfusion despite patency of the epicardial vessels.

Although microvascular (arteriolar) spasm[3,4] and platelet aggregation have been proposed as putative mechanisms, neither arteriolar vasodilators nor platelet glycoprotein inhibitors[5] have proven effective at preventing these complications. In fact, the only therapies that have been able to reduce the incidence of these complications have been devices that protect against distal atherosclerotic embolization. This suggests that atheroembolization is the root cause of these complications (perhaps compounded by secondary microvascular spasm and platelet aggregation). Moreover, preliminary data suggest that similar embolization and distal organ complications also occur in native coronary arteries (particularly during primary angioplasty for acute myocardial infarction), carotid stenting, and renal artery stenting, in that the use of embolic protection devices both retrieves significant atherosclerotic debris and reduces the incidence of end-organ complications.

Three types of embolic protection devices have being evaluated and will be discussed, in turn, in this chapter (Figure 36-1).

DISTAL OCCLUSION BALLOONS

The first approach to embolic protection was *distal occlusion,* performed using a low-pressure balloon mounted on a hollow guidewire shaft (Figure 36-2). The initial device was the PercuSurge Guard Wire (Medtronic), but balloons filled with carbon dioxide rather than dilute liquid contrast material are being developed (Possis and Kensey-Nash). The devices in this class can have deflated profiles as low as 0.026 in, and are passed across the target lesion in a manner similar to a conventional guidewire. Once positioned in a relatively free distal "landing zone" of suitable diameter, the balloon is inflated to occlude antegrade flow. Any debris liberated by intervention during the period of balloon inflation thus remains trapped in the stagnant column of blood, and can be aspirated before the occlusion balloon is deflated and antegrade flow is restored.

Preliminary data in saphenous vein grafts showed that embolic debris (size range 25 μm to 2 mm) was recovered in more than 95% of such procedures, that the histology of the debris (cholesterol clefts, foam cells) resembled that of the treated lesion, and that the incidence of cardiac enzyme elevation was much lower (4%) than expected.[6] This benefit was confirmed in the 801-patient SAFER (Saphenous Vein Graft Angioplasty Free of Emboli, Randomized) trial[7] in which patients undergoing saphenous vein graft (SVG) intervention were randomized to stenting over the occlusion wire or a conventional guidewire, showing substantial reduction in the 30-day rate of major adverse cardiac events (from 16.9% to 9.6%) and no reflow (from 8.3% to 3.3%); refer to Table 36-1. This result was predominantly due to a reduction in creatine kinase elevations of all magnitudes (Figure 36-3)

Strong evidence is available for the distal occlusion devices supporting debris recovery and clinical benefit in SVG and carotid stenting, with the major advantage of retrieving both particles of all sizes and humoral mediators of no reflow. They also have the lowest crossing profile of current embolic protection devices (absent an external constraining catheter as required with virtually all distal filter devices). On the other hand, they are subject to

- Distal occlusion

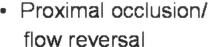

- Distal filters

- Proximal occlusion/
  flow reversal

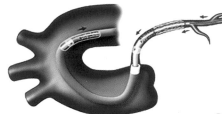

FIGURE 36-1. Depictions of the three basic types of embolic protection devices. Top to bottom: Distal occlusion, distal filter, and proximal occlusion.

various limitations, including distal ischemia resulting from prolonged antegrade, shunting of emboli into side branches or collaterals originating proximal to the point of occlusion (especially in non-SVG applications), incomplete aspiration of debris marginated in the stagnant section, potential vessel injury at the point of balloon inflation, and generally greater procedural complexity that the distal filter devices.

DISTAL FILTERS

The second class of embolic protection devices are *distal filters,* which are mounted on a conventional 0.014-in guidewire shafts[8] (Figure 36-4). The filter is passed across the target lesion in its smaller collapsed state (usually constrained by an outer delivery sheath) and then opened to allow the edges of the filter to approximate against the vessel wall. The filter then remains in place to catch any liberated embolic material larger than the filter pore size (usually 100 μ), until the filter is collapsed following stent deployment using a purpose-specific retrieval sheath.

The first such filter to complete a pivotal clinical trial was the FilterWire (EPI/Boston Scientific), which was evaluated against the distal occlusion device in the 656-patient FIRE (Functional Improvement through Revascularization of the Extremities) trial.[9] That trial showed that the distal filter was noninferior (equivalent or better) than the distal occlusion device in 30-day MACE, suggesting that the distal filter mechanism provides effective embolic protection to distal occlusion and aspiration (Table 36-2, Figure 36-5). One clear limitation recognized in the early development of the FilterWire was incomplete apposition of the filter loop to the vessel wall, potentially allowing embolic debris to pass beside rather than through the filter loop. Better procedural attention to this possibility (by confirming loop apposition to the vessel wall in at least two orthogonal views), accounted for the better performance of the FilterWire in the pivotal FIRE trial than in the earlier SPARK registry. A subsequent modification to the device (FilterWire EZ) attaches the filter loop to a freely rotating suspension arm rather than directly to the wire, as in the FilterWire EX design used in FIRE. This modification resulted in a further reduction in MACE to 5.7% in the BLAZE registry. Food and Drug Administration approval of the EZ design is now pending. Even with only the EX design available in the United States, preliminary experience since its release in early 2003 shows that the greater ease of use and ability to maintain antegrade flow throughout the procedure have caused it to nearly replace the PercuSurge distal occlusion device in clinical practice.

Additional distal embolic filters from various manufacturers are currently completing clinical testing, and should be available by early 2004. One of these, the Rubicon filter, makes use of a novel filter constraint system during delivery,

FIGURE 36-2. The PercuSurge GuardWire consists of a hollow 0.014-in nitinol hypotube equipped with a low-pressure occlusion balloon at its tip. It is passed across the target lesion (**A**) and inflated with dilute contrast to occlude antegrade flow (**B**), so that any debris liberated during stent deployment is trapped in the stagnant column of blood (**C**), which is aspirated with a separate Export catheter prior to deflation of the distal occlusion balloon and restoration of antegrade flow. Bottom inserts show the gross (*left*) and microscopic (*right*) appearance of recovered debris, the latter including cholesterol clefts and foam cells typical of the histology of degenerated saphenous vein graft lesions.

TABLE 36-1

Findings in the SAFER Trial[a]

	GUARDWIRE	CONTROL	P VALUE
Patients (n)	406	395	
Graft age (median, y)	10.4	10.9	NS
Reference diameter (mm)	3.44	3.42	NS
Lesion length (mm)	15.6	16.6	NS
30-d MACE (%)	9.6	16.5	.004
Death	1.0	2.3	NS
Q-wave MI	1.2	1.3	NS
Non–Q-wave MI (CK-MB > 3×)	7.4	13.7	.008
Emergency CABG	0	0.5	NS
No reflow (%)	3	9	.001

CABG = coronary artery bypass grafting; CK-MB = creatine kinase, myocardial bound; MACE = major adverse cardial event; MI = myocardial infarction; NS = not significant; SAFER = Saphenous Vein Graft Angioplasty Free of Emboli, Randomized (trial).
[a]See reference 7.

reducing the profile and stiffness considerably, until the filter is released in the distal vessel by a central pull-wire. Retrieval of this filter, however, still requires advancement of a retrieval sheath across the deployed stent.

This type of device has the advantages of maintaining antegrade flow during the procedure, allowing intermittent contrast injection to visualize underlying anatomy, and potentially causing less diversion of debris into proximal side branches than the distal occlusion devices. On the other hand, the filters have potential inherent disadvantages, including allowing debris with a diameter less than the filter pore size to pass through, reliance on complete apposition of the filter to the vessel wall to prevent "blow-by" of debris (a challenging task in tortuous vessels), the possibility of filter clogging by platelet fibrin thrombi, or overloading of filter capacity by heavy embolic volumes. The somewhat larger crossing profile (3.5–4.0 Fr, or 0.035–0.040 in) and stiffness of the delivery sheath, compared with the smallest distal occlusion devices, may increase crossing difficulty or increase the chance of embolization during device crossing.

PROXIMAL OCCLUSION DEVICES

The third type of embolic protection device involves creating *proximal occlusion* of the treated vessel upstream of the target lesion. This can be achieved with a low-pressure balloon located on the tip or just beyond the tip of the guiding catheter. During such inflow occlusion, antegrade flow is interrupted so that any liberated potential embolic material remains suspended rather than making its way into the distal microcirculation. In fact, adequate distal collateral vessels can usually propel any liberated debris back into the lumen of the guiding catheter via retrograde flow. Alternatively, absent sufficient collaterals, saline infusion through a distally positioned "rinsing" catheter, combined with gentle suction through the lumen of the guiding catheter, can motivate suspended debris back into the guiding catheter.

The initial device in this class was the Parodi Arteria device for use in the carotid circulation. In the coronary circulation, the Proxis device (Velocimed, ev3) makes use of a custom, short-sleeve catheter that is positioned between within the distal portion of the guiding catheter and the proximal portion of the vessel being treated[10] (Figure 36-6). Inflation of low-pressure (< 1 atm) balloons located at either end of this sleeve occludes antegrade flow and "couples" the vessel lumen to the guiding catheter lumen. This allows the intervention to proceed normally through the 0.060-in lumen of the sleeve, visualized by stagnant contrast that was injected and trapped following inflation of the sleeve balloon but before crossing with the guidewire or stent. Once the intervention begins, antegrade injection of contrast through the guiding catheter obviously should be avoided, until aspiration is performed through the guiding catheter to remove any suspended debris created by the intervention.

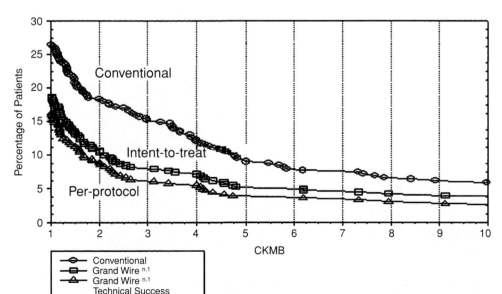

FIGURE 36-3. Cumulative distribution curves from the SAFER trial (see reference 7) show the percent of patients who had myocardial-bound creatine kinase (CK-MB) levels greater than the multiple of the upper limit of normal shown on the X-axis, in three groups: those randomized to stenting over a conventional guidewire, those randomized to the GuardWire (intent-to-treat), and those in which the GuardWire as able to be advanced across the lesion, inflated to occlude flow, and deflated only after aspiration of the proximal vessel (per-protocol). It is clear from the downward shift of these curves that use of the GuardWire reduces the frequency of CK-MB elevation of all magnitudes compared with conventional stenting.

> ### TABLE 36-2

Findings in the FIRE Trial[b]

	FILTERWIRE	GUARDWIRE	P VALUE
Patients (n)	304	283	
Graft age (median, y)	10.5	10.8	NS
Reference diameter (mm)	3.36	3.36	NS
Lesion length (mm)	13.2	14.1	NS
30-d MACE (%)	9.5	11.0	.002 for equivalence
Death	1.0	0.7	NS
Q-wave MI	0.7	0.7	NS
Non–Q-wave MI (CK-MB > 3×)	7.9	9.2	NS
Emergency CABG	0.7	2.1	NS
No reflow (%)	2.3	3.6	NS

CABG = coronary artery bypass grafting; CK-MB = creatine kinase, myocardial bound; FIRE = Functional Improvement through Revascularization of the Extremities (trial); MACE = major adverse cardial event; MI = myocardial infarction; NS = not significant.

[b]See reference 9.

Filter Devices for Distal Protection

AngioGuard (Cordis)

AccuNet (Guidant)

FilterWire (EPI-BSC)

NeuroShield/Cardio-Shield (MedNova)

The Trap VFS (MicroVena)

Interceptor (Medtronic)

Rubicon

Spyder (eV3)

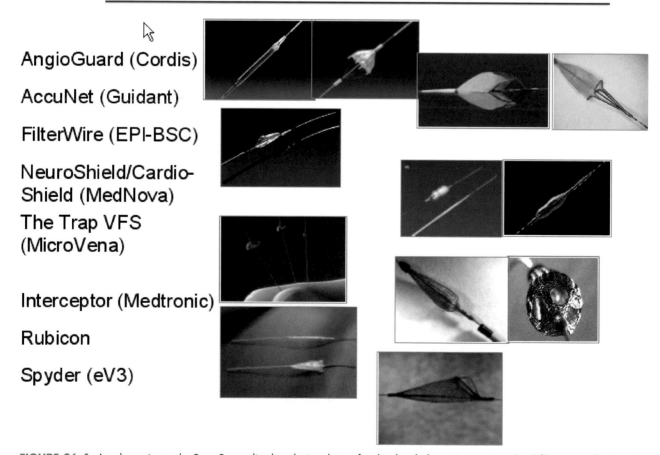

FIGURE 36-4. An alternative to the PercuSurge distal occlusion device for distal embolic protection is a distal filter, several examples of which are shown. Most use a perforated polymeric sheet (pore size ~100 μm), supported by a self-expanding nitinol armature. Others (ev3 Spyder, Trap, Interceptor) use a fine weave of nitinol wire as the filter material.

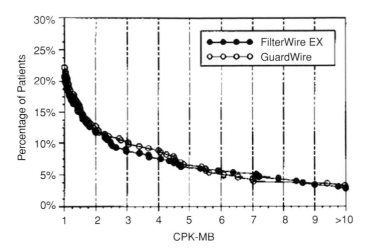

FIGURE 36-5. The FIRE trial (see reference 9) was an equivalence (noninferiority) study that compared the EPI-FilterWire to the PercuSurge GuardWire in 650 patients with saphenous vein grafts undergoing stenting (see reference 8). This figure shows an overall rate of major adverse cardiac events (MACE) of 9.5% in the FilterWire patients, with an 11.0% MACE rate in the GuardWire patients, giving a probability (P) less than .002 that the distal filter device is equivalent or better than the distal occlusion device. (CK-MB = creatine kinase, myocardial bound.)

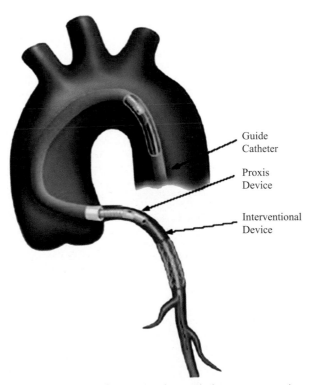

FIGURE 36-6. Another approach to embolic protection is the concept of proximally occluding the vessel to be treated (shown here for an internal carotid lesion, but also applicable to saphenous vein graft lesions). This proximal occlusion can be created with a balloon-tipped guiding catheter (Kerberos) or an inflatable sleeve within a conventional guiding catheter (Velocimed), and removal of the forward-driving pressure allows any liberated debris to move retrograde into the guiding catheter lumen rather than antegrade to the myocardial bed. One unique advantage of this approach is that protection is established before the target lesion is instrumented.

Another device in this category is the Kerberos device, which uses a custom guiding catheter with a low-pressure occlusion balloon at it tip. This provides a potentially larger lumen for intervention than the Velocimed sleeve approach, although the need for a range of custom guiding catheters may be an issue. Another difference is that the Kerberos device uses an active pressure-washing catheter, whose infusion rate is linked to the rate of aspiration through the guiding catheter lumen. This removes the reliance on collateral vessels, and can potentially more effectively motivate debris adherent to the vessel wall back into the guiding catheter before antegrade flow is restored.

Both devices of this type have thus far undergone only limited clinical testing. In the 35-patient FASTER (Feasibility And Safety Trial, European Registry) pilot trial, the Velocimed Proxis device recovered debris and had a 4% MACE rate.[10] Similar preliminary findings have been reported using the Kerberos proximal occlusion system. Larger clinical trials to show equivalence to one of the approved embolic protection devices are in progress.

The proximal occlusion approach has a potential to reduce the overall incidence of MACE compared with the distal protection approaches, in that protection is established before the first wire crosses the target lesion. The active pressure-washing by the Kerberos device may also retrieve debris that has marginated into the low-flow boundary layer at the vessel wall, or that is loosely attached through the stent cells (so-called *cheese-grater material*), preventing subsequent embolization after brisk antegrade flow is restored. Theoretically, the proximal occlusion approach could be used to protect proximal side branches and bifurcation lesions, if the collateral inflow to all such branches was adequate and balanced. On the other hand, the need for flow interruption, dependence on collateral inflow, and need for carefully coordinated actions by a second operator would be disadvantages of proximal occlusion compared with the distal filter technology unless a greater reduction in embolic events can be demonstrated.

NEWER INDICATIONS BEYOND SAPHENOUS VEIN GRAFTS

Although the initial proof of principle and clinical approval trials were done in patients with embolic-prone diseased saphenous vein grafts, there is at least preliminary evidence that embolization occurs and produces end-organ damage during intervention in other vascular territories. Devices of all three types are thus being evaluated for other anatomic and clinical situations.

In native coronaries of patients experiencing acute myocardial infarction, liberation of thrombi and underlying atherosclerotic debris may contribute to no reflow, limited myocardial reperfusion, impaired resolution of ST-segment elevation, and limited myocardial salvage.[11] Preliminary studies using both the distal occlusion PercuSurge and the distal filter EPI devices[12] have recovered debris and improved myocardial perfusion compared with historical controls of primary angioplasty without such embolic protection. But the large randomized EMERALD trial[13] failed to show significant improvements in myocardial blush, ST-segment resolution, or radionuclide infarct size, even though significant embolic debris was recovered.

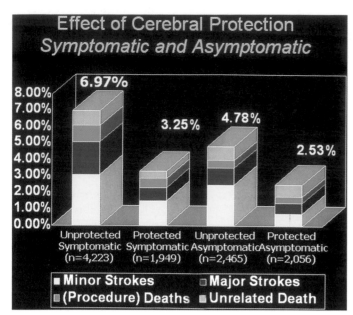

FIGURE 36-7. Summary of major adverse event rates in carotid stenting, based on symptomatic status and the use of distal protection, demonstrating a significant reduction in event rates with embolic protection (see reference 17).

It is not clear if this negative result in an adequately conducted trial indicts the strategy of embolic protection in lipid-rich acute myocardial infarct lesions, or reflects limitations of distal occlusion in that setting (eg, shunting of embolic debris into more proximal side branches, offsetting any benefit to the territory beyond the occlusion balloon). Future studies using distal filters in this setting are in the planning stages. If positive, it is likely that acute myocardial infarction will be a second major use of these devices. Follow-on studies in unstable angina or vulnerable plaque (all of which contain potentially embolizable superficial lipid pools), along with more deliverable devices customized for smaller native vessel diameters (2.5–3.5 mm),[14] could make embolic protection the standard in all coronary interventions.

Although carotid artery stenting is still investigational, there is ample evidence from transcranial Doppler monitoring that stent placement is associated with cerebral embolization that likely contributes to the 3% to 5% incidence of post-procedural stroke.[15,16] Embolic protection devices of all three types have been effective in recovering emboli and reducing the neurologic complication rate (Figure 36-7), making them part of all ongoing carotid stenting protocols.[17–19] Similar preliminary data are available for distal occlusion devices and distal filters in stenting of atherosclerotic renal artery stenosis,[20–21] with definitive clinical trials to follow.

SUMMARY

Contrary to earlier beliefs that atheroembolization is a "nonissue" during percutaneous catheter interventions, mounting evidence now indicates that distal atherosclerotic debris *commonly* embolizes from lesions in many vascular territories during percutaneous intervention, that it can be recovered using any of the three types of embolic protection device, and that use of those devices reduces the incidence of end-organ injury. Distal embolic protection devices

are thus likely to become an important part of catheter based intervention, used either alone or in combination with active thrombectomy[22] to improve the safety and predictability of acute procedural outcomes in high-risk lesions on the arterial supply to ischemia-sensitive end-organs such as the heart, brain, and kidneys.

REFERENCES

1. Topol EJ, Yadav JS. Recognition of the importance of embolization in atherosclerotic vascular disease. *Circulation.* 2000;101:570.
2. Hong MK, Mehran R, Dangas G, et al. Creatine kinase-MB enzyme elevation following successful saphenous vein graft intervention is associated with late mortality. *Circulation.* 1999;100:2400.
3. Piana RN, Paik GY, Moscucci M, et al. Incidence and treatment of "no-reflow" after percutaneous coronary intervention. *Circulation.* 1994;89:2514.
4. Galiuto L, DeMaria AN, Balzo U, et al. Ischemia-reperfusion injury at the microvascular level-treatment by endothelin A selective antagonist and evaluation by myocardial contrast echocardiography. *Circulation.* 2000;102:3111.
5. Ellis SG, Linkoff AM, Miller D, et al. Reduction in complications of angioplasty with abciximab occurs largely independently of baseline lesion morphology. *J Am Coll Cardiol.* 1998;32:1619.
6. Webb JG, Carere RG, Virmani R, et al. Retrieval and analysis of particulate debris following saphenous vein graft intervention. *J Am Coll Cardiol.* 1999;34:461.
7. Baim DS, Wahr D, George B, et al. Randomized trial of a distal embolic protection device during percutaneous intervention of saphenous vein aorto-coronary bypass grafts. *Circulation.* 2002;105:1285.
8. Muller-Hulsbeck S, Jahnke T, et al. In vitro comparison of four cerebral protection filters for preventing human plaque embolization during carotid interventions. *J Endovasc Ther.* 2002;9:793.
9. Stone GW, Rogers C, Hermiller J, et al. Randomized comparison of distal protection with a filter-based catheter and a balloon occlusion and aspiration system during percutaneous intervention of diseased saphenous vein aortocoronary bypass grafts. *Circulation.* 2003;108:548.
10. Sievert H, Wahr DW, Schuler G, et al. Effectiveness and safety of the Proxis system in demonstrating retrograde coronary blood flow during proximal occlusion and in capturing embolic material. *Am J Cardiol.* 2004;94:1134.
11. Kotani J, Mintz GS, Pregowski J, et al. Volumetric intravascular ultrasound evidence that distal embolization during acute infarct intervention contributes to inadequate myocardial perfusion grade. *Am J Cardiol.* 2003;92:728.
12. Limbruno U, Micheli A, De Carlo M, et al. Mechanical protection of distal embolization during primary angioplasty: Safety, feasibility, and impact on myocardial reperfusion. *Circulation.* 2003;108:171.
13. Stone G. Presentation at the American College of Cardiology annual meeting, March 2004; New Orleans.
14. Chen WH, Lee PY, Ng W, Lau CP. Safety and feasibility of the use of a distal filter protection device in percutaneous revascularization of small coronary arteries. *Cathet Cardiovasc Interv.* 2004;61:360.
15. Okhi T, Marin ML, Lyon RT, et al. Ex vivo human carotid artery bifurcation stenting: Correlation of lesion characteristics with embolic potential. *J Vasc Surg.* 1998;27:463.
16. Jordan WD, Voellingeer DC, Doblar DD, et al. Microemboli detected by transcranial Doppler monitoring in patients during carotid angioplasty versus carotid endarterectomy. *Cardiovasc Surg.* 1999;7:33.
17. Wholey MH, Al-Mubarek N, Whole MW. Updated review of the global carotid stent registry. *Cathet Cardiovasc Intervent.* 2003;60:259.
18. Cremonesi A, Mannetti R, Setacci F, et al. Protected carotid stenting: Clinical advantages and complications of embolic protection devices in 442 consecutive patients. *Stroke.* 2004;34:1936.
19. Al-Moubarak N, Roubin GS, Vitek JJ, et al. Effect of distal balloon protection system on microembolization during carotid stenting. *Circulation.* 2001;104:1999.
20. Holden A, Hill A. Renal angioplasty and stenting with distal protection of the main renal artery in ischemic nephropathy: Early experience. *J Vasc Surg.* 2003;38:962.
21. Henry M, Henri I, Klonaris C, et al. Renal angioplasty and stenting under protection: The way of the future? *Cathet Cardiovasc Interv.* 2003;60:299.
22. Ho PC, Leung CY. Rheolytic thrombectomy with distal filter embolic protection as adjunctive therapies to high-risk saphenous vein graft intervention. *Cathet Cardiovasc Interv.* 2004;61:202.

CHAPTER (37)

Intervention in Venous and Arterial Grafts

John S. Douglas, Jr, MD

HISTORICAL DEVELOPMENT

The surgeon's use of saphenous veins and a variety of arterial conduits (left internal mammary artery [LIMA], right internal mammary artery [RIMA], gastroepiploic artery, and radial artery) to bypass obstructive coronary atherosclerotic disease preceded percutaneous revascularization by about a decade. In that relatively short period of time, the inferiority of venous compared with arterial grafts and the potential for atheroembolization with vein graft manipulation at surgery had become apparent. When Andreas Gruentzig reported the first 50 patients treated with percutaneous coronary angioplasty in 1979, 5 had undergone saphenous vein graft (SVG) dilation and 3 (60%) developed restenosis, leading him to surmise "the different kind of disease may explain the high incidence of recurrence in graft stenosis" and to question the wisdom of percutaneous SVG intervention.[1]

In the nearly 30 years since that observation, interventional cardiologists have struggled with the indications for SVG intervention because of higher acute complications, more restenosis than was observed in native coronary arteries and arterial grafts, and high late-event rates. By 1983, outcomes of SVG intervention had been more completely characterized, and the first LIMA intervention reported.[2] In several thousand reported cases of balloon angioplasty in SVGs, procedural mortality was less than 1%, Q-wave infarction occurred in less than 2%, and emergency surgery was required in 0.3% to 4%.[3] A gradient was observed in SVG restenosis rates, with very high rates approaching 70% at proximal anastomoses and progressively less in more distal locations (refer to the discussions of mid-graft and distal anastomosis lesions, later in this chapter).

【 】 BARE-METAL STENTS

Use of stents in SVG intervention was supported by the report in 1995 of the Palmaz-Schatz multicenter registry experience involving more than 500 patients with favorable outcomes. The following findings were reported: procedural success in 97% of patients, stent thrombosis in 1.4%, in-hospital mortality in 1.7%, urgent surgery in 0.9%, and restenosis in 18% of de novo lesions and 46% of restenotic lesions.[4]

In the Saphenous Vein De Novo (SAVED) trial, 220 patients with SVG stenosis of at least 50% and angina or objective evidence of ischemia were randomized to deployment of Palmaz-Schatz stent or balloon angioplasty.[5] Patients with lesion lengths requiring more than two stents, myocardial infarction within 7 days, or graft thrombus were excluded. Patients who underwent stent implantation had a higher procedural efficacy, defined as a reduction in stenosis to less than 50% of the vessel diameter with the assigned therapy (92% vs 69%; $P < .001$). Patients assigned to receive stents had a larger increase in lumen diameter immediately (1.92 mm vs 1.21 mm; $P < .001$), and a greater net gain in lumen diameter at 6 months (0.85 mm vs 0.54 mm; $P = .002$). There was more bleeding in stented patients as a result of warfarin anticoagulation. Major in-hospital complications were otherwise similar in the two groups, although there was a trend toward fewer non-Q-wave myocardial infarctions (MIs) in the stent group (2% vs 7%). This observation has led some operators to prefer a strategy of direct stenting in SVGs, attempting to minimize distal atheroembolization.[6]

In the SAVED trial, restenosis occurred in 37% of stented patients and in 46% of patients treated with balloon angioplasty

($P = .24$). Event-free survival at 240 days (freedom from death, MI, or repeat revascularization) was significantly higher in stented patients (73% vs 58%; $P < .03$). It was noted that late lumen loss was significantly greater in patients who had high-pressure stent deployment (> 16 atm), suggesting that high-pressure stent expansion may be undesirable in SVGs. Less aggressive stent expansion was also supported by an intravascular ultrasound study of over 200 SVGs that showed that stent expansion to more than 100% of the reference cross-sectional area was associated with significantly more non-Q-wave MIs (29% vs 17%; $P = .05$) and similar rates of target vessel revascularization at 1 year (31% vs 26%; $P = .3$).[7]

Observational reports of intervention in SVGs suggest that outcomes were somewhat better in 1995–1998 compared with 1990–1994 (1-year event-free survival of 71% vs 59%; $P < .001$) and that use of stents had a protective effect.[8] However, in an analysis of more than 600 patients with SVGs included in five large randomized trials, rates of major adverse coronary events (MACE) were twice that observed in native vessel intervention and use of glycoprotein IIb/IIIa platelet receptor inhibitors did not reduce MACE in SVG patients at 30 days or 6 months.[9]

[ ] EMBOLIC PROTECTION

In the past decade, the importance of atheroembolic MI complicating percutaneous coronary intervention (PCI) has become increasingly apparent, especially in SVG interventions. In relatively simple SVG lesions, stenting resulted in MI in about 20% of patients. The rate of MI increased with lesion complexity, length, and estimated plaque volume,[10] and in approximately 1000 patients who underwent SVG intervention, creatine kinase, myocardial bound (CK-MB) elevation was the best independent predictor of late mortality.[11] Strategies to prevent atheroembolic infarction include transient occlusion of the SVG during stent deployment followed by aspiration and the use of filters. The first atheroembolic protection method tested, the PercuSurge Guardwire system, uses a 0.014-in percutaneous transluminal coronary angioplasty wire with a compliant distal occlusion balloon followed by aspiration. Use of this system was found to prevent infarction in 23 of 24 SVG stent procedures, and 95% of aspirates had typical atherosclerotic debris.[12] However, it was the Saphenous Vein Graft Angioplasty Free of Emboli, Randomized (SAFER) trial that unequivocally demonstrated the value of distal protection during SVG intervention. In 801 patients randomized to PercuSurge or unprotected stent implantation, the 30-day MACE rate was reduced by 42% with use of the GuardWire (from 16.9% to 9.6%; $P < .001$, primarily due to reduced infarction (from 14.7% to 8.6%; $P = .008$).[13] Advantages of this technique include its low crossing profile, which permits crossing severe stenoses, and the ability to capture small particles and soluble vasoactive molecules such as endothelin and serotonin and coagulation components such as tissue factor, plasminogen activator inhibitor, prothrombin fragments, and thrombin-antithrombin complexes, which have been shown to be liberated during SVG interventions.[14]

The effectiveness of filter-based distal protection during SVG stent implantation was evaluated in the FIRE (Functional Improvement through Revascularization of the Extremities) trial, a randomized study of 656 patients in 65 centers[15] (Figure 37-1). Thirty-day MACE was 9.9% with the FilterWire and 11.6% with PercuSurge, and virtually identical rates were observed for MI (9% vs 10%) and death (0.9% vs 0.9%). Advantages of the FilterWire included ease of use, maintenance of flow, and avoidance of ischemia during stenting and good visualization. A variety of filters are currently being tested.

A second form of occlusion-aspiration known as Proxis, which uses a proximal occluding balloon, is being tested in randomized trials. Advantages of proximal occlusion include protection during wire passage, side-branch protection, and no need for a distal parking segment, a problem that, in many patients, prevents use of the FilterWire and PercuSurge.

[ ] ATHERECTOMY-THROMBECTOMY

Debulking procedures in SVGs using directional atherectomy, the Transluminal Extraction Catheter, and excimer laser have been shown to have increased costs without evidence of improved outcomes. Mechanical thrombectomy is currently feasible with a variety of techniques, including aspiration with guide catheter, Export (AVE Medtronic, Santa Rosa, CA), or Pronto (Vascular Solutions, Minneapolis, MN), AngioJet (Possis Medical, Minneapolis, MN), or X-Sizer (ev3, Plymouth, MN). Although proof of benefit is lacking, anecdotal experiences of seasoned operators have convinced most that proceeding with PCI in the face of a large thrombus burden is rarely advisable when mechanical thrombectomy or some other strategy to eliminate or reduce thrombi is feasible.

[ ] DRUG-ELUTING STENTS IN SAPHENOUS VEIN GRAFTS

Although no randomized, controlled trials of the use of drug-eluting stents in SVGs have been performed, preliminary observational studies suggest efficacy. Data from an observation trial, which involved compassionate use of sirolimus-eluting stents in patients with recurrent stenoses who were not candidates for other procedures, showed similar outcomes in SVGs and native coronary arteries. In 19 consecutive patients with de novo SVG lesions treated with 1.6 sirolimus-eluting stents per patient, only one lesion required retreatment and event-free survival was 84% at 1 year.[16]

[ ] COVERED STENTS

The results of two trials comparing polytetrafluoroethylene (PTFE)-covered stents with bare-metal stents in SVGs were not encouraging.[17,18] In patients receiving covered stents, the 6-month MACE rates were higher—the result of more MIs and late occlusion. However, PTFE-covered stents remain an important, potentially lifesaving adjunct for treatment of patients with SVG perforation.

[ ] BRACHYTHERAPY IN SAPHENOUS VEIN GRAFTS

Although brachytherapy for treatment of in-stent restenosis in SVGs is not a Food and Drug Administration (FDA)-approved indication, it has been shown to be effective in a randomized, controlled trial.[19] In 120 randomized patients, restenosis at 6 months

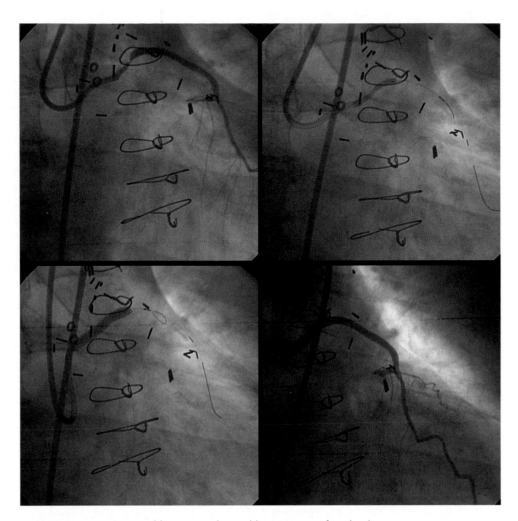

FIGURE 37-1. A 79-year-old woman with unstable angina was found to have severe stenosis in a saphenous vein graft (SVG) to the left anterior descending coronary artery (*upper left*), which had been placed 24 years earlier. The right coronary artery was occluded. The patient was somewhat forgetful and was not judged to be a good candidate for repeat surgery. Following placement of a FilterWire for distal protection, and using an Amplatz left guide catheter, the lesion was predilated safely (*upper right*). A stent was selected to extend from the SVG ostium well beyond the lesion (*lower left*). Note the position of the filter. Following stent deployment, an excellent angiographic result was obtained (*lower right*). There was a moderate amount of atherosclerotic debris in the filter and no evidence of periprocedural myocardial ischemia or infarction. Had the patient been younger and better suited for repeat surgery, this option might have been used. The current ability to offer distal protection, enhancing procedural safety, and use of drug-eluting stents to ameliorate restenosis have significantly improved outcomes in such cases.

was markedly reduced (21% vs 44%; P = .005), and MACE at 3 years was significantly lower (38% vs 63%; P = .006). Randomized trials comparing drug-eluting stents and brachytherapy for treatment of in-stent restenosis in SVGs have not been done.

PATIENT AND LESION CHARACTERISTICS

[ ] LENGTH OF TIME SINCE CORONARY ARTERY BYPASS GRAFTING

The types of SVG lesions encountered are determined by the length of time that has passed since the patient underwent coronary bypass surgery. The longer the interval, the higher the probability of encountering bulky, friable, atherosclerotic lesions with high atheroembolic potential. Recurrent myocardial ischemia within days of coronary artery bypass grafting is commonly due to acute SVG thrombosis, but venous or arterial anastomotic lesions or uncorrected native coronary disease may be encountered. Among 145 patients with early postoperative ischemia evaluated with coronary angiography, 60% had graft stenosis or occlusion, 10% had incomplete revascularization, and no cause was apparent in the remainder.[3] Seventy-four patients underwent repeat revascularization. PCI in this setting is a class I indication, according to guidelines of the American College of Cardiology (ACC) and American Heart Association (AHA), and can be lifesaving. The need for treatment of anastomotic lesions early after surgery is more common with off-pump and minimally invasive surgery in my experience.

【 】 PROXIMAL GRAFT LESIONS

Lesions at the origin of LIMA or RIMA grafts are quite rare, but stent implantation at these sites has been described.[3] Aorto-ostial SVG lesions are much more common and are difficult to treat effectively due to elastic recoil and restenosis. In a study of 320 consecutive patients with stent implantation for SVG aorto-ostial stenoses, about half of whom had debulking with atherectomy, 1-year target lesion revascularization was about 20% and event-free survival 70%.[20] Atherectomy prior to stenting conferred no benefit. Results of the use of drug-eluting stents at this site have not been reported. Aorto-ostial lesions in older SVGs carry a high risk of distal embolization, and use of filters is recommended for embolic protection.

【 】 MID-GRAFT LESIONS

Internal mammary artery (IMA) grafts are "immune" to atherosclerosis; mid-RIMA or mid-LIMA graft lesions are rare and most likely the result of operative trauma. Atherosclerotic lesions in the shaft portion of SVGs appear with increasing frequency beginning about 3 years after coronary bypass surgery.[3] Data from the SAFER trial showed that even with the shortest lesions (< 10 mm length), a 77% reduction in 30-day MACE was experienced when embolic protection with PercuSurge was utilized (2.2% vs 8.1%).[21] Although the risk of atheroembolic MI is highest with complex lesions,[10] this observation in simple lesions strongly supports routine use of a distal protection strategy during stent implantation in virtually all de novo SVG lesions where the anatomy permits it. An exception is the lesion appearing within 1 or 2 years of surgery, a time frame in which intimal hyperplasia is the usual pathology and embolic complications are rare. Most operators use drug-eluting stents in mid-SVG lesions.[16]

【 】 DISTAL ANASTOMOSIS LESIONS

Lesions occurring at the distal anastomosis of arterial and venous grafts within a year of surgery ("favorite" timing is 3 months) respond well to balloon angioplasty alone; restenosis occurs in about 20%, with no apparent advantage of bare-metal stenting. Lesions occurring later after surgery are increasingly atherosclerotic, and stent implantation is preferred. Results of studies using drug-eluting stents for this site have not been reported, but most operators use them routinely in older lesions. When a bulky and presumably atherosclerotic distal anastomosis lesion is encountered, Proxis is the only applicable distal protection strategy.

【 】 LARGE THROMBUS

Lesion-associated thrombus is a predictor of complications, especially periprocedural infarction. In the SAFER trial, baseline SVG thrombus was associated with higher mortality (3.0% vs 0.9%; $P = .04$), more no-reflow (9.9% vs 3.4%; $P = .001$), and higher 30-day MACE (17.4% vs 10.4%; $P = .006$).[22] This striking difference in outcomes occurred despite of the fact that 50% of patients in SAFER received distal protection with PercuSurge, which reduced complications (OR 0.625; $P = .02$). Some experienced operators attempt to reduce lesion-associated thrombus prior to stent implantation by administration of antithrombotic therapy along with glycoprotein IIb/IIIa platelet receptor inhibitors for a few days, or by infusing thrombolytic agents locally. However, mechanical thrombectomy was shown to be superior to urokinase and is the most common approach, combined with a distal protection strategy if possible.

【 】 RESTENOSIS LESIONS

Restenosis following stent implantation in a SVG is common. When disease in the SVG appears to be confined to the in-stent restenosis lesion, repeat intervention can be conducted with such a low risk of atheroembolization that distal protection is not routinely implemented.[23] Because repeat restenosis occurs subsequently in almost one half of such patients, treatment with either brachytherapy (see earlier discussion) or deployment of drug-eluting stents has become the usual treatment.

【 】 TOTALLY OCCLUDED SAPHENOUS VEIN GRAFTS

If the clinical history suggests recent SVG occlusion, recanalization with mechanical thrombectomy followed by stent implantation may yield good long-term results. However, complications are more frequent and serious. Prolonged infusion of thrombolytic agents has been associated with major bleeding, including intracranial hemorrhage, and MI infarction and low SVG patency rates have been reported. The ACC/AHA guideline statement considers a chronically occluded SVG to be a class III indication for PCI (not useful, may be harmful).

【 】 "STRING-LIKE" ARTERIAL GRAFTS

Occasionally one encounters a "string-like" arterial graft that has failed due to competitive flow, and this requires no action. However, if ischemia is present in the distribution of such a graft, balloon dilation and placement of stents throughout the length of the graft may be a consideration, especially when the graft is a relatively thick-walled radial artery and is not very long. Drug-eluting stents have also been used in the reconstruction of "string-like" radial artery and IMA grafts. Several "string-like" in-situ LIMA grafts have also been rehabilitated by balloon dilation of severe stenoses or occlusions in the distal graft, in my experience.

【 】 DIABETIC PATIENTS

A study of more than 2000 thousand patients who underwent PCI of SVG lesions at Emory University pointed out the poor 5-year survival of diabetic compared with nondiabetic patients (60% vs 82%; $P = .001$). Event-free survival at 5 years was also significantly lower (23% vs 37%; $P = .001$).[24] Drug-eluting stents were not utilized during this experience.

EQUIPMENT

The guidewires, balloon catheters, stents, atherectomy and thrombectomy devices, and available distal protection equipment are described in detail in other chapters of this text. The reader is referred to these chapters for discussion of the devices themselves. Recommendations for use of these devices in saphenous vein and arterial grafts appear elsewhere in this chapter.

STEP-BY-STEP INTERVENTION

【 】 PREPARATION OF THE PATIENT

The author premedicates patients with clopidogrel (600 mg loading dose), aspirin (325 mg), diphenhydramine ([Benadryl] 50 mg orally), a calcium-blocking drug such as diltiazem (60 mg orally), and a thrombin inhibitor. Patients with obvious thrombi, insulin-dependent diabetes, or other factors that place them at high risk may receive glycoprotein IIb/IIIa platelet receptor inhibitors.

【 】 GUIDE CATHETER SELECTION AND MANIPULATION

For in-situ LIMA or RIMA interventions, 7 French (Fr) IMA catheters are utilized from a femoral approach, if possible. Use of an 0.035-in angle-tip glide wire facilitates entering the subclavian artery or innominate artery, if needed. If entry into the IMA is difficult, a straight lateral view is obtained, and the tip of the IMA catheter rotated anteriorly. Extreme care is taken to avoid traumatizing the ostium of the IMA, especially when balloon catheters are withdrawn.

For SVG and free arterial graft intervention, 7-Fr multipurpose guide catheters are used for down-going grafts to the right coronary artery, hockey-stick or Amplatz shapes are used for grafts that arise from the anterior aorta and supply LAD or diagonal (see Figure 37-1), and Amplatz shapes are favored for grafts to the circumflex distribution, especially when their initial portion is superiorly oriented. Amplatz guide catheters provide superior "backup," which becomes especially important when distal protection strategies are applied. If ostial narrowing is present, or the graft is small, a side-hole guide catheter is preferred.

【 】 SELECTION OF OPTIMAL VIEWS

For LIMA or RIMA interventions at the distal anastomosis with the LAD or diagonal arteries, a straight lateral view, with cranial angulation, if needed, is one of the best views and is frequently coupled with a 30-degree right anterior oblique view to provide two roughly orthogonal views.

When SVG intervention is carried out, at least one and preferably two views are needed that are roughly 90 degrees from the direction of the graft, free of overlap and foreshortening, and displaying the entire length of the lesion. With aorto-ostial lesions, it is difficult but critically important to avoid foreshortening, which prevents the precise placement of the stent required (see Figure 37-1).

【 】 SELECTION OF DISTAL PROTECTION STRATEGY

The reader is referred to the Chapter 36 for a more complete review of this topic. In general, a distal protection strategy is recommended on all interventions on de novo lesions in SVGs that

are 3 years of age or older. PercuSurge is preferred in severely stenotic SVGs supplying moderate or small-sized myocardial segments (where ischemia would be well tolerated). The FilterWire is preferred when it is anticipated ischemia would not be well tolerated. Examples include grafts supplying large myocardial segments, moderate-sized myocardial segments in the presence of left ventricular dysfunction, or last remaining vessel. When there is insufficient room for the PercuSurge GuardWire or FilterWire beyond the lesion, the Proxis device, currently being evaluated, appears to be safe and effective. Whether the Proxis will be superior to the other alternatives remains to be determined.

【 】 GUIDEWIRE SELECTION

In the presence of a very tortuous IMA graft, a 0.014-in floppy guidewire with hydrophilic coating is frequently the best choice and usually permits passage of a balloon catheter. To pass a stent, it may be necessary to use the balloon catheter to exchange for a stiffer guidewire. Use of a stiff wire may straighten and "crimp" the IMA, functionally occluding it. When this happens, it may be necessary to switch back to a less stiff wire once the stent is in the approximate target site, or to deploy the stent using landmarks such as surgical clips. Removal of a stiff guidewire from a straightened IMA is best accomplished via an over-the-wire balloon catheter, with care taken to avoid dragging the guide catheter into the IMA origin. Selection of a guidewire for SVGs follows principles used in native vessel intervention, and middle-weight wires are commonly chosen.

【 】 THROMBECTOMY IN SAPHENOUS VEIN GRAFTS

As previously discussed, when a large thrombus burden is present, PCI is risky. AngioJet thrombectomy is the most effective method for clot removal and is favored when the thrombus is large. Placement of a temporary pacemaker is usually required for treatment of SVGs supplying right and circumflex coronary arteries because of bradycardia caused by adenosine released from red cells. Placement of a filter should be considered in the presence of a large thrombus, but there is some risk of embolizing a clot when placing the filter. Proximal thrombi may be aspirated by a guide catheter, and smaller distal thrombi can be removed by Export, Pronto, or X-Sizer catheters.

【 】 STENT SELECTION

Drug-eluting stents have become the default strategy despite the lack of hard data supporting their use in grafts. Currently, their use in large SVGs is constrained by the geometric expansion limits of the available devices (4.75 mm for Cypher and 4.25 mm for Taxus). As previously noted, data from the SAVED trial and ultrasound studies suggest that in PCI of SVG lesions, stent sizing and expansion pressures should be conservative.[5,7] This strategy also minimizes the risk of SVG perforation, an increasingly frequent complication, in my experience, vand avoids to a degree the extrusion of atheroma through stent struts with subsequent embolization. A "kinder, gentler" approach to SVG PCI, including direct stenting,[6] minimal catheter manipulations, slightly longer stents to trap as much atheroma as possible, and routine use of distal protection are recommended. When distal protection cannot be applied owing to anatomic constraints, use of self-expanding stents without postdilation minimizes the risk of atheroembolization in my experience.

AVOIDING AND TREATING COMPLICATIONS

【 】 SAPHENOUS VEIN GRAFT PERFORATION

The preceding paragraph highlights some of the most important tips to avoid perforation, namely avoiding oversized balloons and stents and unnecessary high-pressure inflations. Despite these cautionary measures, SVG perforations are increasingly encountered, perhaps because of the frequent use of long balloons and stents and the capability of stent balloons to reach pressures as high as 20 atm. Long tears may occur that are difficult and sometimes impossible to seal, even with PTFE-covered stents. Perfusion balloons, covered stents, and coils are invaluable tools in the event of a serious perforation and should be immediately available. When a "free" perforation occurs, it is usually advisable to control it with the balloon that caused the rent while gathering necessary tools to definitively seal it. In some cases, it is advisable to place a second, larger guide catheter from the other leg to accommodate the bulky, covered stent required to seal a large SVG.

【 】 NO REFLOW FOLLOWING SAPHENOUS VEIN GRAFT INTERVENTION

The etiology of the no-reflow phenomenon during SVG intervention is multifactorial and includes vasospasm, but most important is microembolization of plaque and thrombus. As shown in the SAFER trial, effective distal protection significantly reduces no-reflow (from 9.9% to 3.4%; P < .001)[22] and should be routinely used in all PCI procedures involving de novo lesions in SVGs that have been in place for 3 years or more. Participation of microvascular spasm in no-reflow scenarios is strongly suggested by the fact that endothelin and serotonin, both vasoconstrictors, are liberated during PCI of SVG lesions,[25] by reduced incidence of no reflow when calcium channel blockers are administered prior to SVG PCI,[26] by a beneficial treatment effect of microvasculature dilators (nitroprusside, adenosine, and calcium blockers),[27] and by the lack of benefit of nitroglycerin.

When no-reflow occurs, or is anticipated, intracoronary administration of 100 to 300 μg of diltiazem, verapamil, or nitroprusside, or 10 to 30 μg of adenosine, are usual doses, which may be repeated. Based on the work of Kotani,[28] I have adopted a strategy of aspirating the stagnant dye column when no reflow occurs using an Export catheter, with return of some debris. In 75 patients with no reflow, Kotani found direct aspiration of the dye column was more effective than calcium channel blockers in restoring flow and avoiding balloon pumping and death. Aspirates most often contained plaque gruel, and less than 10% contain thrombus. Although glycoprotein IIb/IIIa platelet receptor inhibitors are frequently administered in patients with no reflow,[27] this strategy has not been formally tested.

CONCLUSION

Recurrence of symptoms following CABG is a commonly encountered clinical problem that can often be ameliorated by PCI. The safety of graft PCI has been enhanced by the advent of distal protection strategies and more effective and easily applied thrombectomy devices. Long-term results have been improved by drug-eluting stents and use of brachytherapy in treatment of in-stent restenosis. However, although the interventional cardiologist has never been in a better position to effectively treat this patient subgroup, outcomes remain suboptimal compared with native coronary intervention, engendering caution in selection of this strategy and highlighting the need for further investigation.

REFERENCES

1. Gruentzig AR, Senning A, Siegenthaler WE. Nonoperative dilatation of coronary-artery stenosis. Percutaneous transluminal coronary angioplasty. N Engl J Med. 1979;301:61.
2. Douglas JS, Gruentzig AR, King SB, et al. Percutaneous transluminal coronary angioplasty in patients with prior coronary bypass surgery. J Am Coll Cardiol. 1983;2:745.
3. Douglas JS Jr. Percutaneous intervention in patients with prior coronary bypass surgery. In: Topol EJ, ed. Textbook of Interventional Cardiology, 4th ed. Philadelphia, PA: Saunders; 2003, p 317.
4. Wong SC, Baim DS, Schatz RA, et al. Acute results and late outcomes after stent implantation in saphenous vein graft lesions: The multicenter USA Palmaz-Schatz stent experience. J Am Coll Cardiol. 1995;26:704.
5. Savage MP, Douglas JS Jr, Fischman DL, et al. Stent placement compared with balloon angioplasty for obstructed bypass grafts. Saphenous Vein De Novo Trial Investigators. N Engl J Med. 1997;337:740.
6. Leborgne L, Chemeau E, Pichard AD, et al. Effect of direct stenting on clinical outcome in patients treated with percutaneous coronary intervention on saphenous vein graft. Am Heart J. 2003;146:501.
7. Iakovau I, Dangas G, Mintz GS, et al. Relation of final lumen dimensions in saphenous vein grafts after stent implantation to outcome. Am J Cardiol. 2004;93:963.
8. Hong MK, Mehran R, Dangas G, et al. Are we making progress with percutaneous saphenous vein graft treatment? J Am Coll Cardiol. 2001;38:150.
9. Roffi M, Mukherjee D, Bhatt DL, et al. Percutaneous interventions of coronary bypass grafts have doubled major adverse events. J Am Coll Cardiol. 2001;37(suppl A):6A.
10. Liu MW, Douglas JS Jr, Lembo NJ, et al. Angiographic predictors of a rise in serum creatine kinase (distal embolization) after balloon angioplasty in saphenous vein coronary artery bypass grafts. Am J Cardiol. 1993;72:514.
11. Hong MK, Mehran R, Dangas G, et al: Creatine kinase-MB enzyme elevation following successful saphenous vein graft intervention is associated with late mortality. Circulation. 1999;100:2400.
12. Webb JG, Carere RG, Virmani R, et al. Retrieval and analysis of particulate debris following saphenous vein graft intervention. J Am Coll Cardiol. 1999;34:461.
13. Baim DS, Wahr D, George B, et al. Randomized trial of a distal embolic protection device during percutaneous intervention of saphenous vein aorto-coronary bypass grafts. Circulation. 2002;105:512.
14. Salloum J, Reddy B, Vaughan DE, et al. Elimination of soluble vasoactive factors by the PercuSurge Guardwire distal protection device during percutaneous coronary intervention of saphenous vein graft. J Am Coll Cardiol. 2004;43:71A.
15. Stone G, Rogers C, Hermiller J, et al. Randomized comparison of distal protection with filter-based catheter and a balloon occlusion and aspiration system during percutaneous intervention of diseased saphenous vein aorto-coronary bypass grafts. Circulation. 2003;108:548.
16. Hoye A, Lemos PA, Arampatzis CA, et al. Effectiveness of the sirolimus-eluting stent in the treatment of saphenous vein graft disease. J Invas Cardiol. 2004;16:230.
17. Stankovic G, Colombo A, Presbitero P, et al. Randomized evaluation of polytetrafluoroethylene-covered stent in saphenous vein grafts. Circulation. 2003;108:37.
18. Schachinger V, Hamm CW, Munzel T, et al. A randomized trial of polytetrafluoroethylene-covered stents compared with conventional stents in aortocoronary saphenous vein grafts. J Am Coll Cardiol. 2003;42:1360.

19. Rha SW, Waksman R, Kuchulakanti PK, et al. Three-year follow-up after intracoronary gamma radiation for in-stent restenosis in saphenous vein grafts. *J Am Coll Cardiol.* 2004;104A.

20. Wong SC, Popma JJ, Hong MK, et al. Procedural results and long term clinical outcome in aorto-ostial saphenous vein graft lesions after new device angioplasty. *J Am Coll Cardiol.* 1995;25(suppl A):394A.

21. Giugliano GR, Prpic R, Cutlip, et al. Does the beneficial effect of distal protection in saphenous vein graft interventions vary with lesion length? A SAFER (Saphenous Vein Graft Angioplasty Free of Emboli Randomized) substudy. *J Am Coll Cardiol.* 2002;39:9A.

22. Giri S, Kuntz RE, Eisenhauer C, et al. Effect of baseline thrombus in the SAFER (Saphenous Vein Graft Angioplasty Free of Emboli Randomized) trial. *J Am Coll Cardiol.* 2002;39:52A

23. Assali AR, Sdringola S, Moustapha A, et al. Percutaneous intervention in saphenous vein grafts: In-stent restenosis lesions are safer than de novo lesions. *J Invas Cardiol.* 2001;13:446.

24. Ashfaq S, Malki Q, Weintraub W, et al. The outcome of percutaneous coronary interventions of saphenous vein grafts in diabetic patients compared to nondiabetic patients. *J Am Coll Cardiol.* 2003;41:47A.

25. Salloum J, Reddy B, Vaughan DE, et al. Elimination of soluble vasoactive factors by the PercuSurge Guardwire distal protection device during percutaneous coronary intervention of saphenous vein graft. *J Am Coll Cardiol.* 2004;43:71A.

26. Michaels AD, Appleby M, Otten MH, et al. Pretreatment with intragraft verapamil prior to PCI of saphenous vein graft lesions: Results of the VAPOR trial. *J Invas Cardiol.* 2002;14:299.

27. Klein LW, Kern MJ, Berger P, et al. Society of cardiac angiography and interventions: Suggested management of the no-reflow phenomenon in the cardiac catheterization laboratory. *Cathet Cardiovasc Interv.* 2003;60:194.

28. Kotani J, Fujita M, Higo S, et al. Direct coronary aspiration improved stagnated coronary flow due to no-reflow during angioplasty for acute coronary syndrome–compared with pharmacological treatment. *Circulation.* 2001;104:II-417.

CHAPTER (38)

Special Considerations: Acute Myocardial Infarction

Bruce R. Brodie, MD, and William O'Neill, MD

Mechanical reperfusion therapy has recently been accepted as the preferred reperfusion strategy for ST-segment elevation myocardial infarction (STEMI). Few other interventions in clinical medicine require the complex organization of health care delivery systems and the high level of technical expertise necessary to achieve optimum outcomes. The outstanding clinical results achieved in randomized trials, which validated the superiority of mechanical intervention over thrombolytic therapy, can be duplicated in clinical practice only with dedicated medical leadership and comprehensive programs to implement and manage mechanical reperfusion strategies.

In this chapter, we review the evidence for the use of emergency percutaneous coronary intervention (PCI) in the management of STEMI and examine patient subsets who are likely to benefit most from this approach. We discuss the use of stents and adjunctive pharmacologic therapies, the triage of patients presenting at non-interventional hospitals, cost considerations, technical aspects of primary PCI, and new therapies to optimize microvascular reperfusion and reduce reperfusion injury.

MECHANICAL VERSUS PHARMACOLOGIC REPERFUSION STRATEGIES

[ ] CLINICAL OUTCOMES

In 23 randomized trials that involved 7739 patients, primary PCI was compared with thrombolytic therapy for acute myocardial infarction (AMI). These trials were summarized in a 2003 meta-analysis,[1]

which showed that primary PCI was superior to thrombolytic therapy in reducing short term mortality, nonfatal reinfarction, and stroke (Figure 38-1). These results were maintained at long-term follow-up and were independent of the type of thrombolytic agent used (streptokinase vs fibrin-specific thrombolytics) and whether patients were transferred emergently for primary PCI. The incidence of intracranial hemorrhage was significantly less with primary PCI, although the overall risk of major bleeding (mostly related to access site bleeding) was higher with primary PCI (Figure 38-2). The risk of access site bleeding with primary PCI appears to be less in more recent trials with better management of anticoagulation and earlier femoral artery sheath removal.

The survival benefit of primary PCI compared with thrombolytic therapy reported in this meta-analysis was substantial (21 lives saved per 1000 patients treated) and compares favorably with the survival benefit of thrombolytic therapy compared with placebo reported by the Fibrinolytic Therapy Trialists' (FTT) Collaborative Group (19 lives saved per 1000 patients treated), as illustrated in Figure 38-3.[2] The relative reduction in death and nonfatal reinfarction is similar across all subgroups of patients treated, including the elderly, women, diabetics, patients with anterior or nonanterior infarction, patients with prior infarction, and those classified as low risk or not low risk.[3] The greatest absolute benefit occurs in patients at highest risk, and several randomized trials have specifically evaluated these high-risk subgroups. The SHOCK trial (SHould we emergently revascularize Occluded Coronaries for cardiogenic shocK), which randomized 302 patients with cardiogenic shock to emergency revascularization versus medical stabilization, found lower mortality with emergency revascularization at 6 months (50% vs 63%; $P = .03$).[4]

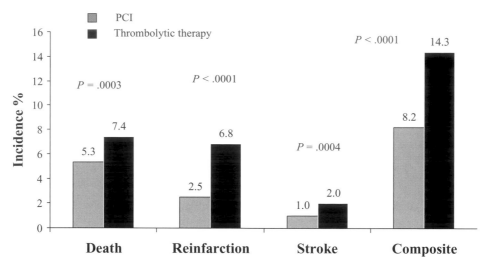

FIGURE 38-1. Meta-analysis of 23 randomized trials comparing short term outcomes with primary PCI versus thrombolytic therapy for acute myocardial infarction. Adapted from Keeley et al with permission.[1]

The survival benefit was especially pronounced in patients treated within 6 hours of symptom onset and was seen only in patients younger than 75 years of age. Garcia and colleagues randomized 220 patients with anterior infarction to primary PCI versus alteplase and found substantially lower mortality with primary PCI (2.8% vs 10.8%; $P = .02$).[5] The Zwolle group randomized 87 elderly patients (older than 75 years) to primary PCI versus streptokinase and found a lower incidence of the composite end point of death, nonfatal reinfarction, or stroke at 30 days with primary PCI (8.7% vs 29.3%; $P = .01$).[6]

Primary PCI is capable of achieving much higher rates of TIMI 3 flow than thrombolytic therapy[7,9,10] (Figure 38-4), and this probably explains most of the mortality advantage with primary PCI. Newer thrombolytic strategies using combination therapy with low-dose thrombolytics and platelet glycoprotein IIb/IIIa inhibitors have shown improved TIMI 3 flow rates in small pilot trials,[9] but these rates are well below the TIMI 3 flow rates achieved with primary PCI and have not shown any mortality advantage in the large GUSTO V (Global Use of Strategies To Open occluded arteries in acute myocardial infarction) and ASSENT-3 (ASessement of the Safety and Efficacy of a New Thrombolytic regimen) trials.[11,12]

【 】 ACUTE ANGIOGRAPHIC OUTCOMES

Achieving normal (Thrombolysis in Myocardial Infarction [TIMI] 3) antegrade flow in the infarct artery is critical to optimizing clinical outcomes with both thrombolytic therapy and primary PCI.[7,8]

【 】 LATE CLINICAL AND ANGIOGRAPHIC OUTCOMES AND MYOCARDIAL SALVAGE

The initial clinical benefit of primary PCI over thrombolytic therapy in reducing death and reinfarction appears to be maintained at

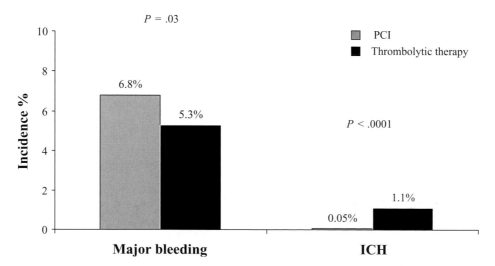

FIGURE 38-2. Meta-analysis of 23 randomized trials comparing hemorrhagic complications with primary PCI versus thrombolytic therapy for acute myocardial infarction. (ICH = intracerebral hemorrhage.) Adapted from Keeley et al with permission.[1]

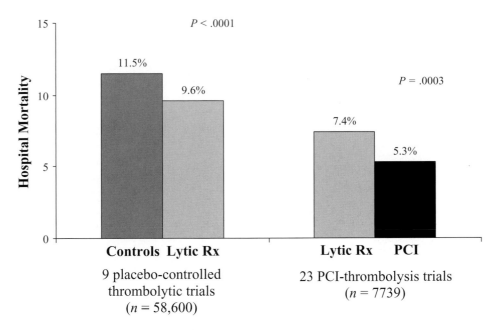

FIGURE 38-3. Comparison of mortality reduction with thrombolytic therapy versus placebo[2] and primary PCI versus thrombolytic therapy.[1]

late follow-up. The PAMI (Primary Angioplasty in Myocardial Infarction) investigators and the Zwolle investigators found that death or reinfarction was lower at late follow-up with primary PCI versus thrombolytic therapy[13,14] (Figure 38-5). Keeley's meta-analysis, discussed earlier, also showed that the initial benefit with primary PCI was maintained at late follow-up (6 to 18 months).[1]

Infarct artery patency rates at late angiographic follow-up have been much higher with primary PCI compared with thrombolytic therapy, and patency rates have improved with the use of stents[10,15,16] (Table 38-1). Late reocclusion rates following throm-

bolytic therapy have been high (20–28%) due to frequent high-grade residual stenosis when adjunctive PCI is not employed.[17–19]

Randomized trials have shown that myocardial salvage and myocardial salvage index as assessed by paired technetium-99 sestamibi scintigraphy are better with mechanical reperfusion using stents and platelet glycoprotein IIb/IIIa inhibitors compared with pharmacologic reperfusion using half-dose alteplase plus IIb/IIIa inhibitors.[20,21] The greater myocardial salvage with primary PCI is probably related to higher patency rates, less reocclusion, and possibly better myocardial reperfusion.

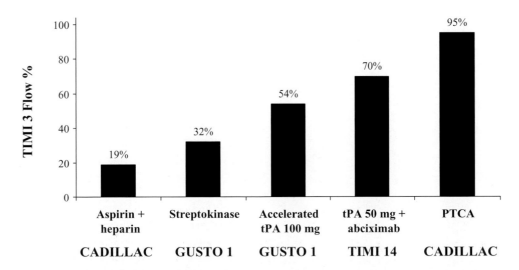

FIGURE 38-4. Frequency of achieving TIMI 3 flow in the infarct artery with aspirin and heparin,[10] several thrombolytic regimens,[7,9] and primary PCI.[10] (ASSENT = ASessment of the Safety and Efficacy of a New Thrombolytic regimen; CADILLAC = Controlled Abciximab and Device Investigation to Lower Late Angioplasty Complications; GUSTO = Global Use of Strategies To Open occluded arteries in acute myocardial infarction); tPA = tissue plasminogen activator.)

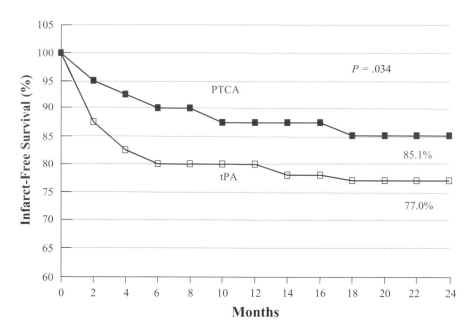

FIGURE 38-5. Actuarial infarction-free survival curves for patients with acute myocardial infarction treated with primary angioplasty (PTCA) (*solid boxes*) versus tissue plasminogen activator (tPA) (*open boxes*). Reproduced with permission from Nunn et al.[13]

ADJUNCTIVE THERAPIES WITH MECHANICAL REPERFUSION

【 】 STENTS

The Stent PAMI trial documented a clear benefit with stenting versus balloon angioplasty in reducing restenosis, reocclusion, and the need for target vessel revascularization after primary PCI for AMI[15] (see Table 38-1). However, using the first-generation Palmaz-Schatz

TABLE 38-1

Infarct Artery Restenosis and Reocclusion and Target Vessel Revascularization (TVR) at 6 to 7 Months After Primary PCI for Acute Myocardial Infarction

	PTCA (%)	STENT (%)	P VALUE
Restenosis			
Stent PAMI trial[15]	33.5	20.3	<.001
CADILLAC trial[10]	40.8	22.2	<.001
Reocclusion			
Stent PAMI trial[15]	9.3	5.1	.04
CADILLAC trial[10]	11.3	5.8	.02
TVR			
Stent PAMI trial[15]	17.0	7.7	<.001
CADILLAC trial[10]	14.7	6.8	<.001

CADILLAC = Controlled Abciximab and Device Investigation to Lower Late Angioplasty Complications; PAMI = Primary Angioplasty in Myocardial Infarction.

heparin-coated stent, stented patients had lower TIMI 3 flow rates post-PCI and a disturbing trend toward higher mortality at 1 year. Consequently, stenting had not been recommended for routine use and was reserved for selected patients. Subsequently, the CADILLAC (Controlled Abciximab and Device Investigation to Lower Late Angioplasty Complications) trial evaluated the role of stenting and platelet glycoprotein IIb/IIIa inhibition with abciximab in 2082 patients with AMI treated with primary PCI[10] (see Table 38-1). Patients were randomized to one of four treatment strategies: percutaneous transluminal coronary angioplasty (PTCA) alone, PTCA plus abciximab, stenting alone, and stenting plus abciximab. As in the Stent PAMI trial, a clear benefit was demonstrated for stenting over balloon angioplasty alone in reducing 6-month restenosis (22.2% vs 40.8%; $P < .001$), reocclusion (5.7% vs 11.3%; $P = .01$), ischemic target vessel revascularization (6.8% vs 14.7%; $P < .001$), and major adverse cardiac events (MACE) (10.9% vs 18.3%; $P < .001$). In contrast to Stent PAMI, using the newer generation MultiLink stent (Guidant, Santa Clara, CA), there was no degradation of TIMI flow post-stenting and no difference in 6-month mortality (3.6% with stenting vs 3.5% with PTCA). Based on these data from CADILLAC, stenting can now be recommended for routine use in eligible patients with AMI treated with mechanical intervention.

Drug-eluting stents (DES) have proven very effective in reducing restenosis and target vessel revascularization (TVR) compared with bare metal stents (BMS) following elective and urgent PCI, but their role in treating patients with STEMI undergoing primary PCI has not been established. There is concern that the incidence of stent thrombosis with DES may be higher in the setting of STEMI, and the benefits of DES may not be as great as with elective PCI, since the incidence of TVR is relatively low with the use of BMS in patients with STEMI. Two recent randomized trials have found conflicting results with DES versus BMS in STEMI. The TYPHOON

(A Multi-center Randomized Trial Comparing Sirolimus-eluting Stents to Bare Metal Stents in Primary Angioplasty for Acute Myocardial Infarction) Trial found less TVR with SES ($n = 355$) versus BMS ($n = 350$) (5.6% vs 13.4%, $P < 0.001$)[21a] while the PASSION (Randomized Comparison of Paclitaxel-eluting Stent versus Conventional Stent in ST-elevation Myocardial Infarction) Trial found no difference in target lesion revascularization between paclitaxel-eluting stents (PES, $n = 309$) and BMS ($n = 310$) (6.2% vs 7.4%, $P = .23$).[21b] In a large observational experience from the STENT Group, Brodie and colleagues found no significant difference in TVR between DES ($n = 520$) and BMS ($n = 304$) (3.9% vs 5.3% $P = 0.38$) and a low incidence of stent thrombosis with DES (0.8%),[21c] The HORIZONS trial is currently enrolling patients with STEMI target for primary PCI and will randomize 3400 patients to PES versus BMS in a 3:1 ratio and will hopefully clarify the role of DES in patients with STEMI.

【 】 PLATELET GLYCOPROTEIN IIB/IIIA INHIBITORS

To date, five randomized trials evaluated platelet glycoprotein inhibition with abciximab as adjunctive therapy with primary PCI [22–26,26a]. All showed a reduction in the composite end point of death, reinfarction, or urgent target vessel revascularization at 30 days (Table 38-2). The greatest benefit was seen in the ADMIRAL (Abciximab before Direct angioplasty and stenting in Myocardial Infarction Regarding Acute and Long-term follow-up) trial, in which abciximab was given early at the time of randomization or prior to angiography.[24] In addition to better clinical outcomes, the ADMIRAL trial found improved infarct artery patency prior to PCI and improved left ventricular ejection fraction at 6 months with abciximab. The CADILLAC trial showed improvement in 30-day outcomes with abciximab, but most of the benefit with abciximab versus placebo in reducing the composite end point was seen in patients treated with PTCA alone (4.8% vs 8.4%; $P = .02$), with less benefit seen in stented patients (4.5% vs 5.7%; $P = $ NS).[10] There was no benefit in left ventricular ejection fraction at 7 months. However, abciximab reduced acute thrombosis in stented patients (0% vs 1.0%; $P = .03$) as well as in all patients (0.4% vs 1.4%; $P = .01$). Currently, abciximab has a Class IIa indication by ACC/AHA Guidelines for use with primary PCI for STEMI.[26b] There are little data with eptifibitide or tirofiban. Because many of the trials showing benefit of abciximab with primary PCI were performed before the routine use of stents, and because the largest trial, CADILLAC, showed little benefit in stented patients, the role of glycoprotein IIb/IIIa platelet inhibitors with primary PCI has remained controversial. Although most trials have not shown an increased incidence of major bleeding with abciximab when used with primary PCI, bleeding is still a major problem when primary PCI is performed with unfractionated heparin, clopidogrel, and platelet glycoprotein IIb/IIIa inhibitors. The HORIZONS (Harmonizing Outcomes with Revascularization and Stents) Trial will compare bivalirudin, a direct thrombin inhibitor, with unfractionated heparin plus glycoprotein IIb/IIIa inhibition in STEMI patients undergoing primary PCI and may provide data which will help to determine

TABLE 38-2

Randomized Trials Comparing 30-Day Outcomes with Abciximab versus Placebo in Primary PCI for Acute Myocardial Infarction[a]

	ABCIXIMAB (%)	PLACEBO (%)	P VALUE
RAPPORT ($n = 483$)[22]			
Death	2.5	2.1	NS
Reinfarction	3.3	4.1	NS
Urgent TVR	1.7	6.6	.006
Composite	5.8	11.2	.03
ADMIRAL ($n = 300$)[24]			
Death	3.4	6.6	NS
Reinfarction	1.3	2.6	NS
Urgent TVR	1.3	6.6	.02
Composite	6.0	14.6	.01
ISAR-2 ($n = 401$)[23]			
Death	2.5	4.5	NS
Reinfarction	0.5	1.5	NS
Urgent TVR	3.0	5.0	NS
Composite	5.0	10.5	.04
CADILLAC ($n = 2,082$)[25]			
Death	1.9	2.2	NS
Reinfarction	0.8	0.9	NS
Urgent TVR	2.5	4.4	0.02
Stroke	0.1	0.2	NS
Composite	4.6	7.0	0.01
ACE ($n = 400$)[26]			
Death	3.5	4.0	NS
Reinfarction	0.5	4.5	.01
Urgent TVR	0.5	1.5	NS
Stroke	0.0	0.5	NS
Composite	4.5	10.5	.02

ACE = Abciximab and carbostent evaluation; ADMIRAL = Abciximab Before Direct Angioplasty and Stenting in Myocardial Infarction Regarding Acute and Long Term Follow-up; CADILLAC = Controlled Abciximab and Device Investigation to Lower Late Angioplasty Complications; ISAR = Intracoronary Stenting and Antithrombotic Regimen; RAPPORT = ReoPro in Acute myocardial infarction and Primary PTCA Organization and Randomized Trial.

[a]Patients in the ADMIRAL, ISAR-2, and ACE trials were treated with primary stenting; half of CADILLAC patients were treated with stents.

the optimum anticoagulant therapy and the role of glycoprotein IIb/IIIa inhibitors with primary PCI.

ROLE OF CARDIAC SURGERY IN THE PRIMARY PCI APPROACH

Approximately 10% of patients brought to the catheterization laboratory with the intent to perform primary PCI are triaged to either medical treatment or coronary bypass surgery. Bypass surgery is indicated when there is severe left main artery disease, coronary anatomy that is unsuitable for PCI, or in selected patients with severe three-vessel coronary artery disease with preserved (TIMI 3) flow in the infarct artery. Medical therapy is indicated for patients with (1) no myocardial infarction (mistaken diagnosis), (2) no significant stenosis in the infarct artery (resolution of spasm or thrombus), (3) inability to identify the infarct artery, and (4) unsuitable anatomy or sometimes a very small infarct artery.

Bypass surgery may be selected as the primary reperfusion strategy but also may be performed emergently after failed angioplasty, urgently for reinfarction or recurrent ischemia, and electively following primary PCI for definitive treatment of multivessel coronary disease. In experienced centers and with the availability of stents, emergency bypass surgery after failed PCI is rare (about 0.4%), and the need for urgent bypass surgery for reinfarction or recurrent ischemia that cannot be managed with repeat PCI is also rare (0.1%).[15] Elective bypass surgery for treatment of residual coronary artery disease after initial successful primary angioplasty has been used in about 2% to 5% of patients.[15,27] Altogether, bypass surgery is performed in about 6% to 10% of patients with the primary angioplasty approach.[15,28] Considering the severity of illness of these patients, surgical mortality has been very acceptable (6.4% with emergency or urgent bypass surgery and 2.0% with elective bypass surgery in the PAMI-2 trial).[28]

Cardiac surgery is also used in patients with mechanical complications of AMI. Patients with ventricular septal rupture, acute mitral regurgitation due to papillary muscle rupture, and contained myocardial rupture with tamponade usually develop cardiogenic shock and have a very poor outcome without surgical intervention, and these patients are candidates for emergent surgery. Patients with cardiogenic shock with severe left main artery disease (without mechanical complications) may also be candidates for emergent bypass surgery.

REPERFUSION STRATEGIES FOR PATIENTS WITH ACUTE MYOCARDIAL INFARCTION WHO PRESENT AT NONINTERVENTIONAL HOSPITALS

The use of primary PCI for AMI has been limited because most hospitals do not have interventional facilities and skilled personnel to perform PCI. Until recently, the transfer of patients presenting at community hospitals with AMI has not been widely recommended because of the potential deleterious effects of treatment delay on clinical outcomes and myocardial salvage. However, recent randomized trials have shown that transferring patients from non-

interventional hospitals to interventional hospitals may be a viable strategy.[29–32]

[ ] TRANSFER FROM NONINTERVENTIONAL HOSPITALS FOR PRIMARY PCI

The results from randomized trials (predominantly from Europe) indicate that outcomes are better when patients with STEMI who present to noninterventional hospitals are transferred to an interventional facility for primary PCI compared with being given fibrinolytic therapy at the local hospital (Table 38-3).[33–37] The additional treatment delays of primary PCI compared with fibrinolytic therapy (door-to-balloon time minus door-needle time) in these trials have ranged from 55 to 103 minutes. Unfortunately, in the United States transfer delays are much longer than this. Recent data from the National Registry of Myocardial Infarction (NRMI) found median delays of 180 minutes from arrival at the noninterventional hospital to balloon inflation at the primary PCI hospital with only 4.2% of transferred patients achieving door-to-balloon times <90 minutes.[37a] Consequently, many patients presenting to nonprimary PCI hospitals in the United States may not be eligible for primary PCI because of the long potential treatment delays. There are currently nationwide and many statewide efforts to improve door-to-balloon times, including for patients presenting to noninterventional hospitals. It has been shown that with well-defined goals, commitment from administrative and clinical leaders, standardized protocols, integrated systems of transfer, and data feedback to monitor progress, door-to-balloon times for patients presenting to noninterventional hospitals can be dramatically reduced and can often approach and meet guidelines for timely treatment with primary PCI.[37b,37c]

However, there are situations where this is not possible, and recommendations regarding triage of patients with STEMI for fibrinolytic therapy versus transfer for primary PCI have been controversial. Boersma's meta-analysis of randomized trials comparing fibrinolytic therapy versus primary PCI have suggested that primary PCI has a mortality advantage even with additional delays to PCI (door-to-balloon minus door-needle time) up to two hours.[37d] Data evaluating the impact of treatment delay with primary PCI on mortality suggest that treatment delay impact mortality most in patients presenting early after the onset of symptoms but have much less impact in patients presenting late after the onset of symptoms but have much less impact in patients presenting late after the onset of symptoms.[37e,37f,37g] Currently, ACC/AHA guidelines recommend that patients with cardiogenic shock and patients who are ineligible for fibrinolytic therapy should be transferred for primary PCI.[26b] Decisions regarding triage of remaining STEMI patients should depend on an assessment of time and risk—time to presentation, time delay to PCI, risk of bleeding from fibrinolytic therapy, and risk of STEMI. Patients with anterior infarction who present early and who have long delays to primary PCI should preferentially be treated with fibrinolytic therapy while patients presenting later should preferentially be transferred for primary PCI, even with longer delays to PCI.

There has been hope that facilitated PCI (early pharmacologic reperfusion therapy followed by transfer for emergent PCI) may provide a solution to the problem of time delays with primary

TABLE 38-3

Randomized Trials Comparing 30-Day Outcomes in Patients Transferred for Primary PCI versus Treatment Locally with Thrombolytic Therapy

	DEATH	REINFARCTION	STROKE	COMPOSITE	P VALUE[a]	TREATMENT DELAY[b] (min)
Vermeer et al (n = 150)[33]						
PCI	6.7	1.3	2.7	10.7	.25	90
Alteplase	6.7	9.3	2.7	18.7		
PRAGUE-1(n = 200)[34]						
PCI	6.9	1.0	0	7.9	.005	88
Streptokinase	14.1	10.1	1.0	23.2		
AR-PAMI(n = 137)[35]						
PCI	8.4	1.4	0	8.5	.33	104
Alteplase	12.1	0	4.5	13.6		
DANAMI-2(n = 1572)[36]						
PCI	6.6	1.6	1.1	8.0	.0004	61
Alteplase	7.5	6.3	2.0	13.5		
PRAGUE-2(n = 850)[37]						
PCI	6.8			8.4	.003	92
Streptokinase	10.0			15.2		

Air-PAMI = Air Primary Angioplasty in Myocardial Infarction; DANAMI = DANish trial in Acute Myocardial Infarction; PRAGUE = Primary Angiography in patients transferred from General community hospitals to specialized PTCA Units with or without Emergency thrombolysis.

[a]Compares composite end points.

[b]Treatment delay is the difference between symptom onset to balloon inflation with PCI and symptom onset to thrombolytic therapy.

PCI. Unfortunately, recent trials with facilitated PCI have not shown benefit.[37h] This will be discussed in a later section.[38]

[ ] PRIMARY PCI AT HOSPITALS WITHOUT ON-SITE CARDIAC SURGERY

An alternative approach to expanding the use of mechanical reperfusion for AMI is performing primary PCI at hospitals without on-site cardiac surgery. The C-PORT (Atlantic Cardiovascular Patient Outcomes Research Team) trial evaluated primary PCI at hospitals with catheterization laboratories but without cardiac surgery or elective PCI.[39] Using skilled operators who perform PCI at nearby tertiary centers, the C-PORT investigators randomized patients with AMI to primary PCI versus lytic therapy and documented lower 6-month composite event rates of death, reinfarction, or stroke with primary PCI (12.4% vs 19.9%; P = .03). Wharton and colleagues reported outcomes from a multicenter registry in high-risk patients with AMI presenting to hospitals with catheterization facilities but no on-site cardiac surgery who were treated with primary PCI.[40] Outcomes were similar to outcomes in comparable high-risk patients from the Air-PAMI (Air Primary Angioplasty in Myocardial Infarction) trial who were transferred from noninterventional hospitals for primary PCI, but with shorter treatment times.

Current American College of Cardiology (ACC)/American Heart Association (AHA) guidelines provide a class IIb indication for primary PCI at hospitals without on-site surgery when the procedure can be performed by experienced operators (> 75 procedures per year) in a timely fashion (90 + 30 minutes of arrival), if at least 36 primary PCI procedures are performed per year at the hospital, and if stringent guidelines are in place.[41]

COSTS AND COST-EFFECTIVENESS OF MECANICAL REPERFUSION STRATEGIES

Data from early randomized trials[42–44] have shown a shorter length of hospital stay and lower hospital costs with primary PCI compared with thrombolytic therapy. Initial catheterization laboratory costs with primary PCI are more than offset by higher drug charges for thrombolytic agents and costs related to high utilization of catheterization and PCI in thrombolytic treated patients. A strategy of early discharge with primary PCI may reduce costs further.[27]

The impact of adjunctive treatment with coronary stents on costs with primary PCI was evaluated in the Stent PAMI and CADILLAC trials.[45,46] The initial increased costs of stenting versus angioplasty alone were partially recovered in the Stent PAMI trial and completely recovered in the CADILLAC trial by decreased posthospital costs in the stented group due to less target vessel revascularization.[45,46] The narrow cost differences and the improved quality of life with stenting, as a result of the reduced need for repeat revascularization procedures, make stenting with primary PCI highly cost-effective.

The CADILLAC investigators found that the platelet glycoprotein IIb/IIIa inhibitor abciximab increased aggregate costs at 1 year by about $1200 compared with standard therapy.[46] Abciximab was not cost-effective unless nonsignificant differences in 1-year mortality were incorporated in the analysis.

TECHNICAL ASPECTS OF PRIMARY PCI

【 】 TREATMENT IN THE EMERGENCY DEPARTMENT

When primary PCI is planned for patients with known or suspected AMI, only a limited history and physical examination should be performed to avoid delays in initiating the catheterization procedure. Patients are given 325 mg of soluble chewable aspirin, 70 u/kg of intravenous unfractionated heparin, sublingual nitroglycerin, intravenous beta-blockers unless contraindicated, and supplemental oxygen, and are transported promptly from the emergency department to the catheterization laboratory. Clopidogrel 300–600 mg should also be given in the emergency department based on evidence from multiple trials[46a,46b,46c] (though not specifically STEMI–treated with primary PCI) and since the need for emergent CABG following primary PCI for STEMI is very low.

【 】 CARDIAC CATHETERIZATION AND ANGIOGRAPHY

Femoral access is usually preferred because this allows for the use of larger devices if necessary and facilitates the use of adjunctive therapy with intra-aortic balloon pumping or transvenous pacing when indicated. An activated clotting time (ACT) is measured, and additional heparin is given to prolong the ACT to more than 300 seconds or 200 to 300 seconds if platelet glycoprotein IIb/IIIa inhibitors are used. Left ventriculography should be performed prior to intervention to assess the severity of ventricular and valvular dysfunction, to help in identification of the infarct artery (if this is uncertain), and to aid in making decisions regarding the necessity for adjunctive therapy, such as intra-aortic balloon pumping and pulmonary artery catheter insertion. Occasionally, papillary muscle rupture, ventricular septal defect, or rarely even frank free wall rupture will be demonstrated when not previously suspected, prompting urgent surgery. Alternatively, demonstration of normal left ventricular function may raise early concerns of nonischemic diagnoses such as aortic dissection or pericarditis. A femoral venous sheath may be helpful in patients with occlusion of the right coronary artery to allow access for temporary transvenous pacing if necessary. In patients with hypotension or hemodynamic instability, placement of a pulmonary artery catheter is important to define and monitor hemodynamics. The use of a pulse oximeter to monitor oxygen saturation is also helpful.

Following diagnostic coronary and left ventricular angiography, patients are triaged to the most appropriate therapy. About 10% of patients who undergo emergency coronary angiography do not undergo primary angioplasty and are triaged to bypass surgery or medical therapy using criteria described earlier.

【 】 PRIMARY PCI PROCEDURE

Primary PCI is generally performed with 6 French (Fr) or 7-Fr standard guiding catheters and soft or floppy-tipped 0.014-in steerable guidewires. The soft tip can almost always cross the soft fresh thrombus (in contrast to chronic total occlusions) and is less traumatic than stiffer wires. The guidewire is advanced well down the infarct artery to ensure that it is located in the true lumen and not in a small side branch or under an intimal dissection, because navigation is usually performed blindly distal to the occlusion. If the infarct-related artery is initially totally occluded, reperfusion will often be established after crossing with the guidewire. If not, it may be preferable to cross the occlusion with a balloon and then withdraw the balloon without inflating it ("Dottering" the lesion) to establish reperfusion. The more gradual reperfusion provided with the wire or Dottering technique may result in less reperfusion arrhythmias than rapidly inflating the balloon immediately after crossing.

Balloon angioplasty or stenting of the infarct lesion is performed with techniques similar to conventional PCI. If stenting is planned, clopidogrel (300–600 mg) should be given prior to PCI if not previously given in the emergency department. At one time operators were taught that primary PCI should be performed only on the infarct artery, because dilating a noninfarct artery might place too much myocardium acutely in jeopardy. More recently, with the availability of stents and with the recognition that there may be rupture of multiple plaques in the setting of AMI, PCI of more than one vessel is sometimes performed. However, this should be done only with careful judgment when the risk of recurrent ischemia or infarction from a second ruptured plaque is judged to be more than the immediate risk of a second vessel intervention.

【 】 MANAGEMENT OF NO REFLOW

No reflow (TIMI 0-1 flow) or slow reflow (TIMI 2 flow) may occur transiently or may persist after primary PCI for AMI in 10% to 25% of patients. This is generally due to microvascular dysfunction from spasm, distal embolization, or endothelial injury and is associated with poorer recovery of left ventricular function and a higher incidence of post-MI complications.[47,48] When slow reflow or no reflow occurs, TIMI 3 flow usually can be reestablished with the use of intracoronary verapamil (100–200 μg boluses), adenosine (10–20 μg boluses), or nitroprusside (50–100 μg boluses) given through the guiding catheter (for slow reflow) or through an infusion catheter or the distal lumen of the balloon catheter (for no reflow).[49] The no-reflow phenomenon may sometimes be prevented by early administration of platelet glycoprotein IIb/IIIa inhibitors (abciximab) or by preadministation of adenosine or verapamil.[50] Caution should be used in stenting lesions with no reflow, because poor run-off may increase the likelihood of stent thrombosis.

【 】 CATHETERIZATION LABORATORY COMPLICATIONS

With increasing operator experience, improved equipment and patient selection, and the availability of stents, major catheterization laboratory complications with primary PCI have become

TABLE 38-4

Acute Catheterization Laboratory Complications with Primary Angioplasty (PTCA) and Primary Stenting from the Stent PAMI Trial[15]

COMPLICATION	STENT (N = 451) (%)	PTCA (N = 448) (%)	COMBINED (N = 899) (%)
Laboratory death	0.2	0	0.1
Emergency bypass surgery	0.2	0.2	0.2
Cardiac arrest			
Ventricular tachycardia/fibrillation[a]	3.1	4.7	3.9
Cardiopulmonary resuscitation[b]	0.9	0.4	0.7
Intubation	0.2	0.7	0.4
Asystole/Bradycardia[c]	9.3	8.5	8.9
Sustained hypotension[d]	7.8	8.3	8.0

[a]Requiring electric cardioversion.
[b]Requiring chest compression.
[c]Requiring atropine or temporary pacing.
[d]Requiring vasopressors or intra-aortic balloon counterpulsation.

infrequent. Acute catheterization laboratory complications from the Stent PAMI trial in nonshock patients are shown in Table 38-4.[15] Laboratory death and emergency bypass surgery for failed PCI are rare. Ventricular tachycardia or fibrillation, asystole and bradycardia (including second- and third-degree atrioventricular block), and hypotension are the most common complications and often occur immediately after reperfusion. With increased operator experience and with anticipation, these complications can usually be managed effectively and often prevented.

[ ] MANAGEMENT OF CARDIOGENIC SHOCK

The management of patients with cardiogenic shock remains one of the great challenges in the treatment of AMI. Dopamine or noradrenaline (when necessary) should be initiated in the emergency department to maintain adequate arterial pressure and prevent neurologic and renal sequelae. Arterial oxygen saturation should be monitored, and mechanical ventilation should be initiated when needed. Ventricular tachycardia and fibrillation should be promptly treated with DC cardioversion and intravenous amiodarone.

On arrival to the catheterization laboratory, an intra-aortic balloon pump should be placed immediately. Although no randomized trials have been performed, observational studies have documented the benefit of this approach.[51,52] A pulmonary artery catheter should generally be placed early to help guide the management of intravascular volume and exclude hypovolemia as a contributing cause of hypotension. Left ventriculography should be performed to assess regional and global left ventricular function and to evaluate for mechanical causes of shock. If ventricular septal rupture, papillary muscle rupture with severe mitral regurgitation, or subacute free wall rupture are noted, urgent surgery is generally indicated. Shock resulting from right ventricular infarction can be identified by occlusion of the proximal right coronary artery, preserved left ventricular function, absence of mechanical

complications, and elevation of right atrial pressure. This complication is treated with intravenous fluids, vasopressors, and usually intra-aortic balloon pumping in addition to mechanical reperfusion of the infarct artery.

In most patients, cardiogenic shock results from severe left ventricular dysfunction with left ventricular pump failure. Primary PCI of the infarct artery is performed similar to nonshock patients, but reperfusion rates (TIMI 3 flow) are substantially lower compared with those in nonshock patients (77% vs 94%; $P = .001$),[53] possibly related to poor systemic and coronary perfusion pressure and altered plaque characteristics in shock patients. Observational data suggest that the use of stents and glycoprotein IIb/IIIa inhibitors may improve outcomes with primary PCI in shock patients.[54–56] If shock remains refractory after treatment with intra-aortic balloon pumping and PCI of the infarct lesion, PCI of a critical lesion in a second or third vessel may sometimes provide hemodynamic improvement.

[ ] POST-PCI CARE

Post-procedure care has been standardized in the Stent PAMI and CADILLAC trials.[10,15] Following the interventional procedure, heparin should be held until the ACT is less than 170 seconds, at which time the sheath should be removed. Heparin should not be routinely resumed except perhaps in patients who undergo balloon angioplasty only and do not receive a glycoprotein IIb/IIIa inhibitor.[57] In these patients heparin may be resumed 2 hours after sheath removal without a bolus, continued for 48 hours, decreased to one-half dose for 12 hours to prevent a rebound hypercoagulable state, and then discontinued.

Low-risk patients can be transferred from the catheterization laboratory directly to the subacute unit and can be targeted for discharge on day 2 or 3 (day 0 = day of admission).[27] Aspirin should be given routinely, and clopidogrel should be used in

TABLE 38-5

Randomized Trials Evaluating Rescue PCI for Failed Fibrinolysis

	CONTROL (%)	RESCUE PCI (%)	REPEAT LYTICS	P VALUE
RESCUE Trial (n = 151)[60]				
Death	9.6	5.1		.18
CHF	7.0	1.3		.11
Death or CHF	16.6	6.4		.05
MERLIN Trial (n = 136)[60a]				
Death	19.3	16.2		.60
Reinfarction	12.9	5.4		.10
Stroke	1.6	6.8		.20
TVR	22.6	5.4		.003
CHF	38.7	29.7		.30
Composite	62.9	48.6		.09
REACT Trial (n = 427)[60b]				
Death	12.8	6.2	12.7	.12
Reinfarction	8.5	2.1	10.6	<.01
Stroke	0.7	2.1	0.7	.63
CHF	7.8	4.9	7.0	.58
Composite	29.8	15.3	31.0	<.01

stented patients for year.[46a,46b] Beta-blockers, angiotensin-converting enzyme (ACE) inhibitors, and statins should be given according to current standards. Patients who develop symptoms or electrocardiographic changes of recurrent ischemia or reinfarction should undergo emergency repeat catheterization and intervention when indicated.

RESCUE PCI

Rescue PCI is the mechanical reopening of an infarct artery after unsuccessful fibrinolytic therapy. Rescue PCI should be differentiated from facilitated PCI (described later), which is the use of pharmacologic therapy followed by planned emergent PCI. Rescue PCI is generally not planned. With current fibrinolytic therapy, successful reperfusion (TIMI 3 flow) is achieved in only 55% to 60% of patients.[7] Consequently, almost half of patients who undergo fibrinolytic therapy may be candidates for rescue PCI.

【 】 EVIDENCE SUPPORTING RESCUE PCI

In the initial experience with rescue PCI procedural outcomes were often suboptimal, but with the introduction of stents and platelet inhibitors procedural outcomes have improved, and there are now several randomized trials documenting improved outcomes with rescue PCI (Table 38–5).[58,59,60,60a,60b] The RESCUE (Randomized Evaluation of Salvage Angioplasty with Combined Utilization of Endpoints) Trial Investigators randomized 151

patients with first anterior wall myocardial infarction treated with fibrinolytic therapy who had an occluded infarct artery within 8 hours of symptom onset to rescue PCI versus conservative care.[60] The rescue PCI group had a lower composite event rate of death or congestive heart failure and better exercise left ventricular ejection fraction (43 vs. 38%, P = .04). These benefits occurred despite the fact that stents were not yet available and despite, what the authors felt, was a strong investigator bias not to randomize patients presenting very early in the course of their infarction. The MERLIN (Middlesbrough Early Revascularization to Limit Infarction) Trial Investigators randomized patients with STEMI and failed thrombolysis (<50% ST-segment resolution at 60 minutes) to rescue PCI versus conservative care.[60a] There was no difference in 30-day mortality (the primary endpoint), but event-free survival was better with rescue PCI (P = .02). The REACT (Rescue Angioplasty versus Conservative Treatment or Repeat Thrombolysis) Trial randomized patients with STEMI and failed fibrinolysis (<50% ST-segment resolution at 90 minutes) to rescue PCI, repeat fibrinolysis or conservative care.[60b] Patients treated with rescue PCI had a lower incidence of the composite endpoint (death, re-infarction, stroke, or heart failure) than patients treated with either repeat fibrinolytic therapy or conservative care.

【 】 USE OF GLYCOPROTEIN IIB/IIIA PLATELET INHIBITORS IN RESCUE PCI

The use of glycoprotein IIb/IIIa platelet inhibitors with rescue PCI is controversial.[61–64,64a] Small observational studies have suggested better

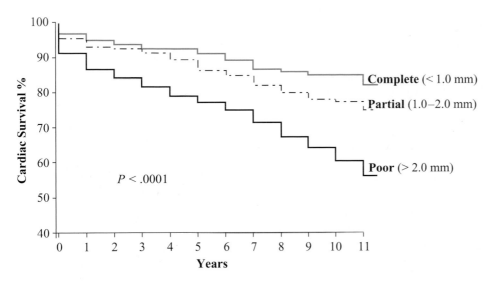

FIGURE 38-6. Actuarial survival curves for patients with complete, partial, and poor ST-segment resolution following primary PCI for acute myocardial infarction.[71]

outcomes with IIb/IIIa inhibitors, but the risk of bleeding when IIb/IIIa inhibitors are used in conjunction with thrombolytic therapy, aspirin, and heparin is high.[65,66] There are no randomized data evaluating IIb/IIIa inhibitors with rescue PCI. A reasonable approach may be to use IIb/IIIa inhibitors with rescue PCI in high risk patients (anterior infarction, Killip class 3–4) who have a low risk of bleeding (eg, avoid elderly patients, low weight patients, and possibly women).

[ ] DETECTION OF FAILED THROMBOLYSIS

A major limitation of the rescue PCI approach is the lack of a reliable noninvasive method to detect reperfusion after thrombolytic therapy. The electrocardiogram is very specific in predicting patency of the infarct artery when there is complete (> 70%) resolution of ST-segment elevation, but this occurs in only a minority of patients.[67] In most patients there is partial or no resolution of ST-segment elevation, and the patency status of the infarct artery is uncertain. Consequently, acute angiography is often required to determine infarct artery patency.

Based on data from the randomized trials described above, acute angiography with rescue PCI should be considered in patients with STEMI who are thought to have failed thrombolysis, as evidenced by persistent chest pain, lack of resolution of ST-segment elevation, or hemodynamic compromise persisting more than 90 minutes after treatment.

FUTURE DIRECTIONS

[ ] BEYOND TIMI FLOW: OPTIMIZING MICROVASCULAR REPERFUSION

Primary PCI is effective in restoring normal epicardial coronary flow (TIMI 3 flow) in more than 90% of patients with AMI, but more than half of these patients will have suboptimal flow at the tissue level as evidenced by suboptimal myocardial contrast by echocardiography, poor angiographic blush scores, or lack of complete electrocardiographic ST-segment resolution.[68–70] Although achieving TIMI 3 flow in the epicardial coronary artery is important, optimal outcomes with reperfusion therapy also require optimum reperfusion of the microvasculature or optimum myocardial reperfusion[71] (Figure 38-6).

One potential cause for suboptimal myocardial reperfusion is distal embolization of thrombus and fragments of atherosclerotic plaque at the time of PCI, resulting in obstruction of the distal microcirculation. The role of platelet glycoprotein IIb/IIIa inhibitors in preventing distal embolization and enhancing microvascular reperfusion has been controversial. Abciximab was shown to improve ST-segment resolution in the ACE trial,[26] but the large CADILLAC (Controlled Abciximab and Device Investigation to Lower Late Angioplasty Complications) trial did not find any benefit from abciximab in improving ST-segment resolution or angiographic blush scores.

There have been great expectations that distal protection devices may enhance microvascular reperfusion and improve outcomes in patients with AMI. The GuardWire (Medtronic PercuSurge, Sunnyvale, CA) has been shown to be effective in reducing distal embolization during elective PCI of saphenous vein grafts[72] and has recently been evaluated in patients with AMI in the EMERALD (Enhance Myocardial Efficacy and Recovery by Aspiration of Liberalized Debris) trial (Figure 38-7). Unfortunately, the EMERALD trial failed to show any improvement in microvascular reperfusion or reduction in infarct size with the GuardWire (see also Chapter 36).[73]

Thrombus plays a major role in the pathogenesis of AMI and can result in distal embolization as well as compromising procedural results. The AngioJet Rheolytic Thrombectomy Catheter (Possis Medical, Minneapolis, MN) is currently approved for thrombus removal and is commonly used to treat thrombotic lesions during PCI. The AiMI (AngioJet Rheolytic Thrombectomy in Patients Undergoing Primary Angioplasty for Acute MI) trial recently evaluated the role of thrombectomy in improving outcomes in patients undergoing primary PCI for STEMI.[73a] Unfortunately, thrombectomy did not improve myocardial blush or ST-segment resolution and, surprisingly, was associated with slightly larger infarct size (12.5% vs 9.8% $P = .02$). Consequently, thrombectomy is not recommended for routine use with primary PCI, although there may be a role for thrombectomy in patients with large thrombus burden.

[ ] REPERFUSION INJURY

There is evidence that deleterious effects to the myocardium, other than from distal embolization, may occur at the time of reperfusion resulting in suboptimal myocardial reperfusion. The pathogenesis of this reperfusion injury is poorly understood but may be related to a complement-dependent inflammatory response, to the formation of oxygen free radicals, or to several other mechanisms.

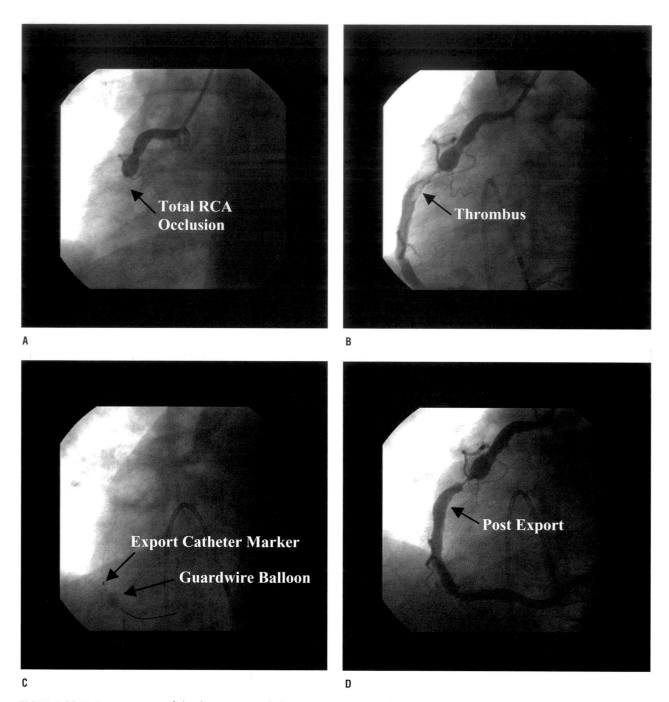

FIGURE 38-7. Demonstration of distal protection with the PercuSurge system during primary PCI for acute myocardial infarction. **A.** Total occlusion of the right coronary artery (RCA). **B.** Thrombus evident in the RCA after crossing with the GuardWire. **C.** Aspiration thrombectomy with the Export catheter while distal protection is achieved with inflation of the GuardWire balloon. **D.** Most of the thrombus is removed. **E.** Stent deployment with distal protection. **F.** Aspiration thrombectomy with the Export catheter while distal protection is maintained with the GuardWire. **G.** Final result with a widely patent artery and TIMI 3 flow. **H.** Demonstration of grade 3 myocardial blush.

Trials evaluating agents to reduce reperfusion injury have generally been disappointing, but several studies have shown promise. Adenosine could potentially reduce reperfusion injury by suppressing free radical formation and by preventing neutrophil activation. AMISTAD I (Acute Myocardial Infarction Study of Adenosine) found a 33% reduction in infarct size in patients with anterior wall infarction treated with adenosine, but no benefit in inferior infarction.[74] AMISTAD II, which evaluated only patients with anterior wall infarction, found a trend toward reduction in infarct size and clinical events at 6 months with adenosine, and, in the subgroup of patients with successful reperfusion, found a significant reduction in clinical events at 6 months.[75] In another reperfusion injury trial, the investigational complement inhibitor, pexelizumab (Alexian Pharmaceuticals and Proctor and Gamble),

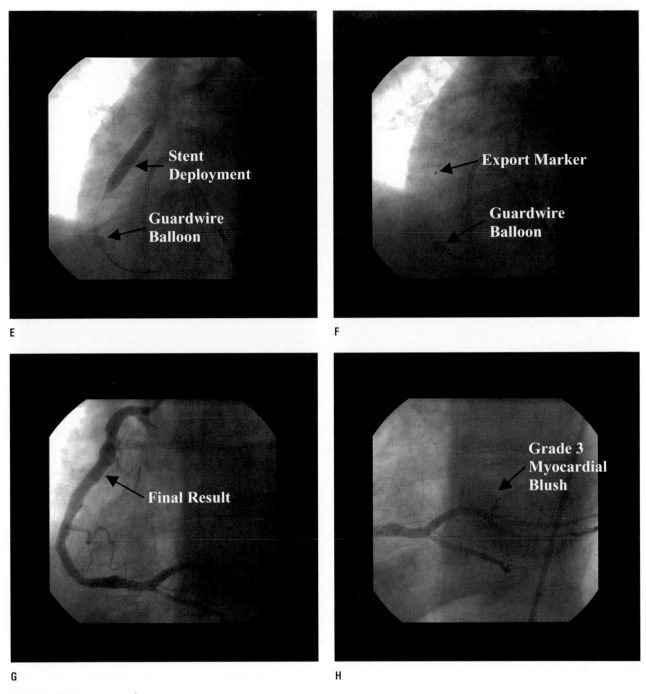

FIGURE 38-7. (continued)

showed a surprising mortality benefit in patients with AMI treated with primary PCI.[76] This surprising result occurred despite no reduction in infarct size, and has raised questions regarding the potential mechanisms of this mortality benefit.

These results have stimulated the initiation of the large APEX trial which was designed to evaluate the effect of pexelizumab on survival in patients with STEMI undergoing primary PCI. Unfortunately, the study was stopped early for financial reasons, but the results, which are not currently available, may still provide useful information. Systemic hypothermia initiated prior to reperfusion may potentially reduce reperfusion injury. New cooling systems have been developed using catheters with coils placed in the inferior vena cava via the femoral vein through which cold saline is circulated. These systems can provide rapid cooling and have been evaluated in the COOL MI (Hypothermia as an Adjunctive Therapy to PCI in Patients with Acute Myocardial Infarction) and ICE-IT (Intravascular Cooling AdjunctivE to Percutaneous Coronary InTervention) Trials.[76a,76b,77] Neither trial met its primary endpoint (reduction in infarct size) but both trials suggested that hypothermia reduced infarct size in patients with anterior infarction who are cooled to target temperature prior to reperfusion. Currently, COOL MI-2 is evaluating the effects of

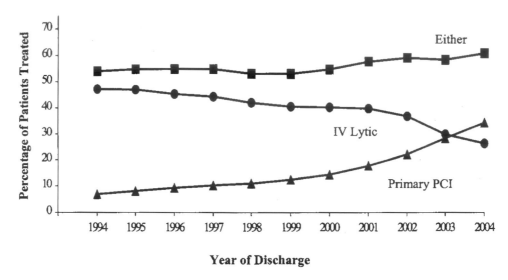

FIGURE 38-8. Temporal trends in the use of reperfusion therapy for patients with ST-elevation acute myocardial infarction of less than 12 hours' duration. (*Presented by Dr William French at Transcatheter Therapeutics (TCT), Washington, DC, 2005*).

systemic hypothermia in patients with anterior infarction who are cooled to target temperatures prior to reperfusion.

【 】 FACILITATED PCI

Most patients with AMI present to hospitals without interventional facilities, and the time delay required to transfer patients for primary PCI has led to a great deal of interest in pharmacologic reperfusion combined with mechanical reperfusion or facilitated PCI. Facilitated PCI is the use of pharmacologic therapy to establish reperfusion as rapidly as possible followed by immediate PCI to maximize TIMI 3 flow rates and to stabilize the ruptured plaque. Several pieces of evidence suggest that facilitated PCI may prove to be beneficial. Patients undergoing primary PCI for AMI who arrive at the catheterization laboratory with an open versus closed infarct artery have higher procedural success rates, better recovery of left ventricular function, and lower early and late mortality.[78,79] Pharmacologic agents used in facilitated PCI trials (half-dose thrombolytic agents plus platelet glycoprotein IIb/IIIa inhibitors) have been shown to be synergistic with PCI. Unfotunately, the ASSENT-4 PCI (Assessment of the Safety and Efficacy of a New Treatment Strategy with Percutaneous Coronary Intervention) trial, which randomized patients to tenecteplase-facilitated PCI versus PCI alone found a higher incidence of death, reinfarction, and stroke with facilitated PCI.[79a] In a recent meta-analysis performed by Keeley and Grines, facilitated PCI using lytic therapy or combination therapy also was associated with higher rates of death, reinfarction, stroke and bleeding compared with primary PCI alone.[79b] Consequently, facilitated PCI cannot be currently recommended as a reperfusion strategy. Facilitated PCI would be expected to help most in patients who present early after the onset of symptoms and who have long delays to PCI. It is possible that facilitated PCI may be helpful in these patients when adequate platelet inhibition is used, but this remains to be proven in randomized trials. The FINESSE Trial, which is ran-

domizing patients to facilitated PCI with half-dose reteplase plus abciximab or abciximab alone versus primary PCI alone, will provide further data that may help define the role of facilitated PCI with STEMI.

【 】 NEW ANTICOAGULANTS AND DRUG-ELUTING STENTS

Unfractionated heparin is the current standard of care for anticoagulation with primary PCI for AMI. Low-molecular-weight heparin has been found to be superior to unfractionated heparin in some studies and equivalent in other studies in high risk acute coronary syndromes but has not been studied extensively with primary PCI for STEMI. Bivalirudin (Angiomax), a direct thrombin inhibitor, recently was found to have equivalent efficacy with less bleeding compared with unfractionated heparin in high risk patients with unstable angina and NSTEMI most of whom were pretreated with clopidogrel in the ACUITY (Acute Catheterization and Urgent Intervention Triage Strategy) trial.[79c] Bivalirudin is currently being compared with heparin plus IIb/IIIa inhibition in STEMI patients in the HORIZONS trial.

CONCLUSION

Mechanical reperfusion therapy has become the preferred reperfusion strategy for patients with STEMI when it can be performed by skilled operators in a timely fashion. Outcomes have improved with the use of stents, platelet inhibitors, and with increased experience, and there is promise that outcomes can become even better with new methods to enhance *myocardial* reperfusion and reduce reperfusion injury and with new anticoagulants and drug-eluting stents. Recent treands from the National Registry of Myocardial Infarction (NRMI) have shown that the frequency of use of primary PCI has increased and has surpassed lytic therapy, but primary PCI is still only used to treat a minority of patients with STEMI[80] (Fig. 13–8). The major challenge for clinicians in the next decade will be to find new ways to make mechanical reperfusion more available, especially for patients presenting at noninterventional hospitals. The American Heart Association has accepted this challenge and has launched a nationwide effort to reduce door-to-balloon times at interventional and noninterventional hospitals with the goal of making primary PCI more available to patients with STEMI.

REFERENCES

1. Keeley EC, Boura JA, Grines CL. Primary angioplasty vs. intravenous thrombolytic therapy for acute myocardial infarction, a quantitative review of 23 randomized trials. *Lancet.* 2003;361:13.

2. Fibrinolytic Therapy Trialists' (FTT) Collaborative Group. Indications for fibrinolytic therapy in suspected acute myocardial infarction: Collaborative overview of early mortality and major morbidity results from all randomized trials of more than 1000 patients. *Lancet.* 1994;343:311.

3. Grines CL, Ellis S, Jones M, et al. Primary coronary angioplasty vs. thrombolytic therapy for acute myocardial infarction: Long term follow up of ten randomized trials [abstract]. *Circulation.* 1999;100:I-499.

4. Hochman JS, Sleeper LA, Webb JG, et al. Early revascularization in acute myocardial infarction complicated by cardiogenic shock. *N Engl J Med.* 1999;341:625.

5. Garcia E, Elizaga J, Perez-Castellano N, et al. Primary angioplasty vs. systemic thrombolysis in anterior myocardial infarction. *J Am Coll Cardiol.* 1999;33:605.

6. de Boer M-J, Ottervanger JP, van't Hof AW, et al. Reperfusion therapy in elderly patients with acute myocardial infarction: A randomized comparison of primary angioplasty and thrombolytic therapy. *J Am Coll Cardiol.* 2002;39:1729.

7. GUSTO Angiographic Investigators. The effects of tissue plasminogen activator, streptokinase, or both, on coronary artery patency, ventricular function, and survival after acute myocardial infarction. *N Engl J Med.* 1993;329:1615.

8. Stone GW, O'Neill WW, Jones B, et al. The central unifying concept of TIMI-3 flow after primary PTCA and thrombolytic therapy in acute myocardial infarction [abstract]. *Circulation.* 1996;94(suppl I):I-515.

9. Antman EM, Giugliano RP, Gibson CM, et al. Abciximab facilitates the rate and extent of thrombolysis: Results of the thrombolysis in myocardial infarctions (TIMI) 14 trial. *Circulation.* 1999;99:2720.

10. Stone GW, Grines CL, Cox DA, et al. Comparison of angioplasty with stenting, with or without abciximab, in acute myocardial infarction. *N Engl J Med.* 2002;346:957.

11. The GUSTO V Investigators. Reperfusion therapy for acute myocardial infarction with fibrinolytic therapy or combination reduced fibrinolytic therapy and platelet glycoprotein IIb/IIIa inhibition: The GUSTO V randomized trial. *Lancet.* 2001;357:1905.

12. The ASSENT-3 Investigators. Efficacy and safety of tenecteplase in combination with enoxaparin, abciximab, or unfractionated heparin: ASSENT-3 randomized trial in acute myocardial infarction. *Lancet.* 2001;358:605.

13. Nunn CM, O'Neill WW, Rothbaum D, et al. Long-term outcome after primary angioplasty: Report from the primary angioplasty in myocardial infarction (PAMI-1) trial. *J Am Coll Cardiol.* 1999;33:640.

14. Zijlstra F, Hoorntje JCA, de Boer M-J, et al. Long-term benefit of primary angioplasty as compared with thrombolytic therapy for acute myocardial infarction. *N Engl J Med.* 1999;341:1413.

15. Grines CL, Cox DA, Stone GW, et al. for the stent primary angioplasty in myocardial infarction study group. Coronary angioplasty with or without stent implantation for acute myocardial infarction. *New Engl J Med.* 1999;341:1949.

16. Brodie BR, Grines CL, Ivanhoe R, et al. Six month clinical and angiographic follow-up after direct angioplasty for acute myocardial infarction: Final results from the primary angioplasty registry. *Circulation.* 1994;25:156.

17. Veen G, de Boer M-J, Zijlstra F, et al. Improvement in three-month angiographic outcome suggested after primary angioplasty for acute myocardial infarction (Zwolle Trial) compared with successful thrombolysis (APRICOT Trial). *Am J Coll Cardiol.* 1999;84:763.

18. White HD, French JK, Hamer AW, et al. Frequent re-occlusion of patent infarct-related arteries between four weeks and one year: Effects of antiplatelet therapy. *J Am Coll Cardiol.* 1995;25:218.

19. Brouwer MA, van den Bergh PJ, Aengevaeren WR, et al. Aspirin plus coumarin versus aspirin alone in the prevention of reocclusion after fibrinolysis for acute myocardial infarction: Results of the antithrombotics in the prevention of reocclusion in coronary thrombolysis (APRICOT-2) trial. *Circulation.* 2002; 106:659.

20. Schömig A, Kastrati A, Dirschinger J, et al. Coronary stenting plus platelet glycoprotein IIb/IIIa blockade compared with tissue plasminogen activator in acute myocardial infarction. *N Engl J Med.* 2000;343:385.

21. Kastrati A, Mehilli J, Dirschinger J, et al. Myocardial salvage after coronary stenting plus abciximab vs. fibrinolysis plus abciximab in patients with acute myocardial infarction: A randomized trial. *Lancet.* 2002;359:920.

21a. Spaulding C. Final results of the TYPHOON study, a multi-center randomized trial comparing the use of sirolimus-eluting stents to bare metal stents in primary angioplasty for acute myocardial infarction. Presented at the American College of Cardiology Scientific Sessions, Atlanta, Georgia, March 2006.

21b. Dirksen MT. Randomized comparison of paclitaxel eluting stent versus conventional stent in ST-segment elevation myocardial infarction: Results of the PASSION trial. Presented at the American College of Cardiology Scientific Sessions, Atlanta, Georgia, March 2006.

21c. Brodie BR, Stuckey TD, Pulsipher M, et al. Stent thrombosis and target vessel revascularization following primary percutaneous coronary intervention with drug-eluting stents versus bare metal stents for ST elevation myocardial infarction. Results from the STENT registry. *J Am Coll Cardiol* 2006;47 (Suppl B): 41B.

22. Brener SJ, Barr LA, Burchenal JEB, et al. Randomized placebo-controlled trial of platelet glycoprotein IIb/IIIa blockade with primary angioplasty for acute myocardial infarction. *Circulation.* 1998;98:734.

23. Neumann FJ, Kastrati A, Schmitt C, et al. Effect of glycoprotein IIb/IIIa receptor blockade with abciximab on clinical and angiographic restenosis rate after the placement of coronary stents following acute myocardial infarction. *J Am Coll Cardiol.* 2000;35:915.

24. Montalescot G, Barragan P, Wittenberg O, et al. Platelet glycoprotein IIb/IIIa inhibition with coronary stenting for acute myocardial infarction. *N Engl J Med.* 2001;344:1895.

25. Tcheng JE, Kandzari DE, Grines CL, et al. Benefits and risks of abciximab use in primary angioplasty for acute myocardial infarction: The controlled abciximab and device investigation to lower late angioplasty complications (CADILLAC) trial. *Circulation.* 2003;108:1316.

26. Antoinucci D, Rodriquez A, Hempel A, et al. A randomized trial comparing primary infarct artery stenting with or without abciximab in acute myocardial infarction. *J Am Coll Cardiol.* 2003;42:1879.

26a. De Luca G, Suryapranata H, Stone GW, et al. Abciximab as adjunctive therapy to reperfusion in acute ST-segment elevation myocardial infarction: a meta-analysis of randomized trials. *JAMA* 2005;293:1759.

26b. Antman EM, Anbe DT, Armstrong PW, et al. ACC/AHA guidelines for the management of patients with ST-elevation myocardial infarction. ACC/AHA guidelines for the management of patients with ST-elevation myocardial infarction—executive summary: a report of the American College of Cardiology/American Heart Association Task Force on Practice Guidelines (Writing Committee to Revise the 1999 Guidelines for the Management of Patients With Acute Myocardial Infarction). *Circulation,* 2004;110:558. Etratum in: *Circulation.* 2005;111:2013.

27. Grines CL, Marsalese DL, Brodie BR, et al. Safety and cost-effectiveness of early discharge after primary angioplasty in low risk patients with acute myocardial infarction. *J Am Coll Cardiol.* 1998;31:967.

28. Stone GW, Brodie BR, Griffin JJ, et al, for the PAMI-2 Investigators. The role of cardiac surgery in the hospital phase management of patients treated with primary angioplasty for acute myocardial infarction. *Am J Cardiol.* 2000;85:1292.

29. Brodie BR, Stuckey TD, Hansen CJ, et al. Effect of treatment delay on outcomes in patients with acute myocardial infarction transferred from community hospitals for primary percutaneous coronary intervention. *Am J Cardiol.* 2002;89:1243.

30. Goldberg RJ, Mooradd M, Gurwitz JH, et al. Impact of time to treatment with tissue plasminogen activator on morbidity and mortality following acute myocardial infarction (the Second National Registry of Myocardial Infarction). *Am J Cardiol.* 1998;82:259.

31. Brodie BR, Stuckey TD, Wall TC, et al. Importance of time to reperfusion for 30-day and late survival and recovery of left ventricular function after primary angioplasty for acute myocardial infarction. *J Am Coll Cardiol.* 1998;32: 1312.

32. Brodie BR, Stone GW, Cox DA, et al. Impact of time to presentation, door-to-balloon time, and total reperfusion time on outcomes of primary percutaneous coronary intervention for acute myocardial infarction: The CADILLAC Trial. *Circulation.* 2006;151:1231.

33. Vermeer F, Oude Ophuis AJ, vd Berg EJ, et al. Prospective randomized comparison between thrombolysis, rescue PTCA, and primary PTCA in patients with extensive myocardial infarction admitted to a hospital without PTCA facilities: A safety and feasibility study. *Heart.* 1999;2:426.

34. Widimsky P, Groch L, Zelizko M, et al. Multi-center randomized trial comparing transport to primary angioplasty vs. immediate thrombolysis vs. combined strategy for patients with acute myocardial infraction presenting to a community hospital without a catheterization laboratory. *Eur Heart J.* 2000;21:823.

35. Grines CL, Westerhausen DR Jr, Grines LL, et al. A randomized trial of transfer for primary angioplasty vs. on-site thrombolysis in patients with high-risk myocardial infarction: The air primary angioplasty in myocardial infarction study. *J Am Coll Cardiol.* 2002;39:1713.

36. Andersen HR, Nielsen TT, Rasmussen K, et al. A comparison of coronary angioplasty with fibrinolytic therapy in acute myocardial infarction. *N Engl J Med.* 2003;349:733.

37. Widimsky P, Budesinsky T, Vorac D, et al. Long distance transport for primary angioplasty vs immediate thrombolysis in acute myocardial infarction. *Eur Heart J.* 2003;24:94.

37a. Nallamothu BK, Bates ER, Herrin J, et al. Times to treatment in transfer patients undergoing primary percutaneous coronary intervention in the United States: National Registry of Myocardial Infarction (NRMI)-3/4 analysis. *Circulation* 2005;111:718.

37b. Henry TD, Unger BT, Sharkey SW, et al. Design of a standardized system for transfer of patients with ST-elevation myocardial infarction for percutaneous coronary intervention. *Am Heart J* 2005;150:373.

37c. Bradley EH, Curry LA, Webster TR, et al. Achieving rapid door-to-balloon times: How top hospitals improve complex clinical systems. *Circulation* 2006;113:1079.

37d. Boersma E. The Primary Coronary Angioplasty vs. Thrombolysis (PACT)—M2 trialists' collaborative group. *Eur Heart J* 2006; 27:779–788.

37e. Brodie BR, Hansen C, Stuckey TD, et al. Door-to-balloon time with primary percutaneous coronary intervention for acute myocardial infarction impacts late cardiac mortality in high-risk patients and patients presenting early after the onset of symptoms. *J Am Coll Cardiol* 2006;47:289.

37f. Brodie BR, Stone GW, Cox DA, et al. Impact of treatment delays on outcomes of primary percutaneous coronary intervention for acute myocardial infarction: analysis from the CADILLAC trial. *Am Heart J* 2006; 151:1231.

37g. Gersh BJ, Stone GW, White HD, et al. Pharmacological facilitation of primary percutaneous coronary intervention for acute myocardial infarction. Is the slope of the curve the shape of the future? *JAMA* 2005;293:979.

37h. Assessment of the Safety and Efficacy of a New Treatment Strategy with Percutaneous Coronary Intervention (ASSENT-4 PCI) investigators. Primary versus tenecteplase-facilitated percutaneous coronary intervention in patients with ST–segment elevation acute myocardial infarction (ASSENT-4 PCI): randomized trial. *Lancet* 2006;367:569.

38. Steg PG, Bonnefoy E, Chabaud S, et al. Impact of time to treatment on mortality after prehospital fibrinolysis or primary angioplasty. *Circulation.* 2003;108:2851.

39. Aversano T, Aversano LT, Passamani E, et al. Thrombolytic therapy vs. primary percutaneous coronary intervention for myocardial infarction in patients presenting to hospitals without on-site cardiac surgery: A randomized control trial. *JAMA.* 2002;287:1943.

40. Wharton TP, Grines LL, Turco MA, et al. Primary angioplasty in acute myocardial infarction at hospitals with no surgery on-site (PAMI No SOS) versus transfer to surgical centers for primary angioplasty. *J Amer Coll Cardiol.* 2004;43:1943.

41. Antman EM, Anbe DT, Armstrong PW, et al. ACC/AHA guidelines for the management of patients with ST-elevation myocardial infarction. ACC/AHA guidelines for the management of patients with ST-elevation myocardial infarction—executive summary: a report of the American College of Cardiology/American Heart Association Task Force on Practice Guidelines (Writing Committee to Revise the 1999 Guidelines for the Management of Patients With Acute Myocardial Infarction). *Circulation,* 2004;110:558. Etratum in: *Circulation.* 2005;111:2013.

42. Reeder GS, Bailey KR, Gersh BJ, et al. Cost comparison of immediate angioplasty versus thrombolysis followed by conservative therapy for acute myocardial infarction: A randomized prospective trial. *Mayo Clin Proc.* 1994;69:5.

43. Stone G, Grines C, Rothbaum D, et al. Analysis of the relative cost and effectiveness of primary angioplasty vs. tissue type plasminogen activator: The Primary Angioplasty in Myocardial Infarction (PAMI) Trial. *J Am Coll Cardiol.* 1997;29:901.

44. Le May MR, Davies RF, Labinaz M, et al. Hospitalization costs of primary stenting versus thrombolysis in acute myocardial infarction. *Circulation.* 2003;108:2624.

45. Cohen DJ, Taira DA, Berezin R, et al. Cost-effectiveness of coronary stenting in acute myocardial infarctions: Results from the Stent PAMI Trial. *Circulation.* 2001;104:3039.

46. Bakhai A, Stone GW, Grines CL, et al. Cost-effectiveness of coronary stenting and abciximab for patients with acute myocardial infarction. *Circulation.* 2003;108:2857.

46a. Mehta SR, Yusuf S, Peters RJ, et al. Effects of pretreatment with clopidogrel and aspirin followed by long-term therapy in patients undergoing percutaneous coronary intervention: the PCI-CURE study. *Lancet* 2001;358:527.

46b. Steinhubl SR, Berger PB, Mann JT, et al. Early and sustained dual oral antiplatelet therapy following percutaneous coronary intervention: a randomized controlled trial. *JAMA* 2002;288:2411.

46c. Sabatine MS, Cannon CP, Gibson CM, et al. Effect of clopidogrel pretreatment before percutaneous coronary intervention in patients with ST-elevation myocardial infarction treated with fibrinolytics: the PCI-CLARITY study. *JAMA* 2005;294:1224.

47. Morishima I, Sone T, Okumura K, et al. Angiographic no-reflow phenomenon as a predictor of adverse long-term outcome in patients treated with percutaneous transluminal coronary angioplasty for first acute myocardial infarction. *J Am Coll Cardiol.* 2000;36:1202.

48. Mehta RH, Harjai KJ, Boura J, et al. Prognostic significance of transient no-reflow during primary percutaneous coronary intervention for ST-elevation acute myocardial infarction. *Am J Cardiol.* 2003;92:1445.

49. Taniyama Y, Ito H, Iwakura K, et al. Beneficial effect of intracoronary verapamil on microvascular and myocardial salvage in patients with acute myocardial infarction. *J Am Coll Cardiol.* 1997;30:1193.

50. Marzilli M, Orsini E, Marraccini P, et al. Beneficial effects of intracoronary adenosine as an adjunct to primary angioplasty in acute myocardial infarction. *Circulation.* 2000;101:2154.

51. Brodie BR, Stuckey TD, Hansen C, et al. Intra-aortic balloon counterpulsation before primary percutaneous transluminal coronary angioplasty reduces catheterization laboratory events in high risk patients with acute myocardial infarction. *Am J Cardiol.* 1999;84:18.

52. Chen EW, Canto JG, Parsons LS, et al. Relation between hospital intra-aortic balloon counterpulsation volume and mortality in acute myocardial infarction complicated by cardiogenic shock. *Circulation.* 2003;108:951.

53. Brodie BR, Stuckey TD, Muncy DB, et al. Importance of time-to-reperfusion in patients with acute myocardial infarction with and without cardiogenic shock treated with primary percutaneous coronary intervention. *Am Heart J.* 2003;145:708.

54. Zeymer U, Vogt A, Niederer W, et al. Primary PTCA with and without stent implantation in 671 patients with acute myocardial infarction complicated by cardiogenic shock. Results of the ALKK primary-PTCA registry. *J Am Coll Cardiol.* 2000;35:363A.

55. Antoniucci D, Valenti R, Migliorini, et al. Abciximab therapy improves survival in patients with acute myocardial infarction complicated by early cardiogenic shock undergoing coronary artery stent implantation. *Am J Cardiol.* 2002;90:353.

56. Chan AW, Chew DP, Bhatt DL, et al. Long-term mortality benefit with the combination of stents and abciximab for cardiogenic shock complicating acute myocardial infarction. *Am J Cardiol.* 2002;89:132.

57. Harjai KJ, Grines CL, Stone GW, et al. Does the use of heparin after primary angioplasty for acute myocardial infarction in patients not receiving glycoprotein IIb/IIIa antagonists alleviate recurrent cardiac ischemia? Insights from the CADILLAC study. *Am J Cardiol.* 2003;92:42L.

58. Mukherjee D, Ellis SG. "Rescue" angioplasty for failed thrombolysis. *Cleve Clin J Med.* 2000;67:341,345,349.

59. Califf RM, Topol EJ, Stack RS, et al. Evaluation of combination thrombolytic therapy and timing of cardiac catheterization in acute myocardial infarction: Results of thrombolysis and angioplasty in myocardial infarction-phase 5 randomized trial. *Circulation.* 1991;83:1543.

60. Ellis SG, da Silva ER, Heyndrickx G, et al. Randomized comparison of rescue angioplasty with conservative management of patients with early failure of thrombolysis for acute anterior myocardial infarction. *Circulation.* 1994; 90:2280.

60a. Sutton AGC, Campbell PG, Graham R, et al. A randomized trial of rescue angioplasty versus a conservative approach for failed fibrinolysis in ST-segment elevation myocardial infarction. *J Am Coll Cardiol,* 2004;44:287.

60b. Gershlick AH, Stephens-Lloyd A, Hughes S, et al. Rescue angioplasty after failed thrombolytic therapy for acute myocardial infarction. *N Engl J Med* 2005;353:2758.

61. Moreno R, Garcia E, Abeytua M, et al. Coronary stenting during rescue angioplasty after failed thrombolysis. *Catheter Cardiovasc Interv.* 1999;47:1.

62. Dirschinger J, Pocat J, Kastrati A, et al. Clinical outcome after rescue stenting in patients with acute myocardial infarction [abstract]. *J Am Coll Cardiol.* 1999;33(Suppl A):30A.

63. Miller JM, Smalling R, Ohman EM, et al. Effectiveness of early coronary angioplasty and abciximab for failed thrombolysis (reteplase or alteplase) during acute myocardial infarction (results from the GUSTO-III trial). Global Use of Strategies. To Open occluded coronary arteries. *Am J Cardiol.* 1999;84:779.

64. Petronio AS, Musumeci G, Limbruno U, et al. Abciximab improves 6-month clinical outcome after rescue coronary angioplasty. *Am Heart J.* 2002; 143:334.

64a. Gruberg L, Suleiman M, Kapeliovich M, et al. Glycoprotein IIb/IIIa inhibitors during rescue percutaneous coronary intervention in acute myocardial infarction. *J Invasive Cardiol* 2006;18:59.

65. Cantor WJ, Kaplan AL, Velianou JL, et al. Effectiveness and safety of abciximab after failed thrombolytic therapy. *Am J Cardiol.* 2001;87:439.

66. Jong P, Cohen EA, Batchelor W, et al. Bleeding risks with abciximab after full-dose thrombolysis in rescue or urgent angioplasty for acute myocardial infarction. *Am Heart J.* 2001;141:218.

67. Zeymer U, Schröder R, Molhoek P, et al. Non-invasive detection of early infarct vessel patency by resolution of ST-segment elevation in patients with thrombolysis for acute myocardial infarction; results of the angiographic substudy of the hirudin for improvement of thrombolysis (HIT)-4 trial. *Eur Heart J.* 2001;22:769.

68. Ito H, Maruyama A, Iwakura K, et al. Clinical implications of the 'no reflow' phenomenon: A predictor of complications and left ventricular remodeling in reperfused anterior wall myocardial infarction. *Circulation.* 1996; 93:223.

69. van 't Hof AWJ, Liem A, Suryapranata H, et al. Angiographic assessment of myocardial reperfusion in patients treated with primary angioplasty for acute myocardial infarction. *Circulation.* 1998;97:2302.

70. van 't Hof AWJ, Liem A, de Boer M-J, et al. Clinical value of 12-lead electrocardiogram after successful reperfusion therapy for acute myocardial infarction. *Lancet.* 1997;350:615.

71. Brodie BR, Stuckey TD, Kissling G, et al. Electrocardiographic ST-segment resolution is an independent predictor of late cardiac survival after primary percutaneous coronary intervention for acute myocardial infarction [abstract]. *Am J Cardiol.* 2002;90(suppl 6A):47H.

72. Baim DS, Wahr D, George B, et al. A randomized trial of a distal embolic protection device during percutaneous intervention in saphenous vein aortocoronary bypass grafts. *Circulation.* 2002;105:1285.

73. Ali A, Cox D, Dib N, et al. Rheolytic thrombectomy with percutaneous coronary intervention for infarct size reduction in acute myocardial infarction: 30 day results from a multicenter randomized study. *J Am Coll Cardiol* 2006;48:244.

74. Mahaffey KW, Puma JA, Barbagelata NA, et al. Adenosine as an adjunct to thrombolytic therapy for acute myocardial infarction: Results of a multi-center randomized, placebo controlled trial: The acute myocardial infarction study of adenosine (AMISTAD) trial. *J Am Coll Cardiol.* 1999;34:1711.

75. Ross A. Acute myocardial infarction study of adenosine (AMISTAD-II) [abstract]. *J Am Coll Cardiol.* 2002;39:338A.

76. Granger CB, Mahaffey KW, Weaver D, et al. Pexelizumab, an anti-C5 complement antibody, as adjunctive therapy to primary percutaneous coronary intervention in acute myocardial infarction. *Circulation.* 2003;108:1184.

76a. O'Neill WW. Hypothermia as an Adjunctive Therapy to PCI in Patients with Acute Myocardial Infarction. Presented at TCT (Transcatheter Therapeutics), Washington, DC, 2003.

76b. Grines C. Intravascular cooling adjunctive to percutaneous coronary intervention. Presented at TCT (Transcatheter Therapeutics), Washington, DC, 2004.

77. van der Horst ICC, Zijlstra F, van 't Hof AWJ, et al. Glucose-insulin-potassium infusion in patients treated with primary angioplasty for acute myocardial infarction. *J Am Coll Cardiol.* 2003;42:784.

78. Brodie BR, Stuckey TD, Hansen C, et al. Benefit of coronary reperfusion before intervention on outcomes after primary angioplasty for acute myocardial infarction. *Am J Cardiol.* 2000;85:13.

79. Stone GW, Cox D, Garcia E, et al. Normal flow (TIMI-3) before mechanical reperfusion therapy is an independent determinant of survival in acute myocardial infarction: Analysis from the primary angioplasty in myocardial infarction trials. *Circulation.* 2001;104:636.

79a. ASSENT-4 PCI Investigators. Primary versus tenecteplase-facilitated percutaneous coronary intervention in patients with ST-segment elevation acute myocardial infarction (ASSENT-4 PCI): Randomised trial. *Lancet* 2006;367:569.

79b. Keeley EC, Boura JA, Grines CL. Comparison of primary and facilitated percutaneous coronary intervention for ST-elevation myocardial infarction: Quantitative review of randomized trials. *Lancet* 2006;367:579.

79c. Stone GW. Prospective, randomized comparison of heparin plus IIb/IIIa inhibition and bivalirudin with or without IIb/IIIa inhibition in patients with acute coronary syndromes: The ACUITY Trial. Presented at the Annual Scientific Session of the American College of Cardiology, Atlanta, Ga, March, 2006.

80. Rogers WJ, Canto JG, Lambrew CT, et al. Temporal trends in the treatment of over 1.5 million patients with myocardial infarction in the U.S. from 1990 through 1999. *J Am Coll Cardiol.* 2000;36:2054.

CHAPTER (39)

Complex Lesion Intervention: Bifurcation, Left Main Coronary Artery, and Ostial Lesions

Seung-Jung Park, MD, PhD, and
Young-Hak Kim, MD

Lesions involving bifurcations, ostium, or the left main coronary artery have often been associated with increased procedural complications and poor long-term outcome owing to lesion complexity and technical difficulties. However, recent advancements in techniques and equipment make these lesions inviting targets for interventional cardiology. In this chapter, I offer procedural tips, describe published results, and project future perspectives on interventions involving such lesions.

INTERVENTION FOR BIFURCATION LESIONS

Although the treatment of bifurcation lesions has been reported to represent 4% to 16% of all percutaneous coronary intervention (PCI), it is a challenging area because of the increased risk of side-branch occlusion.[1] Moreover, occlusion of major side branches ($\geq$ 2.0 mm) represents a major cause of complications (non–Q-wave myocardial infarction) after stent placement. With the extensive use of coronary stents, high-pressure balloon dilation to maximize the lumen gain may compromise the flow in the side branches originating from the treated segment. In addition, the presence of a large atheromatous plaque at the site of bifurcation has been associated with deterioration (the so-called *snow-plow effect*) or even occlusion of the side branch after stent placement. The snow-plow effect represents the shifting of atheromatous plaque, resulting in occlusion of the side branch. Therefore, side-branch occlusion has been shown to be more frequent after stent placement than after balloon angioplasty.[2,3]

[ ] CLASSIFICATION OF BIFURCATION LESIONS

To facilitate PCI, bifurcation coronary lesions have been classified in terms of the angulation of the bifurcation and the plaque burden.[4] These factors may have an impact on both the technical approach and the immediate result.

In Y-shaped lesions (ie, side-branch and main-branch angulation < 70%), the risk of a snow-plow effect seems to be higher than in T-shaped lesions (ie, angulation > 70%). Furthermore, it is difficult to achieve the perfect coverage of the side-branch ostium using T-stenting. Conversely, T-shaped lesions are generally perfectly treated using T-stenting.

Location of the plaque burden is also crucial, and four main types of lesions have been described[4] (Figure 39-1). Type 1 lesions are defined as true bifurcation lesions involving the main branch, proximal and distal, and the ostium of the side branch. Type 2 lesions involve only the main branch at the bifurcation site and not the ostium of the side branch. Nevertheless, severe ostial stenosis or sometimes occlusion of the side branch as a result of the snow-plow phenomenon may be observed after stent implantation. Type 3 lesions are located in the main branch proximal to the bifurcation. They are frequently associated with a deterioration of the ostium of one or two branches when the stent is placed only at the site of the lesion proximal to the bifurcation. In type 4 lesions, only the ostium of each branch of the bifurcation is involved, and there is no proximal disease, whereas in type 4a and 4b lesions, the ostium of either the main (4a) or the side branch (4b) is involved. For all "pseudobifurcational" lesions (types 2 through 4), treating

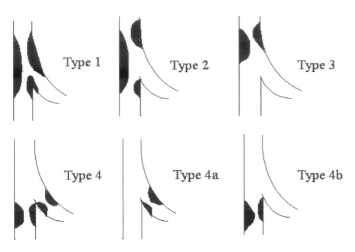

FIGURE 39-1. Classification of bifurcation lesions according to their morphology.

the main vessel often results in plaque shifting into the side branch, thus converting the original lesion into a true bifurcation lesion.

【 】 SIDE-BRANCH PROTECTION

When interventional cardiologists treat a bifurcation lesion with PCI, the vessel size of the side branch and the severity of the side-branch ostial stenosis should be considered. Side branches that are less than 2.0 mm in diameter and supply a small amount of viable myocardium are rarely considered for side-branch protection.[1] However, vessels with a lumen diameter of 2.5 mm or larger can be considered for the balloon dilation or stenting.[5] Although dedicated stents for vessels less than 2.5 mm are not often developed, small- to moderate-sized side branches (2.0–2.5 mm) also require careful planning in PCI.

The risk of side-branch occlusion has often been thought to depend on the severity of the side-branch ostial stenosis. For side branches that originate from the main branch, the risk of occlusion is lowest if the side branch contains an ostial stenosis less than 50%, intermediate if the side branch contains a nonostial stenosis

greater than 50%, and highest if the side branch contains an ostial stenosis greater than 50%. In one study, the risk of progressive narrowing was 12% if the side-branch ostial stenosis was 50% or less versus 41% if stenosis was greater than 50%.[6] Therefore, relatively large side branches ($\geq$ 2.5 mm in diameter) with severe (diameter stenosis $\geq$ 50%) narrowing of the side-branch ostial stenosis are considered for side protection with two-wire placement and specific treatment with elective balloon percutaneous transluminal coronary angiography (PTCA) or stenting.

【 】 BALLOON DILATION TECHNIQUE

Double Guidewire Placement

This approach involves placing two guidewires in the main branch and the side branch. The main advantage of this technique is that it maintains continuous access to both limbs of the bifurcation in the event acute closure occurs or balloon exchange is needed. This technique is also very useful in bifurcation stenting. In a side branch with ostial narrowing, predilation often decreases the risk of side-branch occlusion during main-branch stenting. Moreover, the "jailed" guidewire in the side branch can act as a marker of the occluded side branch, as well as straightening the angle between the side branch and the main branch to facilitate access after stent implantation in the main branch.

"Kissing" Balloon Dilation

Simultaneous "kissing" balloon dilation is preferable to prevent plaque shifting and snow-plow injury. By performing simultaneous inflations, adequate dilation of the proximal vessel can be achieved without oversizing the balloon relative to the smaller distal vessels. Moreover, kissing balloon inflation after stent placement in the bifurcation has been recommended to counteract any stent deformation.[4,5]

【 】 STENTING TECHNIQUES

Single Stent Placement Covering the Side Branch

The easiest way to treat a bifurcation lesion is to stent the main branch covering the ostium of the side branch (Figure 39-2). Although this treatment strategy may be very useful in type 2 and 3 bifurcation lesions involving normal side-branch ostium, it can also be used in lesions involving side-branch ostial stenosis after predilation in the side branch. In the event of significant flow impairment of the side branch after stent implantation in the main branch, treatment of the side branch should be performed. In moderate lesions (diameter stenosis < 70% to 80%) of the side branches that are associated with good flow, long-term patency and clinical outcome are excellent.[7,8] Therefore, treatment of such lesions with stent implantation should be resisted.

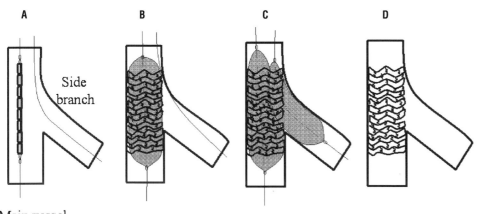

FIGURE 39-2. Single stent implantation covering the side branch. Stent implantation in the main vessel (**B**) was performed using the double-wire technique (**A**). After retrieval of the wire in the side branch a new wire is inserted into the side branch through the stent strut. Optional "kissing" balloon dilation can then be performed (**C**). Final result (**D**).

If significant flow impairment develops, a second wire should be crossed into the side branch for treatment. Kissing balloon dilation, described earlier, can be performed if required. Alternatively, implantation of a second stent may be performed if the result of kissing balloon dilation is suboptimal. If the decision to perform final kissing balloon dilation or second stent implantation is made, recrossing a new wire into the side branch is a mandatory step. The technique is sometimes very complex, and success is sometimes greater with a wire having a stiffer tip or a hydrophilic coating (Scimed Choice PT, Cordis Shinobi). If the wire recrossing is successful, balloon passage is another complex step. A very low-profile balloon should be selected to cross the stent strut, and stepwise balloon dilation may be required in some cases.

Because complex procedures using multiple stents for bifurcation lesions potentially require greater time, heavier metal component, and higher cost than single stent procedures, recent reports suggested that complex procedure have no long-term advantage over single stent implantation in the era of bare-metal stent implantation.[9,10] Pan and colleagues found that the rate of major adverse cardiac events (MACE) was higher in patients undergoing multiple stent implantation ($n = 23$) as compared with single stent implantation ($n = 47$) (75% vs 44%; $P < .05$).[9] Yamashita and colleagues reported similar results when they compared patients who received multiple stent implantation ($n = 53$) with those receiving single stent implantation ($n = 39$): Both in-hospital MACE (13% vs 0%; $P < .05$) and 6-month angiographic restenosis (62% vs 48%; $P = $ NS) were more common in the multiple stent group.[10]

Recent studies using a drug-eluting stent also showed that complex stenting may not be superior to simple stenting. Pan and colleagues[10a] evaluated outcomes of simple stenting ($n = 47$) versus complex stenting ($n = 44$) by a randomized study. Although they were not statistically different, restenosis rates of both the main vessel (2% vs 10%) and the side branch (5% vs 15%) tend to be lower in a simple stenting strategy than in a complex stenting strategy.

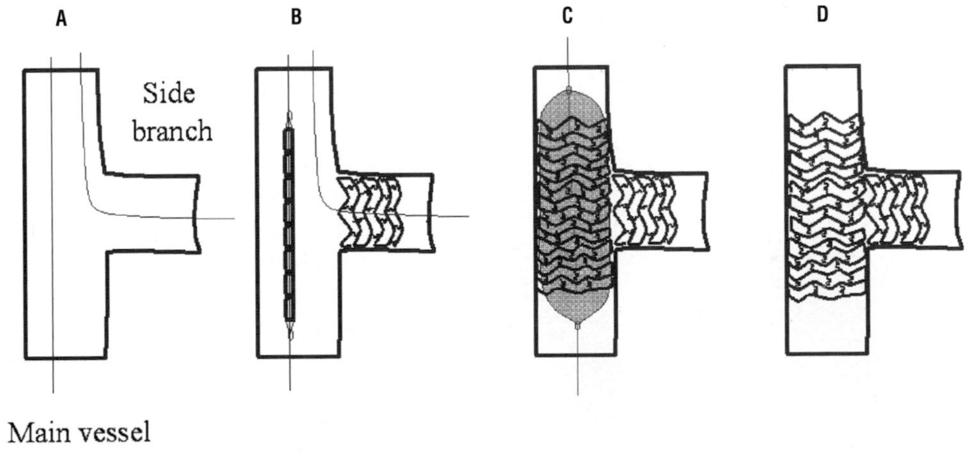

T-Stenting Technique

The technique of T-stenting is better suited to treat side branches that originate at an angle of 90 degrees or close to 90 degrees. The deployment of the two stents in the side branch and the main vessel can be performed in different phases. To avoid recrossing the stent strut in the main vessel, deployment of the side branch stent before that of the main vessel is preferred (Figure 39-3). This technique is safer and eliminates the difficulties involved in advancing the second stent through the first. However, this strategy also carries a risk of achieving incomplete coverage of the side branch ostium.

With the advent of drug-eluting stents, complete coverage of the entire diseased segment has become one of the most important technical considerations. The potential gap at the side branch ostium may create an easy target for recoil and late restenosis. Conversely, if the stent protrudes into the main vessel, further treatment of the artery may be difficult. The limitations of the T-stenting technique thus warrant development of new techniques using drug-eluting stents. The so-called *stent crush technique*, described later, is one example.

Sheiban and colleagues reported the initial and long-term results of T-stenting of 54 bifurcation lesions.[11] Despite achieving complete initial procedural success in both branches, the overall 6-month angiographic restenosis rate was 63% (27/43). Restenosis occurred in the main vessel, only, in 14% of patients, in the side branch, only, in 19%, and in both main vessel and side branch in 30%. In a comparison of T-stenting with other multiple stenting techniques, Al Suwaidi and colleagues noted a lower 1-year MACE rate in T-stenting ($n = 33$) than in Y-stenting (n = 19) (30.4% vs 86.3%; $P = .004$).[12] They surmised that the worse outcome seen in Y-stenting may be attributable to overlapped segments of stents and a greater frequency of trauma during stent deployment, possibly simulating the formation of neointimal hyperplasia. This hypothesis may also be applicable to the implantation of bare-metal stents in bifurcation lesions.

A recent nonrandomized study revealed that the T-stenting technique with drug-eluting stent might be associated with worse clinical outcomes compared to the crush technique, which was a new bifurcation stenting strategy with drug-eluting stent.[12a] At one year follow-up, the T-stenting technique ($n = 61$) required higher rate of target lesion revascularization compared to the crush technique ($n = 121$) (14.0% vs 31.1%, $P = 0.01$). They suggested that incomplete lesion coverage by the T-stenting might be related with worse clinical outcomes.

Y-Stents or "Culotte" Stenting Technique

As first introduced, the Y-stenting technique was a very complex procedure that involved implantation of stents in both branch ostia and a third stent in the main vessel, followed by a

FIGURE 39-3. T-stent implantation technique. The first stent is advanced into the side branch but not expanded, and a second stent is advanced into the main vessel, covering the ostium of the side branch. Covering the ostium of the side branch **(A)**. The first stent is carefully positioned at the ostium of the side branch or slightly within the main vessel and then dilated **(B)**. The balloon and wire are removed from the side branch, and the stent in the main vessel is deployed **(C)**. The side branch is then rewired, and "kissing" balloon dilation of both branches is performed. Final result **(D)**.

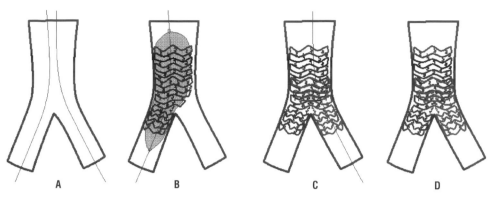

FIGURE 39-4. "Culotte" or inverted Y-stenting technique. After predilation, the wire is removed from the straighter branch and the more angulated branch is stented **(A,B)**. After removing the wire from the stented branch, a wire is recrossed through the stent strut. The stent strut should be dilated toward the nonstented branch with a balloon. A second stent is advanced and expanded into the nonstented branch **(C)**. The first stented branch is then rewired, and final "kissing" balloon inflation is performed. Final result **(D)**.

final kissing balloon dilation.[13] This technique was soon abandoned, replaced by modified techniques that include the so-called *inverted Y-stenting* or *"culotte" stenting.*

The "culotte" technique was first described by Chevalier and colleagues,[14] and it is summarized in Figure 39-4. In this technique, the more angulated branch is the first to be stented. However, if an important dissection or occlusion has occurred in one branch, implantation of a stent in that branch should be performed first, because wire removal might be risky.

This technique is useful for all angles of bifurcation lesions, and it can be applied when the initial plan to stent only one branch has resulted in deterioration of another branch. The potential limitations are the heavy metal component in the proximal part of the bifurcation and possible difficulties in advancing the wire through the stent strut several times. Two reports using this technique with bare-metal stents were not encouraging.[12,14]

These complex stenting techniques have also been used in drug-eluting stent implantation. However, the efficacy has not been elucidated.

"Kissing" Stents

This two-stent implantation technique, which is similar to kissing balloon inflation, is shown in Figure 39-5. A minimum 8 French (Fr) guiding catheter is needed for the procedure. The two stents are deployed simultaneously, which creates a double lumen in the main vessel proximal to the bifurcation site. Adjunctive sequential alternative balloon dilation with final kissing balloon dilation may be required to ensure optimal stent expansion, especially in the distal part of bifurcation. This technique is useful in bifurcation lesions that involve two large side branches, with a large diameter of the vessel proximal to the bifurcation. A practical concern when using the kissing stent technique is the difficulty of reaccessing both branches if restenosis occurs. If a wire passes through the proximal overlapped stent strut, subsequent balloon dilation may destroy the implanted stents. Because of this limitation, the kissing stent technique has not been widely used in bifurcation lesions. However, in the era of drug-eluting stents, it has been reintroduced as an appropriate stenting technique for bifurcation lesions with a very large proximal vessel to the bifurcation, such as left main bifurcation lesion.

Speed and ease of execution are two major advantages of this technique. The technique is very safe, because access to both branches is always maintained, and it allows complete lesion coverage.

Bifurcated Stents

Several bifurcated stents were developed in the late 1990s to provide complete coverage of bifurcation lesions. These included the Bard XT Carina stent (Billerica, MA), AVE bifurcation stent (Arterial Vascular Engineering, Santa Rosa, CA), and NIR Side Royal stent (Medinol, Tel Aviv, Israel). Preliminary studies using these bifurcated stent were reported[16,17]; however, the stents were not used widely due to procedural complexity and poor long-term outcomes.

The AST SLK-View Bifurcation Stent System (Advanced Stent Technologies, San Francisco, CA) was developed for use in bifurcation lesions. It incorporates a stainless-steel stent with a hole located between the proximal and distal section, as shown in Figure 39-6. The purpose of this hole is to allow access to the side branch vessel after deployment. The delivery system is constructed of a proximal dual lumen section; one lumen is skived away at this distal end and an inner member is inserted through that lumen and attached to a balloon. The second lumen is used to carry a moveable side

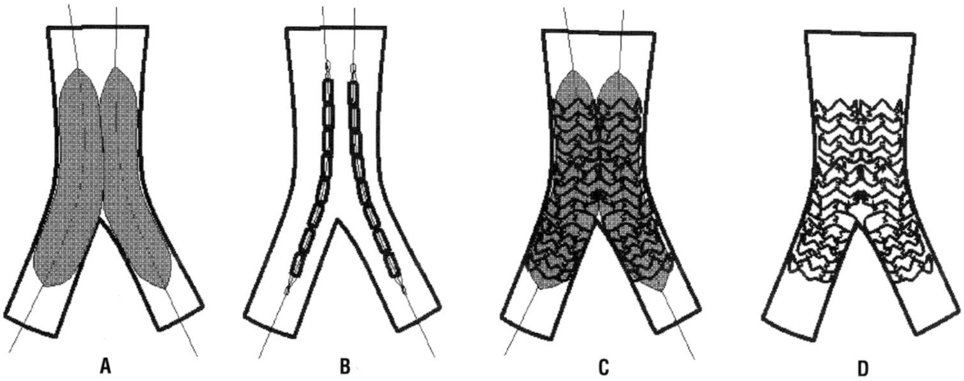

FIGURE 39-5. "Kissing" stenting technique. Both branches are wired and dilated **(A)**. The two unexpanded stents are positioned at the bifurcation with parallel proximal stent edges **(B)** and are then deployed simultaneously **(C)**. Final result **(D)**.

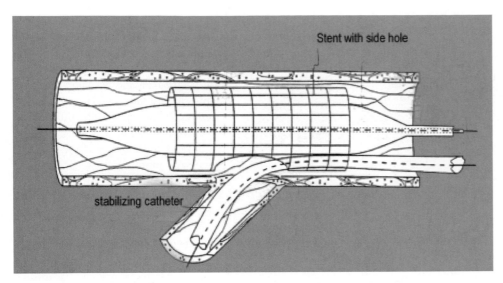

FIGURE 39-6. Stent design of the SLK-View Bifurcation Stent system. The main catheter system consists of a main stent with a side hole and a stabilizing catheter. This stent has an expandable side opening with a radiopaque marker. The illustration shows the expanded stent advanced on the two wires in both branches.

sheath. The SLK-View system has several advantages. The second lumen of its delivery system protects the ostium of the side branch during stent deployment, with the result that plaque shifting and protrusion are less likely to occur. Furthermore, because access to the side branch is easy and safe, without risk of destruction of the stent strut in the parent vessel, the additional treatment of the side branch can be performed optimally. Preliminary data using this stent system showed an excellent initial outcome.[18,19]

Ikeno and colleagues reported outcomes of multicenter experience with the SLK-View bifurcated stent.[19a] For 84 native bifurcation lesions, binary restenosis rate was 28.3% in the main vessel and 37.7% in the side branch, which were comparable to the previous studies using a bare metal stent. The addition of drug-eluting properties to the bifurcated stents is an investigational research method for overcoming the limitations of a simple drug-eluting stent for bifurcation lesions.

DEBULKING ATHERECTOMY

Directional coronary atherectomy (DCA) has unique advantages in the treatment of bifurcation coronary lesions because it removes atheromatous plaque, limiting both elastic recoil and plaque shifting. Analysis of data from the CAVEAT I (Coronary Angioplasty Versus Excisional Atherectomy) trial indicated a larger post-procedure lumen in main vessels when bifurcation lesions were treated with DCA as opposed to PTCA. The investigators also noted an increased risk of side-branch occlusion associated with an increase in small, non–Q-wave myocardial infarction and no difference in restenosis at 6 months.[20]

Furthermore, DCA followed by coronary stenting has been regarded as having a synergistic benefit, combining removal of atheromatous plaque and prevention of elastic recoil and remodeling. One nonrandomized control study showed that DCA followed by stenting (*n* = 31) decreased the incidence of 6-month restenosis compared with stenting alone (*n* = 31), but without statistical

significance (29% vs 44%; *P* = .13).[21] More recently, subgroup analysis of an unpublished, randomized Atherectomy before Multi-link Improves lumen Gain and clinical Outcomes (AMIGO) trial showed that debulking followed by stenting may be beneficial for bifurcation lesions. In this study, the 6-month angiographic restenosis rate was significantly lower in patients who received DCA followed by stenting (*n* = 45) than in those who received stenting alone (*n* = 43) (9.8% vs 20.9%; *P* < .05). To date, however, the benefit of debulking with or without stenting has not been evaluated by a large randomized study.

After the wide application of drug-eluting stent, use of debulking atherectomy has rapidly decreased by the remarkable reduction of restenosis by drug-eluting stent. However, the role of debulking in the future coronary intervention has to be evaluated further.

DRUG-ELUTING STENTS

Having produced excellent results in de novo coronary lesions,[22–24] drug-eluting stents are emerging as a promising therapeutic modality for bifurcation lesions. The US Multicenter, Randomized, Double Blind Study of the SIRolImUS-eluting stent in de novo native coronary lesions (SIRIUS) was a multicenter randomized trial to assess the safety and efficacy of sirolomUS-eluting stents for the treatment of bifurcation lesions.[25,25a] Eighty-five patients were randomly assigned to either stenting of both branches (group A) or stenting of the main branch with provisional stenting of the side branch (SB) (group B). By the high rate of crossover, ultimately, 63 patients and 22 patients were treated with two-stent implantation and single-stent implantation. The total restenosis rate at 6 months was not statistically different between the two groups A (28.0%) and B (18.7%). This study gave important information: (1) the drug-eluting stent significantly decreased the overall restenosis rate for bifurcation coronary lesions compared to the bare metal stent. (2) However, restenosis at the side branch remained a problem even in drug-eluting stent implantation. Therefore, a new bifurcation stenting technique such as the crush technique has been introduced to improve the outcomes of bifurcation interventions through complete lesion coverage with two stents overlapped.[26]

BIFURCATION STENTING WITH DRUG-ELUTING STENTS: MODIFIED T-STENTING TECHNIQUE WITH CRUSHING

This technique, introduced by Colombo and colleagues in 2003,[26] is illustrated in Figure 39-7. Both the side and main branches are wired and alternatively dilated. The first stent is advanced into the

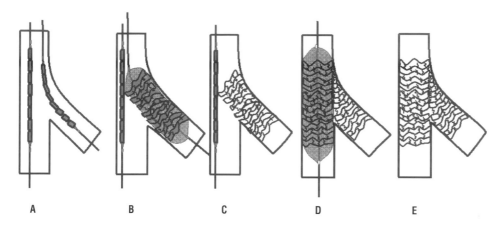

FIGURE 39-7. Modified T-stenting with crushing. A first stent is advanced into the side branch but not expanded, and a second stent is advanced into the main branch to cover fully the bifurcation **(A)**. At this time, the proximal marker of this stent in the main vessel is always more proximal in the coronary tree than the proximal marker of the stent for the side branch. When the side-branch stent is appropriately positioned, the balloon is inflated and the stent is deployed **(B)**. After stent implantation in the side branch, the delivery balloon and the wire are removed from the side branch **(C)**. The stent in the main branch is then expanded, and the protruding struts of the stent implanted in the side branch are crushed against the wall of the main vessel **(D)**. Final result **(E)**.

side branch but not expanded; then the second stent is advanced into the main branch to cover fully the bifurcation. The proximal marker of the side-branch stent must be situated in the main branch 4 to 5 mm proximal to the carina of the bifurcation. The stent in the side branch will protrude in the main branch. When the side-branch stent is appropriately positioned, the balloon is inflated and the stent is deployed. After stent implantation in the side branch, the delivery balloon and the wire are removed from the side branch. The stent in the main branch is then expanded. During balloon inflation and stent implantation in the main branch, the protruding struts of the stent implanted in the side branch are crushed against the wall of the main vessel. In this way, there are no floating struts; instead, there are three layers of struts in the proximal part of the bifurcation and near the ostium of the side branch.

This technique has demonstrated several advantages in the era of drug-eluting stents. First, it ensures the complete circumferential coverage of the side-branch ostium. Moreover, it may deliver a high dosage of rapamycin near the bifurcational site owing to the presence of multiple struts. A practical advantage is that the technique is quite safe and relatively simple to execute. It provides an immediate, successful result–patency of both branches–without particular technical difficulties.

One important concern when using this technique has been whether or not to perform a final kissing balloon dilation at the conclusion of the procedure. Recent experimental and clinical observations showed a clear benefit of final kissing balloon inflation in performing the crush technique.[26a, 26b] The implantation of final kissing balloon inflation allows better strut contact against the ostium of the side branch and therefore better drug delivery to the target lesions (reference 1 of the following references). Ge L et al showed that restenosis rate at the side branch was significantly decreased by final kissing inflation (11.1% vs 37.9%, $P < .001$). Thus, final kissing inflation was an independent predictor of target

lesion revascularization (hazard ratio 4.17; 95% confidence interval 1.14 to 2.80, $P = .001$).

Colombo and colleagues reported the immediate and 30-day outcome of this technique in 20 bifurcation lesions.[26] They performed final kissing balloon dilation in selected cases ($n = 7$) when the ostium of the side branch appeared unsatisfactory. The angiographic result was successful in all cases. In-hospital complications were as follows: one Q-wave myocardial infarction and two non–Q-wave infarctions. One patient with a Q-wave myocardial infarction developed acute procedural stent thrombosis, which was treated successfully with repeat intervention. During the 30-day follow-up period, no other major adverse cardiac events were noted.

CONCLUSION

The stenting technique for bifurcation lesions has improved considerably over the past decade. Several investigators have proposed many new techniques with a theoretical basis. Moreover, new bifurcated stents designed for treatment of specific bifurcation lesions have been developed by many manufacturers. However, use of these complex procedures and dedicated bifurcation stents did not dramatically decrease the restenosis rate until the emergence of drug-eluting stents. The introduction of these stents should overcome the primary limitation of the bare-metal stent, restenosis. Despite such advances, however, bifurcation lesions may remain a challenge to the interventional cardiologist. Further research to find the best approach for true bifurcation lesions using the current drug-eluting stents or a new dedicated bifurcated technique with a drug-eluting property is warranted.

INTERVENTION FOR UNPROTECTED LEFT MAIN CORONARY ARTERY STENOSIS

Several etiologies contribute to left main coronary artery (LMCA) stenosis (Table 39-1). Although LMCA stenosis might be considered an attractive target for balloon angioplasty because of its large caliber, short lesion length, and lack of tortuosity, the results initial procedures were not favorable, with a high rate of procedural complications and early mortality.[27–29] Histologically, the LMCA has the most elastic tissue of all the coronary vessels, accounting for the poor response of the LMCA to simple balloon angioplasty.

Use of coronary stents has been shown to reduce the immediate need for coronary artery bypass surgery (CABG) to treat abrupt vessel closure as well as the likelihood of restenosis after balloon angioplasty.[30] At present, new devices are widely used to overcome

TABLE 39-1

Etiology of Left Main Coronary Artery Disease

Atherosclerosis

Nonatherosclerotic Causes
    Idiopathic
    Radiation
    Takayasu arteritis
    Syphilitic aortitis
    Rheumatoid arthritis
    Aortic valve disease
    Kawasaki disease
    Injury after left main coronary intervention or cardiac
        surgery

the limitations of balloon angioplasty, and these may also be useful to treat unprotected LMCA stenosis in particular groups of patients. Thus, stenting of unprotected LMCA stenosis is, today, a therapeutic option in selected patients.[31–41e]

[ ] STENTING TECHNIQUES

Ostial Lesion

The ostial LMCA lesion is dilated and stented with the guide tip positioned in the aortic sinus. The proximal end of the stent is left protruding outside the ostium and expanded against the aortic wall, as in any standard stenting of an aorto-ostial lesion. My colleagues and I usually deploy the stent slightly to protrude into the aorta (1–2 mm) for treatment of LMCA ostial lesions. After the deployment of the stent, the stented segment is further dilated with high-pressure balloon inflation to achieve angiographic optimization. Slotted-tube stents are preferred over coil stents for LMCA ostial disease because of their strong radial force. Stent size is selected based on the reference artery size and lesion length. The balloon inflation is brief (< 30 seconds) and multiple (> 3 seconds) to avoid prolonged global ischemia and ischemia-related complications.

[ ] SHAFT LESION

The lesion at the midshaft can be predilated and then stented, as for any discrete lesion in other branches. As in the ostial LMCA lesion, a debulking procedure is also recommended in suitable lesions.

Bifurcation Lesion

Because of the technical difficulties, stenting for LMCA bifurcation disease should be restricted to highly skilled interventionalists working with patients who understand the risk/benefit ratio of the percutaneous approach. During the procedure, side-branch occlusion resulting from plaque shifting or stent strut can produce acute closure of the ostium of the left anterior descending artery or left circumflex artery. This can lead to disastrous clinical events.

In a group of 80 selected patients, my colleagues and I found that stenting with or without debulking for LMCA bifurcation stenosis was safe and technically feasible.[39] The stenting techniques used

were stenting across the left circumflex ostium, T (Y)-shaped stenting, kissing stenting, or bifurcation stenting. In this study, the left circumflex ostium was covered by a stent without risk of occlusion if it was diminutive or normal, showing that a small or nondiseased left circumflex artery in the vicinity of a stenotic lesion does not prohibit the use of a stent. Furthermore, 54% of patients were successfully treated with stent placement across the left circumflex ostium, suggesting that this technique may be widely applicable to the treatment of LMCA bifurcation lesions. However, progression of the side-branch lesion spanned by a stent may be difficult to treat, and a possible risk of side-branch occlusion remains an important limitation of this strategy.

[ ] INTRAVASCULAR ULTRASOUND

Intravascular ultrasound (IVUS) provides important quantitative and qualitative information about coronary artery lesions. It is often difficult to evaluate the actual size of the LMCA using angiography alone.[47] Often the left main trunk is short and lacks a normal segment for comparison. In addition, contrast in the aortic cusp sometimes obscure the ostium, and "streaming" of contrast may result in a false impression of luminal narrowing. Furthermore, angiography underestimates stenosis severity. IVUS before stenting, therefore, provides useful information about the selection of adequately sized balloons and stents. In one report, the accurate information on amounts and extent of calcification provided by IVUS contributed to a change in treatment modalities in 40% of non-LMCA lesions.[43] My colleagues and I documented negative remodeling (defined as external elastic membrane CSA of the lesion site less than that of the distal reference segment) in 91% in IVUS-guided stenting of ostial LMCA lesions.[34] In these cases of ostial lesions with negative remodeling and consequently small amounts of plaques volumes, the treatment strategies should be changed from debulking with stenting to stenting only. In addition, quantitative IVUS measurements should be used as guidelines of intervention. Although absolute ultrasound criteria for "critical" left main stenosis intervention are lacking, suggested IVUS criteria for significant left main disease are as follows: Greater than 50% diameter stenosis, greater than 60% area stenosis, an absolute cross-sectional area < 7 mm^2 in patients with symptoms, or < 6 mm^2 in asymptomatic patients.

Abizaid and colleagues evaluated 122 patients with intermediate LMCA disease (~42% diameter stenosis by quantitative coronary angiography).[44] My colleagues and I reported the data comparing the final result of stenting for unprotected LMCA with or without IVUS guidance.[34] The lumen diameter after stenting was significantly larger in the IVUS-guided group (4.2 ± 0.6 mm in IVUS guidance vs 4.0 ± 0.6 mm in angiographic guidance; P = .003). But angiographic restenosis rate and target lesion revascularization rate were not different between IVUS-guided and angiography-guided procedures in this study (18.6% vs 19.5%; P = NS).

[ ] DEBULKING ATHERECTOMY

Several clinical trials have shown that IVUS-guided optimal debulking coronary atherectomy (DCA) leads to reduction of restenosis in non-LMCA diseases.[45–47] In addition, by removing the plaque, DCA might facilitate successful stent placement. In our nonrandomized comparison study of LMCA stenosis, described earlier, my colleagues and I, using univariate analysis, showed that debulking before stenting resulted in significant reduction of angiographic restenosis ($P = .034$) and target lesion revascularization ($P = .049$).[34] Reduction of restenosis rate was most striking in LMCA ostial stenosis (1/17 [6%] in the debulking group vs 20/60 [33%] in the nondebulking group; $P = .025$). However, the benefit of debulking atherectomy was not found to be significant on multivariate analysis.

Bifurcation lesions have been considered good targets for debulking. One report showed that restenosis at the parent vessel occurred less frequently in the debulking group than in the non-debulking group (5% vs 33%; $P = .02$).[39] Another study also showed that IVUS-guided aggressive debulking produced favorable long-term outcomes.[48] In this study, stent implantation was necessary in 17 cases (25.4%) to achieve an optimal result, and the 6-month restenosis rate was 20%.

[ ] INTRA-AORTIC BALLOON PUMP

Patients with normal left ventricular function are tolerant of global ischemia during the balloon occlusion. Although an intra-aortic balloon pump is not routinely recommended during the procedure, it should be used to prevent hemodynamic collapse in patients with severely depressed left ventricular function.

[ ] IMMEDIATE AND LONG-TERM RESULTS OF UNPROTECTED LMCA STENTING

Several trials have evaluated the procedural safety and initial outcome of PCI for LMCA stenosis. Careful patient selection may be crucial to achieving favorable outcomes. In the later report of the Unprotected Left Main Trunk Intervention Multi-center Assessment (ULTIMA) registry ($n = 279$), 46% of patients were deemed inoperable or at high surgical risk. Among this group, 38 patients (14%) died during hospitalization.[37] The 1-year incidence rates were 24.2% for all-cause mortality, 20.2% for cardiac mortality, 9.8% for myocardial infarction, and 9.4% for CABG. The independent correlates of all-cause death during and after hospi-

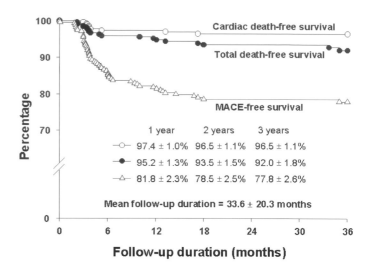

FIGURE 39-8. Three-year survival curves for unprotected left main coronary artery (LMCA) stenting in patients with normal left ventricular function from the Asian Pacific Multicenter Registry. (MACE = major adverse cardiac events, including total death, myocardial infarction, and target lesion revascularization.) From Park et al.[41]

talization are shown in Table 39-2, using multivariate analysis. Decreasing left ventricular function was related to events in an inverse fashion but not linearly, with an apparent inflection point at the 30% LVEF cutoff level. Similar data have also been reported by other investigators.[36,38,41b,41c]

On the other hand, using the low subset of 89 patients from the ULTIMA registry, the 1-year actuarial incidence of death was 3.4%, and the incidence of myocardial infarction, 2.3%. Of note, there were no periprocedural deaths in this subgroup, and no additional deaths or myocardial infarction beyond 4 months after discharge (up to 35 months).[37] My colleagues and I reported data from LMCA stenting procedures performed in selected patients who were good surgical candidates with normal left ventricular function.[34,39,41] The procedural success rate was 99.1%, and the 6-month restenosis rate, 19%. Three-year event rates from the Asian Pacific Multicenter Registry data are shown in Figure 39-8.

LMCA bifurcation disease is a controversial target of PCI. My colleagues and I found that elective stenting for LMCA bifurcation ($n = 63$) in highly selected patients with normal LVEF and a large reference vessel might be safe and effective and had good initial and long-term outcomes.[39] In this report, the procedure was successful in all patients, and major in-hospital events did not occur in any patients. The overall angiographic restenosis rate was 28%. Moreover, no significant differences were noted in the rates of 2-year freedom from target lesion revascularization among LMCA ostial, shaft, and bifurcation stenting (82%, 86%, and 85%, respectively), as illustrated in Figure 39-9.

From these data, we can conclude that judicious patient selection may be essential to achieve favorable results in LMCA stenting. Unfortunately, patients with poor surgical

TABLE 39-2

Correlates of All-Cause Mortality (In-Hospital and During Follow Up) After Unprotected LMCA Intervention

EVENT	% OF STUDY POPULATION	HAZARD RATIO	95% CI	P
LVEF ≤ 30%	14.3	4.21	2.27–7.81	.001
MR grade 3 or 4	4.1	3.66	1.61–8.30	.001
Cardiogenic shock	13.7	3.56	1.73–7.34	.001
Creatinine ≥ 2 mg/dL	5.8	3.10	1.30–7.39	.011
Severe lesion calcification	8.9	2.32	1.13–4.76	.022

LMCA = Left main coronary artery; LVEF = Left ventricular ejection fraction; MR = mitral regurgitaton.

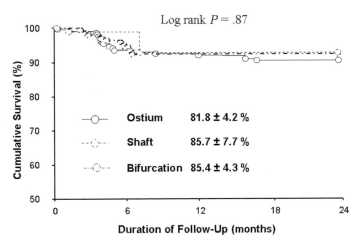

FIGURE 39-9. Two-year freedom from target lesion revascularization according to the location of left main coronary artery (LMCA) stenosis. There was no statistical difference according to the location of LMCA stenosis. Unpublished data from Park et al.[34]

risks are also poor candidates for PCI. Therefore, LMCA stenting should be reserved for selected patients who have normal left ventricular function, are not candidates for CABG, or refuse CABG.

[ ] IN-STENT RESTENOSIS AFTER LMCA INTERVENTION

In spite of the good initial and long-term outcomes of PCI for LMCA stenosis, in-stent restenosis remains a challenging problem. Until now, elective CABG has been recommended for treatment of in-stent restenosis. In general, prior stenting in the LMCA does not interfere with subsequent coronary bypass grafting. Repeated PCI using rotational atherectomy or radiation therapy, or both, in selected patients who refuse surgery has been performed successfully.

Takagi and colleagues have suggested that the gradual increase in MACE noted after stenting may be attributable to restenosis.[40] However, drug-eluting stents have emerged as a solution for restenosis. Recent randomized studies have shown that use of drug-eluting stents dramatically reduces restenosis with safety. In the Rapamycin-Eluting Stent Evaluated At Rotterdam Cardiology Hospital (RESEARCH) registry evaluating the efficacy of sirolimus-eluting stents in the "real world" of interventional cardiology, the intermediate clinical outcome of 31 patients with LMCA disease was excellent.[49] Repeat revascularization for LMCA restenosis post-procedure was not required in any patient. It is expected that ongoing studies will extend the dramatic impact of drug-eluting stents to patients with LMCA disease.

UNPROTECTED LMCA INTERVENTION WITH DRUG-ELUTING STENT

The drug-eluting stent remarkably decreases in-stent restenosis in elective patients with relatively simple coronary lesions. Along with these results, some studies report early clinical experience of unprotected LMCA-stenting with a drug-eluting stent. The study of Park SJ and colleagues[41a] represents a prospective ongoing registry

of patients with de novo unprotected LMCA stenosis and preserved left ventricular function undergoing elective percutaneous coronary intervention using a sirolimus-eluting stent. The outcomes of the first 102 patients treated with the sirolimus-eluting stent have been analyzed and compared to 121 patients treated with the bare metal stent as an historical control. The procedural success rate was 100% in both sirolimus-eluting stent and bare metal stent groups. There were no incidents of death, stent thrombosis, Q-wave myocardial infarction, or emergent bypass surgery during hospitalization in either group. Quantitative angiographic and IVUS results after the procedures showed that the minimal lumen diameter (4.08 ± 0.57 vs 3.36 ± 0.47 mm, $P < .001$) and IVUS lesion lumen area (12.41 ± 3.20 vs 9.62 ± 2.57 mm, $P < .001$) after the procedure were larger due to greater acute lumen gain (2.73 ± 0.73 vs 2.06 ± 0.56 mm, $P < .001$) in the bare metal stent group compared to the sirolimus-eluting stent group. However, at follow-up angiography, lumen loss (0.05 ± 0.57 vs 1.27 ± 0.90 mm, $P < 0.001$) and the overall angiographic restenosis rate (7.0% vs 30.3%, $P < .001$) were significantly lower in the sirolimus-eluting stent group than the bare metal stent group. At 1 year, there were no deaths or acute myocardial infarctions in either group. Target lesion revascularization at 1 year was performed in 2 sirolimus-eluting stent patients (2.0%) and 21 bare metal stent patients (17.4%) ($P < 0.001$). At 12 months, the major adverse cardiac events-free survival rate was $98.0 \pm 1.4\%$ in the sirolimus-eluting stent group and $81.4 \pm 3.7\%$ in the bare metal stent group ($P = .0003$).

Chieffo and colleagues[41b] reported the outcome of 85 patients treated with a drug-eluting stent (41 with a sirolimus-eluting stent, and 44 with a paclitaxel-eluting stent) were compared with 64 received a bare metal stent. At the 6-month clinical follow-up from the study of Chieffo et al, the incidence of major adverse cardiac events was significantly lower in the drug-eluting stent group (17 of 85) than in the bare metal stent group (23 of 64) (20.0% vs 35.9%, respectively, $P = .039$). The mortality rate is lower in the drug-eluting stent group (3 patients, 3.5%) than in the bare metal stent group (9 patients, 14.1%, $P = 0.03$). Cardiac deaths were also lower in the drug-eluting stent group (3 patients, 3.5%) than in the bare metal stent group (6 patients, 9.3%) without statistical significance ($P = .17$). Interestingly, target lesion revascularization rate did not decrease significantly with drug-eluting stent implantation (14.1%) as compared to the bare metal stent implantation (24.2%, $P = .13$). At follow-up angiography, late loss was significantly lower in the drug-eluting stent than in the bare metal stent group (0.58 vs 1.08 mm, respectively, $P = .01$). However, restenosis rate occurred in 12 drug-eluting stent patients (19%) and in 15 bare metal stent patients (30.6%, $P = .18$).

Valgimigli and colleagues[41c] included 95 patients with drug-eluting stent implantation and 86 patients with bare metal stent implantation. There were no significant differences between the drug-eluting stent and the bare metal stent groups in the incidence of major adverse cardiovascular events during the first 30 days. After a median follow-up of 503 days (range, 331–873 days), the cumulative incidence of major adverse cardiovascular events (death, myocardial infarction, or target vessel revascularization) was significantly lower in the drug-eluting stent patients than in the bare metal stent patients (24% vs 45%; hazard ratio [HR], 0.52; 95% CI, 0.31–0.88; $P = .01$). Mortality was similar in the drug-eluting stent (14%) and bare metal stent cohort (16%; HR, 0.79; 95% Cl both the rate of myocardial infarction as well as in the need for target vessel revascularization (6% vs 23%; HR, 0.26; 95% Cl, 0.10–0.65; $P = .004$) in the drug-eluting stent group.

[ ] EMERGENCY INTERVENTION FOR UNPROTECTED LMCA STENOSIS

Procedure-related Complications

LMCA dissection following coronary angiography or PCI procedures is a rare but serious complication. Careful observation or elective CABG may be a reasonable approach for a non–flow limiting dissection. However, emergent CABG or bail-out stenting should be performed for a flow-limiting dissection of the LMCA. A recent retrospective observational study showed that bail-out stenting for LMCA dissection was successful in all cases ($n = 10$) and had very favorable long-term outcomes.[50]

Acute Myocardial Infarction

Because there is a paucity of data reporting outcomes of acute myocardial infarction in patients with acute closure of the LMCA, the role of primary angioplasty remains uncertain. Most patients initially present with cardiogenic shock, requiring aggressive mechanical support. These patients, unlike those with other forms of acute myocardial infarction, have high in-hospital mortality and morbidity because of left ventricular pump failure. In the ULTIMA registry, the rate of in-hospital cardiac death rate was high (> 50% of patients undergoing primary angioplasty), because of the inability to prevent acute left ventricular failure.[51] However, a recent study showed that 10 surviving patients of 18 patients with LMCA infarction at discharge lived well during 39 ± 22 months, with the exception of one patient with target lesion revascularization.[52] Therefore, new approaches, such as early catheter-based reperfusion therapy plus left ventricular assisted device insertion, may offer an alternative to emergent bypass surgery.

[ ] CONCLUSION

Stenting may be a novel therapeutic strategy in patients with unprotected LMCA stenosis; however, it should be reserved for patients who are poor candidates for or refuse CABG, or selected patients with normal left ventricular function. Considering the large size of left main coronary artery, drug-eluting stents may, in the near future, provide an excellent therapeutic option for patients with LMCA stenosis, along with the prospect of negligible in-stent restenosis. The next step will be to undertake prospective randomized trials comparing the clinical outcomes of elective stenting with drug-eluting stents and CABG in the treatment of patients with unprotected LMCA stenosis.

Currently, two large randomized studies comparing drug-eluting stent with CABG for unprotected LMCA stenosis are being conducted. The SYNergy between percutaneous coronary intervention with TAXus and cardiac surgery (SYNTAX) trial is randomizing 1700 patients with de novo triple-vessel disease or LMCA disease (either isolated or with single-, double-, or triple-vessel disease) to either percutaneous coronary intervention with TAXUS stents or CABG. At least 810 patients will have unprotected LMCA disease. The COMparison of Bypass surgery versus AngioplasTy using sirolimus-eluting stent in patients with left main coronary artery disease (COMBAT) trial is planning to randomize 1730 patients with unprotected LMCA stenoses with or without disease in other epicardial vessels to revascularization using sirolimus-eluting stents versus CABG.

INTERVENTION FOR OSTIAL DISEASE

Ostial coronary lesions pose a special management problem for interventional cardiologists. These lesions are associated with suboptimal results and poor long-term outcomes due to lesion rigidity and elastic recoil. Ostial coronary lesions can be classified into two categories: aorto-ostial and branch-ostial lesions.[53] An aorto-ostial lesion is usually defined as a lesion that involves the junction between the aorta and the orifice of the right coronary artery, LMCA, or saphenous vein graft. A branch-ostial lesion is defined as a lesion that involves the junction between a large epicardial vessel and the orifice of a major branch. In some studies, these are referred as "origin" lesions. In many studies, the term *ostial lesion* was extended to include a lesion located within 3 to 5 mm of the vessel orifice but which does not necessarily involve the ostium.

[ ] AORTO-OSTIAL LESIONS

With the advancement of both PCI techniques and coronary devices, the immediate procedural result of PCI for aorto-ostial lesions, as for nonostial lesions, is now excellent.[54–57, 57a] Previously, lesion rigidity, high elastic recoil, or dissection from catheter manipulation often led to suboptimal results when using balloon angioplasty. The development of the coronary stent has overcome these limitations.

Technical Considerations

Before beginning the ostial intervention, the presence of stenosis should be ensured with intracoronary nitroglycerin administration to rule out catheter-induced spasm. Most aorto-ostial lesions can be successfully approached with Judkins guiding catheters. If pressure damping occurs, a side-hole catheter should be used. In general, coaxial alignment minimizes ostial injury, permits proper positioning of interventional devices, and facilitates angiographic assessment of the ostium.

Once the balloon is properly positioned, the guiding catheter can be gently retracted into the aorta. The balloon should not be fully inflated inside the guiding catheter, because of the risk of balloon rupture and air embolism, as illustrated in Figure 39-10.

After balloon angioplasty, stent implantation is recommended in nearly all cases because of the specific lesion characteristics, high elastic recoil, and lesion rigidity. Optimal visualization of the ostial lesion is essential for positioning the device. Frequent test injections are required to verify proper stent positioning and to ensure that the guiding tip does not inadvertently engage beyond the ostium. To ensure proper positioning of the stent, the housing of the guiding catheter should partially extend into the aorta. The proximal 1 to 2 mm of the stent should extend into the aorta to ensure complete coverage of the lesion (Figure 39-11). IVUS performed at this point in the procedure is useful to identify the ves-

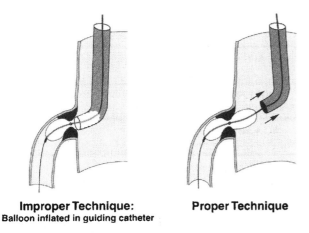

Improper Technique:
Balloon inflated in guiding catheter

Proper Technique

FIGURE 39-10. Comparison of proper and improper balloon dilation technique in aorto-ostial lesions. Proper technique requires gentle retraction of the guiding catheter 1 to 2 cm into the aorta prior to balloon inflation.

sel reference size and stent optimization. In general, slotted-tube stents are preferable to coil or self-expanding stents because of greater radial strength, less stent distortion, and less chance of guiding catheter damage to the stent.

Procedural Results

Aorto-ostial lesions have not been associated with poor initial and long-term results since the development of coronary stents. Two small studies evaluated the role of newer interventional devices, including excimer laser, directional atherectomy, and rotational atherectomy, for treatment of ostial right coronary artery lesions.[58,59] The results were not encouraging, and neither studies found the plaque reduction devices to be superior to stenting.

Iakovou I and colleagues[57a] present the benefit of aorto-ostial intervention with sirolimus-eluting stent ($n = 32$), as compared to the historical controls of bare metal stent implantation ($n = 50$). They show that sirolimus-eluting stent decreases the need of target lesion revascularization (6.3% vs 28%, $P = .01$) and angiographic restenosis rate (11% vs 51%, $P = .001$).

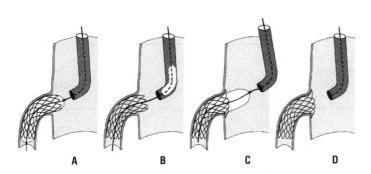

FIGURE 39-11. Proper stenting technique in aorto-ostial lesions. **(A)** The proximal 1 mm of the stent should be extended into the aorta. The guiding catheter should be retracted 1 to 2 cm before stent implantation. **(B)** After stent deployment, the delivery balloon is removed while maintaining backward tension of the guide to prevent it from advancing into the ostium and damaging the stent. **(C)** Adjunctive balloon dilation is performed using a high-pressure balloon. **(D)** Final result.

[ ] BRANCH-OSTIAL LESIONS

Branch-ostial lesions tend to be more angulated, and compromise of the side branch or the parent vessel increases the complexity and complication rate of the procedure. Several studies have shown that coronary stent implantation produces acceptable immediate and long-term results in branch-ostial lesions.[60,61] However, ostial lesions of the left anterior descending artery (LAD) often involve the distal LMCA and the circumflex artery. For this reason, bypass surgery is often considered as a therapeutic option for the treatment of ostial LAD stenosis.

Despite concern that ostial lesions of left anterior descending artery (LAD) often involve the distal LMCA and the circumflex artery, advent of drug-eluting stent improves the outcomes of a complex lesion subset.[61a, 61b]

Technical Considerations in Ostial LAD Stenting

Precise positioning of the stent is of the utmost importance. The stent should be deployed so that the most proximal part of the lesion is covered without protrusion of the stent into the LMCA. Superzooming technique (magnification ×8) at the lesion site is very useful in the right and left inferior oblique views to facilitate exact positioning of the devices. Proper positioning can be confirmed by a small test injection and by multiple projections.

Sometimes, motion of the heart away from the angioplasty catheter causes the stent to withdraw into the LMCA. The stent becomes subject to an oscillating or rocking motion in time with the cardiac cycle, and this makes exact positional deployment impossible. In this case, use of a large guiding catheter, with deeper intubation of the guide catheter and with use of a stiffer guidewire, may allow the whole angioplasty apparatus to swing with cardiac motion. A further option would be to attempt to match balloon inflation to coincide with diastole.

Some interventionists recommend partial inflation technique to overcome cardiac-cycle–related motion of the stent.[62,63] A slight predilation with 2 atm would reduce stent oscillation, making it possible to advance or withdraw the stent several millimeters without difficulty to optimize its position. However, abrasion of the coronary intima by the stent and possible deformation of the stent strut in the process cannot completely be avoided. Moreover, inadequate stent implantation or stent loss is possible with this technique.

The angle between the circumflex artery and the LAD is an important determinant of circumflex narrowing after stent implantation. Asakaura and colleagues proposed that the narrow angle is a predictor of circumflex narrowing after ostial LAD stenting,[64] surmising that when the LAD-circumflex angle is 80 degrees or less, ostial LAD balloon dilation directly affects the ostial circumflex due to snowplow plaque and mechanical compression of the stent. In a later study, however, a narrow angle was not found to be a determinant of circumflex jail.[65]

A study using the sirolimus-eluting stent shows that a simpler stenting technique crossing the circumflex artery is an effective stenting strategy in more complex ostial LAD lesions, such a plaque involvement in LMCA, a narrow angle, and difficult stent positioning.[61a]

Procedural Results

Several studies have reported that ostial LAD stenting could be performed with safety and favorable initial and long-term outcomes.[65,66] Some authors hypothesize that debulking atherectomy may be very beneficial for ostial LAD lesions. Registry data analyzed in one study showed that the angiographic restenosis rate was 14.5% after DCA followed by stenting in 80 patients with ostial LAD lesions.[66] However, a more recent randomized study conducted to evaluate the role of DCA before stenting did not find DCA plus stenting to be superior to stenting alone.[67] In this study, 86 patients with ostial LAD stenoses were randomly assigned to DCA followed by stenting (group A) or stenting alone (group B). Aggressive DCA or optimal stenting was performed in both groups under the guidance of IVUS. The post-procedural minimal lumen diameter was larger in group A than in group B (4.0 ± 0.4 mm vs 3.5 ± 0.5 mm; $P < .001$). However, the angiographic restenosis rates were not significantly different between the two groups (28.1% in group A vs 36.7% in group B; $P = .472$) due to the tendency for greater late loss in group A. With IVUS analysis, the authors suggested that the negative result might be explained in part by the insufficient reduction of atheromatous plaque with conventional DCA devices.

Seung KB and colleagues[61a] present the effectiveness of ostial LAD stenting with the sirolimus-eluting stent ($n = 68$) as compared to the historical control of bare metal stent implantation ($n = 77$). Rates of angiographic restenosis (5.1% vs 32.3%, $P < .001$) and target lesion revascularization (0% vs 17%) are lower in sirolimus-eluting stent implantation than bare metal stent implantation. Also, in patients with distal LMCA involvement, stent implantation across the left circumflex ostium achieves complete lesion coverage and leads to favorable clinical outcomes. These results suggest that the sirolimus-eluting stent implantation with complete lesion coverage may achieve excellent outcomes in ostial LAD lesions, and may be the preferred technique to treat ostial LAD disease with distal LMCA involvement. Tsagalou E and colleagues[61b] also shows similar findings in that the drug-eluting stent ($n = 43$) reduces the restenosis rate (5.7% vs 31.3%, $P = .01$) and the need of target lesion revascularization (7% vs 25.6%, $P = .038$) as compared to the bare metal stent ($n = 43$).

[ ] CONCLUSION

Recent advances in devices and techniques, especially coronary stents, may allow the techniques of PCI to be extended to lesions involving ostial stenosis. The procedural and long-term outcomes of coronary ostial stenting have been reported to be comparable to those of other coronary lesions. Moreover, the expanded use of drug-eluting stents leads to a dramatic reduction in the rate of the repeat revascularization in patients with ostial coronary lesions.

REFERENCES

1. Safian RD. Bifurcation stenosis. In: Safian RD, Freed MS, eds. *Manual of Interventional Cardiology*. Royal Oak, 41: Physician Press, 2001;2:221.
2. Arora RR, Raymond RE, Dimas AP, et al. Side branch occlusion during coronary angioplasty: Incidence, angiographic characteristics, and outcome. *Cathet Cardiovasc Diagn*. 1989;18:210.
3. Iniguez A, Macaya C, Alfonso F, et al. Early angiographic changes of side branches arising from a Palmaz-Schatz stented coronary segment: Results and clinical implications. *J Am Coll Cardiol*. 1994;23:911.
4. Lefevre T, Louvard Y, Morice MC, et al. Stenting of bifurcation lesions: Classification, treatments, and results. *Catheter Cardiovasc Interv*. 2000;49:274.
5. Di Mario C, Airoldi F, Reimers B, et al. Bifurcational stenting. *Semin Interv Cardiol*. 1998;3:65.
6. Boxt LM, Meyerovitz MF, Taus RH, et al. Side branch occlusion complicating percutaneous transluminal coronary angioplasty. *Radiology*. 1986;161:681.
7. Arora RR, Raymond RE, Dimas AP, et al. Side branch occlusion during coronary angioplasty: Incidence, angiographic characteristics, and outcome. *Cathet Cardiovasc Diagn*. 1989;18:210.
8. Mazur W, Grinstead WC, Hakim AH, et al. Fate of side branches after intracoronary implantation of the Gianturco-Roubin flex-stent for acute or threatened closure after percutaneous transluminal coronary angioplasty. *Am J Cardiol*. 1994;74:1207.
9. Pan M, Suarez de Lezo J, Meding A, et al. Simple and complex stent strategies for bifurcated coronary arterial stenosis involving the side branch origin. *Am J Cardiol*. 1999;83:1320.
10. Yamashita T, Nishida T, Adamian MG, et al. Bifurcation lesions: Two stents versus one stent-immediate and follow-up results. *J Am Coll Cardiol*. 2000;35:1145.
10a. Pan M, de Lezo JS, Medina A, et al. Rapamycin-eluting stents for the treatment of bifurcated coronary lesions: A randomized comparison of a simple versus complex strategy. *Am Heart J*. 2004;148:857.
11. Sheiban I, Albiero R, Marsico F, et al. Immediate and long-term results of "T" stenting for bifurcation coronary lesions. *Am J Cardiol*. 2000;85:1141.
12. Al Suwaidi J, Berger PB, Rihal CS, et al. Immediate and long-term outcome of intracoronary stent implantation for true bifurcation lesions. *J Am Coll Cardiol*. 2000;35:929.
12a. Ge L, Iakovou I, Cosgrave J, et al. Treatment of bifurcation lesions with two stents: one year angiographic and clinical follow up of crush versus T stenting. *Heart*. 2006;92:371–6.
13. Fort S, Lazzam C, Schwartz L. Coronary 'Y' stenting: A technique for angioplasty of bifurcation stenoses. *Can J Cardiol*. 1996;12:678.
14. Chevalier B, Glatt B, Royer T, Guyon P. Placement of coronary stents in bifurcation lesions by the "culotte" technique. *Am J Cardiol*. 1998;82:943.
15. Colombo A, Gaglione A, Nakamura S, Finci L. "Kissing" stent for bifurcation coronary lesions. *Cathet Cardiovasc Diagn*. 1993;22:1642.
16. Carlier SG, van der Giessen WJ, Foley DP, et al. Stenting with a true bifurcated stent: Acute and mid-term follow-up results. *Catheter Cardiovasc Interv*. 1999;47:361.
17. Cervinka P, Foley DP, Sabate M, et al. Coronary bifurcation stenting using dedicated bifurcation stents. *Catheter Cardiovasc Interv*. 2000;49:105.
18. Kim YH, Lee JH, Lee CW, et al. Initial clinical experience with the new AST SLK-View stent for bifurcation coronary lesions. *Am J Cardiol*. 2002;90(Suppl 1):H13.
19. Toutouzas K, Stankovic G, Takagi T, et al. A new dedicated stent and delivery system for the treatment of bifurcation lesions: Preliminary experience. *Catheter Cardiovasc Interv*. 2003;58:34.
19a. Ikeno F, Kim YH, Luna J, et al. Acute and long-term outcomes of the novel side access (SLK-View trademark) stent for bifurcation coronary lesions: A multicenter nonrandomized feasibility study. *Catheter Cardiovasc Interv*. 2006;67:198.
20. Brener SJ, Leya FS, Apperson-Hansen C, et al. A comparison of debulking versus dilatation of bifurcation coronary arterial narrowings (from the CAVEAT I Trial). Coronary Angioplasty Versus Excisional Atherectomy Trial-I. *Am J Cardiol*. 1996;78:1039.
21. Karvouni E, Di Mario C, Nishida T, et al. Directional atherectomy prior to stenting in bifurcation lesions: A matched comparison study with stenting alone. *Catheter Cardiovasc Interv*. 2001;53:12.
22. Morice MC, Serruys PW, Sousa JE, et al. A randomized comparison of a sirolimus-eluting stent with a standard stent for coronary revascularization. *N Engl J Med*. 2002;346:1773.
23. Park SJ, Shim WH, Ho DS, et al. A paclitaxel-eluting stent for the prevention of coronary restenosis. *N Engl J Med*. 2003;348:1537.
24. Moses JW, Leon MB, Popma JJ, et al. SIRIUS Investigators. Sirolimus-eluting stents versus standard stents in patients with stenosis in a native coronary artery. *N Engl J Med*. 2003;349:1315.
25. Colombo A, Louvard Y, Raghu C, et al. Sirolimus eluting stents in bifurcation lesions: 6 month angiographic result according to the implantation technique. *J Am Coll Cardiol*. 2003;41:53A.
25a. Colombo A, Moses JW, Morice MC, et al. Randomized study to evaluate sirolimus-eluting stents implanted at coronary bifurcation lesions. *Circulation*. 2004;109:1244.
26. Colombo A, Stankovic G, Orlic D, et al. Modified T-stenting technique with crushing for bifurcation lesions: Immediate results and 30-day outcome. *Catheter Cardiovasc Interv*. 2003;60:145.
26a. Ormiston JA, Currie E, Webster MW, et al. Drug-eluting stents for coronary bifurcations: insights into the crushing technique. *Catheter Cardiovasc Interv*. 2004;63:332.

26b. Ge L, Airoldi F, Iakovou I, et al. Clinical and angiographic outcome after implantation of drug-eluting stents in bifurcation lesions with the crush stent technique: Importance of final kissing balloon post-dilation. *J Am Coll Cardiol.* 2005;46:613.

27. O'Keefe JH, Hartzler GO, Rutherford BD, et al. Left main coronary angioplasty: Early and late results of 127 acute and elective procedures. *Am J Cardiol.* 1989;64:144.

28. Hartzler GO, Rutherford BD, McConohay DR, et al. High-risk percutaneous transluminal coronary angioplasty. *Am J Cardiol.* 1988;61:33G.

29. Eldar M, Schulhoff RN, Hertz I, et al. Results of percutaneous transluminal coronary angioplasty of the left main coronary artery. *Am J Cardiol.* 1991; 68:255.

30. Bittl JA. Advances in coronary angioplasty. *New Engl J Med.* 1996;335:1290.

31. Ellis SG, Tamai H, Nobuyoshi M, et al. Contemporary percutaneous treatment of unprotected left main stenoses: Initial results from a multicenter registry analysis 1994-1996. *Circulation.* 1997;96:3867.

32. Park SJ, Park SW, Hong MK, et al. Stenting of unprotected left main coronary artery stenoses: Immediate and late outcome. *J Am Coll Cardiol.* 1998;31:37.

33. Kosuga K, Tamai H, Ueda K, et al. Initial and long-term results of angioplasty in unprotected left main coronary artery. *Am J Cardiol.* 1999;83:32.

34. Park SJ, Hong MK, Lee CW, et al. Elective stenting of unprotected left main coronary artery stenosis: Effect of debulking before stenting and intravascular ultrasound guidance. *J Am Coll Cardiol.* 2001;38:1054.

35. Laruelle CJ, Brueren GB, Ernst SM. E, et al. Stenting of "unprotected" left main coronary artery stenoses: Early and late results. *Heart.* 1998;79:148.

36. Silvestri M, Barragan P, Sainsous J, et al. Unprotected left main coronary artery stenting: Immediate and medium-term outcomes of 140 elective procedures. *J Am Coll Cardiol.* 2000;35:1543.

37. Tan WA, Tamai H, Park SJ, et al; ULTIMA Investigators. Long-term clinical outcomes after unprotected left main trunk percutaneous revascularization in 279 patients. *Circulation.* 2001;104:1609.

38. Black A Jr, Cortina R, Bossi I, et al. Unprotected left main coronary artery stenting: Correlates of midterm survival and impact of patient selection. *J Am Coll Cardiol.* 2001;37:832.

39. Park SJ, Lee CW, Kim YH, et al. Technical feasibility, safety and clinical outcome of stenting of unprotected left main coronary artery bifurcation narrowing. *Am J Cardiol.* 2002;104:1609.

40. Takagi T, Stankovic G, Finci L, et al. Results and long-term predictors of adverse clinical events after elective percutaneous interventions on unprotected left main coronary artery. *Circulation.* 2002;106:698.

41. Park SJ, Park SW, Hong MK, et al. Long-term (3-years) outcomes after stenting of unprotected left main coronary artery stenosis in patients with normal left ventricular function. *Am J Cardiol.* 2003;91:12.

41a. Park SJ, Kim YH, Lee BK, et al. Sirolimus-eluting stent implantation for unprotected left main coronary artery stenosis: comparison with bare metal stent implantation. *J Am Coll Cardiol.* 2005;45:351.

41b. Chieffo A, Stankovic G, Bonizzoni E, et al. Early and mid-term results of drug-eluting stent implantation in unprotected left main. *Circulation.* 2005;111:791.

41c. Valgimigli M, van Mieghem CA, Ong AT, et al. Short- and long-term clinical outcome after drug-eluting stent implantation for the percutaneous treatment of left main coronary artery disease: Insights from the Rapamycin-Eluting and Taxus Stent Evaluated At Rotterdam Cardiology Hospital registries (RESEARCH and T-SEARCH). *Circulation.* 2005;111:1383.

41d. de Lezo JS, Medina A, Pan M, et al. Rapamycin-eluting stents for the treatment of unprotected left main coronary disease. *Am Heart J.* 2004;148: 481.

41e. Kim YH, Park SW, Hong MK, et al. Comparison of simple and complex stenting techniques in the treatment of unprotected left main coronary artery bifurcation stenosis. *Am J Cardiol.* 2006;1597.

42. Hermiller JB, Buller CE, Tenaglia AN, et al. Unrecognized left main coronary artery disease in patients undergoing interventional procedures. *Am J Cardiol.* 1993;71:173.

43. Mintz GS, Pichard AD, Kovach JA, et al. Impact of preintervention intravascular ultrasound imaging on transcatheter treatment strategies in coronary artery disease. *Am J Cardiol.* 1994;73:423.

44. Abizaid AS, Mintz GS, Abizaid A, et al. One-year follow-up after intravascular ultrasound assessment of moderate left main coronary artery disease in patients with ambiguous angiograms. *J Am Coll Cardiol.* 1999;34:707.

45. Baim DS, Cutlip DE, Sharma SK, et al for the BOAT Investigators. Final results of the Balloon vs Optimal Atherectomy Trial (BOAT). *Circulation.* 1998;97:322.

46. Suzuki T, Hosokawa H, Katoh O, et al. Effects of the adjunctive balloon angioplasty after intravascular ultrasound-guided optimal directional coronary atherectomy study: The results of Adjunctive Balloon Angioplasty After Coronary Atherectomy Study (ABACAS). *J Am Coll Cardiol.* 1999;34:1028.

47. Tsuchikane E, Sumitsuji S, Awata N, et al. Final results of the Stent versus directional coronary Atherectomy Randomized Trial (START). *J Am Coll Cardiol.* 1999;34:1050.

48. Hu FB, Tamai H, Kosuga K, et al. Intravascular ultrasound-guided directional coronary atherectomy for unprotected left main coronary stenoses with distal bifurcation involvement. *Am J Cardiol.* 2003;92:936.

49. Arampatzis CA, Lemos PA, Tanabe K, et al. Effectiveness of sirolimus-eluting stent for treatment of left main coronary artery disease. *Am J Cardiol.* 2003;92:327.

50. Lee SW, Hong MK, Kim YH, et al. Bail-out stenting for left main coronary artery dissection during catheter-based procedure: Acute and long-term results. *Clin Cardiol.* 2004;27:393.

51. Marso SP, Steg G, Plokka T, et al. Catheter-based reperfusion of unprotected left main stenosis during an acute myocardial infarction (the ULTIMA experience). *Am J Cardiol.* 1999;83:1513.

52. Lee SW, Hong MK, Lee CW, et al. Early and late clinical outcomes after primary stenting of the unprotected left main coronary artery stenosis in the setting of acute myocardial infarction. *Int J Cardiol.* 2004;97:73.

53. Pritchard CL, Mudd JG, Barner HB. Coronary ostial stenosis. *Circulation.* 1975;52:46.

54. Tan K, Sulke N, Taub N, Sowton E. Clinical and lesion morphologic determinants of coronary angioplasty success and complications: Current experience. *J Am Coll Cardiol.* 1995;25:855.

55. Rocha-Singh K, Morris N, Wong SC, et al. Coronary stenting for treatment of ostial stenoses of native coronary arteries or aortocoronary saphenous venous grafts. *Am J Cardiol.* 1995;75:26.

56. Jain SP, Liu MW, Dean LS, et al. Comparison of balloon angioplasty versus debulking devices versus stenting in right coronary ostial lesions. *Am J Cardiol.* 1997;79:1334.

57. Motwani JG, Raymond RE, Franco I, et al. Effectiveness of rotational atherectomy of right coronary artery ostial stenosis. *Am J Cardiol.* 2000;85:563.

57a. Iakovou I, Ge L, Michev I, Sangiorgi GM, et al. Clinical and angiographic outcome after sirolimus-eluting stent implantation in aorto-ostial lesions. *J Am Coll Cardiol.* 2004;44:967.

58. Jain SP, Liu MW, Dean LS, et al. Comparison of balloon angioplasty versus debulking devices versus stenting in right coronary ostial stenosis. *Am J Cardiol.* 1997;79:1334.

59. Motwani JG, Raymond RE, Franco I, et al. Effectiveness of rotational atherectomy of right coronary artery ostial stenosis. *Am J Cardiol.* 2000;85:563.

60. Mathur A, Liu MW, Goods CM, et al. Results of elective stenting of branch ostial lesions. *Am J Cardiol.* 1997;79:472.

61. Tan RP, Kini A, Shalouh E, et al. Optimal treatment of nonaorto-ostial coronary lesions in large vessels: Acute and long-term results. *Catheter Cardiovasc Interv.* 2001;54:283.

61a. Seung KB, Kim YH, Park DW, et al. Effectiveness of sirolimus-eluting stent implantation for the treatment of ostial left anterior descending artery stenosis with intravascular ultrasound guidance. *J Am Coll Cardiol.* 2005;46:787.

61b. Tsagalou E, Stancovic G, Iakovou I, et al. Early outcome of treatment of ostial de novo left anterior descending coronary artery lesions with drug-eluting stents. *Am J Cardiol.* 2006;97:187–191.

62. Webster MW, Dixon SR, Ormiston JA, et al. Optimal stent positioning in coronary arteries: partial balloon inflation to overcome cardiac cycle-related motion of the stent/delivery system. *Catheter Cardiovasc Interv.* 2000;49:102.

63. Hildick-Smith DJ, Shapiro LM. Ostial left anterior descending coronary artery stent positioning: Partial preinflation prevents stent oscillation and facilitates accurate deployment. *J Interv Cardiol.* 2001;14:439.

64. Asakaura Y, Takagi S, Ishikawa S, et al. Favorable strategy for the ostial lesion of the left anterior descending coronary artery: Influence on narrowing of circumflex coronary artery. *Cathet Cardiovasc Diagn.* 1998;43:95.

65. Park SJ, Lee CW, Hong MK, et al. Stent placement for ostial left anterior descending coronary artery stenosis: Acute and long-term (2-year) results. *Catheter Cardiovasc Interv.* 2000;49:267.

66. Bramucci E, Repetto A, Ferrario M, et al. Effectiveness of adjunctive stent implantation following directional coronary atherectomy for treatment of left anterior descending ostial stenosis. *Am J Cardiol.* 2002;90:1074.

67. Kim YH, Hong MK, Lee SW, et al. Randomized comparison of debulking followed by stenting versus stenting alone for ostial left anterior descending artery stenosis: Intravascular ultrasound guidance. *Am Heart J.* 2004;148:663.

CHAPTER (40)

Special Considerations: Small Vessel and Diffuse Disease

James B. Hermiller, MD

Since the inception of angioplasty, small vessel coronary disease and diffuse coronary disease have been particularly challenging subsets for treatment with transcatheter coronary interventional therapies. Often associated with other higher risk comorbidities, small vessel disease more frequently is associated with diabetes, female gender, and diffuse coronary involvement.[1] As a result, a higher incidence of acute complications, including significant vessel dissection, acute vessel closure, myocardial infarction, and emergent coronary bypass grafting, has historically complicated intervention in small and diffusely diseased vessels.[2,3] Furthermore, these lesions are frequently technically challenging. Their often noncompliant and calcified character, frequent tortuous nature, and distal location impair device delivery. Along with poorer acute outcomes, these subsets are plagued by high restenosis rates, often necessitating repeat intervention or bypass surgery.[4,5] Despite the challenges and complexities inherent to small vessel intervention, the problem is common; between 30% and 67% of all interventions involve small vessels, depending on the definition of a small vessel.[6–9]

This chapter will review the definition and diagnostic approach to small and diffuse coronary disease. Acute and long-term outcomes associated with balloon angioplasty and bare metal stenting will be reviewed. Finally, the favorable impact of drug-eluting stents and their future role in the treatment of these subsets will be examined.

DEFINITION OF SMALL VESSEL AND DIFFUSE DISEASE

The definition of what constitutes a small vessel in the context of coronary interventional therapy has been quite variable. A number of studies examining small vessel intervention have defined vessels less than 3.0 mm in reference size as being small, and this criterion is in part derived from early stent trials in which vessels less than 3.0 mm were excluded from enrollment.[10,11] Other studies have defined small vessels as those less than 2.5 to 2.8 mm in diameter.[9,12–14] Certainly, less than 3.0 mm is the most sensitive descriptor, although necessarily less specific. Despite whatever arbitrary cutoff is utilized, the relationship between vessel size and outcome is not a step function; instead, a continuous inverse relationship exists between outcomes and size.[8,15] Consequently, differences in the definition and enrollment criterion frequently help explain apparently conflicting results from various studies of small vessel intervention. Like the small vessel, diffuse disease has had various definitions; however, the most consistent definition is lesion length greater than 20 mm.[16]

The definition of small vessel has been based on angiography; nevertheless, results of intravascular ultrasound (IVUS) have demonstrated that many angiographically small vessels are in fact "pseudosmall" as a result of angiographically undetected disease in the reference segment and positive remodeling at the lesion site.[17] Briguori and colleagues compared 344 consecutive patients having 419 lesions in small vessels (angiographic reference vessel ≤ 2.75 mm) with 953 patients having 1161 lesions in large vessels (> 2.75 mm); all underwent concomitant IVUS. The difference in angiographic and IVUS reference vessel dimension Delta (IVUS-angiography) was calculated for all lesions.[18] The tendency to underestimate vessel size was significantly greater for small vessels (difference between IVUS and angiography, 1.3 ± 0.5 mm vs 1.0 ± 0.6 mm; $P < .001$). Angiography underestimated vessel size by more than 1.0 mm in 71% of small vessels and in only 49% of large vessels ($P < .001$). There was a stronger correlation between plaque burden and the Delta (IVUS-angiography) in small vessels

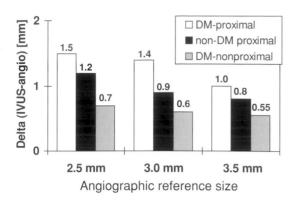

FIGURE 40-1. Graph demonstrating predictors of large discrepancies between intravascular ultrasound (IVUS) and angiography as reported in one study. Independent predictors of greater than a 1.0-mm delta were small vessel size (< 3.0 mm), location of the lesion in the proximal vessel, and diabetes. DM = diabetes mellitus; IVUS-angio = IVUS-angiography. *(From Moussa I, Kobayashi Y, Adamian M, et al.[19])*

(r = 0.80; P < .001) than in large vessels (r = 0.59; P < .001). Predictors of Delta (IVUS-angiography) were proximal or middle lesion location and female gender.[19] Extending these observations, Moussa et al examined the predictors of large discrepancies between IVUS and angiography. Independent predictors of greater than a 1.0 mm Delta (IVUS-angiography) were small vessel size (< 3.0 mm), location of the lesion in the proximal vessel, and diabetes (Figure 40-1). The authors suggested that IVUS might be particularly helpful in small vessel intervention when the lesion was proximally located or the patient had diabetes.

NONSTENT INTERVENTION

Early studies of PTCA demonstrated the higher risks associated with small vessel intervention.[20] Shunkert and colleagues compared 813 patients with vessel diameters ≤2.5 mm with 1493 patients with vessel sizes greater than 2.5 mm.[1] Those with smaller vessels were older and more frequently female, and they more often presented with diabetes mellitus, heart failure, and multivessel disease (<.001 for each variable). Overall procedural success was significantly less for small vessels compared to the larger vessel group (92% vs 98%; P = .006). Furthermore, major adverse cardiac events occurred more frequently in the small vessel cohort (3.4% vs 2.0%; P = .03). Hypotheses explaining the higher event rates include the association of small vessels with other high-risk comorbidities, greater lesion complexity, and the higher incidence of diffuse plaquing. The combination of small vessel size and diffuse disease is particularly difficult, with a much higher incidence of abrupt closure compared to focal lesions. To limit the frequency of dissection and improve outcomes, longer balloons have been utilized in diffuse disease. Tenaglia et al studied the use of long balloon angioplasty in 89 patients with diffuse, predominantly small vessel disease.[21] The use of 30 and 40 mm balloons in 93 stenoses in this study was associated with a high rate of procedural success of 97% and major dissection rate of only 11%. Angiographic restenosis was however 55%. Umeda and colleagues examined a strategy of gradual and prolonged balloon angioplasty (GPBA) in

small arteries. They randomized 263 patients to GPBA, cutting balloon (CB) or plain old balloon angioplasty (POBA).[22] Compared to POBA, a strategy of gradual and prolonged inflation (cumulative inflation times of > 10 minutes) was associated with a lower final residual stenosis (27.3% vs 34.2%; P = .31) and decreased need for stent placement (8.0% vs 22.2%; P = .034). Restenosis rates were lower with GPBA compared to POBA (31.3% vs 50.6%; P = .043).

More recently, the cutting balloon has been used in the setting of diffuse and small vessel disease.[22–25] Registry and randomized comparisons have suggested that CB compared to POBA reduces the frequency of dissections and need for bailout stenting.[23] In the Restenosis Reduction by Cutting Balloon Evaluation (REDUCE) 1 trial, 800 patients were randomized to either CB or POBA. Major dissections were noted in 25.2% of CB patients and in 38.9% of POBA patients (P < .0001). In the REDUCE IVUS substudy of 89 patients, vessel dissection was significantly less in those with vessel calcification undergoing CB angioplasty.[24] In the Cutting Balloon Angioplasty Versus Plain Old Balloon Angioplasty Randomized Study (CAPAS), 248 patients with small vessel disease were randomized to cutting balloon or POBA. Reference diameters were 2.17 ± 0.43 and 2.2 ± 10.42 in the CB and POBA groups respectively. Acute gains were similar, but 6-month minimum lumen diameter was significantly greater in the CB group (1.31 ± 0.48 vs 1.18 ± 0.58; P = .08), leading to significantly lower binary restenosis rate in CB group (25.2% vs 41.5%; P = .009).[23] The application of CB may allow for more complete dilation. In Umada's study, the cutting balloon in vessels less than 2.5 mm in size reduced restenosis (32.9% vs 50.6%; P = .059) and target lesion revascularization (TLR) (20% vs 37.6%; P = .033).[22] These data suggest that in small vessels where the intention is to avoid stenting, a strategy of CB dilation or gradual prolonged balloon inflation are reasonable ones, with a lower probability of significant dissection necessitating bailout stenting.

ABLATIVE TECHNIQUES: ROTATIONAL ATHERECTOMY AND LASER

Ablative techniques have been applied to small vessel and diffuse disease, as intuitively these subsets seem suited to these adjunctive therapies because the short- and long-term results with balloon angioplasty have been suboptimal.[26,27] In a study of 226 lesions in 159 patients with small vessel stenoses (mean vessel diameter = 2.36 + 0.49 mm), Tsubokawa et al reported no reflow/slow flow in 12.4% of patients and acute closure in 3.5% of patients. Restenosis rates at 6 months were 44.2% and TLR was 33%.[26] The high restenosis and TLR during follow-up were comparable among patients who underwent rotational atherectomy with balloon angioplasty or rotablator plus stenting. Bittl et al completed a meta-analysis of trials examining percutaneous intervention versus atherectomy or laser angioplasty. Ablative techniques were associated with a higher acute complications and no restenosis benefit.[27] Despite no data to suggest plaque ablative techniques should be routinely used in small vessel or diffuse disease, rotational atherectomy continues to have a niche role in heavily calcified vessels, where it facilitates complete dilation and may assist device delivery.[28]

STENTS

Early reports of stenting in small vessels suggested higher rates of complications, and no improvement in restenosis.[29–31] Furthermore, diffuse disease treated with multiple or long stents was associated with a higher risk of stent thrombosis as well. A meta-analysis of the Belgian-Netherlands Stent (BENESTENT) study and the Stent Restenosis Study (STRESS) suggested no improvement in restenosis in small vessels when elective stenting was compared with balloon angioplasty.[32] These reports led to the ACC/AHA consensus panel recommendation that small vessels should not be routinely stented.[33]

Despite these mediocre early results, subsequent reports of bailout stenting in the setting of abrupt or threatened closure in small vessels were encouraging.[34,35] In addition, an analysis of small vessel lesions enrolled in STRESS I and II suggested that in vessels less than 3.0 mm, elective stenting was beneficial.[10] Angiographic restenosis was significantly less in those receiving elective stenting (34% restenosis vs 55% stent vs balloon, $P <$ .0001), and there was no difference in abrupt closure between the POBA and stent group (3.6% in both groups). Many other elective registries also suggested favorable outcomes with stenting when compared to historical controls.[36–45]

Following these early reports, there have subsequently been a large number of randomized trials comparing bare metal stenting to PTCA.[9,13,45–53] There has been considerable variability in the results of these studies. The disparate outcomes of these randomized trials have been problematic. Further analysis suggests that differences could potentially result from the quality of outcomes in the percutaneous transluminal coronary angioplasty (PTCA) group, the type of stent used, and differences in the sizes of vessel included in these studies. In those trials in which the residual stenosis after PTCA was lower, the benefit of stenting was less (Figure 40-2). In addition and although controversial, strut thickness may play a role with less restenosis in those studies using thinner-strutted stents.[54]

Moreno and colleagues recently performed a meta-analysis of these randomized trials. Overall, 3541 patients were included in these studies, with 1672 allocated to balloon angioplasty and 1869 to bare metal

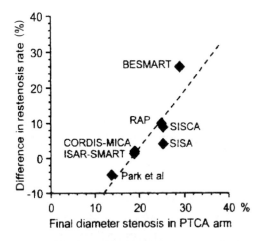

FIGURE 40-2. Graph demonstrating that a lower residual stenosis after percutaneous transluminal coronary angioplasty (PTCA) is associated with a reduced relative benefit of stenting. *(From Kastrati A, Mehilli J, Dirschinger J, et al.[54])*

stenting.[55] Of these, 84% had angiographic follow-up. The pooled restenosis rate was 25.8% assigned to stenting and 34.2% in patients allocated to balloon angioplasty (RR, 0.75; 95% CI, 0.67–0.84; $P <$ .001). A smaller reference vessel diameter at baseline was associated with higher risk reduction of restenosis in the stent group ($P =$ 0.012). In summary, these studies suggest that stenting improves restenosis in small vessels particularly when PTCA outcomes are not optimal and possibly when reference vessel size is smaller.

〔 〕 STENT STRATEGIES

Initially, the treatment of diffuse disease, particularly in small vessels, was discouraging because of higher rates of stent thrombosis and restenosis. Subsequent studies suggested more favorable results. In long lesions, Serruys showed the superiority of IVUS-guided stenting compared to optimal balloon angioplasty in the Additional Value of NIR stents for treatment of long Coronary lEsions (ADVANCE) trial.[56] In this study, 437 patients with lesions 20 to 50 mm in length were angioplastied with long balloons; 149 (34%) of the patients required bailout stenting for flow-limiting dissections. The remaining 288 patients who achieved an optimal PTCA result were randomized to IVUS-directed stenting or no further therapy. The restenosis rate in the stent group was significantly lower than the PTCA-only group (27% vs 42%; $P =$ .022), with no difference in early complications. Using IVUS guidance, Colombo described a technique whereby the vessel was aggressively dilated and segments within the lesion with minimal lumen areas less than 5.5 mm received spot stenting.[57] Compared to usual stenting, spot stenting was associated with no difference in 30-day major adverse cardiac events (MACE) but with significantly less restenosis (25% vs 39%, $P <$ .05). Although single center reports of spot-stenting have been encouraging, the time-consuming and operator-dependent technique has not been embraced as a mainstream strategy.

Another strategy examined in the setting of small vessel intervention has been direct stenting.[58] Garcia and colleagues randomized 350 patients with reference vessel sizes between 2.2 and 2.7 mm to either direct stenting or predilation followed by stenting using the Pixel stent.[59] Of those assigned to direct stenting, 83% were successfully stented without predilation. Binary angiographic restenosis at 180-day follow-up was 16% for direct stenting versus 25% for the control ($P =$ NS). Target lesion revascularization was low in both groups (3.4% vs 4.3% direct stent vs control; $P =$ NS).

Finally, the use of 2b/3a inhibitors as a routine strategy in small vessels intervention has not been shown to reduce restenosis. Hausleiter and colleagues randomized 502 patients in a 2 × 2 factorial design to stent (phosphochlorine-coated) versus PTCA and abciximab versus control.[48] There was no difference in 30-day MACE, restenosis or TVR between the abciximab and control groups.

〔 〕 DRUG-ELUTING STENTS

The fundamental problem with stenting in small arteries is that on average, the amount of neointimal hyperplasia is independent of vessel size, with small arteries suffering on average the same amount of late loss (0.8 mm) as larger vessels.[8] Because of lower postprocedure stent area, small vessels are less able to accommodate neointimal accumulation than larger arteries. Lesion length

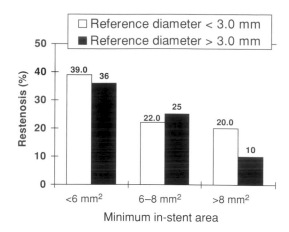

FIGURE 40-3. Graph demonstrating results of one study demonstrating that even when the in-stent minimal vessel areas are large, small vessels have higher rates of target vessel revascularization than larger vessels with similar postprocedural minimal in-stent lumen areas. *(From Moussa I, Kobayashi Y, Adamian M, et al.[19])*

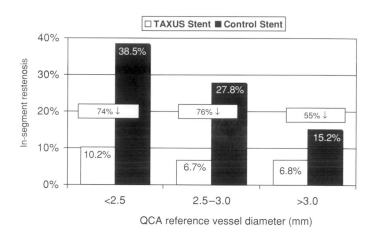

FIGURE 40-5. Results from TAXUS IV, which demonstrate substantial reductions in in-segment restenosis with no edge restenosis with concomitant reductions in target vessel and target lesion revascularization. QCA = quantitative coronary angiography. *(From Grube E, Silber S, Hauptmann KE, et al.[63])*

independently exacerbates the negative impact of smaller vessel size.[8] Even when the in-stent minimal vessel areas are large, small vessels have higher rates of TVR than larger vessels with similar postprocedural minimal in-stent lumen areas (Figure 40-3).[60]

The solution to improving long-term outcomes in small and diffuse vessel stenting is to reduce neointimal proliferation, thereby attenuating late lumen loss. The site-specific application of antiproliferative agents such as sirolimus and paclitaxel dramatically and unequivocally reduce restenosis in larger vessels.[61–65] Subset analysis from randomized trials and subsequent small vessel-specific studies have demonstrated remarkable effectiveness in the setting of small vessel disease as well. Their impact on diffuse disease has been equally favorable.

The SIRolImUS (SIRIUS) trial demonstrated that the sirolimus-eluting Bx-velocity stent (SES) dramatically reduced in-stent late loss in smaller vessels with some attenuation of the effect over the analysis segment due to proximal edge restenosis (Figure 40-4).[62] TVR was reduced in a similar fashion, although

the relative reduction was somewhat less for smaller vessels. Results from the e-SIRIUS and c-SIRIUS trials, where considerable attention was paid to avoiding geographic miss, also examined the CYPHER stent in small vessels compared to the Bx-VELOCITY bare metal stent.[65] The in-segment late loss was uniformly decreased across all vessel sizes with late loss in the small (−2.2 mm), medium (2.8 mm) and large (−3.0 mm) vessels being 0.12 mm, 0.18 mm, and 0.19 mm respectively. The lack of edge restenosis in these more contemporary studies suggests that avoiding geographic miss and stenting "normal to normal" is particularly important in small vessels. Holmes recently reported an analysis of SES versus balloon angioplasty.[66] In vessels with reference size less than 3.0 mm, he evaluated the effectiveness of the sirolimus-eluting stent in the SIRIUS trial and compared it to the results of balloon angioplasty in patients treated in BENESTENT I and II and STRESS. Subacute occlusion was 0.4% versus 1.4% (SES vs POBA), and the SES reduced TLR from 24% to 5.1% (difference −18.9%, 95% CI (−23.5%, −14.3%) difference, suggesting that the drug-eluting stent was far more effective than balloon angioplasty.

Like the sirolimus-eluting stent, the paclitaxel-eluting stent appears very effective in small vessel disease.[64] Results from TAXUS

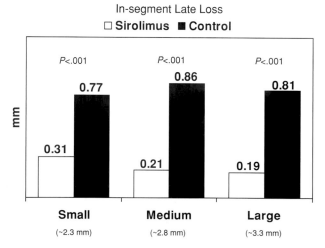

FIGURE 40-4. The SIRIUS trial demonstrated that the sirolimus-eluting Bx-velocity stent dramatically reduced in-stent late loss in smaller vessels. *(From Moses JW, Leon MB, Popma JJ, et al.[62])*

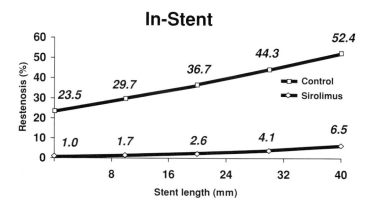

FIGURE 40-6. Graph demonstrating the dramatic reduction in restenosis as a function of stent length in the SES and bare metal stent groups. *(From Moses JW, Leon MB, Popma JJ, et al.[62])*

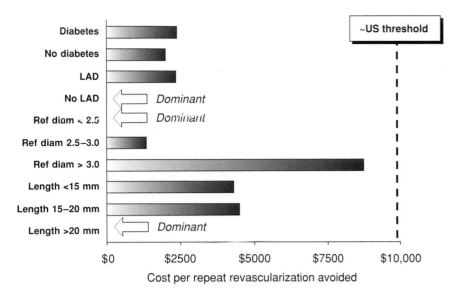

FIGURE 40-7. In a substudy of the SIRIUS trial, the authors analyzed the relative cost-effectiveness of using the sirolimus-eluting stent and calculated the cost per repeat revascularization avoided as a function of vessel diameter and lesion length. LAD = left anterior descending (coronary artery); ref diam = reference diameter. *(From Greenberg D, Bakhai A, Cohen DJ, et al.[70])*

ization associated with CYPHER was significantly lower overall in small vessels and long lesions.[69]

Finally, are drug-eluting stents worth their high cost in the setting of small vessel or diffuse disease? In a substudy of the SIRIUS trial, Greenberg et al analyzed the relative cost-effectiveness of using the sirolimus-eluting stent and calculated the cost per repeat revascularization avoided as a function of vessel diameter and lesion length.[70] The typical US threshold for accepting a technology as cost effective is $10,000 or less per event avoided. Treating small or diffuse disease with drug-eluting stents was particularly cost effective/cost saving (Figure 40-7).

SUMMARY

Small vessel and diffuse coronary disease continue to be challenging subsets even in the era of advanced transcatheter therapies. Frequently, what is thought to be a small vessel by angiographic criterion is often incorrect, because unsuspected disease in the reference areas and positive remodeling at the lesion promotes the underestimation of vessel size, particularly in the proximal coronary segments and in patients with diabetes. The acute risks and technical problems associated with percutaneous intervention of these lesions can be higher, although advances in stent design have attenuated these challenges. Multiple randomized trials have not uniformly demonstrated that the elective use of bare metal stents is superior to balloon angioplasty, with many studies demonstrating no difference in acute major adverse cardiac events, restenosis, and repeat revascularization. The comparative benefits of bare metal stents seems to be least effective when an optimal angiographic result is obtained after balloon angioplasty. Finally, drug-eluting stents have revolutionized the treatment of small and diffuse disease. Although the restenosis rates with DES in small vessels may be incrementally higher than in larger vessels, drug-eluting stents dramatically improve angiographic outcomes, reduce repeat revascularization, and decrease total cost in small and diffuse vessel coronary intervention. As a result, DES has become the dominant technology utilized for these lesions and has broadened the indication for transcatheter therapy in many untreatable patients who suffer from the difficult problem of small and diffuse coronary disease.

IV demonstrate substantial reductions in in-segment restenosis, with no edge restenosis with concomitant reductions in target vessel and target lesion revascularization (Figure 40-5). One issue arising from the TAXUS IV trial was that the rates of small vessel restenosis were lower than many anticipated, because a late loss of 0.3 mm historically seen with the TAXUS stent would have translated into higher restenosis rates in small vessels than were observed. To better understand this issue, Stone and colleagues examined late loss as a function of stent size.[67] In the TAXUS IV trial, the late loss noted with 3.5-mm, 3.0-mm, and 2.5-mm TAXUS stents was 0.28 mm, 0.22 mm, and 0.17 mm, respectively. One hypothesis explaining these results is that potentially with less expansion of the TAXUS stent-struts, there is greater paclitaxel delivered per unit area, resulting in lower neointimal accumulation.

Like in small vessels, both SES and TAXUS effectively reduce restenosis in diffuse disease. Figure 40-6 demonstrates the dramatic reduction in restenosis as a function of stent length in the SES and bare metal stent groups.[62] Similar observations were noted in TAXUS IV.[64]

In the setting of small vessel and diffuse disease, trials comparing paclitaxel-eluting and sirolimus-eluting stents have been inconsistent. The results of the A Prospective, Randomized, Multi-Center Comparison Study of the CYPHER Siroliumus-Eluting and TAXUS Paclitaxel-eluting Systems (REALITY) trial randomized patients having a mean vessel diameter of 2.4 mm and a lesion length of 17 mm to either the TAXUS or CYPHER SES stent.[68] Although the in-stent late loss was significantly less in the CYPHER group, there was no overall significant difference in binary angiographic restenosis and target lesion revascularization; in particular, neither stent was superior in the subgroups of "long lesions" and "small vessel." In contradistinction, Windecker and colleagues in the Randomized Comparison of SIRoliumus with PacliTAXel-eluting Stents for Coronary Revascularization in all Comers (SIRTAX) trial found that the angiographic restenosis and target lesion revascular-

REFERENCES

1. Schunkert H, Harrell L, Palacios IF. Implications of small reference vessel diameter in patients undergoing percutaneous coronary revascularization. *J Am Coll Cardiol.* 1999;34:40.
2. Ellis SG, Vandormael MG, Cowley MJ, et al. Coronary morphologic and clinical determinants of procedural outcome with angioplasty for multivessel coronary disease. Implications for patient selection. Multivessel Angioplasty Prognosis Study Group. *Circulation.* 1990;82:1193.
3. Akiyama T, Moussa I, Reimers B, et al. Angiographic and clinical outcome following coronary stenting of small vessels: a comparison with coronary stenting of large vessels. *J Am Coll Cardiol.* 1998;32:1610.
4. Elezi S, Kastrati A, Neumann FJ, et al. Vessel size and long-term outcomes after stent placement. *Circulation.* 1998;98:1875.

5. Hausleiter J, Kastrati A, Mehilli J, et al. Predictive factors for early cardiac events and angiographic restenosis after coronary stent placement in small coronary arteries. *J Am Coll Cardiol.* 2002;40:882.

6. Hirshfeld JW, Schwartz JS, Jugo R, et al. Restenosis after coronary angioplasty: a multivariate statistical model to relate lesion and procedure variables to restenosis. *J Am Coll Cardiol.* 1991;18:647.

7. Boaurassa MG, Lesperance J, Eastwood C, et al. Clinical, physiologic, anatomic and procedural factors predictive of restenosis after percutaneous transluminal coronary angioplasty. *J Am Coll Cardiol.* 1991;18:368.

8. Foley DP, Melkert R, Serruys PW. Influence of coronary vessel size on renarrowing process and late angiographic outcome after successful balloon angioplasty. *Circulation.* 1994;90:1239.

9. Kastrati A, Schomig A, Dirschinger J, et al. A randomized trial comparing stenting with balloon angioplasty in small vessels in patients with symptomatic coronary artery disease. ISAR-SMART Study Investigators. Intracoronary Stenting or Angioplasty for Restenosis Reduction in Small Arteries. *Circulation.* 2000;102:2593.

10. Savage MP, Fischman DL, Rake R, et al. Efficacy of coronary stenting versus balloon angioplasty in small coronary arteries. Stent Restenosis Study (STRESS) Investigators. *J Am Coll Cardiol.* 1998;31:307.

11. Lau KW, He Q, Ding ZP, et al. Safety and efficacy of angiography-guided stent placement in small native coronary arteries of < 3.0 mm in diameter. *Clin Cardiol.* 1997;20:711.

12. Huang P, Levin T, Kabour A, et al. Acute and late outcome after use of 2.5-mm intracoronary stents in small (< 2.5 mm) coronary arteries. *Catheter Cardiovasc Intervent.* 2000;49:121.

13. Haude M, Konorza TF, Kalnins U, et al, for the Heparin-COAted STents in small coronary arteries Trial Investigators. Heparin-coated stent placement for the treatment of stenoses in small coronary arteries of symptomatic patients. *Circulation.* 2003;107:1265.

14. Suwaidi JA, Garratt KN, Berger PB, et al. Immediate and one-year outcome of intracoronary stent implantation in small coronary arteries with 2.5-mm stents. *Am Heart J.* 2000;140:898.

15. Kuntz R, Gibson C, et al. Generalized model of restenosis after conventional balloon angioplasty, stenting and directional atherectomy. *J Am Coll Cardiol.* 1993;21;155.

16. Cohen DJ, Dauerman. Treatment of diffuse coronary lesions: a time for randomized trials. *Am Heart J.* 1999;137:193.

17. Mintz GS. Painter JA. Pichard AD, et al. Atherosclerosis in angiographically "normal" coronary artery reference segments: an intravascular ultrasound study with clinical correlations. *J Am Coll Cardiol.* 1995;25:1479.

18. Briguori C, Tobis J, Nishida T, et al. Discrepancy between angiography and intravascular ultrasound when analysing small coronary arteries [see comment]. *Eur Heart J.* 2002;23:247.

19. Moussa I, Kobayashi Y, Adamian M, et al. Characteristics of patients with a large discrepancy in coronary artery diameter between quantitative angiography and intravascular ultrasound. *Am J Cardiol.* 2001;88:294.

20. Meier B. How to treat small coronary vessels with angioplasty. *Heart.* 1998; 79:215.

21. Tenaglia AN, Zidar JP, Jackman JD Jr, et al. Treatment of long coronary artery narrowings with long angioplasty balloon catheters. *Am J Cardiol.* 1993; 71:1274.

22. Umeda H, Iwase M, Kanda H, et al. Promising efficacy of primary gradual and prolonged balloon angioplasty in small coronary arteries: a randomized comparison with cutting balloon angioplasty and conventional balloon angioplasty. *Am Heart J.* 2004;147:E4.

23. Lee MS, Singh V, Nero TJ, et al. Cutting balloon angioplasty. *J Invasive Cardiol.* 2002;14:552.

24. Okura H, Hayase M, Shimodozono S, et al, for the REDUCE (Restenosis Reduction by Cutting Balloon Evaluation) Investigators. Mechanisms of acute lumen gain following cutting balloon angioplasty in calcified and noncalcified lesions: an intravascular ultrasound study. *Catheter Cardiovasc Intervent.* 2002; 57:429.

25. Orford JL, Fasseas P, Denktas AE, et al. Safety and efficacy of cutting balloon angioplasty: the Mayo Clinic experience. *J Invasive Cardiol.* 2002;14:720.

26. Tsubokawa A, Ueda K, Sakamoto H, Iwase T, Tamaki S. Acute and long-term outcomes of rotational atherectomy in small (< 3.0 mm) coronary arteries. *J Intervent Cardiol.* 2003;16:315.

27. Bittl JA, Chew DP, Topol EJ, Kong DF, Califf RM. Meta-analysis of randomized trials of percutaneous transluminal coronary angioplasty versus atherectomy, cutting balloon atherotomy, or laser angioplasty. *J Am Coll Cardiol.* 2004;43:936.

28. Kwon K, Choi D, Choi SH, et al. Coronary stenting after rotational atherectomy in diffuse lesions of the small coronary artery: comparison with balloon angioplasty before stenting. *Angiology.* 2003;54:423.

29. Schuhlen H, Kastrati A, Dirschinger J, et al. Intracoronary stenting and risk for major adverse cardiac events during the first month. *Circulation.* 1998;98:104.

30. Chan CN, Tan AT, Koh TH, et al. Intracoronary stenting in the treatment of acute or threatened closure in angiographically small coronary arteries (< 3.0 mm) complicating percutaneous transluminal coronary angioplasty. *Am J Cardiol.* 1995;75:23.

31. Fishman D, Savage M, et al. Angiographic predictors of subacute thrombosis following coronary stenting. *Circulation.* 1991;84(suppl 2):588.

32. Azar A, Detre K, et al. A meta-analysis on the clinical and angiographic outcomes of stents vs. PTCA in the different coronary vessel sizes in the Benestent-1 and STRESS 1/2 trials. *Circulation.* 1995;92(suppl 1):475.

33. Holmes DR Jr, Hirshfeld J Jr, Faxon D, et al. ACC expert consensus document on coronary artery stents. *J Am Coll Cardiol.* 1998;32:1471.

34. Kawagishi N, Tsurumi Y, Ishii Y, et al. Clinical and angiographic outcome of stenting following suboptimal results of percutaneous transluminal coronary angioplasty in small (< 2.5 mm) coronary arteries. *Catheter Cardiovasc Intervent.* 1999;47:269.

35. Eeckhout E, Grobety M, Vogt P, et al. Corrective use of the 2.5-mm GFX stent for suboptimal angioplasty results in small coronary arteries. *Catheter Cardiovasc Interv.* 1999;48:157.

36. Koning R, Chan C, Eltchaninoff H, et al. Primary stenting of de novo lesions in small coronary arteries: a prospective, pilot study. *Cathet Cardiovasc Diagn.* 1998;45:235.

37. Casella G, Prati F. Stenting small coronary arteries: the Multi-Link PIXEL Multicenter Italian Registry. *J Invasive Cardiol.* 2003;15:371.

38. Kinsara AJ, Niazi K, Patel I, et al. Effectiveness of stents in small coronary arteries. *Am J Cardiol.* 2003:92:584.

39. Grenadier E, Roguin A, Hertz I, et al. Stenting very small coronary narrowings (< 2 mm) using the biocompatible phosphorylcholine-coated coronary stent. *Cathet Cardiovasc Intervent.* 2002;55:303.

40. Moer R, Myreng Y, Molstad P, et al. Stenting small coronary arteries using two second-generation slotted tube stents: acute and six-month clinical and angiographic results. *Cathet Cardiovasc Intervent.* 2000;50:307.

41. Ruygrok PN, Webster MW, Ardill JJ, et al. Vessel caliber and restenosis: a prospective clinical and angiographic study of NIR stent deployment in small and large coronary arteries in the same patient. *Cathet Cardiovasc Intervent.* 2003;59:165.

42. Cohen MG, Kong DF, Warner JJ, et al. Outcomes following interventions in small coronary arteries with the use of hand-crimped Palmaz-Schatz stents. *Am J Cardiol.* 2000;85:446.

43. Lau KW, Ding ZP, Sim LL, Sigwart U. Clinical and angiographic outcome after angiography-guided stent placement in small coronary vessels. *Am Heart J.* 2000;139:830.

44. Briguori C, Nishida T, Adamian M, et al. Coronary stenting versus balloon angioplasty in small coronary artery with complex lesions. *Cathet Cardiovasc Intervent.* 2000;50:390.

45. Lemos PA, Martinez EE, Quintella E, et al. Stenting vs. balloon angioplasty with provisional stenting for the treatment of vessels with small reference diameter. *Cathet Cardiovasc Intervent.* 2002;55:309.

46. Park SW, Lee CW, Hong MK, et al. Randomized comparison of coronary stenting with optimal balloon angioplasty for treatment of lesions in small coronary arteries. *Eur Heart J.* 2000;21:1785.

47. Koning R, Eltchaninoff H, Commeau P, et al, for the BESMART (BeStent in Small Arteries) Trial Investigators. Stent placement compared with balloon angioplasty for small coronary arteries: in-hospital and 6-month clinical and angiographic results. *Circulation.* 2001;104:1604.

48. Hausleiter J, Kastrati A, Mehilli J, et al, for the ISAR-SMART Trail investigators. Comparative analysis of stent placement versus balloon angioplasty in small coronary arteries with long narrowings (the Intracoronary Stenting or Angioplasty for Restenosis Reduction in Small Arteries [ISAR-SMART] Trial). *Am J Cardiol.* 2002;89:58.

49. Moer R, Myreng Y, Molstad P, et al. Stenting in small coronary arteries (SISCA) trial. A randomized comparison between balloon angioplasty and the heparin-coated beStent. *J Am Coll Cardiol.* 2001;8:1598.

50. Doucet S, Schalij MJ, Vrolix MC, et al, for the Stent In Small Arteries (SISA) Trial Investigators. Stent placement to prevent restenosis after angioplasty in small coronary arteries. *Circulation.* 2001;104:2029.

51. Rodriguez AE. Rodriguez Alemparte M, Fernandez Pereira C, et al. LASMAL II Investigators. Latin American randomized trial of balloon angioplasty versus

coronary stenting in diabetic patients with small vessel reference size (Latin American Small Vessel [LASMAL II] Trial): immediate and long-term results. *Am Heart J* 2005;150:188.

52. Garcia E, Gomez-Recio M, et al. Stent reduces restenosis in small vessels. Results of the RAP Study. *J Am Coll Cardiol.* 2001;37(suppl A):495.

53. Muramatsu T, Iwasaki K, Inoue N, et al. Coronary heart disease stenting in small vessels versus balloon angioplasty study (CHIVAS): A randomized prospective multicenter trial (abstr). *J Am Coll Cardiol.* 2002;39(Suppl A):50A.

54. Kastrati A, Mehilli J, Dirschinger J, et al. Intracoronary stenting and angiographic results: strut thickness effect on restenosis outcome (ISAR-STEREO) trial. *Circulation.* 2001;103:2816.

55. Moreno R, Fernandez C, Hernaneez-Antolin R, et al. The benefit of coronary stenting in small vessels is dependent on reference vessel diameter: results from a meta-analysis of 11 randomized trials. *J Am Coll Cardiol.* 2004;43:58A.

56. Serruys PW, Foley DP, Suttorp MJ, et al. A randomized comparison of the value of additional stenting after optimal balloon angioplasty for long coronary lesions: final results of the additional value of NIR stents for treatment of long coronary lesions (ADVANCE) study. *J Am Coll Cardiol.* 2002;39:393.

57. Colombo A, De Gregorio J, Moussa I, et al. Intravascular ultrasound-guided percutaneous transluminal coronary angioplasty with provisional spot stenting for treatment of long coronary lesions. *J Am Coll Cardiol.* 2001;38:1427.

58. Caputo RP, Flately M, Ho KK, Baim DS. Safety and effectiveness of stent implantation without predilation for small coronary arteries. *Cathet Cardiovasc Intervent.* 2003;59:455.

59. Garcia E. Randomized Trial of Direct Stenting with the Pixel Stent in Small Vessels. Transcatheter Cardiovascular Therapeutics (TCT), 2003. (Cited Feb 5, 2005.) Available from: http://www.tctmd.com/expert-presentations/slides.html.

60. Moussa I, Moses J, Di Mario C, et al. Does the specific intravascular ultrasound criterion used to optimize stent expansion have an impact on the probability of stent restenosis? *Am J Cardiol.* 1999;83:1012.

61. Morice M-C, Serruys PW, Sousa JE, et al. A randomized comparison of a sirolimus-eluting stent with a standard stent for coronary revascularization. *N Engl J Med.* 2002;346:1773.

62. Moses JW, Leon MB, Popma JJ, et al. Sirolimus-eluting stents versus standard stents in patients with stenosis in a native coronary artery. *N Engl J Med.* 2003;349:1315.

63. Grube E, Silber S, Hauptmann KE, et al. TAXUS I: six- and twelve-month results from a randomized, double-blind trial on a slow-release paclitaxel-eluting stent for de novo coronary lesions. *Circulation.* 2003;107:38.

64. Stone GW, Ellis SG, Cox DA, et al. A polymer-based, paclitaxel-eluting stent in patients with coronary artery disease. *N Eng J Med.* 2004;350:221.

65. Schampaert E, Cohen EA, Schluter M, et al, for the C-SIRIUS Investigators. The Canadian study of the sirolimus-eluting stent in the treatment of patients with long de novo lesions in small native coronary arteries (C-SIRIUS). *J Am Coll Cardiol.* 2004;43:1110.

66. Holmes DR, Moses J, Leon M, et al. Sirolimus versus plain old balloon angioplasty small vessels. *J Am Coll Cardiol.* 2005;43:35A.

67. Stone GW, Ellis SG, O'Shaughnessy C, et al. Reduction in late loss and restenosis in patients with small vessels treated with the slow rate-release, polymer-based paclitaxel-eluting stent: results from TAXUS-IV. *J Am Coll Cardiol.* 2005;43:87A.

68. Morice MC, Colombo A, Meier B, et al. REALITY Trial Investigators. Sirolimus- el. vs paclitaxel-eluting stents in de novo coronary artery lesions: the REALITY trial: a randomized controlled trial: *JAMA* 2006;295:895.

69. Windecker S, Remondino A, Eberli FR, et al. Sirolimus-eluting and paclitaxel-eluting stents for coronary revascularization. *N Eng J Med* 2005;353:653.

70. Greenberg D, Bakhai A, Cohen DJ. Can we afford to eliminate restenosis? Can we afford not to? *J Am Coll Cardiol.* 2004;43:513.

CHAPTER (41)

Special Patient Subsets: Patients with Diabetes and the Elderly

Zoran S. Nedeljkovic, MD, Clifford J. Berger, MD, and Alice K. Jacobs, MD

PATIENTS WITH DIABETES

Diabetes mellitus is a major contributor to the morbidity and mortality of cardiovascular disease, and its prevalence is growing steadily. Between 1980 and 2002, the number of Americans with diabetes more than doubled, from 5.8 to 13.3 million.[1] It is also estimated that an additional 5.2 million people in the United States have undiagnosed diabetes mellitus.[2] Both type 1 and type 2 diabetes are not only independent risk factors for the development of coronary artery disease, but they are also associated with other comorbidities such as renal insufficiency and peripheral vascular disease.[3–5]

Approximately 23% of patients undergoing percutaneous coronary intervention (PCI) in the first two waves of the Dynamic Registry of the National Heart Lung and Blood Institute (NHLBI) had diabetes.[6] This proportion will continue to increase as the prevalence of diabetes increases in the general population.

[ ] PERCUTANEOUS CORONARY INTERVENTION

Patients with diabetes undergoing PCI are more likely to have advanced coronary artery disease, with more multivessel disease, total occlusions, and diffuse disease, compared with their nondiabetic counterparts (Figure 41-1).[6–8] In the NHLBI Dynamic Registry, the patients with diabetes were more often women and had a higher prevalence of hypertension, hypercholesterolemia, renal insufficiency, peripheral vascular disease, and congestive heart failure in comparison to patients without diabetes.[6] In general, acute procedural success and complications are similar in diabetic

and non-diabetic patients undergoing PCI.[6,9,10] An analysis of the NHLBI Dynamic Registry demonstrated significantly higher in-hospital mortality in patients with diabetes compared with patients without diabetes (2.3% vs 1.3%, respectively; $P = .02$) undergoing contemporary PCI.[6] However, after adjustment for baseline concomitant risk factors, there remained a trend towards increased in-hospital mortality (OR 1.46, 95% CI 0.80–2.66). Additionally, patients with diabetes who undergo PCI are at increased risk of angiographic restenosis, repeat revascularization, and myocardial infarction (MI) and death during subsequent follow-up.[6,11,12] Despite use of coronary stents and glycoprotein IIb/IIIa platelet receptor antagonists, diabetes is still a significant and independent predictor of adverse events after PCI.[6,13] Furthermore, following MI, patients with diabetes are also at significantly higher risk of acute and long-term mortality and reinfarction.[14]

[ ] RESTENOSIS

The presence of diabetes represents a consistent risk factor for restenosis following balloon angioplasty (Figure 41-2). The biology and pathophysiology of restenosis following coronary intervention is discussed more extensively in Section 1, Chapter 7. However, there is evidence that the metabolic abnormalities associated with the diabetic state (hyperglycemia and hyperinsulinemia) can lead to enhanced platelet adhesion, activation, and aggregation, in addition to thrombus formation, endothelial cell dysfunction, and alterations in local growth factor production.[15] Smooth muscle cell proliferation and extracellular matrix deposition, crucial elements in the cellular response to vessel injury and subsequent development of restenosis following coronary intervention, are also enhanced in patients with diabetes.[15]

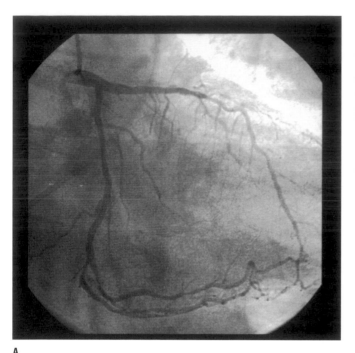

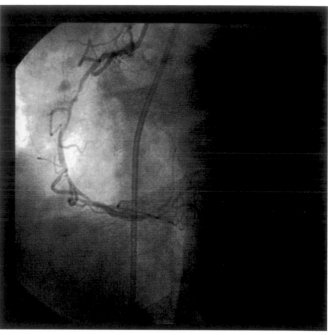

A

B

FIGURE 41-1. Selective angiography of the left (right anterior oblique, caudal projection) and right (left anterior oblique projection) coronary arteries in a patient with diabetes. Left coronary angiography (**A**) demonstrates diffuse narrowing of the mid to distal left anterior descending artery, occlusion of a second diagonal branch, and diffuse disease of a branching second obtuse marginal branch. The right coronary artery (**B**) is diffusely narrowed in the mid and distal portions.

Among patients with diabetes studied in the first report from the NHLBI Percutaneous Transluminal Coronary Angioplasty Registry, restenosis occurred in 47%, compared with 32% in patients without diabetes.[16] More contemporary data from the NHLBI Dynamic

Registry demonstrated a more frequent need for subsequent revascularization procedures in patients with diabetes compared with those without diabetes.[6] Alternative angioplasty devices, including directional coronary atherectomy, similarly showed higher rates of restenosis among patients with diabetes compared with those without diabetes.[10,17] By serving as an endovascular scaffold, coronary artery stenting prevents elastic recoil and vasospasm, resulting in a better acute gain in vessel size, when compared with balloon angioplasty alone.[18,19] Accordingly, restenosis following coronary stent placement is largely due to neointimal hyperplasia and can be further quantified angiographically as late loss (defined as the difference minimum lumen diameter [MLD] immediately postprocedure from MLD at follow-up). Carrozza et al observed that the mechanism of increased restenosis in patients with diabetes compared with those without diabetes following coronary stent placement was due to increased late loss of MLD, suggesting more aggressive neointimal hyperplasia in diabetes.[19] The potential of drug-eluting stents, regarding reduction in late loss and restenosis is discussed below.

【 】 PERCUTANEOUS CORONARY INTERVENTION VERSUS CORONARY ARTERY BYPASS SURGERY

The optimal method of revascularization in patients with diabetes and multivessel coronary artery disease remains controversial. The available data from a number of randomized clinical trials and registries provide conflicting results.

The Bypass Angioplasty Revascularization Investigation (BARI) trial randomized 1829 patients with symptomatic multivessel coronary artery disease to either multivessel balloon angioplasty with percutaneous transluminal coronary angioplasty (PTCA) or

FIGURE 41-2. Selective angiography of the left coronary artery (right anterior oblique, caudal projection) demonstrates diffuse restenosis within a previously placed stent in the proximal left anterior descending artery.

coronary artery bypass graft (CABG) surgery.[20] The overall trial results showed no difference in mortality between the two revascularization strategies. However, a subsequent post hoc analysis of the 353 patients with diabetes revealed a significantly lower 5-year survival in the group treated with PTCA compared with CABG (65.5% vs 80.6%).[21] The benefit of surgery was greater in the patients treated with insulin compared with those treated with oral hypoglycemic agents and appeared to be limited to patients receiving internal mammary artery grafts and to those with more diffuse disease defined by four or more lesions.[21,22]

One possible explanation for the improved survival seen in BARI in patients with diabetes undergoing CABG may be the increased progression of disease in patients with diabetes undergoing PTCA. One retrospective analysis of 248 patients referred for diagnostic angiography more than 1 month after successful PTCA found a significantly higher rate of new lesions on the follow-up angiogram in patients with diabetes compared with those without the disease (22% vs 12%, $P < .004$).[23] Angioplasty appeared to increase the risk of new lesions distant from the treatment site, and the risk was additive in patients with diabetes. This may, in part, account for the possible survival advantage of CABG, especially using the internal mammary artery, because the grafts would be presumed to be more protective than PTCA in the event of future plaque rupture.

The Coronary Angioplasty versus Bypass Revascularization Investigation (CABRI) and Emory Angioplasty versus Surgery Trial (EAST) trials were similar trials of PTCA versus CABG in patients with multivessel coronary artery disease.[24,25] Both trials showed a trend toward improved survival with CABG in the diabetic subset, but the number of patients with diabetes in these trials was small and the differences did not reach statistical significance.

However, not all studies have confirmed the findings reported in BARI of improved survival of patients with diabetes treated with CABG. BARI also included a registry of an additional 2010 patients with multivessel disease who were eligible for the trial but did not consent to randomization.[26] In the registry, nearly twice as many patients were selected by their physicians for PTCA compared with CABG. When treating physicians chose the revascularization method for their patients with diabetes and multivessel disease, the 7-year survival was similar for patients undergoing PTCA or CABG. Patients selected for CABG tended to have more lesions, proximal disease of the left anterior descending artery, and type C lesions.

Furthermore, other databases such as the Duke University registry have not found mortality differences among patients with diabetes undergoing PTCA compared with those treated with CABG.[27] Patients with diabetes receiving either PTCA or CABG had significantly higher mortality compared with patients without the disease, after adjustment for baseline characteristics, but the effect of diabetes on prognosis was similar in both treatment groups.

PERCUTANEOUS CORONARY INTERVENTION WITH STENTS VERSUS CORONARY ARTERY BYPASS SURGERY

All of the above mentioned trials compared PTCA with CABG, but clinical practice has evolved such that the vast majority of PCI procedures now involve the implantation of coronary stents, which result in lower rates of emergency CABG and restenosis.[28,29]

To determine whether the use of stents would decrease the difference in outcomes between patients treated with PTCA and CABG, 1205 patients with multivessel disease were randomly assigned to bare metal stents or CABG in the Arterial Revascularization Therapy Study (ARTS).[30] Although the overall mortality was similar in this trial between the two revascularization strategies, the subgroup of patients with diabetes had a lower 1-year event-free survival rate with multivessel stenting compared with CABG (63% vs 84%)[30,31] that was driven by a higher rate of repeat revascularization in the group treated with stents. There was a trend toward a higher mortality in the patients with diabetes treated with multivessel stents compared with CABG (6.3% vs 3.1%), but this difference did not reach statistical significance.

BARI-2D is another ongoing trial in which patients with diabetes are randomized in a 2×2 design to revascularization (with PCI or CABG) with intensive medical therapy to an initial strategy of intensive medical therapy alone.[32] The second arm of the trial is comparing the use of insulin providing to an insulin-sensitizing regimen for optimal glycemic control. This trial should be an important addition to our understanding of the optimal treatment strategies for patients with diabetes and coronary artery disease.

DRUG-ELUTING STENTS

Following the introduction of drug-eluting stents into clinical practice, there has been increasing enthusiasm for their use in the majority of patients receiving PCI. There is still a relative paucity of data examining the differential benefits of drug-eluting stents in patients with diabetes.

Of the 1058 patients in the SIRolImUS (SIRIUS) trial comparing the sirolimus-eluting Cypher stent to a bare metal stent, 279 patients had diabetes.[33] Target lesion revascularization and major adverse cardiac events were reduced in the patients with diabetes receiving the sirolimus-eluting stent compared with the bare metal stent. After 9 months, 22.3% of the patients with diabetes receiving bare metal stents compared with only 6.9% of those receiving drug-eluting stents required repeat PCI. Major adverse cardiac events (death, MI, repeat revascularization) were also reduced from 25% in the patients receiving bare metal stents compared with 9.2% in the patients receiving drug-eluting stents. There was also some suggestion that patients with insulin-requiring diabetes had more restenosis than those who did not require insulin, but the numbers were too small to be conclusive.[33] The sirolimus-eluting Cypher stent was clearly superior to bare metal stents even in patients with diabetes, but we eagerly await additional randomized trial data to guide us on optimal patient selection for PCI compared with CABG in patients with diabetes and multivessel disease.

Another trial was designed to test the efficacy of two different paclitaxel-eluting stent formulations, a slow-release and moderate-release, compared with a bare metal stent in 536 patients.[34] The main objective of the study was to assess the percentage of in-stent neointimal obstruction at 6 months using intravascular ultrasound. Other secondary end points included the rate of restenosis at 6 months as well as the incidence of major adverse cardiac events at 6 and 12 months. Both the slow- and moderate-release formulations demonstrated a similar percentage of neointimal obstruction (7.8 %) that was significantly lower than the obstruction associated with bare metal stents (23.2% and 20.5%, respectively). Six-month binary restenosis rates were significantly improved in both the slow-release (20.1% vs 5.5%, $P = .0004$) and moderate-release (23.8% vs 8.6%, $P = .001$) formulations, when compared with bare metal stents. Clinical event rates (death, MI, or target vessel revascularization [TVR]) were also lower at 6 months in the slow-release versus control group (8.5% vs 19.5%, $P = .01$) and in the moderate-release versus control group (7.8% vs 20.0%, $P = .006$). These improved clinical event rates were largely driven by lower rates of target lesion revascularization among patients receiving paclitaxel-eluting stents, and were consistent at 12-months follow-up. Unpublished data similarly show lower 6-month binary restenosis with paclitaxel-eluting stents compared to bare metal stents, not only in patients without diabetes (18.4% vs 1.4%, $P < .0001$) but also in those with diabetes (20.5% vs 0%, $P = .0059$) (JB Hermiller, MD; Transcatheter Cardiovascular Therapeutics, September 29, 2004, Washington, DC).

The TAXUS IV trial enrolled 1314 patients and included a broader range of lesion subsets (2.5–3.75-mm diameter and 10-28-mm length) to examine the efficacy of a polymer-based paclitaxel-eluting stent in reducing the risk of clinical and angiographic restenosis.[35] This study reported a 61% relative risk reduction in TVR at 9 months with implantation of a paclitaxel-eluting stent compared with a bare metal stent (4.7% vs 12%, $P < .001$). This significant reduction in TVR resulted in a similar reduction in major adverse cardiac events (death, MI, TVR) at 9 months (8.5% vs 15%, $P < .001$). Unpublished data examining the subset of patients with diabetes in TAXUS IV demonstrated consistent reductions in binary restenosis. Compared with bare metal stents, paclitaxel-eluting stents resulted in a lower rate of binary restenosis at 9 months in both patients without diabetes (22.5% vs 5.6%, $P < .001$) and those with diabetes (31.6% vs 5.1%, $P < .001$) (JB Hermiller, MD; Transcatheter Cardiovascular Therapeutics, September 29, 2004, Washington, DC).

The Future Revascularization Evaluation in Diabetic patients: Optimal management of Multivessel disease (FREEDOM) trial is an ongoing multicenter trial randomizing patient with diabetes to multivessel PCI with drug-eluting stents or CABG and should provide further guidance to the best method of revascularization in diabetics with coronary disease.

【　】GLYCOPROTEIN IIB/IIIA PLATELET RECEPTOR ANTAGONISTS

The glycoprotein IIb/IIIa inhibitors have been shown to reduce the incidence of acute ischemic complications after elective or urgent PCI by 30% to 50%.[36,37] Patients with diabetes tend to have larger platelets with increased platelet aggregation and adhesiveness and greater thromboxane synthesis, glycoprotein IIb/IIIa expression, and mitogenic activity.[38–42] Diabetes has also been associated with increased levels of circulating fibrinogen, thrombin, as well as factor VII, diminished antithrombin III, and fibrinolytic activity.[37,41,42]

One meta-analysis examined the subset of diabetic patients in six large, randomized, double-blind trials of glycoprotein IIb/IIIa inhibitors in the setting of acute coronary syndromes.[43] The trials included in this analysis were Platelet Receptor Inhibition in Ischemic Syndrome Management (PRISM),[44] Platelet Receptor Inhibition in Ischemic Syndrome Management in Patients Limited

by Unstable Signs and Symptoms (PRISM-PLUS),[45] Platelet IIb/IIIa Antagonism for the Reduction of Acute Coronary Syndrome Events in a Global Organization Network (PARAGON) A,[46] Platelet IIb/IIIa Antagonism for the Reduction of Acute Coronary Syndrome Events in a Global Organization Network (PARAGON) B,[47] Platelet Glycoprotein IIb/IIIa in Unstable Angina: Receptor Suppression Using Integrilin Therapy (PURSUIT),[48] and Global Utilization of Strategies To Open Occluded Coronary Arteries (GUSTO)-IV.[49] The analysis included several different agents (tirofiban in PRISM and PRISM-PLUS, lamifiban in PARAGON A and PARAGON B, eptifibatide in PURSUIT, and abciximab in GUSTO-IV). A total of 6458 patients with diabetes and 23,072 patients without diabetes were included in these six trials. Among the patients with diabetes, the use of glycoprotein IIb/IIIa inhibitors was associated with a significant reduction in mortality at 30 days (6.2% vs 4.6%, $P = .007$), whereas the patients without diabetes showed no survival benefit (3.0% vs 3.0%). The most marked benefit of the glycoprotein IIb/IIIa inhibitors was seen in the 1279 patients with diabetes in these trials who underwent PCI during the index hospitalization. This group had a reduction in mortality at 30 days from 4.0% in the placebo group to 1.2% in the active treatment group ($P = .002$). The magnitude of the survival benefit appeared similar across all patients with diabetes, regardless of the use of insulin, oral hypoglycemic drugs, or diet control alone. However, whether there is a significant advantage of one glycoprotein IIb/IIIa agent compared with the others in patients with diabetes who have acute coronary syndromes is unclear.

Lincoff performed a meta-analysis of five randomized trials of glycoprotein IIb/IIIa inhibitors during PCI and reported detailed outcomes for patients with and without diabetes.[37] These trials included Evaluation of c7E3 for Prevention of Ischemic Complications (EPIC),[50] Evaluation in PTCA to Improve Long-term Outcome with abciximab GP IIb/IIIa blockade (EPILOG),[51] Evaluation of Platelet Inhibition in STENTing (EPISTENT),[52] Enhanced Suppression of the Platelet IIb/IIIa Receptor with Integrilin Therapy (ESPRIT),[53] and do Tirofiban And ReoPro Give similar Efficacy Trial (TARGET).[54] Abciximab versus placebo was used in EPIC, EPILOG, and EPISTENT; eptifibatide versus placebo in ESPRIT; and tirofiban versus abciximab in TARGET. The four placebo-controlled trials comparing abciximab or eptifibatide to placebo showed similar benefits in the 30-day end point of death, MI, or urgent revascularization in both diabetic and nondiabetic patients (Figure 41-3). Furthermore, the 30-day event rates were not higher in patients with diabetes compared with those without diabetes, consistent with other trials that have shown similar risk for early ischemic complications after PCI. The TARGET trial also showed the benefits of abciximab over tirofiban for 30-day major adverse cardiac events was similar in patients with and without diabetes.

The rate of TVR was higher at 6 months (Figure 41-4) in patients with diabetes versus those without diabetes in all trials except EPILOG, but the effects of glycoprotein IIb/IIIa inhibition on TVR appear to be less consistent in these studies. Only the EPISTENT trial showed a significant reduction in TVR in patients with diabetes after stenting when a glycoprotein IIb/IIIa inhibitor was used. In EPISTENT, the use of abciximab in patients with diabetes undergoing stent implantation was associated with a 50% decrease in TVR rates only in patients with the disease, and this

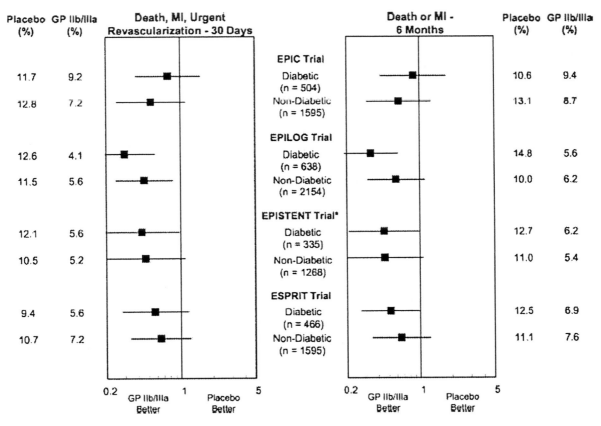

FIGURE 41-3. Odds ratio and 95% confidence intervals for 30-day (*left*) and 6-month (*right*) ischemic end points among diabetic and nondiabetic patients in placebo-controlled trials of abciximab (EPIC, EPILOG, and EPISTENT) or eptifibatide (ESPRIT). Stent arms (placebo vs abciximab) only in EPISTENT. GP = glycoprotein; MI = myocardial infarction. (*Reproduced with permission from Lippincott Williams & Wilkins; Lincoff AM.[37]*)

effect was not seen in those without the disease.[52] However, in the TARGET trial, there was no difference in TVR rates among diabetics randomized to abciximab compared with tirofiban.[54]

The Prevention of REStenosis with Tranilast and its Outcomes (PRESTO) trial enrolled 11,482 patients randomized to receive tranilast (an investigational drug with the potential to reduce restenosis) versus placebo.[13] This study revealed no difference between groups with respect to the primary end point, but a subgroup analysis found that the patients with diabetes had a higher rate of death, MI, and TVR at 9 months after PCI than those without diabetes. However, in the 43% of patients with the disease who received abciximab, there was no reduction in TVR. This contradicts the findings in the EPISTENT trial of a reduction in TVR with abciximab in the group with diabetes.[52] Overall, there is no consistent evidence that patients with diabetes have a reduction in restenosis with the use of abciximab.

【 】 PRACTICAL CONSIDERATIONS

As described above, patients with diabetes undergoing PCI are at increased risk of periprocedural and long-term complications.[6] Careful periprocedural and intraprocedural management can often mitigate some of the acute risk. Representative strategies that have been helpful to consider are described below.

Patients with diabetes should be in a euvolemic state prior to receiving iodinated contrast agents. Volume depletion increases the

risk of contrast-medicated renal insufficiency, which is a particular concern in patients with diabetes. We recommend that diuretics be held the morning of the scheduled procedure and if there is any baseline renal impairment, consider withholding angiotensin-converting enzyme inhibitors and administering *N*-acetylcysteine. Our practice is to withhold metformin at least 24 hours prior to the procedure, if possible, and to withhold it for a minimum of 72 hours postprocedure. In addition, we routinely hold oral hypoglycemic agents and short-acting insulin preparations. Long-acting insulin can be administered at a reduced (half) dose. Our patients also routinely receive 0.9% isotonic saline (with dextrose added if insulin is administered) at a rate of 1 ml/kg/h prior to the start of the procedure.

Although there is lack of compelling data to suggest any major differences in outcomes, we routinely use low- or iso-osmolar iodinated contrast agents and monitor total intake and output during the course of the cardiac catheterization. Continuous monitoring of right heart filling pressures is often helpful in this regard. Because patients with diabetes are at increased risk of repeat revascularization, intracoronary stents (particularly drug-eluting) are our preferred revascularization strategy. A few studies suggest that glycoprotein IIb/IIIa inhibitors are particularly helpful in patients with diabetes and result in reduced immediate and long-term complications.[43]

In the postprocedure setting, attention to volume status remains critical. We routinely administer 2 to 3 liters of isotonic saline

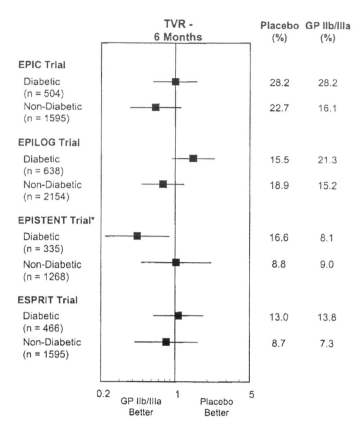

TVR - 6 Months	Placebo (%)	GP IIb/IIIa (%)
EPIC Trial		
Diabetic (n = 504)	28.2	28.2
Non-Diabetic (n = 1595)	22.7	16.1
EPILOG Trial		
Diabetic (n = 638)	15.5	21.3
Non-Diabetic (n = 2154)	18.9	15.2
EPISTENT Trial*		
Diabetic (n = 335)	16.6	8.1
Non-Diabetic (n = 1268)	8.8	9.0
ESPRIT Trial		
Diabetic (n = 466)	13.0	13.8
Non-Diabetic (n = 1595)	8.7	7.3

FIGURE 41-4. Odds ratio and 95% confidence intervals for 6-month target vessel revascularization end point in patients with and without diabetes in placebo-controlled trials of abciximab (EPIC, EPILOG, and EPISTENT) or eptifibatide (ESPRIT). Stent arms (placebo versus abciximab) only in EPISTENT. GP = glycoprotein; TVR = target vessel revascularization. *(Reproduced with permission from Lippincott Williams & Wilkins; Lincoff AM.[37])*

postprocedure and monitor intake and output. Measurement of serum electrolytes and creatinine is also routine in our patients on the day after the procedure. Implementing some of these practical maneuvers may decrease the overall procedural risks of PCI in patients with diabetes.

【 】 RECOMMENDATIONS

We prefer PCI in patients with diabetes and single- or double-vessel coronary artery disease, if the anatomy is suitable. However, deciding on a revascularization strategy in a patient with diabetes and multivessel (and multilesion) coronary artery disease is more of a challenge. We strongly consider CABG for patients with diabetes and multivessel diffuse disease, particularly if left ventricular systolic function is reduced and renal function is impaired. However, emerging data on drug-eluting stents in diabetic patients may reveal PCI to be as durable as CABG.

ELDERLY PATIENTS

According to the US Census Bureau, there were 34 million Americans over the age of 65 in 1990.[55] This group represents the fastest growing segment of the US population, and by 2030, it is projected that the group will make up 25% of the population.[55] The prevalence of coronary artery disease is higher in the elderly and as this population grows, the number with symptomatic coronary artery disease will also increase. Accordingly, elderly patients will increasingly be referred for invasive evaluation and treatment of coronary artery disease.[56]

【 】 REVASCULARIZATION VERSUS MEDICAL THERAPY

Coronary revascularization, with either PCI or CABG, is appropriate for relieving ischemic symptoms in patients with obstructive coronary artery disease.[57,58] Medically treated patients can further be stratified into "high-risk" or "low-risk" for mortality, based on certain clinical features, and may benefit from earlier revascularization (predominantly surgical).[59–61] Prior randomized studies of coronary revascularization compared with medical therapy included mostly younger patients, and these findings might not be applicable to the elderly. However, an earlier report from the Coronary Artery Surgery Study (CASS) registry of nearly 1500 nonrandomized patients older than 65 years of age demonstrated an improvement in survival and symptoms with surgical versus medical therapy. This survival benefit, however, was limited to "high-risk" patients, not those with mild angina, relatively preserved left ventricular systolic function, and no left main coronary obstruction.[62]

More recently, the Trial of Invasive versus Medical therapy in Elderly patients with symptomatic coronary artery disease (TIME) investigators prospectively compared an invasive revascularization strategy versus optimized medical therapy, in patients aged 75 years or older (n = 301), with chronic angina pectoris (Canadian Cardiac Society class 2 or more) despite treatment with at least two anti-anginal medications.[63] Subjects in the invasive arm underwent cardiac catheterization followed by either PCI or CABG. Those randomized to optimum medical therapy had an increase in the number and dose of antianginal medications, with 44% requiring three or more drugs to decrease symptoms. The primary end points of the study were quality of life and the presence of a major adverse event (death, nonfatal MI, or hospitalization for acute coronary syndrome). Among the group randomized to the invasive approach, 109 (74%) underwent revascularization procedures, of which 79 (72%) were PCI and 30 (28%) were CABG. The remaining patients (n = 43) were medically treated, either because they refused revascularization, had anatomy unsuitable for revascularization, or had no significant coronary artery disease. At 6-month follow-up, angina severity decreased and quality of life increased in both groups, but these two conditions improved more significantly in the group assigned to invasive treatment. Major adverse events occurred more frequently in the medical group compared to the invasive group (49% vs 19%, $P < .0001$), predominantly due to higher rates of hospitalization for acute coronary syndromes and nonfatal MI. Six-month mortality was lower in the medical group (6.2%) but twice as high in the invasive group (13%), although it did not reach statistical significance.

Among elderly patients, improvements in symptom and quality of life measures may take more precedence to survival end points. The results of this study suggest that coronary revascularization (here primarily achieved with PCI) in patients 75 years of age or older, results in less angina, a better quality of life, and fewer hospital readmissions, when compared with optimized medical therapy.

【 】 PERCUTANEOUS CORONARY INTERVENTION

Older patients referred for PCI are more likely to manifest multivessel or diffuse disease, have calcified coronary arteries, and have a prior history of MI and baseline left ventricular dysfunction, placing them at higher risk of periprocedural morbidity and mortality (Figure 41-5).[64] An earlier report of a cohort of elderly patients undergoing balloon angioplasty similarly reported higher procedural, particularly vascular, complications.[65] Age was also found to be an independent risk factor for death and MI. These elderly patients were more likely to be female and present with unstable coronary syndromes, both features associated with higher complication rates. As operator experience and procedural technique have improved over time, the rates of procedure-related

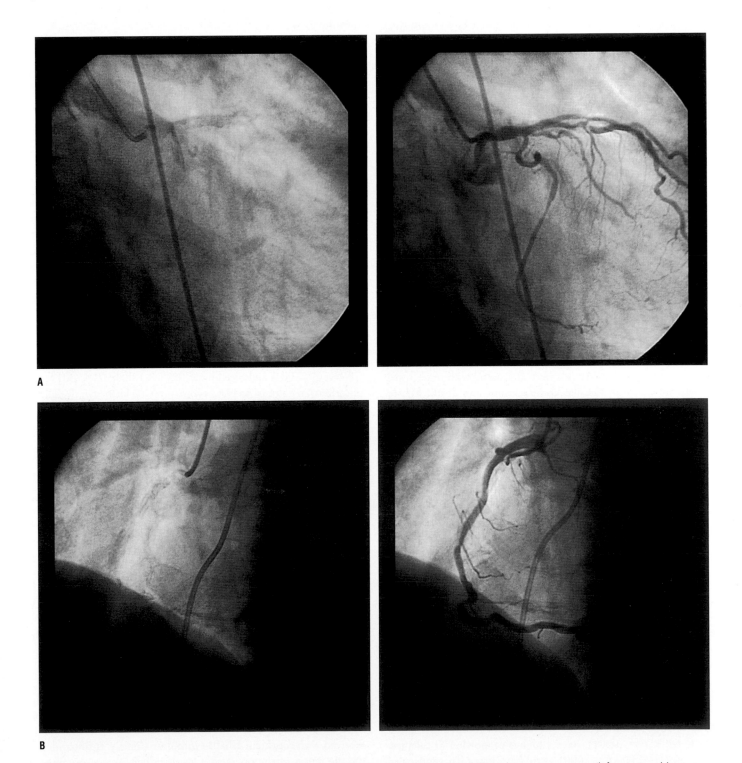

FIGURE 41-5. Fluoroscopy of the (**A**) left coronary artery (anterior posterior projection) and (**B**) right coronary artery (left anterior oblique projection) immediately prior to contrast injection demonstrates moderate vessel calcification.

complications have decreased, even in the elderly.[66] Advances in interventional techniques, particularly intracoronary stent deployment and adjunctive glycoprotein IIb/IIIa inhibitor use, have improved procedural success rates and ischemic complications, and data in the elderly are emerging.[67]

Using the National Cardiovascular Network database (NCN), Batchelor et al examined the contemporary outcomes of octogenarians undergoing PCI compared with patients younger than 80 years of age over a 4-year period (1994–1997).[68] This multicenter database represents the largest procedural outcomes study in the stent era and includes 7472 octogenarians and 102,236 nonoctogenarians. Octogenarians in this series were more likely to be female and have their procedure performed on an urgent basis. They were also more likely to have other comorbidities, including peripheral vascular and cerebrovascular disease and renal insufficiency. This older cohort was also more likely to have multivessel disease and moderate to severely reduced left ventricular systolic function (ejection fraction < 35 %), consistent with prior reports in the elderly. The use of balloon angioplasty and stenting was similar between the two groups, although octogenarians were more likely to undergo atheroablative procedures using rotational atherectomy, presumably due to a higher prevalence of calcified coronary arteries. Procedural success was achieved in both groups at a fairly high rate, although somewhat less in the octogenarian group (84% vs 89%, $P < .001$). Clinical outcomes, however, were uniformly inferior in the octogenarians, including a higher mortality (3.8% vs 1.1%, OR 3.6, 95% CI 3.2–4.1), a higher composite of death, MI, or stroke (4.9% vs 1.9%, OR 2.6, 95% [CI 2.3–2.9]), and a higher incidence of vascular complications (6.7% vs 3.3%, OR 2.1, 95% CI 1.9–2.4). During the 4 years of the study, procedural outcomes improved for all patients, and even more in octogenarians, possibly explained by the increased use of coronary stents. Favorable trends were also noted with respect to a decreased incidence of vascular complications and death, MI, or stroke when comparing data from 1997 with 1994. Using multivariate logistic regression analysis, the investigators were able to identify seven clinical features associated with increased mortality in octogenarians. In order of decreasing importance, these were cardiogenic shock, acute MI, ejection fraction less than 35%, renal insufficiency, first PCI, age of 85 years or more, and diabetes mellitus. This suggests that one may be able to identify a "low risk" octogenarian, namely one younger than 85 years of age who does not have diabetes or renal impairment and who is undergoing a PCI in the nonurgent setting (not for acute MI or cardiogenic shock). In summary, these data suggest that in appropriately selected patients, contemporary PCI can be performed with high rates of procedural success and relatively low mortality.

DeGregorio and colleagues examined a group of 137 elderly patients older than 75 years of age who underwent coronary stent procedures at their center between March 1993 and July 1997.[64] They were compared with a group of patients younger than 75 years of age (n = 2551) who underwent similar procedures during the same period. Compared with the younger group, elderly patients were more likely to present with unstable angina (47% vs 28%, $P = .0001$), have a higher prevalence of multivessel disease (78% vs 62%, $P = .0001$), have a higher proportion of calcified lesions (30% vs 13%, $P = .0001$), and have lower left ventricular ejection fractions (54% vs 58%, $P = .0001$). Procedure-related

complications were also higher in the elderly group, including MI, defined as an elevation in creatine kinase levels to twice normal with or without the development of pathologic Q waves (2.9% vs 1.7%, $P = .2$), emergency CABG (3.7% vs 1.4%, $P = .04$), and procedural death (2.2% vs 0.1%, $P = 0.0001$). Thrombotic events and bleeding complications did not differ significantly between the two groups. Similarly, vascular complications were also equal between the two groups (0.8% vs 0.9%, $P = NS$), representing a marked reduction when compared with a decade ago. During follow-up, restenosis and TVR rates were higher in the elderly group, most likely explained by the elderly populations' higher-risk clinical (unstable angina, lower ejection fraction) and angiographic (more complex and calcified lesions) presentation. Clinical follow-up of only the elderly group during a mean period of 12 months demonstrated an event-free survival (survival free from death, MI, revascularization, and angina) of 54%, and an overall survival of 91%. Despite higher rates of periprocedural complications, a higher incidence of restenosis, and lower event-free survival, this elderly group of patients undergoing PCI with coronary stents demonstrated a favorable overall 1-year survival.

Chauhan et al reported on the largest series of pooled data from a cohort of elderly patients (≥ 80 years) enrolled in six major trials of coronary stent procedures between September 1995 and March 1999.[69] These elderly patients (n = 301) were more likely to present with unstable angina and have multivessel disease when compared with the nonelderly patients (n = 5885). Procedural success was achieved at a rate greater than 97%, despite smaller reference vessel diameters and more prevalent vessel calcification in this cohort. The in-hospital mortality was significantly higher in the aged population (1.33% vs 0.1%, $P = .001$), although lower than previously reported by DeGregorio et al (2.2%).[64] In this series, elderly patients had a higher incidence of vascular (4.98% vs 1.19%, $P < .001$) and bleeding (4.98% vs 1.00%, $P < .001$) complications, in contrast to DeGregorio's report. However, overall, the elderly patients in this series had favorable outcomes with regard to restenosis and no difference in target lesion revascularization, when compared to the nonelderly patients at 1-year follow-up (8.30% vs 10.90%, $P = .19$). The investigators concluded that aged patients may safely undergo PCI using coronary stents, with excellent short- and long-term outcomes, although with higher vascular and bleeding complications, and higher in-hospital and 1-year mortality.

Numerous randomized controlled clinical trials have demonstrated the benefits of adjunctive glycoprotein IIb/IIIa inhibitor administration in patients undergoing PCI with respect to periprocedural ischemic complications (mainly cardiac enzyme elevations and nonfatal MI).[50–52,70–72] Although shown to be safe, with low rates of bleeding complications, the elderly were in general underrepresented, and the safety and efficacy of these agents in this group are less well established. Many interventional cardiologists have reservations using potent intravenous antiplatelet regimens in the elderly, particularly if the risk of bleeding (especially intracranial hemorrhage) may outweigh the potential benefit. Sadeghi et al examined 1392 consecutive patients, 80 years of age and older, who underwent PCI at a single center between January 1998 and June 2001.[73] Of this unselected cohort, 459 (33%) received a glycoprotein IIb/IIIa inhibitor (mostly eptifibatide), at the discretion of the operator. Octogenarians in the glycoprotein IIb/IIIa inhibitor group had higher rates of access-site and non-access-site bleeding compared with those in the nonglycoprotein IIb/IIIa inhibitor group. However, there was no increase in the risk of intracranial or retroperitoneal hemorrhage. Consistent with higher bleeding rates, hospital length-of-stay in the glycoprotein IIb/IIIa inhibitor group was longer than in the nonglycoprotein IIb/IIIa inhibitor group. It is interesting to note that there was a higher incidence of postprocedural non-Q-wave MI in the glycoprotein IIb/IIIa inhibitor group, which can be explained by their higher-risk clinical and procedural profile (more unstable clinical presentations or multivessel interventions). In-hospital mortality rates in the patients treated with and without glycoprotein IIb/IIIa inhibitors were 3.1% versus 3.0%, respectively. This relatively high mortality may also be explained by the higher-risk profile of octogenarians referred for coronary revascularization in the current era. These data should be interpreted cautiously before being applied broadly to all octogenarians, because patients were selected for glycoprotein IIb/IIIa inhibitor use at the discretion of the operator performing the PCI, and not in a randomized or blinded fashion. It is reassuring, however, that these potent antiplatelet agents can be used safely in selected elderly patients.

【 】 ACUTE CORONARY SYNDROMES

Results of several key randomized trials have demonstrated that a routine invasive strategy (coronary angiography followed by revascularization) is superior to a conservative strategy (angiography and revascularization driven by recurrent symptoms or inducible ischemia on stress testing) in the management of moderate-risk patients with acute coronary syndrome without ST-segment elevation.[74–77] Although the trend is shifting, elderly patients have traditionally been underrepresented in randomized controlled trials of acute coronary syndrome and MI. A recent analysis of the published literature demonstrated that patients older than 75 years of age made up only 2% of all subjects studied prior to 1990, but increased to 9% in the decade from 1991 to 2000.[78] Despite some of these more recent trials having no explicit exclusion criteria with respect to age, these figures are still low in relation to the number patients in the United States with MI who are elderly (37%). Others have also found that elderly patients are less likely to receive standard therapy for unstable angina, including cardiac catheterization, compared with their younger counterparts.[79]

Although increasing age is a powerful predictor of adverse events in the setting of acute coronary syndrome, some physicians may be reluctant to offer the elderly invasive cardiac procedures due to the increased incidence of periprocedural complications. To further clarify the impact of age on outcomes comparing an early invasive strategy with one of conservative management in patients with acute coronary syndrome, Bach and colleagues analyzed data from the recent Treat Angina with Aggrastat and Determine Cost of Therapy with an Invasive or Conservative Strategy-Thrombolysis in Myocardial infarction (TACTICS-TIMI) 18 trial.[80] Patients enrolled in TACTICS-TIMI 18 were treated with aspirin, heparin, and tirofiban and randomly assigned to an early invasive or conservative treatment arm. The primary end point was a composite of death, nonfatal MI, or rehospitalization for acute coronary syndrome. As prespecified in the study protocol, end point comparisons were stratified on the basis of age (< 65 vs ≥ 65 years). The patients 65 years of age and older (n = 962, representing 43% of

the entire study group) were more likely to be women and have features associated with higher baseline risk, including ST-segment changes on electrocardiogram, elevated serum troponin T, and a history of diabetes mellitus and congestive heart failure. In TACTICS-TIMI 18, patients 65 years of age or older more often had Thrombolysis in Myocardial Infarction (TIMI) risk scores greater than or equal to 3 (intermediate or high risk[81]) when compared with the younger group (90.6% vs 63%, $P < .001$). The results comparing the early invasive with the conservative strategy between the two age strata were impressive. The composite rate of death and MI in patients younger than 65 years of age did not differ significantly between the groups assigned to either invasive or conservative treatments at 30 days (3.9% vs 4.9%) or 6 months (6.1% vs 6.5%). However, in patients 65 years of age or older, an early invasive strategy conferred a 44% relative risk reduction in the composite of death and nonfatal MI compared with a conservative strategy at 30 days (5.7% vs 9.8%, $P = .019$). Findings in this group between the two strategies were similar at 6 months (8.8% vs 13.6%, $P = .018$). A post hoc analysis of patients stratified according to age (≤ 55, > 55–65, > 65–75, and > 75 years) found progressively increasing benefit from an early invasive strategy with regard to the end point of death and nonfatal MI in older patients. Compared with conservative management, patients older than 75 years of age assigned to an early invasive strategy had a 56% relative risk reduction in death or MI (10.8% vs 21.6%, $P = .016$). In none of the other three age groups was there any statistical difference in an early invasive versus a conservative, ischemia-driven strategy in these patients with acute coronary syndrome.

Several findings should be emphasized. First, this study represents more contemporary management of patients who present with unstable angina and non-ST segment elevation MI, including upstream use of a glycoprotein IIb/IIIa inhibitor and use of coronary stents during PCI (in > 80% of patients). Second, when elderly patients present with acute coronary syndrome, they tend to have a higher clinical risk profile and a higher TIMI risk score compared with younger patients. Finally, a routine early invasive strategy offers more reduction in the cumulative incidence of death and MI among older patients, compared with a conservative strategy especially in the subgroup older than 75 years of age.

Methods to establish patency of an occluded infarct-related artery rapidly and effectively are of paramount importance in the management of patients with ST-segment elevation MI (STEMI). Typically, this can be achieved with either fibrinolysis or primary PCI with or without coronary stent placement. The elderly, in particular, are at increased risk of hemorrhagic complications from receiving fibrinolytic therapy, and primary PCI may be a more attractive strategy.[82] The largest contemporary trial to examine the outcomes of the elderly undergoing primary PCI for acute MI, the Controlled Abciximab and Device Investigation to Lower Late Angioplasty Complications (CADILLAC) trial, recently reported their findings in the elderly.[83] Although elderly patients had more baseline comorbid conditions compared with their younger counterparts (history of hypertension and cerebrovascular and peripheral vascular disease) and tended to present later during the course of their MI, procedural success was similar across all age groups. Specifically, final angiographic measures (percent residual stenosis and postprocedural TIMI grade 3 flow) were similar among all age groups. Despite similar procedural success rates, 30-day and 1-year rates of mortality, stroke, and major bleeding were increased in elderly patients compared with their younger counterparts.

[ ] CARDIOGENIC SHOCK

Cardiogenic shock represents one of the most devastating complications and is the leading cause of death from MI. The SHould we emergently revascularize Occluded Coronaries for cardiogenic shocK (SHOCK) trial was designed to determine whether emergency revascularization for cardiogenic shock complicating STEMI would reduce 30-day mortality when compared with a strategy of initial medical stabilization (IMS) with the use of intra-aortic balloon pump support and subsequent revascularization as appropriate.[84] The investigators found no difference in 30-day mortality between the group assigned to emergency revascularization (ERV) and the group assigned to IMS (46.7% vs 56%, $P = .11$). However, by 6 months and 12 months, there was a statistically significant survival advantage for those assigned to ERV.[84,85]

An important finding from the SHOCK study, particularly with regard to the elderly, was that ERV was associated with a 15.4% absolute risk reduction in 30-day mortality compared with IMS (41.4% vs 56.8%, $P < .01$) in the prespecified subgroup of patients younger than 75 years of age. However, no benefit in those older than 75 years of age (n = 56) was noted (Figure 41-6). This finding is reflected the updated ACC/AHA Guidelines for the Management of Patients with ST-Elevation MI by assigning a class I recommendation to "…early revascularization for patients less than 75 years old with ST elevation or LBBB who develop shock within 36 hours of MI and who are suitable for revascularization that can be performed within 18 hours of shock . . ." potentially restricting invasive strategies to younger patients.[86] This study may have included too few elderly patients to draw definitive conclusions from. The much larger SHOCK registry found that patients 75 years of age or older who underwent ERV (n = 257) had a higher survival compared to those not receiving ERV (n = 213).[87] This suggests that in selected elderly patients (ie, those with good functional status and fewer comorbid conditions), ERV can be accomplished safely and with reasonable clinical outcomes.

[ ] CORONARY ARTERY BYPASS GRAFT SURGERY

Previous reports of outcomes among the elderly undergoing coronary bypass surgery, limited by small numbers of patients and single-center experiences, have found variable morbidity and mortality rates.[88–90] Alexander et al compiled the largest contemporary data on in-hospital morbidity and mortality among 67,764 patients undergoing cardiac surgery at 22 centers in the National Cardiovascular Network between 1994 and 1998.[91] Octogenarians (n = 4306) who underwent CABG had a significantly higher operative mortality compared to younger patients (8.1% vs 3.0%, $P < .05$), with mortality rising in a linear fashion with advancing age. Similar trends of increased mortality were seen among octogenarians undergoing combined CABG/valve surgery when compared with younger patients. Using multivariate logistic regression, it was found that patients both young and old share many predictors for in-hospital mortality following CABG. These include the need for an emergency procedure, recent MI, and reduced ejection fraction. Mortality among octogenarians in this series (8.1%) was lower than that reported in the largest prior series using Medicare data for CABG between 1987 and 1990 (11.5%).[92] Rates of renal failure (6.9% vs 2.9%, $P < .05$) and stroke were somewhat higher in the octogenarian group but lower when compared with previous series. The rates of stroke (3.9% vs 1.8%, $P < .05$) were also higher in the octogenarian group but comparable with previous reports. These improvements in outcomes from earlier series may be attributed to better selection of elderly patients for CABG, coupled with improvements in operator experience and surgical technique.

[ ] PERCUTANEOUS CORONARY INTERVENTION VERSUS CORONARY ARTERY BYPASS GRAFT SURGERY

Trials comparing balloon angioplasty with CABG for multivessel coronary artery disease have consistently demonstrated no difference in death or MI between the two strategies, although CABG tends to offer better relief of angina and a reduced need for subsequent revascularization procedures.[93] Coronary stents have improved on some of the limitations of early stand-alone balloon angioplasty, namely acute or threatened vessel closure and late restenosis.[28,94,95] Recent trials comparing multivessel stenting with CABG similarly demonstrate a greater need for subsequent revascularization procedures in the stent group but at lower rates compared to balloon angioplasty.[30,96] A limitation of these studies is that they generally included younger patients, with a mean age of 61 years, so extrapolating these conclusions to the elderly might not be accurate. A retrospective case-control analysis of nearly 400 patients older than 70 years of age undergoing bypass surgery and balloon angioplasty found a higher in-hospital mortality in the surgical group compared with the angioplasty group (9% vs 2%, $P = .007$).[97] Patients undergoing

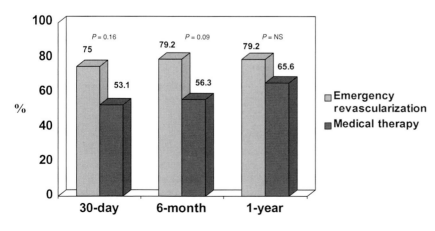

FIGURE 41-6. Mortality among patients 75 years of age and older in the SHOCK Trial. There was no significant difference in 30-day, 6-month, or 1-year mortality with emergency revascularization compared with medical therapy.

CABG also had a higher incidence of stroke (5% vs 0%, $P <$ .0001) and Q-wave MI (6% vs 1%, $P =$ .01). Five-year survival was similar between the two groups (63% in the angioplasty group vs 65% in the CABG group, $P =$ NS), but the surgical group had less recurrent angina and required fewer revascularization procedures in follow-up. The future will likely include more elderly patients in trials comparing multivessel stent implantation with CABG. We eagerly await further trials comparing these two revascularization modalities in the current era of drug-eluting stents.

[ ] PRACTICAL CONSIDERATIONS

As outlined above, elderly patients are at increased risk of periprocedural complications following PCI. However, several strategies can be implemented to reduce this risk (Figure 41-7).

We are particularly careful with ensuring that elderly patients' volume status is optimized prior to cardiac catheterization. In particular, congestive heart failure should be treated as aggressively as possible with diuretics, and strong consideration should be given to right heart catheterization for invasive monitoring of filling pressures. Conversely, volume depletion should be avoided, because the added contrast load can further increase the risk of nephrotoxicity. Elderly patients may be more sensitive to the effects of sedatives and anxiolytics, so adjusting the dose of these medications is appropriate. Additionally, elderly patients' creatinine clearance may also be lower despite a serum creatinine within the normal reference range, necessitating that other medication dosages be reduced accordingly. We prefer using 6-Fr sheaths and guiding catheters to minimize any increase risk of femoral complications from larger systems. In our experience, elderly patients, particularly females with a small body habitus, are at increased risk of bleeding, so judicious use of glycoprotein IIb/IIIa is recommended. When diffuse aortoiliac disease is present, we favor exchanging our catheters and equipment over a guidewire. A final caveat to consider in improving acute procedural success is the use of atherectomy to debulk heavily calcified coronary lesions.

[ ] RECOMMENDATIONS

Elderly patients are increasingly being referred for evaluation of symptomatic coronary artery disease. Medical therapy is effective in ameliorating ischemic symptoms but may offer incomplete relief and often is poorly tolerated in the elderly. Data suggest that although complication rates are higher, PCI can be performed with acceptable risk in appropriately selected patients and may avoid some of the complications associated with CABG. Depending on the level of risk, "culprit" lesion PCI is often undertaken as a palliative approach. Drug-eluting stents have brought much excitement to the world of interventional cardiology, and it remains to be seen whether their benefit extends across all patient groups, including the elderly. The optimal approach in deciding

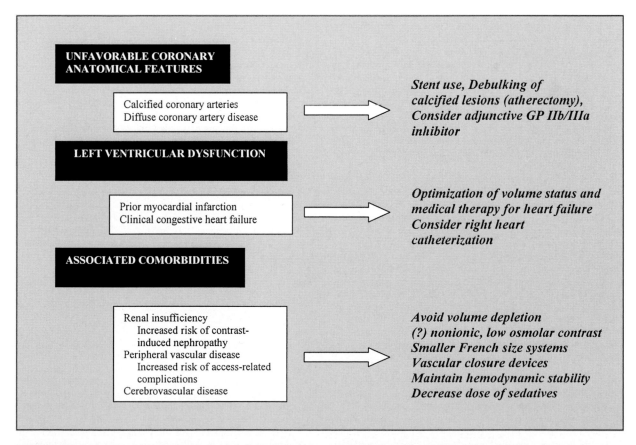

FIGURE 41-7. Factors associated with decreased procedural success and increased complications in elderly patients undergoing percutaneous coronary intervention and strategies to minimize risk. GP = glycoprotein.

on revascularization in the elderly is one that utilizes appropriate clinical judgment, taking into account the patient's overall functional status, desires, and expectations, rather than dismissal solely on the basis of age. Collaboration with surgical colleagues concerning the relative risks and benefits of PCI versus CABG, completeness of revascularization, and surgical back-up of the PCI procedure is critically important to allow the selection of the most appropriate revascularization procedure in the individual patient.

REFERENCES

1. Centers for Disease Control and Prevention, Diabetes Public Health Resource. Available at: http://www.cdc.gov/diabetes/statistics. Accessed January 19, 2005.

2. King H, Aubert RE, Herman WH. Global burden of diabetes. 1995–2025: prevalence, numerical estimates, and projections. *Diabetes Care.* 1998;21:1414.

3. Wilson PW, D'Agostino RB, Levy D, et al. Prediction of coronary heart disease using risk factor categories. *Circulation.* 1998;97:1837.

4. Wilson PW. Diabetes mellitus and coronary heart disease. *Am J Kidney Dis.* 1998;32:S89.

5. Nelson RG, Knowler WC, Pettitt JD, Bennett PH, National Diabetes Data Group. Kidney diseases in diabetes. In: *Diabetes in America.* Bethesda, Md: National Institutes of Health, National Institute of Diabetes and Digestive and Kidney Diseases. 1995;349.

6. Laskey WK, Selzer F, Vlachos HA, et al. Comparison of in-hospital and one-year outcomes in patients with and without diabetes mellitus undergoing percutaneous catheter intervention (from the National Heart, Lung, and Blood Institute Dynamic Registry). *Am J Cardiol.* 2002;90:1062.

7. American Diabetes Association. Consensus development conference on the diagnosis of coronary artery disease in people with diabetes. *Diabetes Care.* 1998;21:1551.

8. Natali A, Vichi S, Landi P, et al. Coronary atherosclerosis in type II diabetes: angiographic findings and clinical outcome. *Diabetologica.* 2000;43:632.

9. Stein B, Weintraub WS, Gebhart SPG, et al. Influence of diabetes mellitus on early and late outcome after percutaneous transluminal coronary angioplasty. *Circulation.* 1995;91:979.

10. Levine GN, Jacobs AK, Keller GP, et al. Impact of diabetes mellitus on percutaneous revascularization (CAVEAT-1). *Am J Cardiol.* 1997;79:748.

11. Elezi S, Kastrati A, Pache J, et al. Diabetes mellitus and the clinical and angiographic outcome after coronary stent placement. *J Am Coll Cardiol.* 1998; 32:1866.

12. Abizaid A, Kornowski R, Mintz GS, et al. The influence of diabetes mellitus on acute and late clinical outcomes following coronary stent implantation. *J Am Coll Cardiol.* 1998;32:584.

13. Mathew V, Gersh BJ, Williams BA, et al. Outcomes in patients with diabetes mellitus undergoing percutaneous coronary intervention in the current era: a report from the Prevention of REStenosis with Tranilast and its Outcomes (PRESTO) trial. *Circulation.* 2004;109:476.

14. Behar S, Boyko V, Reicher-Reiss H, Goldbourt U. Ten-year survival after acute myocardial infarction: comparison of patients with and without diabetes. *Am Heart J.* 1997;133:290.

15. Aronson D, Bloomgarden Z, Rayfield EJ. Potential mechanisms promoting restenosis in diabetic patients. *J Am Coll Cardiol.* 1996;27:528.

16. Holmes DR Jr, Vietstra RE, Smith HC, et al. Restenosis after percutaneous transluminal coronary angioplasty (PTCA): a report from the PTCA Registry of the National Heart, Lung, and Blood Institute. *Am J Cardiol.* 1984; 53:77C.

17. Popma JJ, Mintz GS, Satler LF, et al. Clinical and angiographic outcomes after directional coronary atherectomy. *Am J Cardiol.* 1993;88:975.

18. Schatz RA, Baim DS, Leon M, et al. Clinical experience with the Palmaz-Schatz coronary stent. Initial results of a multicenter study. *Circulation.* 1991; 83:148.

19. Carrozza JP, Kuntz RE, Fishman RF, et al. Restenosis after arterial injury caused by coronary stenting in patients with diabetes mellitus. *Ann Intern Med.* 1993; 118:344.

20. The Bypass Angioplasty Revascularization Investigation (BARI) Investigators. Comparison of coronary bypass surgery with angioplasty in patients with multivessel disease. *N Engl J Med.* 1996;335:217.

21. The BARI Investigators. Influences of diabetes on 5-year mortality and morbidity in a randomized trial comparing CABG and PTCA in patients with multivessel disease: the Bypass Angioplasty Revascularization Investigation (BARI). *Circulation.* 1997;96:1761.

22. Schwartz L, Kip KE, Frye RL, et al. Coronary bypass graft patency in patients with diabetes in the Bypass Angioplasty Revascularization Investigation (BARI). *Circulation.* 2002;106:2652.

23. Rozenman Y, Sapoznikov D, Mosseri M, et al. Long-term angiographic follow-up of coronary balloon angioplasty in patients with diabetes mellitus. A clue to the explanation of the results of the BARI study. *J Am Coll Cardiol.* 1997; 30:1420.

24. Kurbann AS, Bowker TJ, Iisley CD, et al. Differences in the mortality of the CABRI diabetic and nondiabetic populations and its relation to coronary artery disease and revascularization mode. *Am J Cardiol.* 2001;87:947.

25. King SB, Kosinski AS, Guyton RA, et al. Eight-year mortality in the Emory Angioplasty versus Surgery Trial (EAST). *J Am Coll Cardiol.* 2000;35:1116.

26. Feit F, Brooks MM, Sopko G, et al. Long-term clinical outcome in the Bypass Angioplasty Revascularization Investigation Registry. Comparison with the randomized trial. *Circulation.* 2000;101:295.

27. Barsness GW, Peterson ED, Ohman EM, et al. Relationship between diabetes mellitus and long-term survival after coronary bypass and angioplasty. *Circulation.* 1997;96:2551.

28. Fischman DL, Leon MB, Baim DS, et al. A randomized comparison of coronary-stent placement and balloon angioplasty in the treatment of coronary artery disease. Stent Restenosis Study Investigators. *N Engl J Med.* 1994; 331:496.

29. Serruys PW, de Jaegere P, Kiemeneij F, et al. A comparison of balloon-expandable-stent implantation with balloon angioplasty in patients with coronary artery disease. Benestent Study Group. *N Engl J Med.* 1994;331:489.

30. Serruys PW, Unger F, Sousa JE, et al. Comparison of coronary-artery bypass surgery and stenting for the treatment of multivessel disease. *N Engl J Med.* 2001;344:1117.

31. Abizaid A, Costa MA, Centemero M, et al. Clinical and economic impact of diabetes mellitus on percutaneous and surgical treatment of multivessel coronary artery disease patients: insights from the Arterial Revascularization Therapy Study (ARTS) trial. *Circulation.* 2001;104:533.

32. Sobel BE, Frye R, Detre KM. Bypass Angioplasty Revascularization Investigation 2 Diabetes Trial. Burgeoning dilemmas in the management of diabetes and cardiovascular disease: rationale for the Bypass Angioplasty Revascularization Investigation 2 Diabetes (BARI 2D) Trial. *Circulation.* 2003; 107:636.

33. Moussa I, Leon MB, Baim DS, et al. Impact of drug-eluting stents on outcome in diabetic patients. A SIRIUS substudy. *Circulation.* 2004;109:2273.

34. Colombo A, Drzewiecki J, Banning A, et al. Randomized study to assess the effectiveness of slow- and moderate-release polymer-based paclitaxel-eluting stents for coronary artery lesions. *Circulation.* 2003;108:788.

35. Stone GW, Ellis SG, Cox DA, et al. A polymer-based, paclitaxel-eluting stent in patients with coronary artery disease. *N Engl J Med.* 2004;350:221.

36. Topol EJ, Lincoff AM, Kereiakes DJ, et al. Multi-year follow-up of abciximab therapy in three randomized placebo-controlled trials of percutaneous coronary revascularization. *Am J Med.* 2002;113:1.

37. Lincoff AM. Important Triad in Cardiovascular Medicine. Diabetes, Coronary Intervention, and Platelet Glycoprotein IIb/IIIa Receptor Blockade. *Circulation.* 2003;107:1556.

38. Shukla SD, Paul A, Klachko DM. Hypersensitivity of diabetic human platelets to platelet activating factor. *Thromb Res.* 1992;66:239.

39. Davi G, Gresele P, Violi F, et al. Diabetes mellitus, hypercholesterolemia, and hypertension but not vascular disease per se are associated with persistent platelet activation in vivo: evidence derived from the study of peripheral arterial disease. *Circulation.* 1997;96:69.

40. Knobler H. Savion N, Shenkman B, et al. Shear-induced platelet adhesion and aggregation on subendothelium are increased in diabetic patients. *Thromb Res.* 1998;90:181.

41. Jokl R, Colwell JA. Arterial thrombosis and atherosclerosis in diabetes. *Diabetes Rev.* 1997;5:316.

42. Tschoepe D. The activated megakaryocyte-platelet system in vascular disease: focus on diabetes. *Semin Thromb Hemost.* 1995;21:152.

43. Roffi M, Chew DP, Mukherjee D, et al. Platelet glycoprotein IIb/IIIa inhibitors reduce mortality in diabetic patients with non-ST-segment-elevation acute coronary syndromes. *Circulation.* 2001;104:2767.

44. The Platelet Receptor Inhibition in Ischemic Syndrome Management (PRISM) Study Investigators. A comparison of aspirin plus tirofiban with aspirin plus heparin for unstable angina. *N Engl J Med.* 1998;338:1498.

45. The Platelet Receptor Inhibition in Ischemic Syndrome Management in Patients Limited by Unstable Signs and Symptoms (PRISM-PLUS) Study Investigators. Inhibition of the platelet glycoprotein IIb/IIIa receptor with tirofiban in unstable angina and non-Q-wave myocardial infarction. *N Engl J Med.* 1998;338:1488.

46. The PARAGON Investigators. International, randomized, controlled trial of lamifiban (a platelet glycoprotein IIb/IIIa inhibitor), heparin, or both in unstable angina. Platelet IIb/IIIa Antagonism for the Reduction of Acute coronary syndrome events in a Global Organization Network. *Circulation.* 1998; 97:2386.

47. Moliterno DJ. Patient-specific dosing of IIb/IIIa antagonists during acute coronary syndromes: rationale and design of the PARAGON B study. The PARAGON B International Steering Committee. *Am Heart J.* 2000; 139:563.

48. The PURSUIT Trial Investigators. Inhibition of platelet glycoprotein IIb/IIIa with eptifibatide in patients with acute coronary syndromes. Platelet glycoprotein iib/iiia in unstable angina: receptor suppression using integrilin therapy. *N Engl J Med.* 1998;339:436.

49. Simoons ML. Effects of glycoprotein IIb/IIIa receptor blocker abciximab on outcome in patients with acute coronary syndromes without early coronary revascularisation: the GUSTO IV-ACS randomised trial. *Lancet.* 2001; 357:1915.

50. EPIC Investigators. Use of a monoclonal antibody directed against the platelet glycoprotein IIb/IIIa receptor in high-risk coronary angioplasty. *N Engl J Med.* 1994;330:956.

51. EPILOG Investigators. Platelet glycoprotein IIb/IIIa receptor blockade and low-dose heparin during percutaneous coronary revascularization. *N Engl J Med.* 1997;336:1689.

52. EPISTENT Investigators. Randomised placebo-controlled and balloon-angioplasty-controlled trial to assess safety of coronary stenting with use of platelet glycoprotein IIb/IIIa blockade. Evaluation of Platelet IIb/IIIa Inhibitor for Stenting. *Lancet.* 1998;352:87.

53. ESPRIT Investigators. Novel dosing regimen of eptifibatide in planned coronary stent implantation (ESPRIT): a randomised, placebo-controlled trial. *Lancet.* 2000;356:2037.

54. Topol EJ, Moliterno DJ, Hermann HC, et al. Comparison of two platelet glycoprotein IIb/IIIa inhibitors, tirofiban and abciximab, for the prevention of ischemic events with percutaneous coronary revascularization. *N Eng J Med.* 2001;344:1888.

55. US Bureau of the Census, US Interim Projections by Age, Sex, Race, and Hispanic Origin. Available at: http://www.census.gov. Accessed January 19, 2005.

56. Rady MY, Johnson DJ. Cardiac surgery for octogenarians: is it an informed decision? *Am Heart J.* 2004;147:347.

57. Gibbons RJ, Abrams J, Chatterjee K, et al. ACC/AHA 2002 Guideline Update for Management of Patients with Chronic Stable Angina: A report of the American College of Cardiology/American Heart Association Task Force on Practice Guidelines (Committee to update the 1999 Guidelines for the Management of Patients with Chronic Stable Angina). 2002. Available at: http://www.acc.org/clinical/guidelines/stable/stable_pdf. Accessed January 19, 2005.

58. Smith SC, Jr, Dove JT, Jacobs AK, et al. ACC/AHA guidelines for percutaneous coronary intervention: a report of the American College of Cardiology/American Heart Association Task Force on Practice Guidelines (Committee to Revise the 1993 Guidelines for Percutaneous Transluminal Coronary Angioplasty). *J Am Coll Cardiol.* 2001;37:2239i.

59. Weiner DA, Ryan TJ, McCabe CH, et al. Prognostic importance of a clinical profile and exercise test in medically treated patients with coronary artery disease. *J Am Coll Cardiol.* 1984;3:772.

60. Myers WO, Schaff HV, Gersh BJ, et al. Improved survival of surgically treated patients with triple vessel coronary artery disease and severe angina pectoris. A report from the Coronary Artery Surgery Study (CASS) registry. *J Thorac Cardiovasc Surg.* 1989;97:487.

61. Yusuf S, Zucker D, Peduzzi P, et al. Effect of coronary artery bypass graft surgery on survival: overview of 10-year results from randomized trials by the Coronary Artery Bypass Graft Surgery Trialists Collaboration. *Lancet.* 1994;344:563.

62. Gersh BJ, Kronmal RA, Schaff HV, et al. Comparison of coronary artery bypass surgery and medical therapy in patients 65 years of age or older. A nonrandomized study from the Coronary Artery Surgery Study (CASS) registry. *N Engl J Med.* 1985;313:217.

63. TIME Investigators. Trial of invasive versus medical therapy in elderly patients with chronic symptomatic coronary artery disease (TIME): a randomized trial. *Lancet.* 2001;358:951.

64. DeGregorio JD, Kobayashi Y, Albiero R, et al. Coronary artery stenting in the elderly: short-term outcome and long-term angiographic and clinical follow-up. *J Am Coll Cardiol.* 1998;32:577.

65. Lindsay J Jr, Reddy V, Pinnow EE, et al. Morbidity and mortality rates in elderly patients undergoing percutaneous transluminal coronary angioplasty. *Am Heart J.* 1994;128:697.

66. Thompson RC, Holmes DR, Grill DE, et al. Changing outcome of angioplasty in the elderly. *J Am Coll Cardiol.* 1996;27:8.

67. Lefevre T, Morice MC, Eltchminoff H, et al. One-month results of coronary stenting patients ≥ 75 years of age. *Am J Cardiol.* 1998;82:17.

68. Batchelor WB, Anstrom KJ, Muhlbaier LH, et al. Contemporary outcome trends in the elderly undergoing percutaneous coronary interventions: results in 7,472 octagenerians. *J Am Coll Cardiol.* 2000;36:723.

69. Chauhan MS, Kuntz RE, Ho KKL, et al. Coronary artery stenting in the aged. *J Am Coll Cardiol.* 2001;37:856.

70. IMPACT II Investigators. Randomised placebo controlled trial of eptifibatide on complications of percutaneous coronary interventions: IMPACT II. Integrilin to Minimise Platelet Aggregation and Coronary Thrombosis-II. *Lancet.* 1997;349:1422.

71. Karvouni E, Katritsis DG, Ioannidis JPA. Intravenous glycoprotein IIb/IIIa receptor antagonists reduce mortality after percutaneous coronary interventions. *J Am Coll Cardiol.* 2003;41:26.

72. Lincoff AM, Califf RM, Moliterno DJ, et al, for the Evaluation of Platelet IIb/IIIa Inhibition in Stenting Investigators. Complementary clinical benefits of coronary artery stenting and blockade of platelet glycoprotein receptors. *N Engl J Med.* 1999;341:319.

73. Sadeghi HM, Grines CL, Chandra HR, et al. Percutaneous coronary interventions in octogenarians: glycoprotein IIb/IIIa receptor inhibitors' safety profile. *J Am Coll Cardiol.* 2003;42:428.

74. Invasive compared with non-invasive treatment in unstable coronary-artery disease: FRISC II prospective randomised multicentre study. Fragmin and Fast Revascularisation during InStability in Coronary artery disease Investigators. *Lancet.* 1999;354:708.

75. Wallentin L, Lagerqvist B, Husted S, et al. Outcome at 1 year after an invasive compared with a non-invasive strategy in unstable coronary-artery disease: the FRISC II invasive randomized trial. FRISC II Investigators. Fast Revascularisation during Instability in Coronary artery disease. *Lancet.* 2000; 356:9.

76. Cannon CP, Weintraub WS, Demeopoulos LA, et al. Comparison of early invasive and conservative strategies in patients with unstable coronary syndromes treated with the glycoprotein IIb/IIIa inhibitor tirofiban. *N Engl J Med.* 2001;344:1879.

77. Fox KA, Poole-Wilson PA, Henderson RA, et al. Interventional versus conservative treatment for patients with unstable angina or non-ST-elevation myocardial infarction: the British Heart Foundation RITA 3 randomised trial. Randomised Intervention Trial of unstable Angina. *Lancet.* 2002;360:743.

78. Lee PY, Alexander KP, Hammill BG, et al. Representation of elderly persons and women in published randomized trials of acute coronary syndromes. *JAMA.* 2001;286:708.

79. Giugliano RP, Camargo CA Jr, Lloyd-Jones DM, et al. Elderly patients receive less aggressive medical and invasive management of unstable angina: potential impact of practice guidelines. *Arch Intern Med.* 1998;158:1113.

80. Bach RG, Cannon CP, Weintraub WS, et al. The effect of routine, early invasive management on outcome for elderly patients with non-ST-segment elevation acute coronary syndromes. *Ann Intern Med.* 2004;141:186.

81. Antman EM, Cohen M, Bernink PJ, et al. The TIMI risk score for unstable angina/non-ST elevation MI: A method for prognostication and therapeutic decision making. *JAMA.* 2000;284:835.

82. Berger AK, Schulman KA, Gersh BJ, et al. Primary coronary angioplasty vs. thrombolysis for the management of acute myocardial infarction in elderly patients. *JAMA.* 1999;282:341.

83. Guagliumi G, Stone GW, Cox DA, et al. Outcome in elderly patients undergoing primary coronary intervention for acute myocardial infarction. Results from the Controlled Abciximab and Device Investigation to Lower Late Angioplasty Complications (CADILLAC) Trial. *Circulation.* 2004;110:1598.

84. Hochman JS, Sleeper LA, Webb JG, et al. Early revascularization in acute myocardial infarction complicated by cardiogenic shock. SHOCK Investigators. Should We Emergently Revascularize Occluded Coronaries for Cardiogenic Shock. *N Engl J Med.* 1999;341:625.

85. Hochman JS, Sleeper LA, White HD, et al. One-year survival following early revascularization for cardiogenic shock. *JAMA.* 2001;285:190.

86. Antman EM, Anbe DT, Armstrong PW, et al. ACC/AHA guidelines for the management of patients with ST-elevation myocardial infarction: a report of the American College of Cardiology/American Heart Association Task Force on Practice Guidelines (Committee to Revise the 1999 Guidelines for the Management of Patients With Acute Myocardial Infarction). 2004. Available at: www.acc.org/clinical/guidelines/stemi/index.pdf. Accessed January 19, 2005.

87. Dzavik V, Sleeper LA, Cocke TP, et al. Early revascularization is associated with improved survival in elderly patients with acute myocardial infarction complicated by cardiogenic shock: a report from the SHOCK Trial Registry. *Eur Heart J.* 2003;24:828.

88. Weintraub WS, Clements SD, Ware J, et al. Coronary artery surgery in octogenarians. *Am J Cardiol.* 1991;68:1530.

89. Edmunds LH, Stephenson LW, Edie RN, et al. Open-heart surgery in octagenerians. *N Engl J Med.* 1988;319:131.

90. Mullany CJ, Darling GE, Pluth JR, et al. Early and late results after isolated coronary artery bypass surgery in 159 patients aged 80 years and older. *Circulation.* 1990;82(suppl 4):229.

91. Alexander KP, Anstrom KJ, Muhlbaier LJ, et al. Outcomes of cardiac surgery in patients age ≥ 80 years: results from the National Cardiovascular Network. *J Am Coll Cardiol.* 2000;35:731.

92. Peterson ED, Copwer PA, Jollis JG, et al. Outcomes of coronary artery bypass graft surgery in 24,461 patients aged 80 years or older. *Circulation.* 1995;92(suppl 2):85.

93. Pocock SJ, Henderson RA, Rickards AF, et al. Meta-analysis of randomised trials comparing coronary angioplasty with bypass surgery. *Lancet.* 1995; 346:1184.

94. Roubin GS, Cannon AD, Agrawal SK, et al. Intracoronary stenting for acute and threatened closure complicating percutaneous transluminal coronary angioplasty. *Circulation.* 1992;85:916.

95. George BS, Voorhees WB 3rd, Roubin GS, et al. Multicenter investigation of coronary stenting to treat acute or threatened closure after percutaneous transluminal coronary angioplasty: clinical and angiographic outcomes. *J Am Coll Cardiol.* 1993;22:135.

96. The SoS Investigators. Coronary artery bypass surgery versus percutaneous coronary intervention with stent implantation in patients with multivessel coronary artery disease (the Stent or Surgery trial): a randomised controlled trial. *Lancet.* 2002;360:965.

97. O'Keefe JH Jr, Sutton MB, McCallister BD, et al. Coronary angioplasty versus bypass surgery in patients > 70 years old matched for ventricular function. *J Am Coll Cardiol.* 1994;24:425.

CHAPTER (42)

Inoue-Balloon Mitral Valvuloplasty

Jui-Sung Hung, MD, and Kean-Wah Lau, MBBS

The introduction of percutaneous balloon mitral valvuloplasty (BMV) by Inoue et al[1] in 1982 has opened a new dimension in the treatment of patients with mitral stenosis. The body of data accrued to date has clearly established this invasive, nonsurgical procedure as the treatment of choice in symptomatic patients with moderate to severe mitral stenosis (mitral valve area < 1.5 cm^2) and favorable valve morphology (noncalcified, pliable valve with minimal subvalvular disease and no or mild mitral regurgitation.[2-5] The presence of severe ($\geq$ grade 3+) angiographic mitral regurgitation and left atrial thrombus are considered to be two contraindications for BMV. However, several controversial issues in the use of this procedure exist, because the selection of patients for BMV in clinical practice continues to be a complex decision involving consideration of multiple variables, including clinical profile, operator skill, valve morphology, and severity of associated mitral regurgitation.

Among the multiple variables, valve morphology and severity of associated mitral regurgitation have to a large extent remained the principal determinants in patient selection. In patients with favorable valve morphology (pliable, noncalcified valve with minimal subvalvular disease) and no or mild mitral regurgitation, BMV predictably yields excellent results and a low risk of resultant severe mitral regurgitation. With successful balloon valve enlargement, there is generally a 2-fold increase in the mitral valve area and an associated dramatic fall in transmitral valve gradient, left atrial pressure, and pulmonary artery pressure.[2-5] These hemodynamic benefits are mirrored in clinical improvements in the patients' symptoms and exercise tolerance.

This is not entirely surprising, considering the fact that BMV enlarges the stenosed mitral valve in the same manner as that afforded by surgical commissurotomy—namely that of commissural split. Several randomized trials[6-11] comparing BMV and closed and/or open surgical commissurotomy in patients with favorable valve morphology have demonstrated that BMV is as efficacious, if not more so, than surgical mitral commissurotomy in acutely relieving the obstructed valve and achieving favorable clinical outcome. The long-term results of BMV are excellent, especially when the acute results are optimal and valve morphology is good. Long-term data in BMV have also indicated that after optimal mitral valve dilation, the restenosis rate is low and the acute symptomatic benefits are sustained.[12-16] When restenosis is defined as mitral valve area less than 1.5 cm^2, the restenosis rate in patients with favorable valve morphology at 7-year follow-up in the randomized trial by Farhat et al[11] was 6.6% in patients who underwent BMV; this rate was similar in those who underwent open surgical commissurotomy and was far superior to the restenosis rate of 37% observed after closed surgical commissurotomy. Hernandez and associates[16] found that survival free of major events (cardiac death, mitral surgery, repeat BMV, or functional impairment) was 69% at 7 years, ranging from 88% to 40% in different subgroups of patients. Mitral area loss, although mild (0.13 ± 0.21 cm^2), increased with time and was greater than or equal to 0.3 cm^2 in 12%, 22%, and 27% of patients at 3, 5, and 7 years, respectively.

In contrast to the usually excellent results obtained with the procedure in patients with favorable valve anatomy, the results of BMV in those with adverse valve morphology (heavily calcified leaflets and commissures and extensive subvalvular disease) are less predictable.[17-20] BMV in the latter compared with the former patient subset tends to produce inferior acute and long-term results. Therefore, patients with unfavorable mitral morphology are in general better served with mitral valve replacement (but not surgical commissurotomy). Having said that, there remains a significant minority of patients with adverse valve morphology in whom BMV may yield acceptable hemodynamic outcome and

TABLE 42-1

Recommended Treatment Strategies for Various Subsets of Patients

PATIENT SUBSET	RECOMMENDED TREATMENT
Pliable, noncalcified mitral valve with absent or mild subvalvular disease, and	
a) absent or mild MR	BMV
b) moderate MR	Trial of BMV
c) with left atrial cavity thrombus	OSC with thrombectomy
Nonpliable, grossly calcified mitral valve with significant subvalvular disease, and	
a) with or without moderate MR	MVR
b) in special clinical settings:	BMV
– High-surgical risk patients	
– Urgent noncardiac surgery required	
– Bridge procedure to mitral surgery	
– Patient refusal for surgery	
– Shortened life-span from medical comorbidities	

BMV = percutaneous balloon mitral valvuloplasty; MR = mitral regurgitation; MVR = mitral valve replacement; OSC = open surgical commissurotomy.

may continue to gain long-term symptomatic improvement. It is thus reasonable to perform BMV in these patients if they refuse surgery as a bridge to surgery at a later stage, particularly if urgent noncardiac surgery is required or if the risk of cardiac surgery is deemed to be prohibitively high because of other major medical comorbidities (Table 42-1). In fact, BMV may occasionally be the only option for some of these patients.

Many centers performing BMV exclude patients with moderate (angiographic grade 2+) mitral regurgitation from the procedure for fear of increasing the severity of the mitral regurgitation and the need for emergency mitral valve surgery. In our centers, these patients with moderate mitral regurgitation but with otherwise favorable valve characteristics are not excluded from BMV. In our experience, the risk of resultant severe mitral regurgitation is minimal with the use of cautionary balloon sizing approach and the controlled stepwise dilation technique.[21–23] However, should the procedure fail to provide optimal clinical results, the patients can still be subjected to elective surgery without exposing them to any additional risk.

The presence of left atrial thrombus has traditionally been considered a contraindication to BMV because of the heightened risk of cardioembolism with the procedure. In patients with nonpedunculated thrombi in the left atrial cavity, one may elect to administer long-term (3–6 months) warfarin therapy (targeting the international normalized ratio between 2 and 2.5), if their clinical and hemodynamic status does not warrant immediate surgery and the mitral valves are deemed suitable for BMV. When the thrombus is observed to have resolved with transthoracic echocardiographic reassessments performed at 3-month intervals, BMV can then be performed safely after confirmation of the absence of thrombi in the left atrial cavity with transesophageal echocardiography.[23,24] Patients with lytic-resistant or mobile thrombi should be considered for open surgical commissurotomy with direct visual clot removal. Despite our safe and successful experience in performing Inoue-BMV in patients with left atrial thrombi confined to the appendage,[23,25] the subject has remained controversial even among experienced operators of Inoue-BMV. Therefore, the alternative approach is either to subject patients with appendage thrombi to mitral valve surgery, or to defer BMV for stable patients until resolution of the thrombi under warfarin treatment.[23,26]

The best choice of technique for BMV remains a contentious issue. Beside the original Inoue technique using size-adjustable, self-positioning balloon catheters, various other techniques for performing BMV have been developed that use fixed-sized balloon catheters. These include the antegrade (transvenous) approaches with one or two balloon catheters through one or two interatrial septal punctures[27,28] or the retrograde (transarterial) approaches with transseptal wiring or without transseptal access.[29] An overview of the various comparative studies, both randomized and nonrandomized, does not reliably indicate that either the double-balloon or the Inoue-balloon technique is superior to the other in achieving a larger final mitral valve area. There is, however, persuasive evidence that the Inoue-balloon approach is technically less demanding and clearly simpler to perform; hence it has a shorter irradiation and procedural time, and it is safer than the double-balloon approach.[30–32] These advantages are vital in pregnant patients in whom the hazards of irradiation to the fetus are of paramount importance and for patients with pulmonary edema in whom swift and expeditious BMV is clearly desirable. Therefore, the transvenous Inoue-balloon approach has obtained its current position as the principal BMV technique.

Subsequent sections of the present chapter are drawn largely from our incremental experience in Inoue-BMV techniques and evolving technical refinements in BMV techniques. These have resulted in a nearly 100% technical success rate and a significant diminution in complications despite the presence of a significant number of technically demanding scenarios and high-risk comorbid conditions.[12,22–23] Mainly discussed are the technical aspects of Inoue-BMV, the pitfalls and tricks to facilitate a successful procedure, and how to minimize procedure-related complications.

TRANSSEPTAL ACCESS

Transseptal catheterization is a vital component of BMV. Transseptal puncture must not only be executed safely to avoid cardiac perforation but also made at an appropriate interatrial septal site to facilitate balloon crossing of the stenosed mitral valve.[33] To avert cardiac perforation, some operators have resorted to routine intraprocedural transesophageal echocardiography to facilitate optimal transseptal needle placement; however, even with the echocardiographic guidance, cardiac perforation may still occur.[34] Recently developed intracardiac echocardiography is useful, but it is not widely available and its use adds to more cost. Therefore, acquisition of basic transseptal skill is essential. To perform transseptal procedure, biplane fluoroscopic equipment is preferable, but single-plane fluoroscopy is usually sufficient.

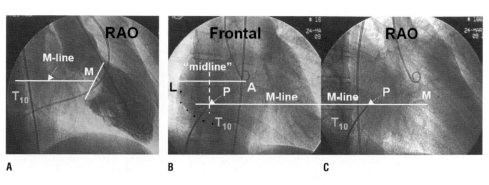

FIGURE 42-1. Defining M-line and "midline." **(A)** Defining M-line using stop frame left ventriculogram (RAO view). **(B)** Defining vertical "midlines" in fluoroscopic frontal view. **(C)** Puncture site (P) on M-line in RAO view. A = pigtail catheter tip; L = left atrial lateral border; RAO = right anterior oblique; T_{10} = 10th thoracic vertebra. The dotted line in **B** indicates left atrial silhouette. See text for discussion. *(Courtesy of www.ptmv.org.)*

The instruments used for the procedure include a Brockenbrough needle and a 7-Fr or 8-Fr transseptal catheter. The use of an outer sheath is optional, but its utility is recommended, especially for inexperienced operators for two reasons: (1) to prevent inadvertent perforation of the dilator by the needle during its insertion, and (2) to prevent left atrial perforation during insertion of the catheter/needle into the left atrium; the sheath tip works as a safety stopper at the septum.

【 】 LANDMARKS FOR OPTIMAL PUNCTURE SITE

The puncture target site is usually located at the cross point of (1) a horizontal line crossing the center of the mitral annulus (M-line) and (2) a vertical line, assumed to divide the inter-atrial septum into anterior and posterior halves ("midline"). However, in individual cases, the puncture site may have to be adjusted. For example, in patients with giant left atria, the operator is often forced to make the interatrial septal puncture more caudal to the horizontal M-line. In patients with a more vertically oriented left ventricle and a relatively small left atrium, the operator may need to make the puncture site slightly more cephalad to the M-line and lateral to the vertical "midline."

Definition of Horizontal "M-Line" (Figure 42-1)

The line is derived from a diastolic stop frame of diagnostic left ventriculography obtained in 30-degree right anterior oblique (RAO) view. This horizontal line level is memorized in relation to the vertebral body. The angiogram is also used as a road map during transseptal puncture and balloon catheter manipulation.

Definition of Vertical "Midline"

Inoue devised a specific transseptal puncture technique designed for the Inoue balloon BMV, incorporating the concept of a vertical "midline," a line assumed to divide the interatrial septum into anterior and posterior halves.[35] The "midline" is a vertical line crossing the midpoint of a horizontal line spanning the anterior and posterior limits of the septum. The upper end of the tricuspid is assumed to be the anterior septal limit in Inoue's angiographic method, corresponding to the aortic valve in our modified fluoroscopic method.

Because the septum lies within the superimposed area between the two atria in both methods, the medial atrial silhouette (usually the left atrium) is used as the posterior limit (not necessarily the posterior border) because there is no septum beyond this silhouette. Infrequently, such as in patients with giant left atria or distorted cardiac anatomy, the right atrial border is medial to that of the left atrium, and thus the right atrial border is used as the posterior limit.

1. Angiographic method (Figure 42-2A, B): The "midline" is defined based on the landmarks obtained from frontal plane right atrial angiography during normal respiration.

2. Fluoroscopic method (Figure 42-2C): In this method, the aortic valve is used to substitute the upper end of the tricuspid valve as the anterior septal limit because the two structures are in close proximity to each other. Therefore, a pigtail catheter is placed with its tip in the noncoronary sinus of Valsalva, touching the aortic valve. The "midline" thus derived is usually identical to that from Inoue's angiographic method.

Because in most cases of mitral stenosis, the left and right atrial silhouettes are visible under fluoroscopy (see Figure 42-2C), the angiographic method is infrequently used and is reserved for the following situations: (1) for operators inexperienced with the transseptal puncture technique, (2) in cases in which atrial silhouettes are not well visualized under fluoroscopy, and (3) in extremely difficult cases of transseptal puncture (eg, in the presence of a giant left atrium[33] and kyphoscoliosis).[36] In these cases, it may be necessary to perform biplane (frontal and lateral) right angiography to properly visualize the atrial septal orientation and relative anatomic relationships of the atria, the tricuspid valve, and the aorta.

【 】 CONFIRMATION OF OPTIMAL PUNCTURE SITE

Frontal View

Under frontal view, the needle-fitted transseptal catheter placed in the superior cava inserted from the right femoral vein is slowly withdrawn to align the catheter/needle on the "midline." Reshaping of the distal Brockenbrough needle to make it more curved may be necessary to align the catheter tip with the "midline." The needle tip should be constantly kept concealed slightly (2–3 mm) within the catheter tip before needle puncture.

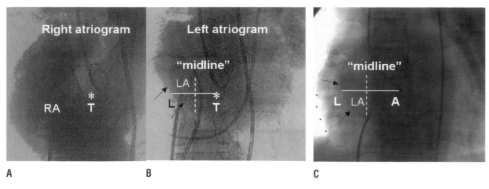

FIGURE 42-2. Definition of "midline." Angiographic method (**A** and **B**): the upper end of the tricuspid valve at systole (*point T,* marked as asterisk) is determined on a stop-frame frontal right atrial (RA) image (**A**) and translated to a stop-frame left atrial (LA) image (**B**). On the latter image, a horizontal line is drawn from point T until point L, where the line intersects the LA silhouette. The "midline" (broken line) is the vertical line crossing at the midpoint between T and L. Fluoroscopic method (**C**): a horizontal line is drawn from the tip of the pigtail catheter *(point A)* to L, the LA silhouette *(black arrows),* to define the "midline." The dotted line indicates the right atrial silhouette. *(Courtesy of www.ptmv.org.)*

The catheter tip should not be set medial to the "midline" to avoid puncturing the aorta, tricuspid valve, or coronary sinus. More importantly, the puncture site thus made is too close to the mitral valve, and this makes balloon crossing of the mitral valve difficult or even impossible. Slight lateral deviation of the puncture site to the "midline" is permissible, especially in patients with relatively small left atria. It is important to note that there may not be septum in an area near the inferior (caudal) border of the left atrium because the atrium often bulges caudally beyond the true septal boundary.

Thirty-Degree Right Anterior Oblique View

The catheter tip site is further examined in this view to confirm its optimal position (see Figure 42-1B), also using the left ventriculogram as a road map (see Figure 42-1A). The tip position is usually in front of the spinal column, and the distance between the intended puncture site and the mitral orifice (P to M in Figure 42-1C) should exceed 1.3 times the vertebra width for easy catheter balloon crossing of the mitral valve. Because the catheter tip is away from the aorta, tricuspid valve, coronary sinus, and the left atrial posterior border, needle puncture at this point pierces only the septum unless puncture is made too caudally near the caudal edge of the left atrium in frontal view.

【 】 CONFIRMATION OF CATHETER TIP AT SEPTUM

When setting of the catheter/needle at the septum is in doubt, septal flush or stain method may be used to examine the catheter/needle tip position. This is done by injecting a small amount of pure contrast medium contained in a 5-mL syringe attached to the proximal needle end.

Septal Flush Method

The contrast medium flushing outlines the right atrial margin of the septum,[33] and the optimal puncture site is at the curving segment of the septal outline (Figure 42-3A, right panel).

Septal Stain Method

After needle puncture is made, the needle is aspirated and contrast medium is injected to confirm its entry into the left atrium. If no blood is aspirated, the needle either has dissected the higher septum or is caught in the thickened septum (usually, in the muscular septum). Staining of the septum with injection of contrast medium[33] easily distinguishes the two (Figure 42-3B, C). If the catheter/needle is caught in the septum, it should be carefully forced across the septum. With pressure monitoring, it is not possible to differentiate high septal dissection from needle entrapment in the thick septum. This is another reason why the authors perform the transseptal puncture without constant pressure monitoring.

【 】 CONFIRMATION OF LEFT ATRIAL ENTRY

After entry of the needle in the left atrium is confirmed, first by contrast medium injection followed by pressure recording, the needle direction is set toward 3 o'clock (left side of the patient). If there is no or little resistance, the catheter/needle is advanced forward slightly into the left atrium. Then, the catheter alone is advanced until the tip of the sheath meets a resistance at the septum, while the needle is being withdrawn.

On needle removal, heparin, 100 U/kg body weight, is given immediately through the catheter. After baseline hemodynamic studies, BMC is performed. If the patient has been on warfarin prior to BMV, the drug is discontinued 2 to 3 days before the procedure and substituted with intravenous unfractionated or subcutaneous low-molecular weight heparin until before the procedure.

SELECTION OF BALLOON CATHETER

Selection of an appropriate-sized balloon catheter for the controlled stepwise dilation technique is extremely important in order to avoid creating severe mitral regurgitation during BMV. Our balloon catheter selection methods have evolved from our continuing efforts to minimize this complication.[12,21–23]

【 】 CATHETER SELECTION

Selection guidelines are based on balloon reference size (RS) derived from patient height, transthoracic echocardiographic findings of the mitral valve, fluoroscopic presence of valvular calcification, and degree of angiographic mitral regurgitation before the procedure. The RS is calculated according to the simple formula:[12,22] patient height (cm) is rounded to the nearest zero and divided by 10, and 10 is added to the ratio to yield the RS (mm). (For example, if the patient's height is 167 cm, then RS = 170/10 + 10 = 27 mm [see Table 42-2].) In patients with pliable and noncalcified valves, and with mitral regurgitation less than or equal to

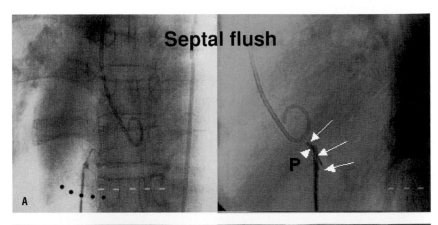

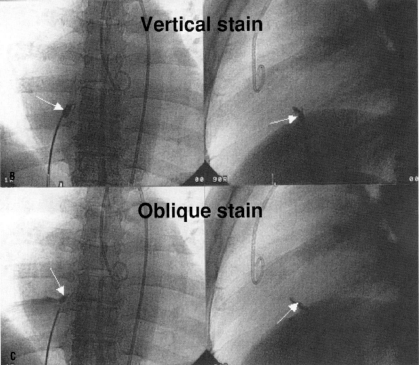

FIGURE 42-3. Septal flush/stain method in frontal (left panel) and lateral (right panel) views. (**A**) Flushing of contrast medium outlines the right atrial margin of the septum *(white arrows, lateral view)*. The optimal puncture site *(P, arrowhead)* is at the curved segment of the septal outline *(right)*. The dotted line shows the left atrial caudal border. (**B**) Needle puncture at higher septum results in septal dissection as evidenced by staining of the septum in a more vertical orientation *(arrow)*, and the catheter direction is aligned with the septal outline *(lateral view)*. (**C**) Contrast staining of the septum after needle puncture made at more caudal site shows obliquely directed staining *(arrow)*, indicating that the puncture is made at an optimal site at the curved segment of the septum. *(Courtesy of www.ptmv.org.)*

1+, a catheter with a nominal balloon size at least that of the RS (an RS-matched catheter) is used. In contrast, in patients at high risk for creating severe mitral regurgitation (valvular calcification and/or severe subvalvular lesions, baseline 2+ mitral regurgitation), a balloon catheter one size smaller than an RS-match is selected. Therefore, in the above example with an RS of 27 mm, a PTMC-28 catheter would be selected for a pliable, noncalcified valve, and a PTMC-26 catheter for a calcified valve and/or a valve with severe subvalvular disease.

【 】 PRETESTING FOR BALLOON-SYRINGE MISMATCH

Although the volume predefined by red marks on the syringe and its corresponding balloon size at full inflation have been tested by the manufacturer, balloon-syringe mismatch may occur. Although this mismatch is usually mild, gross mismatch may take place when the catheter and the syringe are from different packages. The mismatch, if undetected, may result in either underinflation or overinflation of the balloon. Therefore, before inserting the balloon catheter into each patient, the diameters of balloon inflated by injection of diluted contrast medium should be confirmed using a test; the balloon diameter chosen for the first inflation and the nominal diameter of the balloon should be compared. If there is a mismatch, the difference should be noted and adjusted.

CATHETER PLACEMENT

【 】 BALLOON CATHETER ADVANCEMENT

Resistance at Groin Access Site

To avoid creating a long subcutaneous tunnel, which may pose some resistance during insertion of the balloon catheter, the puncture needle is angled more vertically than usual during the initial vascular access (at about 60° to the skin surface). After insertion of the coiled-tip guidewire into the left atrium, the shorter subcutaneous

TABLE 42-2

Catheter Selection and Balloon Sizing Based on Patient Height and Valvular Status

Reference Size (mm)

Height (cm) (rounded to nearest 0) × 1/10 + 10
 (eg, height = 167 cm)

RS = 170 × 1/10 + 10 = 27 mm

Catheter Selection

VALVULAR STATUS	BALLOON CATHETER
Pliable	RS matched (eg, PTMC-28 for RS 27 mm)
Calcified/SL	One-size < RS matched (eg, PTMC-26 for RS of 27 mm)
MR 2+	One-size < RS matched

Balloon Sizing

VALVULAR STATUS	INITIAL	INCREMENTS
Pliable	RS − 2 mm	1 mm, or 0.5 mm in [a]high pressure zone (if MR or unilateral commissural split)
Calcified/SL/MR 2+	RS − 4 mm	1 mm ([b]low–pressure zone) 0.5 mm ([a]high–pressure zone)

[a]High-pressure zone, balloon diameter within 2 mm of nominal balloon size.
[b]Low-pressure zone, balloon diameter < 2 mm of nominal balloon size.
MR = mitral regurgitation, preexisting or increased; RS = reference size; RS matched = catheter with its nominal balloon size ≥ RS; SL = severe subvalvular lesions.

track is then well stretched with an artery forceps alongside the wire. This is followed by use of the 12-Fr dilator, which is also used to dilate the atrial septum. When inserting the stretched balloon catheter, the guidewire should be held taut by an assistant. Use of a 14-Fr intravascular sheath for balloon catheter insertion is optional. During insertion of the catheter into the femoral vein, the catheter should never be twisted or the metal stretching tube or the guidewire will bend, thereby requiring replacement.

Septal Passage and Resistance

After placement of the coiled-tip guidewire in the left atrium, there may be some difficulty at times in advancing the balloon catheter across the septum, particularly when the latter is markedly thickened at the puncture site. When this occurs, forceful action is to be avoided. Rather, the balloon catheter should be turned slightly, usually in a clockwise direction, as it is pushed forward to overcome septal resistance. In the rare instances when this method also fails, the septum is redilated with the dilator. After passage across the septum, it is also important not to push the catheter tip up against the left atrial roof, or the guidewire may be bent into an acute angle.

【 】 DEEP CATHETER PLACEMENT IN LEFT ATRIUM

The balloon catheter is introduced under frontal fluoroscopic view into the atrium over the coiled-tip guidewire to form a large loop with the tip medial to the mitral valve (Figure 42-4). This placement has the following advantages: (1) the catheter thus posi-

tioned is less likely to flip to the left atrial appendage area when the stylet is inserted to the catheter tip; (2) the catheter does not enter the pulmonary veins; and (3) in subsequent manipulations to cross the valve, the catheter has already been advanced deep into the atrium, and it will need only to be withdrawn. Thus, the mitral valve crossing is attempted first with the vertical method, and potential catheter entrapment by a tough septum is avoided.

MITRAL VALVE CROSSING (SEE FIGURE 42-4)

Catheter manipulation is done in the 30° RAO view using the left ventriculogram as a road map. In difficult cases, such as in patients with giant left atria, additional use of lateral fluoroscopic view may be needed to facilitate valve crossing.

With the stylet inserted to the catheter tip, the partially inflated distal balloon is directed toward the anteriorly located mitral orifice. The balloon is directed anteriorly by applying a counterclockwise twist (usually 180°) to the stylet with one hand (usually the right), thus controlling the axial movement of the catheter balloon (see Figure 42-4). The catheter is then withdrawn gradually, using the other hand, thus to control the vertical motion of the balloon. Mitral valve crossing is then attempted using four methods in the order that they are described below.

【 】 VERTICAL METHOD (SEE FIGURE 42-4)

On further slight retraction of the catheter, the balloon is observed to move in (during diastole) and out of the left ventricle even

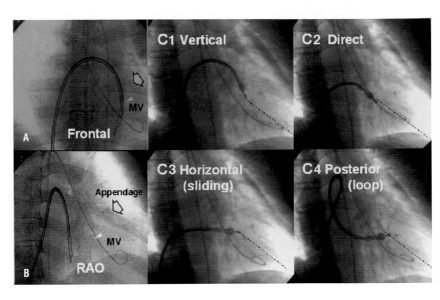

FIGURE 42-4. Deep catheter placement in left atrium and mitral valve crossing. A balloon catheter is introduced under frontal view into the atrium over a coiled-tip guidewire to form a large loop with the tip medial to the mitral valve (MV), pointing downward to a 6 to 7 o'clock direction (**A**). The catheter thus positioned is less likely to flip to the left atrial appendage area (*open arrowhead*). Subsequent catheter manipulations are done in 30° right anterior oblique (RAO) view. (**B**) Mitral valve crossing is attempted in order of vertical, horizontal, direct and posterior loop method (**C1 to C4**). The broken line indicates mitral orifice to left ventricular apex orientation. (*Courtesy of www.ptmv.org.*)

though the catheter is not aligned with the orifice-apex axis of the left ventricle (black broken line). Coincident with diastole, only the stylet is withdrawn. This allows the distal segment of the catheter to take on a more horizontal orientation to cross the valve and enter deep in the left ventricle.[37] Having replaced the originally used direct method, the vertical method is now the most frequently used successful crossing method.

DIRECT METHOD (SEE FIGURE 42-4)

When the vertical method fails, the balloon catheter is further withdrawn until the catheter balloon is near the valve and the catheter is well aligned with the orifice-apex axis. At this time, a "woodpecking" sign is observed as the balloon moves away from the mitral orifice in systole and toward it in diastole along the axis between the mitral orifice and the left ventricular apex (orifice-apex axis). Once this sign is evident, the operator jerks the stylet back slightly as the balloon approaches the orifice and simultaneously advances the catheter with the left hand to drive the balloon across the valve and deep into the left ventricle.

HORIZONTAL (OR SLIDING) METHOD (SEE FIGURE 42-4)

This method has proved to be effective, especially in cases in which the septal puncture is made too caudally and/or the left ventricle assumes a more horizontal orientation. The balloon is first directed toward the mitral valve by keeping the stylet twisted counterclockwise. The distal catheter segment is then made more flexible by withdrawing the stylet clear out of the balloon segment. Once the slightly inflated balloon is at the mitral orifice, cardiac contractions cause the balloon segment to tilt upwards during systole. In diastole, the balloon segment aligns with the catheter shaft. With the operator carefully watching the rhythmic motion of the cardiac cycle, only the catheter is advanced forward (with the stylet kept fixed) during diastole to cross the valve. The stylet is then advanced to help align the catheter with the orifice-apex axis.

POSTERIOR LOOP METHOD (SEE FIGURE 42-4)

First, a vertical loop is made (as in Figure 42-4B) and the stylet is then withdrawn to a point 2 to 3 cm proximally to make the balloon segment more flexible. With the stylet twisted clockwise, the balloon tip is brought toward the posterior and inferior wall of the left atrium; thus the catheter forms a loop in the left atrium.

With the stylet held firmly, only the balloon catheter is advanced, allowing the balloon to move forward to the mitral orifice. When the balloon enters the left ventricle, its tip usually points upwards. The loop is then reduced by carefully withdrawing the catheter and slightly advancing the stylet to the balloon segment to align the distal catheter with the orifice-apex axis.[35] This method is infrequently used in the authors' experience.

DISCUSSION OF THE METHODS

In the vertical and direct methods, the major causes of valve crossing failure are (1) bending of the distal balloon segment, resulting in malalignment of the balloon segment with the mitral orifice, and (2) insufficient counterclockwise rotation of the stylet, thus failing to bring the catheter balloon segment sufficiently anteriorly to align toward the mitral orifice. Therefore, it is important to insert the stylet all the way to the balloon catheter tip to straighten the latter. Occasionally, however, the stylet may be too short to reach the catheter tip, thus making a slight bend in the catheter tip. If this occurs, the rubber grip at the proximal end of the stylet can be pulled further back to lengthen the exposed segment of the stylet or, failing that, the rubber grip can be cut at 1 to 2 mm from its distal end and removed. In addition, the stylet must be kept twisted at all times. An extra counterclockwise twist is occasionally needed to direct the catheter tip anteriorly. Less commonly, inappropriate stylet tip curving may also contribute to the failure. If this occurs, the stylet should be reshaped according to the positional relationship between the septal puncture site and the valve orifice.

In the catheter sliding or the posterior loop method, the catheter has a propensity to enter the left atrial appendage region during a failed valve-crossing attempt because the distal balloon catheter is more horizontally oriented. Therefore, the stylet should not be pulled back too vigorously to avoid excessive forward movement of the catheter towards the appendage region.

BALLOON INFLATION PROCEDURES

【 】 ENSURING FREE BALLOON MOVEMENT IN LEFT VENTRICLE

Once the mitral valve has been crossed, the free movements of the partially inflated distal balloon in the left ventricle should be ascertained to prevent disastrous consequences (ie, rupture of chordae, papillary muscles, or leaflets) stemming from its subsequent full inflation within the chordae. This is done by simultaneously pushing the catheter and pulling the stylet slightly in opposite directions ("accordion" maneuver)[22] to ensure that the partially inflated distal balloon slides freely along the orifice-apex axis.

After crossing the mitral valve, the catheter balloon may point more vertically and deviate away from the orifice-apex axis. This suggests that the catheter has strayed among the chordae. To correct this situation, the distal balloon is inflated larger to prevent the balloon from being inadvertently retracted into the atrium, and the catheter is carefully pulled back to assume a more horizontal orientation. After satisfactory alignment of the catheter with the orifice-apex axis, the catheter is advanced toward the apex, and the previously described accordion maneuver is performed before initiating the inflation procedure. Similarly, a twist in the balloon during the inflation process may also indicate that the catheter has tethered among the chordae. In this case, the inflation should be promptly aborted and the balloon repositioned.

【 】 REASSESSMENT OF SUBVALVULAR STATUS

Before BMV, mitral valvular status is determined by preprocedural transthoracic echocardiography and fluoroscopy (for the presence of valvular calcification), and an appropriate balloon catheter is then chosen accordingly. Extensive subvalvular disease has been found by various investigators to be a predictor of significant mitral regurgitation. Because echocardiography often underestimates the severity of subvalvular disease,[22] severe mitral regurgitation may be created during BMV despite the presence of apparently favorable valve morphology. Therefore, during the actual balloon dilations, vigilance is required to identify the presence of previously undetected severe subvalvular disease. We and others have found other more reliable signs of significant subvalvular involvement.[12,38,39] The most commonly encountered sign is a distorted balloon due to compression by severe subvalvular disease when it is being inflated.[22] Even in patients in whom no severe subvalvular disease is demonstrated by echocardiography, when the presence of severe subvalvular disease is suspected during the balloon inflation process, the balloon dilation protocol should be altered accordingly as described below (see Balloon Sizing).

【 】 CONTROLLED STEPWISE DILATIONS

To avoid or minimize the complication of severe mitral regurgitation, the selection of an appropriate balloon catheter and the con-

trolled stepwise dilation technique are mandatory. In addition, one should be familiar with the pressure-volume relationship and inflation limit of the catheter balloon.[22]

Balloon Pressure–Volume Relationship

The intraballoon pressure transits from the "low-pressure" to the "high-pressure" zone as the balloon is inflated to within 2 mm of its nominal size (eg, the 24–26-mm zone in a 26-mm-balloon catheter). Each catheter can be safely inflated to a maximal diameter of 1 mm above the nominal size because of the built-in safety margin. Initial balloon inflation is never to be performed with balloon diameter in the high-pressure zone, regardless of the valvular morphology.

Balloon Sizing (Table 42-2)

As indicated earlier, balloon sizing for the stepwise dilation technique is crucial in avoiding the complication of severe mitral regurgitation. By adhering to the cautionary methods outlined below, especially in patients with severe subvalvular disease, creation of significant mitral regurgitation (increase of $\geq 2+$ angiographically) can be minimized.[23]

1. Pliable, noncalcified valves. In patients with pliable, noncalcified valves and no severe subvalvular lesions, as determined by the subvalvular reassessment outlined above, an RS-matched balloon catheter is selected as stated previously. The initial inflated balloon diameter is RS minus 2 mm. In subsequent dilations, the balloon size is increased by 1 mm. When there is preexisting mitral regurgitation or any question of increase in the degree of mitral regurgitation, the increment should be 0.5 mm in the high-pressure zone. This approach also applies when unilateral commissural splitting occurs during the previous dilation, as observed by asymmetrical balloon waists on fluoroscopy. The final diameter is best kept within 1 mm above the RS to avoid oversizing; that is a risk factor for creating severe mitral regurgitation in this group of patients.[12]

2. Calcified valves and/or with severe subvalvular disease. In patients with either fluoroscopically visible valvular calcification, or severe subvalvular lesions as observed by transthoracic echocardiography, instead of an RS-match, a balloon catheter one size smaller than the RS-match is selected at the outset. For those whose subvalvular lesions are not detected by preprocedural echocardiography, the RS-matched catheter already placed in the patient may still be used if the dilation procedures are carried out with extra care. Ideally, the catheter should be exchanged for a smaller one, but this is quite costly.

For the first dilation, a balloon diameter 4 mm less than the RS is used. For subsequent dilations, the balloon size is increased by 1 mm in the low-pressure zone and by 0.5 mm in the high-pressure zone until satisfactory results are obtained or until mitral regurgitation develops or worsens. In cases where the gradient has already been reduced to one half and several more dilation attempts have failed to reduce it further, the procedure is terminated to avoid creating severe mitral regurgitation. Reducing the mitral valve gradient by one half should result in a 41% increase in the mitral valve area, as calculated by the Gorlin formula, provided that heart rate and cardiac output remain the same. Our previous study[21] suggests that a 40% increase in the valve area is sufficient for symptomatic improvements in patients with a more sedentary life style.

[ ] EXCHANGE FOR DIFFERENT-SIZED BALLOON CATHETERS

Exchange of balloon catheters is carried out for two reasons. The first is to downsize the catheter in the presence of severe subvalvular disease that may have evaded detection by echocardiography but was noted during the BMV procedure itself. The second occurs in the rare instance when there is a need to upsize the balloon catheter to one that is one size larger because of inadequate hemodynamic improvement with the initial balloon catheter. In such a situation, before exchanging for a larger catheter, it is vital that the initial catheter's final balloon diameter be remeasured and reverified after its complete removal from the patient, particularly when it has been inflated beyond its nominal size. This precautionary exercise is essential because, not uncommonly, despite pretesting, the balloon size is smaller than what it is supposed to be after in vivo usage. When this occurs, the original balloon catheter is retested to determine the actual volume of diluted contrast in the syringe necessary to achieve maximum balloon size (the balloon tolerates about 1–2 mm) in excess of its nominal size before rupturing), the original balloon catheter is reintroduced into the patient, and the dilation process is repeated. However, if the balloon matches its predefined size, an exchange for a larger-sized catheter is made and dilations with the larger balloon are performed. Failing to reverify the maximum balloon size before inflating a much larger balloon may risk the creation of severe mitral regurgitation.

Balloon "Popping" to Left Atrium

When the mitral valve has already been enlarged by dilations, the balloon may occasionally slip into the left atrium during subsequent inflations with larger balloon diameters. To prevent the latter from occurring, the stylet is advanced far into the balloon segment to stiffen the catheter, and before the catheter is retracted to anchor the balloon at the orifice, the distal balloon is inflated to a diameter slightly larger than the previous one. As soon as the balloon assumes an hourglass configuration, the catheter is advanced slightly to prevent it from jerking out into the left atrium, and full balloon expansion is then executed. With this extra dilation, although the mitral gradient may be unchanged, enhanced splitting of the commissures, as assessed by echocardiography, is often observed.

The balloon "popping" signals enlargement of the mitral orifice with wide splitting of the commissures. It is usually encountered in patients with pliable, noncalcified valves and foretells excellent BMC results. However, suboptimal hemodynamic results are occasionally observed despite the balloon "popping" sign, especially in the presence of atrial fibrillation. In these cases, although the mitral valve with split commissures can be forced to accommodate the fully inflated balloon, the effective mitral valve area is, in reality, limited by the thickened and stiff leaflets, and by ineffective atrial contractions in the beating heart.

Assessment After Each Valve Dilation Procedure

After each balloon inflation procedure, the catheter balloon is withdrawn to the left atrium. The effects of the balloon dilation is assessed by observing the left atrial pressure waveforms, by measuring the transmitral gradient and also by auscultation. If mitral regurgitation is suspected by the appearance of a large or giant "v" wave and by a new or worsening systolic murmur, echocardiography or left ventriculography may be performed. Although not essential, transthoracic or online transesophageal echocardiography is an excellent tool to assess and monitor the valve status after each balloon dilation if the logistics permit its use. However, the tool is too sensitive for detection of new or increase in the degree of mitral regurgitation, and thus sole dependence on the echocardiography findings may result in premature termination of the procedure.

AVOIDING LEFT ATRIAL APPENDAGE

Left atrial appendage thrombus may be unsuspected when BMV candidates are screened only with insensitive transthoracic echocardiography. Balloon catheter encroachment on the left atrial appendage region must thus be avoided in order to minimize the risk of inadvertent thrombus dislodgement and systemic embolism. Under 30-degree right anterior oblique fluoroscopic view, the anterolaterally located appendage is cephalad to and right of the pigtail catheter segment in the left ventricle (see Figure 42-4B). Therefore, the balloon catheter tip should always be kept to the left of the pigtail catheter during catheter manipulation in the left atrium by adopting the following steps:

1. Deep placement of balloon catheter in the left atrium (see Figure 42-4A).
2. Mitral valve crossing. The balloon catheter tip is more horizontally orientated when performing the catheter sliding or the posterior loop method (see Figure 42-4) in crossing the mitral valve. The catheter tip is thus more prone to entering the left atrial appendage region during a failed valve-crossing attempt. Therefore, the stylet should not be pulled back too vigorously during the crossing attempt to avoid excessive forward movement of the catheter toward the appendage region.
3. Catheter withdrawal to the left ventricle. After each balloon inflation procedure, in order to exert better control over the catheter tip, the stylet is advanced halfway into the balloon segment and the catheter is withdrawn just out of the mitral orifice from the left ventricle. Then, a slight clockwise twist to the stylet is applied to direct the catheter tip posteriorly. The balloon catheter can then be safely retrieved to the atrium by cautiously withdrawing the catheter and the stylet in steps until the catheter stands straight upwards.
4. Mitral valve gradient measurement. After each valve dilation procedure, a transmitral valve gradient measurement is performed without fluoroscopy. Thus, care should be exercised to avoid pushing the catheter forward into the appendage.

After the precautions have become rote, it is possible to perform BMV safely even in the presence of left atrial appendage thrombi. Despite our safe and successful experience in performing BMV in patients with thrombi confined to the appendage,[23] the subject has remained controversial even among experienced operators of Inoue-BMV. Therefore, the alternative approaches are either to subject patients with appendage thrombi to mitral valve surgery or to defer BMC for stable patients until resolution of the thrombi after warfarin treatment.[23,24]

REFERENCES

1. Inoue K, Owaki T, Nakamura T, et al. Clinical application of transvenous mitral commissurotomy by a new balloon catheter. *J Thorac Cardiovasc Surg.* 1984;87:394.

2. Arora R, Kalra GS, Murty GSR, et al. Percutaneous transatrial mitral commissurotomy: immediate and intermediate results. *J Am Coll Cardiol.* 1994;23:1327.

3. Ruiz EC, Zhang HP, Macaya C, et al. Comparison of Inoue single-balloon versus double-balloon technique for percutaneous mitral valvotomy. *Am Heart J.* 1992;123:942.

4. A report from the National Heart, Lung, and Blood Institute Balloon Valvuloplasty Registry. Complications and mortality of percutaneous balloon mitral commissurotomy. *Circulation.* 1992;85:2014.

5. Iung B, Cormier B, Ducimetiere P, et al. Immediate results of percutaneous mitral commissurotomy. *Circulation.* 1996;94:2124.

6. Turi ZG, Reyes VP, Raju S. Percutaneous balloon versus closed commissurotomy for mitral stenosis. A prospective, randomized trial. *Circulation.* 1991;83:1179.

7. Patel JJ, Shama D, Mitha AS, et al. Balloon valvuloplasty versus closed commissurotomy for pliable mitral stenosis: a prospective hemodynamic study. *J Am Coll Cardiol.* 1991;125:1318.

8. Arora R, Nair M, Kalra GS, et al. Immediate and long-term results of balloon and surgical closed mitral valvotomy: a randomized comparative study. *Am Heart J.* 1993;125:1091.

9. Bueno R, Andrade P, Nercolini D, et al. Percutaneous balloon mitral valvuloplasty versus open mitral commissurotomy. A randomized clinical trial. *J Am Coll Cardiol.* 1993;21:429A.

10. Reyes VP, Raju BS, Wynne J. Percutaneous balloon valvuloplasty compared with open surgical commissurotomy for mitral stenosis. *N Engl J Med.* 1994;331:961.

11. Farhat MB, Ayari M, Maatouk F, et al. Percutaneous balloon versus surgical closed and open mitral commissurotomy. Seven-year follow-up resultsw of a randomized trial. *Circulation.* 1998;97:245.

12. Hung JS, Chern MS, Wu JJ, et al. Short- and long-term results of catheter balloon percutaneous transvenous mitral commissurotomy. *Am J Cardiol.* 1991;67:854.

13. Pan M, Medina A, de Lezo JS, et al. Factors determining late success after mitral balloon valvulotomy. *Am J Cardiol.* 1993;71:1181.

14. Iung B, Cormier B, Ducimetiere P, et al. Functional results 5 years after successful percutaneous mitral commissurotomy in a series of 528 patients and analysis of predictive factors. *J Am Coll Cardiol.* 1996;27:407.

15. Dean LS, Mickel M, Bonan R, et al. Four-year follow-up of patients undergoing percutaneous balloon mitral commissurotomy. *J Am Coll Cardiol.* 1996;28:1452.

16. Hernandez R, Banuelos C, Alfonso F, et al. Long-term clinical and echocardiographic follow-up after percutaneous mitral valvuloplasty with the Inoue balloon. *Circulation.* 1999;99:1580.

17. Yoshida Y, Kubo S, Tamaki S, et al. Percutaneous transvenous mitral commissurotomy for mitral stenosis patients with markedly severe mitral valve deformity: immediate results and long-term clinical outcome. *Am J Cardiol.* 1995;76:406.

18. Dean LS, Mickel M, Bonan R, et al. Four-year follow-up of patients undergoing percutaneous balloon mitral commissurotomy. *J Am Coll Cardiol.* 1996;28:1452.

19. Hung JS, Lau KW. Percutaneous transvenous mitral commissurotomy is an acceptable therapeutic alternative in patients with calcified mitral valve. *J Invasive Cardiol.* 1999;11:362.

20. Wahl A, Meier B. Percutaneous mitral balloon valvuloplasty in non-ideal patients: go for it without expecting too much. *J Invasive Cardiol.* 1999;11:359.

21. Lau KW, Hung JS. A simple balloon-sizing method in Inoue balloon percutaneous transvenous mitral commissurotomy. *Cathet Cardiovasc Diagn.* 1994;33:120.

22. Hung JS, Lau KW. Pitfalls and tips in Inoue-balloon mitral commissurotomy. *Cathet Cardiovasc Diagn.* 1996;37:188.

23. Hung JS, Lau KW, Lo PH, et al. Complications of Inoue-balloon mitral commissurotomy-Impact of operator experience and evolving technique. *Am Heart J.* 1999;138:114.

24. Hung JS. Mitral stenosis with left atrial thrombi: Inoue balloon catheter technique. In: Cheng TO, ed. *Percutaneous Balloon Valvuloplasty.* New York, NY: Igaku-Shoin Medical Publishers; 1992:280.

25. Yeh KH, Hung JS, Wu CJ, et al. Safety of Inoue balloon mitral commissurotomy in patients with left atrial appendage thrombi. *Am J Cardiol.* 1995;75:302.

26. Tsai LM, Hung JS, Chen JH, et al. Resolution of left atrial appendage thrombus in mitral stenosis after warfarin therapy. *Am Heart J.* 1991;121:1232.

27. Lock JE, Khalilullah M, Shrivastava S, et al. Percutaneous catheter commissurotomy in rheumatic mitral stenosis. *N Engl J Med.* 1985;313:1515.

28. Al Zaibag M, Ribeiro PA, Al Kasab S, et al. Percutaneous double-balloon mitral valvotomy for rheumatic mitral valve stenosis. *Lancet.* 1986;1:757.

29. Stefanadis C, Toutouzas P. Retrograde nontransseptal mitral valvuloplasty. In: Topol EJ, ed. *Textbook of Interventional Cardiology.* 2nd ed. Philadelphia, PA: WB Saunders; 1994:1253.

30. Park SJ, Kim JJ, Park SW, et al. Immediate and one-year results of percutaneous mitral balloon valvuloplasty using Inoue and double-balloon techniques. *Am J Cardiol* 1993;71:939.

31. Sharma S, Loya YS, Desai DM, et al. Percutaneous mitral valvotomy using Inoue and double balloon technique: comparison of clinical and hemodynamic short-term results in 350 cases. *Cathet Cardiovasc Diagn.* 1993;29:18.

32. Arora R, Kalra GS, Murty GSR, et al. Percutaneous transatrial mitral commissurotomy: immediate and intermediate results. *J Am Coll Cardiol.* 1994;23:1327.

33. Hung JS. Atrial septal puncture technique in percutaneous transvenous mitral commissurotomy: mitral valvuloplasty using the Inoue balloon catheter technique. *Cathet Cardiovasc Diagn.* 1992;26:275.

34. Goldstein SA, Campbell A, Mintz GS, et al. Feasibility of on-line transesophageal echocardiography during balloon mitral valvulotomy: experience with 93 patients. *J Heart Valve Dis.* 1994;3:136.

35. Inoue K, Lau KW, Hung JS. Percutaneous transvenous mitral commissurotomy. In: Grech ED, Ramsdale DR. *Practical Interventional Cardiology.* 2nd ed. London, UK: Martin Dunitz Ltd; 2002:373.

36. Ramasamy D, Zambahari R, Fu M, Yeh KH, et al. Percutaneous transvenous mitral commissurotomy in patients with severe kyphoscoliosis. *Cathet Cardiovasc Diagn.* 1993;30:40.

37. Hung JS, Lau KW. Vertical approach: a modified method in balloon crossing of mitral valve in Inoue balloon mitral valvuloplasty. *J Invasive Cardiol.* 1998;10:548.

38. Lau KW, Hung JS. "Balloon impasse:" a marker for severe mitral subvalvular disease and a predictor of mitral regurgitation in Inoue balloon percutaneous transvenous mitral commissurotomy. *Cathet Cardiovasc Diagn.* 1995;35:310.

39. Hernandez R, Macaya C, Banuelos C, et al. Predictors, mechanisms and outcome of severe mitral regurgitation complicating percutaneous mitral valvotomy with the Inoue balloon. *Am J Cardiol.* 1992;70:1169.

CHAPTER (43)

Aortic Valvuloplasty and Future Solutions to Aortic Valve Disease

Alain Cribier, MD, Helene Eltchaninoff, MD, and Christophe Tron, MD

For the vast majority of patients with degenerative calcific aortic valve stenosis, aortic valve replacement, which offers symptomatic relief and improving long-term survival, is the treatment of choice.[1-3] However, surgical valve replacement is still associated with a high mortality and morbidity rates in growing subsets of elderly patients with poor cardiac and noncardiac conditions.[4-9] For those patients with high surgical risk or no option for surgery, balloon aortic valvuloplasty (BAV), introduced by our group in 1986,[10] can efficiently palliate the symptoms of congestive heart failure and diminish the need for rehospitalization.[11,12] BAV has been recognized by the American College of Cardiology/American Heart Association (ACC/AHA) guidelines as a class 2B indication in this subset of patients.[13] The technique has become simpler and is associated with a low complication rate. However, the duration of hemodynamic and clinical benefits remains unpredictable and is rarely more than 1 year, precluding BAV to be more commonly performed. Although this procedure has not been shown to confer survival benefit in large registries,[14,15] it may be beneficial for individual patients. In our group, repeat procedures are commonly performed in selected patients (up to five times), with subsequent prolonged survival.

In the past years, there have been exciting developments in the field of percutaneous treatment of valvular diseases, with the first reported cases of catheter-based heart valve implantation in animals[16-20] and in humans[21-24]; this opens a new era for the management of these patients. In our group, the concept of catheter-based aortic valve replacement emerged in the 1990s with the goal of improving the results of BAV. In April 2002, we successfully performed the first human implantation of a percutaneous heart valve (PHV) in a patient with end-stage aortic stenosis and cardiogenic shock.[23] Since then, several improvements to the PHV device have been made, and the clinical experience enriched by additional patients with end-stage aortic stenosis and multiple comorbidities, in whom the technique was applied on a compassionate basis. Our intermediate clinical experience on 6 patients has been published.[24]

This chapter will report the standard technique currently used for BAV in our institution, where 40 to 50 cases are still performed each year, and where BAV currently remains the only therapeutic option for the majority of nonoperable patients with aortic stenosis. We will then describe the techniques used for PHV implantation and briefly overview the preliminary results observed.

TECHNIQUE OF BALLOON AORTIC VALVULOPLASTY IN OUR INSTITUTION

With an experience of more than 1000 patients and with the current BAV technique used, it is possible to perform the procedure in less than 1 hour, with few complications. In this population of very ill and fragile elderly patients, the technical tips are crucial to make the procedure fast and safe. After the baseline hemodynamic measurements are obtained, a coronary arteriography is usually performed, and if indicated, angioplasty and stenting are undertaken in the same session, after BAV has been completed.

The procedure requires local anesthesia and mild sedation. A dose of 5000 IU of heparin is administered intravenously at the beginning of the procedure.

[ ] CROSSING THE NATIVE VALVE

Proper technique permits negotiation of the stenotic aortic valve within a few minutes in all cases. This is achieved with the use of a 7-Fr Sones (B type) catheter (or an Amplatz left coronary artery catheter in case of enlarged ascending aorta), advanced in the femoral artery through a 8-Fr sheath over a 0.035-inch straight-tip guidewire. In the 40-degree left anterior oblique view, the catheter's tip is first positioned at the upper limit of the valve. The catheter is then slowly pulled back while a strong clockwise rotation is maintained, and the straight guidewire is sequentially advanced out and retrieved inside the catheter. After the valve has been crossed with the wire, the catheter is advanced in the left ventricle. The transvalvular gradient is obtained, using the lateral sheath connector to record the aortic pressure.

[ ] TECHNICAL ASPECTS OF VALVE DILATION

With regard to the dilation procedure itself, the major aspects that need to be stressed are: (1) use of a very rigid guidewire for advancing the balloon catheter up to the aortic valve and keeping it stable during dilation, (2) use of a 14-Fr arterial sheath for arterial access, and (3) use of temporary fast cardiac pacing to maintain the balloon stable across the valve during inflation.

Guidewire

A 0.035-inch, 270-cm long, extra-stiff guidewire (Cook, Denmark) is inserted into the Sones (or Amplatz) catheter, and the diagnostic catheter is removed. Before use, the flexible distal end of this wire must be reshaped in an exaggerated pigtail curve in order to decrease the risk of left ventricular trauma or perforation and the incidence of ventricular ectopies or ventricular tachycardia. The 8-Fr sheath is removed and replaced by a 14-Fr sheath.

14-French Arterial Sheath

The use of a 14-Fr arterial introducer (Cook, Denmark) has markedly decreased the rate of local complications at the femoral puncture site. The proximal diaphragm of this introducer is watertight and prevents blood loss around the guidewire during catheter exchange procedures. Preclosure of the femoral puncture site is now routinely performed at the beginning of the procedure using a 10-Fr Perclose device (Abbots Vascular, United States) and this has further decreased the rate of bleeding complication after removal of the sheath.[25,26]

Balloon Catheter

Until last year, all cases were performed with a 9-Fr, three-lumen, pigtail catheter (Boston Scientific, United States) that we specially designed for this procedure. The advantage of this device was the ability to produce sequential dilation of the valve without exchanging catheters. Because the manufacturer has stopped making peripheral balloon catheters, our choice has turned to the Z-Med II balloon catheter (NuMed, Canada), which is a single 9-Fr double-lumen catheter with a 30-mm length balloon. In the majority of cases, we use the 23-mm balloon size in first intention, whereas sequential inflations starting with smaller size (20-mm) are preferred in case of very calcified valves or a small size annulus. Despite being particularly resistant to high inflation pressure, the balloon is carefully purged of air before use to avoid any air embolization in case of balloon rupture.

After being prepared, the balloon catheter is advanced through the 14-Fr sheath over the stiff guidewire while a negative pressure is maintained with a 20-mL syringe filled with a solution of 10/90 contrast/saline. This dilution is enough to visualize the balloon on fluoroscopy and facilitates hand balloon inflation/deflation (Figure 43-1A).

Fast Heart Pacing During Balloon Inflation

Whereas an excellent stability during balloon inflation could be easily obtained with the Boston Scientific catheter due to the longer balloon length and the distal pigtail tip, it was more challenging to maintain the NuMed balloon in position across the valve during inflation. The procedure has been considerably facilitated by the use of a brief period of rapid cardiac pacing (200–220/min) during the 3 to 4 seconds required for fast and maximal balloon inflation (Figure 43-1B). The pacing lead is placed in the right ventricle at the beginning of the procedure and the pacing rate able to decrease the blood pressure to 30/40 mm Hg is assessed. In the majority of cases, a rate of 220/min is required. The pacemaker used must allow a sudden increase of heart rate to the desired level. Fast pacing is started at the time balloon inflation is initiated and stopped at maximal inflation. Just as the process of deflation begins, the balloon is withdrawn from the valve while keeping the guidewire in the left ventricle. This maneuver is crucial to promptly restore the antegrade blood flow. It may be noted that the temporary pacemaker is also useful in case of transient complete heart block, which can occur during manipulation of the hardware in the left ventricle (it is more frequent in patients with preexisting conduction abnormalities).

The same procedure is generally repeated before withdrawal of the balloon catheter. Even in case of suboptimal results, a larger balloon size (25 mm) is never used in our practice, in order to avoid the risk of valvular or aortic annulus disruption. The results are assessed on the residual transvalvular gradient obtained with a pigtail catheter advanced over the wire in the left ventricle and the sidearm of the sheath (Figure 43-1C) and during the pullback maneuver. The Gorlin formula is used to evaluate the final aortic valve area. The results are considered "optimal" when the valve area has doubled in comparison to baseline.

[ ] POSTPROCEDURE MANAGEMENT

Immediately after the procedure, the balloon catheters and arterial sheaths are removed. The femoral artery entry site is closed using the predelivered percutaneous sutures, which is successfully performed in 90% of the cases. In case of technical failure, pneumatic compression devices are used. When BAV is applied in the context of severely impaired left ventricular function or cardiogenic shock, inotropic support may be transitorily required in the days following the procedure. In other uncomplicated cases, the patients can be discharged after 2 days.

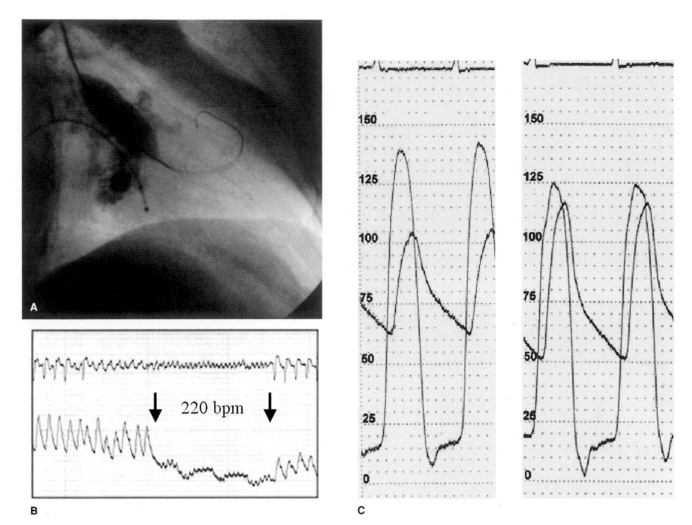

FIGURE 43-1. (A) The Z-Med II balloon valvuloplasty catheter at full inflation during valve dilation. **(B)** Aortic blood pressure recording during the percutaneous heart valve (PHV) delivery phase showing the effect of a 220/min fast right ventricular pacing. The induced decrease of blood flow allows optimal balloon stabilization at the time of PHV delivery. **(C)** Transaortic pressure gradient at baseline and after balloon valvuloplasty. The mean residual gradient has decreased to 12 mm Hg with an increase in valve area from 0.48 to 1.00 cm^2 in this patient.

Long-term follow-up is sequentially assessed on clinical and echocardiographic evaluations. Only in patients in whom the recurrence of symptoms is delayed by at least 6 months, repeat BAV can be indicated and generally leads to similar results.

COMPLICATIONS

The complications associated with the BAV have markedly decreased over time. However, if the local complications at the femoral entry site have been significantly reduced to below 2% with the use of arterial introducers and the preclosing device, it seems unlikely to decrease the rate of death (2.5%) and neurologic complication (2%) reported in 1995[27] in patients with severely compromised hemodynamic status or cardiogenic shock, or diseased cerebral vessels and previous cerebrovascular events. Strokes generally occur during hypotension induced by manipulation of the hardware across the diseased valve or balloon inflation. Heparinization and short balloon inflation/deflation time are highly recommended in this regard.

PERCUTANEOUS VALVE IMPLANTATION

DEVICE DESCRIPTION

The PHV currently used in humans comprises a stainless steel balloon-expandable stent with an integrated trileaflet tissue valve made of three equal sections of equine pericardium (Figure 2A) preserved in low concentration solution of glutaraldehyde. The valve is securely attached by sutures to the stent frame. The stent is 14 mm in length, with a maximal external diameter of 23 mm; to date, this is the only size available. The PHV durability passed 200 millions cycles (5 years) in bench testing.

A crimper (Figure 43-2B) has been specially developed to symmetrically reduce the diameter of the PHV from its expanded size to its collapsed size over the delivery balloon catheter (Figure 43-2C). The crimping is performed manually by means of a rotary knob located on the housing. A check gauge is used to verify that

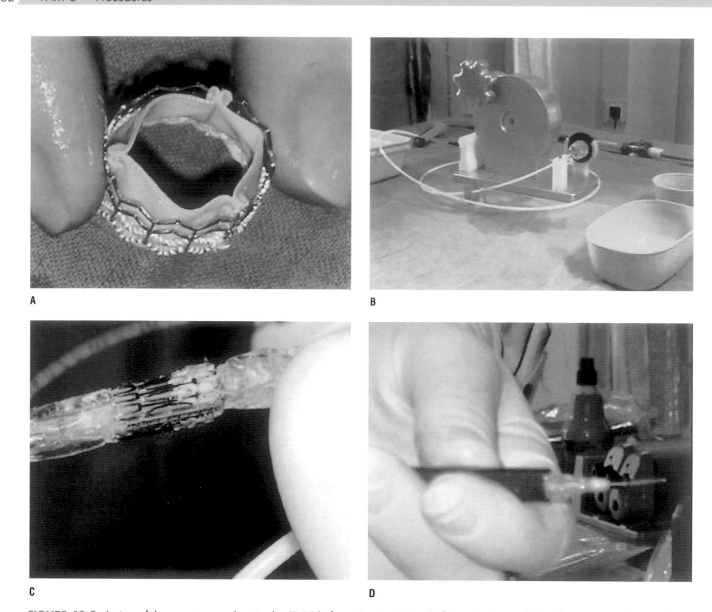

A

B

C

D

FIGURE 43-2. A view of the percutaneous heart valve (PHV) before crimping (**A**) and of the crimping tool (**B**). After crimping, the PHV/ balloon assembly (**C**) can be advanced with no friction through a 24-Fr tubular calibration gauge (**D**).

the balloon assembly is suitable for introduction in a 24-Fr sheath (Figure 43-2D).

The delivery valvuloplasty balloon catheter is similar to the one used for BAV, a 9-Fr Z-MED II (NuMed, United States), 120 cm in length. The noncompliant balloon is 30 mm in length and 22 mm in maximal diameter.

[ ] PREPROCEDURAL EVALUATION

The patients are selected on the basis of complete clinical evaluation, transthoracic and transesophageal echocardiography (TTE and TEE), cardiac catheterization with left ventricular and aortic angiograms, and coronary arteriography. The following criteria are taken into account when considering the patients for inclusion and the method used for PHV implantation: the type and severity of aortic stenosis, the amount and distribution of valvular calcification, the aortic annulus diameter, the left ventricular function, the diameter, tortuousities and disease of the peripheral arteries, the association between coronary disease and other valvular diseases. A surgical risk score (Parsonnet's score) is obtained.[28]

[ ] TECHNIQUES OF PERCUTANEOUS HEART VALVE IMPLANTATION

The PHV can be implanted using either the antegrade transseptal or the retrograde approaches. The antegrade approach was the first used in humans, in a patient who had no patent femoral arteries. Because PHV implantation was easily performed in this patient, and because PHV implantation requires a large 24-Fr introducer that can always be inserted in the femoral vein, the same approach was repeated in the following cases. However, since mid-2003, the retrograde approach was also successfully attempted in selected patients with healthy and large femoroiliac arteries. Both techniques have advantages and limitations.

Whatever the technique used, the procedure is performed under local anesthesia and mild sedation. Aspirin (160 mg) and clopidogrel (300 mg) are administered 24 hours before the procedure. In all cases, the procedure starts with the reassessment of baseline parameters (right and left side pressures, transvalvular aortic gradient, and aortic valve area using the Gorlin formula). The same measurements will be obtained after PHV implantation.

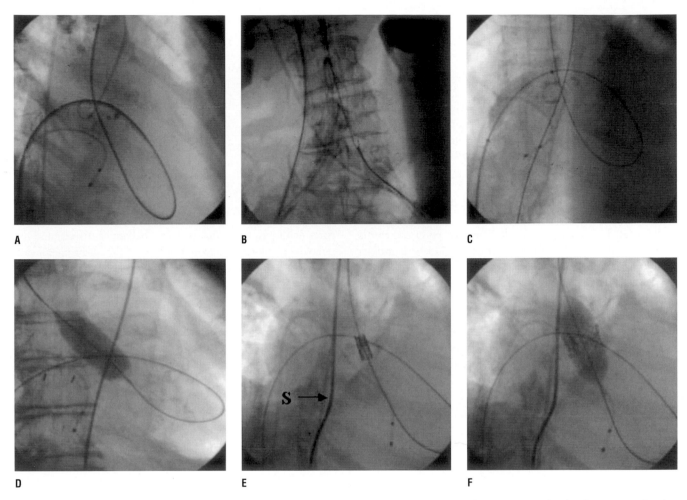

FIGURE 43-3. Phases of percutaneous heart valve (PHV) implantation via the antegrade route. After the aortic valve has been crossed with the Swan-Ganz catheter, a long stiff guidewire is advanced in the descending aorta (**A**), and snared and externalized through the right femoral artery with a lasso (**B**). The transatrial septum puncture site is dilated with a 10-mm balloon (**C**), and the native valve is predilated with a 23-mm valvuloplasty balloon advanced from the femoral vein (**D**). Accurate PHV positioning at midpart of the native aortic valve (**E**) is obtained with the help of a 7-Fr Sones catheter (*S, arrow*) advanced through the femoral artery. The delivery balloon is fully inflated (**F**) under rapid cardiac pacing.

Supra-aortic angiograms showing the aortic valvular apparatus perpendicular to the screen with the coronary ostia clearly visible are performed in order to select the optimal view. The anteroposterior view is generally selected, and a frame frozen on another screen will be one of the markers used at the time of PHV implantation. A 5-Fr pacemaker lead is placed into the right ventricle. The stimulation parameters are controlled and the pacemaker set on demand at 80 beats/min.

[ ] ANTEGRADE TRANSSEPTAL APPROACH

Transseptal Catheterization, Guidewire Placement, and Dilation of the Transatrial Septum

Through the right femoral vein, the usual technique of transseptal catheterization is undertaken, using an 8-Fr Mullins sheath. After completion of the transseptal puncture, heparin (5000 IU) is administered intravenously. Through the Mullins sheath in the left atrium, a 7-Fr Swan-Ganz catheter (Edwards Lifesciences, United States) is advanced in the left ventricle and used to cross the aortic valve with the help of a 0.035-inch straight guidewire. With the catheter in place in the ascending aorta, the guidewire is removed

and replaced by a 0.035-inch, 360-cm long stiff guidewire (Amplatz, Cook, Denmark), advanced in the descending aorta (Figure 43-3A), down to the onset of the iliac arteries. Through a 8-Fr sheath in the left femoral artery, a catheter snare (Microvena, Amplatz Goose Neck, United States) is used to catch and externalize the long guidewire (Figure 43-3B). The externalized parts of the wire should be equivalent on both sides (about 100 cm out of the right femoral vein and the left femoral artery). Through a 10-Fr sheath in the right femoral vein, a balloon septostomy catheter (Owens, Boston-Scientific Scimed, United States), 10 mm in diameter, is advanced over the stiff guidewire, positioned within the interatrial septum, and inflated with a 30/70 contrast/saline solution to dilate the transseptal puncture site (Figure 43-3C).

Balloon Predilation of the Aortic Valve

After removal of the septostomy catheter from the right femoral vein, the 10-Fr sheath is replaced by a 14-Fr sheath (Cook, Denmark) and a 23-mm Z-Med II balloon valvuloplasty catheter (NuMED, Canada) is prepared, purged of air, advanced over the stiff guidewire, and positioned across the aortic valve. Using a technique similar to the one described above for retrograde BAV, the balloon is fully inflated and deflated under rapid cardiac pacing (Figure 43-3D). Two to three balloon inflations are generally performed. The balloon catheter is then withdrawn.

Percutaneous Heart Valve Implantation

The PHV is meticulously rinsed in a saline solution, and the balloon prepared. A 10/90 contrast/saline solution is used to inflate the balloon, purge it of air, and determine the exact amount of solution able to obtain a 22-mm balloon diameter at full inflation using a measuring ring. The balloon is then totally deflated and the PHV crimped over it. Before use, it is checked that the PHV/balloon assembly slides smoothly inside the 24-Fr size measuring gauge.

From the left femoral artery, A 7-Fr Sones (B type) catheter is advanced over the stiff 360-cm long 0.035-inch guidewire until its distal tip is positioned about 2 cm above the aortic valve (Figure 43-3E). This catheter will be later used for accurate PHV positioning.

The 14-Fr introducer is removed from the right femoral vein and replaced by a 24-Fr introducer (Cook, Denmark). Additional local anesthesia is administered before sheath insertion and the puncture site is sufficiently enlarged with forceps.

The PHV/balloon assembly is then introduced inside the 24-Fr and advanced over the guidewire, successively across the interatrial septum, the left atrium, the mitral valve, the left ventricle, and the native diseased aortic valve. Using the calcification of the native valve on fluoroscopy and the frozen selected frame of the supra-aortic angiogram as markers, the PHV is accurately

positioned at mid-part of the native valve (see Figure 43-3E). The Sones catheter, placed in contact with the delivery catheter tip, is helpful to obtain the ideal PHV positioning, to prevent any uncontrolled ejection of the device in the ascending aorta, and to push the device backward if necessary. The balloon can then be maximally inflated for PHV delivery (Figure 43-3F) and immediately deflated and removed from the valve. A brief period of rapid cardiac pacing (220/min) is undertaken during valve deployment, starting just prior to balloon inflation and discontinued at maximal inflation.

Hemodynamic/Angiographic Controls Post-Percutaneous Heart Valve Implantation

After withdrawal of the delivery balloon catheter and before removing the long guidewire from the PHV, a 6-Fr pigtail catheter is advanced over it to the mid-left ventricle from the femoral vein. The long guidewire can then be safely withdrawn by traction from the femoral vein, with no risk of mechanical injury to the mitral valve.

Using the pigtail catheter in the left ventricle and one catheter in the ascending aorta (pigtail or Sones catheters), the trans-PHV systolic pressure gradient is measured (Figure 43-4). A supra-aortic angiogram is then performed to assess any aortic regurgitation and visualize the coronary ostia (see Figure 43-4). A selective coronary arteriography can be performed if the coronary ostia are not clearly visible (Figure 43-5).

All the catheters are removed. The arterial entry sites are closed with puncture closing devices (Angio-Seal, St Jude Medical,

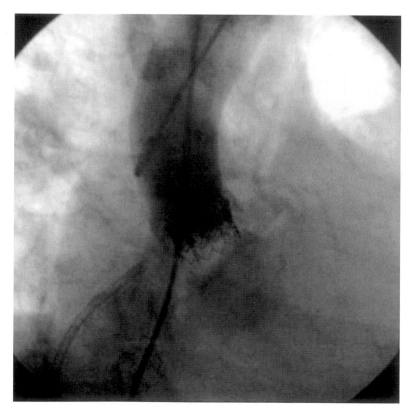

A

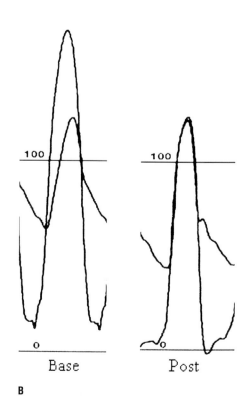

B

FIGURE 43-4. Assessment of the post-percutaneous heart valve implantation results by supra-aortic angiogram (**A**) and simultaneous aortic and ventricular pressures recording (**B**), showing no aortic regurgitation, and no residual gradient.

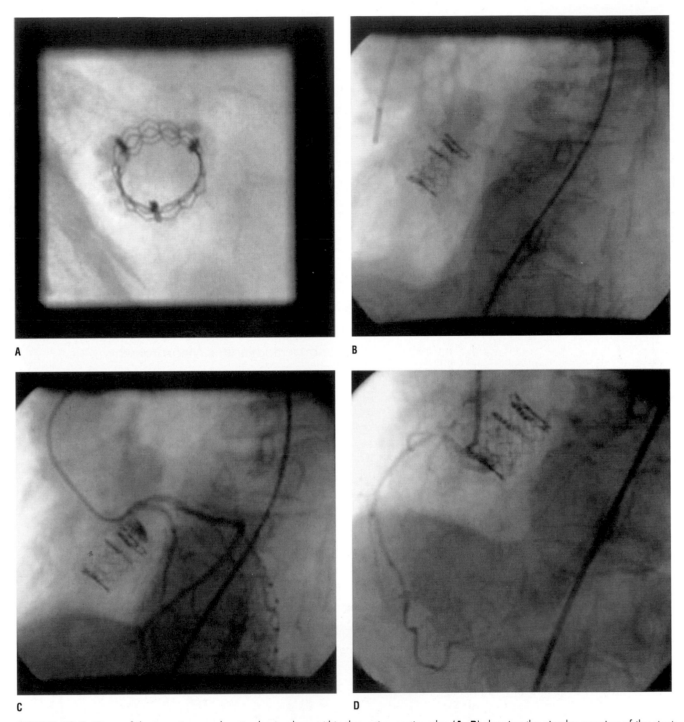

A

B

C

D

FIGURE 43-5. Views of the percutaneous heart valve in place within the native aortic valve (**A**, **B**) showing the circular opening of the stent frame in spite of severe valvular calcifications. Selective coronary arteriography confirming the patency of the left (**C**) and right (**D**) coronary arteries.

Belgium). The venous entry sites are closed by pneumatic or manual compression.

Advantages and Limitations of the Antegrade Transseptal Approach

The antegrade approach offers several advantages: (1) the large 24-Fr introducer can be introduced in all cases in the femoral vein and removed without surgery; (2) the risk of arterial complication is low, similar to the one associated with regular left-side catheterization in elderly patients with often diseased femoroiliac arteries; and (3) the

PHV crosses the native aortic valve through the less diseased surface of the aortic leaflets, in a direction coincident with blood flow.

The limitations are: (1) the need for transseptal catheterization, which carries its own potential risks; (2) the need for transatrial septum dilation with a 10-mm balloon; and (3) the risk of transient collapse during the procedure due to the traction exerted by the stiff guidewire on the mitral valve with subsequent massive mitral regurgitation. In this regard, a constant attention to the position of the guidewire in the left ventricle (to maintain a large loop) and to the blood pressure is required at each step of the procedure (Figure 43-6).

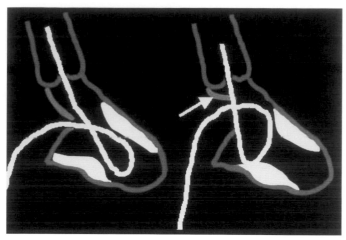

FIGURE 43-6. The incidental loss of the large guidewire loop into the left ventricle (*left*) can lead to acute mitral regurgitation by traction (*arrow*) of the mitral valve leaflet (*right*).

【 】 RETROGRADE APPROACH

In the course of our experience, the retrograde approach appeared a possible alternative to the antegrade route, with the potential advantage of being simpler and faster. The retrograde approach should be limited to patients with no significant tortuousities and atheroma of the femoral and iliac vessels, with femoral artery internal diameter greater than 7 mm, on angiography or scanner assessment, and with mild or at the most moderate aortic valve calcification. The potential limitations are the risks of femoral artery occlusion, rupture of femoroiliac vessels, atheromatous plaque dislodgment with distal embolization, and hemorrhagic complication at the arterial entry site. Because a large 24-Fr introducer is needed, preclosure of the femoral puncture site is performed at the beginning of the procedure using two 10-Fr Perclose devices.

Balloon Predilation of the Aortic Valve

The technique used for predilating the aortic valve is strictly similar to the one described for BAV, using a 23-mm Z-Med II balloon catheter, inserted into the selected most suitable femoral artery, through a 14-Fr introducer, over a 270-mm stiff guidewire. One or two balloon inflations are generally performed under rapid cardiac pacing.

Percutaneous Insertion of the 24-French Sheath

After removal of the balloon catheter, leaving the stiff guidewire in place in the left ventricle, the 14-Fr sheath is removed while hemostasis is obtained with manual compression. After additional local anesthesia has been administered, the femoroiliac axis is carefully predilated using three polyethylene dilators (18-, 20-, and 24-Fr), sequentially and cautiously advanced inside the vessels under fluoroscopic control. Thereafter, the 24-Fr sheath is introduced and slowly advanced over the wire.

Percutaneous Heart Valve Implantation and Hemodynamic Measurements

After the sheath's dilator has been removed, the PHV/balloon assembly is introduced inside the 24-Fr sheath, advanced over the guidewire, pushed across the aortic valve, and positioned as previously described. Rapid cardiac pacing and valve delivery are then performed (Figure 43-7). After PHV delivery, the deflated balloon is rapidly withdrawn from the PHV. Before withdrawing the wire from the left ventricle, a pigtail catheter can be advanced over it and used to measure the trans-PHV gradient, using the sidearm of the sheath to measure the aortic pressure (see Figure 43-7). As in the antegrade technique, a supra-aortic angiogram (see Figure 43-7), a coronary arteriography, and an assessment of the aortic valve area are obtained before removal of all catheters. The femoral artery entry site is closed using the predelivered percutaneous sutures or

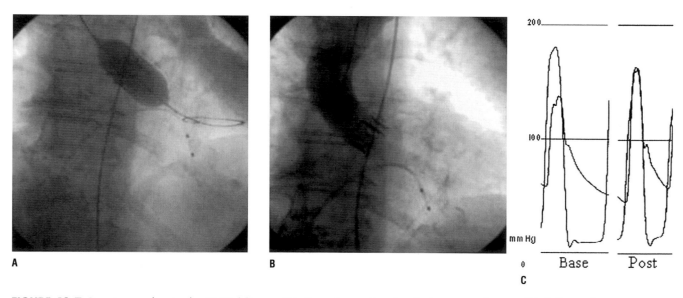

FIGURE 43-7. Percutaneous heart valve (PHV) delivery within the native aortic valve via the retrograde route (**A**). Balloon inflation is performed under rapid cardiac pacing. Supra-aortic angiogram post-PHV implantation showing no regurgitation and patent coronary arteries (**B**). No residual trans-PHV pressure gradient is observed after implantation (**C**).

a surgical repair in case of failure, preferentially in a sterile operative room. A pneumatic device or hand pressure is applied on the other vascular entry sites.

Advantages and Limitations of the Retrograde Approach

The main advantage of the retrograde approach is its technical ease for investigators used to the similar technique of retrograde BAV. However, this advantage is counterbalanced by the limitation of percutaneous femoral artery catheterization with the large 24-Fr size introducer, in a population of elderly patients with often fragile, small size, tortuous and diseased femoroiliac arteries. If the sheath introduction is feasible in selected patients, its removal is more challenging. The entry site closure with the preinserted eight sutures of two 10-Fr Perclose deserves a significant learning curve. Surgical repair of the artery carries the risk of local infection when performed in a less sterile environment such as the cardiac catheterization laboratory. Finally, failing to cross the calcific native valve retrogradely with the PHV/balloon assembly remains to date the main limitation to the retrograde approach. This can occur when the stiff guidewire cannot be dislodged from a severely calcific valvular commissure.

〖 〗 CLINICAL AND ECHOCARDIOGRAPHIC FOLLOW-UP AFTER PERCUTANEOUS HEART VALVE IMPLANTATION

The patients are closely monitored during follow-up, with clinical assessment and TTE, TEE, and Doppler examinations at day 1. TTE and Doppler are repeated at day 7 and every month thereafter. Postprocedural treatment includes aspirin (160 mg) and clopidogrel (75 mg) daily. Subcutaneous low-molecular-weight heparin is administered during the hospitalization stay. Oral anticoagulants are given only in patients with chronic atrial fibrillation and started two days before discharge.

〖 〗 CLINICAL EXPERIENCE

In our institution, PHV implantation has been attempted to date on a compassionate basis in 18 patients, mean age 78 ± 10 years, with end-stage severe calcific aortic stenosis (mean gradient: 43 ± 12 mm Hg, mean valve area: 0.56 ± 0.06 cm^2). According to French regulations, the inclusion criteria were strictly restricted to patients with impending death. According to New York Heart Association functional class IV, surgery had been formally declined by two cardiac surgeons owing to hemodynamic instability and associated severe cardiac and/or extracardiac comorbidities. Mean Parsonnet's score was 52 ± 7 (42–66). The most frequent associated cardiac factors were major left ventricular dysfunction or cardiogenic shock, and severe coronary artery disease or recent myocardial infarction, whereas noncardiac factors were headed by evolving cancer, major pulmonary insufficiency, end-stage renal failure, and recent stroke. The goals were to assess the feasibility of PHV implantation, the risk of PHV dislodgement and of coronary occlusion, and the degree of valvular and hemodynamic/clinical improvement.

The detailed results obtained in this first series of patients will be later published and have been partially reported.[24] Briefly, PHV was attempted using the antegrade approach in 11 patients (one

failure) and the retrograde approach in 7 patients (three failures, with subsequent successful transseptal implantation in one case, in the same session). PHV was successfully and accurately implanted in 15 patients, with no impairment of the coronary ostia, no residual transvalvular gradient, and an increase in valve area to 1.70 ± 0.1 cm^2. Periprocedure major complications were one stroke (during aortic valve predilation), one pericardial tamponade (during pacing lead placement), and three deaths. Deaths occurred in two patients in cardiogenic shock (one during predilation of the aortic valve, one after immediate PHV migration in a patient with associated grade IV aortic regurgitation), and in one patient who developed intractable collapse after relief of a severe prolonged ischemia of the leg (crush syndrome) with no other cause found on autopsy. In four patients in whom the antegrade approach was used, a brief period of hemodynamic collapse occurred during the intracardiac maneuvers due to guidewire-induced mechanical acute mitral regurgitation. Postimplantation paravalvular aortic regurgitation was frequently noted (grade 3/4 in three patients, 2/4 in two patients), with no consequences on left ventricular and clinical improvement.

An immediate dramatic clinical improvement was observed in all patients after PHV implantation associated with lasting valvular (unchanged aortic valve area and transvalvular gradient) and left ventricular functions improvement. Left ventricular ejection fraction was increased at 8 days from 42 + 18% to 55 + 12%.

Ten noncardiac related deaths occurred during follow-up (between 1 and 5 months) due to the worsening of multiple life-threatening comorbidities, metabolic disorders, aggravation of the renal or pulmonary conditions, or complication of noncardiac surgery. No PHV dislodgement or deterioration of the valvular function were observed on TEE and TTE assessment. To date, the longest follow-up in a surviving patient is 8 months. In this 83-year-old woman, the PHV function remains unchanged and is associated with remarkable clinical improvement.

〖 〗 FUTURE OF THE PROCEDURE

This preliminary clinical experience in nonoperable patients with end-stage aortic stenosis confirmed the feasibility of PHV implantation, even in the worst clinical life-threatening circumstances. An orifice valve area of 1.7 cm^2 with minimal transvalvular gradient was consistently achieved and remained unchanged during follow-up; it was associated with dramatic relief of signs of heart failure. There were no impairments of the coronary ostia and no secondary PHV dislodgement. Some degree of paravalvular leak was frequently observed due to imperfect apposition of the stent frame within the asymmetric calcified native valvular structures. When severe, this might impair the long-term outcome and warrants further improvement in stent size and design.

In this subset of elderly patients with no surgical option, the superiority of PHV implantation over balloon aortic valvuloplasty on short-term results is already confirmed. In the near future, technical refinement and inclusion of less severely ill patients with less potentially fatal comorbidities should allow assessment of PHV function stability and long-term clinical benefit. This is required to determine the role of this promising new therapeutic approach in this growing population of patients not amenable to surgical valve replacement.

REFERENCES

1. Kvidal P, Bergström R, Hörte L-G, et al. Observed and relative survival after aortic valve replacement. *J Am Coll Cardiol.* 2000;35:747.

2. Culliford AT, Galloway AC, Colvin SB, et al. Aortic valve replacement for aortic stenosis in persons aged 80 years and over. *Am J Cardiol.* 1991;67:1256.

3. Lytle BW, Cosgrove DM, Taylor PC, et al. Primary isolated aortic valve replacement. Early and late results. *J Thorac Cardiovasc Surg.* 1989;97:675.

4. Morris JJ, Schaff HV, Mullany CJ, et al. Determinants of survival and recovery of left ventricular function after aortic replacement. *Ann Thorac Surg.* 1993;56:22.

5. Connolly HM, Oh JK, Schaff HV, et al. Severe aortic stenosis with low transvalvular gradient and severe left ventricular dysfunction. Results of aortic valve replacement in 52 patients. *Circulation.* 2000;101:1940.

6. Logeais Y, Langanay T, Roussin R, et al. Surgery for aortic stenosis in elderly patients. A study of surgical risk and predictive factors. *Circulation.* 1994;90:2891.

7. Sharony R, Grossi EA, Saunders PC, et al. Aortic valve replacement in patients with impaired ventricular function. *Ann Thorac Surg.* 2003;75:1808.

8. Iung B, Baron G, Butchart E, et al. A prospective survey of patients with valvular heart disease in Europe: The Euro Heart Survey on Valvular Heart Disease. *Eur Heart J.* 2003;24:1231.

9. Pereira JJ, Lauer MS, Bashir M, et al. Survival after aortic valve replacement for severe aortic stenosis with low transvalvular gradients and severe left ventricular dysfunction. *J Am Coll Cardiol.* 2002;39:1356.

10. Cribier A, Savin T, Saoudi N, et al. Percutaneous transluminal valvuloplasy of acquired aortic stenosis in elderly patients: an alternative to valve replacement? *Lancet.* 1986;1:63.

11. Safian RD, Berman AD, Diver DJ, et al. Balloon aortic valvuloplasty in 170 consecutive patients. *N Eng J Med.* 1988;319:125.

12. The NHLBI Participants. Percutaneous balloon aortic valvuloplasty. Acute and 30-day follow-up results in 674 patients from the NHLBI Balloon Valvuloplasty Registry. *Circulation.* 1991;84:2383.

13. ACC/AHA guidelines for the management of patients with valvular heart disease. A report from the American College of Cardiology/American Heart Association. Task Force on Practice Guidelines (Committee on Management of Patients with Valvular Disease). *J Am Coll Cardiol.* 1998;32:1486.

14. Otto CM, Mickel MS, Kennedy W, et al. Three-year outcome after balloon aortic valvuloplasty. Insights into prognosis of valvular aortic stenosis. *Circulation.* 1994;89:642.

15. Lieberman EB, Bashore TM, Hermiller JB, et al. Balloon aortic valvuloplasty in adults: failure of procedure to improve long term survival. *J Am Coll Cardiol.* 1995;26:1522.

16. Andersen HR, Knudsen LL, Hasemkam JM. Transluminal implantation of artificial heart valves: description of a new expandable aortic valve and initial results with implantation by catheter techniques in closed chest pigs. *Eur Heart J.* 1992;13:704.

17. Bonhoeffer P, Boudjemline Y, Saliba Z, et al. Transcatheter implantation of a bovine valve in pulmonary position: a lamb study. *Circulation.* 2000;102:813.

18. Boudjemline Y, Bonhoeffer P. Steps toward percutaneous aortic valve replacement. *Circulation.* 2000;13:704.

19. Boudjemline Y, Bonhoeffer P. Percutaneous implantation of a valve in the descending aorta in lambs. *Eur Heart J.* 2002;23:1045.1049.

20. Cribier A, Eltchaninoff H, Borenstein N, et al. Transcatheter implantation of balloon expandable prosthetic heart valves: early results in an animal model. *Circulation.* 2001;104(suppl 2):552.

21. Bonhoeffer P, Boudjemline Y, Saliba Z, et al. Percutaneous replacement of pulmonary valve in a right-ventricle to pulmonary-artery conduit with valve dysfunction. *Lancet.* 2000;356:1403.

22. Sachin K, Coats L, Taylor A, et al. Percutaneous pulmonary valve implantation in humans. Reasults in 59 consecutive patients. *Circulation.* 2005;112:1189.

23. Cribier A, Eltchaninoff H, Bash A, et al. Percutaneous transcatheter implantation of an aortic valve prosthesis for calcific aortic stenosis: first human description. *Circulation.* 2002;106:3006.

24. Cribier A, Eltchaninoff H, Tron C, et al. Early experience with percutaneous transcatheter implantation of heart valve prosthesis for the treatment of end-stage inoperable patients with calcific aortic stenosis. *J Am Coll Cardiol.* 2004;43:698.

25. Feldman T. Percutaneous suture closure for management of large French size arterial and venous puncture. *J Intervent Cardiol.* 2000;13:237.

26. Solomon LW, Fusman B, Jolly N, et al. Percutaneous suture closure for management of large French size in aortic valvuloplasty. *J Invasive Cardiol.* 2001;13:592.

27. Eltchaninoff H, Cribier A, Tron C, et al. Balloon aortic valvuloplasty in elderly patients at high risk for surgery, or inoperable. Immediate and mid-term results. *Eur Heart J.* 1995;16:1079.

28. Parsonnet V, Dean D, Bernstein AD. A method of uniform stratification of risk for evaluating the results of surgery in acquired adult heart disease. *Circulation.* 1989;79(suppl 1):3.

CHAPTER (44)

Balloon Pulmonary Valvuloplasty

Susan P. Tourner, MD, and Jeffrey A. Feinstein, MD

Isolated valvar pulmonic stenosis (PS) accounts for between 7% and 12% of all congenital heart defects.[1–4] Although the annulus size is most often normal, the valve is usually thickened and has limited excursion due to the fusion of two or more leaflets. Other congenital cardiac defects that may be associated with valvar PS include atrial and ventricular septal defects, tetralogy of Fallot, transposition of the great arteries, double-outlet right ventricle, and ventricular inversion.[5]

Patients with PS are usually asymptomatic, and the diagnosis is made when a murmur is noted on a routine physical examination. When present, symptoms occur most commonly with advancing age and are due to right ventricular hypertrophy, decreased ventricular compliance, and right-sided heart failure. They are manifested by exercise intolerance and dyspnea.

The First Natural History Study of Congenital Heart Defects followed patients evaluated between 1958 and 1969 with various forms of congenital heart disease, including PS. Most of the patients with an initial gradient of less than 50 mm Hg were managed medically, and surgical valvotomy was performed in those with a gradient greater than 80 mm Hg. Patients with a gradient of 50 to 79 mm Hg were managed both medically and surgically. The authors found that trivial or mild PS seldom progressed, whereas moderate or severe PS generally progressed and required/received treatment. The patients with the greatest increase in pressure gradients were younger (ie, younger than 11 years of age) and had more significant initial obstruction.[6]

In 1993, 15 years after the initial natural history study, a second natural history study revisited the original cohort and reported the long-term results of medical and surgical management. The probability of survival was similar to the general population, and the majority of patients, regardless of medical or surgical management, remained asymptomatic. The chance of a child with a transpulmonary valve gradient greater than 25 mm Hg needing intervention was less than 5% during childhood and adolescence and virtually 0% thereafter. Patients with an initial gradient of 25 to 49 mm Hg subsequently required valvotomy 20% of the time. The vast majority of patients with a gradient of 50 to 70 mm Hg underwent valvotomy.[7] It was believed that individuals with PS mild enough not to warrant intervention and those who had successful relief of moderate or severe PS could expect a normal life span.

Currently, the degree of obstruction is defined by echocardiographic measurements of the gradient across the valve, and mirror the natural history study categories: trivial, less than 25 mm Hg; mild, 25 to 49 mm Hg; moderate, 50 to 79 mm Hg; and severe or critical, greater than 80 mm Hg.[5,26] This gradient (or pressure drop) is calculated using the simplified Bernoulli equation ($P = 4 \times V^2$, where P is the peak instantaneous pressure gradient [mm Hg] and V is the peak flow velocity [meters per second] in the main pulmonary artery). Good correlation has been documented between echocardiographic and catheterization derived pressure gradients.[8]

In 1997, a multicenter database review evaluating PS based on echocardiographic measurements substantiated the conclusions from the natural history studies. In most patients with mild PS, the initial gradient was not significantly different in repeat measurements over a period of 1 month to 5 years.[1] Patients younger than 1 to 2 years of age, however, were the most likely to progress, with a 15% to 28% chance of evolving from mild to moderate or severe stenosis.[1,3,9] No patients older than 2 years of age with an initial gradient less then 50 mm Hg progressed to severe PS. Patients with an initial diagnosis of severe PS, regardless of age at initial diagnosis, did not have spontaneous regression of their obstruction. Rather, moderate to severe PS patients had progression of the disease with worsening stenosis and an increased pulmonary valve (PV) gradient.[9]

TREATMENT OPTIONS

Surgical correction of PS may be performed as either an open (ie, using cardiopulmonary bypass) or closed procedure. First performed in 1947, the closed procedure, however, was found to provide poor long-term relief of obstruction and led to the use of open procedures with direct visualization. The technique of inflow occlusion was introduced in 1950 and in some reports was documented to be successful, as safe as, and more cost-effective than cardiopulmonary bypass. In the recent surgical era, however, the morbidity and mortality associated with cardiopulmonary bypass has been reduced to a point where surgical valvotomy is now routinely performed using cardiopulmonary bypass.

The first successful transcatheter treatment of PS was reported by Semb when he relieved the obstruction by pulling a carbon dioxide-filled balloon from the pulmonary artery to the right ventricle.[11] Kan then described the current method using static balloon dilation,[12] which was modeled on the surgical techniques of inflow occlusion and manual dilation.[13] Since that initial report, the tools have changed dramatically but the technique and mechanism of success have remained the same: the obstruction is alleviated by tearing or rupturing the weakest part of the valve mechanism when the circumferential pressure produced by balloon inflation is applied. The weakest part is usually the fused commissure; however, the valve cusps may also be torn or the valve leaflet may be avulsed.

The balloon-to-annulus ratio (BAR) and valve morphology have been found to be predictors of success with balloon pulmonary valvuloplasty (BPV). The annulus size is determined by carefully calculating the valve hinge point diameter using echocardiographic dimensions and measurements during catheterization (Figure 44-1). A BAR greater than 1 is associated with an immediate and long-term decrease in peak systolic gradient across the PV as well as lower RV systolic pressures. In one study, the optimum BAR was found to be 1.25.[14] There were improved short-term as well as long-term results with respect to the peak systolic gradient and right ventricular (RT) systolic pressure. A BAR less than 1 is less effective and has a higher incidence of restenosis. A BAR of 0.98 ± 0.2 resulted in approximately 15% restenosis. Repeat valvuloplasty using a BAR of 1.19 ± 0.12 was shown to be successful.[15] BAR greater than 1.5 is related to increased complications, including damage to the RV outflow tract as well as the valve apparatus.[14–16] In this study, BARs greater than 1.25 were less effective in relief of obstruction in the immediate and long-term postcatheterization periods. It was theorized that the larger balloon size triggers greater infundibular spasm immediately following the procedure and this spasm prevents adequate valve opening in the long-term. Also, it was believed that larger balloons may cause valvar injury resulting in restenosis.

Thick, immobile valve leaflets with angiographic appearance of uneven thickening or nodules, valve ring hypoplasia, absence of doming, and no post-stenotic dilation define pulmonary valve dysplasia. PS in mildly dysplastic valves may be resolved using a larger BAR during repeat BPV. A severely dysplastic valve could not be ballooned successfully in one study.[15] However, a separate study used a larger BAR of 1.37 ± 0.22 with dysplastic valves and had a success rate similar to that of nondysplastic valves.[16] Discrepancies in the results reported after BPV of dysplastic valves may be attributed to varying degrees of valve dysplasia, interpretation of data in categorizing dysplasia, or concurrence of commissural fusion. According to the authors of the Valvuloplasty and Angioplasty of Congenital Anomalies (VACA) registry results, "The most practical solution is to define a dysplastic pulmonary valve as one that fails to respond to balloon dilation."[17]

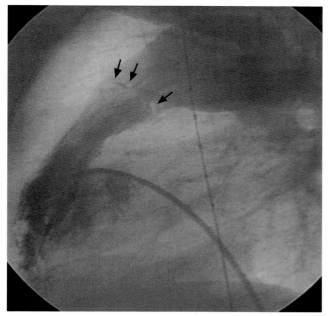

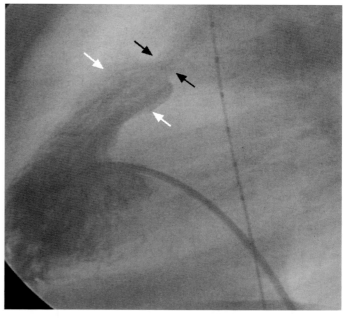

A

B

FIGURE 44-1. Angiograms in the lateral projection demonstrate the doming pulmonary valve leaflets (*black arrows*, [**A**]), pulmonary annulus (*white arrows*, [**B**]), and effective orifice (*black arrows*, [**B**]). A wire with radio-opaque markers is used as a reference grid.

In a study of 40 adult patients, the RV to pulmonary arterial (PA) peak systolic gradient immediately improved with BPV from 107 ± 29 mm Hg to 37 ± 25 mm Hg.[18] In several patients, a high residual gradient was ascribed to subvalvar obstruction or infundibular spasm. Relieving a more severe distal obstruction, caused by the narrow orifice of the PV, could uncover the more proximal obstruction. In a separate study, propranolol was administered intravenously with resolution of the systemic level pressures in the right ventricle. These patients were treated for several months with oral propranolol and did not require surgical resection of the infundibular obstruction.[16] Significant residual gradients immediately postcatheterization have also been attributed to infundibular hyper-reactivity that also subsides with time.[18,19]

Intermediate and long-term studies of adult patients with PS demonstrate continued success after BPV, and regression of residual PV gradient was seen at follow-up. In the aforementioned study with 40 adult patients, the peak RV-to-PA systolic pressure gradient decreased from 107 ± 29 mm Hg to 31 ± 13 mm Hg in the 24.5 ± 11.5 months following catheterization. Eight patients had significant residual mean gradients of 74.5 mm Hg that decreased to 33.5 mm Hg at long-term follow-up.[18] The results were comparable in a separate study of 24 adult patients. The mean pressure gradient decreased from 92 ± 36 mm Hg to 43 ± 19 mm Hg immediately following BPV, to 33 ± 10 mm Hg at the 3 month follow-up, and to 30 ± 7 mm Hg at 1 year. Seven patients had a significant residual gradient of greater than 50 mm Hg, with a mean of 70 mm Hg. After 3 to 12 months, the gradient abated to a mean gradient of 35 mm Hg.[19] The residual gradient in one patient was demonstrated to be due to subvalvar muscle hypertrophy that spontaneously receded in the ensuing months.

In a recent study comparing the long-term results of surgery versus balloon valvuloplasty for pulmonary valve stenosis in infants and children, both surgical and transcatheter techniques were successful in reducing the mean transvalvar gradient to less than 30 mm Hg.[2] Surgical correction reduced the mean pressure gradient from 64.8 ± 30.8 mm Hg to 17.4 ± 14.7 mm Hg immediately postoperatively and to 12.8 ± 9.8 mm Hg after an average of 10 years of follow-up. Although differences between the surgical and BPV groups were statistically significant, the BPV group demonstrated comparable clinical results, reducing the mean gradient from 66.2 ± 21.4 mm Hg to 23.8 ± 15.8 mm Hg immediately postcatheterization and 21.5 ± 15.9 mm Hg after an average follow-up of 5-1/2 years.

The incidence of restenosis was less in the surgical group (5.6% vs 14.1%), but the incidence of moderate pulmonary insufficiency was higher (44% vs 10%). In a meta-analysis-type review, the operative mortality was reported as 3% to 14%, whereas while that for BPV was 0%.[16] This review also corroborated the higher incidence of pulmonary insufficiency in the surgical group and higher occurrence of restenosis in the catheterization group.

Because BPV is far less invasive and significantly less costly when compared to surgical correction, and given the comparable relief of obstruction with less insufficiency, balloon valvuloplasty is thought to be the treatment of choice for valvar PS in patients of all ages.

PATIENT SELECTION, PROCEDURE INDICATION, AND TIMING

It is generally accepted that patients with moderate to severe degrees of stenosis (PV gradient > 50 mm Hg) or symptoms of angina, fatigue, dyspnea, or syncope should have BPV. The exception to this rule is patients with cardiac pathology who require additional surgical intervention. As described previously, patients with dysplastic pulmonary valves are less likely to respond to balloon dilation and the decision to try BPV is operator- and institution-dependent. However, it is most often attempted.

Controversy arises with management of mild stenosis (PV gradient 30–50 mm Hg). A 1988 review by Rao[9] verified that valvuloplasty improves the PV gradient in mild PS (38 ± 6 mm Hg, 20 ± 11 mm Hg, 24 ± 12 mm Hg, measured before, immediately after, and several months after valvuloplasty, respectively); however, there was only a modest reduction in RV pressures at follow-up several months later (with final RV pressures measuring 75 ± 18% of prevalvuloplasty pressures). Based on the second natural history study, only 20% of patients with mild stenosis required intervention, and most were asymptomatic, free of dysrhythmia, had no RVH on electrocardiogram, and had normal to mildly depressed RV function on echocardiography.[7] Given the benign natural course of mild PS, BPV is not warranted.

PS severe enough to impair RV output in the neonatal period requires immediate attention. Severe cyanosis and death may ensue without urgent relief of the RV outflow obstruction or initiation of prostaglandin. The RV pressures are suprasystemic, and there is often an atrial level right-to-left shunt leading to cyanosis. Because of the smaller patient size and critically ill state, it is technically more difficult, and the complication rate and failure rate for BPV are higher in neonatal critical PS compared to pediatric and adult experience.

After valvuloplasty, infundibular obstruction may necessitate continuation of prostaglandins for an additional time. Failure rates after BPV range from 6% to 45% in various institutions, although they tend toward the lower end of the spectrum. Some patients had improvement of gradient after repeat valvuloplasty, whereas others required surgical valvotomy after failure of BPV.[4,20]

TECHNIQUE

BPV can safely be performed using local anesthesia and either conscious sedation, deep sedation, or general anesthesia. The choice of technique to be used depends on the patient status, operator and anesthesiologist preferences, and the complexity of the procedure. This tends to vary from institution to institution. In adolescents and adults, BPV is most often performed using generous local anesthesia and conscious sedation and is an outpatient procedure.

Typically, the right, left, or both femoral veins are accessed percutaneously using the modified Seldinger technique to perform BPV. Although the femoral route is generally preferred, crossing the pulmonary valve from this approach in patients with a dilated right atrium, severe tricuspid regurgitation, and RV failure can be challenging.

The right internal jugular has also been safely and effectively accessed for use in BPV.[21] Large size (14 Fr) and multiple (side-by-side 9 Fr) sheaths have been introduced into the internal jugular vein without complications. However, balloon instability can be a problem because of the 180-degree course of the catheter. In addition, working from "above" (ie, the head of the table) may be more difficult, because most laboratories are designed for femoral approaches.

Although arterial access is not required for successful treatment of isolated PS, it may be indicated if left heart or coronary artery pathology are to be investigated during the same procedure. Also, some operators prefer to have invasive, real-time hemodynamic monitoring during interventional procedures.

A Berman angiographic catheter (Arrow International; Reading, PA) is used to perform a limited right-sided heart catheterization consisting of saturation measurements in the high superior vena cava, low superior vena cava, right atrium, and possibly the inferior vena cava and right ventricle as well as pressure measurement in the right atrium and ventricle. Angiography is then performed in the right ventricle. In single-plane catheterization laboratories, the straight lateral projection (90° LAO) is the preferred camera position (see Figure 44-1). When biplane angiography is available, the anterior-posterior camera is oriented in a straight antero-posterior or slightly cranially angulated fashion. A calibrated grid placed externally or markers embedded in a catheter (eg, Royal Flush II Angled Sizing Catheter, Cook, Bloomington, IN, or Accu-Vu Sizing Pigtail, AngioDynamics, Queensbury, NY) or wire (eg, Graduate Measuring Guide Wire, Cook, Bloomington, IN) are used as reference to account for image magnification when measuring the annulus size. The pulmonary annulus size can be calculated as follows:

$$\frac{\text{Measured pulmonary annulus}}{\text{Actual pulmonary annulus}} = \frac{\text{Measured reference size}}{\text{Actual reference size}}$$

which can be simplified to:

$$\text{Actual annulus} = \frac{\text{Measured annulus} \times \text{actual reference size}}{\text{Measured reference size}}$$

The Berman catheter is then removed and a diagnostic end-hole (eg, multipurpose) or wedge pressure catheter (Arrow International, Reading, PA) is advanced through the right side of the heart and across the PV and into the left pulmonary artery. Balloon flotation catheters reduce the risk of passing through the interchordal spaces of the tricuspid valve on the way to the pulmonary artery. Although the right pulmonary artery may be used, the catheter course to the left pulmonary artery makes the remainder of the procedure technically easier. A 0.035-inch diameter J-guidewire is inserted through the wedge catheter and directed to the lower lobe of the pulmonary artery (Figure 44-2). The catheter is removed, leaving the guidewire in place. Balloons are chosen to be 100% to 140% of the annulus size. Larger balloons are associated with an increased risk of RV outflow tract or pulmonary valve annulus damage, whereas balloons smaller than 100% of the annulus size are not as likely to achieve adequate gradient reduction.[16]

Balloons 20 to 30 mm in length are generally used for pediatric cases (20 mm for neonates) and 30 to 40 mm in length for adolescents and adults. Short balloons are difficult to keep positioned across the pulmonary valve during inflation, whereas long balloons may impinge on the tricuspid valve mechanism, possibly resulting in injury and subsequent tricuspid insufficiency.[16]

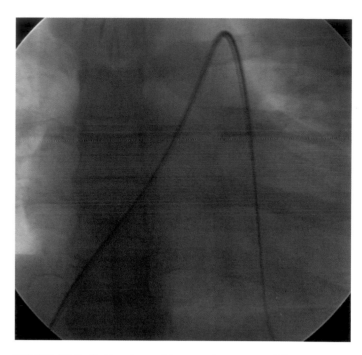

FIGURE 44-2. Stable wire position is vital to a successful intervention. Securing the exchange length wire in the distal left lower lobe pulmonary artery makes the remainder of the procedure technically easier.

The balloon is flushed and prepared in a standard fashion to remove as much air as possible from it and the catheter. The balloon port is then attached to a pressure gauge filled with diluted contrast (1 part contrast and 4 parts normal saline) to allow for rapid inflation and deflation. The balloon catheter is guided over the wire and the balloon is positioned across the pulmonary valve. Under fluoroscopy, the balloon is inflated by hand pressure until the waist (the indentation on the balloon caused by the valve) disappears (Figure 44-3).

The entire RV outflow is occluded when the balloon is inflated, resulting in cessation of pulmonary blood flow and consequently cardiac output. Transient systemic hypotension and bradycardia occur consistently during balloon inflation when the single balloon technique is used. A shorter period of balloon inflation, 5 seconds rather than 10 seconds, is effective in reducing systemic hypotension, yet does not compromise success. The inflation pressure should be noted. Typically, the waist disappears with a pressure of 6 atm or less, whereas higher pressures are associated with increased chance of rupture.[16]

The balloon is deflated and removed. Pressure measurements can be made without losing wire position using either a MultiTrack catheter (B. Braun Medical, Bethlehem, PA) or Royal Flush II Angled Sizing Catheter (Cook, Bloomington, IN) in combination with a Tuey-Borst adapter hooked up to a pressure transducer.

Repeat inflations with increased balloon diameters may be used until there is no significant valvar gradient (generally believed to be 25 mm Hg). Echocardiography can be used during the procedure to estimate the size of the PV annulus, the gradient across the valve, as well as the degree of PV insufficiency before and after valvuloplasty. The single balloon technique is limited by the size of balloons commercially available and kept in catheterization labo-

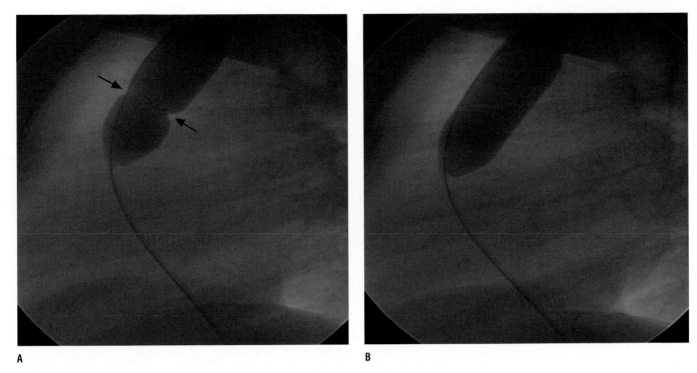

A   **B**

FIGURE 44-3. The balloon is inflated slowly until a waist (*arrows*) is seen (**A**) and it is centered across the valve; full inflation to 4-5 atm eliminates the waist (**B**).

ratory stock, and by the difficulty in maintaining a large balloon's position across the valve during inflation.

DOUBLE BALLOON TECHNIQUE

Double balloon valvotomy in adults is slightly more difficult technically, but some authors advocate the use of the double-balloon technique as the procedure of choice in adults. The use of the double balloon technique or Trefoil balloons[22,23] when available reduces the occurrence of systemic hypotension by providing a "venting area" to prevent complete occlusion of pulmonary flow.

The double balloon technique requires two venous access sites to accommodate the two balloon catheters. The sum of the diameters of the catheters should be 3 to 5 mm more than the PV annulus[24] or the diameters of the balloons may be calculated using a formula suggested by Rao et al.[25,26]

$$\text{Effective balloon diameter} = \frac{D1 + D2 + \Pi\ (D1/2 + D2/2)}{\Pi}$$

where D1 and D2 are the diameters of the balloons used and the effective balloon diameter is 1.0 to 1.4 times the annulus size, as is the case with the single balloon technique. It is useful to have effective dilating diameter tables available in the catheterization laboratory for reference during the procedure.[27]

The balloons can be inflated simultaneously or sequentially. If the sequential option is chosen, the first balloon is nearly completely inflated before the second is started. Once the second balloon has stabilized the position of both balloons across the valve, the inflation of the balloons is completed and the waist disappears (Figure 44-4). The incidence of hypotension and bradycardia is

significantly reduced using the double balloon technique because the obstruction to pulmonary blood flow is not complete. Inflation can be maintained for up to 8 to 10 seconds. The combined diameter of the two balloons, rather than the cross-sectional area, is the determining factor for success,[24] and there is no difference in results when compared to the single balloon technique.[16]

Postcatheterization Care

Postcatheterization care usually includes 4 to 6 hours of bed rest and observation. A chest x-ray is performed a few hours after the procedure to look for pleural effusions or mediastinal widening, and an echocardiogram may be performed as a new "baseline" if it was not done in the catheterization laboratory. Electrocardiograms may be required if significant arrhythmias were seen during the procedure. Most patients older than 1 year of age can be safely discharged the same day.

PROCEDURAL COMPLICATIONS

Although rare but serious complications have been cited, the most common complications are those associated with cardiac catheterization in general and include cardiac perforation, arrhythmias, and venous thrombosis. Additional complications reported with the internal jugular approach include pneumothorax, hydrothorax, superior sagittal sinus thrombosis, thoracic duct injury, vertebral artery pseudoaneurysm, and injury to the phrenic or vagus nerve.[21]

Mortality associated with BPV is exceptionally uncommon and most often occurs in neonates and young infants. Rupture of the PV annulus and subsequent tamponade have been reported in the BPV literature for critical PS. A neonate with critical PS died from

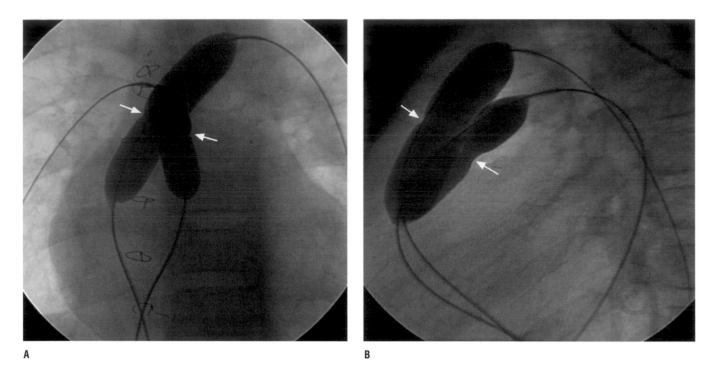

FIGURE 44-4. For the double balloon technique, two venous access sites are required. One wire is secured in the left pulmonary artery and the other in the right pulmonary artery. *Arrows* indicate the waists in the balloons in the anteroposterior (**A**) and lateral (**B**) projections prior to full inflation.

pericardial tamponade after rupture of the PV annulus and RV outflow tract.[28]

Perforation of the RV outflow tract occurs in 0.1% of patients undergoing BPV.[18] A report of a neonate with critical PS who died during BPV describes a significant narrowing at the infundibulum that was much smaller than the pulmonary artery annulus. Using a balloon catheter that cannot be accommodated by the infundibulum results in myocardial damage and increased risk of RV perforation.[29] As a result, when there is a discrepancy between the size of the annulus and infundibulum, the infundibular size should guide the selection of the initial balloon size.

During balloon valvotomy, especially when oversized balloons are used, incomplete tears may occur along the pulmonary artery in addition to those at the valve site. The pulmonary trunk is rich in elastic fibers but loses much of its elasticity as it enters the infundibular myocardium. The supravalvar annulus is devoid of elastic fibers. The absence of fibers makes this area susceptible to tearing and subsequent dissection during BPV. It is postulated that using oversized balloons to dilate dysplastic valves is effective because tearing of the pulmonary artery and annulus aids in additional relief of obstruction. In a case report of three pediatric patients undergoing BPV, cineangiography revealed a linear radiolucency in the wall adjacent to the anterior pulmonary valve leaflet. There was no extravasation of contrast, and the postvalvuloplasty clinical course was uncomplicated.[30]

Pulmonary insufficiency (PI) is less common and less severe with balloon valvuloplasty as compared to surgical valvotomy; nevertheless, the incidence of PI is reported to be as high as 79%.[16] PI is generally mild and is not of clinical significance. Normal exercise tolerance has been reported after balloon valvuloplasty in patients with mild PI.[31] However, exercise impairment in patients

with severe PI after surgical valvotomy has been documented.[32] Previous reports showed no evidence of RV volume overload secondary to PI on follow-up,[16] but more and more anecdotal cases of volume overload necessitating valve placement are being reported. For this reason, many interventionalists are being less aggressive at the time of initial valvuloplasty, choosing balloons 1 to 1.2 times the pulmonary annulus with the hope of reducing the likelihood and amount of PI, but realizing a second procedure may be required in the future.

Post-BPV tricuspid insufficiency is rare, with an estimated incidence of 0.2%.[18] A pediatric case report of acute onset of tricuspid regurgitation after BPV revealed that there was rupture of the tricuspid valve papillary muscle. The distal third of a long (60-mm) balloon catheter was positioned across the pulmonary valve. The proximal third was located at the apical portion of the anterior tricuspid papillary muscle. During inflation, pressures were transmitted to the papillary muscle and resulted in avulsion, as confirmed by surgery for a separate defect.[33]

Acute pulmonary edema following BPV is extremely rare, but has been reported.[34] In chronic, severe PS, the pulmonary vascular bed has long-standing poor perfusion and undergoes remodeling. The smooth muscles in the pulmonary arterioles are diminished, causing the cardiopulmonary vasculature to be more susceptible to leakage. The vascular bed cannot adapt to the acute increase in pulmonary blood flow after resolution of the stenosis, resulting in pulmonary edema. Resolution of the pulmonary edema with diuretics and ventilatory support is rapid.

An alternative mechanism for acute pulmonary edema is overload of the left ventricle. Preexisting impairment of the left side of the heart may be obscured by the limited pulmonary blood flow. After an acute increase in RV output, the left side of the heart may be unable to accommodate the increased flow. The ensuing elevation in left atrial and pulmonary venous pressures also results in acute pulmonary edema.[34]

FOLLOW-UP

Traditionally, repeat catheterization several months after BPV has been used to evaluate success of the procedure. Recent innovations, specifically echocardiography, now allow for less invasive follow-up, while maintaining reliability of the postcatheterization monitoring.

Echocardiogram with Doppler can be used in follow-up to evaluate RV outflow gradient, PV gradient, RV hypertrophy, PI, and tricuspid regurgitation (TR). Evidence suggests that Doppler can be used to accurately predict the PV gradient. There is excellent correlation between Doppler and catheterization data obtained within 24 hours of each other during follow-up at 6 months to 3 years. However, this correlation was not as strong in the immediate postcatheterization period, likely secondary to RV outflow tract hyperreactivity.[16]

Electrocardiographic testing can be useful in the intermediate term follow-up to evaluate residual PV gradient. Normal electrocardiograms were found in patients with PV gradients of less than 30 mm Hg. Electrocardiograms before and after BPV were compared. After successful valvuloplasty with PV gradients less than 30 mm Hg, the immediate postcatheterization electrocardiogram may not be changed, but the electrocardiograms obtained after 6 months were significantly improved. If RV hypertrophy was found on the electrocardiogram 6 months after BPV, there was likely residual gradient across the PV.

ANEURYSMAL POST-STENOTIC DILATION

Post-stenotic dilation of the pulmonary arteries is common in congenital pulmonary valvar stenosis, but progression to aneurysm, dissection, and rupture are rare.[35] Typical post-stenotic dilation diameter measures 3 to 3.5 cm and involves the main and left pulmonary arteries. Aneurysms are defined as greater than 5 cm in diameter; they occur more commonly with absent pulmonary valve leaflets and where left-to-right shunt is present. The natural history of pulmonary artery aneurysms is unknown because the condition is rare; however, rupture and dissection are possible, especially with coexisting cardiac disease, left-to-right shunt, or pulmonary hypertension. Percutaneous pulmonary balloon valvuloplasty is a conservative option when there is no evidence of pulmonary hypertension or left-to-right shunt. It serves to relieve the stenosis and prevent further post-stenotic dilation. Recommended modifications include administering beta blockade to minimize infundibular hyper-reactivity, using a smaller initial BAR of 1 and progressive dilation with larger balloon diameter, and using a shorter balloon to minimize risk of injury to the main pulmonary artery.

SUMMARY

The short, intermediate, and long-term results of balloon pulmonary valvuloplasty are excellent when compared with surgical valvotomy, and clinically significant complications are rare in the adult population. In addition, there are many benefits of transcatheter intervention: (1) the recovery period and cost are significantly more favorable, (2) there is less morbidity and mortality when compared with surgery and cardiopulmonary bypass, and (3) there is no exposure to blood products and no surgical scars. Lastly, BPV reduces the average length of stay from 3 to 5 days to 24 hours or less.

Surgical valvotomy should be reserved for patients with dysplastic valves who have failed transcatheter intervention or patients requiring cardiopulmonary bypass for concomitant lesions. Balloon pulmonary valvuloplasty is a safe and effective method for treating moderate to severe valvar pulmonary stenosis in the adolescent and adult population and should be regarded as the treatment of choice.

REFERENCES

1. Rowland DG, et al. Natural course of isolated pulmonary valve stenosis in infants and children utilizing Doppler echocardiography. *Am J Cardiol.* 1997;79:344.
2. Peterson C, et al. Comparative long-term results of surgery versus balloon valvuloplasty for pulmonary valve stenosis in infants and children. *Ann Thorac Surg.* 2003;76:1078, 1082.
3. Anand R, Mehta AV. Natural history of asymptomatic valvar pulmonary stenosis diagnosed in infancy. *Clin Cardiol.* 1997;20:377.
4. Wang JK, et al. Balloon dilatation for critical pulmonary stenosis. *Int J Cardiol.* 1999;69:27.
5. Rao PS. Transcatheter treatment of pulmonary outflow tract obstruction: a review. *Prog Cardiovasc Dis.* 1992;35:119.
6. Nugent EW, et al. Clinical course in pulmonary stenosis. *Circulation.* 1977;56(suppl 1):38.
7. Hayes CJ, et al. Second natural history study of congenital heart defects. Results of treatment of patients with pulmonary valvar stenosis. *Circulation.* 1993;87(suppl 2):28.
8. Lima CO, et al. Noninvasive prediction of transvalvular pressure gradient in patients with pulmonary stenosis by quantitative two-dimensional echocardiographic Doppler studies. *Circulation.* 1983;67:866.
9. Rao PS. Indications for balloon pulmonary valvuloplasty. *Am Heart J.* 1988;116:1661.
10. Shumacker H. *The Evolution of Cardiac Surgery.* Bloomington, IN: Indiana University Press; 1992.
11. Semb BK, et al. "Balloon valvulotomy" of congenital pulmonary valve stenosis with tricuspid valve insufficiency. *Cardiovasc Radiol.* 1979;2:239.
12. Kan JS, et al. Percutaneous balloon valvuloplasty: a new method for treating congenital pulmonary-valve stenosis. *N Engl J Med.* 1982;307:540.
13. Blalock A, Kieffer RF Jr. Valvulotomy for the relief of congenital valvular pulmonic stenosis with intact ventricular septum; report of 19 operations by the Brock method. *Ann Surg.* 1950;132:496.
14. Narang R, et al. Effect of the balloon-annulus ratio on the intermediate and follow-up results of pulmonary balloon valvuloplasty. *Cardiology.* 1997;88:271.
15. Ali Khan MA, et al. Results of repeat percutaneous balloon valvuloplasty for pulmonary valvar restenosis. *Am Heart J.* 1990;120:878.
16. Rao PS. Balloon pulmonary valvuloplasty: a review. *Clin Cardiol.* 1989;12:55.
17. McCrindle BW. Independent predictors of long-term results after balloon pulmonary valvuloplasty. Valvuloplasty and Angioplasty of Congenital Anomalies (VACA) Registry Investigators. *Circulation.* 1994;89:1751.
18. Kaul UA, et al. Long-term results after balloon pulmonary valvuloplasty in adults. *Am Heart J.* 1993;126:1152.
19. Sievert H, et al. Long-term results of percutaneous pulmonary valvuloplasty in adults. *Eur Heart J.* 1989;10:712.
20. Thanopoulos B, Triposkiadis F, Tsaousis GS. Single-stage balloon valvuloplasty for critical pulmonary valve stenosis in the neonate. *Cathet Cardiovasc Diagn.* 1997;40:322.
21. Joseph G, et al. Right internal jugular vein approach as an alternative in balloon pulmonary valvuloplasty. *Cathet Cardiovasc Interv.* 1999;46:425.
22. Meier B, et al. Trefoil balloon for percutaneous valvuloplasty. *Cathet Cardiovasc Diagn.* 1986;12:277.

23. Thanopoulos BD, et al. Valvuloplasty with large trefoil balloons for the treatment of congenital pulmonary stenosis. *Acta Paediatr Scand.* 1989;78:742.

24. Al Kasab S, Ribeiro P, Al Zaibag M. Use of a double balloon technique for percutaneous balloon pulmonary valvotomy in adults. *Br Heart J.* 1987;58:136.

25. Rao PS. Influence of balloon size on short-term and long-term results of balloon pulmonary valvuloplasty. *Tex Heart Inst J.* 1987;14:57.

26. Rao PS. How big a balloon and how many balloons for pulmonary valvuloplasty? *Am Heart J.* 1988;116:577.

27. Yeager SB, Flanagan MF, Keane JF. Catheter intervention: balloon valvotomy. In: Lock JE, Keane JF, Perry SB, eds. *Diagnostic and Interventional Catheterization in Congenital Heart Disease.* Boston, MA: Kluwer Academic Publishers; 2000:154.

28. Schroeder VA, et al. Surgical emergencies during pediatric interventional catheterization. *J Pediatr.* 2002;140:570.

29. Gildein HP, et al. Treatment of critical pulmonary valve stenosis by balloon dilatation in the neonate. *Am Heart J.* 1996;131:1007.

30. Burrows PE, et al. Pulmonary artery tears following balloon valvotomy for pulmonary stenosis. *Cardiovasc Intervent Radiol.* 1989;12:38.

31. O'Connor BK, et al. Intermediate-term outcome after pulmonary balloon valvuloplasty: comparison with a matched surgical control group. *J Am Coll Cardiol.* 1992;20:169.

32. Yetman AT, et al. Comparison of exercise performance in patients after pulmonary valvulotomy for pulmonary stenosis and tetralogy of Fallot. *Am J Cardiol.* 2002;90:1412.

33. Attia I, et al. Rupture of tricuspid valve papillary muscle during balloon pulmonary valvuloplasty. *Am Heart J.* 1987;114:1233.

34. Cheng TO. Acute pulmonary edema complicating percutaneous balloon valvuloplasty for pulmonic stenosis. *J Cardiothorac Vasc Anesth.* 2002;16:391.

35. Fernandes V, et al. Successful balloon valvuloplasty in an adult patient with severe pulmonic stenosis and aneurysmal poststenotic dilatation. *Cathet Cardiovasc Intervent.* 2002;55:376.

CHAPTER (45)

Percutaneous Closure of Atrial Septal Defect and Patent Foramen Ovale

David P. Lee, MD, and Stanton B. Perry, MD

Over the course of the past decade, there has been a burgeoning interest in closing septal defects percutaneously. To date, there are now percutaneous closure devices available for the intended closure of ostium secundum atrial septal defects (ASDs) as well as patent foramen ovale (PFO). With the increased interest in these percutaneous procedures, the interventional cardiologist now has an additional set of procedures to master outside the coronary vasculature. This chapter will review the current techniques and devices employed during these specialized procedures.

ATRIAL SEPTAL DEFECT

ASDs are the most common adult congenital cardiac abnormality,[1] occurring in about 8% of the adult congenital heart disease population with a slight female predominance (3:2). They are classified by the anatomic location as well as their associations with other local anatomic structures. ASDs can be classified as: (1) ostium primum, in which the defect is located inferiorly and is often associated with tricuspid and or mitral valve abnormalities as well as a ventricular septal defect; (2) ostium secundum, in which the defect is related to persistent separation at the midatrial level due to failed fusion during cardiac development; and (3) sinus venosus, in which there is partial anomalous pulmonary venous return due to the septal defect extending superiorly along the atrial septum to include the incoming pulmonary veins. Of these three types of ASDs, transcatheter repair is tenable at this time only with the secundum-type defect.

In general, the threshold for closure is dictated by hemodynamic findings. Historical data, largely from the surgical literature, suggest that ASD closure is warranted in patients with a Qp/Qs of 1.5 or greater. Closure may also be warranted if pulmonary hypertension or early echocardiographic evidence of right ventricular enlargement and/or failure is present. A paradoxical embolus may also be considered to be an indication for closure. Clinically, patients often present with dyspnea on exertion or evidence of right-sided heart failure. It is generally rare to see a cryptogenic neurologic event with an ASD, given that most of the flow early in the process involves left-to-right shunting; as the right heart fails, however, the shunting becomes mixed and even reversed in late-stage disease, with predominantly right-to-left shunting. An electrocardiogram showing incomplete right bundle branch block is common is patients with secundum ASD.

A transesophageal echocardiogram (TEE) is critical in defining the anatomy of the ASD and is useful in determining the potential success of percutaneous closure of a secundum-type defect. An adequate (≥ 1 mm) anterosuperior aortic rim is important to allow adequate anchoring of the ASD closure device. In addition, the size of the defect and an estimate of the shunt fraction may be helpful in determining the eligibility for closure as well as appropriate balloon sizing. Right ventricular enlargement of at least a mild degree is usually observed. Other important features revolve around the definition of the type of defect and the relationship of the mitral valve annulus to the ASD. An investigation of the left atrial appendage to rule out thrombus and a bicaval view to assess inflow into the atrium is important to exclude a sinus venosus-type defect.

【 】 PERCUTANEOUS ATRIAL SEPTAL DEFECT CLOSURE

Percutaneous closure of a secundum ASD has been performed for many years in both pediatric and adult populations. The first attempt at transcatheter ASD closure was in 1974 by King and Mills.[1] The techniques have been refined over time, and there are now a number of commercially available devices outside the United States. Within the United States, one device, the Amplatzer Septal Occluder (AGA Medical, Golden Valley, MN) has received approval from the Food and Drug Administration for secundum ASD closures (Figure 45-1).

The Amplatzer Septal Occluder (ASO) consists of two attached circular disks—a larger left atrial disk separated by a small space on top of a smaller right atrial disk. These disks are made of polyester fabric encasing a wire mesh made of a nitinol. The device is screwed onto a delivery cable and delivered via a long sheath. In the typical ASO, the left atrial disk is 6 to 8 mm larger than the right atrial disk and a central space ("waist") consisting of a small mesh tube, which also promotes self-centering. The device is sized per the right atrial disk.

Screening for potential percutaneous closure candidates consists of the tests noted above to diagnose and confirm a secundum-type ASD. In addition, tests to exclude concurrent infection, pregnancy, and a hypercoagulable state should be performed prior to closure. It is important to also administer intravenous (IV) antibiotics at the time of closure to prevent any potential infectious risk. This is performed usually just prior to obtaining venous access. The procedure in the catheterization laboratory is relatively straightforward and has recently been reviewed.[2]

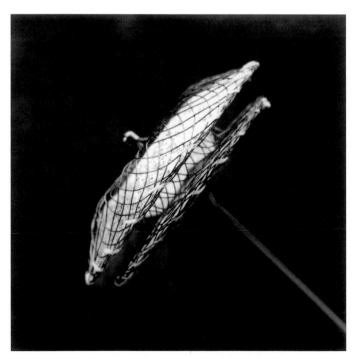

FIGURE 45-1. The Amplatzer Septal Occluder (AGA Medical, Golden Valley, MN) is composed of two nitinol disks covered by polyester. It is approved for use in the United States for appropriate secundum-type atrial septal defects.

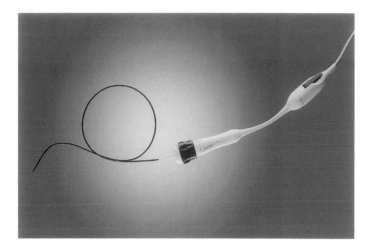

FIGURE 45-2. AcuNav Intracardiac echocardiographic catheter (Siemens Medical Solutions, Malvern, PA). It images at 10 MHz and is 10-Fr sheath compatible.

Two venous sheaths are placed in the right femoral vein. Unfractionated heparin (100 U/kg) is then administered intravenously with an aim to keep an activated clotting time of greater than 200 seconds. To confirm the hemodynamic significance of the ASD, a saturation run with pressure measurements should be performed prior to the planned closure. Once the shunting has been confirmed, one of the sheaths can be replaced with a 10-Fr sheath to allow the passage of a 10 MHz intracardiac echocardiography (ICE) probe (AcuNav; Siemens Medical Solutions, Malvern, PA; Figure 45-2), which allows direct visualization of the atrial chambers and atrioventricular valves during closure. An alternative is to use TEE during the procedure, but recent studies have suggested a greater benefit for using ICE over TEE.[3,4] In addition, there is also another commercially available ICE catheter (ICE; Boston Scientific, Fremont, CA), but this device differs from the AcuNav in several ways: (1) most significantly, it does not harbor the capability for Doppler imaging; (2) it cannot be easily manipulated along different planar views; (3) it images at 9 MHz; and (4) it is 9 Fr-compatible.

Once the probe has been guided into the right atrium at the level of the ASD, a 6-Fr multipurpose diagnostic coronary catheter is directed over a 260 cm J-tipped (Rosen) wire to the right atrium. The catheter is then manipulated toward the ASD, and the wire is guided across the ASD into the left atrium and anchored within the pulmonary veins, preferably the left superior pulmonary vein. Once the wire is anchored, the catheter is removed. Using the ICE and previous TEE data as a guide, a 24- or 34-mm sizing balloon (AGA Medical, Golden Valley, MN) can be guided across the ASD and its position confirmed by ICE and/or fluoroscopy. Typically, the stretched diameter of the ASD is 30% larger than the unstretched diameter. The sizing balloon is then inflated with a 1:4 mixture of contrast and saline and a balloon "waist" appears fluoroscopically as well as on the ICE. This "waist" is then measured as the stretched diameter of the ASD using predefined markers on the balloon catheter for calibration (Figure 45-3). Once the ASD size is confirmed, the balloon is then removed.

Typically, the chosen ASD closure device size with the ASO is 1 to 4 mm larger than the stretched diameter. Because of the variety

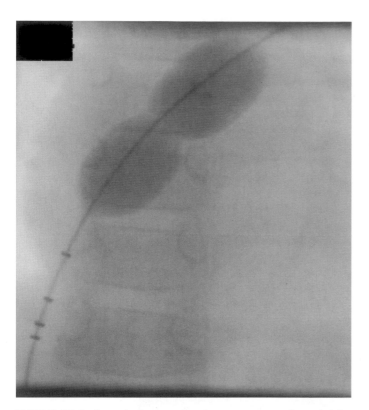

FIGURE 45-3. Sizing balloon used in the measurement of septal defect size. In this photograph, the sizing balloon has been inflated to reveal the atrial septal defect size when stretched, allowing appropriate sizing for a septal occluder device. Markers on the sizing balloon allow accurate estimation of defect size.

of ASD closure device sizes (4–40 mm), the delivery sheath size may vary. For example, for a 22-mm ASO, an 9-Fr delivery sheath is adequate, whereas a 36-mm ASO requires at least a 12-Fr delivery sheath. Once the proper delivery sheath size is chosen, the femoral sheath is exchanged for a long (80 cm) curved delivery sheath. The introducer should be placed into the pulmonary vein and then removed along with the wire once the sheath has been anchored within the pulmonary vein. Great care should be taken to expunge any air from the sheath by carefully removing fluid and potential air from the sheath and then gently flushing with saline.

The ASO is screwed in a clockwise fashion until tight onto the delivery cable. A 180-degree counterclockwise turn is then used to slightly loosen the device and prevent locking of the ASO onto the delivery cable. A small introducer sheath included in the packaging should then be used to expunge any air from the delivery cable and device while pulling back in a pool of saline. This short sheath with the ASO on the distal end of the delivery cable is then connected onto the proximal end of the delivery sheath and pushed into the delivery sheath with care taken to avoid kinking of the cable or sheath. It is common to experience some mild initial resistance with the introduction of the ASO into the delivery sheath.

Fluoroscopy can then be used to visualize the delivery cable and ASO within the sheath as it approaches the tip of the delivery sheath. When the device is at the tip of the sheath, the entire system is then retracted back into the upper portion of the left atrium. When this is accomplished the sheath is gently retracted from the delivery cable and the left atrial disk should be deployed (Figure 45-4). Under ICE and fluoroscopic guidance, the left atrial

disk, delivery cable, and sheath are then retracted as a unit until the left atrial disk is flush against the left atrial side of the ASD. Once this is established, the sheath is then further retracted to allow deployment of the right atrial disk (Figure 45-5). The device should be well-seated across the atrium with both respective atrial disks fully expanded on either side of the septum. A gentle to-and-fro motion ("Minnesota wiggle"[5]) can be used to gauge the positional stability of the ASO while using ICE or TEE. This can be confirmed with ICE and Doppler imaging of the ASD on either side of the device. Contrast or bubbles may be injected through the delivery sheath to image the right atrium and detect contrast across the ASD with the device, still held in place by the delivery cable, in the defect. If these methods detect minimal or no leakage, the device is then detached from the delivery cable by attaching the rotator knob on the back end of the delivery cable and using a counterclockwise rotation of the knob. It is imperative to maintain a very slight and gentle constant traction on the device as the knob is rotated until the device is released. The device may "jump" or slightly reorient/recenter itself as the device is released (Figure 45-6).

Prior to release, if positioning is unsatisfactory, the sheath can be readvanced into the left or right atrium to recover the right and/or left atrial disk, and the deployment process can begin again. If the deployments remain unsatisfactory, some operators have advanced a second catheter to help better align the device as it is deployed by using a constant upward pressure on the device and/or sheath as it is deployed across the ASD.[6] This obviously requires another venous sheath to be placed. For larger ASDs, a novel technique[7] has recently been described in 14 patients using the sizing balloon inflated within the right atrium to help support large ASOs as they are deployed.

Once the device has been released, ICE should be used to scan along the atrium from the superior vena cava (SVC) to the inferior aortic border to confirm the positioning of the device as well as the elimination of the shunt itself by Doppler (Figure 45-7). In addition, a scan of the atrioventricular valves should be performed to exclude impingement on either of these structures. Alternatively, some operators inject bubbles through the now empty venous delivery sheath and image as the bubbles are in the right atrium to see if any bubbles are able to cross the ASD. Residual shunting through the device is not uncommon immediately after release. Significant residual shunting usually suggests device malposition of the device or a second defect. A second device can be used depending on the size and location of the defect. If there are significant bubbles or Doppler-detected flow across the ASD on either side of the device, a second device can be placed by recrossing the ASD with a multipurpose catheter and stiff J-wire and eventual deployment of a smaller second ASO without the use of a sizing balloon. Alternatively, some operators who have noted moderate persistent defects on one end of the device have used coronary catheters to "adjust" the positioning along the end of the device with a persistent residual shunt. Once the final result has been deemed to be satisfactory, the sheaths are removed.

In addition, clopidogrel is administered after device closure, with a loading dose of 600 mg in the laboratory, with plans for a maintenance dose of 75 mg qd for 3 to 6 months with concomitant aspirin. Ticlopidine may be used as an alternative for patients who are clopidogrel-sensitive.

The issue of thrombus formation and its significance is interesting and controversial. The devices are thought to acutely close

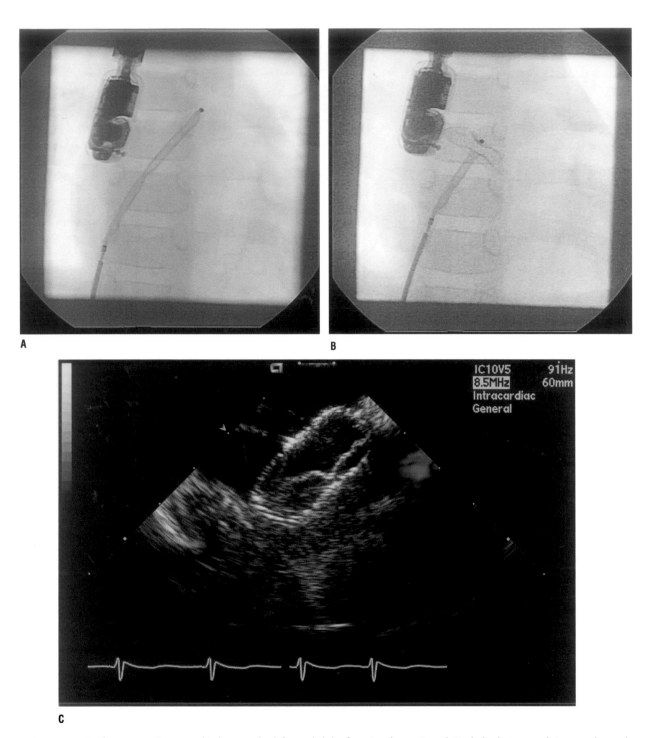

FIGURE 45-4. Fluoroscopy (*top panels*) showing the left atrial disk of an Amplatzer Septal Occluder being used. Intracardiac echocardiography (*bottom*) shows the left atrial disk used within the left atrium.

septal defects by mechanical obstruction of the defect as well as thrombosis with long-term closure secondary to endothelialization.

【 】 POSTPROCEDURAL CARE

In addition to the postprocedure aspirin and clopidogrel for 3 to 6 months, our standard of practice in the hospital has been to continue IV antibiotics (cefazolin 1 g IV q8h; for penicillin-sensitive patients, vancomycin 1 g IV q12h) through the course of the hospitalization postprocedure.

The patient is usually discharged on the following morning after a transthoracic echocardiogram (TTE) with contrast. This is done for two reasons: (1) to reconfirm proper device positioning (Figure 45-8); and (2) to establish the degree of shunting, if any, across the device. In addition, an anteroposterior and lateral chest x-ray is taken. The ultrasound imaging studies are repeated at 1 month, 6 months, 12 months, and then at yearly intervals. The use of contrast during the TTE follow-up studies is reserved for those patients with persistent residual shunts. Chest x-rays are performed at the first 6-month visit and at subsequent annual evaluations.

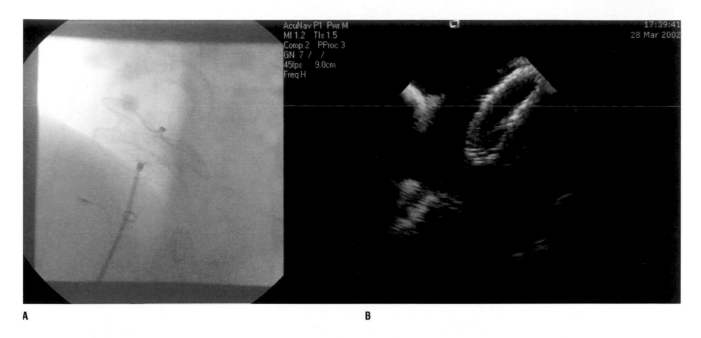

FIGURE 45-5. Deployment of the right atrial disk under fluoroscopy and intracardiac echocardiographic (ICE) guidance. The ICE imaging also shows the Doppler signal at the aortosuperior rim of the device.

The patient should allow at least 4 weeks to allow complete endothelialization of the device. In our program, no lifting of objects that weigh more than 20 pounds is recommended for the first month postprocedure. Gentle walking is allowed immediately postprocedure and until the patient returns for follow-up at 1 month. An important reminder involves the prevention of device infection: the patient should follow American College of Cardiology/American Heart Association (ACC/AHA) guidelines for bacterial endocarditis prophylaxis for 6 months postprocedure.

[ ] COMPLICATIONS

The delivery of a septal defect closure device has a particular set of complications of which every operator should be aware. Beyond the rare complication of vascular access issues, there are a number of unique potential complications related to these devices. These include transient bradyarrhythmias and tachyarrhythmias, ST-segment elevation, device embolization, device erosion, thrombosis and embolism, and pericardial effusion.

The incidence of bradyarrhythmias, such as complete heart block, is rare. In a recent review,[8] 162 patients underwent percutaneous ASD closure. Periprocedural atrioventricular (AV) block was noted in 3 patients (1.9%). During the postprocedure follow-up at 1 week, an additional 7 patients developed AV block. Four of these 10 patients had first-degree AV block. All had no symptoms or hemodynamic compromise. All patients with higher-degree AV block completely recovered within 6 months. Two patients had residual first-degree block at 12 and 33 months postprocedure. Interestingly, those patients with a larger defect and hence larger shunt fraction and ASO (>19 mm) had a much higher incidence of AV block. In a series from Italy,[9] the incidence of AV block was 1/417 (0.2%). In this patient, complete heart block developed, and the operators then removed the device with complete cessation of the AV block. One year later, the patient underwent an uneventful percutaneous ASD closure. In another study, 41 patients were studied for electrocardiographic abnormalities,[10] and 3 patients (7%) were found to have intermittent second-degree heart block or complete AV-dissociation postclosure.

Tachyarrhythmias, such as atrial tachycardia and atrial fibrillation, have also been reported. In a recent series from the Mayo Clinic[11] using ICE-directed ASD or PFO closure, the incidence of atrial tachyarrhythmia was 4.3% (4/94). Three of these patients had atrial fibrillation, whereas one had a supraventricular tachycardia. Two of these four cases resolved spontaneously, whereas the other two were cardioverted without incidence. There were no cases of ventricular arrhythmias. In another study,[10] 9 of 41 patients (22%) exhibited nonsustained supraventricular tachycardia; no patients had atrial fibrillation or other atrial tachycardias. Five of the 199 patients (2.5%) in Wang's study experienced supraventricular tachycardia, but all of these were terminated with administration of IV adenosine.[12]

ST-segment elevation is an interesting development peri- and post-ASD closure. This usually occurs in the inferior leads, and the mechanism postulated has been inadvertent air embolism during device deployment. It is usually transient and resolves spontaneously within 20 minutes. Clinically, the patient may complain of chest discomfort and nausea, but this usually subsides in a short period.

Device dislodgement and embolization is a known complication of ASD closure. This is an operator-driven error and can be the result of many possible errors, most commonly incomplete attachment to the delivery cable, sizing and device error, malpositioning, and premature device release. In an Italian series of ASD closure[9] with a variety of devices, 1 patient (0.2%) had device embolization. In a more generalized survey of ASO operators by Levi and Moore,[13] a 0.6% incidence of device embolization was noted. In general, larger devices are thought to be associated with a higher incidence of device embolization because of the inadequacy

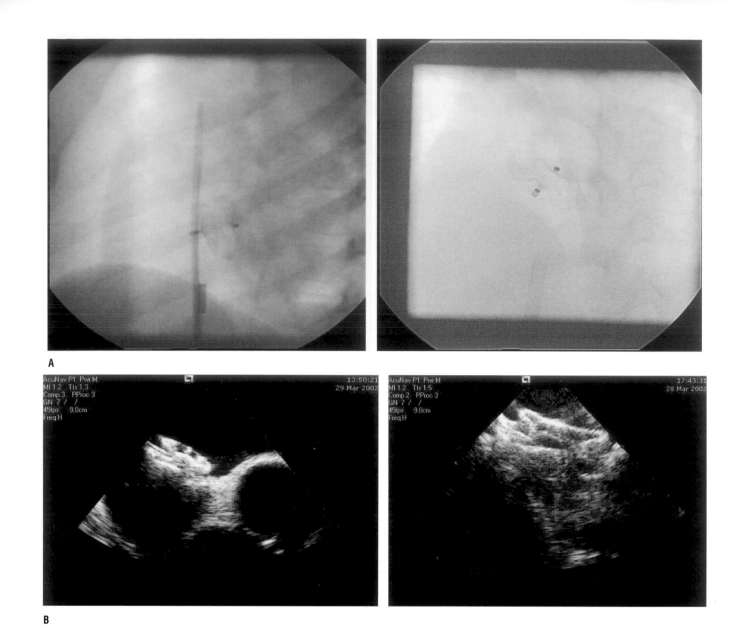

FIGURE 45-6. (A) Immediate result of device release (*left*) compared with the final result (*right*). Please note the orientation change of the Amplatzer Septal Occluder after it has settled into position. This is considered normal and can be further investigated with intracardiac echocardiography, seen in (**B**), which shows excellent device placement and apposition.

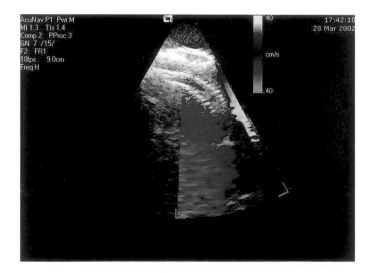

FIGURE 45-7. Intracardiac echocardiography: Doppler investigation of an Amplatzer Septal Occluder after deployment.

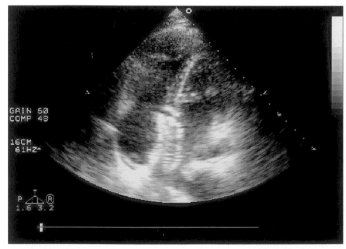

FIGURE 45-8. Transthoracic echocardiogram image of a large Amplatzer Septal Occluder 1 day after placement across a secundum defect.

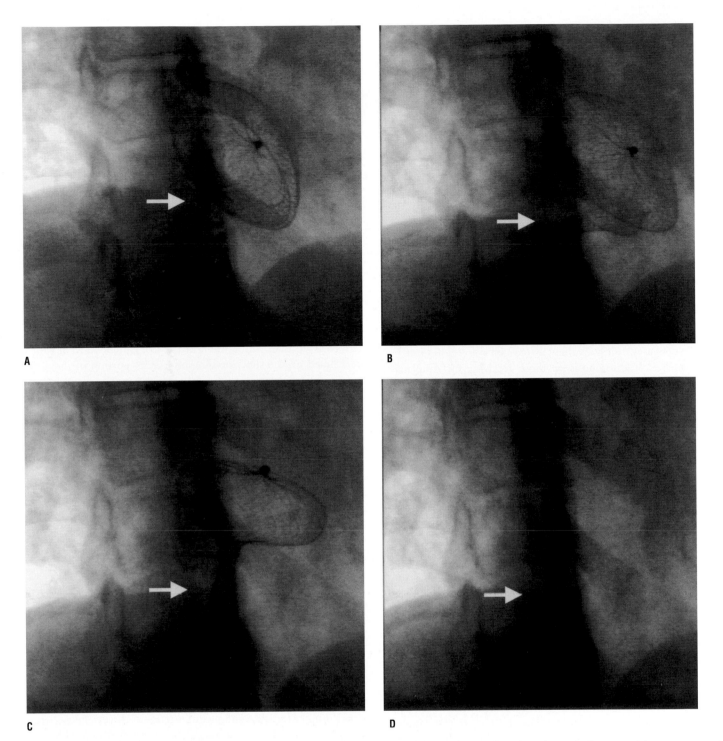

FIGURE 45-9. Retrieval of an Amplatzer Septal Occluder after embolization into the right atrium. The *arrow* shows the location of the snare around the screw-type interface between the original delivery catheter and device. The snare is used to grab (**A**) and retract the device back into the capture sheath. Note that the right atrial disk is first collapsed (**B**) and withdrawn into the sheath (**C**), followed by the left atrial disk. Eventually, the entire device is captured within the sheath (**D**) and removed.

of a rim to anchor the device in a large defect. Indeed, in several series,[9,12–14] larger (or undersized) devices were shown to be more prone to malpositioning and dislodgement/embolization. Device embolization was noted in 7/417 Italian patients (1.7%) and 1/191 (0.5%) in the Taiwanese experience.

Techniques to retrieve the ASO vary but all involve a gooseneck snare and the use of an oversized venous sheath. The review by Levi and Moore[13] in which they surveyed a number of expe-

rience ASO operators suggests that a stiffer sheath with a beveled tip may be advantageous when recapturing a dislodged ASO. The technique to retrieve a device involves snaring the right atrial disk screw and pulling the device back into a sheath (Figure 45-9). A bioptome generally cannot sufficiently "grab" a device by its right atrial screw for removal. In some cases, however, a bioptome may be used to pull the device into the inferior vena cava (IVC) with the snare holding the right atrial disk screw.

Once there, a stiff J-wire can be advanced across the device in the IVC to stabilize its position.[15] The ASO can then be pulled more easily into the retrieval sheath and removed. In their survey, 15/21 (71%) device embolizations were successfully retrieved via a percutaneous route from a total cohort of 3824 patients. The other 6 patients underwent surgical removal. Chessa et al[9] successfully retrieved 4 of 11 embolized or malpositioned devices. The other 7 patients underwent successful surgical retrieval and closure.

There is a growing interest in the thrombosis rate for any septal defect closure device. In the case of the ASO, this has been examined in a small study by Anzai and colleagues.[16] In their study, 66 patients underwent septal defect closure with either a CardioSeal, an Amplatzer PFO occluder, or an ASO. TEE was performed in 50 patients 1 month postclosure, and the incidence of detectable thrombus on the 27 patients with the Amplatzer devices was 0%. A recent review by Krumsdorf and colleagues[17] of the incidence of thrombosis induced by septal closure devices (including both ASD and PFO devices) in 1000 patients undergoing septal defect closure suggested that the mean incidence of thrombosis in the 407 ASD closure cases, using a variety of devices, was 1.2% (5/407). The incidence of thrombosis in those receiving an Amplatzer device was 0%. These thrombi were detected at the planned 30-day and/or 6-month follow-up, which included a TEE. Interestingly, 14/221 (6.3%) ASD patients had a coagulation disorder; in these patients, there was a higher incidence of a precedent embolic event prior to closure. In addition, of the 326 Amplatzer devices used in this study, there were no cases of detected thrombus by echocardiographic imaging. This reduced incidence of detectable thrombosis in the Amplatzer patients may be due to the covering of the nitinol mesh with polyester. Other devices, because of a difference in the covering, may be more prone to thrombus formation. However, a recent review and meta-analysis of seventeen reports found 54 patients with device thrombosis and no device was spared from this complication.[18] Predictors of thrombus formation include hypercoagulability, presence of atrial fibrillation, and presence of a persistent atrial septal aneurysm in PFO patients. The presence or absence of a residual shunt does not appear to predict thrombus formation, nor does diabetes, hypertension, or concomitant coronary heart disease.[17]

Overt cardiac rupture is heretofore unheard of, but the development of significant pericardial effusion leading to pericardial tamponade has been reported in a number of studies. The report by Chessa et al[9] included two pericardial effusions (0.5%), one of which required emergent surgical drainage in the catheterization laboratory because of a guidewire perforation. The other effusion resolved with medical therapy after 20 days. Four (2.0%) of the 199 patients in the series described by Wang et al[12] developed pericardial effusions, one of which required pericardiocentesis for relief of tamponade. In a recent registry review of ASO erosions,[19] 28 cases (14 in the United States) were examined. All erosions were near the aortic root, and the large majority of these patients had a deficient aortic rim (89%) or superior rim. In addition, oversizing of the defect with aggressive balloon sizing and a subsequent oversized device may have played a role in these perforations. Early recognition is the key to avoid any poor outcome. Serial echocardiograms are recommended for those patients who develop a pericardial effusion at the time of the procedure and early postprocedure.

RESULTS

The results of percutaneous ASD closure[5,9,12,20–22] are very encouraging. The earliest report of using the Amplatzer device for secundum ASD closure[20] was a small pediatric study of 16 patients, and these procedures were performed without complication. An acute closure without residual shunting was achieved in 13 of the 16 patients (81%), and 2 of these 3 patients had no TEE-detectable shunt at 3 months for an overall success rate of 94%. In another study of ASD closure,[21] 200 patients were closed using the ASO device. At 3 months postprocedure, 98.1% of patients had no detectable shunt, with only trivial residual shunting noted in the remaining patients. In a review of 3580 ASD closures in 3535 patients,[22] Omeish and Hijazi reported a 97.4% acute success rate for closure based on TEE findings of minimal or no shunt at the time of closure. At 3 months, the closure rate per the TTE was 99.2%, and at 3 years, it was 100%. There were no device-related deaths, and there was a serious complication rate of 0.3%. In a recent study from Taiwan,[12] 197 patients underwent ASD closure with the Amplatzer device and the use of TEE. A deficient rim, defined as less than 5 mm, was noted in 114 patients, 113 of which were noted on the superior-anterior (aortic) portion of the atrial septum. Interestingly, the presence of a deficient rim was not associated with an increase in procedural failure. A total of 191 procedures were successful; repositioning (redeployment) of the device was needed in 28 patients. Of the 6 failures, 4 were in adults with an ASD stretched diameter of greater than 34 mm and 2 were in young children younger than 4 years of age with stretched ASDs of greater than 20 mm. Complications were noted in 3 patients; 1 had complete AV block that eventually resolved after 3 days, 1 experienced cardiac tamponade requiring pericardiocentesis, and 1 had embolization of the device and required emergent surgery after failed attempts to retrieve the device. The follow-up on these patients included TEE, and residual shunts were seen in 4% of patients at 2 years.

SUMMARY

The development of a percutaneous device to close secundum ASDs has advanced the use of these devices in the adult cardiac catheterization laboratory. Experience with these devices is growing and these devices have become commonplace in many centers in the United States and around the world as a true alternative to surgical closure. The acute and medium-term (<10 years) experience has been very positive, and percutaneous ASD closure will continue to grow as the devices and operators improve. Early recognition of problems in ASD closure is important and may obviate the need for surgical intervention in a large number of complicated cases.

PATENT FORAMEN OVALE

PFO is a common congenital heart finding that can be an incidental finding in 10% to 30% of autopsies but can have a much higher incidence in patients with a neurologic event unascribed to another cause ("cryptogenic"). A PFO is a residual of a failed closure of the fossa ovalis, a remnant of the fetal circulation. In most people, the foramen ovale closes shortly after birth. In patients with a PFO, this closure fails to occur, and the heart is left with a persistent potential shunt between the right and left atrium (Figure 45-10). In the large majority of patients with PFO, no neurologic events ensue. This is likely due to the adequacy of atrial flow and turbulence, which prevent thrombi from forming, and to the small chance of passage of embolic material through a small shunt.

[ ] RELATIONSHIP OF THE PATENT FORAMEN OVALE TO NEUROLOGIC EVENTS

As noted above, a large percentage of the general population harbors a PFO. An evolving interest in PFO has been driven by the finding that 40% of ischemic stroke patients have no defined cause ("cryptogenic"). In many of these patients, especially young patients, a PFO is discovered. The mechanisms postulated for the development of a cryptogenic stroke with PFO are (1) passage of thromboemboli from the right heart circulation across a PFO into the left atrium and thus into the cerebral circulation, and (2) in situ thrombosis across the PFO and thromboembolism from the PFO itself into the left atrium and into the cerebral circulation. Although there is no absolute proof that a PFO is a cause of

cryptogenic neurologic events, there are several series suggesting that there is a higher incidence of PFOs in patients with cryptogenic stroke.[23–26]

Mas et al[27] performed a retrospective study of 132 patients with a cryptogenic neurologic event and a PFO and/or atrial septal aneurysm (ASA). The findings suggested that the annual rate of recurrent stroke was 1.2%, with a 3.4% annual rate for any neurologic event. The risk was highest for patients with both a PFO and ASA with an annual stroke recurrence rate of 4.4%. Another study by Nedeltchev et al[28] examined 318 patients with a cryptogenic neurologic event (stroke or transient ischemic attack [TIA]) and PFO. A total of 159 patients underwent medical therapy; this consisted of vitamin K antagonists with a targeted international normalized ratio of 2.0 to 3.0 in 79 patients and platelet inhibitors (aspirin or clopidogrel) in 80 patients. At a mean follow-up period of 29 months, 21 patients (13.4%) had had a recurrent neurologic event (7 stroke, 14 TIA). Based on this, the mean annual rate of stroke recurrence was 1.8% (5.5% for recurrent stroke or TIA). The Patent Foramen Ovale in Cryptogenic Stroke Study[29] (PICSS) was a substudy of the 630-patient Warfarin-Aspirin Recurrent Stroke Study (WARSS), in which 203 patients had a documented PFO. In this medical therapy comparison, there was no difference in outcomes of recurrent stroke or death between warfarin or aspirin treatment, and the presence of a PFO did not affect outcomes. In addition, the size of the PFO or the presence of an ASA also did not affect outcomes. A meta-analysis of several studies[30] in secondary prevention of recurrent neurologic events in PFO patients, however, suggested that warfarin is superior to aspirin and may be equivalent to surgical closure of a PFO.[31]

Standard medical therapy has thus not been concretely defined but generally consists of warfarin with or without concomitant antiplatelet therapy. Within the neurology community, the actual "best practice" regarding medical therapy remains controversial;[32] thus, patients may be taking aspirin, aspirin and Persantine, clopidogrel with or without aspirin, or warfarin for secondary prevention of a cryptogenic stroke. With the development of devices for mechanical closure of a PFO, this has generated a great interest in mechanical closure of PFOs in patients with cryptogenic stroke.

[ ] SPECIAL INTEREST: PATENT FORAMEN OVALE AND MIGRAINE HEADACHES

An interesting relationship, albeit not a proven causal one, has suggested that PFOs may be implicated in migraine headaches. From observational studies,[33–36] it appears that patients with migraine headaches have about twice the incidence of PFOs, especially with ASA, than the general population. PFO closure may help alleviate the frequency of migraine headaches,[36] as suggested by a study of migraine headache attacks in a population undergoing PFO closure for cryptogenic neurologic events. Based on these findings, a randomized clinical trial in the United Kingdom studying the role of PFO closure with the StarFlex device in patients with migraine headaches (MIST = Migraine Intervention with StarFlex Technology) without cryptogenic neurologic events has recently been reported at the 2006 American College of Cardiology Scientific Sessions. In this important study,

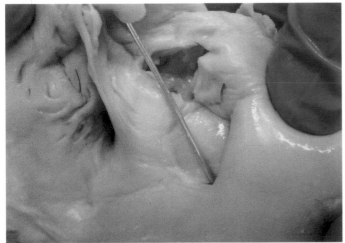
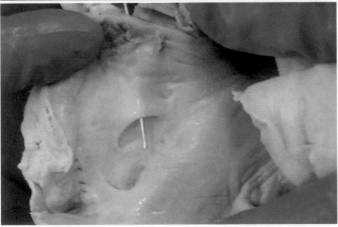

FIGURE 45-10. Patent foramen ovale from a cadaver shows the probe patency from the right atrial (*top*) and left atrial (*bottom*) sides of the defect.

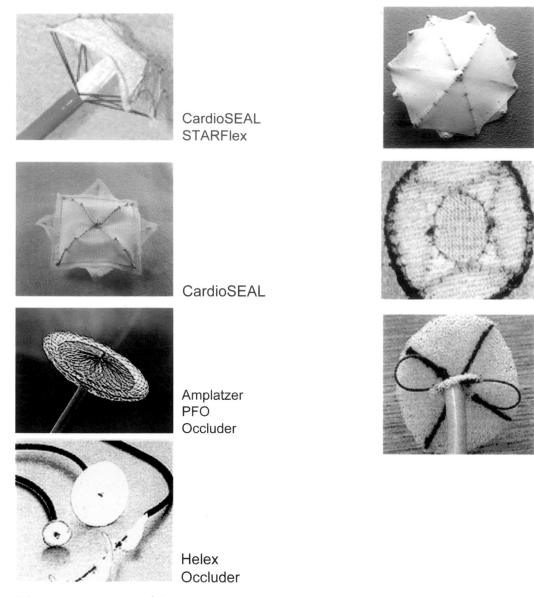

CardioSEAL
STARFlex

CardioSEAL

Amplatzer
PFO
Occluder

Helex
Occluder

Intracept

Guardian
Angel

Sideris
Buttoned
Device

FIGURE 45-11. A variety of devices are available outside the United States for percutaneous closure of a patent foramen ovale. Within the United States, only the CardioSeal and Amplatzer PFO Occluder have humanitarian device exemption from the Food and Drug Administration for secondary prevention of cryptogenic stroke.

147 patients were randomized to either device closure of their PFO or medical management with a sham procedure. The primary endpoint of the trial, complete cessation of migraine headaches, was achieved in 3/74 patients in the device group and 3/73 patients in the medical treatment (sham procedure) group. However, the device group had a significant improvement in their headache burden score (frequency × duration; $P = .033$) and in experiencing a 50% or greater reduction in headache days (42% of patients in the procedure arm and 23% in the sham arm; $P = .038$). This trial, with its small number but promising results, should prompt further interest and study into the relationship between PFOs and migraines as well as potential device therapy. There are now at least four planned randomized clinical trials investigating the utility of percutaneous PFO closure in migraineurs.

[ ] THE DECISION TO CLOSE A PATENT FORAMEN OVALE

The decision to percutaneously close a PFO is often a difficult one. Currently, in the United States, there are two available devices specifically indicated for PFO closure: the NMT CardioSeal and the Amplatzer patent foramen ovale occluder (APO). Several other devices are under trial in the United States as well. Outside the United States, there are a number of commercially available devices (Figure 45-11), and there are several other PFO closure devices under development examining the use of energy (radiofrequency/thermal), sutures and/or clips, as well as biodegradable technology. Both the CardioSeal and the APO are restrained by a Humanitarian Device Exemption (HDE) from the Food and Drug Administration (FDA). The HDE is specific in the indication for mechanical closure; it

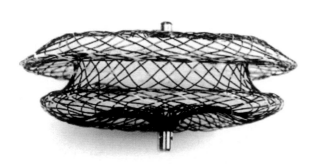
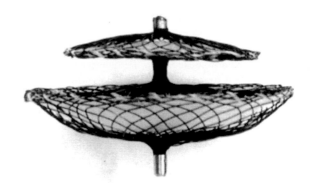

FIGURE 45-12. The differences between the Amplatzer Septal Occluder (ASO; *left*) for secundum-type atrial septal defects and Amplatzer Patent Foramen Ovale Occluder (*right*) are evident with both devices oriented with the left atrial disk at the top: the ASO has a larger left atrial disk and a larger "waist" in the middle.

states that the device may be used under the HDE only for patients who have suffered a cryptogenic stroke and who have failed warfarin therapy. This has led to a difficult decision-making tree for many physicians, in part because of the widely held belief that mechanical closure is superior and in many cases preferable to medical therapy. In addition, patients may believe that they are at risk for a recurrent cryptogenic event while on warfarin therapy, which by itself may be objectionable because of the required monitoring. As a result, a number of closures are performed outside of the HDE ("off-label"), driven both by physician and patient preferences regarding mechanical closure and avoiding warfarin or other medical therapy. This is occurring despite the lack of concrete data suggesting that mechanical closure confers any advantage over medical therapy.

【 】 PERCUTANEOUS PATENT FORAMEN OVALE CLOSURE

Percutaneous PFO closure can be accomplished easily with either of the two above-approved devices in the United States. The APO differs from the ASO in that the APO has a larger right atrial disk than left atrial disk–opposite that of the ASO–and the APO has a very thin, 3-mm long, "waist" compared to the ASO (Figure 45-12). The APO size is reported by the right atrial disk size and the APO comes only in 18-, 25-, and 35-mm sizes. The 18-mm device is 8-Fr sheath–compatible, whereas the 35-mm device requires a 9-Fr sheath. Similar to the ASO, the APO is retrievable while still on the delivery cable and may be redeployed to achieve a satisfactory closure.

The technique for deploying the APO is very similar to the previously described technique using the ASO, with the exception that no right-sided heart catheterization is necessary. The sizing for PFO closure is based not on the stretched PFO diameter but rather on anatomic measurements. The proper APO size for PFO closure is based on the shortest distance of (1) the distance between the aortic root to the defect or (2) the distance between the defect and the SVC. In addition, the ASA length should be considered. For instance, a 9-mm PFO with a distance of 12 mm from the farther edge of the PFO to the aortic root and 14-mm SVC–PFO length would dictate an 18-mm device. For a 6-mm PFO and an aortic root–PFO distance of 15 mm, SVC–PFO distance of 20 mm, the

size should be 25 mm. If any of the measured distances are less than 6 mm, the device should not be used.

With the devices from NMT Medical, the technique is significantly different. The CardioSeal is available under an HDE in the United States and the StarFlex is available in the United State only in a randomized clinical trial (CLOSURE I = evaluation of the StarFlex septal closure system in patients with a stroke and /or ischemic attack due to presumed paradoxical embolism through a PFO.). The devices are similar, in that both use a nitinol skeleton within a polyester umbrella with a small "waist" in the middle separating the umbrellas. The StarFlex has the added advantage of harboring a tiny spring, which allows self-centering of the device within a defect. The major disadvantage of these particular devices is that they are not retrievable (ie, if both umbrella arms have been released prematurely, it is difficult to retrieve them even while still on the delivery cable).

To be a candidate for closure, all patients should have a thorough workup, including hypercoagulability studies, carotid and magnetic resonance imaging studies, as well as a TEE to diagnose a PFO and cryptogenic stroke. Once the decision to close the PFO has been reached, the patient should cease taking warfarin at least 3 days prior to the procedure. Just prior to starting the procedure, antibiotics should be administered.

In the catheterization laboratory, the sizing of the defect is identical to the procedure described in the ASD section above. No right-sided heart catheterization is necessary, and ICE may be employed for imaging.

Once the size of the PFO has been established, the choice of device size ensues, and this is dictated by the size of the defect. For CardioSeal or StarFlex devices, the general rule is to use a device twice the measured PFO size. The device is available in several sizes: 17, 23, 28, and 33 mm. For instance, a 9-mm PFO should be closed with a 23-mm CardioSeal. Delivery of the CardioSeal requires either a 10-Fr or a 11-Fr sheath. For the StarFlex, the available sizes are 23, 28, and 33 mm, and the delivery sheath sizes are the same.

The protocol for device preparation and delivery of either the CardioSeal or StarFlex differs significantly from that of the Amplatzer devices. The CardioSeal comes packaged with the device and a loading kit. This kit consists of a funneled opening at one end, with a clear plastic covering at the other end. The CardioSeal is attached to its delivery cable by a pin mechanism. This pin mechanism must be precisely aligned to secure the device to the delivery system. The pin on the delivery cable is retractable and extendable; it should be extended to lock the corresponding pin on the device and then gently retracted and locked onto the delivery cable. Once the device is attached, it is stretched to collapse the right atrial umbrella through the clear portion of the plastic loading kit and then pulled again to collapse the left atrial umbrella. The device should be pulled within the clear plastic section with the collapsed left atrial umbrella at its tip, and the device should be well flushed to expunge any air from the system. The device and delivery cable can then be placed through the 10-Fr or 11-Fr delivery sheath and guided forward until it is fluoroscopically visible near the tip of the delivery sheath. Within the left atrium, the sheath should be pulled back into the midportion of the atrium, and then retracted to open the left atrial umbrella. Care should be taken to avoid premature delivery of the right atrial umbrella. Using ICE or TEE guidance, the left atrial umbrella and delivery sheath can be retracted until it reaches the interatrial septum. Once satisfactory positioning has been established, the delivery sheath can be retracted again, allowing the expansion of the right atrial umbrella. Again, care should be taken to avoid premature delivery of the right atrial arms within the PFO tunnel. Once expanded, the umbrellas should be on opposite sides of the atrium. At this point, proper positioning is confined with the echo, and the Minnesota wiggle can be used to establish device stability and, if satisfactory, the device can be detached from the delivery cable by unlocking the pin mechanism while gentle traction is applied. Once released, the device often "settles" into a slightly different orientation along the interatrial septum. It should be investigated with ICE or TEE with Doppler imaging and/or bubbles to establish the position and function of the device.

It should be noted that some investigators use no extrafluoroscopic imaging; rather, they use the use of contrast "puffs" through the delivery sheath to establish the location of the PFO and then use fluoroscopic guidance to place the left and right umbrellas across the septum appropriately. An atrial angiogram is performed prior to device release; a final right atrial angiogram is performed after release to gauge the acute efficacy of the seal.

POSTPROCEDURE CARE

The postprocedure care does not differ from that of ASD closures (see above).

COMPLICATIONS

Complications associated with PFO closure are similar to those of ASD closure. In one of the earlier studies, Windecker et al[37] reported their experience in 80 patients, 8 (10%) experienced a periprocedural complication. Air embolization occurred in 2 patients, resulting in a transient neurologic deficit in one case and inferior ST-segment elevation in the other. An intraprocedural cerebrovascular accident (CVA) occurred in 1 patient, also presumed due to air embolism. Cardiac tamponade requiring pericardiocentesis after puncture of the right atrium by the delivery sheath was seen in 1 patient. Three device embolization events occurred, 2 of which were successfully retrieved by percutaneous method, and in 1, the device used was a reversed button

device in which the occluder portion remained in the proper position in the PFO. In another report,[38] Hung and colleagues closed 63 PFOs using the Clamshell, CardioSeal, or Buttoned devices. The only periprocedural complication was four episodes of periprocedural or postprocedural new-onset atrial fibrillation, all of which resolved within the 2.6-year mean follow-up. In another series of 152 patients with PFO and cryptogenic neurologic events,[39] 1 patient had a femoral artery laceration that necessitated surgery and eventual surgical PFO closure. Ten procedural complications were seen: device embolization in 4 patients, cardiac tamponade requiring pericardiocentesis in 1 patient, symptomatic air embolism in 3 patients, and arteriovenous fistula at the puncture site in 1 patient. None of these 10 patients had any permanent disability due to the complications. Braun et al[40] reported their findings in 276 patients, with 11 patients (4%) suffering a periprocedural complication. Transient atrial fibrillation was seen in 2 patients, TIAs in 2 patients, reversible ST-segment elevation in 4 patients, and transient third-degree heart block in 1 patient. Device embolization occurred in two patients. The experience at the Massachusetts General Hospital[41] in 110 patients revealed a periprocedural complication in 2 patients: pericardiocentesis was necessary in case, and a device embolism occurred in another. A significant shunt or device malposition requiring a repeat procedure was needed by 4 (3.6%) patients in this study. In a phase 1 trial with the APO in 50 patients,[42] an arteriovenous fistula that required surgical treatment occurred in 1 patient. There were no APO-related complications.

RESULTS

PFO closure for the secondary prevention of neurologic events in patients with cryptogenic stroke has been generally positive. The incidence of an acute residual shunt post-closure ranges from 17% to 55%;[37–43] a large majority of these are trivial or mild in grade. Larger shunts (moderate or greater in degree) had an incidence of 3% to 12%, with the general experience that most will close fully by 6 months. It is currently a topic of debate whether a residual shunt is related to a higher risk of recurrent neurologic events.

Windecker et al[37] reported the 5-year follow-up on patients and found the annual risk of a recurrent TIA of 2.5%, 0% for CVA, and 0.9% for peripheral embolism. They also found that a residual shunt was a predictor for an event. The experience of Hung and colleagues[38] in Boston revealed 3 TIAs and 1 CVA in 63 patients at the mean 2.6-year follow-up, for a 3.2% calculated annual risk of TIA or stroke after device placement.

Wahl and colleagues[39] found 9 patients (6%) in their 150 patient series with a neurologic event within a mean follow-up of 1.7 years after device placement. The risk of a neurologic event was significantly higher ($P = .02$) in the 21% of patients with a residual shunt. In the United States, the small 18-patient study by Du[43] showed acute complete closure in 12 patients (67%) and complete closure by 2 years. No neurologic events were seen within the mean follow-up of 2.2 years. In the study by Braun et al,[40] 276 patients were followed for a mean of 15 months post-PFO closure, and the annual risk of thromboembolic events was 1.7% for TIA, 0% for stroke, and 0% for peripheral emboli. There was no significant difference between patients with and without a residual shunt. Interestingly, 8 patients (2.9%) were noted to have thrombus adhering to the device; this prompted warfarin treatment, and follow-up TEE showed no thrombus in any of these patients. In yet another study[41] involving 110 patients at a mean follow-up of 2.3 years, there was an annual neurologic event rate post-PFO closure of 0.9%. The initial experience of Hong and colleagues[42] with the APO in 50 patients revealed no neurologic events post-closure at a mean follow-up of 16.5 months.

The major weakness of the data generated thus far has been the lack of a prospective randomized control trial of device versus medical therapy. A recent meta-analysis of several reports of closure or medical therapy[44] included 10 studies of transcatheter closure and 6 studies of medical therapy, with 1355 patients undergoing device therapy and 895 patients treated medically for the secondary prevention of cryptogenic neurologic events. The findings included an annual rate of recurrent neurologic events in the device group of 0% to 4.9%, whereas the medical group had an annual rate of 3.8% to 13.0%. The conclusion from this study was that transcatheter closure was safe and provided a benefit in the prevention of secondary neurologic events but that a firm recommendation about therapy could not be made in the absence of randomized controlled clinical trials comparing device and medical therapy. Indeed, a report from the American Academy of Neurology[45] made the same recommendation regarding clinical trials to investigate the benefits of medical versus device therapy. This report noted that medical therapy itself was inconclusive as to whether warfarin or aspirin should be the recommended therapy for secondary prevention. In addition, the findings noted that PFO by itself did not increase the risk of a subsequent event in patients treated medically but that patients with a PFO and an ASA were possibly at a higher risk of subsequent events in patients medically treated.

As a result of the above recommendations and the desire to move beyond HDE status, at least 3 companies are currently moving forward with randomized trials comparing their PFO device to medical therapy. The CLOSURE I study is currently enrolling 1600 patients in a randomized trial comparing device closure using the StarFlex device to warfarin therapy. Similarly, the Amplatzer PFO device is also under investigation in the secondary prevention of cryptogenic stroke with a similar randomized trial called Randomized Evaluation of Recurrent Stroke Comparing PFO Closure to Established Current Standard of Care Treatment (RESPECT PFO); the trial involves comparing the APO against best medical therapy (antiplatelet or warfarin). Another trial, using the Intrasept device, the fourth generation of the PFO-Star device (Cardia, Burnsville, MN), is also currently underway. It is hoped that all of these trials will be completed sometime during 2007.

REFERENCES

1. King TD, Mills NL. Nonoperative closure of atrial septal defects. *Surgery.* 1974;75:383.
2. Harper RW, Mottram PM, McGaw DJ. Closure of secundum atrial septal defects with the Amplatzer septal occluder device: techniques and problems. *Cathet Cardiovasc Intervent.* 2002;57:508.
3. Hijazi ZM, Wang Z, Cao Q-L, et al. Transcatheter closure of atrial septal defects and patent foramen ovale under intracardiac echocardiographic guidance: feasibility and comparison with transesophageal echocardiography. *Cathet Cardiovasc Intervent.* 2001;52:194.
4. Bartel T, Konorza T, Arjumand J, et al. Intracardiac echocardiography is superior to conventional monitoring for guidance device closure of interatrial communications. *Circulation.* 2003;107:795.
5. Masura J, Gavora P, Formanek A, et al. Transcatheter closure of secundum atrial defects using the new self-centering Amplatzer septal occluder. *Cathet Cardiovasc Intervent.* 1997;42:388.
6. Wahab HA, Bairam AR, Cao Q-L, et al. Novel technique to prevent prolapse of the Amplatzer septal occluder though large atrial septal defect. *Cathet Cardiovasc Intervent.* 2003;60:543.
7. Dalvi BV, Pinto RJ, Gupta A. New technique for device closure of large atrial septal defects. *Cathet Cardiovasc Intervent.* 2005;64:102.
8. Suda K, Raboisson M-J, Piette E, et al. Reversible atrioventricular block associated with closure of atrial septal defects using the Amplatzer device. *J Am Coll Cardiol.* 2004;43:1677.
9. Chessa M, Carminati M, Butera G, et al. Early and late complications associated with transcatheter occlusion of secundum atrial septal defect. *J Am Coll Cardiol.* 2002;39:1061.
10. Hill SL, Berul CI, Patel HT, et al. Early ECG abnormalities associated with transcatheter closure of atrial septal defects using the Amplatzer septal occluder. *J Intervent Cardiol Electrophysiol.* 2000;4:469.
11. Earing MG, Cabalka AK, Seward JB, et al. Intracardiac echocardiographic guidance during transcatheter device closure of atrial septal defect and patent foramen ovale. *Mayo Clin Proc.* 2004;79:24.
12. Wang J-K, Tsai S-K, Wu M-H, et al. Short and intermediate-term results of transcatheter closure of atrial septal defect with the Amplatzer Septal Occluder. *Am Heart J.* 2004;148:511.
13. Levi DS, Moore JW. Embolization and retrieval of the Amplatzer septal occluder. *Cathet Cardiovasc Interv.* 2004;61:543.
14. Butera G, Carminati M, Chessa M, et al. Cardioseal/Starflex versus Amplatzer devices for percutaneous closure of small to moderate (up to 18 mm) atrial septal defects. *Am Heart J.* 2004;148:507.
15. Peuster M, Boekenkamp R, Kaulitz R, et al. Transcatheter retrieval and repositioning of an Amplatzer device embolized into the left atrium. *Cathet Cardiovasc Interv.* 2000;51:297.
16. Anzai H, Child J, Natterson B, et al. Incidence of thrombus formation on the CardioSeal and Amplatzer interatrial closure devices. *Am J Cardiol.* 2004;43:426.
17. Krumsdorf U, Ostermayer S, Billinger K, et al. Incidence and clinical course of thrombus formation on atrial septal defect and patent foramen ovale closure in 1,000 consecutive patients. *J Am Coll Cardiol.* 2004;43:302.
18. Sherman JM, Hagler DJ, Cetta F. Thrombosis after septal closure device placement: a review of the current literature. *Cathet, Cardiovasc Intervent.* 2004;63:486.
19. Amin Z, Hijazi ZM, Bass JL, et al. Erosion of the Amplatzer septal occluder device after closure of secundum atrial septal defects: review of registry of complications and recommendations to minimize future risk. *Cathet Cardiovasc Intervent.* 2004;63:496.
20. Thanopoulos BD, Laskari CV, Tsaousis GS, et al. Closure of atrial septal defects with the Amplatzer occlusion device: preliminary results. *J Am Coll Cardiol.* 1998;31:1110.
21. Berger F, Ewert P, Bjornstad PG, et al. Transcatheter closure as standard treatment for most interatrial defects: experience in 200 patients treated with the Amplatzer Septal Occluder. *Cardiol Young.* 1999;9:468.
22. Omeish A, Hijazi ZM. Transcatheter closure of atrial septal defects in children and adults using the Amplatzer Septal Occluder. *J Intervent Cardiol.* 2001;14:37.
23. Lechat P, Mas JL, Lascault G, et al. Prevalence of patent foramen ovale in patients with stroke. *N Engl J Med.* 1988;318:1148.
24. Webster MW, Chancellor AM, Smith HJ, et al. Patent foramen ovale in young stroke patients. *Lancet.* 1988;2:11.
25. Hausmann D, Mugge A, Becht I, et al. Diagnosis of patent foramen ovale by transesophageal echocardiography and association with cerebral and peripheral embolic events. *Am J Cardiol.* 1992;70:668.
26. Kerut EK, Norfleet WT, Plodnick GD, et al. Patent foramen ovale: a review of associated conditions and the impact of physiological size. *J Am Coll Cardiol.* 2001;38:613.
27. Mas JL, Zuber M. Recurrent cerebrovascular events in patients with patent foramen ovale, atrial septal aneurysm, or both and cryptogenic stroke or transient ischemic attack. French Study Group on Patent Foramen Ovale and Atrial Septal Aneurysm. *Am Heart J.* 1995;130:1083.
28. Nedeltchev K, Arnold M, Wahl A, et al. Outcome of patients with cryptogenic stroke and patent foramen ovale. *J Neurol Neurosurg Psychiatry.* 2003;72:347.
29. Homma S, Sacco RL, Di Tullio MR, et al, for the PICSS Investigators. Effect of medical treatment in stroke patients with patent foramen ovale: patent foramen ovale in cryptogenic stroke study. *Circulation.* 2003;105:2625.

30. Orgera MA, O'Malley PG, Taylor AJ. Secondary prevention of ischemia in patent foramen ovale: systematic review and meta-analysis. *South Med J.* 2001;94:699.

31. Dearani JA, Ugurlu BS, Danielson GK, et al. Surgical patent foramen ovale closure for the prevention of paradoxical embolism-related cerebrovascular ischemic events. *Circulation.* 1999;100(Suppl 2):171.

32. Lamy C, Giannesini C, Zuber M, et al. Clinical and imaging findings in cryptogenic stroke patients with and without patent foramen ovale: the PFO-ASA Study. Atrial Septal Aneurysm. *Stroke.* 2002;33:706.

33. Anzola GP, Magoni M, Guindani M, et al. Potential source of cerebral embolism in migraine with aura: a transcranial Doppler study. *Neurology.* 1999;52:1622.

34. Anzola GP, Del Sette M, Rozzini L, et al. The migraine-PFO connection is independent of sex. *Cerebrovasc Dis.* 2000;10:163.

35. Sztajzel R, Genoud D, Roth S, et al. Patent foramen ovale, a possible cause of symptomatic migraine: a study of 74 patients with acute ischemic stroke. *Cerebrovasc Dis.* 2002;13:102.

36. Schwerzmann M, Wiher S, Nedeltchev K, et al. Percutaneous closure of patent foramen ovale reduces the frequency of migraine attacks. *Neurology.* 2004;62:1399.

37. Windecker S, Wal A, Chatterjee T, et al. Percutaneous closure of patient foramen ovale in patients with paradoxical embolism. Long-term risk of recurrent thromboembolic events. *Circulation.* 2000;101:893.

38. Hung J, Landzberg MJ, Jenkins KJ, et al. Closure of patent foramen ovale for paradoxical emboli: intermediate-term risk of recurrent neurological events following transcatheter device placement. *J Am Coll Cardiol.* 2000;35:1311.

39. Wahl A, Meier B, Haxel B, et al. Prognosis after percutaneous closure of patent foramen ovale for paradoxical embolism. *Neurology.* 2001;57:1330.

40. Braun MU, Fassbender D, Schoen SP, et al. Transcatheter closure of patent foramen ovale in patients with cerebral ischemia. *J Am Coll Cardiol.* 2002;39:2019.

41. Martin F, Sanchez PL, Doherty E, et al. Percutaneous transcatheter closure of patent foramen ovale in patients with paradoxical embolism. *Circulation.* 2002;106:1121.

42. Hong TE, Thaler D, Brorson J, et al, for the Amplatzer PFO investigators. Transcatheter closure of patent foramen ovale associated with paradoxical embolism using the Amplatzer PFO occluder: initial and intermediate results of the US multicenter clinical trial. *Cathet Cardiovasc Intervent.* 2003;60:524.

43. Du Z-D, Cao Q-L, Joseph A, Koenig P, et al. Transcatheter closure of patent foramen ovale in patients with paradoxical embolism: intermediate-term risk of recurrent neurologic events. *Cathet Cardiovasc Intervent.* 2002;55:189.

44. Khairy P, O'Donnell CP, Landzberg MJ. Transcatheter closure versus medical therapy of patent foramen ovale and presumed paradoxical thromboemboli. *Ann Intern Med.* 2003;139:753.

45. Messé SR, Silverman IE, Kizer JR, et al. Practice parameter: recurrent stroke with patent foramen ovale and atrial septal aneurysm. Report on the Quality Standards Subcommittee of the American Academy of Neurology. *Neurology.* 2004;62:1042.

CHAPTER (46)

Alcohol Septal Ablation for Obstructive Hypertrophic Cardiomyopathy

Christopher D. Nielsen, MD, and
William H. Spencer III, MD

Hypertrophic cardiomyopathy (HCM) is a condition in which there is abnormal hypertrophy of the ventricular myocardium out of proportion to conditions known to cause hypertrophy such as valvular aortic stenosis and hypertension. In the obstructive form of HCM, which is often called hypertrophic obstructive cardiomyopathy, there is relatively more hypertrophy in the interventricular septum, leading to asymmetric septal hypertrophy. This leads to obstruction of outflow from the left ventricle. Although the hypertrophy most often disproportionately involves the proximal portion of the interventricular septum, other anatomic variants can be seen involving other walls alone, the apex, or the entire myocardium. HCM is usually genetically transmitted, but sporadic cases may occur. Multiple different genetic mutations encoding for sarcomeric contractile proteins have been identified as causes of this condition.[1] Histologically, there is myocyte hypertrophy, myocyte disorganization and disarray, and myocardial fibrosis.

The signs and symptoms of obstructive HCM arise from the left ventricular outflow tract (LVOT) obstruction and left ventricular diastolic dysfunction. Patients may present with dyspnea, angina, congestive heart failure, dizziness, and syncope. Sudden death remains the most devastating complication of HCM and may occur in the absence of other symptoms. Recent data suggest that the risk of sudden death may be correlated to septal thickness and LVOT gradient.[2]

Treatment of obstructive HCM involves decreasing the LVOT obstruction, improving diastolic function, and decreasing the risk of sudden death. Outflow tract obstruction is a dynamic process that is affected by the preload, afterload, and contractility, and it

has been shown that gradients taken at different times can vary widely.[3] Medical therapy usually begins with negative inotropes and negative chronotropes. Beta-blockers, negatively inotropic calcium channel blockers, and disopyramide have been shown to decrease outflow tract gradients and improve symptoms in some patients.[4–6] Avoidance of volume depletion, hypotension, and inotropic medications are also essential for adequate treatment. Many patients remain symptomatic despite medical therapy, whereas some have only a short-lived response to medical therapy or have side effects making maximal medical therapy intolerable. Ventricular pacing from the right ventricular apex has been used in an attempt to decrease LVOT gradient and symptoms. The theory is that by pacing the right side of the interventricular septum, paradoxical motion of the septum occurs, pulling it away from the outflow tract during early systole. This creates less systolic anterior motion of the mitral valve, thereby decreasing outflow obstruction. Early reports of pacing therapy seemed to show improvement in LVOT gradients as well as symptoms; however, these improvements were largely in nonrandomized, uncontrolled studies.[7,8] More recent randomized trials have shown less of an improvement in objective measurements but a large placebo effect.[9,10]

Surgical therapy with septal myectomy is an effective therapy for patients who fail medical therapy.[11–13] Although results of surgical myectomy are good and the procedure has many years of follow-up results showing sustained improvements in symptoms, the attendant morbidity of an open heart surgical procedure is undesirable in many patients.

Alcohol septal ablation (ASA) is a relatively new percutaneous technique used to create a controlled septal infarct to decrease septal thickness and therefore decrease LVOT gradient and symptoms. This procedure has been referred to by multiple names: ASA, non-surgical septal reduction therapy (NSRT), transcoronary ablation of septal hypertrophy (TASH), and percutaneous transluminal septal myocardial ablation (PTSMA). ASA was first performed in 1994[14] and has now been performed in thousands of patients worldwide.

PATIENT SELECTION

Patients should be symptomatic despite adequate medical therapy. Currently accepted criteria for ASA include asymmetric septal hypertrophy with a septal thickness of at least 1.5 cm and a septal-to-posterior wall ratio of at least 1.3:1, a resting Doppler LVOT gradient of more than 30 mm Hg, or a provoked gradient of more than 60 mm Hg using the Valsalva maneuver or after a premature ventricular contraction.

PROCEDURE

Patients are taken to the cardiac catheterization laboratory, where coronary angiograms are performed to rule out significant coronary artery disease that may produce similar symptoms. The septal perforator arteries are identified, usually arising from the left anterior descending (coronary artery; LAD), but occasionally arising from the left main coronary artery (LMCA), ramus intermedius, or diagonal branches. The first septal perforator is usually the largest and is usually the one chosen for septal ablation (Figure 46-1A). If the patient does not already have a permanent pacemaker or implantable cardioverter defibrillator (ICD), a temporary transvenous pacemaker is placed. If the patient has a previously placed pacemaker or ICD, then the output of the ventricular lead is increased to a maximum output temporarily to ensure ventricular capture if needed during the procedure. A second arterial access site should be obtained for placement of a 4- or 5-Fr pigtail catheter in the left ventricle. This allows continuous beat-to-beat monitoring of the gradient during the procedure. Unfractionated heparin is then administered at a dose of 70 mg/kg. Heavy conscious sedation is given to allow adequate anesthesia and amnesia, because significant pain may be felt during alcohol injection.

A 6- or 7-Fr left coronary artery guiding catheter is then selected that will provide the most coaxial engagement of the LMCA to avoid dissection of the coronary artery. This is especially important in these often young patients with normal coronary arteries. An over-the-wire balloon is then selected, which should be as short as possible (6–10 mm) and should be slightly oversized for the septal artery (usually 1.5–2.5 mm). Wiping the exterior of the uninflated balloon with an alcohol swab can rid the balloon of its hydrophilic coating and prevent slippage of the balloon (watermelon-seeding) on inflation. A medium support guidewire is then selected. The guidewire is shaped to give it an almost 90-degree primary curve at the tip, with a smooth 45-degree secondary curve about 3 cm back from the tip—where the floppy tip joins the stiffer shaft of the wire. Optimal variations on the wire shape depend on the anatomy of the septal artery. The guidewire is then advanced into

the septal artery, and the balloon is tracked over the wire into the septal artery such that the proximal portion of the inflated balloon is inside the septal artery and not protruding into the LAD. The balloon is inflated to nominal pressure, and a repeat coronary angiogram is performed to ensure that the balloon is entirely within the septal artery (Figure 46-1B). The guidewire is then withdrawn, and contrast solution is injected through the wire lumen of the balloon to show a selective angiogram of the septal artery to be infarcted (Figure 46-1C). This is done to ensure that (1) there is no leakage of contrast into the LAD (which could be disastrous when alcohol is injected); (2) the entire septal is adequately opacified and that the balloon is not selectively placed in a branch or excluding a major branch of the septal artery; and (3) there are no visible collaterals communicating with other arteries, which would risk creating an infarction remote from the septum during alcohol injection.

Echocardiography is performed with injection of contrast into the septal artery through the balloon (Figure 46-1D and E). Although there are commercially available echocardiographic contrast agents, we have found that "agitated" radiographic contrast dye works well in this situation. Agitated contrast is made by vigorously injecting air into or vigorously stirring a container of contrast to induce microbubbles within the contrast. The myocardium supplied by the septal becomes echodense after contrast administration and ensures proper localization of alcohol injection. This allows one to determine if undesirable areas such as the papillary muscles or another wall of the heart are highlighted by echocardiographic contrast indicating the possibility of a remote infarct. The desired effect is to see that the area of maximal echodensity within the septum is matched with the area of maximal Doppler flow velocity acceleration and/or the area of septal and anterior mitral leaflet contact.

Once the proper area has been localized by angiography and echocardiography, pure desiccated alcohol is injected. The volume of alcohol used is 1 to 4 mm, depending on the size of the septal artery. Although the optimal volume of alcohol has not been determined, one good rule of thumb is to measure the septal thickness in centimeters and to inject that number of milliliters of alcohol. Alcohol is injected slowly through the central lumen of the balloon catheter at 1 mL/min. If heart block or arrhythmias develop, then the injection is slowed or stopped. The balloon is left inflated for a total of 5 minutes from the time of the start of the alcohol injection (or for at least 2 minutes after completion of the injection) to ensure that the alcohol has time to diffuse into the myocardium and cause the desired damage to this segment of myocardium. When the balloon is deflated, the central balloon lumen is simultaneously aspirated to withdraw any remnants of alcohol (obviously, this means that the guidewire cannot be placed back through the balloon). When the balloon is completely deflated and with continued aspiration of the central lumen, the balloon catheter is withdrawn into the guiding catheter and quickly removed from the body. One must not pull the balloon out prior to full deflation, thereby preventing pulling the guiding catheter deeper into the coronary artery, which will increase the risk of coronary dissection. Allowing free back bleeding through the guiding catheter removes any potential small traces of alcohol.

An angiogram is then performed to make sure that the LAD and other vessels remain patent and to show the occluded septal

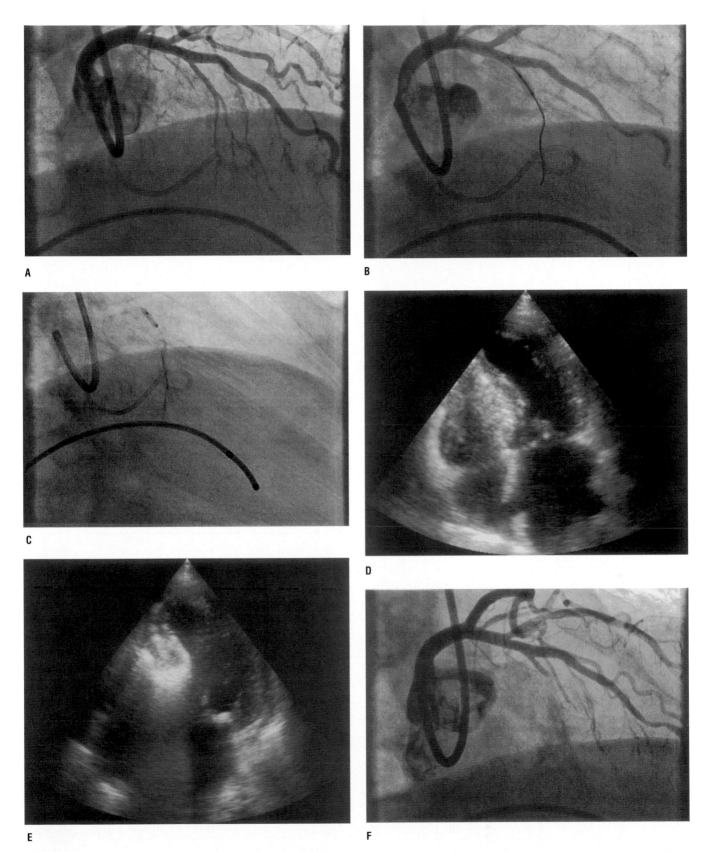

FIGURE 46-1. A. Coronary arteriogram in right anterior oblique-cranial projection showing large first septal perforator off the proximal left anterior descending coronary artery. **B.** Balloon inflated within the first septal perforator artery. **C.** Selective septal angiogram through balloon central lumen. **D.** Echocardiographic image in the apical 4-chamber view showing markedly hypertrophied interventricular septum. **E.** Echocardiographic image showing echogenic area within the interventricular septum after contrast injection through the septal artery. **F.** Coronary arteriogram in right anterior oblique–cranial projection showing occluded septal perforator artery after alcohol injection.

artery. Often the septal artery is completely occluded without any flow, but occasionally the infarcted septal artery fills slowly with slow runoff (Figure 46-1F). Catheter pressure gradients (Figure 46-2A and B) and Doppler LVOT gradients are obtained, and the two-dimensional echocardiogram shows the echodense infarct area. If a significant gradient remains, further septal arteries may be treated using the same steps above.

Once the gradient has been satisfactorily decreased, or if there are no further suitable septal arteries available in the proper area of the septum to inject, the procedure is complete. The temporary pacing wire is left in place for at least several hours after the procedure. If the patient requires transient pacing during the proce-

dure or in the early period after the procedure, the pacing wire is left in place for at least 24 hours. If the patient becomes pacemaker-dependent or requires intermittent pacing after 24 to 48 hours, a permanent pacemaker is implanted. Patients are transferred to the cardiac care unit after the procedure where serum creatine kinase (CK) is measured every 4 hours until the peak is reached, usually within 12 to 24 hours. Most patients ambulate the day after the procedure and are discharged home 48 hours after the procedure. Many patients can be discharged on fewer medications, and often we decrease the doses of both calcium channel blockers and beta-blockers. Patients are told to perform only light activities for 2 weeks after the procedure.

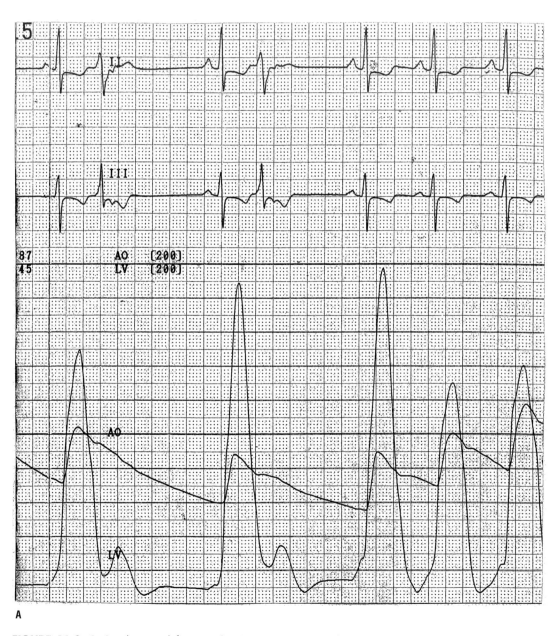

A

FIGURE 46-2. A. Simultaneous left ventricular–Ao pressure tracing showing resting left ventricular outflow tract (LVOT) gradient as well as increased gradient after a premature ventricular contraction (PVC).
B. Simultaneous left ventricular-Ao pressure tracing showing no resting or post-PVC LVOT gradient after alcohol injection.

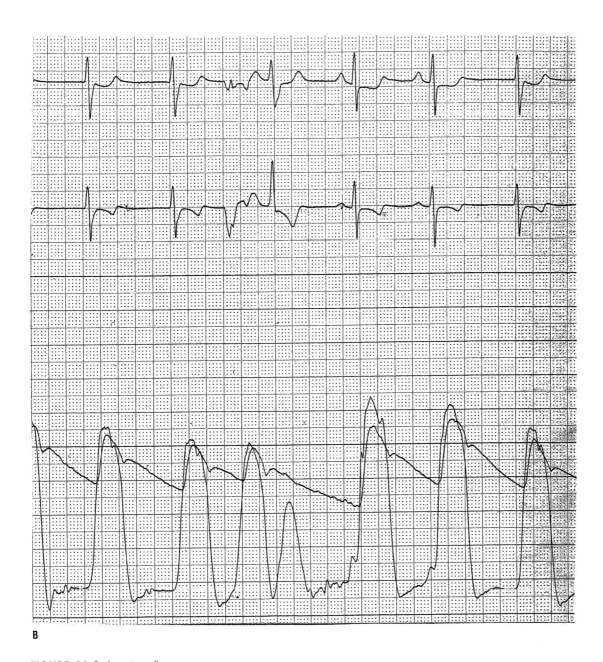

B

FIGURE 46-2. (continued)

RESULTS

Multiple reports of the successful results of ASA have been made since the first case series was reported. Seggewiss et al[15] reported a series of 25 patients with symptomatic obstructive HCM who underwent ASA. The mean LVOT gradient measured invasively decreased from a mean of 61.8 mm Hg preprocedure to 19.4 mm Hg postprocedure. The mean increase in CK was 780 mg/dL. Clinical and echocardiographic improvement was sustained in 22 patients (88%) at 3 months. In a subsequent report,[16] this same group of patients was followed for almost 3 years. The patients remained improved symptomatically. Three patients (9%) underwent a second procedure due to residual LVOT gradient and symptoms. The mean LVOT gradient on long-term follow-up was 3 mm Hg at rest and 12 mm Hg with provocation. None of the patients had a decrease in ejection fraction at follow-up.

Lakkis et al[17] published a series of 33 patients treated with echocardiography-guided ASA. The mean preprocedure LVOT gradient was 49 mm Hg at rest and 96 mm Hg with dobutamine. The mean increase in CK was 1964 mg/dL after the procedure. At 6 weeks, the mean LVOT gradient was 9 mm Hg at rest and 24 mm

Hg with dobutamine. At 6 months, the mean LVOT gradient was 3 mm Hg at rest and 40 mm Hg with dobutamine. There was a significant improvement in New York Heart Association (NYHA) class in all patients after the procedure. In addition to subjective measures, exercise time was used as an objective measurement of clinical improvement before and after the procedure. The preprocedure exercise time was 286 seconds, and at 6 weeks postprocedure, the exercise time was 422 seconds. No patients died during the procedure or follow-up period.

Lakkis et al[18] reported 1-year outcome in a subsequent series of 50 patients. The mean LVOT gradient in these patients decreased from 74 mm Hg at baseline to 6 mm Hg at 1 year. Seven patients (14%) underwent more than one ASA procedure due to a significant residual gradient and symptoms. Six of these procedures were successful in reducing the residual gradient. One patient went on to surgical myectomy, which was successful in reducing the gradient. Nearly all patients reported improvement in symptoms based on NYHA class. The mean exercise time prior to the procedure was 271 seconds and improved to 407 seconds at follow-up. There was no change in ejection fraction as measured by echocardiogram at 1 year. There was a decrease in septal thickness from a mean of 2.1 cm before the procedure to 1.5 cm 1 year later, without any change noted in posterior wall thickness.

COMPLICATIONS

The most common complication of ASA is complete heart block (CHB) requiring permanent pacemaker insertion. In early series, this complication was very common and occurred in up to one third of patients.[19] With further refinements in the procedure and with slower injection of alcohol, the frequency of this complication has decreased dramatically. In a recent series, CHB requiring permanent pacemaker occurred in 6.7% of patients.[20] Several studies have looked at the electrocardiographic changes after ASA.[21,22] The most common change is induction of a right bundle branch block (RBBB), and this occurs in about two thirds of patients after the procedure. Because of this, patients with a preexisting left bundle branch block (LBBB) are at the highest risk of developing CHB because of the addition of a RBBB to a LBBB.

In younger patients, the coronary arteries are thin-walled and do not have any significant plaques. These arteries may have a higher risk of dissection or perforation. This makes coaxial guide catheter placement and careful advancement of guidewires important. Several series have reported young patients who had coronary dissections during the procedure.

Procedure-related death is rare and usually relates to coronary dissection or escape of alcohol to undesired areas of myocardium. Patients with HCM have an increased risk of sudden cardiac death. A recent study showed that the risk of sudden death increases with increasing LVOT gradient,[2] and although it stands to reason that decreasing the LVOT gradient by ASA might decrease this risk, this has not been definitively proven. The only therapy that has been proven to decrease the risk of sudden death to date is implantation of an ICD.[23] One should use the risk factors for sudden death prior to ASA to decide if an ICD is indicated. There is a theoretical concern that the creation of a septal scar with ASA will create an arrhythmogenic focus, but this has not been validated in the studies to date.

The risk of remote infarct is rare, but several case reports have described infarcts in the apex and papillary muscles. Therefore the injection of contrast into the septal artery, ensuring that there is no leakage of dye into the parent artery or through collaterals, is an essential step in the procedure. Also, the intraprocedure echocardiogram is essential for showing potential remote infarct areas during contrast injection before injection of alcohol. Although there has been one case report of a ventricular septal defect that occurred after ASA,[24] this seems to be a rare complication and has not been seen in any of the large series of patients reported.

CELLULAR AND MOLECULAR CHANGES AFTER ALCOHOL SEPTAL ABLATION

In addition to the decrease in gradient seen after ASA, other alterations in myocardial structure and function may help explain the dramatic improvement in symptoms in these patients. Patients with symptomatic obstructive HCM have altered diastolic function due to many mechanisms. Left ventricular end diastolic pressure is usually increased, and left ventricular ejection fraction is often augmented by mitral regurgitation. Nagueh et al[25] showed that 6 months after successful ASA, there was a decrease in left atrial size, reduction in mitral regurgitation volume, decrease in the left ventricular passive filling pressure (pre-A pressure), and an increase in passive filling volume as measured by echocardiography, all indicating improved diastolic function.

Regression of left ventricular hypertrophy has been demonstrated in patients after ASA and likely plays a role in improved diastolic function in these patients. Mazur et al[26] studied 26 patients who underwent NSRT at baseline, 1 year, and 2 years after the procedure. The left ventricular end-diastolic dimension increased significantly and the left ventricular end-systolic dimension similarly increased, whereas the ejection fraction did not change at 2 years. Echocardiographically calculated left ventricular mass decreased significantly (a mean left ventricular mass of 301 g at baseline that decreased to 223 g at 1 year and to 190 g at 2 years).

There are changes at the cellular and molecular level as well that may contribute to symptom improvement after ASA. Tumor necrosis factor-alpha (TNF-α) is a cytokine involved in myocardial hypertrophy and fibrosis. Collagen is present in the interstitial matrix surrounding myocytes, and specifically collagen I is known to be a very stiff form of collagen that contributes abnormal left ventricular stiffness. Nagueh et al[27] performed endomyocardial biopsies on 15 patients before and 6 weeks after ASA to compare TNF-α levels, collagen I levels, and myocyte size in these patients compared to normal controls. There was a significant reduction in the levels of TNF-α, myocyte size, and collagen I levels at 6 weeks postprocedure.

COMPARISON TO SURGERY

There are currently no randomized studies comparing ASA with surgical myectomy. Qin et al[28] reported an observational study of 25 patients treated with ASA and 26 treated with surgical myectomy, who were followed for 3 months. LVOT gradient decreased from 64 mm Hg to 24 mm Hg at follow-up in the ASA group and from 62 mm Hg to 11 mm Hg in the surgery group. Septal thickness and NYHA class decreased similarly in both groups. One limitation of this study was that the selected treatment was not randomized; therefore, patients who were older or had other comorbidities tended to be treated with ASA (mean age: 63 years), whereas younger patients with fewer concomitant illnesses tended to have surgical myectomy (mean age: 48 years). Another limitation is that the follow-up time was brief, so that no long-term conclusions can be drawn from this study.

In an attempt to alleviate bias associated with age, Nagueh et al[29] performed an age- and gradient-matched analysis of 41 patients who underwent ASA and 41 who underwent surgical myectomy. The mean age in both groups was 49 years. At 1 year, the mean LVOT gradient decreased from 76 mm Hg to 8 mm Hg in the ASA group and from 78 mm Hg to 4 mm Hg in the surgery group. NYHA class improved and the septal thickness decreased similarly in both groups. The mean exercise time improved from 289 to 417 seconds in the ASA group and from 330 to 480 seconds in the surgery group. One patient in the ASA group died after a coronary dissection during the procedure. No patients in the surgery group died. Nine patients in the ASA group (22%) and 1 patient in the surgery group (2.4%) required a permanent pacemaker due to CHB. In the ASA group, only 3 patients developed new aortic regurgitation, all of which were classified as mild. In the surgery group, 10 patients developed mild aortic regurgitation, and 1 patient developed moderate aortic regurgitation. No other major complications were noted in either group. Although this was not a randomized comparison of ASA and myectomy surgery, it showed that these 2 procedures have similar effectiveness at 1 year.

CONCLUSION

In the studies reported to date, ASA has been shown to be an effective procedure that improves symptoms in patients with obstructive HCM. A variety of hemodynamic, cellular, and molecular changes account for the effectiveness of this procedure, and the procedure has been favorably compared with surgical myectomy.

REFERENCES

1. Burch M, Blair E. The inheritance of hypertrophic cardiomyopathy. *Pediatr Cardiol.* 1999;20:331.
2. Maron MS, Olivotto I, Betochhi S, et al. Effect of left ventricular outflow tract obstruction on clinical outcome in hypertrophic cardiomyopathy. *N Engl J Med.* 2003;348:295.
3. Kizilbash AM, Heinle SK, Grayburn PA. Spontaneous variability of left ventricular outflow tract gradient in hypertrophic obstructive cardiomyopathy. *Circulation.* 1998;97:461.
4. Thompson DS, Naqvi N, Juul SM, et al. Effects of propranolol on myocardial oxygen consumption, substrate extraction, and hemodynamics in hypertrophic obstructive cardiomyopathy. *Br Heart J.* 1980;44:488.
5. Bonow RO, Dilsizian V, Rosing DR, et al. Verapamil-induced improvement in left ventricular diastolic filling and increased exercise tolerance in patients with hypertrophic cardiomyopathy. *Circulation.* 1985;72:853.
6. Pollick C. Muscular subaortic stenosis: hemodynamic and clinical improvement after disopyramide. *New Engl J Med.* 1982;307:997.
7. Fananapazir L, Epstein ND, Curiel RV, et al. Long-term results of dual chamber (DDD) pacing in obstructive hypertrophic cardiomyopathy: evidence for progressive symptomatic and hemodynamic improvement and reduction of left ventricular hypertrophy. *Circulation.* 1994;90:2731.
8. Jeanrenaud X, Goy JJ, Kappenberger L. Effects of dual-chamber pacing in hypertrophic obstructive cardiomyopathy. *Lancet.* 1992;339:1318.
9. Maron BJ, Nishimura RA, McKenna WJ, et al. Assessment of permanent dual-chamber pacing as a treatment for drug-refractory symptomatic patients with obstructive hypertrophic cardiomyopathy. A randomized, double-blinded, crossover study (M-PATHY). *Circulation.* 1999;99:2927.
10. Linde C, Gandler F, Kappenberger L, et al. Placebo effect of pacemaker implantation in obstructive hypertrophic cardiomyopathy. Pacing in cardiology (PIC) study group. *Am J Cardiol.* 1999;83:903.
11. Robbins RC, Stinson EB. Long-term results of left ventricular myotomy and myomectomy for obstructive hypertrophic cardiomyopathy. *J Thorac Cardiovasc Surg.* 1996;111:586.
12. McCully RB, Nishimura RA, Tajik AJ, et al. Extent of clinical improvement after surgical treatment of hypertrophic obstructive cardiomyopathy. *Circulation.* 1996;94:467.
13. Schulte HD, Borisov K, Gams E, et al. Management of symptomatic hypertrophic obstructive cardiomyopathy: long-term results after surgical therapy. *J Thorac Cardiovasc Surg.* 1999;47:213.
14. Sigwart U. Non-surgical myocardial reduction for hypertrophic obstructive cardiomyopathy. *Lancet.* 1995;346:211.
15. Seggewiss H, Gleichmann U, Faber L, et al. Percutaneous transluminal septal myocardial ablation in hypertrophic obstructive cardiomyopathy: acute results and 3-month follow-up in 25 patients. *J Am Coll Cardiol.* 1998;31:252.
16. Faber L, Meissner A, Ziemssen P, et al. Percutaneous transluminal septal myocardial ablation for hypertrophic obstructive cardiomyopathy: long-term follow-up of the first series of 25 patients. *Heart.* 2000;83:326.
17. Lakkis NM, Nagueh SF, Kleiman NS, et al. Echocardiography-guided ethanol septal reduction for hypertrophic obstructive cardiomyopathy. *Circulation.* 1998;98:1750.
18. Lakkis MN, Nagueh SF, Dunn JK, et al. Nonsurgical septal reduction therapy for hypertrophic obstructive cardiomyopathy: one-year follow-up. *J Am Coll Cardiol.* 2000;36:852.
19. Gietzen FH, Leuner CJ, Raute-Kreisen U, et al. Acute and long-term results after transcoronary ablation of septal hypertrophy (TASH). Catheter interventional treatment for hypertrophic obstructive cardiomyopathy. *Eur Heart J.* 1999; 20:1342.
20. Nielsen CD, Killip D, Spencer WH III. Nonsurgical septal reduction therapy for hypertrophic obstructive cardiomyopathy: results in 50 consecutive patients. *Clin Cardiol.* 2003;26:275.
21. Runquist LH, Nielsen CD, Killip D, et al. Electrocardiographic findings after alcohol septal ablation therapy for obstructive hypertrophic cardiomyopathy. *Am J Cardiol.* 2002;90:1020.
22. Qin JX, Shiota T, Lever HM, et al. Conduction system abnormalities in patients with obstructive hypertrophic cardiomyopathy following septal reduction interventions. *Am J Cardiol.* 2004;93:171.
23. Maron BJ, Shen WK, Link MS, et al. Efficacy of implantable cardioverter-defibrillator for the prevention of sudden death in patients with hypertrophic cardiomyopathy. *N Engl J Med.* 2000;342:365.
24. Aroney CN, Goh TH, Hourigan LA, et al. Ventricular septal rupture following nonsurgical septal reduction for hypertrophic cardiomyopathy: treatment with percutaneous closure. *Cathet Cardiovasc Intervent.* 2004;61:411.
25. Nagueh SF, Lakkis NM, Middleton KJ, et al. Changes in left ventricular filling and left atrial function six months after nonsurgical septal reduction therapy for hypertrophic obstructive cardiomyopathy. *J Am Coll Cardiol.* 1999; 34:1123.
26. Mazur W, Nagueh SF, Lakkis NM, et al. Regression of left ventricular hypertrophy after nonsurgical septal reduction therapy for hypertrophic obstructive cardiomyopathy. *Circulation.* 2001;103:1492.
27. Nagueh SF, Stetson SJ, Lakkis NM, et al. Decreased expression of tumor necrosis factor alpha and regression of hypertrophy after nonsurgical septal reduction therapy for patients with hypertrophic obstructive cardiomyopathy. *Circulation.* 2001;103:1844.
28. Qin JX, Shiota T, Lever HM, et al. Outcome of patients with hypertrophic obstructive cardiomyopathy after percutaneous transluminal septal myocardial ablation and septal myectomy surgery. *J Am Coll Cardiol.* 2001;38:1994.
29. Nagueh SF, Ommen SR, Lakkis NM, et al. Comparison of septal reduction therapy with surgical myectomy for the treatment of hypertrophic obstructive cardiomyopathy. *J Am Coll Cardiol.* 2001;38:1701.

CHAPTER (47)

Coronary Vein Device Insertion

Todd J. Brinton, MD, Ali Hassan, MD, and Alan C. Yeung, MD

Although there is extensive knowledge of the anatomy and physiology of the coronary artcrics and knowledge of the established impact of catheter- and surgery-based manipulation of this system, the coronary veins have been incompletely described and there is limited experience at manipulation. Not until the eighteenth century did anatomists and physiologists first establish the role of the coronary venous system.[1] The first human cannulation of the coronary sinus (CS) was not performed until 1947, but complications and poor outcomes quickly blunted further investigation.[2] However, the development of retroperfusion for circulatory support during cardiac surgery utilizing the coronary veins quickly accelerated past stagnating investigation. In the past 4 decades, methods for intermittent CS occlusion, retroperfusion of oxygenated blood, and retroinfusion of myocardially active substances have expanded to form the foundation for modern circulatory support.[3–6]

In the early 1960s, cardiologists began to perform percutaneous cannulation of the CS during electrophysiology studies and ablation of the left-sided bypass tracks.[7] Investigation of left-sided pacing and the placement of pacing leads via the CS and its tributaries has further expanded percutaneous cannulation procedures.[8] The combination of a left ventricular lead placed percutaneously through the CS and right ventricular lead has shown superiority to maximum medical management alone in patients with heart failure.[9] A recent trial has also demonstrated that right ventricle pacing alone in patients with a defibrillator for heart failure may be harmful.[10] Both of these trials have lead to more widespread use pacing via the CS. The increasing clinical indications and improvement in available technology have facilitated the development of new catheter systems with improved ease of sinus cannulation and improved targeting of lead placement.

Increasing utilization of the coronary veins for electrophysiologic applications has generated increasing enthusiasm for new therapies that may also use this conduit. The potential for using the venous conduit as an in vivo arterial bypass graft has been an exciting but challenging field of investigation. Percutaneous placement of devices for mitral valve disease due to the proximity of the coronary venous system to the valve apparatus has generated recent enthusiasm. However, the discovery of potent angiogenic biologic products along with more recent advances in our knowledge of the regenerative properties of pluripotent stem cells has fueled probably the most exciting potential application for the coronary venous system. The coronary venous route may serve as ideal conduit for potential therapeutic intervention due to the nature of this low-pressure conduit and resistance to the atherosclerotic process.

CORONARY VENOUS ANATOMY

The coronary venous system is an intricate network of meshlike venules and sinusoids, which lead to the larger veins to drain the arterial circulation of the heart. Much like the arterial circulation, a nomenclature for the venous system has been established (Figure 47-1). Approximately 75% of the arterial blood flow is drained via the CS, and the remaining amount is drained via non-CS routes (15%) or through the thebesian system (10%).[10] The thebesian system provides a direct conduit to the endocardial surface of the ventricle for venous drainage. The entire coronary venous system is contiguous with the coronary sinus in fewer than 11% of cases. In the remaining majority of cases, there is only incomplete drainage of the right ventricle via the CS.

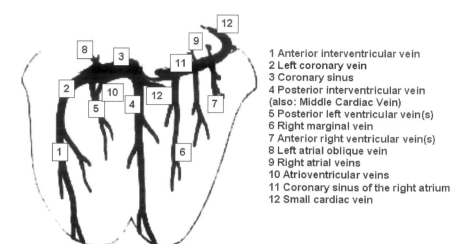

1 Anterior interventricular vein
2 Left coronary vein
3 Coronary sinus
4 Posterior interventricular vein
   (also: Middle Cardiac Vein)
5 Posterior left ventricular vein(s)
6 Right marginal vein
7 Anterior right ventricular vein(s)
8 Left atrial oblique vein
9 Right atrial veins
10 Atrioventricular veins
11 Coronary sinus of the right atrium
12 Small cardiac vein

FIGURE 47-1. Anatomic nomenclature of coronary veins.

The venous system parallels the arterial circulation but with flow directed in a retrograde direction. There is great variability in the distribution of the coronary venous anatomy from individual to individual, but major regions of the circulation are conserved. The left anterior descending artery is paralleled by the anterior interventricular vein (Figure 47-2). This vein drains the entire anterior region of the left ventricle and the anterior half of the septum. The left circumflex artery is paralleled by the great cardiac vein (GCV) and its tributaries. These provide venous drainage for the lateral region of the left ventricle. The proximal right coronary artery is paralleled by the small cardiac vein. The posterior interventricular vein, also called the middle cardiac vein, drains the posterior left

ventricle and posterior half of the septum, as well as segments of right ventricle in varying extents. It is usually paralleled by the posterior descending artery system, and it forms an anastomosis with the CS at an acute angle in the proximal region. The GCV forms the transition conduit between the anterior interventricular vein and CS. The posterior and marginal (lateral) veins exit the GCV at subacute angles on the lateral region of the left ventricle. In the minority of cases, where the CS is contiguous with the small cardiac vein, the right ventricle is drained directly by this conduit.

The entry port for the interventionalist is the orifice of the CS, which is positioned in the posterior medial aspect of the right atrium. The thebesian valve is present in the proximal region in the majority of cases. However, this valve is complete in only 30% of cases. The length of the sinus itself varies.[11] In an anatomical evaluation of 140 human hearts,[10] the CS was defined as moderate in length in 74% of the cases (20–60 mm), long in 18% of cases (60–82 mm), and short in 7% of cases (15–20 mm). The diameter ranged from 6 to 10 mm. The CS follows closely the peripheral curvature of the posterior leaflet of the mitral valve (Figure 47-3). However, in only 12% of the cases does the vein lie at the same elevation as the annulus fibrosis. The CS was found to be elevated (above the annulus fibrosis) by 3 mm in 16% of cases, 7 mm in 50% of cases, and 8 mm and higher in 22% of cases (Figure 47-4). The transition from the CS to the GCV is marked by the valve of Vieussenii. This valve is present in a large majority of cases. The valve is unicuspid in 62% of cases and bicuspid in 25% of cases.

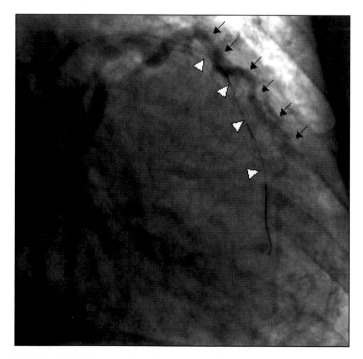

FIGURE 47-2. Topographical relationship between major veins and arteries of the heart, showing the topographical position of the anterior interventricular vein (*black arrows*) and a guidewire positioned in the left anterior descending artery (*white arrows*).

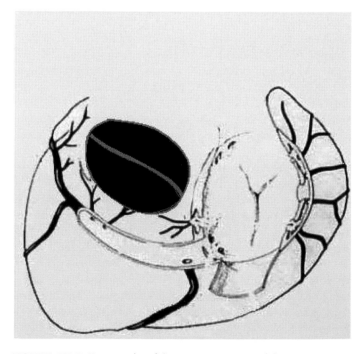

FIGURE 47-3. Topography of the coronary sinus and the posterior leaflet of the mitral valve.

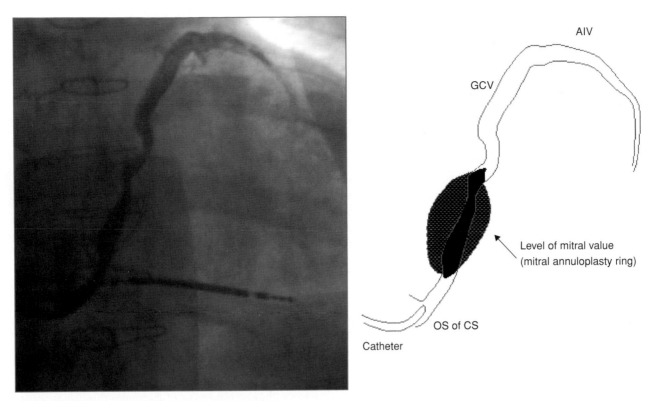

FIGURE 47-4. Topographical elevation of coronary sinus from the atrioventricular level. This retrograde coronary venogram in left anterior oblique projection shows the proximity of the coronary sinus (CS) and great cardiac vein (GCV) to the mitral valve (indicated by the opacity of a surgically implanted annuloplasty ring). In this case, the midportion of CS and proximal GCV show topographical elevation from the level of mitral valve. AIV = anterior interventricular vein; OS = ostium of the coronary sinus.

APPROACHES TO CORONARY SINUS ACCESS

There are two main components to performing interventions in the coronary venous system. The first technical challenge is localization of the CS and successful cannulation. The second challenge is navigation of the tortuous venous conduits and tributaries. The ability to accomplish both of these challenges ultimately determines whether a device can be localized to the targeted region.

The first technical challenge is localization of the CS. The sinus is usually located in the posterior medial fossa of the right atrium. However, congenital anomalies and pathologic modification of the atria structure may alter this anatomy. Although fluoroscopic images have traditionally been the mainstay for localizing the sinus, several new ultrasound technologies have been developed to assist in localization of the CS. Transesophageal echocardiography and intracardiac echocardiography have both been used successfully to assist in identifying the sinus orifice. The recent development of an optical catheter-based device that allows for visualization of the sinus through blood may represent a significant advancement for this technical challenge as well.

After the sinus has been localized, cannulation is modulated by several factors. The presence of a valve at the proximal sinus, although rare, is a critical factor in many failed procedures. This is also a likely the etiology for sinus dissections. Those proceduralists with coronary experience tend to utilize a guidewire to cannulate the ostium directly. Careful manipulation of the guidewire is an important factor for passing the valve, avoiding trauma and potential complications, and ultimately performing successful venous

intervention. We have found that despite interventionalists' familiarity with 0.014-in guidewires, a 0.035-in straight or angle-tip glidewire can be very useful for cannulation. An alternative method utilized by many electrophysiologists is the use of a traditional pacing catheter for cannulation. Either of these methods can lead to success. The angle of the sinus "takeoff" is likely the most important mitigating factor in the majority of cases. As previously mentioned, there is large variation in the position of the sinus and GCV in relation to the annulus fibrosis. Sometimes the sinus can take an acute superior turn, complicating cannulation. Although guide catheter and wire selection are important, the venous access point may influence the angle of approach to the sinus for improved cannulation success.

The coronary venous system can be accessed through three different percutaneous approaches. Due to the increased indications for left ventricular pacing, the left subclavian approach has become the most common entry for the CS intervention. This approach offers convenience, because the pacer or defibrillator pocket sits above the subclavian vein. However, the subclavian approach often positions the catheter on the opposite side of the atrium and can make reaching the sinus difficult, particularly in patients with a large atrium due to heart failure. A host of directable catheters has simplified this challenge. The femoral approach is likely the most familiar for interventional cardiologists. Entry through the femoral vein and approach to the sinus via the inferior vena cava positions the catheter superior to sinus. This can be challenging for the sinus with an acute "takeoff" but also advantageous for the sinus, which is parallel to the atrioventricular groove. Selection of catheter shapes such as Amplatz may facilitate cannulation from this position. Lastly, the internal jugular approach likely is the most advantageous, positioning the catheter in midatrium and facilitating cannulation for most variations of anatomical variation.

Navigation of the coronary venous system can also be challenging. Depending on the goals for venous intervention, such as placement of pacing leads versus positioning of a delivery catheter, the targeted region varies. The CS makes gradual caliber transitions into the GCV and then the anterior interventricular vein as it approaches the anterior wall of the heart. We prefer the previously mentioned 0.035-in straight or angle-tip guidewire for placement into the anterior interventricular vein. On the other hand, the lateral and posterior tributaries of the venous system often bifurcate into small branches that are difficult to cannulate even when using a 0.014-in guidewires. One of the greatest challenges for left ventricular pacing applications has been the ability to place the leads at the mid ventricle lateral wall for this same reason.

POTENTIAL PROBLEMS AND COMPLICATIONS

In patients with severe malformation of the right atrium due to congenital disease or longstanding right-sided heart failure, cannulation of the CS can be quite challenging. This is usually due to changes in the entry angle of the CS. Valvular obstruction can also add to the complexity of intervention. Although the thebesian valve is only complete in a minority of cases, traumatic wire injury to this region can be a source for sinus dissection. However, the valve of Vieussenii is a more common source for difficulty in catheter navigation and complications (Figure 47-5). Additionally, an intramural venous course or scarring due to a neighboring site

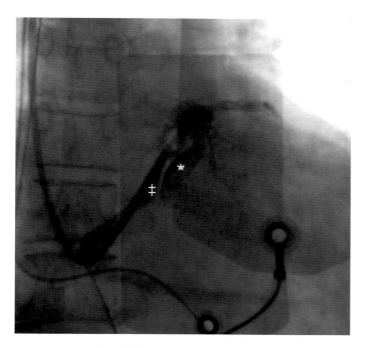

FIGURE 47-5. Valves of the coronary veins: anatomical considerations during catheterization of coronary sinus. This figure shows major dissection during catheterization of the coronary sinus. The dissection appears to have occurred at the position of the Vieussenii valve (transition between coronary sinus and great cardiac vein). A major contrast deposit (*) is seen, which tends to compress the lumen coronary sinus (‡).

of previous coronary artery intervention may also contribute to difficulty in navigating the venous conduit. Finally, coronary vein perforation, potentially leading to pericardial effusion or tamponade, may be a major area of concern.

CURRENT CORONARY VEIN APPLICATIONS

【 】 LEFT VENTRICULAR PACING APPLICATION

Cardiac resynchronization therapy (CRT) has become an important treatment modality for heart failure. Several studies have demonstrated the benefits of CRT on quality of life; 6-minute walking distance; New York Heart Association functional class; peak oxygen consumption and exercise treadmill time; favorable changes in cardiac structure and function[9,12,13]; and most recently, long-term mortality.[14] Left ventricular pacing is a critical component of CRT. Left ventricular pacing is performed epicardially but most commonly is accomplished using an endovascular approach. Based on studies using epicardial electrodes, the best hemodynamic response to left ventricular pacing is achieved through pacing in the midlateral or posterior left ventricle.[15] The challenge is to achieve optimal placement of electrodes through an endovascular approach.

Optimal left ventricular pacing is usually accomplished through placement of a lead in the lateral or posterior venous branches via the CS (Figure 47-6). However, these positions may cause diaphragmatic stimulation due to phrenic nerve stimulation. Often optimal hemodynamic positioning cannot be accomplished due to diaphragmatic stimulation, and the lead must be repositioned in a less desirable position. The development of new guide sheaths to cannulate the CS and leads to reach and stay within the venous branches have assisted in reaching optimal position for pacing with minimal side effects. The sheaths come in either a straight or angled tip to engage a range of CS anatomy. Two different types of lead systems have been designed; stylet-driven or guidewire-directed. The stylet-driven leads are characterized by a preformed tip that can be modified using the stylet such that it can negotiate and track along the tributaries in the CS. The guidewire-directed leads may be useful in reaching a more distal location for lead placement. Due to the risk of perforation, active screw-in fixation is undesirable; therefore, passive fixation systems have been developed using either a bend or spiral tip device.

Registry data are available on the success rate of several of the commercially available lead systems. A success rate of 90% to 93% has been noted with the Medtronic stylet-driven system. Implantation time ranged from 0.9 to 7.3 hours, with a dislodgement rate of 4% to 12%.[12,16,17] The Guidant lead system has demonstrated similar results with a success rate of 92%, an implantation time ranging from 0.9 to 8 hours, with a dislodgement rate of 2%.[18] Although serious complications are rare, they are not insignificant. The Multicenter Insync Randomized Clinical Evaluation (MIRACLE) trial noted 1 fatality due to hypotension from assumed tamponade. One additional patient required aggressive resuscitation following the procedure. Less serious complications included a 4% rate of CS dissection and 2% rate of venous perforation.[9]

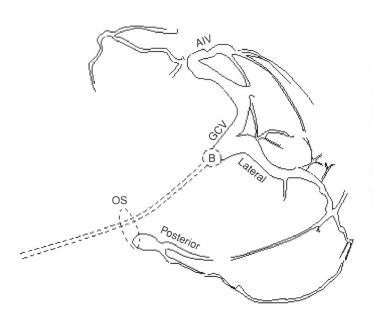

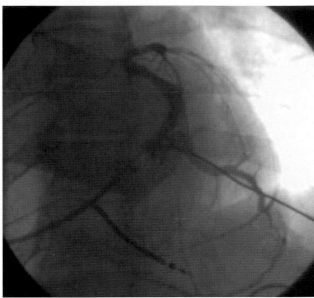

FIGURE 47-6. Veins of the lateral left ventricle. AIV = anterior interventricular vein; B = inflated Swan-Ganz balloon catheter; GCV = great cardiac vein; lateral = lateral vein of the left ventricle; posterior = posterior vein of the left ventricle; OS = ostium of the coronary sinus.

Despite the development of improved tools for placements and lead positioning, the inability to cannulate the CS due to pathologic anatomic anomalies is the most common cause of implant failure. The introduction of steerable guide catheters, improved lead delivery systems, and easier sheath removal systems will further improve implant success rates and further minimize complications. Areas of current development include multiple site left ventricle pacing and tools to assist in improving CS cannulation as well as the negotiation of the venous tributaries. We anticipate that CRT will continue to expand, resulting in greater needs for left ventricle lead placement expertise and technologies.

【 】 MITRAL VALVE APPLICATIONS

Mitral valve disease is a common medical problem. There are approximately 500,000 discharge diagnoses annually for mitral valve disease in the United States alone.[19] Surgical treatment for mitral valve disease approaches almost 40,000 cases annually worldwide.[20] However, this likely underrepresents the number of patients who could benefit from mitral valve treatments, because many patients are deemed nonsurgical due to comorbidities and others are likely too well for such an invasive strategy. In fact, most patients with a diagnosis of mitral regurgitation never need traditional surgical intervention.[21] Causes of mitral regurgitation include degenerative (20%–70%), ischemic (1%–30%), rheumatic (3%–40%, and infectious etiologies (10%–12%).[22] Current surgical options for treatment include valve replacement with or without preservation of the subvalvular apparatus and repair. Because morbidity and mortality rates of an open procedure as well a cost for such a hospitalization are not insignificant, an impetus for percutaneous methods has developed in recent years.

Several new catheter-based implant systems utilize the coronary venous system for device placement due to the close proximity to the curvature of the mitral valve annulus. These devices are designed to reshape the annulus and therefore improve leaflet coaptation for reduction of regurgitation. The ev3/Mitralife system is placed percutaneously through a 10-Fr delivery guide catheter into the CS and cinched around the annulus. Device feasibility has been tested both acutely and in chronic implantation for 180 days.[23] In the acute phase of the study, 11 C-cure devices were placed in 7 healthy 50- to 60-kg sheep. Using intracardiac echocardiography, the degree of actuation of the device was modified and results of valve function recorded. The effects of chronic implantation were evaluated in 8 healthy 55- to 60-kg pigs in which the C-cure device was used in the CS, resulting in a significant change in the mitral annular diameter (2.55 vs 1.83 cm; P = .004; 28% reduction in size). Importantly, follow-up angiography at 6 months demonstrated patent coronary arteries and sinus without evidence of thrombus, whereas echocardiography evaluation demonstrated no change in ventricular size or valve function.

Studies have also been performed to assess the feasibility of new percutaneous technologies within the CS in animal models of specific types of mitral regurgitation. The Viacor annuloplasty device is placed via a specialized 7-Fr delivery catheter to modify the septal lateral annular diameter. In a feasibility study of acute ischemic mitral regurgitation, 6 sheep were studied, and mitral regurgitation was reduced from 3–4+ to 0–1+ by a significant reduction in diameter (30 ± 2.1 mm vs 24 ± 1.7 mm; P < .03).[24] Similar results have also been demonstrated utilizing a different percutaneous mitral valve device in an animal model of functional mitral regurgitation. In a study of 12 dogs, the device that was placed via the CS reduced the mitral annular dimension and severity of regurgitation significantly 4 weeks after placement (MR jet/LA area: 26 ± 1%–7 ± 2%; P <.05).[25]

Results of early animal studies have been met with great enthusiasm. However, two major potential problem areas exist. First, the CS does not provide access to the anterior leaflet. Second, as previously described, the course of the CS in the majority of cases is above the atrioventricular groove. Both of these anatomic challenges may limit the potential applicability of these devices for clinical use. These concerns aside, further animal experiments as well as early human trials of the devices are underway.

Additionally, combination devices that address pacing technologies with mitral valve treatments are currently in development.

[ ] VENOUS DELIVERY METHODS

The coronary venous system is a complex network that has great anatomic variation, much like the veins in other areas of the body. In addition, the physiology of this system is extremely sophisticated. Widespread application of coronary venous delivery for myocardial treatment has been limited because of features such as the complexity of venous drainage, significant differences in microvascular flow, anastomoses between the arterial and venous systems, and the variable effects of cardiac cycle on venous flow.[26] However, recent technical advances have been made to mediate these complexities in order to facilitate use of the coronary venous system as a conduit for biologic therapeutic delivery.

Simple injection of products into the venous system has resulted in poor efficiency of delivery. This was originally tested using radionuclide-labeled 15-μm microspheres. Simple low-pressure injection into the coronary venous system of ischemic canine hearts demonstrated that 95% of the material bypassed the intramyocardial microcirculation to directly enter the right heart chamber.[26] Backflow into the CS, venovenous collateral washout, and drainage through the thebesian system all are the likely contributors to poor efficiency. Efforts to evaluate the potential benefit of coronary venous occlusion has included a study of coronary vein hemodynamics during delivery. Occlusion within the GCV during infusion resulted in an increase of systolic and diastolic pressure in the GCV from $7 \pm 3/1 \pm 0.6$ to $29 \pm 11/5 \pm 3$ mm Hg. Occlusion of the distal anterior interventricular vein (AIV) resulted in increases in mean pressure within the proximal AIV from 17 ± 6 to 28 ± 9 mm Hg without significant changes in mean arterial pressure, left ventricular end-diastolic pressure (LVEDP), or coronary wedge pressure.[27] Importantly, coronary blood flow is not compromised during venous occlusion. No significant hemodynamic changes, including LVEDP or coronary blood flow, within the left anterior descending artery were observed during balloon tip catheter occlusion of the distal AIV in a porcine study.[28]

Pressurized retroinfusion can be used to augment delivery by overcoming the pressure for drainage. This can cause not only flow reversal but also disruption of small venous plexuses without trauma to larger, more critical, venous branches.[29] Extravasation through the small channels results in direct exposure to the interstitium and cardiomyocytes. Investigation of the effects of retroperfusion in the AIV in ischemic pigs demonstrated that regional myocardial function increased linearly with increasing retroperfusion flow rates up to 200% that of arterial flow.[30] Maximum intraluminal AIV pressure was 132 ± 57 mm Hg.

Single "high"-pressure retroinfusion into a branch of the coronary venous system may be a very effective mode of delivery. Early studies utilizing an occlusion balloon for selective branch delivery with a delivery rate of 0.5 to 1.0 mL/sec, equating to intraluminal pressures of 100 to 200 mm Hg, demonstrated that delivery of radiographic contrast selectively infiltrates targeted myocardial regions.[31] Videodensitometric analysis demonstrated that contrast persisted for up to 30 minutes. In a study of fibroblast growth factor-2 (FGF-2) delivery in a chronic ischemic pig model for angiogenesis, AIV delivery with selective proximal balloon occlusion demonstrated higher retention values of FGF-2 within the left ventricle at 1-hour postdelivery compared to the same amount of protein delivered through the intracoronary route (1.3 vs 0.82 μg).[32]

Application of this same delivery modality for cell transplant has also yielded interesting results. In a study comparing endomyocardial catheter-based delivery and retrograde venous delivery using a single "high"-pressure injection into the AIV with proximal occlusion, both methods demonstrated successful transplantation of fibroblasts in a porcine infarct model at 21 days ($17.3 \pm 24.3\%$ vs $15.7 \pm 11.6\%$). However, the distribution pattern was quite different. Percutaneous endocardial delivery demonstrated 96% of fibroblasts localized to the endocardial surface in satellite regions within the anterior septal ventricle. Retrograde venous delivery demonstrated 60% of fibroblasts within the endocardial half and a more homogeneous delivery throughout the anterior septal and lateral territories.[33]

Although proximal occlusion has been demonstrated to improve delivery hemodynamics and therefore augment effective delivery, venovenous channels remain a challenge for improved efficacy of delivery. The development of a novel double (proximal and distal) balloon occlusion system that minimizes venovenous collateral "washout" should minimize this factor. We are currently focusing ongoing work on optimizing delivery mechanics for maximum venule disruption and maximum delivery of biological product or cell transplantation without larger vessel injury. This will continue to be an ongoing area of investigation for our group in therapeutic treatments of the diseased heart.

In an effort to combat the effects of myocardial contraction with each cardiac cycle on venous blood flow, a system was developed to augment retroperfusion during diastole.[34] The electrocardiogram-synchronized, gas-actuated pump injects perfusate through a balloon catheter. When positioned in the drainage area of an ischemic territory, the approach demonstrated localization of delivery material to the ischemic area with a 3-fold higher content than that of nonischemic territories.[35] Recently, this method has been utilized to promote myocardial gene transfer in animal models.[36] Selective retrograde gene delivery into the anterior cardiac vein during brief ischemia substantially increased reporter gene expression in the targeted left anterior descending artery territory when compared to percutaneous transluminal gene delivery in the coronary artery. When compared to both surgical and percutaneous intramyocardial delivery, selective pressure-regulated gene delivery has demonstrated a substantial increase and more homogenous reporter gene expression in the targeted left anterior descending artery territory.[37] This same method has been utilized to delivery liposomes containing NFkappaB decoy oligonucleotides to minimize reperfusion injury in animal models.[38] In an animal model of chronic ischemia, selective pressure-regulated retroinfusion of FGF-2 was superior to antegrade infusion for regional myocardial function and blood flow.[39] The animal study concluded that in chronic ischemia, selective pressure-regulated retroinfusion increased tissue binding of FGF-2 and enhanced functionally relevant collateral perfusion compared to antegrade delivery.

The introduction of a new method that combines both suction and retroinfusion for selective coronary venous applications has demonstrated significant preservation of myocardial function and further augmentation of oxygen tension when compared to synchronized retroinfusion alone in animal models.[40] This method has been utilized in human studies for protection against ischemia in normal and high-risk percutaneous transluminal coronary angioplasty (PTCA).[41] The results of a recent prospective randomized study that compared outcomes from patients undergoing high-risk PTCA with synchronized selective suction and retroinfusion of oxygenated blood and bypass surgery demonstrated similar outcomes for 28-day and 1-year mortality outcomes. However, event-free survival was higher in the bypass group (71.4 vs 52.3, $P = .2$) due to lower rates of target lesion revascularization, but the percutaneous group compared favorably for length of hospital stay and overall cost.[42]

In contrast to pressurized perfusion methods, delivery of biologic products can be delivered utilizing a needle-based system within the coronary venous circulation. The technology was originally designed to address the need for nonsurgical means of arterial bypass.[43,44] In that application, the catheter-based system was utilized to arterialize the anterior cardiac vein. The phased-array ultrasound imaging system with extending nitinol needle formed a fistula between the proximal portion of the occluded artery and coronary vein. Blockage of the distal cardiac vein provided retroperfusion of the anterior wall. The combination of this technology platform with a microinfusion needle has been utilized to deliver biologic products. In a recent study, the device demonstrated the ability to deliver bone marrow–derived cells to the anterior, lateral, septal, apical, and inferior walls through the anterior interventricular vein without complications.[45] The method and technology appear very promising and have led to the planning of several new trials.

REFERENCES

1. Thebesius A. De circulo sanguines in corde. Leiden, 1708.
2. Beck CS. Revascularization of the heart. *Surgery*. 1949;82.
3. Farcot JC, Meerbaum S, Lang TW, et al. Synchronized retroperfusion of coronary veins for circulatory support of jeopardized ischemic myocardium. *Am J Cardiol*. 1978;41:1191.
4. Meerbaum S. Coronary venous retroperfusion delivery of treatment to ischemic myocardium. *Herz*. 1986;11:41.
5. Mohl W. The momentum of coronary sinus interventions clinically. *Circulation*. 1988;77:6.
6. Mohl W. The relevance of coronary sinus interventions in cardiac surgery. *Thorac Cardiovasc Surg*. 1991;39:245.
7. Gabriele OF. Pacing via coronary sinus. *N Engl J Med*. 1969;280:219.
8. Hunt D, Sloman G. Long-term electrode catheter pacing from coronary sinus. *BMJ*. 1968;4:495.
9. Bristow MR, Saxon LA, Boehmer J, et al. Cardiac-resynchronization therapy with or without an implantable defibrillator. In: Advanced Chronic Heart Failure. *N Engl J Med*. 2004;350:2140.
10. Wilkoff BL, Cook JR, Epstein AE, et al. Dual Chamber and VVI Implantable Defibrillator Trial Investigators. Dual-chamber pacing or ventricular backup pacing in patients with an implantable defibrillator: the Dual Chamber and VVI Implantable Defibrillator (DAVID) Trial. *JAMA*. 2002;288:3115.
11. Mohl W, Wolner E, Glogar D, eds. *Coronary Sinus*. Darmstadt, Germany: Steinkopff Verlag; 1984.
12. Abraham, WT, Fisher WG, Smith AL, et al. Cardiac resynchronization in chronic heart failure. *N Engl J Med*. 2002;346:1845.
13. Auricchio A, Stellbrink C, Block M, et al. Effects of pacing chamber and atrioventricular delay on acute systolic function of paced patients with congestive heart failure. The Pacing Therapies for Congestive Heart Failure Study Group. The Guidant Congestive Heart Failure Study Group. *Circulation*. 1999;99:2993.
14. Cleland JGF, Daubert J, Erdmann E, et al. The effect of cardiac resynchronization on morbidity and mortality. *N Engl J Med*. 2005;352:1539.
15. Auricchio A, Stellbrink C, Sacks S, et al. The pacing therapies for congestive heart failure (PATH-CHF) study: Rationale, design, and endpoints of a prospective randomized multicenter study. *Am J Cardiol*. 1999;83:130D.
16. Cazeau S, Leclercq C, Lavergne T, et al. Effects of multisite biventricular pacing in patients with heart failure and intraventricular conduction delay. *N Engl J Med*. 2001;344:873.
17. Gras D, Leclercq C, Tang AS, et al. Cardiac resynchronization therapy in advanced heart failure the multicenter Insync clinical study. *Eur J Heart Failure*. 2002;4:311.
18. Purerfellner H, Nesser HJ, Winter S, et al. Transvenous left ventricular lead implantation with the EASYTRACK lead system; The European experience. *Am J Cardiol*. 2000;86:K157.
19. Remadi JP, Bizouarn P, Baron O, et al. Mitral valve replacement with the St. Jude Medical prosthesis: a 15-year follow-up. *Ann Thorac Surg*. 1998;66:762.
20. Condado JA, Velez-Gimon M. Catheter-based approach to mitral regurgitation. *J Intervent Cardiol*. 2003;16:523.
21. Otto C. Evaluation and management of chronic mitral regurgitation. *N Engl J Med*. 2001;345:740.
22. Olson LJ, Subramanian R, Ackermann, et al. Surgical pathology of the mitral valve: a study of 712 cases spanning 21 years. *Mayo Clin Proc*. 1987;62:22.
23. Bailey LR, Luna-Guerra J, Sheahan B, et al. A percutaneous approach for the treatment of mitral regurgitation evaluated in the healthy bovine model. *Am J Cardiol*. 2002;90:39H.
24. Liddicoat JR, Mac Neill BD, Gillinov AM, et al. Percutaneous mitral valve repair: a feasibility study in an ovine model of acute ischemic mitral regurgitation. *Cathet Cardiovasc Intervent*. 2003;60:410.
25. Maniu CV, Patel JB, Reuter DG, et al. Acute and chronic reduction of mitral regurgitation in experimental heart failure by percutaneous mitral annuloplasty. *J Am Coll Cardiol*. 2004;44:1652.
26. Villanueva FS, Spotnitz WD, Glasheen WP, et al. Insights into the physiology of retrograde cardioplegia delivery. *Am J Physiol*. 1995;268(4 pt 2):1555.
27. Punzengruber C, Maurer G, Chang BL, et al. Factors affecting penetration of coronary venous injections into normal and ischemic canine myocardium: assessment by contrast echocardiography and digital angiography. *Basic Res Cardiol*. 1990;85:21.
28. Rezaee M, Herity N, Lo S, et al. Therapeutic angiogenesis by selective delivery of basic FGF in the anterior ventricular vein. *J Am Coll Cardiol*. 2001;37:47A.
29. Rezaee M, Price EK, Fitzgerald PJ, et al. The vast potential of the coronary venous system for drug and biological interventions. In: Kipshidze NN, Serruys PW, eds. *Handbook of Cardiovascular Cell Transplantation*. London, England: Martin Dunitz; 2004:323.
30. Oh BH, Volpini M, Kambayashi M, et al. Myocardial function and transmural blood flow during coronary venous retroperfusion in pigs. *Circulation*. 1992;86:1265.
31. Herity NA, Lo ST, Oei F, et al. Selective regional myocardial infiltration by the percutaneous coronary venous route: a novel technique for local drug delivery. *Cathet Cardiovasc Intervent*. 2000;51:358.
32. Fearon WF, Ikeno F, Bailey LR, et al. Evaluation of High Pressure Retrograde Coronary Venous Delivery of FGF-2 Protein. *Cathet Cardiovasc Intervent*. 2004;61:422.
33. Price ET, Ikeno F, Fenn RC, et al. Percutaneous endocardial versus selective coronary venous cellular delivery: comparison of transplant efficiency, distribution, and efficacy in reducing infarct size and improving myocardial function. *J Am Coll Cardiol*. 41;suppl A.
34. Farcot JC, Barry M, Bourdarias JP, et al. New catheter-pump system for diastolic synchronized coronary sinus retroperfusion. *Med Prog Technol*. 1980;8:29.
35. Chang BL, Drury JK, Meerbaum S, et al. Enhanced myocardial washout and retrograde blood delivery with synchronized retroperfusion during acute myocardial ischemia. *J Am Coll Cardiol*. 1987;9:1091.
36. Boekstegers P, Von Degenfeld G, Giehrl W, et al. Myocardial gene transfer by selective pressure-regulated retroinfusion of coronary veins. *Gene Ther*. 2000;7:232.
37. Raake P, Von Degenfeld G, Hinkel R, et al. Myocardial gene transfer by selective pressure-regulated retroinfusion of coronary veins: comparison with surgical and percutaneous intramyocardial gene delivery. *J Am Coll Cardiol*. 2004;44:1124.
38. Kupatt C, Wichels R, Deiss M, et al. Retroinfusion of NfkappaB decoy oligonucleotide extends cardioprotection achieved by CD18 inhibition in a preclinical study of myocardial ischemia and retroinfusion in pigs. *Gene Ther*. 2002;98:518.39.
39. Von Degenfeld G, Raake P, Kupatt C, et al. Selective pressure-regulated retroinfusion of fibroblast growth factor-2 into the coronary vein enhances myocardial blood flow and function in pigs with chronic myocardial ischemia. *J Am Coll Cardiol*. 2003;42:1120.

40. Boekstegers P, Peter W, Von Degenfield G, et al. Preservation of regional myocardial function and myocardial oxygen tension during acute ischemia in pigs: comparison of selective synchronized suction and retroinfusion of coronary veins to synchronized coronary venous retroinfusion. *J Am Coll Cardiol.* 1994;23:459.

41. Boekstegers P, Giehrl W, Von Degenfeld G, et al. Selective suction and pressure-regulated retroinfusion: an effective and safe approach to retrograde protection against myocardial ischemia in patients undergoing normal and high risk percutaneous transluminal coronary angioplasty. *J Am Coll Cardiol.* 1998;31:1525.

42. Pohl T, Giehrl W, Reichart B, et al. Retroinfusion supported stenting in high-risk patients for percutaneous intervention and bypass surgery: results of the prospective randomized myoprotect I study. *Cathet Cardiovasc Intervent.* 2004;62:323.

43. Fitzgerald PJ, Hayase M, Yeung AC, et al. New approaches and conduits: in situ venous arterialization and coronary artery bypass. *Curr Intervent Cardiol Rep.* 1999;1:127.

44. Oesterle SN, Reifart N, Hauptmann E et al. Percutaneous in situ coronary venous arterialization: report of the first human catheter-based coronary artery bypass. *Circulation.* 2001;103:2539.

45. Thompson CA, Nasseri BA, Makower J, et al. Percutaneous transvenous cellular cardiomyoplasty. A novel non-surgical approach for myocardial cell transplantation. *J Am Coll Cardiol.* 2003;41:1964.

CHAPTER (48)

Device Retrieval Systems

Daniel Y. Sze, MD, PhD

CLINICAL BACKGROUND AND HISTORY

Interventionalists are skilled at and comfortable with placing devices permanently into the vascular system. Occasionally, and fortunately, rarely, devices need to be removed from the vascular system. Safe removal of intravascular foreign bodies often requires even more skill and ingenuity than deploying devices. The tools available for such specialized procedures are few and relatively low-technology, but clever use of these tools is consistently successful.

A variety of different unwanted foreign bodies may be found in the vascular system. The most commonly retrieved include catheter fragments, broken or embolized guidewires, misplaced stents and embolization coils, temporary inferior vena cava filters, and the occasional bullet. Many of these are discovered incidentally on radiographs or other imaging studies, but a few may be recognized as acute events, sometimes causing substantial symptoms such as ischemia, infection, or dysrhythmias.

The first reports of percutaneous foreign body retrieval from the vascular system emerged 40 years ago.[1-4] Most of these early practitioners improvised tools from existing guidewires and catheters, most of which were custom-shaped by hand using steam or a Bunsen burner. Modern commercially available devices are recognizable as specially shaped variations of these improvised catheter and wire systems. These devices include snares, baskets, forceps, and balloons.

DEVICES

【 】 SNARES

The simplest improvised retrieval device is the guidewire loop snare. Originally, this configuration was improvised by doubling over a guidewire and inserting the loop through a catheter so that the knuckle emerging from the catheter functioned as a lasso, and some commercially available snares are simply prefabricated versions of this design (Figure 48-1A). Specialized variations of this device include the Amplatz gooseneck snare (ev3, Plymouth, MN), the 3-loop EnSnare (MDTech, Gainesville, FL), and the ExPro (Radius Medical, Maynard, MA). The Amplatz gooseneck snare (Figure 48-1B) consists of a nitinol guidewire with a circular loop fixed to the tip at a right angle to the axis of the wire. The loop itself consists of braided nitinol wire for flexibility, with a gold-plated tungsten wire braided into the loop for radiopacity. These are available in various loop diameters from 5 to 35 mm. The smallest snares are used with a 4-Fr catheter, and the larger ones are used with a 6-Fr catheter; each has a radiopaque band to mark the tip. The EnSnare (Figure 48-1C) consists of 3 loops, each oriented 120° from the other to form a flower-shaped composite loop. These are also used with a 6-Fr radiopaque-tipped catheter and are available in diameters up to 45 mm. Other variations include low-profile snares such as the ExPro (Figure 48-1D), which is available in loop diameters of 5 to 35 mm but fits into a 3-Fr catheter, the equivalent of a 0.035-in guidewire.

【 】 BASKETS

A variation of the loop snare is the basket. These devices are frequently used by interventionalists, gastroenterologists, and urologists to capture calculi in the gastrointestinal, biliary, and urinary systems. Multiple wires are oriented and attached into an ellipsoidal cage with side openings. The size of these apertures can be adjusted in situ by pressure against the tip of the basket, similar to the opening of a coin purse or of a split bamboo tiki lamp. The basket may consist of 3 to 8 wires and the wires may be straight (Figure 48-1E) or spiral (Figure 48-1F). Loop snares and baskets share the characteristic of being able to trap a foreign body by filling the entire cross-section of a vessel, forcing the foreign body into the capture area of the device. Baskets are available as free-standing (Dotter Retriever, Cook) or over-the-wire (Segura, Boston Scientific) configurations and go through guiding catheters as small as 3-Fr (In-Time, Target/Boston Scientific). Both snares and baskets are also being developed specifically to retrieve discrete clots to treat stroke and other thromboembolic diseases.

【 】 FORCEPS

Other devices available include variations of the open mouth biopsy forceps. For foreign body retrieval, the jaws of the forceps are required not to cut tissue with sharp edges but rather to grasp an object with dull, atraumatic edges. Forceps may incorporate a

cable-and-hinge mechanism to open and close, or be a springy open jaw that closes by advancement of a catheter over the open mouth. Some may have three or more barbed jaws that appose when constrained by a catheter (Figure 48-1G). Obviously, these devices need to be used with great caution to avoid injury to the vessel wall.

【 】 MISCELLANEOUS DEVICES

Lastly, standard diagnostic and interventional tools such as pre-shaped catheters, guidewires, tip-deflecting wires, and angioplasty balloons may also be useful, particularly to displace the foreign body from a relatively inaccessible location and position to one where a snare, basket, or forceps can be used effectively. Pigtail

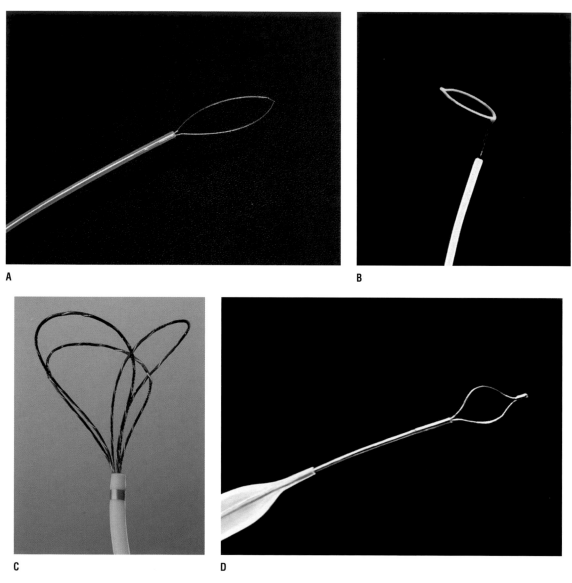

A

B

C

D

FIGURE 48-1. Commercially available devices for device retrieval. **(A)** Wire loop snare, consisting of a guidewire folded and inserted into a guiding catheter. Prefabricated snares usually include a handle to enable one-handed operation. **(B)** Amplatz gooseneck snare, with the snare oriented at 90° to the shaft. **(C)** EnSnare 3-loop snare. **(D)** ExPro microsnare, which fits through standard 0.035-in lumen diagnostic catheters. **(E)** Retrieval basket, designed to retrieve urinary and biliary stones but also useful in the vascular system. **(F)** Spiral basket, which may capture objects more effectively as it is advanced or retracted within a vessel. **(G)** Three-prong forceps, which grasps when the outer catheter is advanced over the tines.

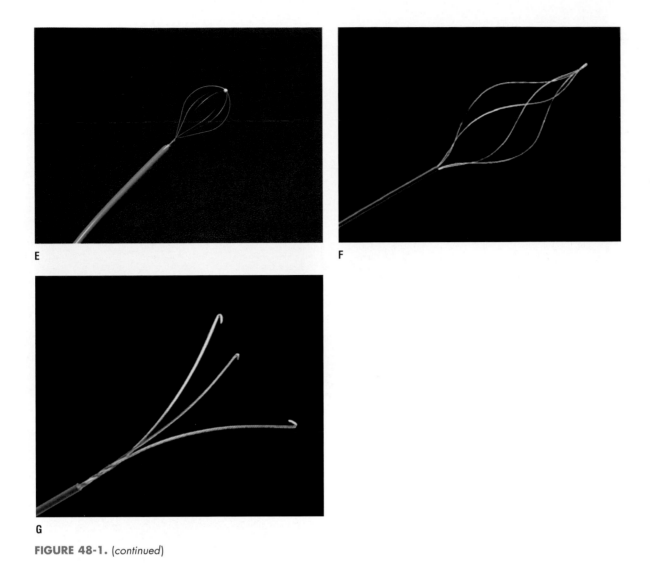

E

F

G

FIGURE 48-1. (continued)

catheters, often stiffened with a tip-deflecting wire (Cook), for instance, can catch the middle of a catheter or wire fragment and help pull the fragment out of a wedged position. Likewise, angioplasty balloons can be used to sweep an object down the lumen of a vessel, or occasionally can be inflated inside a hollow foreign body to capture it.

TECHNIQUES

[ ] SNARING FREE EMBOLIZED CATHETER FRAGMENTS

The use of snares and other devices can be straightforward. Figure 48-2 shows a typical scenario of a female patient after mastectomy for breast cancer who had a ported catheter implanted via the left subclavian vein. After months of use, blood could no longer be withdrawn from the port, and infusion of chemotherapy caused searing pain in the clavicular area. A chest x-ray clearly depicted the catheter fractured at the thoracic inlet from "pinch-off" syn-

drome,[5] and embolization of the fragment into the right pulmonary artery. A pulmonary angiography pigtail catheter (Grollman, Cook, or any flow-directed balloon catheter) was used from a femoral access to traverse the right atrium and right ventricle into the pulmonary artery. The catheter was exchanged over a guidewire for a gooseneck snare, which captured the free end of the fragment. The fragment was then pulled through the heart into the right femoral venous sheath and removed. The sheath size used must be large enough to accommodate the fragment, which is often removed in a doubled-over configuration. Pinch-off syndrome catheter fragments can be avoided by using the right internal jugular vein for access or by performing subclavian venotomy lateral to the thoracic inlet at the time of catheter insertion.

[ ] SNARING FRAGMENTS STILL ON A GUIDEWIRE

When a catheter fragmentation occurs during a procedure, the fragment may still be traversed by the guidewire. Rupture and fragmentation of angioplasty balloon is a typical example of such a situation. The fragment's attachment to the guidewire can be

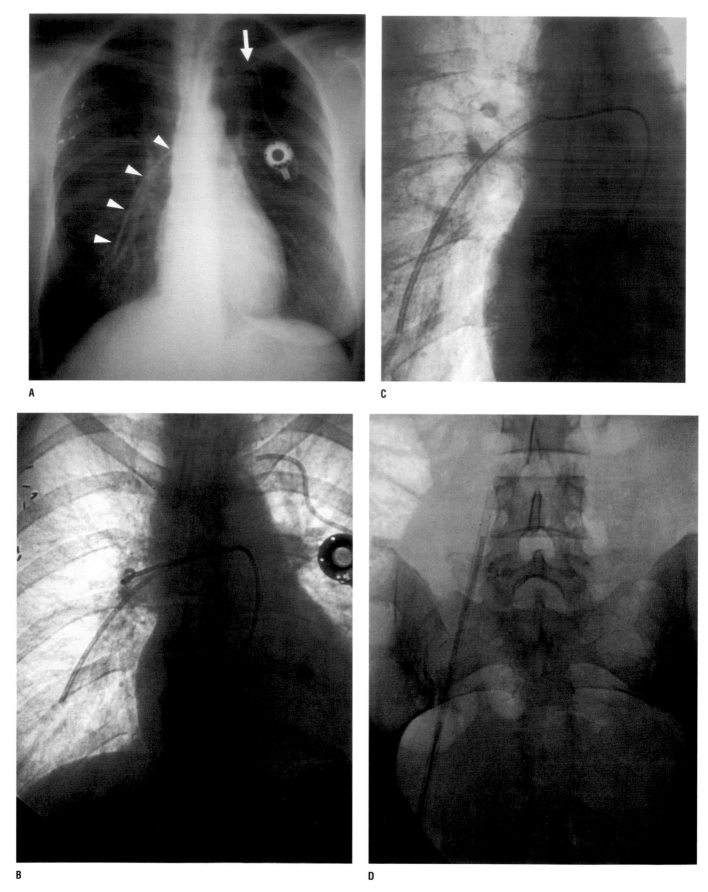

FIGURE 48-2. Retrieval of a venous access catheter fragment. (**A**) Chest x-ray of a woman status post-right mastectomy and nodal dissection. Left subclavian vein ported catheter was inserted with the venotomy at the thoracic inlet (*arrow*). After months of use, blood could no longer be drawn and chemotherapy could no longer be infused due to fracture of the catheter. The fragment migrated into the right pulmonary artery (*arrowheads*). (**B**) A pulmonary artery catheter was used to select the right pulmonary artery. (**C**) The catheter was exchanged over a guidewire for a gooseneck snare, which was able to capture the free end of the fragment. (**D**) The fragment was pulled into the groin sheath and removed.

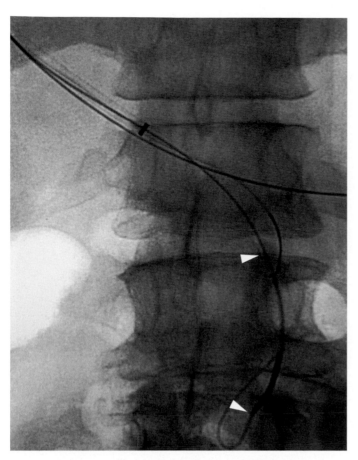

FIGURE 48-3. Catheter fragment on a guidewire. The tip of an angiography catheter was sheared off while still on a guidewire in the portal vein (*between arrowheads*). After upsizing the sheath to 11-Fr, a gooseneck snare was passed over the guidewire to capture the fragment.

exploited by passing the loop snare coaxially over the guidewire and thus over the fragment, allowing removal of the fragment and preservation of access to the target vessel (Figure 48-3).

DISLODGING WEDGED FRAGMENTS

Pigtail and Tip-deflecting Wire

Frequently, multiple tools and techniques are necessary to retrieve a foreign body. Figure 48-4 shows a typical wedged position of another catheter fragment. Initial attempts to snare the fragment were unsuccessful because neither end was free-floating; the distal end was wedged in a pulmonary artery branch and the proximal end was lodged in the wall of the main pulmonary artery. After gaining access to the pulmonary artery, a pigtail catheter was hooked around the middle of the fragment and stiffened with a 1-cm radius tip-deflecting wire (Cook), allowing the fragment to be dragged into the right atrium, where its tips were in the superior and inferior vena cavae. The fragment was then retrieved using a snare.

Braiding Maneuver

Another method to displace a fragment from a lodged position is by wrapping a catheter around the fragment using the "braiding"

maneuver (Figure 48-5).[6] A preshaped catheter such as a pigtail is positioned parallel to the fragment and rotated until the 2 intertwine like a caduceus. The fragment can then be pulled out of the lodged position into a more favorable vessel, where it can be removed with a snare.

LARIAT

Occasionally, the fragment is too stiff or too wedged to be moved by these techniques. Most fragments have at least 2 ends, and if one is inaccessible to retrieval tools, the other end may be targeted. This may require selective catheterization to gain a favorable angle of attack (Figure 48-6). The lower profile snares may be used through standard diagnostic catheters, but care must be taken to avoid damaging the unreinforced tip of such a catheter to avoid snare malfunction and/or damage to the vessel.

SECONDARY LOOP SNARE

Some foreign bodies may be so inaccessible that no commercially available device can be looped around them. However, if a standard guidewire such as a steerable hydrophilic wire (Glidewire, Terumo/Boston Scientific) can be passed around or through the target, the other end of the guidewire can then be captured with a snare, transforming the guidewire itself into a large snare.

SPECIAL CIRCUMSTANCES

PACEMAKER AND IMPLANTABLE CARDIAC DEFIBRILLATOR LEADS

Special circumstances arise in the cases of pacemaker and implantable cardiac defibrillator leads.[7] The shafts of these leads become encased and imbedded in a "fibrin sheath," which is usually composed of collagen and smooth muscle cells. The sheath may be extremely tenacious and may require the use of stiff guiding sheaths to be peeled off the lead, or in the most difficult cases, excimer laser disruption (Spectranetics). Leads may be very elastic, and manipulation to gain maximum mechanical advantage near the cardiac wall fixation site is frequently necessary to remove the lead successfully without further fragmenting the lead or everting the cardiac chamber (Figure 48-7).

INFERIOR VENA CAVA FILTERS

Finally, removable inferior vena cava filters have become commercially available in the past few years and frequently require the use of retrieval devices (Figure 48-8). Long-term implantation of these filters incurs the risk of complete caval thrombosis, a debilitating and sometimes life-threatening situation. When medically advisable, these new generation filters should be removed when they are no longer needed. The Gunther Tulip filter (Cook) requires snaring of the retrieval hook from above to secure the device, to collapse its legs, and to pull it into a sheath. Similarly, the Optease (Cordis/J&J) features a retrieval hook on the caudal end for removal from femoral access. The Recovery (Bard Peripheral

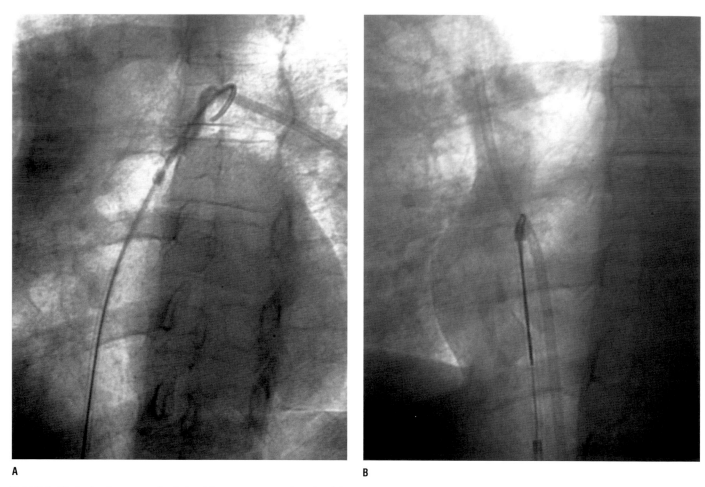

A

B

FIGURE 48-4. Displacement of a lodged fragment. **(A)** Both ends of this Hickman catheter fragment were inaccessible to a snare, so the shaft of the fragment was hooked with a pigtail catheter stiffened with a tip-deflecting guidewire. **(B)** After dragging the fragment into the right atrium, a free end was captured using a 3-loop snare.

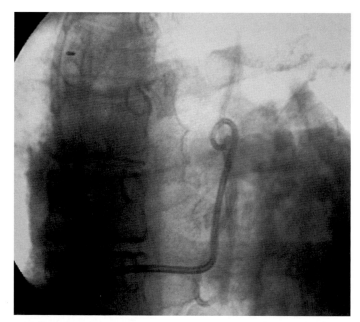

FIGURE 48-5. Braiding technique. A catheter fragment wedged into a pulmonary artery was dragged into a more accessible location by twirling a Grollman catheter next to it, entangling the fragment.

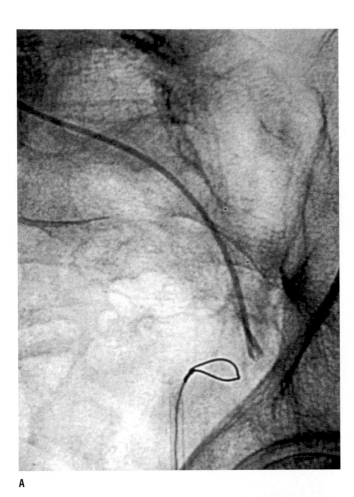

A

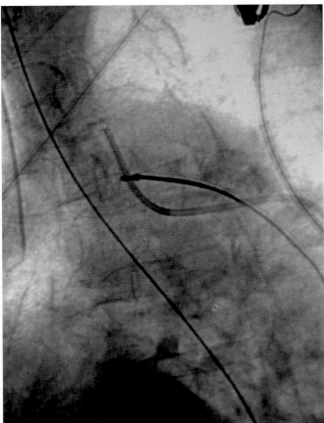

B

FIGURE 48-6. (A) The inferior end of a broken Simmons catheter used for cerebral angiography was inaccessible to a snare in a tortuous iliac artery. **(B)** Puncture of the contralateral common femoral artery and selection of the left subclavian artery allowed a snare to be pulled down over the opposite end of the fragment.

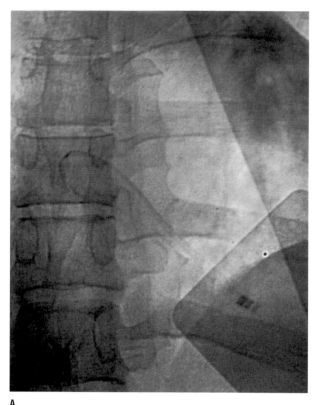

A

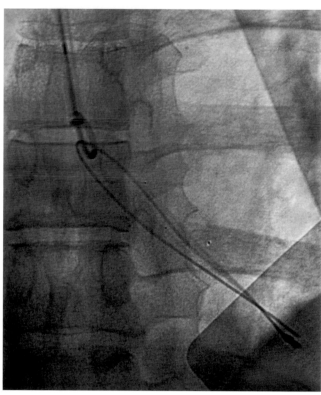

B

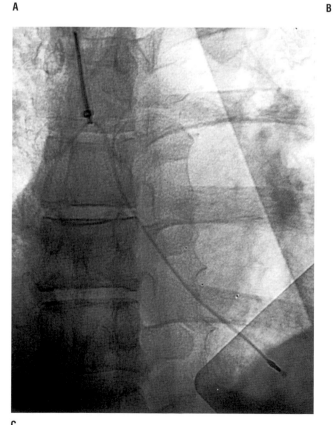

C

FIGURE 48-7. Pacemaker lead removal. (**A**) A chronically imbedded lead was fractured at the time of attempted removal, and the free end folded over and retracted into the right ventricle. (**B**) A pigtail catheter with tip-deflecting wire was introduced from the right internal jugular vein and used to hook the fragment and straighten it. (**C**) The free end was then captured using a gooseneck snare. (**D**) The braid-reinforced sheath was passed over the snare and fragment to the endocardial surface to maximize mechanical advantage. (**E**) Tension on the snare and forward pressure on the sheath allowed successful detachment and removal of the lead without everting the ventricle.

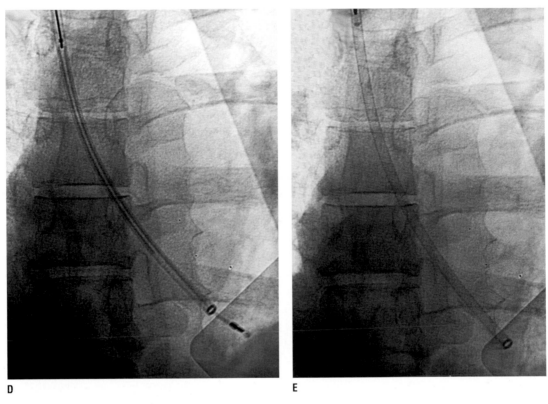

D   E

FIGURE 48-7. (continued)

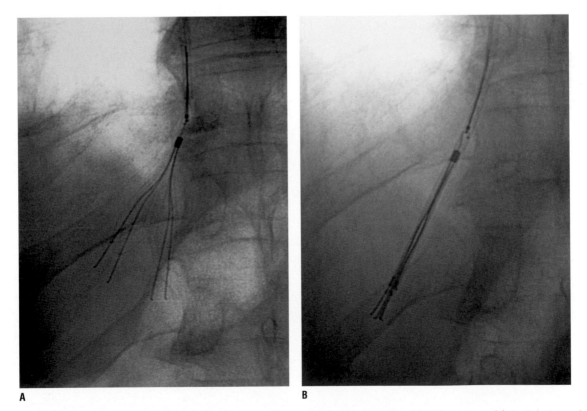

A   B

FIGURE 48-8. Removable inferior vena cava filters. (**A**) The retrieval hook of a Gunther Tulip filter (Cook) was snared from right internal jugular vein access. (**B**) Advancement of the sheath over the filter collapsed the device and detached its retention hooks from the walls of the inferior vena cava.

Vascular) has no hook but is retrievable using a custom umbrella-shaped multiple-tined device, deployed from the cranial aspect of the filter.

CONCLUSION

In the age of nanotechnology, gene therapy, and drug-eluting stents, the crude mechanical devices used for foreign body retrieval seem primitive. However, they work. Intravascular objects, large or small, asymptomatic or life-threatening, can almost always be retrieved percutaneously and redeployed in an innocuous location or removed entirely, precluding drastic open surgical procedures.

REFERENCES

1. Thomas J, Sinclair-Smith B, Bloomfield D, et al. Nonsurgical retrieval of a broken segment of steel spring guide from right atrium and inferior vena cava. *Circulation.* 1964;30:106.
2. Dotter CT, Rosch J, Bilbao MK. Transluminal extraction of catheter and guide fragments form heart and great vessels: 29 collected cases. *AJR.* 1971;111:467.
3. Gabelmann A, Kramer S, Gorich J. Percutaneous retrieval of lost or misplaced intravascular objects. *AJR.* 2001;176:1509.
4. Egglin TK, Dickey KW, Rosenblatt M, et al. Retrieval of intravascular foreign bodies: experience in 32 cases. *AJR.* 1995;164:1259.
5. Hinke DH, Zandt-Stastny DA, Goodman LR, et al. Pinch-off syndrome: a complication of implantable subclavian venous access devices. *Radiology.* 1990;177:353.
6. Ferral H, Kimura Y, Amplatz K. Retrieval of an entrapped guide wire with a braiding maneuver. *J Vasc Intervent Radiol.* 1994;5:649.
7. Kantharia BK, Kutalek SP. Extraction of pacemaker and implantable cardioverter defibrillator leads. *Curr Opin Cardiol.* 1999;14:44.

CHAPTER 49

Percutaneous Treatment of Coronary Artery Fistulae

Mahmood K. Razavi, MD, and Ramin Saket, MD

Coronary artery fistulae (CAFs), first described by Krause in 1865,[1] are shunts created by abnormal connections between a coronary artery and a cardiac chamber or great vessel. These lesions are rare, occurring in only 0.2% of pediatric patients undergoing echocardiographic examinations for heart murmurs[2] and 0.1% to 2.1% of all patients undergoing selective coronary angiography.[3–6] Although CAFs represent only 0.20% to 0.47% of all congenital cardiac abnormalities, they are the most common congenital defects of coronary arteries.[7]

CAFs originate from the right coronary artery (RCA) in 55% of cases, from the left coronary artery (LCA) in 35% of cases, and from both the RCA and LCA in 5% of cases.[8] Most lesions originate from the proximal segment of the coronary artery, facilitating endovascular and surgical closure.[9] These fistulas have a propensity to drain into low-pressure sites, including the right ventricle (42.5%), the right atrium (34%), and the pulmonary artery (15%).[10–12] Only a minority drain into left-sided chambers, with 5% and 3.5% of lesions draining into the left atrium and left ventricle, respectively.[10–12]

ETIOLOGY

The most common etiology of CAFs is congenital. They are thought to arise from abnormal persistence of the intratrabecular vascular network within the fetal myocardium that allows direct communication between arterial and venous structures.[13]

However, with the increasing number of interventional procedures, the incidence of acquired CAFs appears to be on the rise.[14] Acquired CAFs can be grouped into accidental traumatic and iatrogenic traumatic types. Accidental traumatic fistulae tend to occur as a result of deceleration injuries. Iatrogenic traumatic fistulae are more common than accidental, with cardiac surgery being the most frequent cause of all acquired CAFs.[15] Other iatrogenic causes include percutaneous transluminal coronary angioplasty,[16,17] endomyocardial biopsy,[16,18] therapeutic chest irradiation,[19] and placement of permanent ventricular pacing leads.[20]

PRESENTATION

Clinical manifestations of congenital CAFs vary according to age and the size of the shunt. Symptoms arise related to chronic shunting become more common with advancing age, particularly during the fifth and sixth decades of life. Across all ages, 55% to 60% of congenital CAFs are asymptomatic.[14,21] During the first 2 decades of life, only 20% of patients develop symptoms. This percentage, however, increases to 60% for people older than 20 years of age.

During infancy and childhood, most patients present with an asymptomatic continuous heart murmur.[22] When the fistula drains into the right ventricle, the murmur can have a louder mid-diastolic component. When the fistula drains into the pulmonary artery, the murmur may be loudest at the left upper sternal border mimicking a patent ductus arteriosus.

Congestive heart failure (CHF) from large left-to-right shunts is the most common presentation in symptomatic neonates and small infants.[23,24] Older children and young adults have smaller shunts and most commonly present with exercise-induced angina.[5,6,14] This condition results from a coronary steal phenomenon, which lowers the distal intracoronary diastolic pressure, thereby resulting in myocardial ischemia.[25,26] Both CHF and "coronary steal" angina can occur in adulthood with shunt augmentation from progressive enlargement of the fistula.

COMPLICATIONS IN ADULTHOOD

Although adverse clinical outcomes are uncommon in children, patients can suffer from significant complications if CAFs are allowed to persist over time. Many of these patients develop premature atherosclerosis due to shear-induced intimal damage from the turbulent blood flow at the origin of the fistulas.[27] As a result, patients develop angina and may experience myocardial infarctions (MIs) from thromboembolism secondary to plaque rupture.[28,29] Atherosclerotic changes in the vessel wall can also result in saccular aneurysms on rare occasions, occurring concomitantly with CAFs.[30,31] Other reported complications of CAFs include arrhythmias[32,33] and infective endocarditis.[33–35]

DIAGNOSIS

CAFs are traditionally diagnosed by angiography; however, these lesions are increasingly being detected by color Doppler echocardiography.[36] Echocardiography has a high sensitivity for imaging the origin, course, and termination of the fistulas.[37] Additional signs suggestive of CAFs include abnormal high-velocity jets into the recipient chambers or vessels and proximal dilation of affected coronary arteries.[38,39] Computed tomography and MR angiography are other noninvasive methods of detecting these lesions; however, the diagnostic value of these modalities is not yet well studied.

TREATMENT

A treatment decision for an acquired CAF is based on whether it is accidental or iatrogenic in origin. Accidental traumatic fistulas frequently result in long-term complications. Given this unfavorable clinical course, immediate repair is recommended.[16,40] In contrast, most iatrogenic traumatic fistulas heal spontaneously without intervention. Studies indicate that approximately 75% of these lesions resolve on follow-up angiography.[16] Given this relatively benign clinical course, conservative management is recommended.

Congenital lesions should always be repaired when patients are either symptomatic in childhood or develop complications later in life.[9] Additionally, CAFs are generally repaired when the pulmonary-to-systemic flow ratio (Q_p/Q_s) exceeds 1.5, regardless of symptoms. The decision to repair asymptomatic lesions with smaller shunts is controversial. Many argue that these lesions should be treated conservatively. Spontaneous closure, however, occurs only in a minority of cases.[9,41] Surgical repair in symptomatic patients has been associated with an increased rate of perioperative morbidity and mortality.[24] The surgical closure of CAFs in patients older than 20 years of age carries a complication rate of up to 23%,[11] with perioperative MI and mortality rates of 3.6%[42] and 2% to 4%, respectively.[42,43] In contrast, repair in patients younger than 20 years of age has a complication rate of less than 1%[11] and a near 100% closure rate with 100% postoperative survival.[44–46] Given the serious long-term complications that can occur and the associated increased morbidity and mortality with repair in patients who become symptomatic later in life, a number of experts advocate early repair in all asymptomatic patients diagnosed with congenital CAFs, regardless of shunt severity.[3,47,48]

【 】 SURGICAL APPROACHES

There are currently 2 widely accepted surgical techniques for repairing both congenital and acquired CAFs: (1) external ligation and (2) closure from within the recipient chamber. The former was the technique of choice in the 1960s; it is associated with a relatively high recurrence rate of 22% to 28%.[16,21,46] Closure from within the recipient chamber became the technique of choice by the 1980s;[16] it has a lower recurrence rate of 16% to 18%.[16,46]

The most significant complication of surgical repair is postoperative coronary thrombosis. This complication has a greater tendency to occur with distal CAFs due to the resultant reduction in flow through the artery, predisposing it to thrombosis. In contrast, there is a lesser tendency for thrombosis to occur with proximal lesions because closure eliminates the steal phenomenon and increases blood flow through the artery.[23,33] Anticoagulant and antiplatelet therapy is recommended for a period of time after surgery.[49]

【 】 PERCUTANEOUS APPROACHES

Over the past 2 decades, various endovascular techniques have been developed to repair CAFs. These minimally invasive techniques avoid the need for open surgical procedures and can reduce the complication rate, hospital stay, recovery time, and cost associated with CAF repair. Percutaneous approaches are most effective with proximal lesions that have single origins and draining sites. Mavroudis et al[44] recommended performing elective coil occlusion in patients who satisfy the following criteria: absence of multiple fistulas, a single narrow draining site, absence of large branch vessels, and safe accessibility to the coronary artery supplying the fistula. These researchers also recommended that percutaneous closure not be performed for fistulas that arise from the distal portion of the coronary artery, fistulas adjacent to vital coronary branches, and fistulas draining into the left heart system.[44] Recent development of more sophisticated techniques and embolic materials, however, has made the transcatheter therapy for these more difficult lesions possible.

【 】 TRANSCATHETER THERAPY

A successful outcome in percutaneous treatment of CAFs requires thorough familiarity with available embolic materials and embolization techniques. An initial complete diagnostic coronary angiography and delineation of the anatomy of the fistula is the first step. The following key features of the fistula(s) need to be identified: (1) the origin, course, and drainage site(s); (2) the number and intralesional communication patterns, if any; and (3) the approximate diameter and length of the abnormal vessel(s). Based on this information, the appropriate catheter system, embolic material(s), and site(s) of embolization may be selected.

It should be noted that some left CAFs have been reported to occur concomitantly with right coronary artery atresia. In these cases, the fistulae may serve as the supplying artery to the right ventricle.[50] It is therefore recommended that a 5-minute balloon occlusion test be performed prior to embolization of these fistulae to evaluate for possible ischemic or conduction changes.[51]

Embolic Materials

Various permanent and temporary embolic agents are available in the market. For this purpose, temporary embolic agents should not be used and hence will not be considered.

Coils.
Coils are the preferred embolic agents of choice for CAFs. These permanent implantable devices are most commonly made of stainless steel or platinum and come in variety of shapes and sizes. Some are coated with polyester fibers to promote thrombosis and others are made of bare metal, with the main function being to act as space occupiers. Due to the risk of misplacement or inadvertent migration, several coils now allow for controlled release or removal prior to detachment. Advent of these detachable coils has made safe embolization of target vessels in critical areas possible.

An increasing number of medical device companies, including Cook, Boston Scientific (Target), and Johnson & Johnson (Cordis Endovascular) manufacture and market these devices. Similar to stents, each device has its own advantages, disadvantages, and performance characteristics. Operator familiarity with these features is a must.

Detachable Balloons.
In 1983, Reidy et al[52] reported the first successful endovascular CAF occlusion using a detachable balloon. This compliant balloon is placed at the tip of a compatible microcatheter and delivered to the site of embolization. The vessel is then occluded by injection of contrast in the flow lumen of the microcatheter, which inflates the balloon. The detachment mechanism thus allows for precise delivery of the balloon to the target site.

The advantages of this system include immediate occlusion of the target vessel, reversibility until balloon is detached, and the ability to "test occlude" for detection of ischemic changes prior to final detachment. The main disadvantage of detachable balloons is that the delivery is not over-the-wire and requires a coaxial catheter system and large delivery guides. Premature balloon deflation can also occur, leading to reestablishment of flow in the fistula.

Particles.
There are two main varieties of permanent embolic particles: polyvinyl alcohol (PVA) and trisacryl gelatin microsphere (Embosphere). Although there is a role for these agents in arteriovenous malformations, they are not used in the treatment of fistulas because of the high likelihood of passage through the fistula and nontarget embolization.

Liquid Embolic Agents.
These compounds solidify when they come in contact with blood or other ionic solutions, forming a cast inside the vessel. The only agent of its kind commercially available in the United States is N-butyl cyanoacrylate (NBCA), which has approval from the Food and Drug Administration for use in intracranial arteriovenous malformations. The safe use of these agents requires substantial operator experience due to the potential for distal nontarget embolization and/or reflux into the proximal coronary circulation. Once solidified, the effect is permanent, and unlike many coils, they are not retrievable. Their use in the CAFs should be limited to lesions with multiple pathways or relatively long course.

Other Devices.
Various other methods such as the use of vascular occluders or double-umbrella devices have been reported.[53,54] They typically require large and nontortuous feeding vessels but can achieve effective closure.

Stent-grafts such as expanded polytetrafluoroethylene (ePTFE)-covered stents may be used in more proximal lesions where both atherosclerosis and fistula coexist. The potential for occlusion of branch vessels is a disadvantage of the use of these devices.

Technique

After delineation of the anatomy, the projection that best demonstrates the takeoff of the fistula should be selected. For the catheterization of the fistulous tract, we prefer the use of microcatheters through the diagnostic guide in a coaxial fashion (Figure 49-1). This method has several advantages. First is the availability of a wider array of microcatheter-compatible coil sizes and shapes. Second is the improved ability to navigate the microcatheter to a secure location for deposition of coils (see Figure 49-1C), regardless of tortuosity of the vessel. Due to the small size of the microcatheters, there is also reduced risk of compromise of antegrade flow or pericatheter clot formation during the procedure.

The tip of the microcatheter should be placed in a position deep enough to avoid migration back into the feeding coronary artery during coil placement (Figure 49-2). Another important consideration is the length of the fistula and presence or absence of other outflow tracts. Embolization should preferentially be done in a manner to occlude the path to all inflow and outflow vessels.

The choice of coils depends on the diameter and length of the fistula. If there is brisk flow through a large or short tract, deposition of the initial device is critical in the success of embolization. The coil should be slightly oversized for secure attachment. This coil also acts as a barrier against distal embolization of subsequent coils, if necessary. To minimize the risk of either distal or proximal migration of coils, detachable devices can be used. As mentioned previously, this allows for the precise deposition of coils and the ability to remove them prior to final detachment.

Immediate complete cessation of flow in the embolized CAF, although desirable, is not always necessary. Once the effect of procedural anticoagulation is dissipated, the embolized tracts with sluggish flow typically occlude.

【 】 COMPLICATIONS

The most serious complications of CAF embolization stem from either proximal or distal coil migration. Proximal migration is usually due to device recoil during deposition and may cause thrombosis of the parent epicardial vessel. Distal migration is typically due to undersizing of the coil in a high-flow shunt. If this occurs, the patient should be fully anticoagulated immediately and coil retrieval attempted. Coils can be recovered from the pulmonary arteries, the right ventricle, and even the coronary arteries using various snare techniques.

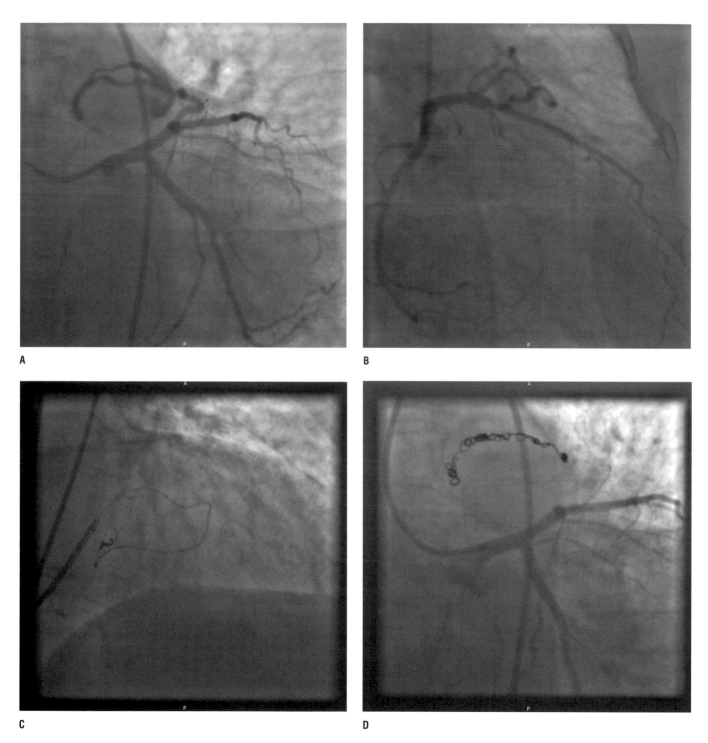

A

B

C

D

FIGURE 49-1. (**A**) and (**B**) Initial left coronary arteriogram in two different projections, revealing an abnormal communication between left anterior descending coronary artery and pulmonary artery. (**C**) A microcatheter has been used to catheterize the fistula to an area just proximal to the pulmonary artery. An appropriately sized coil has been deployed. (**D**) Completion angiogram after coiling of the fistula tract confirms the complete closure of the arteriovenous fistula.

Other less common complications include arrhythmia and endocarditis.

[ ] POSTPROCEDURAL CARE

In the immediate postembolization period, the reduction in flow predisposes the parent coronary artery to thrombosis, especially in the arteries with distal fistula. Conversely, occlusion of more prox- imal fistulae may cause dilation of the distal circulation. In both situations, antiplatelet therapy seems prudent until the normaliza- tion of the coronary arteries occurs. Additional anticoagulation may become necessary if there is progressive coronary dilation over time.

As mentioned previously, endocarditis is a rare complication, and some experts have advocated prophylaxis for at least 1 year postprocedurally.[54]

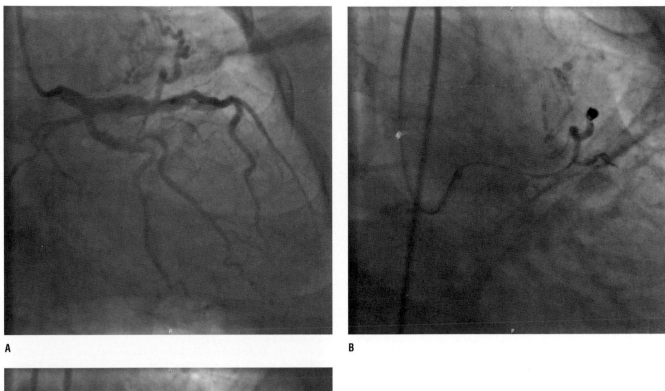

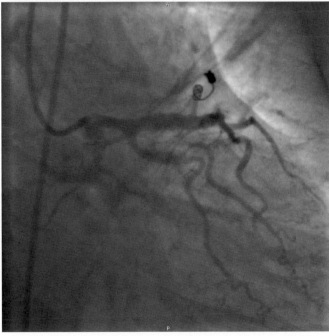

FIGURE 49-2. (A) Left coronary arteriogram shows a fistula in the left anterior descending artery. This tract was too tortuous to catheterize safely beyond the first curvature. **(B)** and **(C)** Repeat angiogram after the deposition of 2 coils reveals complete cessation of flow through the fistula.

REFERENCES

1. Krause W. Uber den Ursprung einerakzessorischen a. coronaria cordis aus der a. pulmonis. *Z Rationelle Med.* 1865;24:225.
2. Hsieh KS, Huang TC, Lee CL. Coronary artery fistulas in neonates, infants, and children: clinical findings and outcome. *Pediatr Cardiol.* 2002;23:415.
3. Lowe JE, Oldham HN Jr, Sabiston DC Jr. Surgical management of congenital coronary artery fistulas. *Ann Surg.* 1981;194:373.
4. Yamanaka O, Hobbs RE. Coronary artery anomalies in 126,595 patients undergoing coronary arteriography. *Cathet Cardiovasc Diagn.* 1990;21:28.
5. Nawa S, Miyachi Y, Shiba T, et al. Clinical and angiographic analysis of congenital coronary artery fistulae in adulthood. Is there any new trend? *Jpn Heart J.* 1996;37:95.
6. Gillebert C, Van Hoof R, Van de Werf F, et al. Coronary artery fistulas in an adult population. *Eur Heart J.* 1986;7:437.
7. Levin DC, Fellows KE, Abrams HL. Hemodynamically significant primary anomalies of the coronary arteries. Angiographic aspects. *Circulation.* 1978;58:25.
8. Oldham HN, Jr., Ebert PA, Young WG, et al. Surgical management of congenital coronary artery fistula. *Ann Thorac Surg.* 1971;12:503.

9. Balanescu S, Sangiorgi G, Castelvecchio S, et al. Coronary artery fistulas: clinical consequences and methods of closure. A literature review. *Ital Heart J.* 2001;2:669.

10. Ogden JA. Congenital anomalies of the coronary arteries. *Am J Cardiol.* 1970;25:474.

11. Liberthson RR, Sagar K, Berkoben JP, et al. Congenital coronary arteriovenous fistula. Report of 13 patients, review of the literature and delineation of management. *Circulation.* 1979;59:849.

12. Baim DS, Kline H, Silverman JF. Bilateral coronary artery-pulmonary artery fistulas. Report of five cases and review of the literature. *Circulation.* 1982;65:810.

13. Grant RT. An unusual anomaly of the coronary vessels in the malformed heart of a child. *Heart.* 1926;13:273.

14. Said SA, el Gamal MI, van der Werf T. Coronary arteriovenous fistulas: collective review and management of six new cases-changing etiology, presentation, and treatment strategy. *Clin Cardiol.* 1997;20:748.

15. Angelini P. Coronary-to-pulmonary fistulae: what are they? What are their causes? What are their functional consequences? *Tex Heart Inst J.* 2000;27:327.

16. Friesen CH, Howlett JG, Ross DB. Traumatic coronary artery fistula management. *Ann Thorac Surg.* 2000;69:1973.

17. Meng RL, Harlan JL. Left anterior descending coronary artery-right ventricle fistula complicating percutaneous transluminal angioplasty. *J Thorac Cardiovasc Surg.* 1985;90:387.

18. Sandhu JS, Uretsky BF, Zerbe TR, et al. Coronary artery fistula in the heart transplant patient. A potential complication of endomyocardial biopsy. *Circulation.* 1989;79:350.

19. Benitez RM. Acquired coronary artery-pulmonary artery connection. *Cathet Cardiovasc Diagn.* 1998;45:413.

20. Saeian K, Vellinga T, Troup P, et al. Coronary artery fistula formation secondary to permanent pacemaker placement. *Chest.* 1991;99:780.

21. Rittenhouse EA, Doty DB, Ehrenhaft JL. Congenital coronary artery-cardiac chamber fistula. Review of operative management. *Ann Thorac Surg.* 1975;20:468.

22. Wong KT, Menahem S. Coronary arterial fistulas in childhood. *Cardiol Young.* 2000;10:15.

23. Wang NK, Hsieh LY, Shen CT, et al. Coronary arteriovenous fistula in pediatric patients: a 17-year institutional experience. *J Formos Med Assoc.* 2002;101:177.

24. Schumacher G, Roithmaier A, Lorenz HP, et al. Congenital coronary artery fistula in infancy and childhood: diagnostic and therapeutic aspects. *Thorac Cardiovasc Surg.* 1997;45:287.

25. Kiuchi K, Nejima J, Kikuchi A, et al. Left coronary artery-left ventricular fistula with acute myocardial infarction, representing the coronary steal phenomenon: a case report. *J Cardiol.* 1999;34:279.

26. Najm HK, Gill IS, FitzGibbon GM, et al. Coronary-pulmonary steal syndrome. *Ann Thorac Surg.* 1996;62:264.

27. Bertinchant JP, Bosc E, Grolleau-Raoux R. Proximal and peripheral coronaro-pulmonary fistulae. Apropos of 10 cases. *Arch Mal Coeur Vaiss.* 1985; 78:601.

28. Hobbs RE, Millit HD, Raghavan PV, et al. Coronary artery fistulae: a 10-year review. *Cleve Clin Q.* 1982;49:191.

29. Yamabe H, Fujitani K, Mizutani T, et al. Two cases of myocardial infarction with coronary arteriovenous fistula. *Jpn Heart J.* 1983;24:303.

30. Koike R, Oku T, Satoh H, et al. Right ventricular myocardial infarction and late cardiac tamponade due to right coronary artery aneurysm–a case report. *Jpn J Surg.* 1990;20:463.

31. Akashi H, Tayama E, Tayama K, et al. Rupture of an aneurysm resulting from a coronary artery fistula. *Circ J.* 2003;67:551.

32. McNamara JJ, Gross RE. Congenital coronary artery fistula. *Surgery.* 1969;65:59.

33. Sakakibara S, Yokoyama M, Takao A, et al. Coronary arteriovenous fistula. Nine operated cases. *Am Heart J.* 1966;72:307.

34. Wilde P, Watt I. Congenital coronary artery fistulae: six new cases with a collective review. *Clin Radiol.* 1980;31:301.

35. Alkhulaifi AM, Horner SM, Pugsley WB, et al. Coronary artery fistulas presenting with bacterial endocarditis. *Ann Thorac Surg.* 1995;60:202.

36. Shakudo M, Yoshikawa J, Yoshida K, et al. Noninvasive diagnosis of coronary artery fistula by Doppler color flow mapping. *J Am Coll Cardiol.* 1989; 13:1572.

37. Ke WL, Wang NK, Lin YM, et al. Right coronary artery fistula into right atrium: diagnosis by color Doppler echocardiography. *Am Heart J.* 1988;116:886.

38. Reeder GS, Tajik AJ, Smith HC. Visualization of coronary artery fistula by two-dimensional echocardiography. *Mayo Clin Proc.* 1980;55:185.

39. Yoshikawa J, Katao H, Yanagihara K, et al. Noninvasive visualization of the dilated main coronary arteries in coronary artery fistulas by cross-sectional echocardiography. *Circulation.* 1982;65:600.

40. Toda S, Nakamura A, Iwamoto T, et al. Successful surgical treatment of aortic regurgitation with coronary artery fistula due to blunt chest trauma–a case report. *Nippon Kyobu Geka Gakkai Zasshi.* 1991;39:1087.

41. Shubrooks SJ Jr, Naggar CZ. Spontaneous near closure of coronary artery fistula. *Circulation.* 1978;57:197.

42. Kriklin JW, Barrart-Boyes BG. Congenital anomalies of the coronary arteries. In: Kriklin JW, Barrart-Boyes BG, eds. *Cardiac Surgery.* New York, NY: Churchill-Livingstone; 1993:945.

43. Perry SB, Keane JF, Lock JE. Pediatric intervention. In: Grossman W, Baim DS, eds. *Cardiac Catheterization, Angiography, and Intervention.* Philadelphia, Pa: Lea & Febiger; 1991:543.

44. Mavroudis C, Backer CL, Rocchini AP, et al. Coronary artery fistulas in infants and children: a surgical review and discussion of coil embolization. *Ann Thorac Surg.* 1997;63:1235.

45. Kamiya H, Yasuda T, Nagamine H, et al. Surgical treatment of congenital coronary artery fistulas: 27 years' experience and a review of the literature. *J Card Surg.* 2002;17:173.

46. Cheung DL, Au WK, Cheung HH, et al. Coronary artery fistulas: long-term results of surgical correction. *Ann Thorac Surg.* 2001;71:190.

47. Said SA, Landman GH. Coronary-pulmonary fistula: long-term follow-up in operated and non-operated patients. *Int J Cardiol.* 1990;27:203.

48. Goto Y, Abe T, Sekine S, et al. Surgical treatment of the coronary artery to pulmonary artery fistulas in adults. *Cardiology.* 1998;89:252.

49. Liotta D, Hallman GL, Hall RJ, et al. Surgical treatment of congenital coronary artery fistula. *Surgery.* 1971;70:856.

50. Farooki ZQ, Nowlen T, Hakimi M, et al. Congenital coronary artery fistulae: a review of 18 cases with special emphasis on spontaneous closure. *Pediatr Cardiol.* 1993;14:208.

51. Moskowitz WB, Newkumet KM, Albrecht GT, et al. Case of steel versus steal: coil embolization of congenital coronary arteriovenous fistula. *Am Heart J.* 1991;121:909.

52. Reidy JF, Sowton E, Ross DN. Transcatheter occlusion of coronary to bronchial anastomosis by detachable balloon combined with coronary angioplasty at same procedure. *Br Heart J.* 1983;49:284.

53. Perry SB, Rome J, Keane JF, et al. Transcatheter closure of coronary artery fistulas. *J Am Coll Cardiol.* 1992;20:205.

54. Okubo M, Nykanen D, Benson LN. Outcomes of transcatheter embolization in the treatment of coronary artery fistulas. *Cathet Cardiovasc Intervent.* 2001;52:510.

CHAPTER (50)

Renal Artery Angioplasty and Stenting

Bhagat K. Reddy, MD

Harry Goldblatt's 1934 classic experimental canine renal artery clamping[1] is the background for understanding the pathophysiology of renal artery stenosis (RAS). Significant renal arterial disease (RAD) causes hemodynamic renal parenchyma flow obstruction, producing "renal ischemia." Detrimental effects of uncontrolled hypertension and renal function impairment are the consequences of untreated RAS.

Accelerated conversion of angiotensin I to II is caused by renal ischemia-induced hyperreninemia. Consequently, profound angiotensin II-mediated vasoconstriction and adrenal release of aldosterone cause significant sodium and water retention, contributing to renovascular hypertension (RVH). RVH accounts for up to 5% of all cases of hypertension and is an important reversible cause of secondary hypertension.

Functionally occlusive RAD causes progressive ischemic nephropathy, leading to chronic renal insufficiency and end-stage renal failure. RAS accounts for a significant proportion of renal disease. Renal ischemia is a powerful activator of the neuroendocrine system. Effects of this activation include endothelial dysfunction, cardiac myocyte hypertrophy, enhanced thrombogenicity, atherosclerotic plaque rupture, inhibition of fibrinolysis, and accelerated atherosclerosis. It is therefore implicated that RAD is an important independent predictor of cardiovascular mortality and overall survival.

Renal revascularization was originally performed surgically. However, it was limited significantly by adverse perioperative morbidity and mortality. Since its inception, endovascular treatment has remained the predominant modality for treatment of RAS. Angioplasty is significantly limited by procedural success and restenosis especially for aorto-ostial lesions such as RAS. Therefore, angioplasty with utilization of endovascular stents has become the primary modality of revascularization, because it significantly improves the acute and long-term outcomes in patients with RAS.[2]

TYPES OF RENAL ARTERIAL DISEASE

【 】 FIBROMUSCULAR DYSPLASIA

Noninflammatory and nonatherosclerotic disease affecting the mid-to-distal renal artery may involve branch renal vessels (Figure 50-1). Common presentation of fibromuscular dysplasia (FMD) is young age and female sex, with worsening hypertension. The condition may involve other vascular beds, especially the extracranial carotid artery. Types of FMD that are characterized by the layer of the vessel wall being affected include the following:

1. Medial fibroplasias (most common; 80% of cases) are characterized angiographically by the classic "string of beads" appearance. The beads are typically larger than the normal reference renal artery.

2. Intimal fibroplasias.

3. Perimedial fibroplasias involve the junction of media and adventitia. The are usually focal, and the beads are smaller than the vessel.

4. Fibromuscular hyperplasias.

5. Periadventitial fibroplasias (rare).

【 】 ATHEROSCLEROSIS

Atherosclerosis is the most common cause of RAD. The majority of lesions (up to 80%) are aorto-ostial in location, making it an abdominal aortic and renal arterial disease. However, they may involve any segment of the renal artery or its branches, including the renal parenchymal vasculature. Aorto-ostial lesions

543

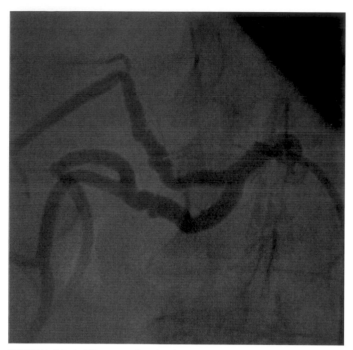

FIGURE 50-1. Fibromuscular dysplasia.

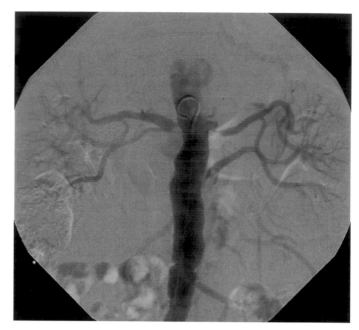

FIGURE 50-2. Multiple renal arteries with renal artery stenosis.

are fibrocalcific; however, severe calcification of this junction is not uncommon. Severe lesions are associated with the presence of post-stenotic dilation, which should not be mistaken for FMD. On occasion, FMD and atherosclerosis may be present together.

SCREENING FOR RENAL ARTERY DISEASE

1. Hypertension is characterized by (a) early onset (< 25 years of age), (b) late onset (> 55 years of age), (c) being medically refractory, (d) malignancy, and (e) associated with clinically evident atherosclerosis.

2. Renal insufficiency is characterized by (a) angiotensin-converting enzyme/angiotensin II blocker-induced azotemia, (b) progressive reduction in kidney size, (c) no known etiology in the elderly, and (d) be associated with clinically evident atherosclerosis.

3. Other factors that may be indicative of RAD are abdominal bruit, flank bruit, recurrent pulmonary edema of unknown etiology, and worsening angina despite appropriate antianginal therapy.

EVALUATION

【 】 NONINVASIVE METHODS

Noninvasive techniques include renal artery duplex scan, captopril renal scan, magnetic resonance (MR) imaging, and computed tomography (CT) angiography.

【 】 INVASIVE METHODS

Renal angiography is the gold standard for evaluation of RAD. Angiography is commonly performed with radiocontrast media in an angiographic suite capable of digital subtraction angiography (DSA) and hemodynamic monitoring.

Abdominal Aortography

Abdominal aortography must be performed before selective renal angiography if possible for the following reasons:

1. Most renal artery lesions are ostial, and if stenosis is critical, selective diagnostic catheter engagement with or without contrast injection may inadvertently cause abrupt vessel closure or unwarranted dissection.

2. This technique provides an anatomic road map of the origin of the renal arteries, which may be widely variable.

3. More than one third of patients have more than one renal artery supplying each kidney. Figure 50-2 shows multiple renal arteries with RAS. Therefore, identification of the number of renal arteries supplying each kidney and their origin from the abdominal aorta is invaluable.

4. This technique allows identification of coexistent abdominal aortic disease (ie, aneurysm, atherosclerotic disease, dissection, ulcers, thrombus). Because RAD is an aorto-ostial disease, evaluation and management of both the renal arterial and abdominal aortic disease should be performed simultaneously.

The disadvantage of flush aortography is the utilization of excessive contrast, which in most circumstances would be justified even in patients with mild to moderate renal impairment, because the information obtained is invaluable for the management of these patients. However, if the patient has moderate to severe renal

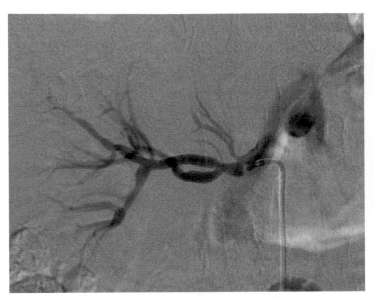
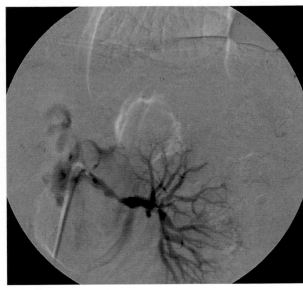

A   **B**

FIGURE 50-3. A and **B.** Bilateral renal artery stenosis with severe intraparenchymal vascular disease.

impairment, where contrast usage is limited, it is advisable to obtain all the anatomic information from noninvasive testing (ie, renal with abdominal duplex scan, MR angiography). Abdominal aortography should be performed in the anterior-posterior projection with DSA utilizing a 28-cm field of view (FOV) on the image intensifier that would accommodate the abdominal aorta, renal arteries, and both kidneys.

Selective Renal Angiography

Selective angiographic imaging of the renal artery is performed to visualize the pathologic characteristics and location of disease in the renal artery and its branches. The nephrogram obtained during selective injections would identify kidney size and intra-parenchymal disease (Figure 50-3). Selective angiography should be performed in the 0- to 15-degree and 10- to 30-degree left anterior oblique projections with DSA for the right and left kidney, respectively, because the renal artery courses caudally and laterally. A 20-cm FOV on the image intensifier is necessary to obtain detailed analysis of the renal artery, branches, and the nephrogram.

Evaluation of Degree of Stenosis

Percentage stenosis of the renal artery is measured using the following formula:

$$1 - \frac{(\text{Minimum luminal diameter})}{\text{Reference vessel diameter}} \times 100$$

Renal ischemia is produced by a hemodynamically significant stenosis. Therefore, evaluation of degree of stenosis and hemodynamic gradient should be performed to delineate the significance of RAD. Published literature suggests that 50% stenosis or more in the renal artery produces a hemodynamic gradient. However, in angiographically intermediate stenosis (50%–79%), a translesional peak systolic pressure gradient of 20 mm Hg or more is necessary to cause renal parenchymal flow limitation.

The accuracy of gradient measurement is invaluable to delineate the significance of a lesion. Pull-back gradients are erroneous as they are inconsistent, nonsimultaneous, and nonreproducible; they are therefore not a true reflection of the true translesional gradient. Thus, they should not be performed for the evaluation of physiologic significance of RAD. Accurate intra-arterial measurement of translesional pressure gradient can be performed using either of the following:

1. Transcatheter, which involves simultaneous placement of catheters distal (≤ 4-Fr) and proximal (≥ 6-Fr) to the stenosis, respectively, utilizing two calibrated transducers.
2. Pressure wire, which uses a pressure-sensing 0.014-in wire distal to the stenosis.

Angiographic and Hemodynamic Criteria for Renal Artery Stenosis Intervention

Criteria include an angiographic diameter stenosis of either:

1. Between 50% and 80%, with 20-mm Hg or greater peak systolic gradient.
2. 80% or greater.

RENAL ARTERY INTERVENTION

【 】 ANTIPLATELET AND ANTICOAGULATION REGIMEN

Preintervention antiplatelet therapy should consist of aspirin 325 mg and clopidogrel 300 mg bolus (ticlopidine 500 mg bolus for clopidogrel-allergic patients). Intravenous (IV) heparin 70 U/kg or

IV bivalirudin should be injected after obtaining vascular access. Target activated clotting time (ACT) should be 250 seconds or more throughout the procedure. Except when using a distal protection device, the ACT should be maintained at 300 seconds due to an increased risk of vessel thrombosis.

【 】 SHEATH AND GUIDE SELECTION

Renal interventions can be performed using 6- to 8-Fr sheaths. Selection of sheath size depends on site of vascular access, size of renal artery, use of adjunctive distal protection devices, utilization of guide versus sheath guides, and stent profile. Vascular access sites consist of radial, brachial, and femoral. Radial and brachial access is useful for steep, inferior, coursing renal arteries, which are commonly seen in patients with abdominal aortic aneurysms. Femoral access is the most favorable access in majority of cases. The majority of patients with RAD have significant coexistent abdominal aortic disease. Therefore, a 25- to 45-cm sheath is appropriate to provide control and stability of the guide catheter and additionally prevents catheter-induced trauma and atheroembolism. Guide catheter or sheath engagement of the renal artery is variable. However, caution should be taken to prevent guide catheter-induced vessel trauma, abrupt vessel closure, dissection, and atheroembolism, because most lesions are ostial.

【 】 TECHNIQUES OF GUIDE CATHETER/ SHEATH ENGAGEMENT

Direct Method

These methods involve guide advancement over a 0.035-in wire into the abdominal aorta, following which direct engagement of the guide into the renal artery is performed. Disadvantages include all the previously mentioned guide-induced complications.

Indirect Methods

These methods are time consuming; however, they are invaluable in preventing serious inadvertent guide-induced complications:

1. Introduction of a diagnostic (4–5 Fr) and a guide catheter (6–8 Fr) in tandem over an 0.035-in wire into the abdominal aorta. Following removal of the 0.035-in wire, the diagnostic catheter is coaxially engaged into the renal ostium. The interventional wire is then introduced through the diagnostic catheter into the distal renal artery. The guide catheter is railed over the diagnostic catheter into the renal ostium; once coaxial, the diagnostic catheter is removed.

2. Guide advancement with a 0.035-in wire into the abdominal aorta. Leaving the 0.035-in wire in place, the guide is gradually maneuvered close to the renal ostium. Then the interventional wire, which is advanced into the distal renal artery, is introduced. The 0.035-in wire is removed, and the guide is railed coaxial to the renal ostium over the interventional wire.

【 】 INTERVENTIONAL WIRES

Renal interventional wires may range from 0.014-in to 0.035-in and should be nonhydrophilic to prevent renal branch vessel

perforation and hematomas. Currently most renal interventions should be performed with the 0.014-in wire for the following reasons:

1. Improved 0.014-in-compatible stent platforms.
2. Minimized wire-induced lesion trauma.
3. Pressure sensing wires are 0.014-in.
4. Distal protection devices are 0.014-in.

【 】 BALLOON ANGIOPLASTY

Initial experience with balloon angioplasty (percutaneous transluminal angioplasty [PTA]) was limited by (1) lower procedural success due to significant residual stenosis, vessel dissection, and abrupt vessel closure; and (2) poor long-term success due to vessel recoil, encroachment of aortic atheroma, and higher restenosis. Therefore, PTA is recommended with less than 1:1 balloon:reference vessel ratio as predilation for atherosclerotic RAD. On the contrary, patients with FMD can be successfully treated with PTA alone, because it successfully alleviates the hemodynamic gradient. PTA is presently the standard of care.

【 】 STENTING

Endovascular stents have emerged as the promising treatment for RAD (Figure 50-4).[2] Primary stenting is recommended if angiography demonstrates the presence of thrombus and absence of calcification. However, the majority of renal lesions are fibrocalcific and have no visible thrombus; therefore, predilation with PTA is advisable to predict dilatability, lesion morphology, and vessel sizing. Nondilatable lesions should be pursued with aggressive PTA prior to stenting. Adequate radial strength and precision placement make balloon expandable stents the endovascular stent of choice. Accurate stent deployment is the key to acute and long-term success in renal interventions. Because most lesions are aorto-ostial, the stent should cover the entire lesion with 1-mm extension into the abdominal aorta. The goal of stenting is to achieve 1:1 sizing with the reference vessel. Risk of vessel rupture during renal interventions can be assessed by presence of significant flank or back pain during vessel dilation with PTA or stenting. Angiographic success in the literature is defined as more than 30% stenosis reduction or less than 50% residual stenosis with normal brisk renal parenchymal arterial flow (Thrombolysis in Myocardial Infarction [TIMI] grade 3). In intermediate lesions with significant gradient prior to stenting, a postintervention gradient of less than 10 mm of Hg is considered a hemodynamically successful result. Postinterventional angiography should be performed in the 20-cm FOV on the image intensifier with DSA to visualize the nephrogram. Assessment should include distal embolization, residual thrombus, vessel perforation, and renal hematoma. The images in Figure 50-5 were created with use of a renal artery distal protection device.

INTRAVASCULAR ULTRASOUND

Intravascular ultrasound (IVUS) is invaluable in the diagnostic and interventional management of RAD (Figure 50-6). Diagnostic uses include stenosis assessment, evaluation of in-stent restenosis, and stent thrombosis. Preintervention uses include

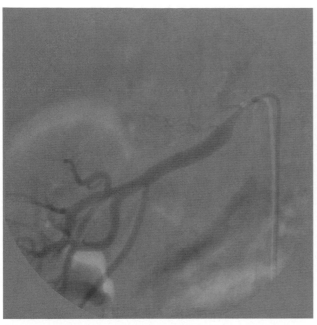

A

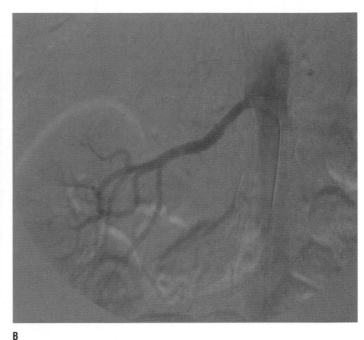

B

FIGURE 50-4. A and **B.** Renal angioplasty and stenting.

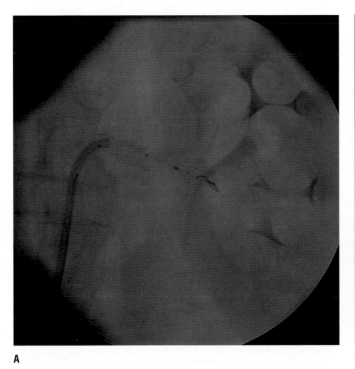

A

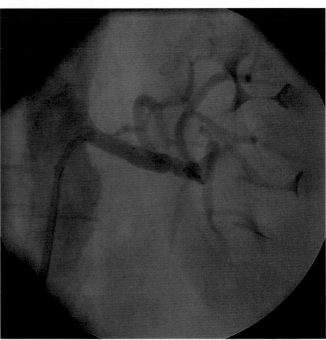

B

FIGURE 50-5. A and **B.** Renal artery distal protection device.

detailed evaluation of lesion morphology, thrombus, atheroma burden, vessel sizing (ie, difficulty is present in aorto-ostial lesions with presence of significant post-stenotic dilation). Postintervention uses include stent analysis consisting of apposition, expansion, lesion coverage, and confirmation of 1-mm extension into the abdominal aorta for ostial lesions. Other related uses for IVUS include evaluation of post-stent dissection, thrombus, hematoma, perforation, and rupture.

RENAL FUNCTION AND DISTAL EMBOLIC PROTECTION

Theoretically, deterioration of renal function following renal artery interventions is multifold and may include the following:

1. Renal atheroembolism. Endovascular filter devices have been designed to capture embolic material produced during the

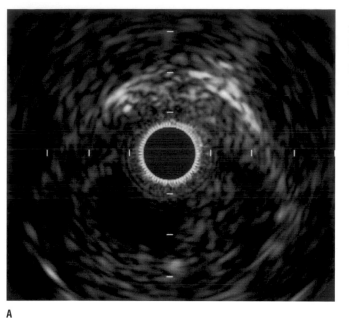

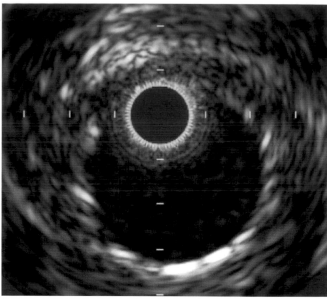

A **B**

FIGURE 50-6. Renal intravascular ultrasound preintervention (**A**) and postintervention (**B**).

interventional procedure to prevent distal embolization.[3] Currently, the devices are investigational and are being tested in 2 clinical trials (RESIST[9] and Cardiovascular Outcomes in Renal Atherosclerotic Lesions [CORAL] trials).[10]

2. Platelet embolism. Theoretically, this condition can be treated with IV glycoprotein IIb/III3a inhibitors and is currently being investigated in the RESIST trial.

3. Preexisting renal parenchymal disease.

4. Contrast nephropathy. Conditions that place patients with RAD at risk of developing contrast nephropathy are chronic renal insufficiency, recent worsening of renal function, diabetes mellitus, congestive heart failure, severe cardiomyopathy, and chronic usage of nonsteroidal anti-inflammatory drugs.

Contrast nephropathy can be reduced by the following:

• Limiting contrast usage. Utilize appropriate information from noninvasive tests, limit and dilute contrast injections, utilize bony landmarks for road maps, stage diagnostic and interventional procedures, and use IVUS to assess preinterventional and postinterventional results.

• IV hydration pre- and post-procedure.

• Periprocedural *N*-acetylcysteine.

• Alternative methods of radiographic imaging (ie, gadolinium,[4] CO_2[5]).

COMPLICATIONS

【 】 VASCULAR ACCESS

As with most endovascular procedures, vascular access complications are the most common complications associated with renal interventions. The complications include access site bleeding, hematoma, vessel injury, retroperitoneal bleed, pseudoaneurysm, atrioventricular fistula, and nerve injury.

【 】 DISSECTION

Dissection may occur inadvertently during diagnostic or guide catheter engagement in critical ostial disease. It commonly occurs distal to the stent edge due to oversizing of the stent. Treatment consists of appropriate stenting.

【 】 THROMBUS

Primary stenting is recommended if there is presence of significant preexisting thrombus and no evidence of calcification. Intraprocedural thrombus generation should be treated with extraction devices, glycoprotein IIb/IIIa inhibitors, or trapping with stent or stent graft.

【 】 DISTAL EMBOLIZATION

Atheromatous and thrombus embolization can be prevented with distal protection devices[3] and glycoprotein IIb/IIIa inhibitors, respectively. However, postinterventional embolization can be treated with IA Nipride and glycoprotein IIb/IIIa inhibitors.

【 】 RUPTURE

Risk is greater in older patients and in those with small vessels, calcified lesions, and post-stenotic dilation. Inappropriate sizing of balloons and/or stents is the commonest etiology of vessel rupture. Procedural mortality is significant if unrecognized and untreated. Treatment consists of immediate balloon tamponade, prompt reversal of anticoagulation, and stent graft placement.

[ ] RENAL HEMATOMA

Renal hematoma occurs commonly due to guidewire-induced vessel perforation; therefore, nonhydrophilic wires are recommended for renal interventions. Postinterventional DSA demonstrates contrast extravasation in the renal parenchyma. Late presentation includes significant flank or abdominal pain with or without hemodynamic compromise, and abdominal CT scan confirms the presence of renal hematoma. Treatment consists of prompt reversal of anticoagulation. If the condition remains uncontrolled, transcatheter vessel embolization or surgical treatment is warranted.

[ ] STENT THROMBOSIS

Etiology is multifold and consists of inappropriate stent sizing, untreated post-stent dissection, intramural hematoma, and noncompliance to antiplatelet therapy or coagulopathy. Treatment should consist of identification of the etiology, thrombus removal with mechanical thrombectomy or extraction devices, distal embolic protection, appropriate antiplatelet therapy, and antithrombotic therapy. IVUS should be used to understand the etiology of stent thrombosis, including detailed assessment of the old stent and persistent vessel morphology to delineate appropriate treatment.

POSTINTERVENTIONAL CARE

Patients are admitted for overnight observation to assess vascular complications, hemodynamic changes, and renal function. Significant hemodynamic changes need prompt evaluation and treatment. It may be reasonable to withhold antihypertensive medications to prevent inadvertent clinical hypotension, which may be caused by renormalization of renal perfusion. The patient should be discharged with aspirin 325 mg lifelong and clopidogrel 75 mg (ticlopidine 250 mg bid) for 1 month.

OUTCOMES OF RENAL REVASCULARIZATION

Such effects include the following:

1. Stabilization and improvement of blood pressure.[6]
2. Decreased usage of antihypertensive medications.
3. Renal function improvement or stabilization.[7]
4. Prevention or delayed progression to end-stage renal disease and preservation of kidney size.[7]
5. Decreased need for dialysis and renal transplantation.
6. Decreased recurrence of pulmonary edema in patients with congestive heart failure.
7. Alleviation of angina in patients with coronary ischemia despite appropriate antianginal treatment.
8. Improved renal related mortality.
9. Improved cardiovascular mortality.
10. Positive effect on quality of life.

FOLLOW-UP EVALUATION

The period of follow-up is 1 month, 3 months, 6 months, and 12 months, and then yearly. Evaluation should consist of assessment and treatment of the following:

1. Blood pressure should be measured. Antihypertensive medications, medication compliance, and side effects should be discussed.
2. Renal function involves measurement of serum creatinine and determination of kidney size.
3. Renal stent patency. A baseline Doppler evaluation should be made, and evaluations should be made at 1 month, 6 months, 12 months, and then yearly.
4. Comorbidities. These conditions include cardiovascular disease, preexisting chronic kidney disease, diabetes mellitus, hyperlipidemia, obesity, and tobacco abuse.

RESTENOSIS

Restenosis is defined as greater than or equal to 50% in-stent diameter stenosis. Restenosis is common in females and people with small vessels (≤ 3.5 mm), calcified lesions, long lesions, diabetes mellitus, stent misadventures (inadequate expansion; malapposition; downsizing; lesion noncoverage; especially at the aorto-ostial junction) [Figure 50-7].

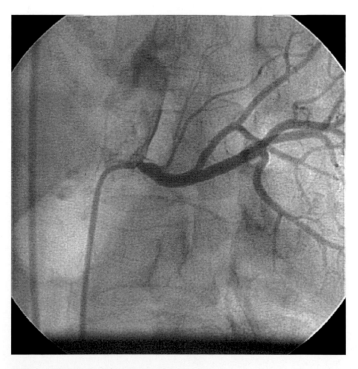

FIGURE 50-7. Renal in-stent restenosis.

【 】 CLINICAL CLUES

Clues include sustained hypertension, worsening hypertension following initial improvement, need for additional antihypertensive medications, and increased postrevascularization serum creatinine (> 50%).

【 】 EVALUATION

Renal angiography is considered the gold standard. A renal Doppler scan, is most commonly used to follow stent patency. Doppler criteria for restenosis include:

- Increase in post-procedure in-stent velocity (> 100 cm/sec) Peak systolic velocity renal/aortic > 3.5.

Other methods of evaluation include captopril renal scanning and CT angiography.

【 】 INDICATIONS FOR TREATMENT

Indications include an angiographic diameter stenosis (≥ 50% to < 80%, with ≥ 20 mm of Hg peak systolic gradient, or ≥ 80%).

【 】 TREATMENT

Methods of treatment include IVUS (see IVUS section), PTA (balloon or cutting balloon), repeat stenting, brachytherapy (investigational), and drug-eluting stents (investigational).

RENAL ARTERY ANEURYSM

Treatment is recommended if the aneurysm is more than 2.5 times the diameter of the reference vessel and based on the location. The majority can be treated with stent grafting.

TRANSPLANT RENAL ARTERIAL DISEASE

RAD has been demonstrated to affect renal transplants. Clinical suspicion is difficult, because antirejection medications and RAS may lead to presentations of either worsening hypertension or renal insufficiency. Duplex scan of the transplanted renal artery can be performed as a screening test. It is invaluable to obtain the operative report for the transplantation, because the arterial anastomosis may vary. Angiographic evaluation should include a complete assessment of the parent vessel, the anastomotic site, and the transplanted renal artery. Long-term outcomes with renal artery angioplasty and stenting in this subset of patients has been studied to be safe and efficacious in improving both blood pressure and renal function.[8]

FUTURE DIRECTIONS

【 】 RESIST TRIAL

This prospective randomized multicenter study is comparing the safety and efficacy of renal artery stenting with and without the use of a distal protection device and with and without use of a platelet aggregator inhibitor.[9]

【 】 CORAL TRIAL

A National Heart, Lung and Blood Institute-sponsored randomized clinical trial of medical therapy versus renal artery angioplasty and stenting with utilization of a distal protection device. Patients have angiographically documented RAS and RVH with blood pressure greater than or equal to 155/90 mm Hg when taking 2 or more antihypertensive medications. Primary end points consist of cardiovascular and renal outcomes including survival with a 5-year follow-up period.[10]

REFERENCES

1. Goldblatt H, et al. Studies on experimental hypertension; production of persistent elevation of systolic blood pressure by means of renal ischemia. *J Exper Med.* 1934;59:347.
2. Van de ven, PJ et al. Arterial stenting and balloon angioplasty in ostial atherosclerotic renovascular disease: a randomised trial. *Lancet.* 1999;353:282.
3. Henry M, et al. Renal angioplasty and stenting under protection: the way for the future? *Catheter Cardiovasc Interv.* 2003;60:299.
4. Harb TS, et al. Renal artery stenting using gadodiamide arteriography in patients with baseline renal insufficiency. *J Endovasc Ther.* 2004 Oct;11:553.
5. Caridi JG, et al. Carbon dioxide digital subtraction angiography for renal artery stent placement. *J Endovasc Ther.* 2004;11:553.
6. Burket MW, et al. Renal artery angioplasty and stent placement: predictors of a favorable outcome. *Am Heart J.* 2000;139(1 pt 1):64.
7. Watson PS, et al. Effect of renal artery stenting on renal function and size in patients with atherosclerotic renovascular disease. *Circulation.* 2000;102:1671.
8. Salvadori M, et al. Efficacy and safety of palmaz stent implantation in the treatment of renal artery stenosis in renal transplantation. *Transplant Proc.* 2005;37:1047.
9. Cooper CJ, et al. RESIST Trial. Available at: http://www.mco.vasculardomain.com.
10. CORAL Trial. Cardiovascular outcomes in renal arterial lesions. Available at: http://www.clinicaltrials.gov and http://www.coralclinicaltrial.org.

CHAPTER (51)

Iliac Angioplasty and Stenting

*Sunil V. Rao, MD, Frank J. Zidar, MD, and
James P. Zidar, MD*

Peripheral arterial disease involving the lower extremities is a common manifestation of systemic atherosclerosis. Epidemiologic studies indicate that up to 5% of men and 2.5% of women older than 60 years of age suffer from symptoms of intermittent claudication as a result of atherosclerotic narrowing or occlusion of the lower extremities.[1] The location of symptoms depends on the site of the obstruction–atherosclerotic narrowing of the iliac arteries (the second most common site of involvement after the superficial femoral arteries) can lead to symptoms of buttock, thigh, and leg claudication and weakness. Although the symptoms of claudication progress slowly in the majority of patients, up to 30% of affected patients have progressive symptoms requiring intervention, and up to 20% develop critical limb ischemia.[2] Perhaps most alarming is that patients with intermittent claudication have a threefold higher cardiovascular mortality when compared with those who do not. The goals of therapy in patients with iliac disease are reduction of cardiovascular mortality, primarily through medical therapy with aspirin and clopidogrel, and symptom relief and prevention of disease progression through revascularization procedures.

The cornerstones of treatment of patients with peripheral arterial disease consist of prudent secondary prevention measures such as exercise for those without contraindications; smoking cessation; antiplatelet therapy with aspirin, ticlopidine, and/or clopidogrel; and lipid-lowering therapy when appropriate to reduce cardiovascular risk. Revascularization, either surgical or endovascular (ie, percutaneous), is reserved for patients with symptoms refractory to medical therapy. Over the past decade, the number of percutaneous procedures to treat iliac disease has increased dramatically. The purpose of this chapter is to review the indications and techniques of percutaneous transluminal angioplasty (PTA) and stenting of the iliac arteries.

HISTORICAL DEVELOPMENT

Endovascular treatment of peripheral arterial disease began in 1964 with the work of Dotter and Judkins who developed a percutaneous technique of superficial femoral artery (SFA) angioplasty using a coaxial system of progressively larger metal dilators.[3] Interestingly, Charles Dotter had his first experience with percutaneous revascularization 1 year earlier when he inadvertently recanalized an occluded right iliac artery by passing a catheter in a retrograde fashion through the iliac artery with the intent of performing an abdominal aortogram in a patient with renal artery stenosis.[4] The most famous of Dotter's reports dealt predominantly with dilation of SFA occlusions, including the first published report that mentioned the famous "do not fix" patient in whom Dotter performed SFA angioplasty against the wishes of the referring surgeon. The initial outcomes of these now crude procedures were excellent, characterized by a famous photograph of Dotter and the "do not fix" patient at the summit of Mount Hood one year after the patient's SFA dilation. Dotter also collaborated with Bill Cook, the chief executive officer of Cook Group Incorporated, to produce some of the first angiography catheters.[5] Since those initial experiences, technology for PTA and stenting has developed exponentially with the helps of many contributors. Julio Palmaz developed the first balloon-expandable stent,[6] and Andreas Gruentzig developed a catheter with a polyvinyl chloride balloon that could be passed over a guidewire in 1974.[7]

Concomitant with the development of catheters, balloons, and guidewires, was the evolution of radiographic imaging to allow accurate visualization of vascular structures. Prior to 1950, x-ray images were still frames that were produced one at a time. Technicians manually changed cassettes quickly to obtain as many images as possible while contrast was still in the vascular structures.

In 1949, the automatic cassette changer and the image intensifier were introduced, permitting the production of angiograms on roll film. In 1950, Dotter invented an x-ray roll-film magazine that could produce images at the rate of 2 frames per second. This was the prototype for what ultimately became the grid-controlled x-ray tube. In the early 1980s, digital imaging was introduced, and now most modern interventional catheterization laboratories have digital imaging with capabilities for biplane imaging, digital subtraction imaging (a process that "subtracts" structures that do not contain contrast from those that do), and flat-plate imaging.

APPROPRIATE SELECTION OF PATIENTS FOR PERCUTANEOUS REVASCULARIZATION

【 】 BASIC ANATOMY

Atherosclerosis affecting the arterial segments distal to the visceral bearing portion of the abdominal aorta is classified into 3 types based on the extent of distal involvement.[8]

1. Type 1 atherosclerosis involves the infrarenal aorta and the common iliac arteries and is present in 5% to 10% of patients with peripheral arterial disease.
2. Type II extends into the external iliac and common femoral arteries and is present in up to 35% of patients.

3. Type III is the most common type and involves the entire vasculature of the lower extremity from the infrarenal abdominal aorta to the tibial arteries.

As discussed previously, symptoms of atherosclerotic obstruction of the lower extremities is a continuum with absence of symptoms at one end and critical limb ischemia at the other. For all patients with signs and symptoms of peripheral arterial disease, the cornerstone of therapy is secondary prevention and medications proven to reduce cardiovascular mortality, such as aspirin and clopidogrel. For those who fail medical therapy, revascularization is required. The two options available are PTA or open surgical revascularization, and the choice is dependent on lesion characteristics. Clinically, the indications for intervention are incapacitating claudication in the face of appropriate medical therapy, limb-threatening ischemia characterized by rest pain, nonhealing ulcers, tissue loss, or gangrene, and vasculogenic impotence.[9] A more recent indication is to allow patients with significant coronary artery disease to achieve acceptable levels of aerobic exercise. For patients with these signs and symptoms and appropriate anatomy, the therapy of choice is PTA.

Because of the importance of lesion anatomy, the TransAtlantic Inter-Society Consensus (TASC) paper on the management of peripheral arterial disease has devised a classification scheme for lesion characteristics.[10] The scheme classifies lesions into 4 groups. Therapeutic recommendations regarding the appropriate revascularization procedure are group-specific (Table 51-1). For type A

TABLE 51-1

Morphological Stratification of Iliac Lesions

TASC ILIAC ARTERY LESION TYPE		TASC TREATMENT RECOMMENDATION
A	• Single stenosis < 3 cm of the CIA or EIA (unilateral/bilateral)	Endovascular
B	• Single stenosis 3–10 cm in length, not extending into the CFA • Total of two stenoses < 5 cm long in the CIA and/or EIA and not extending into the CFA • Unilateral CIA occlusion	"Currently, endovascular treatment is more often used but insufficient evidence for recommendation."
C	• Bilateral 5–10 cm stenosis of the CIA and/or EIA, not extending into the CFA • Unilateral EIA occlusion, not extending into the CFA • Unilateral EIA stenosis extending into the CFA • Bilateral CIA occlusion	"Currently, surgical treatment is more often used but insufficient evidence for recommendation."
D	• Diffuse, multiple unilateral stenoses involving the CIA, EIA, and CFA (usually > 10 cm) • Unilateral occlusion involving both the CIA and EIA • Bilateral EIA occlusions • Diffuse disease involving the aorta and both iliac arteries • Iliac stenoses in a patient with an abdominal aortic aneurysm or other lesion requiring aortic or iliac surgery	Surgical

CIA = common iliac artery; CFA = common femoral artery; EIA = external iliac artery; TASC = Trans Atlantic Inter-Society Consensus.

lesions, endovascular procedures are the treatment of choice. For type D lesions, surgery is the treatment of choice. For types B and C, there appears to be insufficient evidence to recommend specific approaches. At the time of the drafting of the TASC document, it was thought that most clinicians would recommend an endovascular approach for type B lesions and a surgical approach for type C lesions. It should be noted, however, that as percutaneous techniques continue to evolve, these recommendations are bound to change.

Angiography has its limitations, and in cases in which the stenosis does not appear severe in a patient with classic symptoms, there is some utility in assessing the pressure gradient across the stenosis either at rest or after pharmacologic vasodilation. In general, a resting mean pressure gradient across a stenosis of more than 5 to 7 mm Hg and a postvasodilation mean gradient of more than 10 to 15 mm Hg are considered significant.[11] It should be noted that these cutoff values are arbitrary and that the optimal criteria for what constitutes a significant stenosis or what pressure gradient residual after PTA would have better outcomes with stenting is unclear.[12]

[ ] CLINICAL EVIDENCE BEHIND TREATMENT RECOMMENDATIONS

To facilitate the development of guidelines, the American Heart Association has classified levels of evidence into 5 categories based on the rigor of study design (Table 51-2). Using these levels of evidence, the recommendations for treatment can be classified into 3 grades, A, B, and C, with each grade representing successively less support from rigorous clinical data. There are no level I studies supporting iliac PTA or stenting over surgical intervention, but the totality of the evidence provides strong support for the TASC recommendations above.

To measure both short and long-term outcomes, "procedural success" must be based on a uniform standard. The TASC Working Group has developed definitions for primary patency and secondary patency. The former is defined as uninterrupted patency following only the procedure being evaluated, and the latter is defined as patency following the initial procedure or following a repeat intervention to restore patency of an occluded graft or vessel.

[ ] ILIAC ANGIOPLASTY VERSUS SURGERY

As stated previously, there are no large randomized clinical trials comparing PTA with surgical bypass for patients with iliac disease. There are 2 level II studies (randomized, low-power clinical trials), 1 conducted in Sweden and 1 conducted in the United States. Holm and colleagues randomized 102 patients with critical limb ischemia, severe claudication, and a significant ($> 75\%$) stenosis of 6 cm or less in length in the common iliac, external iliac, femoral, or popliteal artery to either bypass surgery (using either a synthetic graft if the stenosis was suprainguinal or vein graft if the stenosis was infrainguinal) or PTA.[13] At 1 year, there was no significant difference in mortality between the two groups. Although there was a higher rate of amputations overall in the group randomized to surgery, this difference was driven by the patients with critical limb ischemia. There was no difference in amputation rates between the treatment groups in patients with intermittent claudication.

The Veterans Study was a randomized trial that was stratified based on symptoms (claudication vs critical limb ischemia) and level of disease (iliac vs distal).[14] Two hundred and sixty-three men with a documented stenosis greater than 80% and less than 10 cm in length in the iliac, superficial femoral, or popliteal arteries, an ankle-brachial index of 0.9 or less, and symptoms of claudication or critical limb ischemia were randomized to either surgery or PTA. At a median follow-up of 4 years, there was no significant difference between the 2 groups in the incidence of death, primary patency, amputations rates, or quality of life.

Complications of either procedure were tracked in the trial by Holm and colleagues. There was no significant difference in the rate of complications between those randomized to surgery or to PTA; complications were defined as bleeding, occlusion, infection, and embolism.[13] However, in the group with critical limb ischemia, the rate of complications was higher in those randomized to PTA. Complications were not systematically recorded in the Veterans Trial. In a prospective study of patients undergoing iliac angioplasty, the periprocedural complication rate was 10% to 20%.[15]

There are several level V case series that report better long-term results of iliac PTA compared with angioplasty of more distal disease. A case series from the University of Toronto of 667 consecutive patients undergoing iliac PTA found that initial success rates were 90% but that long-term (ie, 5-year) patency was only 53%. Further analysis revealed that patients with disease confined to the iliac arteries had a 5-year patency rate of 63% compared with a rate of 51% for those with more extensive involvement. Similarly, a study by Tegtmeyer and colleagues of 200 patients showed an initial success rate of 90% and a long-term patency rate of 88%.[16] Based on the results of the studies mentioned, as well as a case series of iliac PTA in patients with diabetes,[17] it appears that the immediate procedural success rates are excellent. Long-term patency is enhanced by the lack of distal disease and when the procedure is performed for intermittent claudication rather than for limb salvage.

TABLE 51-2

Relation Between Levels of Evidence and Grades of Recommendations

LEVEL OF EVIDENCE	RECOMMENDATION
Level I: Large randomized trials with clearcut results (and low risk of error)	Grade A
Level II: Small randomized trials with uncertain results (and moderate to high risk of error)	Grade B
Level III: Nonrandomized, contemporaneous controls	Grade C
Level IV: Nonrandomized, historical controls	Grade C
Level V: No controls; case series only	

【 】 ILIAC STENTING VERSUS ANGIOPLASTY

Although the rates of complications from iliac PTA are low and the immediate and long-term success rates are good, iliac stenting has been proposed as a more effective means of percutaneous revascularization for iliac arterial disease. Several case series reports of iliac stenting demonstrate procedural success rates of more than 90%, primary patency rates of 70% to 90%, and secondary patency rates of 50% to 80% at 3 to 5 years.[18-21] There is one level 1 study that compared stenting with balloon angioplasty.[22] The Dutch Iliac Stent Trial Study Group randomly assigned 279 patients with intermittent claudication and iliac artery stenosis of 50% or more and lesion length of 5 cm or less to either direct stenting or balloon angioplasty with selective stent placement for a residual mean pressure gradient of more than 10 mm Hg. Stent placement was performed in 43% of the patients assigned to the selective stent group. Initial procedural success rates, complications, and clinical success rates at follow-up did not differ significantly between the 2 groups. At 2 years, 43% of the direct stent group and 35% of the selective stent group still had symptoms, but health-related quality of life measures were significantly improved in both groups after intervention.[23] Moreover, the rates of repeat iliac artery interventions, myocardial infarction, stroke, extracranial bleeding, or death at 5 years were not significantly different between the groups.

Based largely on the results of the Dutch Iliac Stent Trial, it has been proposed that stenting for iliac arterial disease be limited to cases of residual or recurrent stenosis or complications following angioplasty (ie, dissection). However, it was unclear if placing a stent under these circumstances would be associated with a higher rate of complications and perhaps a higher rate of restenosis. In 1 multicenter case series, 25.1% of patients required stenting for residual or recurrent stenosis, residual pressure gradient, long (> 3 cm) occlusions, or dissection.[24] Stent placement was successful in 100% of cases, and the rate of major complications defined as acute thrombosis, residual stenosis, arterial rupture, or acute dissection was 16%. Moreover, secondary patency at 3 years was 57% (similar to iliac PTA). This suggests that there is no increased risk of complications or restenosis with provisional stenting, and that the overall success rate of a provisional stenting strategy is similar to that seen with initially successful PTA of type A lesions. Whether stenting provides advantages over PTA for types B and C lesions is not known.

BASIC EQUIPMENT

Vascular access for iliac intervention can include the ipsilateral common femoral artery, the contralateral femoral artery, as well as the brachial or radial arteries. The ipsilateral femoral approach is often preferred. This approach allows for the most direct sheath position, which provides the most catheter support. Care must be taken in positioning the sheath to avoid disrupting the lesion with the sheath or more often its radiolucent introducer, especially in distal common iliac or external iliac artery interventions. Contralateral femoral access has the advantage of approaching the iliac stenosis or occlusion in an antegrade fashion; however,

catheter support over the iliac bifurcation can be challenging, especially in ostial common iliac lesions. Using a 0.035-in angled Glidewire (Terumo) within a diagnostic catheter with a nearly 180-degree tip (ie, VB, IMA, or pigtail catheter) often facilitates taking a long sheath over the bifurcation to the point of stenosis or occlusion. The proper combination of radial strength and flexibility are necessary characteristics of the long sheath (the 45-cm Terumo Pinnacle Destination or the Cook Balkan sheath) to avoid kinking at the iliac bifurcation. Bilateral common femoral access may be required to provide adequate periprocedural visualization. Bilateral access is required for ostial common iliac or distal aortic disease to perform the "kissing balloon" technique or "double barrel" stenting. Using a 23- or 25-cm sheath provides an adequate lumen to deliver equipment using smaller 6-Fr sheaths. Baseline angiography with an infrarenal abdominal aortogram is a necessary prerequisite. Often, slight left anterior obliquity (~5°) is helpful in the elderly patient who has a "compressed" left iliac system. Additional 30-degree right and left anterior oblique views are helpful in resolving the internal and external iliac bifurcation. Given the relationship between distal run-off and interventional patency, pre- and post-procedural lower extremity angiograms to assess the runoff below the knee are important.

The iliac vessel caliber lends itself to the use of 0.035-in or 0.018-in guidewire-based equipment. Table 51-3 reviews the variety of available wires, which vary in support, tip, coating, and intended use. Peripheral guidewires, like coronary wires, usually have a stainless steel or nitinol core to provide support. The wires vary from extremely flexible, coiled, shapeable to stiffer, straight, or angled ones that maintain the manufactured shape. Lubricious hydrophilic coatings facilitate wire passage through tortuous vessels and severe stenoses. Wires of increasing stiffness are often used in crossing total occlusions; however, these lesions can often be recanalized using the hydrophilic-coated Terumo Glidewire. Alternatively, the Lumend Frontrunner catheter performs blunt microdissection of the chronic iliac occlusion and is often used after an unsuccessful attempt with a guidewire. The use of guidewire support catheters, such as the Quick-Cross Support Catheter (Spectranetics) can facilitate wire crossing. After initial passage through the lesion, exchange from a 0.035-in-based system to a 0.018-in or 0.014-in wire may decrease the risk of distal vessel trauma for the contralateral approach to a distal external iliac lesion.

Accurate assessment of the iliac vessel prior to percutaneous intervention is essential. In a series of male veterans undergoing iliac stenting, the mean balloon diameter was 8.36 plus 0.2 mm.[25] When using a provisional stenting approach, careful assessment of vessel caliber and choice of angioplasty balloon size is critical to avoid dissection. Appropriate device sizing is especially important when intervening on the external iliac, which has a greater propensity to barotrauma and dissection. Periprocedural conscious sedation allows the operator to interact with the patient during balloon inflations in the iliac system. Assessing the patient for flank or back pain during slow inflation of the angioplasty balloon may avoid excessive barotrauma and adventitial injury. Table 51-4 reviews the numerous PTA balloons currently available.

The decision to initially deploy a stent in the iliac artery or in a provisional fashion after balloon angioplasty is based on the lesions angiographic appearance and location. Similarly, the choice of balloon-expandable or self-expanding stent is also determined by

TABLE 51-3

Abbreviated List of Peripheral Guidewires

NAME	DESCRIPTION IN	COATING	TIP	LENGTH (cm)
Cook				
Amplatz (varying stiffness)	0.035	None	Straight and J tip	80, 145, 160, 260, 300
Bentson	0.025, 0.032, 0.035, 0.038	None	Straight tip	145, 180, 300
Roadrunner–Nimble	0.035, 0.038	Hydrophilic	Angled tip	145, 180, 260.
Roadrunner–The Firm	0.035, 0.038	None	Angled tip	145, 180, 260
Rosen	0.035	None	J tip	80, 145, 260
Cordis				
Jindo	0.035	None	Taper to shapeable, 0.022-in	180, 300
eV3				
AQ Wire	0.018/0.035	Hydrophilic	Straight/angled	150, 180, 260
Nitrex	0.014–0.035	None	Straight/angled	145, 180, 260, 400
Guidant				
Spartacore	0.014	None	Straight/shapeable	130, 190, 300
Steelcore	0.018	None	Straight/shapeable and J tip	190, 300
Supracore	0.035	None	Straight/shapeable	145, 190, 300
Mallinkrodt				
Tad II	0.035	None	Taper to shapeable 0.018	140, 260
Wholey	0.035	None	Straight/J tip	145, 175
Terumo/Medi-Tech/Boston Scientific				
Amplatz	0.035	None	Straight/shapeable	145, 180, 260
Glidewire	0.035	Hydrophilic	Straight/angled	150, 180
Glidewire–stiff	0.035	Hydrophilic	Angled tip	150, 180
Magic Torque	0.035	Hydrophilic tip	Straight/shapeable	180, 260
Meier	0.035	None	Angled/J tip	185, 260, 300

OTW = over-the-wire; SS = stainlless steel.

angiographic appearance and location. When additional radial force or precise positioning of the stent is required, balloon-expandable stents are preferred, because some degree of shortening does occur with self-expanding stent deployment. When treating ostial iliac disease or distal aortic disease extending into the iliac arteries, a "double barrel" technique with two balloon expandable stents often yields excellent results. When treating nonostial iliac disease, aneurysmal iliacs and the external iliac artery, self-expanding stents are often preferred. Given the external iliac artery's propensity for dissection with stent deployment, close attention must be paid to stent sizing and length when extending a stent into the external iliac artery. In general, a ratio of 1.1:1 can be used when determining stent size for the iliac artery. The maximum stent size for a woman's iliac artery should rarely exceed 8 mm and

in man's iliac artery should rarely exceed 10 mm. Tables 51-5 to 51-7 review several of the currently available balloon-expandable and self-expanding stents.

Plaque excision or arthrectomy may have a role in the setting of in-stent restenosis in the iliac arteries. The Silverhawk plaque excision catheters (Fox Hollow Technologies) can be used to remove the restenotic tissue prior to PTA. Occasionally, plaque excision alone can provide an adequate residual luminal diameter such that it can be used the sole device for in-stent restenosis.

Covered stents can be useful in the setting of aneurysmal disease and in sealing major dissections. Currently 4 covered stents are available for off-label use in the iliac arteries. The Jostent Peripheral Stent Graft (Abbott Laboratories) utilizes a layer of polytetrafluoroethylene graft material placed between two

TABLE 51-4

Abbreviated List of Peripheral Angioplasty Balloons (> 6 mm)

NAME	DIAMETER (SHEATH COMPATIBILITY)/LENGTH	WIRE SIZE (in)
Abbott		
Fox (OTW)	6–7 mm (5-Fr); 8–9 mm (6-Fr); 10, 12 mm (7-Fr) 20, 30, 40, 60, 80 mm	0.035
Bard		
Centurion Opti-Plast (OTW)	6–7 mm (6-Fr); 8 mm (7-Fr); 9–10 mm (8-Fr) 20, 40 mm	0.035
Conquest (OTW)	6–8 mm (6-Fr); 9–10 mm (7-Fr); 12 mm (8-Fr) 20, 40, 60, 80 mm	0.035
Cordis		
Aviator (monorail)	6–6.5 mm (5-Fr); 7 mm (6-Fr) 15, 20, 30, 40 mm	0.014
Slalom (OTW)	6 mm (5-Fr); 7–8 mm (6-Fr) 20, 40 mm	0.018
Powerflex P3 (OTW)	6–7 mm (6-Fr); 8–10, 12 mm (7-Fr) 10, 15, 20, 30, 40, 50, 60, 80, 100 mm	0.035
Opta Pro (OTW)	6–8 mm (6-Fr); 9–10, 12 mm (7-Fr) 10, 15, 20, 30, 40, 60, 80, 100 mm	0.035
eV3		
Submarine Plus (OTW)	6 mm (4-Fr); 7 mm (5-Fr) 20, 40, 60, 80, 120 mm	0.018
Sailor Plus (OTW)	6–7 mm (5-Fr); 8 mm (6-Fr); 9–12 mm (7-Fr) 20, 40, 60, 80, 120 mm	0.035
Guidant		
Agiltrac-018 (OTW)	6–8 mm (5-Fr); 9–10 mm (6-Fr); 12 mm (7-Fr) 20, 30, 40, 60 mm	0.018
Agiltrac-035 (OTW)	6–9 mm (6-Fr); 10–14 mm (7-Fr) 20, 40, 60, 80 and 100 mm	0.035
Medi-Tech/Boston Scientific		
Peripheral Cutting Balloon (OTW)	6–8 mm (6-Fr) 10-, 20-mm cutting lengths	0.018
Talon (OTW)	6 mm (5-Fr); 7 mm (6-Fr) 15, 20, 40 mm	0.018
Ultrasoft (monorail)	6, 6.5 mm (6-Fr); 7 mm (7-Fr) 15, 20 mm	0.018
Ultrathin SDS/Diamond (OTW)	6 mm (5-Fr); 7 mm (6-Fr); 8–10 mm (7-Fr) 15, 20, 30, 40, 60, 80 mm	0.035
Blue Max 20 (OTW)	6 mm (6-Fr); 7–8 mm (7-Fr); 9–10 mm (8-Fr) 20, 30, 40, 80, 100 mm	0.035
Synergy (OTW)	6–8 (6-Fr); 9–12 mm (7-Fr) 15, 20, 30, 40, 60, 80, 100 mm	0.035

OTW = over-the-wire; SS = stainless steel.

flexible stainless steel balloon-expandable stents. The Wallgraft (Boston Scientific) is a self-expanding stent covered with a proprietary coating, Permalume. The Viabahn stent graft (Gore) also uses a self-expanding design with a nonporous polymer sleeve. As with several self-expanding stents, there may be considerable foreshortening (as much as 20% with the Wallgraft). The iCast stent (Atrium) is the only balloon-expandable covered stent that is large enough for iliac applications. These devices require larger 7- to 10-Fr delivery systems, depending on vessel size and manufacturer.

TABLE 51-5

Abbreviated List of Balloon-Expandable Peripheral Stents (> 6 mm)

NAME	MATERIAL	DIAMETER (SHEATH COMPATIBILITY)/LENGTH	WIRE SIZE (in)
Abbott Medical Devices			
Jostent (bare stent)	SS	2 sizes: "standard" 4–9 mm; "large" 6–12 mm 12, 17, 28, 38, 48, 58 mm	N/A
Wavemax	SS	6–7 mm (6-Fr); 8–9 mm (7-Fr); 10, 12 mm (8-Fr) 17, 28, 38, 58 mm	0.035
EV3			
LD DoubleStrut (bare stent)	SS	9–12 mm (8-Fr) 15, 26, 36, 56, 76 mm	N/A
Primus GPS (OTW)	SS	6–8 mm (6-Fr); 9–10 mm (7-Fr) 12, 17, 27, 37, 57 mm	0.035
Cordis			
Genesis	SS	Available on 0.014-in Aviator platform Available on 0.018-in Slalom platform Available on 0.035-in Opta-Pro platform	0.014 0.018 0.035
Guidant			
Omnilink (OTW)	SS	6–7 mm (6-Fr); 8–9 mm (7-Fr); 10 mm (8-Fr) 12, 16, 18, 28, 38, 58 mm (38–58mm upsize sheath)	0.035
Herculink–Plus (monorail)	SS	6 mm (5-Fr); 6.5, 7 mm (6-Fr) 12, 15, 18 mm	0.014
Medi-Tech/Boston Scientific			
Express Biliary SD (monorail)	SS	4–6 mm (5-Fr); 7 mm (6-Fr)–reinforced proximal one third 15, 20 mm	0.014 0.018
Express Biliary LD (monorail)	SS	5–7 mm (6-Fr); 8–10 mm (7-Fr) 20, 30, 40, 60 mm	0.035
Meditronic AVE			
Bridge Assurant (OTW)	SS	6–8 mm (6-Fr); 9–10 mm (7-Fr) 21, 27, 30, 40, 60 mm	0.035

OTW = over-the-wire; SS = stainless steel.

ADJUNCTIVE PHARMACOLOGY

The evolution of dual antiplatelet therapy for the prevention of periprocedural thrombotic events during coronary interventions has been applied to peripheral arterial interventions. Pretreatment with aspirin and the thienopyridine clopidogrel is the current standard of care for peripheral arterial intervention.

Due to the mechanical plaque disruption and exposure of procoagulant material or the mere presence of a newly deployed stent that is not yet covered by endothelial cells, antithrombotic therapy is required during peripheral intervention. The most widely used antithrombin therapy is unfractionated heparin (UFH). Although not rigorously evaluated in randomized trials during peripheral arterial interventions, a target activated clotting time (ACT) of 200 to 300 seconds balances the benefit of prevention of periprocedural thrombosis with the risk of periprocedural bleeding. Low-molecular-weight-heparins (LMWHs), potent inhibitors of factor Xa, have been studied in surgical revascularization of peripheral arterial disease. Efficacy of LMWHs during percutaneous peripheral arterial interventions has not been assessed in randomized, controlled trials. In a prospective registry (Angiomax Peripheral Procedure Registry of Vascular Events [APPROVE] trial), 505 patients were treated with the direct thrombin inhibitor, bivalirudin, during peripheral arterial intervention.[26] Ischemic events (death, myocardial infarction, unplanned revascularization, and amputation) were low (1.4%); protocol-defined major bleeding and Thrombolysis in Myocardial Infarction (TIMI) major bleeding were 2.2% and 0.4%, respectively. With comparable event rates to UFH, bivalirudin decreased time to sheath removal and ambulation in this nonrandomized, uncontrolled registry.

TABLE 51-6

Abbreviated List of Self-Expandable Peripheral Stents (> 6mm)

NAME	MATERIAL	DIAMETER (SHEATH COMPATIBILITY)/LENGTH	WIRE SIZE (in)
Abbott			
SelfX (OTW)	Nitinol	6, 8, 10 mm (7-Fr), 12 mm (8-Fr) 32, 44, 68, 92 mm	0.035
Xact (monorail)	Nitinol	7–10 mm (7-Fr) (tapered stents also available) 20, 30, 40 mm	0.035
Bard			
Luminexx (OTW)	Nitinol	6–10, 12, 14 mm (6-Fr) 20, 30, 40, 50, 60, 80, 100, 120 mm	0.035
Cook			
Zilver 518 (OTW)	Nitinol	6–9 mm (5-Fr) 20, 30, 40, 50, 60 mm	0.018
Zilver 635 (OTW)	Nitinol	6–10 mm (6-Fr) 20, 30, 40, 50, 60 mm	0.035
eV3			
Protégé GPS (OTW)	Nitinol	6–9 mm (6-Fr); 10–12 mm (7-Fr–0.035-in only) 20, 30, 40, 60, 80, 100, 120, 150 mm	0.018 0.035
Cordis			
Precise (OTW)	Nitinol	5–10 mm (6-Fr) (monorail version available) 20, 30, 40 mm	0.014
SMART control (OTW)	Nitinol	6–10 mm (6-Fr) 20, 40, 60, 80, 100 mm	0.035
Guidant			
Acculink (monorail)	Nitinol	5–10 mm (6-Fr) (tapered stents also available) 20, 30, 40 mm	0.014
Absolute (OTW)	Nitinol	5–10 mm (6-Fr) 20, 30, 40, 60, 80, 100 mm	0.035
Dynalink (OTW)	Nitinol	5–10 mm (6-Fr) 28, 38, 56, 80, 100 mm	0.018 0.035
Medi-Tech/Boston Scientific			
Sentinol (OTW)	Nitinol	5–10 mm (6-Fr) 20, 40, 60, 80 mm	0.035
Wallstent (OTW)	Elgiloy	6–8 mm (9-Fr); 9–11 mm (10-Fr); 12 mm (11-Fr) 20, 30, 50, 70 mm	0.035
Medtronic AVE			
Aurora (OTW)	SS	6–8 mm (6-Fr); 9–10 mm (7-Fr) 20, 40, 60, 80 mm	0.035

OTW = over-the-wire; SS = stainless steel.

COMPLICATIONS

Serious vascular complications, such as arterial rupture or major retrograde aortic dissection, during iliac artery intervention can be catastrophic. A predefined system for emergent surgical backup in the event of a major vascular complication is mandatory. The inability to manually compress the vasculature in the pelvis can lead to rapid hemodynamic collapse. Emergent options should include the possible use of a long balloon proximal to the rupture to tamponade the bleeding or the quick insertion of a covered stent graft. Anticoagulation should be reversed, if heparin is used. Fortunately, in the setting of proper device sizing, the frequency of complications such as vessel rupture is extremely low.[16]

Peripheral embolization is rare and is best assessed by performing pre- and post-procedural lower extremity angiograms to assess

TABLE 51-7

Abbreviated List of Covered Peripheral Stents (> 6mm)

NAME	DELIVERY	MATERIAL	DIAMETER (SHEATH COMPATIBILITY)/LENGTH	WIRE SIZE (in)
Abbott Medical Devices Jostent Stent Graft	Self-expanding	SS; PTFE layer between 2 stents	2 sizes: "standard" 4–9 mm; "large" 6–12 mm 12, 17, 28, 38 48, 58 mm	0.035
Atrium iCast (OTW)	Balloon-expandable	SS (PTFE covered)	5–10 mm (7-Fr); 12 mm (8-Fr) (PTFE covered) 38, 59 mm	0.035
Gore Viabahn (OTW)	Self-exapanding	Nitionl stent (PTFE lined)	6 mm (8-Fr); 7–8 mm (9-Fr); 9–10 mm (11-Fr); 11, 13 mm (12-Fr) 5, 10, 15 mm	0.035 (5–8 mm) 0.025 (9–13 mm)
Medi-Tech/Boston Scientific Wallgraft (OTW)	Self-expanding	Elgiloy stent (PTFE covered)	6–8 mm (9-Fr); 9–11 mm (10-Fr); 12 mm (11-Fr) 20, 30, 50, 70 mm	0.035

OTW = over-the-wire; PTFE = polytetrafluoroethylene; SS = stainless steel.

the run-off below the knee. Mechanical thrombectomy or direct infusion of thrombolytics into the affected limb may be required to prevent an emergent trip to the operating room for a Fogarty embolectomy. With any percutaneous vascular intervention, access site complications such as bleeding, hematoma, infection, or pseudoaneurysm can occur and are best avoided by careful attention to anatomic landmarks and vigilant monitoring of peak ACT and the groin access site during the case. Patients who are appropriate candidates for groin closure devices must be carefully selected, because diffuse atherosclerosis is frequently encountered in these patients' common femoral arteries.

REFERENCES

1. Reunanen A, Takkunen H, et al. Prevalence of intermittent claudication and its effect on mortality. *Acta Med Scand.* 1982;211:249.
2. Cronenwett JL, Warner KG, et al. Intermittent claudication. Current results of nonoperative management. *Arch Surg.* 1984;119:430.
3. Dotter CT, Judkins MP. Transluminal treatment of arteriosclerotic obstruction. Description of a new technic and a preliminary report of its application. *Circulation.* 1964;30:654.
4. Mueller RL, Sanborn TA. The history of interventional cardiology: cardiac catheterization, angioplasty, and related interventions. *Am Heart J.* 1995;129:146.
5. Rosch J, Abrams HL, et al. Memorials: Charles Theodore Dotter, 1920—1985. *AJR Am J Roentgenol.* 1985;144:1321.
6. Palmaz JC, Richter GM, et al. Intraluminal stents in atherosclerotic iliac artery stenosis: preliminary report of a multicenter study. *Radiology.* 1988;168:727.
7. Gruentzig A. Percutaneous transluminal coronary angioplasty. *Lancet.* 1978; 1:263.
8. Green RM, Ouriel K. Peripheral arterial disease. In: Schwartz SI, Shires GT, Spencer FC, Husser WC, eds. *Principles of Surgery,* 6th ed. New York, NY: McGraw-Hill 1994;925.
9. Weitz JI, Byrne J, et al. Diagnosis and treatment of chronic arterial insufficiency of the lower extremities: a critical review. *Circulation.* 1996;94:3026.
10. Dormandy JA, Rutherford RB. Management of peripheral arterial disease (PAD). TASC Working Group. TransAtlantic Inter-Society Consensus (TASC). *J Vasc Surg.* 2000;31(1 pt 2):S1.
11. Bonn J. Percutaneous vascular intervention: value of hemodynamic measurements. *Radiology.* 1996;201:18.
12. Kamphuis AG, van Engelen AD, et al. Impact of different hemodynamic criteria for stent placement after suboptimal iliac angioplasty. Dutch Iliac Stent Trial Study Group. *J Vasc Intervent Radiol.* 1999;10:741.
13. Holm J, Arfvidsson B, et al. Chronic lower limb ischaemia. A prospective randomised controlled study comparing the 1-year results of vascular surgery and percutaneous transluminal angioplasty (PTA). *Eur J Vasc Surg.* 1991;5:517.
14. Wolf GL, Wilson SE, et al. Surgery or balloon angioplasty for peripheral vascular disease: a randomized clinical trial. Principal investigators and associates of Veterans Administration Cooperative Study Number 199. *J Vasc Intervent Radiol.* 1993;4:639.
15. Johnston KW, Rae M, et al. 5-year results of a prospective study of percutaneous transluminal angioplasty. *Ann Surg.* 1987;206:403.
16. Tegtmeyer CJ, Hartwell GD, et al. Results and complications of angioplasty in aortoiliac disease. *Circulation.* 1991;832 (suppl 2):153.
17. Stokes KR, Strunk HM, et al. Five-year results of iliac and femoropopliteal angioplasty in diabetic patients. *Radiology.* 1990;174(3 pt 2):977.
18. Hausegger KA, Cragg AH, et al. Iliac artery stent placement: clinical experience with a nitinol stent. *Radiology.* 1994;190:199.
19. Ballard JL, Sparks SR, et al. Complications of iliac artery stent deployment. *J Vasc Surg.* 1996;24:545.
20. Vorwerk D, Guenther RW, et al. Primary stent placement for chronic iliac artery occlusions: follow-up results in 103 patients. *Radiology.* 1995;194:745.
21. Cikrit DF, Gustafson PA, et al. Long-term follow-up of the Palmaz stent for iliac occlusive disease. *Surgery.* 1995;118:608.

22. Tetteroo E, van der Graaf Y, et al. Randomised comparison of primary stent placement versus primary angioplasty followed by selective stent placement in patients with iliac-artery occlusive disease. Dutch Iliac Stent Trial Study Group. *Lancet.* 1998;351:1153.

23. Bosch JL, van der Graaf Y, et al. Health-related quality of life after angioplasty and stent placement in patients with iliac artery occlusive disease: results of a randomized controlled clinical trial. The Dutch Iliac Stent Trial Study Group. *Circulation.* 1000;99:3155.

24. Treiman GS, Schneider PA, et al. Does stent placement improve the results of ineffective or complicated iliac artery angioplasty? *J Vasc Surg.* 1998;28:104.

25. Lee ES, Steenson CC, et al. Comparing patency rates between external iliac and common iliac artery stents. *J Vasc Surg.* 2000;315:889.

26. Allie DE, Hall P, et al. The Angiomax Peripheral Procedure Registry of Vascular Events Trial (APPROVE): in-hospital and 30-day results. *J Invasive Cardiol.* 2004;16:651.

CHAPTER (52)

Endovascular Abdominal Aortic Aneurysm Repair

Robert S. Dieter, MD, and
John R. Laird, MD

Rupture of abdominal aortic aneurysms (AAAs) accounts for 1% of all deaths and is the tenth leading cause of death in men older than 55 years of age. Out-of-hospital AAA rupture is associated with a mortality of 80% to 90%. Most deaths are preventable by the early diagnosis and treatment of AAA. More than 40,000 surgical procedures for AAA are performed annually in the United States. Despite the excellent results of open surgical repair for the prevention of aneurysm rupture, this procedure is associated with significant morbidity and mortality, especially in high-risk patients. Endovascular aneurysm repair (EVAR), which was developed as a less invasive alternative to open surgical repair, is gaining widespread acceptance, particularly for the high-risk patient.

EPIDEMIOLOGY AND NATURAL HISTORY OF ABDOMINAL AORTIC ANEURYSM

The incidence of AAA increases with age. Approximately 2.6% of men and 0.5% of women between 45 and 54 years of age have an AAA and by 75 to 84 years of age, 19.8% of men and 5.2% of women have an AAA.[1] Men are affected 4 to 6 times more frequently than women.[1] There is thought to be a racial disparity to the incidence of AAA, with the prevalence of AAA more common in whites than in blacks.[2]

Up to 15% of patients with AAA demonstrate a family history of AAA.[3] Because the pathogenesis of AAA is thought to be multifactorial, including disorders of enzymes regulating connective tissue homeostasis, it is not surprising that approximately 5% of patients with an AAA have a concomitant thoracic aneurysm and that approximately 15% have either a femoral artery aneurysm or

a popliteal aneurysm.[4] Synchronous peripheral aneurysms are more common in men. Physical examination has a low sensitivity in detecting these aneurysms, and ultrasound screening may be the preferred method of screening for these aneurysms in patients with AAA. Renal artery involvement is seen in up to 10% of AAAs, and iliac artery involvement in up to 22% of AAAs.[3] Ninety-five percent of AAAs are juxtarenal or infrarenal.

Patients with AAAs often have significant medical and cardiac comorbidities. Coronary artery disease is found in 40% to 70% of patients with AAAs, with evidence of a myocardial infarction in up to 46% of patients.[3] Cerebrovascular disease is present in 25% of patients, claudication is present in 28%,[3] hypertension is present in 55%, and chronic obstructive lung disease in approximately 20% to 25%. A history of blunt abdominal trauma is occasionally found; this can lead to both true aneurysms and pseudoaneurysms of the abdominal aorta. Diabetes is seen only in approximately 10% to 20% of affected patients. The negative correlation between diabetes and AAA has not been adequately explained. Most studies have shown that AAAs are approximately 6 to 7 times more common in smokers, whereas elevated high-density lipoprotein cholesterol (HDL-C) may be protective.[1] Furthermore, 23% have some form of cancer.[3]

Approximately 67% of patients with AAAs die of a cardiovascular etiology.[5]

The aneurysm growth rate, wall tension, and risk of rupture are dependent on aneurysm diameter. Aneurysms less than 5.5 cm in diameter grow at a median rate of 0.2 to 0.3 cm/y, whereas those greater than 5 to 6 cm expand at rates up to 3 cm/y.[6] The strongest predictor of AAA rupture is aneurysm size. Aneurysms between 5.5 and 5.9 cm in diameter have an estimated annual risk of rupture of 9.4%, those between 6.0 and 6.9 cm in diameter have an estimated annual risk of rupture of 10.2%, and those greater than 7 cm have an estimated annual rate of rupture of 32.5%.[3] If AAA size is accounted for, the relationship between aneurysm growth rate and the risk of rupture is reduced in significance. Large aneurysms that rupture also tend to grow more quickly. Eccentric or saccular aneurysms have considerably increased wall stress and are thought to have greater rupture risk than fusiform AAA.[7] Patient age and family history of AAA are not consistent independent predictors of rupture.

TYPES OF ABDOMINAL AORTIC ANEURYSMS

True aortic aneurysms result from the dilation of the intima, media, and adventitial layers of the aorta. Relatively uniform and concentric enlargement results in fusiform aneurysm formation. Saccular aneurysms result from eccentric enlargement of the aorta. As previously noted, saccular aneurysms are thought to have less uniform wall stress distribution and thus an increased risk of rupture.

Although traditionally attributed to atherosclerosis, AAAs more accurately can be attributed to a degenerative process in the arterial wall. Most AAAs result from the imbalance of connective tissue formation and degradation. Some congenital disorders such as Marfan syndrome and Ehlers-Danlos syndrome predispose to aneurysm development. Inflammatory aortitis is a rare cause of AAA formation. Pseudoaneurysms generally result from abdominal trauma or may occur at a graft anastomosis following previous aortic surgery.

Inflammatory AAAs are a subset (5%) of AAAs, which commonly present as abdominal or flank pain, fever, and constitutional symptoms. On computed tomography (CT), these AAAs usually have a "halo" sign with inflammatory tissue predominately anterior and lateral to the AAA. Due to the sometimes extensive inflammation and fibrosis of surrounding structures, including the duodenum, vena cava, left renal vein, and ureters, an endovascular approach may be optimal.[8]

Mycotic AAAs are fortunately rare. Most commonly, *Salmonella* sp or *Staphylococcus aureus* are the etiologic bacteria, although fungal species or other bacteria are sometimes causative. Infected AAAs pose a significant risk to the patient and present many therapeutic challenges. The traditional surgical approach is ligation of the aorta, resection of the infected aneurysm, and extra-anatomic bypass. There have been case reports and small series involving the endovascular treatment of mycotic thoracic and AAAs. Although successful outcomes have been demonstrated in a few cases, the potential for infection of the endoprosthesis raises significant concerns regarding this treatment approach.[9,10] Aorto-enteric fistulae from AAAs have also been successfully excluded using an endograft.[11]

INDICATIONS FOR INTERVENTION

The majority of AAAs are asymptomatic. When an asymptomatic AAA is discovered either during screening, routine physical examination, or incidentally in the evaluation of other pathology, it is important to establish the size of the aneurysm and its growth rate.

The reason to intervene for an asymptomatic AAA is principally to reduce the risk of rupture. The mortality associated with rupture of an AAA is 60% to 80% (30%-65% if the patient reaches the hospital alive).[1]

TREATMENT OF ABDOMINAL AORTIC ANEURYSMS

[ ] MEDICAL THERAPY

Although the basic understanding of the inflammatory and dynamic nature of AAAs has significantly advanced, there is as of yet no effective medical treatment for AAAs. On the premise that aneurysmal growth is dependent in part on the $\delta P/\delta t$ of the aortic pulsation, a trial of the beta-blocker propranolol was carried out. At a mean of 2.5 years, there was no reduction in AAA growth rate or mortality associated with the use of propranolol.[12] Efforts to reduce the activity of the enzymes MMPs directly have been performed with doxycycline in patients with AAAs. Small pilot studies demonstrate that doxycycline reduces the levels of MMP-9 and C-reactive protein (CRP).[13,14] Preliminary investigation suggests that doxycycline may impede aneurysm growth.[14] The effects of raising HDL-C and reducing inflammation with HMG-CoA reductase inhibitors ("statins") on aneurysm growth have not been adequately studied.

Despite the current lack of an adequate medical treatment for AAAs, adjunctive pharmacologic intervention, which is directed at the underlying molecular and enzymatic pathophysiology of AAAs, may ultimately be useful in the long-term treatment of patients who have undergone EVAR. Such therapy could conceivably be of importance because the aneurysm sac is excluded but not removed. Prevention of continued aortic or iliac artery enlargement at the proximal and distal endograft attachment sites is also desirable to prevent late endoleak.

[ ] INVASIVE THERAPY OF ABDOMINAL AORTIC ANEURYSM

The only proven, available method for reduction in mortality from AAA rupture is mechanical aneurysm exclusion. Elective open AAA repair is associated with a mortality of 2.7% to 7% and may be higher depending on patient comorbidities.[1] Indeed, the perioperative cardiac risk is thought to be greater for open AAA exclusion than for coronary artery bypass graft surgery. Thus, the clinician is faced with balancing the interventional risk of AAA repair with that of continued observation and threat of rupture.

Several trials have been performed to determine the size of an AAA that optimizes the trade-off between risk of AAA rupture and perioperative mortality. These studies have suggested that aneurysms less than 5.5 cm that grow at rates less than 0.7 cm/6 mo or 1 cm/12 mo may be safely observed. Surgery can be reserved for aneurysms larger than 5.5 cm without increasing overall mortality or operative risk.[15,16] However, these studies are prefaced on routine AAA surveillance and close patient follow-up.

Despite the equivalent overall survival between surveillance and early repair for aneurysms less than 5.5 cm, caution must be used in extending these criteria to underrepresented study groups. Because women have smaller abdominal aortas than men, criteria for diagnosis of an AAA as well as for intervention for an AAA may not be accurately applied to both genders. Some studies have suggested that a 5.0-cm diameter AAA in women has an equivalent rupture risk to that of a 6.0-cm diameter AAA in men.[7] The application of a single measurement that is not gender specific or referenced to the patient's height may not be entirely valid.

Patients with symptomatic AAAs usually present with abdominal pain that may radiate to the flank or groin, abdominal tenderness to palpation, low back pain, or hemodynamic instability related to the retroperitoneal hemorrhage. In addition to the risk of rupture, aneurysms can be associated with a significant risk of embolic complications. Due to the presence of thrombus or atherosclerotic material within the aneurysm sac, patients may present with evidence of atheroemboli (ie, livedo reticularis), acute renal failure, "blue toe syndrome," or symptoms of lower extremity arterial insufficiency. Enlargement of the AAA can cause a mass effect and obstructive symptoms. Obstructive uropathy can occur and is thought to be more common in inflammatory AAAs.

Contained or frank rupture of an AAA demands emergency intervention. Classically, there is severe pain, abdominal tenderness, and shock. The pain is generally sudden in onset and constant, and it may diffusely involve the abdomen or radiate to the flanks, groin, or legs. Occasionally, a ruptured AAA presents as a gastrointestinal hemorrhage or aortocaval fistula. Expeditious diagnosis with an imaging study (usually CT) or direct transfer to the interventional suite or operating room is necessary to reduce the attendant morbidity and mortality of a ruptured AAA.

In summary, the criteria for intervention on an AAA include an aneurysm diameter greater than 5.5 cm in men (perhaps 5.0 cm in women), rapid expansion of an aneurysm (> 0.5–0.7 cm/6 mo or 1 cm/12 mo), distal embolization from an AAA, aneurysmal mass effect, threatened rupture, or frank rupture.

GENERAL OUTCOMES AFTER ENDOVASCULAR ANEURYSM REPAIR

The goal of EVAR is to prevent aneurysm rupture and reduce the morbidity and mortality associated with exclusion of the AAA. Successful EVAR exclusion is associated with a progressive reduction in aneurysmal volume at a rate of approximately 3 mL/mo and reduction in aneurysm diameter of 4 to 6 mm/y.[17] Regression in aneurysm size may be in part dependent on the type of endograft used.[18]

Technical success rates for device implantation in modern series exceed 90%.[19–22] The currently available modular endograft systems can be successfully delivered in the great majority of cases (Figure 52-1). Modularity allows for customization of the devices for an individual patient's anatomy. Recent randomized trials comparing the results of EVAR with open surgical repair have demonstrated a reduced 30-day mortality rate in those patients undergoing EVAR.[21,22] In addition, perioperative morbidity is significantly reduced with EVAR. There is a 3% to 10% cardiac complication rate in the EVAR group compared with 14% to 21% in the open surgical group.[19–22] Perioperative respiratory complications are seen in approximately 1% to 5% of patients treated by an endovascular approach compared with 12% to 22.5% of patients treated by open repair.[19,20] Avoidance of a laparotomy results in a significant reduction in bowel complications with EVAR. Impotence is also less common after an EVAR than open AAA exclusion.

The mean length of hospital stay after EVAR is 2 to 3 days compared with 6 to 10 days after open AAA repair.[19,20] After EVAR, between 24% and 34% of patients require a stay in the intensive care unit (ICU) for an average of 6 to 24 hours, whereas after open AAA repair, 87% to 96% of patients stay in the ICU for an average of 27 to 67 hours.[19,20] Estimated blood loss is significantly lower during EVAR (300-400 mL) compared with open AAA repair (800–1600 mL).[19,20] Operative time is variable between EVAR and open AAA repair.[19,20] In nearly all cases, open AAA repair is performed under general anesthesia, whereas EVAR is performed under local, epidural, and general anesthesia. The recovery after EVAR is shorter. The time to resumption of an oral diet, ambulation, return to normal activity, and complete recovery all significantly favor EVAR.

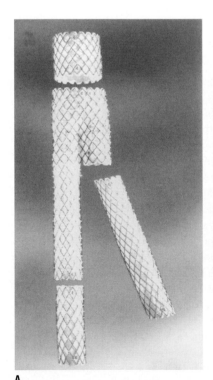
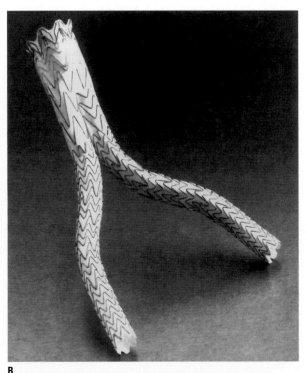

A   **B**

FIGURE 52-1. Modular, bifurcated endovascular graft with one docking limb. **A.** The AneuRx endovascular graft with proximal and distal extension cuffs. **B.** The W.L. Gore Excluder endograft.

Approximately 20% to 40% of patients (approximately 10%-15% per year) undergoing EVAR require reintervention for a variety of indications, including endoleak, stent migration, graft limb occlusion, or infection.[19,23] Late conversion of EVAR to open repair is necessary in approximately 2% to 3% of cases, although the frequency of late conversion may be higher in patients with larger AAAs.[19,23,24] Open conversion often requires a more extensive operation in a higher risk patient population and thus carries a 10% to 20% mortality rate.[25] The incidence of late rupture of an AAA after EVAR is thought to be 0.5% at 3 to 4 years and is perhaps more frequent after use of a tube graft. Rupture after EVAR carries a mortality rate similar to native AAA rupture.[7,26]

[ ] OUTCOMES OF ENDOVASCULAR ANEURYSM REPAIR FOR RUPTURED ABDOMINAL AORTIC ANEURYSMS

The use of EVAR for acutely symptomatic or ruptured AAAs is appealing given the high perioperative morbidity and mortality associated with open repair. Depending on the cohort of patients examined, between 20% and 80% (commonly 60%) of patients with an emergent AAA meet criteria for EVAR. The primary exclusion criteria is typically lack of an adequate aneurysm neck.[27–29] Deviation from the traditional anatomic criteria for EVAR may account for the relatively higher complication and reintervention rate in this patient population compared with elective EVAR. Due to the relative simplicity and rapidity of deployment, aortouni-iliac stent grafts have been used for the treatment of ruptured AAA, despite the requirement for femoral-femoral bypass.

[ ] GENDER DIFFERENCES

There are limited data comparing the outcome of EVAR in women compared with that of men, let alone criteria defining the diameter cutoff at which to repair an AAA in women. Women tend to have smaller peripheral arteries than men, which results in significantly more procedural complications related to arterial access and device delivery.[30] Some reports have suggested a higher frequency of graft limb occlusion and late failures in women.[31,32] Most studies have shown that the mortality rate after EVAR in women is similar to that in men.[30–32]

PREOPERATIVE PATIENT EVALUATION

[ ] PRE-ENDOGRAFT MEDICAL EVALUATION

The patient being scheduled for EVAR should undergo preoperative risk stratification of medical and cardiac comorbidities in accordance to the American College of Cardiology/American Heart Association preoperative risk stratification guidelines. Patients who are at prohibitive risk for open AAA exclusion have an 18% to 43% mortality rate if primary conversion of their EVAR is necessary.[33] However, it is unclear if higher risk patients have more cardiopulmonary complications than lower risk patients after EVAR; indeed, there is some evidence to suggest that EVAR negates the high-risk status of the patient so long as an endovascular repair is performed.[33] Predictors of adverse cardiac events after EVAR include age older than 70 years, history of myocardial infarction, congestive heart failure, and the lack of preoperative beta-blocker use. Patients with an elevated creatinine are also at an increased risk of perioperative complications.

If possible, anesthesia consultation should be obtained prior to undertaking EVAR. The decision regarding the type of anesthesia should be made in concert with the anesthesiologist. Comorbid conditions may dictate one form of anesthesia over another. A potential advantage of EVAR is the ability to use local anesthesia and conscious sedation.

[ ] HIGH-RISK PATIENTS

The application of EVAR to patients who are otherwise high surgical risks is appealing. Comparing results in patients with high-risk comorbidities, such as ischemic coronary artery disease with prior myocardial infarction and congestive heart failure, chronic obstructive pulmonary disease with a forced expiratory volume in 1 second (FEV_1) of less than 1 L/min or a requirement for domiciliary oxygen therapy, chronic liver disease with portal hypertension, or malignancy, with patients without these comorbidities revealed similarities in mortality rates, surgical times, blood loss, postoperative hospital stay, and days in the ICU. In addition, there was no difference in primary and secondary clinical success rates at 2 years.[33] Other patient populations who are better served with an EVAR than open repair are those with a hostile abdomen from multiple prior operations or those with stomas. An EVAR approach in these patients avoids the trauma, time, and complications associated with lysis of adhesions and establishment of adequate surgical exposure.[7,34] EVAR thus represents a viable option for high-risk patients who otherwise would remain untreated and left to the natural history of their AAAs.

LOW-RISK PATIENTS

The place of EVAR in the treatment algorithm of relatively young and healthy individuals with good anatomic substrate is debatable. Currently, the implantation of an endograft requires lifelong surveillance due to the potential for endoleak, endotension, stent migration, and late graft material failure. Such a surveillance program dictates multiple imaging studies over the lifetime of a younger patient. These patients must also realize that there is a 20% to 40% chance of repeat interventions after EVAR. An important concern for some younger patients, however, is the greater risk of erectile dysfunction or retrograde ejaculation after open surgical repair. Up to 83% to 98% of patients develop worsening of erectile function after open AAA exclusion compared with 25% to 50% after EVAR (depending on whether 1 or 2 of the hypogastric arteries are embolized).[35] Some clinicians find that the smaller incision, reduced hospital stay, earlier recovery, and return to full function outweigh the added responsibility of long-term follow-up. Thus, although there is a significant amount of follow-up and reintervention after EVAR, an argument can be made for endovascular repair of AAA in both high- and low-risk populations.

[ ] ANATOMIC DEFINITIONS AND CONSIDERATIONS FOR ENDOVASCULAR ANEURYSM REPAIR

Aneurysm morphology and the status of the iliac and femoral access vessels dictates whether a patient is a candidate for EVAR. Currently, AAA anatomy is the major limiting factor to the application of endografts to AAA repair. Only 50% to 60% of patients with infrarenal AAAs have suitable anatomy (Figure 52-2). The most common cause for exclusion is an inadequate infrarenal aortic neck for proximal fixation of the endograft. Patient anatomy also guides the choice of the endograft device and determines which additional procedures are necessary for successful device deployment and AAA exclusion. The principal proximal considerations are the diameter of the aneurysm neck; the length of the normal aortic neck; the location of the mesenteric arteries, particularly the celiac axis and superior mesenteric artery; and the proximal neck angulation. Distally, anatomic concerns include the size of the iliofemoral arteries, the presence of absence of calcification, the tortuosity of these arteries, and whether there is aneurysmal dilation of the iliac arteries. Successful exclusion of a common iliac artery aneurysm may require embolization of the internal iliac artery and extension of the endograft into the external iliac artery.

Aneurysm Neck

The aneurysm neck is the length from the most inferior (main) renal artery to the onset of the aneurysm. Most endografts that are

commercially available in the United States are designed for infrarenal fixation, with the exception of the Cook Zenith device (investigational: Cordis Fortron, Trivascular, and Medtronic Talent). The maximal diameter of the nonaneurysmal aortic neck that can be sealed is endograft dependent. The device should be oversized by 10% to 20%. The minimal neck length tolerated is also device specific, although generally for infrarenal fixation, the neck length should be at least 15 mm. The angle between the suprarenal aorta and the infrarenal neck (α) and the angle of the flow axis between the infrarenal neck and the body of the aneurysm (β), in which the flow axis is the axis (line) between the distal neck/proximal aneurysm to the aortic bifurcation, should be measured. Calcification and thrombus of the proximal neck should also be noted, because both of these incrementally add to the morphologic complexity of EVAR.

In summary, the neck length should be greater than 15 mm, the neck diameter should be less than 26 to 28 mm, α or β should be greater than 150°, and the degree of calcification or thrombus greater than 2 mm thick should be less than 25% of the neck circumference.[36] The risk of adverse outcome after EVAR is directly related to the proximal aortic neck angulation.

Arterial Branches of the Abdominal Aorta

To anticipate and prevent type II endoleak, it is important to assess for branch arteries off the aneurysm. The lack of patent lumbar arteries, inferior mesenteric artery, or accessory renal artery off the aneurysm sac should reduce the chance of type II endoleak.

Iliac Arteries

The anatomy of the iliac arteries is important with regard to the deliverability and proper sealing of endografts. The preoperative assessment should include measurements of the diameter of the common and external iliac arteries and length of the iliac landing zone. The external iliac artery generally needs to be at least 6 to 6.5 mm in diameter to allow passage of the majority of commercially available devices. The iliac arteries should also be evaluated for the presence of ectasia, stenosis, calcification, and tortuosity. Aortoiliac tortuosity and calcification affect device deliverability and are clearly associated with a more complex EVAR.[36] Maintenance of patency of the internal iliac (hypogastric) arteries is important for to achieve pelvic perfusion and to prevent buttock claudication and intestinal ischemia.

[ ] PREINTERVENTION IMAGING

Preintervention imaging is critical in the planning and assessment of the feasibility of endovascular AAA repair. A variety of different imaging modalities are capable of providing the necessary information for EVAR planning. The most commonly used, and arguably the best, is contrast-enhanced CT with CT angiography. To adequately visualize the aneurysm and make the appropriate measurements, 2- to 3-mm cuts are required. CT angiography can rapidly acquire high-resolution images, which can be postprocessed, producing three-dimensional (3D) models. Valuable data, including aneurysm dimensions, angles, thrombus content, extent of calcification, and iliofemoral artery dimensions can be obtained.[37] Propriety software programs (Medical Media Systems)

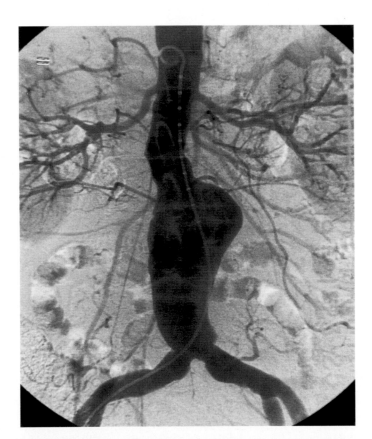

FIGURE 52-2. Favorable anatomy for endovascular aneurysm repair with a long, relatively straight infrarenal aortic neck and suitable landing zones in the common iliac arteries.

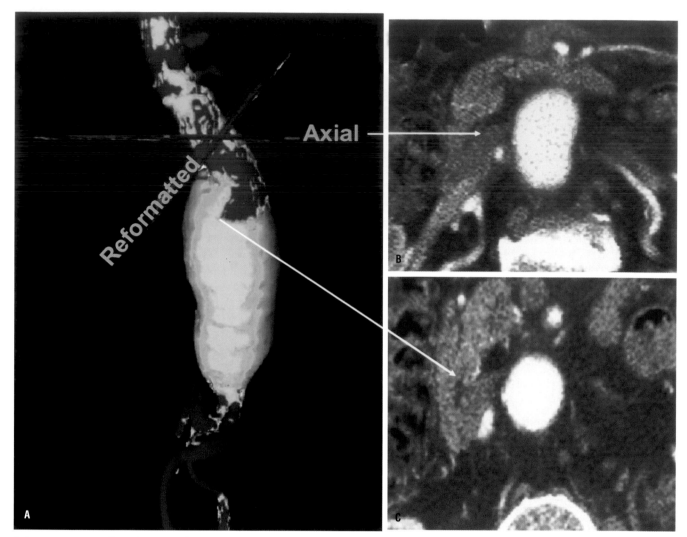

FIGURE 52-3. A. Three-dimensional reconstructed images of abdominal aortic aneurysms using Medical Media Systems software. **B.** Axial slice through angulated aortic neck provides a misleading representation of the aortic lumen. **C.** The reformatted oblique slice provides a true cross-section of the aortic lumen.

provide very accurate measurements of vessel diameter by reformatting raw data to create slices perpendicular to blood flow (Figure 52-3). Accurate length measurements are obtained via a computer-generated graft centerline. Vessel angulation is easily calculated. Virtual Graft technology allows for computer simulation of graft fit for all of the commercially available devices (Figure 52-4). The Medical Media Systems software is also extremely useful for follow-up evaluation after EVAR. Precise measurements of aneurysm diameter and volume are obtained. Endoleaks are modeled as a separate component and can be monitored volumetrically. CT angiography does require iodinated contrast administration and consequently may not be appropriate for patients with severe renal insufficiency.

Other methods for imaging AAAs include magnetic resonance (MR) imaging/angiography, digital subtraction angiography (DSA), and intravascular ultrasound (IVUS). MR imaging/angiography has the advantage of using a non-nephrotoxic contrast agent, gadolinium, and the ability to reconstruct the AAA in 3D. However, MR imaging/angiography does not adequately visualize calcification of the aneurysm wall, and image acquisition time is

much longer. IVUS has also been used as an alternative or adjunct to other imaging modalities. IVUS allows precise diameter measurements, accurate assessment of the quality of the aortic neck (thrombus, calcification, confirmatory length measurements), and precise evaluation of the degree of calcification in the iliac arteries. Angiography (or, DSA) can define the aneurysm length and side branches but cannot adequately define the aneurysm size, extent of thrombus, or calcification.[38] Duplex examination has a very limited role in endovascular planning. Preintervention, ultrasound is best used for diagnosis, whereas postintervention, it has some role in identification of endoleaks and measurement of aneurysm size and pulsatility.

THE ENDOVASCULAR SUITE

Depending on the capabilities of a given institution, EVAR may be performed in an interventional radiology suite, cardiac catheterization laboratory, or in operating room. The specific requirements

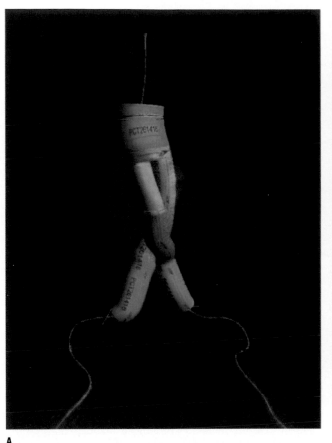
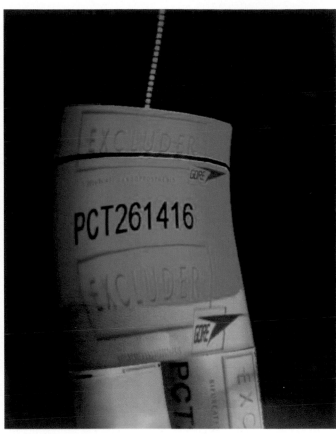

FIGURE 52-4. A. Virtual Graft technology allows computer simulation of endograft fit. **B.** Magnified image of the proximal attachment site simulating placement of a 26-mm W.L. Gore Excluder endograft.

of x-ray equipment, shielding, and dosimetry have previously been covered in this text. In its current stage, the endovascular repair of AAA is essentially a hybrid procedure involving the performance of small surgical incisions for femoral artery access along with extensive catheter-based techniques. Consequently, the ideal endovascular suite accommodates both of these procedures and allows for the possibility of emergency conversion to open surgical repair.

An endovascular suite should have the capabilities of a standard operating theater. This includes the utilization of special air filtration systems and laminar flow. An anesthesiologist and equipment must be available to provide patient sedation both for the surgical cutdown but also in the event of emergent conversion to an open repair. Nurses and technologists capable of functioning as scrub nurses and circulators must be available for operative assistance. Furthermore, surgical instruments necessary for the cutdown and possible emergency repair should be immediately at hand.

The endovascular suite needs to provide optimal radiographic imaging. The image intensifier should ideally provide at least a 12-in field of view. The image processing equipment should be capable of DSA and road mapping, and a power injector needs to be available for aortography. It is debatable how the image intensifier should be mounted. Some experts argue that a ceiling-mounted unit is required for ease of conversion to an open repair if necessary. However, many current cardiac catheterization laboratories use floor-mounted units, which are likely adequate. Portable C-arms have dramatically improved over the years and are now capable of

providing image quality that is comparable to what is achieved with fixed imaging systems.

Whether the endovascular suite is in the cardiac catheterization laboratory, radiology department, or the operating room, catheters, guidewires, balloons, stents, and other equipment necessary for successful EVAR should be readily available. In particular, it should be determined that an aortic occlusion balloon is available in the event of vessel perforation or aneurysm rupture. These balloons are elastomeric and capable of rapidly and relatively atraumatically occluding distal aortic flow, providing temporary control of the situation.

PROCEDURAL OUTLINE

【 】 PREINTERVENTION HYPOGASTRIC ARTERY EXCLUSION PROCEDURES

A significant percentage (20%–30%) of AAAs may extend beyond the aortic bifurcation to involve the iliac arteries. To minimize the chances of type II endoleak at the distal attachment site in the iliac artery, it is occasionally necessary to extend the graft into the external iliac artery. To provide for complete exclusion of the iliac/aortic aneurysm, it is necessary to occlude the ipsilateral hypogastric artery prior to doing so. Some practitioners have taken the approach of coil embolizing the internal iliac artery prior to the endograft deployment procedure. Such a staged approach may allow collaterals to develop and gives the interventionist the chance to observe the patient's response to the hypogastric artery embolization. For those cases in which bilateral common iliac artery aneurysms are present and the patient is clearly not a candidate for open surgical repair, staged occlusion of both hypogastric arteries has been performed.

The practitioner needs to be aware that there may be consequences to hypogastric artery occlusion. With unilateral hypogastric artery occlusion, there is a 13% reduction in the penile brachial index, up to a 38% incidence of erectile dysfunction, and a 39% to 50% chance of hip or buttock claudication.[39,40] The occlusion of bilateral hypogastric arteries is associated with a 28% to 55% incidence of pelvic ischemia. Bilateral hypogastric artery embolization results in a 39% reduction in the penile brachial index, a 50% incidence of erectile dysfunction, and an approximately 50% chance of hip or buttock claudication.[39] Most patients have improvement or resolution of these symptoms over time, but this may occur over a several months (mean, 14 months).[41] Other reported complications after bilateral internal iliac artery embolization include scrotal skin sloughing, sacral decubitus ulceration, and intestinal ischemia.[42] Having a diseased profunda femoris artery with a stenosis greater than 50% was associated with a higher rate of complications.[39]

If the hypogastric artery cannot be spared, and buttock claudication or pelvic ischemia develops, several steps can be taken to help mitigate the symptoms. As noted above, it is possible that if the profunda femoris artery is diseased, profundoplasty may improve symptoms. Regular exercise should be a mainstay of therapy and will prove beneficial. Cilostazol has not been adequately studied in this setting but may be of benefit. Finally, treatment of a diseased contralateral hypogastric artery may be necessary. Surgical hypogastric artery reimplantation may also become necessary in recalcitrant settings. In the event that both hypogastric arteries need to be occluded, sufficient staging should be performed, with at least 3 weeks between each embolization.

Covering the hypogastric artery with the endograft limb without coil embolization is another option if there is no aneurysmal involvement of the distal common and proximal external iliac arteries. By covering, but not coiling the hypogastric artery, the chances of distal embolization into the small branches of the hypogastric artery are reduced and the likelihood of maintaining collaterals is enhanced. There is a trend toward both a reduced rate and severity of complications with this approach. Adequate sealing zones both in the distal common iliac artery and the proximal external iliac artery are necessary. In suitable patients, type II endoleak is similar between covering and embolizing the hypogastric artery.[43] Other procedures such as surgical bypass and proximal ligation of the internal iliac artery, or using an aortouni-iliac endograft and occlusion of the contralateral common iliac artery in conjunction with a femoral-femoral bypass (allowing for retrograde perfusion of the internal iliac artery) are also considerations.

[ ] ARTERIAL ACCESS

For the vast majority of endografting procedures for AAA, a bilateral femoral approach is used. Because of the size of the delivery sheath of the main body (18–24 Fr), a surgical cutdown is generally required. There are two basic types of incisions for the femoral cutdown–vertical and oblique. Small oblique incisions can be used in the great majority of cases and are associated with a lower risk of wound complications. The wound complication rate has been reported to be as high as 7% to 18% for vertical incisions and 0% to 2.8% for oblique incisions.[44] In addition, subsequent femoral access or reoperation is more easily achieved following an oblique incision.

Fully percutaneous EVAR is being performed in a few centers using a "preclose" technique. This requires the preplacement of percutaneous vascular suture closure devices (Prostar XL Percutaneous Vascular Surgery [PVS] Device, Perclose). For larger sheaths (main body), the first closure device is deployed, and then a second device is inserted, 45° to 90° degrees to the first, to avoid duplicate suture entry sites. The arteriotomy is then progressively dilated and the endograft delivery sheath is finally inserted. Success rates with this technique vary between 42% and 96%.[45,46] The contralateral limb is generally deployed through a smaller sheath, and it is generally possible to close the arteriotomy with a "preclose" technique or with more conventional use of an arteriotomy closure device. Advantages to a fully percutaneous procedure include less bleeding, earlier recovery, no incision, and perhaps earlier ambulation. This approach requires proper patient selection with particular attention paid to femoral artery size and the degree of calcification of the femoral artery. Failure of the percutaneous closure mandates prolonged manual compression and possible surgical exploration. The rates of access complications such as pseudoaneurysm, arteriovenous fistula, late stenosis, hematoma, and venous or arterial thrombosis have not been adequately studied.[46]

There are specific technical considerations with percutaneous closure. It has been suggested that rotating the device 90° rather than 45° can allow better separation of the suture needle holes. Using an 8-Fr PVS device followed by 10-Fr PVS device may allow better capture of the tissue with the sutures placed at different tissue levels. Gradual dilation of the arteriotomy is necessary. Finally, prior to cinching and tying the sutures, it is recommended that the guidewire be removed to avoid tying the suture above the artery, on the wire.[45]

[ ] INTRAOPERATIVE IMAGING

Good quality intraoperative fluoroscopy and angiographic technique is required for precise endograft deployment. Accurate localization of the mesenteric and renal arteries is necessary to avoid inadvertent occlusion of these vessels and to document the proximal extent of the aneurysm. This is generally accomplished by placement of an angiographic catheter via contralateral femoral artery or brachial artery. A pigtail or straight multihole angiographic catheter is inserted and advanced to a juxtarenal position. From this position, angiograms are taken during the deployment process to guide precise endograft positioning just below the renal arteries (Figure 52-5). Use of an angiographic "road map" or bony landmarks may be helpful, but neither method is sufficient for precise deployment. Another useful technique is to trace on the monitor with a marker the outline of the aorta and its major branches to serve as a guide. As long as the patient and image

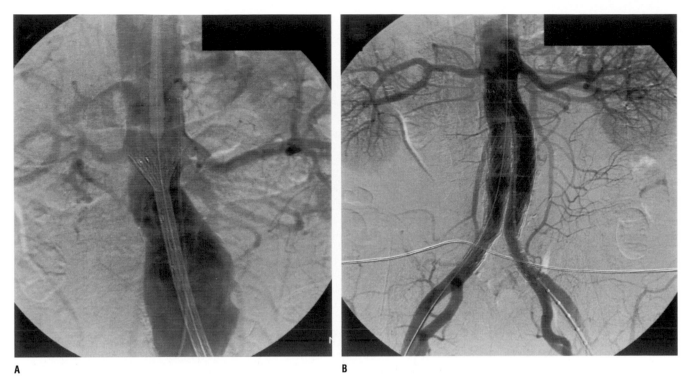

FIGURE 52-5. A. Angiography during deployment of the AneuRx endograft just below the renal arteries. **B.** Completion angiography demonstrating accurate deployment of the endograft below the renal arteries with no evidence of endoleak.

intensifier do not move, this method can assist in positioning of the endograft.

Postdeployment imaging is important to establish if the aneurysm is successfully excluded, to evaluate the patency of the renal and hypogastric arteries, and to evaluate for evidence of dissection of the external iliac arteries. Because the delivery sheaths are large relative to the common femoral artery, they may impede antegrade flow to the lower extremities, and adequate visualization of the iliac and femoral arteries may prove difficult. A retrograde sheath injection may be helpful. Another technique to allow for adequate opacification of the iliac arteries is to attach a 50-mL syringe to both sheath side ports. During aortography, as the contrast is injected, two operators manually aspirate from the syringes. This creates enough antegrade flow in the iliac arteries to allow for adequate visualization.

Inadvertent renal artery occlusion during endograft deployment or subsequent endograft migration across a renal artery can lead to azotemia and ischemic nephropathy. Unless there is a high index of suspicion for endograft occlusion of a renal artery, permanent renal damage may ensue. If the renal artery occlusion is discovered immediately following endograft deployment, the number of options for salvage of the kidney is limited. If the endograft is not completely deployed, either resheathing or manually pulling the graft caudally may be sufficient to uncover the renal artery. Once the endograft is fully deployed, the only option is to use the "dental floss" technique to displace the graft caudally. A guidewire must be advanced across the bifurcation of the endograft, snared from the contralateral iliac artery, and then externalized through the contralateral sheath. Traction on both ends of the wire may be sufficient to pull the endograft down and thus uncover the renal artery. Placing a catheter over the wire across the bifurcation of the

graft and pulling on the catheter may reduce the potential for damage to the graft by the guidewire.

SURVEILLANCE IMAGING

Long-term endograft surveillance is required to document continued exclusion of the aneurysm by the endograft. Imaging protocols vary depending on the institution. Following an uncomplicated EVAR, imaging is usually performed at 1 month, 6 months, and 12 months post-procedure, and annually thereafter. If an endoleak is detected, immediate intervention may be required (as in the case of a type I or III endoleak) or the surveillance protocol may need to be modified. If a type II endoleak is identified, or there is an endoleak of undetermined type, imaging every 6 months or sooner may be necessary.

Helical CT with intravenous contrast and thin slices is the preferred method of post EVAR imaging. The techniques for CT in this setting are well established and standardized. The equipment is readily available in almost all centers, and extensive literature supports its use. As previously described, 3D reconstruction of images using the Medical Media Systems software can be very useful for characterization of endoleaks and for surveillance of the diameter and volume of the aneurysm sac (Figure 52-6). Delayed imaging may be necessary to detect endoleaks in some cases.

Color Doppler ultrasound (CDU) has the advantage of being less expensive and avoiding nephrotoxic contrast agents. The sensitivity of CDU for detecting endoleak ranges from 77% to 97% and may be increased by the use of ultrasound contrast agents. Furthermore, CDU can assess physiologic parameters of the aneurysm such as pulsatility. However, CDU is very operator and patient dependent, and its major limitation is the inability to consistently provide adequate diagnostic images.[47]

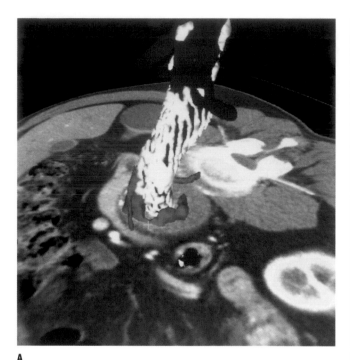

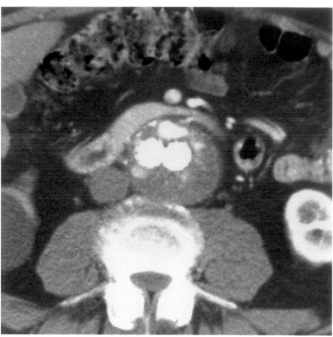

A   B

FIGURE 52-6. A. Three-dimensional imaging demonstrating a type II endoleak (pink) with a lumbar artery communicating with a patent inferior mesenteric artery. **B.** Two-dimensional imaging demonstrating type II endoleak with contrast within the aneurysm sac.

Magnetic resonance (MR) imaging is a less validated method for surveillance of patients following EVAR. Image interpretation may be hampered by artifact caused by the metallic content of the endograft. In the absence of significant artifact from the metal, MR imaging can be useful to evaluate aneurysm sac size and aneurysm morphology. MR angiography allows for the detection and characterization of major endoleak. Future advancements and studies may allow better imaging as well as physiologic assessment of endografts with MR imaging.[47]

COMPLICATIONS OF ENDOVASCULAR ANEURYSM REPAIR

【 】 ENDOLEAK

The term "endoleak" was initially proposed in 1996 by White, Yu, and May in a letter to the editor in *Journal of Endovascular Therapy* and has been referred to as the "Achilles heel" of EVAR.[48,49] Endoleak is the persistent flow of blood into the aneurysm sac after EVAR. There are four types of endoleak (Table 52-1).

1. Type I endoleak results from flow into the sac due to inadequate seal at either the proximal or distal attachment sites.

2. Type II endoleak occurs as a result of retrograde flow into the sac through a branch vessel (eg, accessory renal artery, lumbar artery, internal iliac artery, median sacral artery, gonadal artery, or inferior mesenteric artery).

3. Type III endoleak refers to a leak through the graft itself—either at the junction of modular components or because of a defect in the graft material.

4. Type IV endoleak is not truly an endoleak at all. This just refers to the tendency of some grafts to be porous for a short period of time after insertion in the body. CT scans in the early postoperative period demonstrate contrast in the aneurysm sac due to extravasation of contrast through the interstices of the stent-graft.[49]

Endoleaks can be further categorized as primary or secondary. Primary endoleaks occur in the first 30-days post-EVAR, whereas secondary endoleaks are detected more than 30-days post-EVAR.[50]

Endoleak results in continued pressurization of the aneurysm sac and may increase the risk of rupture following an otherwise successful EVAR. Between 20% and 40% of patients develop endoleaks after EVAR. The rate of endoleaks for aortouni-iliac endografts may be as high as 52.3%.[51] Type I and III endoleaks are thought to result in the highest sac pressures and thus necessitate immediate intervention. Type II endoleaks are generally more benign and can be observed. Many type II endoleaks resolve spontaneously.[50] Close

◗ TABLE 52-1

Endoleak

TYPE	DESCRIPTION
I	Proximal or distal attachment site
II	Side branch
III	Graft tear or leak at modular component
IV	Graft porosity

attention must be paid to the size of the type II endoleak as well as the diameter and volume of the aneurysm sac. If there is growth of the aneurysm sac, consideration should be given to treatment of the type II endoleak. In rare cases, type II endoleaks can result in continued aneurysm pressurization, growth, and ultimate rupture.

Type I Endoleak

Type I endoleak can occur early after EVAR due to failure achieve an adequate proximal or distal seal at the time of the procedure or late due to morphologic changes in the aorta or iliac arteries.[20] Over time, there may be continued dilation of the proximal aortic neck or iliac arteries such that stent graft apposition to the vessel wall may be lost. In addition, as the aneurysm sac diameter and volume decrease, the resultant morphologic changes may lead to endograft migration.

Failure of stent-graft apposition at the proximal or distal attachment sites leads to repressurization of the aneurysm sac, with aneurysmal enlargement and possible rupture. Risk factors for the development of type I endoleak include a short proximal neck (< 15 mm), the use of proximal extender cuffs, AAA diameter greater than 5.5 cm, severe neck angulation (< 120°), and proximal neck calcification.[52,53] Oversizing of the proximal endograft by at least 10% to 20% is thought to reduce the rate of type I endoleak.[54]

There may be differences in the significance of proximal attachment endoleaks (type IA) depending on whether the endograft is supported or unsupported. Type IA endoleaks in fully supported endografts are unlikely to spontaneously resolve and should be treated if present at the time of endograft implantation.[55] Treatment of type IA endoleak can be initially attempted with balloon dilation of the proximal attachment site. If this fails, then deployment of a proximal extension cuff or stent is necessary. There are reports of selectively coiling the gap between endograft and the arterial wall for type I endoleak.[56] This technique should be reserved for cases in which there is an inadequate landing zone for an extension cuff and use of an uncovered stent is not appropriate.

Distal attachment site endoleaks (type IB) occur more commonly in the setting of iliac tortuosity, iliac artery ectasia, or iliac artery calcification. Regardless of the type of endograft (supported or unsupported), type IB endoleaks should be treated at the time of their discovery.[26] Treatment of type IB endoleaks is generally accomplished with either the placement of an uncovered stent or endograft extension.

The use of devices with suprarenal fixation has been recommended for patients with short or angulated infrarenal aortic necks (Figure 52-7). Such devices do not appear to confer a lower type I endoleak rate if the aortic neck anatomy is favorable.[57] For those with inadequate neck length, however, suprarenal fixation may be

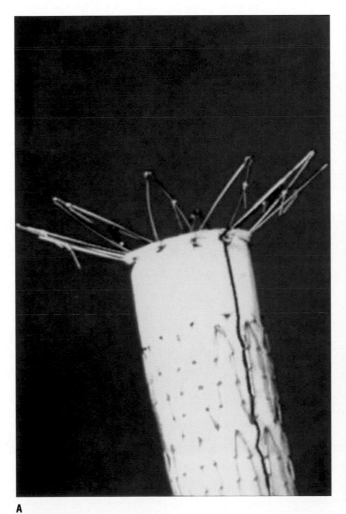

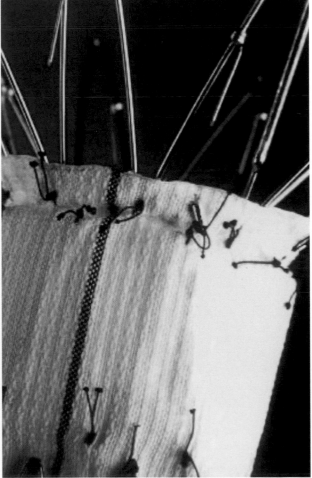

A

B

FIGURE 52-7. A. Cook Zenith endograft with suprarenal fixation. **B.** Magnified view demonstrating the suprarenal fixation system and proximal fixation barbs.

preferred to minimize the risk of late graft migration. Proximal aneurysm neck dilation (> 3 mm) occurs in up to 28% of EVAR in the midterm (2 years), although only 20% of these require intervention.[58] An increased risk of proximal aneurysm neck dilation is related to circumferential thrombus within the neck, pre-EVAR neck diameter, and pre-EVAR AAA diameter.[58] Treatment for neck enlargement includes continued observation unless there is endoleak or suspicion of endotension. In such cases, either proximal extension cuffs are used or the patient may need to undergo conversion to open repair. The initial oversizing of the proximal endograft by 10% to 20% is perhaps the most important preventive strategy to reduce the chances of type I endoleak if aneurysm neck dilation does occur.[58]

Type II Endoleak

As previously described, if there is stabilization or reduction in aneurysm volume, then intervention for type II endoleak is usually not required.[59] In cases where a higher likelihood of type II endoleak is anticipated, some experts have advocated pre-EVAR embolization of branch arteries, use of thrombogenic AAA sac packing at the time of EVAR, or laparoscopically assisted side branch ligation.[59] When prophylactically or primarily treating type II endoleak, it should be kept in mind that type II endoleak is generally benign; its treatment should not be at an excessive risk of morbidity and mortality to the patient.

The diagnosis of type II endoleak can sometimes be challenging. If contrast-enhanced CT imaging is used to identify type II endoleak, it is important to recognize that branch flow into the aneurysm sac can be slow, necessitating delayed enhancement images. CUS is accurate in detecting endoleak and identifying the source artery.[60] Spontaneous sealing often occurs within 12 months. Type II endoleak can be treated with selective arterial coiling, laparoscopic ligation, or translumbar embolization (Figure 52-8). Successful treatment of type II endoleak is associated with a reduction in aneurysm surface area.[61]

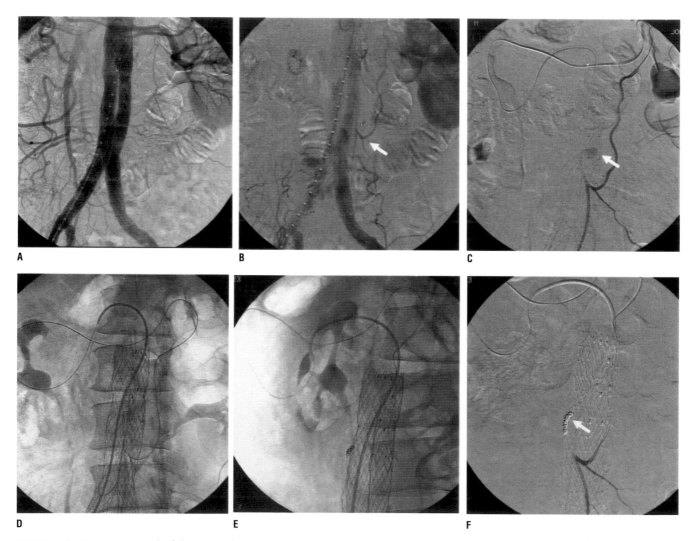

FIGURE 52-8. A. Aortography following endovascular aneurysm repair demonstrating a patent graft with no evidence of type I or III endoleak. **B.** On delayed images, retrograde filling of the inferior mesenteric artery (IMA) is demonstrated (*arrow*). **C.** Selective angiography demonstrates type II endoleak via the IMA (*arrow*). **D.** Guidewire and microcatheter are advanced to the origin of the IMA through branches of the superior mesenteric artery. **E.** Microembolization coils are deployed in the proximal IMA. **F.** Completion angiography demonstrates no evidence of type II endoleak after coil embolization (*arrow*).

Type III Endoleak

Type III endoleak can occur after EVAR due to separation of the modular components (IIIA) or late failure of the graft material (IIIB). Treatment of type IIIA endoleak at the junction of endograft components often requires insertion of an iliac limb or extension cuff within the original graft. Similarly, a hole in the endograft material can be patched from the inside with another iliac limb or cuff. If there is complete separation of the endograft limb from the main body, the endograft limb may be pushed into the aneurysm sac and a new limb inserted.[62] More commonly, the disjointed endograft limb is recannulated and extension cuffs are placed to connect the limb and main body.

During the procedure of placing new endograft extension cuffs, it is critical to confirm intraluminal placement.

Type IV Endoleak

Until the graft becomes impregnated and coated with platelets and fibrin, there may be some contrast "blush" seen in the AAA sac on aortography or contrast CT scan. Type IV endoleak from graft porosity generally resolves within a few weeks post-EVAR. It is essential to distinguish graft porosity (type IV endoleak) from type III microleak. The presence of even very small holes (type III endoleak) in the graft material results in systemic pressurization of the aneurysm sac.[63] The use of color flow duplex imaging can help differentiate these microleaks (type III endoleak) from graft porosity (type IV endoleak).[64]

[ ] ENDOTENSION

The aneurysm sac may be pressurized in the absence of detectable endoleak. The new or persistent pressurization of the aneurysm sac in the absence of endoleak is termed endotension.[50] Endotension may cause sac enlargement and rupture. Proposed mechanisms include aortic pulsatility against thrombus or endoleak that is undetectable by current standards. Endotension is uncommon and its overall clinical significance awaits determination by further studies.

Elegant animal models of isolated canine experimental aortic aneurysms excluded with an endograft demonstrate that the aneurysm sac can develop pressure in the absence of endoleak.[65]

In thrombus-filled aneurysm sacs, the pressure within the sac was highest near the endograft and lowest laterally.[65] The use of finite element models to predict endotension and endograft expansion based on 3D CT measurements and systemic blood pressures are being examined. Furthermore, the use of implantable pressure transducers in an array along the endograft may allow for comprehensive modeling and determination of intrasac pressures. These techniques will ideally be able to predict EVAR failure and potential for rupture. The use of pressure-sensing devices may facilitate the follow-up of patients following EVAR and minimize the need for frequent imaging studies.

[ ] ENDOGRAFT LIMB OCCLUSION

Endograft limb stenosis or occlusion occurs in up to 24% of patients receiving an unsupported endograft. If the limb dysfunction is detected and treated with self-expanding stents, the long

term freedom from recurrence is excellent.[66] Intervention for endograft limb stenosis was required in approximately 10.3% of patients in the Guidant/Endovascular Technologies clinical trials. Limb occlusion occurred in 6.7% of patients. The incidence of graft limb stenosis or occlusion is considerably lower for fully supported endografts. Any endograft deformity, kinking, or stenosis at the time of implantation requires a thorough investigation.[41] Intraoperative evaluation of endograft limbs by IVUS may result in significantly higher utilization of additional interventions but potentially fewer long-term complications.[66]

Limb thrombosis most commonly (but not always) occurs within 2 months of endograft implantation.[41,67] Patients can present with atypical leg discomfort, new-onset claudication, or acute limb ischemia. The decision to intervene on the limb depends on the patient's limitations and the acuity of symptoms. Acutely thrombosed endograft limbs may be treated with open surgical embolectomy (care must be taken to avoid dislocation of modular components during passage of the Fogarty balloon), catheter-directed thrombolysis, or percutaneous thrombectomy with a device such as the Possis Angiojet Rheolytic Thrombectomy catheter. After reestablishing flow through the endograft limb, careful evaluation and treatment of predisposing factors such as limb kink, stenosis, or distal dissection is necessary. Risk factors for developing iliac limb occlusions include smaller limb diameter, limb stenosis, unsupported endografts, and the extension of the graft into the external iliac artery.[67]

A cautionary note to the use of aortouni-iliac endografts with femoral-femoral bypass is the dependence of the entire lower extremity arterial circulation on the inflow from the endograft. Acute occlusion of this graft results in bilateral lower extremity ischemia with its attendant morbidity, risk of reperfusion syndrome, and mortality.

[ ] ENDOGRAFT MIGRATION

Endograft migration occurs in up to 15% to 45% of patients depending on the time frame of evaluation and the definition used for endograft migration (usually, 5–10 mm).[68] The likelihood of endograft migration increases with time with most occurring at a mean of 20 months after EVAR.[68,69] Nearly 50% of patients with endograft migration require repeat interventions, including the placement of proximal extension cuffs.[68] Risk factors for endograft migration include neck dilation of 10% or more and pre-EVAR AAA diameter greater than 5.5 cm.[68,69] The potential for endograft migration emphasizes the need for routine imaging follow-up in patients after EVAR.

[ ] POSTIMPLANTATION SYNDROME

After EVAR, some patients develop fever and leukocytosis with an elevated CRP in the absence of an infectious source. Up to 72% of patients after EVAR compared with 28% of patients after open AAA repair develop temperatures greater than 38°C.[70] Fever, leukocytosis, and elevated CRP have been noted after both thoracic endografting and abdominal EVAR.[71,72] The clinical significance or even presence of postimplantation syndrome is controversial. In a patient after EVAR who develops fever, the first consideration should be infection. Only after the usual causes of postoperative fever have been excluded should the diagnosis of postimplantation syndrome be considered.

CONCLUSION

The endovascular treatment of AAAs has been shown to reduce the morbidity and early mortality associated with aneurysm repair compared with a traditional open surgical approach. Patients at particularly high risk of open repair may benefit the most from EVAR. Proper patient selection with strict attention to the anatomic substrate is necessary for the procedure to be most successful. Further advances in the procedure and the devices will allow the safe application of this technology to a wider range of patients and aneurysm morphologies.

REFERENCES

1. Singh K, Bonaa KH, Jacobsen BK, et al. Prevalence of and risk factors for abdominal aortic aneurysms in a population-based study. *Am J Epidemiol.* 2001;154:236.
2. Lederle FA, Johnson GR, Wilson SE, et al. The aneurysm detection and management study screening program: validation cohort and final results. Aneurysm Detection and Management Veterans Affairs Cooperative Study Investigators. *Arch Intern Med.* 2000;160:1425.
3. Lederle FA, Johnson GR, Wilson SE, for the Veterans Affairs Cooperative Study #417 Investigators. Rupture rate of large abdominal aortic aneurysms in patients refusing or unfit for elective repair. *JAMA.* 2002;287:2968.
4. Diwan A, Sarkar R, Stanley JC, et al. Incidence of femoral and popliteal artery aneurysms in patients with abdominal aortic aneurysms. *J Vasc Surg.* 2000;31:863.
5. Jones K, Brull D, Brown LC, et al. Interleukin-6 and the prognosis of abdominal aortic aneurysms. *Circulation.* 2001;103:2260.
6. Dieter RS. Transluminal endovascular stent-grafting of aortic dissections and aneurysms: a concise review of the major trials. *Clin Cardiol.* 2001;24:358.
7. Brewster DC, Cronenwett JL, Jallett JW Jr, et al. Guidelines for the treatment of abdominal aortic aneurysm. *J Vasc Surg.* 2003;37:1106.
8. Hinchliffe RJ, Macierewicz JA, Hopkinson BR. Endovascular repair of inflammatory abdominal aortic aneurysm. *J Endovasc Ther.* 2002;9:277.
9. Stanley BM, Semmens JB, Lawrence-Brown M, et al. Endoluminal repair of mycotic thoracic aneurysms. *J Endovasc Ther.* 2003;10:511.
10. Berchtold C, Eibl C, Seelig MH, et al. Endovascular treatment and complete regression of an infected abdominal aortic aneurysm. *J Endovasc Ther.* 2002;9:543.
11. Dieter RA Jr, Blum AS, Pozen TJ, et al. Endovascular repair of aortojejunal fistula. *Int Surg.* 2002;87:83–6.
12. The Propranolol Aneurysm Trial Investigators. Propranolol for small abdominal aortic aneurysms: results of a randomized trial. *J Vasc Surg.* 2002;35:72.
13. Baxter BT, Pearce WH, Waltke EA, et al. Prolonged administration of doxycycline in patients with small asymptomatic abdominal aortic aneurysms: report of a prospective (Phase II) multicenter study. *J Vasc Surg.* 2002;36:1.
14. Mosorin M, Juvonen J, Biancari F, et al. Use of doxycycline to decrease the growth rate of abdominal aortic aneurysms: a randomized, double-blind, placebo-controlled pilot study. *J Vasc Surg.* 2001;34:606.
15. The United Kingdom Small Aneurysm Trial Participants. Long-term outcomes of immediate repair compared with surveillance of small abdominal aortic aneurysms. *N Engl J Med.* 2002;346:1445.
16. Lederle FA, Wilson SE, Johnson GR, et al, for the Aneurysm Detection and Management Veterans Affairs Cooperative Study Group. Immediate repair compared with surveillance of small abdominal aortic aneurysms. *N Engl J Med.* 2002;346:1437.
17. Wolf YG, Tillich M, Lee A, et al. Changes in aneurysm volume after endovascular repair of abdominal aortic aneurysm. *J Vasc Surg.* 2002;36:305.
18. Bertges DJ, Chow K, Wyers MC, et al. Abdominal aortic aneurysm size regression after endovascular repair is endograft dependent. *J Vasc Surg.* 2003;37:716.
19. Moore WS, Matsumura JS, Makaroun MS, et al, for the EVT/Guidant Investigators. *J Vasc Surg.* 2003;38:46.
20. Matsumura JS, Brewster DC, Makaroun MS, et al, for the Excluder Bifurcated Endoprosthesis Investigators. A Multicenter controlled trial of open versus endovascular treatment of abdominal aortic aneurysm. *J Vasc Surg.* 2003;37:262.
21. Prinssen M, Verhoeven ELG, Buth J, et al, for the Dutch Randomized Endovascular Aneurysm Management (DREAM) Trial Group. A Randomized Trial Comparing Conventional and Endovascular Repair of Abdominal Aortic Aneurysms. *N Engl J Med.* 2004;351:1607.
22. Greenhalgh RM, Brown LC, Kwong GP, et al; EVAR trial participants. Comparison of endovascular aneurysm repair with open repair in patients with abdominal aortic aneurysm (EVAR trial 1), 30-day operative mortality results: randomised controlled trial. *Lancet.* 2004;364:843.
23. Makaroun MS, Chaikof E, Naslund T, et al, for the EVT Investigators. Efficacy of a bifurcated endograft versus open repair of abdominal aortic aneurysms: a reappraisal. *J Vasc Surg.* 2002;35:203.
24. Ouriel K, Srivastava SD, Sarac TP, et al. Disparate outcome after endovascular treatment of small versus large abdominal aortic aneurysm. *J Vasc Surg.* 2003;37:1206.
25. Bockler D, Probst T, Weber H, et al. Surgical conversion after endovascular grafting for abdominal aortic aneurysms. *J Endovasc Ther.* 2002;9:111.
26. Bernhard VM, Mitchell RS, Matsumura JS, et al. Ruptured abdominal aortic aneurysm after endovascular repair. *J Vasc Surg.* 2002;35:1155.
27. Hinchliffe RJ, Braithwaite BD, Hopkinson BR. The endovascular management of ruptured abdominal aortic aneurysms. *Eur J Vasc Endovasc Surg.* 2003;25:191.
28. Yilmaz N, Peppelenbosch N, Cuypers PWM, et al. Emergency treatment of symptomatic or ruptured abdominal aortic aneurysms: the role of endovascular repair. *J Endovasc Ther.* 2002;9:449.
29. Rose DFG, Davidson IR, Hinchliffe RJ, et al. Anatomical suitability of ruptured abdominal aortic aneurysms for endovascular repair. *J Endovasc Ther.* 2003;10:453.
30. Wolf YG, Arko FR, Hill BB, et al. Gender differences in endovascular abdominal aortic aneurysm repair with the AneuRx stent graft. *J Vasc Surg.* 2002;35:882.
31. Parlini G, Verzini F, Zannetti S, et al. Does gender influence outcome of AAA endoluminal repair? *Eur J Vasc Endovasc Surg.* 2003;26:69.
32. Ouriel K, Greenberg RK, Clair DG, et al. Endovascular aneurysm repair: gender-specific results. *J Vasc Surg.* 2003;38:93.
33. Chaikof EL, Lin PH, Brinkman WT, et al. Endovascular repair of abdominal aortic aneurysms risk stratified outcomes. *Ann Surg.* 2002;235:833.
34. Dieter RS, Stevens SL, Rush DS, et al. Endovascular treatment of bilateral saphenous vein graft aneurysms for renal artery bypass. *Vasc Endovasc Surg.* 2004;38:579.
35. Lee ES, Kor DJ, Kuskowski MA, et al. Incidence of erectile dysfunction after open abdominal aortic aneurysm repair. *Ann Vasc Surg.* 2000;14:13.
36. Chaikof EL, Fillinger MF, Matsumura JS, et al. Identifying and grading factors that modify the outcome of endovascular aortic aneurysm repair. *J Vasc Surg.* 2002;35:1061.
37. Rydberg J, Kopecky KK, Johnson MS, et al. Endovascular repair of abdominal aortic aneurysms assessment with multislice CT. *AJR.* 2001;177:607.
38. Van der Laan M, Milner R, Blankensteijn JD. Preprocedural imaging. *Endovasc Today.* 2002;Nov/Dec:1.
39. Lin PH, Bush RL, Chaikof EL, et al. A prospective evaluation of hypogastric artery embolization in endovascular aortoiliac aneurysm repair. *J Vasc Surg.* 2002;36:500.
40. Lee WA, O'Dorisio J, Wolf YG, et al. Outcome after unilateral hypogastric artery occlusion during endovascular aneurysm repair. *J Vasc Surg.* 2001;33:921.
41. Powell A, Fox LA, Benenati JF, et al. Postoperative management: buttock claudication and limb thrombosis. *Tech Vasc Intervent Radiol.* 2001;4:232.
42. Lin PH, Bush RL, Lumsden AB. Sloughing of the scrotal skin and impotence subsequent to bilateral hypogastric artery embolization for endovascular aortoiliac aneurysm repair. *J Vasc Surg.* 2001;34:748.
43. Wyers MC, Schermerhorn ML, Fillinger MF, et al. Internal iliac occlusion without coil embolization during endovascular abdominal aortic aneurysm repair. *J Vasc Surg.* 2002;36:1138.
44. Slappy ALJ, Hakaim AG, Oldenburg A, et al. Femoral incision morbidity following endovascular aortic aneurysm repair. *Vasc Endovasc Surg.* 2003;37:105.
45. Howell M, Dougherty K, Strickman N, et al. Percutaneous repair of abdominal aortic aneurysms using the AneuRx stent graft and the percutaneous vascular surgery device. *Cathet Cardiovasc Intervent.* 2002;55:281.
46. Londero HF. Percutaneous femoral arterial closure in AAA endograft: advantages and disadvantages. *Catheter Cardiovasc Interv.* 2002;55:288.

47. Golzarian J. Imaging after endovascular repair of abdominal aortic aneurysm. *Abdom Imaging.* 2003;28:236.

48. White GH, Yu W, May J. "Endoleak"—a proposed new terminology to describe incomplete aneurysm exclusion by an endoluminal graft. *J Endovasc Ther.* 1996;3:124.

49. Pacanowski JP Jr, Dieter RS, Stevens SL, et al. Endoleak: the Achilles heel of endovascular abdominal aortic aneurysm exclusion. *WMJ.* 2002;101:59.

50. Chaikof EL, Blankensteijn JD, Harris PL, et al. Reporting standards for endovascular aortic aneurysm repair. *J Vasc Surg.* 2002;35:1048.

51. Clouse WD, Brewster FC, Marone LK, et al, for the EVT/Guidant Investigators. Durability of aortouniiliac endografting with femorofemoral crossover: 4-year experience in the EVT/Guidant trials. *J Vasc Surg.* 2003; 37:1142.

52. Rockman CB, Lamparello PJ, Adelman MA, et al. Aneurysm morphology as a predictor of endoleak following endovascular aortic aneurysm repair: do smaller aneurysm have better outcomes? *Ann Vasc Surg.* 2002;16:644.

53. Parra JR, Ayerdi J, McLafferty R, et al. Conformational changes associated with proximal seal zone failure in abdominal aortic endografts. *J Vasc Surg.* 2003;37:106.

54. Mohan IV, Laheij RJ, Harris PL, for the EUROSTAR Collaborators. Risk factors for endoleak and the evidence for stent-graft oversizing in patients undergoing endovascular aneurysm repair. *Eur J Vasc Endovasc Surg.* 2001;21:344.

55. Dillavou ED, Gupta N, Makaroun MS. Endoleak following AAA repair. *Endo Today.* 2002;Nov/Dec:1.

56. Faries PL, Cadot H, Agarwal G, et al. Management of endoleak after endovascular aneurysm repair: cuffs, coils, and conversion. *J Vasc Surg.* 2003;37:1155.

57. Shames M, Betros F, Dennien B, et al. Transrenal versus infrarenal endograft fixation: influence on type I endoleaks. *Ann Vasc Surg.* 2002;16:556.

58. Cao P, Verzini F, Parlani G, et al. Predictive factors and clinical consequences of proximal aortic neck dilatation in 230 patients undergoing abdominal aorta aneurysm repair with self-expandable stent-grafts. *J Vasc Surg.* 2003;37:1200.

59. Chuter TAM, Faruqi RM, Sawhney R, et al. Endoleak after endovascular repair of abdominal aortic aneurysm. *J Vasc Surg.* 2001;34:98.

60. Parent FN, Meier GH, Godziachvilli V, et al. The incidence and natural history of type I and II endoleak: a 5-year follow-up assessment with color duplex ultrasound scan. *J Vasc Surg.* 2002;35:474.

61. Liewald F, Ermis C, Gorich J, et al. Influence of treatment of type II leaks on the aneurysm surface area. *Eur J Vasc Endovasc Surg.* 2001;21:339.

62. Brouard R, Otal P, Soula P, et al. A useful endovascular technique for treating modular limb disconnection in a bifurcated stent graft. *J Endovasc Ther.* 2002;9:124.

63. White GH, May J, Waugh RC, et al. Type III and IV endoleak: toward a complete definition of blood flow in the sac after endoluminal AAA repair. *J Endovasc Ther.* 1998;5:305.

64. Matsumura JS, Ryu RK, Ouriel K. Identification and implications of transgraft microleaks after endovascular repair of aortic aneurysms. *J Vasc Surg.* 2001;34:190.

65. Pacanowski JP Jr, Stevens SL, Freeman MB, et al. Endotension distribution and the role of thrombus following endovascular abdominal aortic aneurysm (AAA) exclusion. *J Endovasc Ther.* 2002;9:639.

66. Parent EN III, Godziachvili V, Meier GH, et al. Endograft limb occlusion and stenosis after ANCURE endovascular abdominal aneurysm repair. *J Vasc Surg.* 2002;35:686.

67. Carroccio A, Faries PL, Morrissey NJ, et al. Predicting iliac limb occlusions after bifurcated aortic stent grafting: anatomic and device-related causes. *J Vasc Surg.* 2002;36:679.

68. Cao P, Verzini F, Zannetti S, et al. Device migration after endoluminal abdominal aortic aneurysm repair: analysis of 113 cases with a minimum follow-up period of two years. *J Vasc Surg.* 2002;35:229.

69. Conners MS III, Sternbergh WC III, Carter G, et al. Endograft migration one to four years after endovascular abdominal aortic aneurysm repair with the AneuRx device: a cautionary note. *J Vasc Surg.* 2002;36:476.

70. Storck M, Scharrer-Palmer R, Kapfer X, et al. Does a postimplantation syndrome following endovascular treatment of aortic aneurysms exist? *Vasc Surg.* 2001;35:23.

71. Nienaber CA, Fattori R, Lund G, et al. Nonsurgical reconstruction of thoracic aortic dissection by stent-graft placement. *N Engl J Med.* 1999;340:1539.

72. Blum U, Voshage G, Lammer J, et al. Endoluminal stent-grafts for infra-renal abdominal aortic aneurysms. *N Engl J Med.* 1997;336:13.

CHAPTER (53)

Carotid and Vertebral Artery Intervention

Ivan P. Casserly, MD, and
Jay S. Yadav, MD

By applying the skill sets and many of the tools from coronary intervention, interventional cardiologists were among the first to embrace the role of endovascular therapy in the treatment of atherosclerotic disease of the carotid and vertebral arteries. Over the past 10 to 15 years, they have made a major contribution toward making these therapies a reality. Today, the evidence base for carotid intervention has a firm foundation, such that a major shift away from carotid endarterectomy is imminent. Vertebral artery intervention has received considerably less attention but has certainly been demonstrated to be safe and feasible. This chapter will provide perspective on the current status of carotid and vertebral intervention, with an emphasis on the practical aspects of these procedures.

CAROTID INTERVENTION

Carotid artery intervention has evolved largely for the treatment of atherosclerotic disease of the carotid bifurcation.[1] The goal of such therapy is the prevention of atherothrombotic embolism from carotid plaque to the anterior cerebral circulation, thus reducing the incidence of stroke.[2] This mechanism is believed to account for up to 20% of all ischemic strokes, which underscores the potential impact of this therapy on stroke prevention.

Since the first descriptions of carotid artery angioplasty in the early 1980s,[1] carotid artery intervention has faced a number of unique challenges.

- Distal embolization and stroke. At the top of the list is the potential risk of periprocedural stroke caused by distal embolization of

plaque to the anterior cerebral circulation. This risk distinguishes carotid intervention from other peripheral vascular procedures (ie, those not involving the cerebrovascular system) and is largely responsible for the extraordinary scrutiny that carotid intervention has received. The recognition that microembolization of extruded plaque elements is almost universal during carotid angioplasty and stenting prompted investigators to develop techniques and devices that limit or eliminate distal embolization.[3–5] Although no randomized studies of carotid intervention with and without the use of embolic protection have been performed, retrospective observational data support the conclusion that the use of embolic protection has reduced the incidence of procedure-related strokes.[6,7] Given the risk to the patient, embolic protection has been widely embraced and now forms an essential cornerstone of carotid intervention.

- Failure of conventional balloon-expandable stents in the carotid bifurcation. Experience in other vascular territories reinforced the potential advantages of stenting in the carotid location. At these sites, stenting allowed operators to achieve a predictable angiographic result, to treat procedural complications such as abrupt closure and dissection, eliminate vessel recoil, and to improve long-term vessel patency. In the carotid artery, initial attempts to use stiff balloon-expandable stents (eg, Palmaz) were associated with two issues: (1) kinking of the internal carotid artery in the area between the stent and the petrous portion of the artery (Figure 53-1) and (2) a high incidence of (~16%) of stent collapse, where there was loss of wall apposition of all or part of the stent.[8] External compression of the stent in the superficially located carotid artery, together with deformation of the stent from neck movements, was proposed as the likely

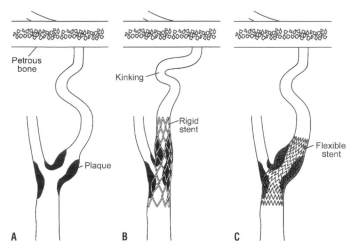

FIGURE 53-1. Schematic illustrating the effect of rigid stainless steel balloon-expandable **(B)** and self-expanding nitinol stents **(C)** in the carotid location **(A)**. Nitinol stents conform to the tortuosity in the carotid artery, minimizing any kinking distally.

mechanism. The development of thrombus in the potential space between the stent and vessel wall was considered possible. These concerns led to the use of self-expanding stents (Wallstent, Boston Scientific) and the development of dedicated low-profile nitinol self-expanding stents that have proven to provide excellent results in the carotid artery.

- A reluctance to abandon the gold standard. Carotid endarterectomy (CEA) has been practiced for more than 50 years for the treatment of obstructive carotid bifurcation disease. In the mid-1980s, considerable uncertainty regarding the efficacy of this therapy prompted the initiation of a large number of randomized trials comparing CEA with medical therapy. These studies provide a solid scientific foundation supporting the benefits of CEA in reducing the incidence of stroke in (1) symptomatic patients with moderate-to-severe carotid artery stenosis[9–11] and (2) asymptomatic patients with severe carotid artery stenosis.[12,13] Such validation of a vascular surgical procedure was unique and may explain the resistance with which the emerging field of carotid intervention was met by sections of the surgical and medical communities.

The result is that a significant burden of proof has fallen on the interventional community to prove that carotid intervention is safe and equally as effective as CEA in all clinical subsets. In addition, many obstacles toward the dissemination of the technique were erected, including the national "noncoverage" policy for carotid intervention by the Center for Medicare and Medicaid Services (formerly the Health Care Financing Administration), restrictions imposed by the Food and Drug Administration (FDA), and the requirement for Investigational Device Exemption outside of the setting of dedicated trials.[14] These challenges have been met but have certainly impeded the availability of this therapy to patients.

【 】 CURRENT INDICATIONS FOR CAROTID INTERVENTION

The randomized CEA trials systematically excluded high-risk patients based on the presence of baseline comorbidities or high-risk anatomic features. It is now apparent that by applying such

exclusion criteria, the conclusions of these trials may not be applicable in clinical practice. For example, in an analysis of outcomes of more than 113,000 Medicare patients undergoing CEA in 1992 to 1993, Wennberg reported 30-day mortality rates that dramatically exceeded those observed in randomized trials.[15] Additionally, in a single-center CEA registry at the Cleveland Clinic, the presence of one or more predefined cardiac, pulmonary, or renal comorbidities defined a high-risk group with a perioperative mortality rate of 4.4% compared with 0.3% in the low-risk group ($P < .001$).[16] Therefore, it seemed reasonable in the initial attempts to demonstrate equipoise between carotid intervention and CEA to choose patients deemed high-risk for CEA as the study population of interest.

There have been two approaches to the study of such a high-risk population using the contemporary approach to carotid intervention of carotid artery stenting (CAS) with embolic protection. Firstly, a large number of prospective single-center, multicenter, and corporate-sponsored registry studies evaluating the outcome of consecutively treated patients have been performed (Table 53-1).[17] Secondly, the Stenting and Angioplasty with Protection in Patients at High Risk for Endarterectomy (SAPPHIRE) trial randomized high surgical risk patients who were deemed eligible for revascularization by surgical or percutaneous methods to treatment with CEA or CAS with embolic protection.[18,19] The patient cohort in this trial is unique in the context of high-risk carotid studies; by virtue of the requirement that carotid revascularization be deemed possible by either surgical or percutaneous techniques, the overall risk was likely somewhat less than registry-type studies where such a requirement did not exist. A separate CAS registry component of the SAPPHIRE trial specifically enrolled patients who were deemed ineligible for CEA by the vascular surgeon reviewing the cases. This group represented a very high-risk group, which likely exceeded that in other "high-risk" registries. These considerations are important in interpreting the data from the SAPPHIRE trial and in comparing outcomes from this trial with other high-risk registries. Although not entirely uniform, the criteria that define "high risk" in these studies have been remarkably similar and are summarized in Table 53-2.

Given the randomized design of the SAPPHIRE trial, the evidence provided by this trial is the most scientifically robust. The outcome at 30 days and 1 year for each of the components of the composite end point are shown in Table 53-3. In the randomized cohort, each of the components of the composite end point trended in favor of the endovascular arm, with a significant reduction in the incidence of myocardial infarction (MI). Not surprisingly, the CAS registry cohort of this trial had a higher frequency of clinical comorbidities and high-risk anatomical features compared with the randomized cohort. Despite this difference, the outcomes in the CAS registry were comparable with the CEA arm of the randomized cohort. Overall, the data support the conclusion that CAS with embolic protection using the Angioguard XP filter is at least equivalent with CEA in high-risk patients. Outcomes from other high-risk registries using a variety of stents and embolic protection devices provide further corroborating evidence by showing a remarkable consistency in the frequency of the composite end point of death/stroke/MI between studies (Figure 53-2).

Based on the results of the SAPPHIRE trial, the FDA Circulatory Systems Devices Panel approved CAS in 2004 using

TABLE 53-1

Summary of "High-Risk" Carotid Artery Stent Registries

STUDY	SPONSOR	SAMPLE SIZE	STENT	EMBOLIC PROTECTION DEVICE	STATUS
SAPPHIRE (CAS registry)	Cordis	409	Precise	Angioguard	30-day and 1-year outcomes presented
ARCHeR 2, 3	Guidant	ARCHeR 2:-278 ARCHeR 3:-145	Acculink (OTW and Rx)	Accunet	30-day outcome ARCHeR 3 and 1-year of outcome ARCHeR 2 presented
SECURITY	Abbott Vascular Devices	320	MedNova Xact	MedNova NeuroShield/ EmboShield	30-day outcomes presented
BEACH	Boston Scientific	480	Wallstent	FilterWire EX and EZ	Enrollment completed
CABERNET	EndoTex	380	NexStent	FilterWire Ex	Enrollment completed CE mark approved
MAVErIC International	Medtronic	51	Exponent	Interceptor	Enrollment completed
MAVErIC II	Medtronic	Phase I:-99 Phase II:399	Exponent	GuardWire	Enrollment completed
PASCAL	Medtronic	115	Exponent	Any CE mark approved device	Enrollment completed
CREATE	ev3	400	Protégé	Spider	Enrollment completed

ARCHeR 2, 3 = ACCULINK for Revascularization of Carotids in High-Risk Patients; BEACH = Boston Scientific EPI-A Carotid Stenting Trial for High-Risk Surgical Patients; CABERNET = Carotid Artery Revascularization Using the Boston Scientific FilterWire and the EndoTex NexStent; CAS = carotid artery stent; CREATE = Carotid Revascularization with ev3 Arterial Technology Evolution; MAVErIC = Evaluation of the Medtronic AVE Self-Expanding Carotid Stent System in the Treatment of Carotid Stenosis; OTW = over-the-wire; PASCAL = Performance And Safety of the Medtronic AVE Self-Expandable Stent in Treatment of Carotid Artery Lesions; Rx = monorail; SAPPHIRE = Stenting and Angioplasty with Protection in Patients at High Risk for Endarterectomy; SECURITY = Registry Study to Evaluate the NeuroShield Bare Wire Cerebral Protection System and X-Act Stent in Patients at High Risk for Carotid Endarterectomy.

TABLE 53-2

Criteria Used to Define High-Risk in Carotid Artery Stent Studies

HIGH-RISK CRITERIA

Clinical
  Age > 80 years
  Congestive heart failure (class III/IV)
  Known severe left ventricular dysfunction, LVEF < 30%
  Open heart surgery needed within 6 wk
  Recent MI (> 24 h and < 4 wk)
  Unstable angina (CCS class III/IV)
  Severe pulmonary disease
  Contralateral largyngeal nerve palsy

Anatomic
  Previous CEA with recurrent stenosis
  High cervical ICA lesions or CCA lesions below the clavicle
  Contralateral carotid occlusion
  Radiation therapy to neck
  Prior radical neck surgery
  Severe tandem lesions

CCA = common carotid artery; CEA = carotid endarterectomy; ICA = internal carotid endartectomy; LVEF = left ventricular ejection fraction; MI = myocardial infarction.

TABLE 53-3

30-Day and 1-Year Outcomes (Based on Actual Treatment Analysis) in the Stenting and Angioplasty with Protection in Patients at High Risk for Endarterectomy (SAPPHIR) Trial

	RANDOMIZED TRIAL	
	CAS	CEA
30-day Outcome		
Death	0.6	2.0
Stroke	3.1	3.3
MI	1.9	6.6
Death/stroke/MI	4.4	9.9
1-year Outcome		
Death	7.0	12.9
Stroke	5.8	7.7
MI	2.5	8.1
30-day death/stroke/ MI plus death and ipsilateral stroke between 31 days and 1 year	12.0	20.1

CAS = carotid artery stenting; CEA = carotid endarterectomy; MACE = major adverse cardiac event; MI = myocardial infarction.

the Precise nitinol stent in conjunction with the Angioguard XP filter for the treatment of symptomatic and asymptomatic patients with at least 50% and at least 80% carotid stenosis, respectively. That same year, the Acculink nitinol stent and Accunet filter received similar approval. It is hoped that these devices will be available to qualified operators for routine clinical use for the approved indications by the end of 2004. Several other carotid

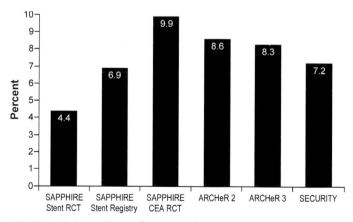

FIGURE 53-2. Incidence of death/stroke/myocardial infarction at 30 days from "high-risk" carotid stent registries and randomized portion of the Stenting and Angioplasty with Protection in Patients at High Risk for Endarterectomy (SAPPHIRE) trial. ARCHeR 2, 3 = ACCULINK for Revascularization of Carotids in High-Risk Patients; CEA = carotid endarterectomy; RCT = randomized controlled trial; SECURITY = Registry Study to Evaluate the NeuroShield Bare Wire Cerebral Protection System and X-Act Stent in Patients at High Risk for Carotid Endarterectomy.

stent-filter combinations will be seeking the same approval and are expected to become available in the next 1 to 2 years.

Carotid intervention remains investigational in patients other than those who have a high risk of CEA. Several clinical trials are currently randomizing symptomatic patients without "high-risk" criteria to either CEA or CAS with embolic protection (Table 53-4).[20–24] These patients will more closely match those enrolled in the initial CEA trials of the 1990s. All patients will receive carotid stents, and embolic protection is either mandatory or strongly encouraged. Enrollment in these studies has been slower than expected and may be further jeopardized by low-risk carotid artery stent registries that are currently being planned. Completion of enrollment and clinical follow-up is projected to take at least 2 to 3 more years, and a meta-analysis of 3 of these studies (Endarterectomy Versus Angioplasty in Patients With Symptomatic Severe Carotid Stenosis [EVA-3S], International Carotid Stenting Study [ICSS], Stent-Supported Percutaneous Angioplasty of the Carotid Artery vs Endarterectomy [SPACE]) is planned. Assuming at least equivalency in outcome between the treatment strategies, the approval process could add a further 1 to 2 years before application into practice of the endovascular strategy in this patient cohort.

Low-risk, asymptomatic patients with carotid artery disease have not been included in carotid intervention studies to date, but randomized and case-controlled studies of CEA versus CAS are planned for this patient population. Any intervention in this group is at best likely to have a narrow therapeutic index, given the low frequency of events in such patients when treated medically. Dedicated trials are required before carotid intervention can be applied in such patients.

TABLE 53-4

Summary of "Low-Risk" Carotid Artery Stent Trials

TRIAL	SAMPLE SIZE	SITES OF ENROLLMENT	FUNDING	CLINICAL ENROLLMENT CRITERIA	LESION ENROLLMENT CRITERIA	ENDOVASCULAR STRATEGY	PRIMARY END POINTS	STATUS OF TRIAL
ICSS (CAVATAS-2)	1500	Europe Australia Canada	Stroke Association Sanofi Synthelabo European Commission	TIA/stroke within 12 months	> 50% by NASCET method or noninvasive equivalent	CAS ± EPD	• 30-day death/ stroke/MI • 3 year death/ disabling stroke	Expect to complete enrollment by 2007
EVA-3S	900	France	National Research Organization	TIA/stroke within 4 months	> 60% by NASCET or noninvasive equivalent	CAS + EPD	• 30-day death/stroke • 30-day death/ stroke + ipsilateral stroke at 2–4 years	300 enrolled in April 2004
SPACE	1900	Germany Austria Switzerland	Federal Ministry of Education and Research German Research Foundation Industry Funding	TIA/stroke within 6 months	> 50% by NASCET or 70% by Doppler	CAS ± EPD	• 30-day death/ ipsilateral stroke • 2 year death/ ipsilateral stroke	667 enrolled in February 2004
CREST	2500	North America Europe	National Institute of Neurological Disorders and Stroke–National Institutes of Health Guidant Corporation	Symptomatic	> 50% by NASCET	CAS + EPD[a]	• 30-day death/stroke/MI • ipsilateral stroke after 30 days	Currently enrolling

[a]Acculink stent and Accunet embolic protection device. CAS = carotid artery stenting; CREST = Carotid Revascularization Endarterectomy versus Stent Trial; EPD = embolic protection device; EVA-3S = Endarterectomy Versus Angioplasty in Patients With Symptomatic Severe Carotid Stenosis; ICSS = International Carotid Stenting Study; MI = myocardial infarction; NASCET = North American Symptomatic Carotid Endarterectomy Trial; SPACE = Stent-Supported Percutaneous Angioplasty of the Carotid Artery versus Endarterectomy; TIA = transient ischemic attack.

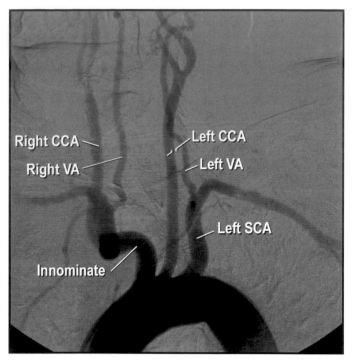

FIGURE 53-3. Normal anatomy of the aortic arch and great vessels. CCA = common carotid artery; SCA = subclavian artery; VA = vertebral artery.

【 】 ANATOMY OF CAROTID ARTERY INTERVENTION

The origin of the right common carotid artery (CCA) is remarkably constant, arising from the bifurcation of the innominate artery. In contrast, the origin of the left CCA is variable. Typically, it is the second great vessel arising directly from the aortic arch (Figure 53-3). However, in 10% to 15% of patients, the origin of the left CCA lies adjacent to the innominate artery (ie, common origin), and in approximately 10% of patients, it arises from the innominate artery (ie, bovine origin) above the level of the arch.

Each CCA bifurcates into an external and internal carotid artery, typically at the level of the C4-C6 vertebral interspace. During diagnostic angiography, the angle of the mandible serves as a useful landmark for the carotid bifurcation. The external carotid artery (ECA) is easily recognized because of its numerous branches to the face, scalp, and thyroid. Under normal conditions, the internal carotid artery (ICA) is recognized by the bulbous dilation at its origin (typically ~ 7 mm in diameter), termed the carotid sinus, which contains the mechanoreceptors responsible for blood pressure regulation. In its proximal portion, the ICA lies posterior and medial to the ECA, and is devoid of branches. By convention, the ICA is divided into four sections (Figure 53-4):

1. Cervical portion, which defines the length of vessel between the CCA bifurcation and the petrous bone.

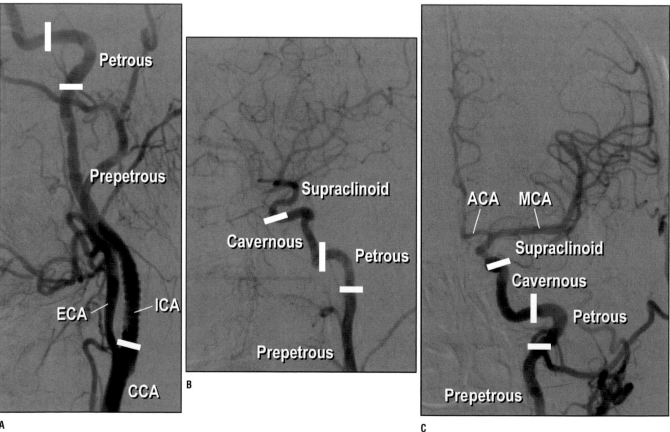

FIGURE 53-4. Anatomy of the internal carotid artery (ICA). **A.** Left anterior oblique view showing the proximal portion of the left ICA. **B.** Lateral view of distal portion of the left ICA. **C.** Posteroanterior cranial view of the distal left ICA and its cerebral branches. ACA = anterior cerebral artery; CCA = common carotid artery; ECA = external carotid artery; ICA = internal carotid artery; MCA = middle cerebral artery.

2. Petrous portion, which defines the L-shaped section of vessel that courses through the petrous bone.

3. Cavernous portion, which courses through the cavernous sinus.

4. Supraclinoid portion, which gives off the important ophthalmic and posterior communicating branches and terminates in the middle and anterior cerebral arteries.

The area of the brain supplied by the anterior and middle cerebral arteries is termed the "carotid" territory.

【 】 DIAGNOSTIC CAROTID ANGIOGRAPHY

Diagnostic carotid angiography should always be preceded by an assessment of the anatomy of the aortic arch. This may be done by performing an arch aortogram at the time of the procedure or an magnetic resonance (MR)/computed tomography (CT) angiogram prior to the procedure. The critical issues that need to be determined are (1) the aortic arch type and (2) the presence any anomalies of the origin of the great vessels. In elderly patients with atherosclerotic disease, the ascending aorta sinks deeper into the thoracic cavity, dragging the origins of the great vessels with it. This results in a progressively greater distance between the apex of the arch and the origin of the great vessels and defines the aortic arch type (types I to III) (Figure 53-5). Type II and III arches significantly increase the difficulty encountered in selectively engaging the great vessels, in delivering a guide or sheath to the CCA, and in delivering equipment through the guide or sheath.

Our practice is to administer low-dose intravenous heparin (~25 U/kg) prior to diagnostic cerebral angiographic studies. In patients with straightforward aortic arch anatomy, a JR 4 diagnostic catheter is typically used. A Vitek catheter is used for most patients with type III arches. Only rarely is a Simmons catheter required.

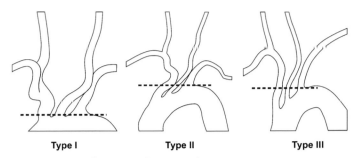

FIGURE 53-5. Illustration of aortic arch types.

Adequate angiography of the left CCA can usually be achieved with the diagnostic catheter at the origin of the vessel. For right CCA angiography, the innominate artery must first be engaged. Using a stiff-angled glide wire to selectively wire the right CCA, the catheter is advanced into the proximal portion of the vessel.

In most circumstances, ipsilateral oblique (30°–45°) and left lateral views of the CCA of interest are adequate to define the anatomy of the carotid bifurcation. However, when the lesion of interest is not defined using this approach, additional views should be performed (eg, straight anteroposterior, contralateral oblique, or adding cranial or caudal angulation to standardized views). Table 53-5 summarizes the angiographic features that require assessment and the impact of those assessments on the carotid intervention.

Additionally, we recommend performing baseline angiography of at least the anterior cerebral circulation prior to planned carotid intervention. This serves to rule out the presence of associated significant intracranial atherosclerotic artery disease or other vascular pathology. In the event of neurologic complications associated with the procedure, it also allows comparison with postprocedural cerebral angiography, facilitating decision-making regarding the likely etiology and management of such events. Posteroanterior

TABLE 53-5

Influence of Assessments Made During Diagnostic Carotid Angiography on Carotid Interventional Procedures

ANGIOGRAPHIC ASSESSMENT	IMPACT ON INTERVENTIONAL PROCEDURE
Assess Lesion Characteristics	
Precise location of the lesion, with definition of the proximal and distal extent of lesion	Influences planned location for stent placement and stent length Influences strategy for delivery of guide/sheath to distal CCA
Approximate length of lesion	Stent length
Complex lesion ulceration	Predict difficulty of crossing lesion with filter device
Severity of stenosis	Predict difficulty of crossing lesion with filter device
	Predict need for predilation of lesion prior to filter delivery
Calcification	Predict ability to achieve good stent expansion
Diameter of CCA and ICA	Influences choice of stent diameter and filter diameter
Assess the entire prepetrous portion of the ICA	Influences the choice of landing zone for the filter device
Tortuosity distal to the lesion and proximal to the landing zone for filter	Favors use of guide to provide support
	Predict degree of difficulty in delivering filter
Patency of external carotid artery	Influences strategy for delivery of guide/sheath to distal CCA

CCA = common carotid artery; ICA = internal carotid artery.

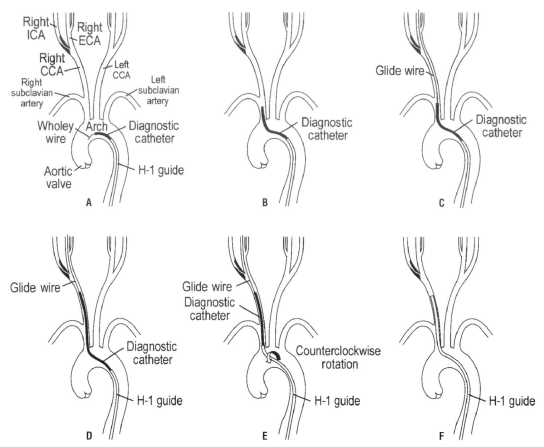

FIGURE 53-6. Schematic of technique used to deliver a guide to the distal common carotid artery internal carotid artery (ICA). See text for details. CCA = common carotid artery; ECA = external carotid artery.

Although the use of a guide or sheath is often determined solely by operator preference and experience, there are advantages and disadvantages to either, as summarized in Table 53-6. Our bias is to use a guide catheter, because it allows for greater flexibility during the procedure. Guides should certainly be considered in situations in which added support is required (eg, significant tortuosity distal to ICA lesion, critical ICA stenosis) and are delivered using a "telescoping technique." Our guide of choice is the H-1 guide. Through a Tuohy-Borst type adaptor at the hub of the guide, a long (125-cm) diagnostic catheter is advanced such that its tip extends beyond the tip of the guide. The diagnostic catheter chosen matches that required to engage the vessel during diagnostic angiography. Therefore, for type I or II arches, a JR 4 is usually chosen, and for type III arches, some type II arches, and

cranial and left lateral views are the standard views used by most operators.

【 】 INTERVENTIONAL TECHNIQUE

Pharmacology

All patients receive aspirin and clopidogrel for at least 3 days prior to CAS. Anticoagulation is typically achieved using unfractionated heparin, with a target activated clotting time of 275 to 300 seconds. In patients with a contraindication to heparin, we have safely performed CAS using the direct thrombin inhibitor, bivalirudin. However, there is currently insufficient data documenting the safety of bivalirudin for routine use during CAS.

Delivery of Sheath or Guide to the Common Carotid Artery

It is impossible within the scope of this chapter to describe the entire array of strategies that are used to perform carotid bifurcation stenting with embolic protection. What follows is a description of the standard techniques that we employ to perform the majority of cases (Figure 53-6).

With rare exception, carotid intervention is performed using femoral arterial access. The first step of carotid intervention is the delivery of a guide or sheath to the distal CCA. With currently available equipment, the inner diameter of an 8-Fr guide or 6-Fr sheath is required to allow easy delivery of required devices.

bovine origins of the left CCA, a Vitek (or rarely Simmons) catheter is selected. The catheter-guide combination is delivered into the aortic arch over an 0.035-in wire. The diagnostic catheter is used to engage the origin of the innominate or left CCA. A stiff-angled glide wire is then advanced through the diagnostic catheter into the ECA. In situations in which the ECA is occluded or severely diseased proximally or the distal CCA is significantly diseased, the stiff-angled glide wire is instead positioned in the distal CCA proximal to any disease. The diagnostic catheter is then slowly advanced over the wire, and the guide is then carefully advanced over the catheter-wire combination to the distal CCA.

Sheaths should be favored in patients with severe peripheral vascular disease because of the smaller arteriotomy required as well as in patients with CCA disease because of the smaller outer diameter of the 6-Fr sheath compared with an 8-Fr guide and the smooth transition between the dilator and sheath catheter. The technique for sheath delivery is similar to that for guides. A 125-cm diagnostic catheter is advanced through a 90-cm sheath and is used to selectively engage the innominate or left CCA. A stiff-angled glide wire is advanced through the diagnostic catheter into the ECA or distal CCA. The diagnostic catheter is then advanced over the glidewire to the ECA or distal CCA. At this point, there are two possible strategies: (1) the sheath may be advanced over the glide wire-catheter combination or (2) the glide wire may be exchanged for a stiff Amplatz wire (6-cm soft tip) and the diagnostic catheter removed. The sheath and its dilator are then delivered to the distal CCA over the stiff Amplatz wire. This approach is advised for

TABLE 53-6

Advantages and Disadvantages of Guide and Sheath-Based Approaches to Carotid Artery Stenting Procedures

	GUIDE	SHEATH
Advantages	• Torque control of tip allows orientation of guide with respect to the ICA • Provides superior support • More resistant to kinking in tortuous vessels or type III arches • Easier to deliver to CCA in presence of ECA occlusion	• 6-Fr sheath adequate for carotid intervention minimizing arteriotomy size, risk of limb ischemia in patients with peripheral vascular disease • Smooth transition between dilator and sheath advantageous in patients with diseased CCA • Easier to deliver through CCA tortuosity
Disadvantages	• 8-Fr guide required for carotid intervention • Transition from diagnostic catheter to guide less optimal than with sheath and dilator	• Provides less support than guide • More likely to be displaced distally into CCA during intervention • Not torquable

CCA = common carotid artery; ECA = external carotid artery; ICA = internal carotid artery.

patients with more complex anatomy where extra support is required to deliver the sheath.

Emboli Protection Devices

Three basic types of emboli protection devices (EPDs) have been developed for carotid intervention.

Filter-Type Device.   The filter-type device is the most popular and user friendly EPD (Table 53-7, Figure 53-7). This type of EPD has been used in the large clinical registries and trials of carotid

artery stenting. The most common filter design is that of a polyurethane membrane containing pores of fixed size (80–140 μm between devices) supported by a nitinol frame, which is integrated with an 0.014-in guidewire with a 3- to 4-cm shapeable floppy tip. The filter EPD is delivered primarily across the carotid lesion on the attached guidewire. Ideally, the filter is positioned in a straight nondiseased portion of the ICA just proximal to the petrous bone (Figure 53-8).

In addition to their ease of use, the major advantage of these devices is that they allow continued antegrade flow during carotid

TABLE 53-7

Summary of Filter-Type Embolic Protection Devices Used During Carotid Intervention

FILTER	MANUFACTURER	DIAMETERS	PORE SIZE	FILTER AND GUIDEWIRE INTEGRATED	FILTER TYPE
Interceptor	Medtronic		100 μm	Yes	Supported
Rubicon	Rubicon Medical	4, 5, 6	100 μm	Yes	Supported
FilterWire EX FilterWire EZ	Boston Scientific	3.5-5.5	80 μm	Yes	Unsupported
Angioguard XP Angioguard RX	Cordis	4, 5, 6, 7, 8	100 μm	Yes	Supported
NeuroShield/ EmboShield	Abbott Laboratories		140 μm	No	Supported
Spider	ev3	3, 4, 5, 6, 7	Variable	Yes	Supported
Accunet OTW Accunet RX	Guidant	4.5, 5.5, 6.5, 7.5	120 μm	Yes	Supported

N/R = not remarkable.

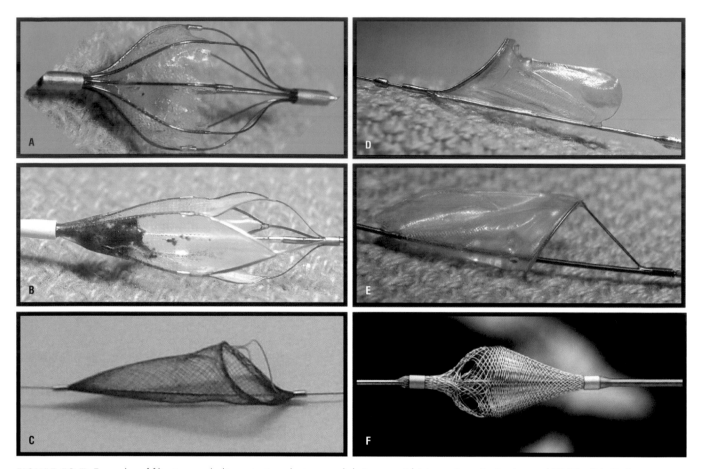

FIGURE 53-7. Examples of filter-type embolic protection devices used during carotid intervention. **A.** Angioguard XP (Cordis). **B.** Accunet (Guidant). **C.** Spider (ev3). **D.** FilterWire EX (Boston Scientific). **E.** FilterWire EZ (Boston Scientific). **F.** Interceptor (Medtronic).

intervention. This is particularly important for patients with compromised collateral flow to the ipsilateral carotid territory (eg, patients with contralateral carotid artery disease or occlusion). Although the crossing profile of these EPDs is slightly greater than distal balloon occlusion devices, predilation of the carotid lesion to facilitate delivery of the filter is rarely required.

Distal Occlusion Balloon Device. The distal occlusion balloon EPD was the first type of EPD used during carotid intervention (~1998). The GuardWire (Medtronic) is currently the sole manufacturer of this type of device.[25,26] Essentially, this device contains a compliant latex balloon that can be inflated and deflated through a hollow nitinol hypotube located in an 0.014-in angioplasty style wire. Similar to a filter-type EPD, the GuardWire is advanced primarily across the carotid lesion, and the balloon maker is positioned in the same location as a filter. Inflation of the balloon then produces complete interruption of antegrade flow. Following the intervention, the column of blood proximal to the filter is aspirated using an export catheter, removing any debris that may have embolized from the carotid plaque. The balloon is then deflated and the wire removed.

The major advantage of the distal occlusion balloon EPD is its lower crossing profile compared with the filter-type EPD. In theory, it should also be able to remove all of the embolized debris, regardless of particle size. Its major limitations are that occlusion of ICA flow may be poorly tolerated in patients with compromised collateral flow to the cerebral circulation and that slight movement

of the balloon may result in loss of occlusion and embolization of the retained particles proximal to the balloon.

Proximal Occlusion Device. The proximal occlusion device is the third and least common type of EPD used during carotid artery intervention. Currently, there are two examples of such devices: The Parodi Anti-Embolism System (PAES) (ArteriA Medical Science) and the MO.MA system (Invatec, Italy). The fundamental principle of these devices is that they generate retrograde flow in the ICA, which theoretically protects the brain from distal embolization during the procedure (Figure 53-9).[27] This is achieved by firstly blocking antegrade flow in the ICA and ECA by inflating compliant balloons in the mid/distal CCA and ECA, respectively. Retrograde flow in the ICA is then produced by connecting the lumen of a catheter whose tip is distal to the occlusive CCA balloon with the femoral vein through a blood return system. The pressure gradient between the carotid artery and femoral vein creates an arteriovenous fistula and allows retrograde flow in the ICA.

In practice, these devices are cumbersome and technically challenging to use. The catheter sizes used are larger than for other types of EPDs, and retrograde flow along the ICA occurs only if the patient has adequate collateral circulation in the circle of Willis. One of the potential advantages of such devices is that they may be used in patients in whom anatomic considerations distal to the carotid bifurcation lesion (eg, tortuosity) prevent the use of filter-type or distal occlusion EPDs. High-risk lesions that contain

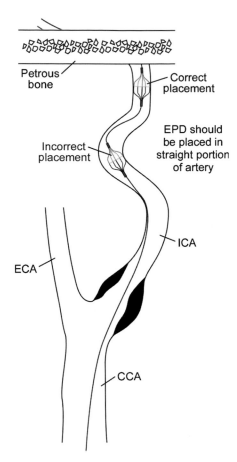

FIGURE 53-8. Schematic of internal carotid artery (ICA) demonstrating correct placement of filter-type embolic protection device (EPD). CCA = common carotid artery; ECA = external carotid artery.

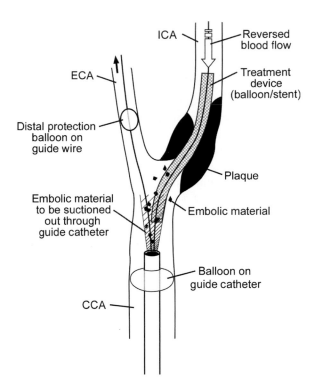

FIGURE 53-9. Illustration of proximal balloon occlusion embolic protection device. See text for details. CCA = common carotid artery; ECA = external carotid artery; ICA = internal carotid artery.

thrombus and friable material may also be better treated with such EPDs. It should be stressed that the clinical data available for proximal occlusion EPDs is very limited,[28] and that their use is currently investigational.

Predilation, Stent Placement, Postdilation

Following placement of the emboli protection device, most operators predilate the lesion prior to stent placement. In our practice, predilation is generally performed using a 4.0-mm diameter coronary balloon (eg, Maverick, Boston Scientific). The primary purpose of predilation is to ensure the subsequent delivery of the stent. In general, the greater the degree of lesion calcification and severity of stenosis, the more likely that predilation is necessary to allow successful stent delivery.

The standard stent for carotid intervention is a self-expanding nitinol stent. Currently, most such stents are cylindrical in shape, although tapered stents are also available. The choice of stent length and diameter is heavily influenced by the location of the lesion (Figure 53-10). The majority of carotid bifurcation lesions involve the ostium of the ICA, and in such situations, a longer stent that extends from the distal CCA into the ICA and whose diameter matches the CCA should be chosen. For lesions that are truly confined to the ICA, a stent confined to the ICA whose diameter matches the ICA is typically chosen.

Most operators dilate the stent following deployment, using 5.5- to 6.0-mm diameter balloons. In contrast to coronary intervention, mild residual stenosis (up to 20%) is generally tolerated following carotid stenting because of the low risk of restenosis. Over time, there is continued expansion of self-expanding stents, which reinforces the general principle of being conservative toward post-stent balloon dilation.

At the completion of the procedure, the EPD is removed. Final angiography of the lesion site is performed, and angiography of the ipsilateral cerebral circulation is repeated to document the absence of angiographic evidence of distal embolization.

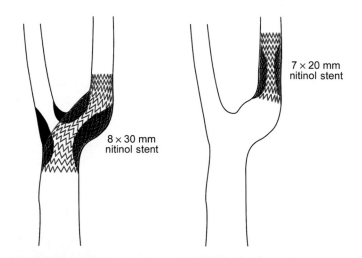

Bifurcation lesion   **Mid-ICA lesion**

FIGURE 53-10. Schematic of internal carotid artery (ICA) demonstrating appropriate nitinol stent placement based on lesion location.

【 】 COMPLICATIONS OF CAROTID INTERVENTION

Hemodynamic Conditions

Hypotension and Bradycardia. Transient hypotension and bradycardia are frequently observed (~40%) during CAS and during the post-procedural period.[29-33] These findings often parallel one another, because they both result from activation of the mechanoreceptors in the carotid sinus due to stretch from the stent and angioplasty balloons. This is consistent with the finding that carotid sinus reflex responses are most commonly seen with bifurcation lesions as opposed to isolated ICA lesions.[29-33] Typically, the maximal effect is seen for seconds to minutes following postdilation of the stent, with more modest persistent effects up to 48 hours following the procedure. For this reason, our practice is to withhold any blood pressure medications on the morning of the procedure. We do not routinely administer atropine prior to stent deployment or postdilation of the stent. This is based on clinical experience that atropine is rarely required, and that in elderly patients, atropine is associated with significant side effects such as urinary retention, severe dry mouth, and confusion. Situations in which we do administer atropine include cases in which there is an exaggerated hypotensive and/or bradycardic response to predilation or stent deployment or in patients with critical aortic stenosis or coronary artery disease. In the latter situations, even brief episodes of bradycardia and hypotension may be poorly tolerated and result in hemodynamic collapse.

Intraprocedurally, hypotension should be managed by aggressive hydration with intravenous fluids. If symptomatic or severe asymptomatic hypotension develops (systolic blood pressure [SBP] < 75 mm Hg), intravenous dopamine is commenced (5 µg/kg) and titrated to achieve an SBP of greater than 90 mm Hg or to alleviate symptoms. During the post-procedural period, persistent hypotension is similarly managed. One must ensure that all blood pressure medications are withheld, and aggressive hydration with intravenous fluids is maintained. Oral pseudoephedrine (Sudafed) may be administered (60 mg q4h) for asymptomatic severe hypotension in an attempt to prevent or eliminate the need for intravenous dopamine. In this situation, one needs to be aware of the risk of inducing coronary ischemia with sympathomimetic agents in patients with associated coronary artery disease. Bradycardia postintervention rarely if ever requires intervention, other than to modify the dose of atrioventricular nodal blocking agents.

Hypertension. Hypertension is common following carotid artery stenting and most commonly reflects a persistence of the patients' baseline condition.[32] The frequency of this event is heavily influenced by the baseline demographics of the patient population, and the attention given to monitoring and aggressively treating post-procedural hypertension. Acute hypertension has been described following carotid endarterectomy and been attributed to transient dysfunction of adventitial baroreceptors at the endarterectomy site.[34] It is unclear if this phenomenon also occurs following CAS. Hypertension following carotid artery stenting is important because it is associated with an increased risk of hyperperfusion to the ipsilateral cerebral hemisphere.[35] First described in patients undergoing carotid endarterectomy, this syndrome is thought to be explained by a loss of autoregulation of cerebral blood flow.[36]

Severe carotid stenosis produces a chronic low-flow state resulting in compensatory dilation of the cerebral vessels distal to the stenosis in an attempt to maintain normal cerebral blood flow. Persistent dilation is believed to lead to loss of the normal vasomotor response of these vessels. As a consequence, following removal of the carotid stenosis during stenting, there is inadequate vasoconstriction, resulting in increased cerebral blood flow (ie, hyperperfusion). Although no dedicated prospective studies of this syndrome have been performed in the setting of carotid artery stenting, retrospective registry data suggest an incidence of between 1% and 5%.[35]

Based on data from CEA and CAS studies, the association of hypertension, critical ipsilateral carotid stenosis (> 90%), and contralateral stenosis (> 80%) or occlusion identifies a high-risk subset of patients for this disorder.[37] Clinically, patients complain of an ipsilateral throbbing headache that may be facial, temporal, or retro-orbital in distribution. Associated symptoms include nausea, vomiting, focal neurologic deficits, or seizures. Ancillary investigations that support the diagnosis include the absence of abnormal findings on CT of the head and increased flow velocities in the ipsilateral middle cerebral artery by transcranial Doppler ultrasound.[38] Management should consist of aggressive treatment with antihypertensive medication. We use beta-blockers as the first-line therapy in this setting due to the risk of associated coronary artery disease in "high-risk" patients and the neutral effect of beta-blockers on cerebral blood flow. Nitroglycerin (intravenous) is also used, although the development of a "nitrate headache" may confuse the clinical picture occasionally. Aggressive reinstitution of the patients' baseline antihypertensive regimen is also important. The feared consequence of inadequate management of hypertension and "hyperperfusion syndrome" is intracranial hemorrhage.[35,39–42] This carries a 30% to 80% mortality rate; among survivors, 20% to 40% have significant residual neurologic deficits.[43] In carotid artery stent registries, the frequency of intracranial hemorrhage is less than 1%, but the morbidity and mortality associated with the condition underscores the importance of meticulous attention to both hypertension management and the prompt diagnosis and aggressive management of "hyperperfusion syndrome."

Stroke

As previously stated, stroke is the major adverse event associated with CAS. Overall, the 30-day incidence of stroke with CAS is less than or equal to 3% in "high-risk" patients,[44,45] which certainly compares favorably to the rate of 3.3% in the CEA arm of the SAPPHIRE trial.[18] Most strokes following CAS are classified as minor (resolution within 30 days or National Institutes of Health Stroke Scale ≤ 3) and are temporally closely related to the procedure. Although the dominant mechanism of stroke is believed to be distal embolization of atherosclerotic debris during angioplasty and stenting, it is important to be aware of other contributing factors, such as manipulation of catheters in the aortic arch and CCA. These manipulations are not "protected" and should particularly be implicated in strokes outside of the territory of the treated carotid artery that are observed following CAS.[46] This phenomenon also explains why even a perfect EPD cannot be expected to reduce the risk of stroke during CAS to zero.

When neurologic deficits occur during the procedure, cerebral angiography should be performed to document the presence or absence of angiographic evidence of distal embolization. If a large artery occlusion is identified, it is reasonable for suitably qualified practitioners to attempt recanalization using a combination of mechanical (ie, angioplasty) and pharmacologic (ie, thrombolytic, glycoprotein IIb/IIIa) therapies. The dosing of pharmacologic agents in this setting is largely empiric. Unfortunately, the therapeutic success with these maneuvers is unpredictable, due in large part to the composition of the emboli (ie, atheromatous debris), which do not respond well to traditional interventional techniques.[47] Distal branch vessel occlusions (vessel diameters < 2 mm) are typically managed noninvasively, although we usually empirically administer a bolus and infusion of glycoprotein IIb/IIIa in an effort to minimize the infarct size. In our experience, the absence of angiographic evidence of distal embolization in the presence of a neurologic deficit is a good prognostic sign and usually associated with full recovery of neurologic function. Such patients should be managed conservatively.

Although uncommon, strokes can occur in the days (usually within the first 2 weeks) following carotid intervention and are typically minor in severity.[48] The mechanism of these strokes is often obscure. Embolization of plaque elements through the interstices of the stent or of platelet thrombi from the stent surface is possible. Alternatively, agitation of atheroma in the aortic arch may result in delayed embolization of plaque elements or of platelet thrombi that form on the irregular traumatized surface. In this circumstance, the first priority should be to rule out intracranial hemorrhage. In the absence of hemorrhage, management is typically conservative.

Adverse Cardiac Events

MI following CAS is uncommon, occurring in < 2% in most series.[45,49] Most are non-Q wave in type. This contrasts markedly with the incidence of MI of 6.6% in the CEA arm of the SAPPHIRE trial and represents a major potential advantage of CAS over CEA.[49] We recommend caution, however, in the use of CAS in patients with critical coronary or cardiac disease awaiting open heart surgery. These patients represent an extremely high-risk subset. Previously, our strategy in this group was to perform CAS, followed by 4 weeks of antiplatelet therapy with aspirin and clopidogrel, followed approximately 5 to 7 days later by open heart surgery. Based on our personal experience of an excess of cardiac mortality in this patient cohort during this waiting period, we have revised our strategy significantly. We now avoid the use of stents and perform carotid angioplasty alone using cutting balloons. Antiplatelet therapy consists of aspirin and one of the small-molecule intravenous glycoprotein IIb/IIIa inhibitors. Following carotid artery angioplasty, the patient proceeds expeditiously to open heart surgery, having stopped the glycoprotein IIb/IIIa inhibitor 4 to 6 hours previously. Postoperatively, the patient is continued on aspirin and clopidogrel is started within 48 hours of the procedure. A carotid ultrasound is performed at 6 to 8 weeks after open heart surgery, and, if needed, a carotid stent is placed at that time.

[ ] POSTPROCEDURAL CARE AND FOLLOW-UP

Patients are admitted to a step-down telemetry floor for overnight observation and typically discharged the following day. As outlined above, the major management issue is blood pressure. The reintro-duction and titration of blood pressure medications must be done carefully. This process requires careful follow-up, including twice-daily blood pressure measurements and daily contact between the patient and health care professional until a stable blood pressure state has been reached. Life-long aspirin therapy is mandatory, and clopidogrel is currently continued for a minimum of 4 weeks following the procedure. Future trials (eg, (Clopidogrel for High Atherothrombotic Risk and Ischemic Stabilization, Management and Avoidance [CHARISMA]) will help determine if more prolonged treatment with clopidogrel offers any clinical benefit in patients with carotid disease. Treatment with "statins" is also warranted in addition to aggressive management of other known risk factors for atherosclerosis.

In longer term follow-up, patients should be monitored for evidence of restenosis or progression of disease in the contralateral carotid artery. Restenosis with CAS is low (2%-5%), with a reported target lesion revascularization rate of less than 1% in both the randomized and registry CAS arms of the SAPPHIRE trial. Reports of ipsilateral stroke or transient ischemic attack (TIA) beyond the initial 2 weeks following CAS are extremely rare. These data certainly underscore the long-term durability and efficacy of the procedure. Management of severe restenosis following CAS is controversial, because the risk of stroke from this process is poorly defined but believed to be low.[50] We typically advocate an aggressive approach to the treatment of high-grade restenosis (> 80%) that includes angioplasty and brachytherapy using gamma radiation.[49] Because of the large diameter of the ICA, beta radiation at this site is unlikely to be effective.

VERTEBRAL ARTERY INTERVENTION

Endovascular intervention of the vertebral artery (VA) has evolved at a considerably slower pace than carotid intervention.[51] There are several reasons for this. Surgical revascularization of VA lesions at the most common sites of atherosclerosis is technically challenging and associated with significant morbidity and mortality. As a consequence, surgical revascularization has traditionally been reserved only for symptomatic patients recalcitrant to medical therapy. Because of the infrequency of the surgical procedure, there was never an impetus to perform randomized trials of surgical therapy versus medical therapy, and hence there is no body of data supporting the role of revascularization in altering the natural history of the disease. Ultrasonography, which is inexpensive and widely available, is unreliable in detecting disease at the ostium and intracranial portions of the VA. MR angiography also has limited utility at these sites.[52] As a result, routine angiography continues to be required for reliable diagnosis, contributing to the underdiagnosis of VA disease. Finally, symptoms attributable to posterior circulation ischemia are more nonspecific than those attributable to anterior circulation ischemia (Table 53-8), contributing further to the underdiagnosis of the disease.

As with carotid intervention, atherosclerosis of the VA is the dominant pathology requiring VA intervention. Angiographic and necropsy studies demonstrate two sites along the VA with a predilection for atherosclerosis: the first 1- to 2-cm of the proximal extracranial VA and the distal intracranial vertebral artery near the

TABLE 53-8

Symptoms Associated with Posterior Circulation Ischemia

Dizziness[a]

Dysarthria

Homonymous hemianopsia

Ataxia

Drop attacks

Vertigo

Diplopia

Bilateral leg weakness

Alternating paresthesia

Perioral numbness

[a]Usually associated with other symptoms.

junction with the basilar artery. In a rigorous prospective registry of 407 patients with posterior circulation stroke or TIA, VA atherosclerosis at these sites figured prominently as the primary or contributory mechanism in a significant proportion of patients.[53] For example, embolism from atherosclerotic plaque and occlusive disease in the proximal extracranial VA and the intracranial VA was believed to represent the primary mechanism of ischemia in approximately 24% and 32% of patients, respectively. These data clearly underscore the importance of VA atherosclerosis in patients with posterior circulation ischemia and as a potential target for therapy in the primary and secondary prevention of posterior circulation ischemic events.

Endovascular intervention at the proximal extracranial VA and the intracranial VA are distinctly different entities. Intervention to the proximal extracranial VA is technically straightforward in most cases, is associated with a low rate of procedural complication, and is certainly within the realm of most suitably qualified interventional cardiologists.[54–56] In contrast, intervention to the intracranial VA can be technically very challenging, may be associated with devastating neurologic complications, and should be practiced only by interventional cardiologists with dedicated intracranial cerebrovascular training.[51,57–59] For this reason, we will confine our discussion to endovascular treatment of proximal extracranial VA disease.

【 】 INDICATIONS FOR VERTEBRAL ARTERY INTERVENTION

There is no clear consensus regarding the indications for proximal VA intervention. The lack of comparative data between medical therapy and either percutaneous or surgical revascularization is primarily responsible for this uncertainty. Interventionists are thus faced with balancing their assessment of the risk associated with an intervention against the risk associated with the natural history of the lesion. The assessment of procedural risk is derived exclusively from retrospective single-center registry experiences of the treatment of symptomatic patients.[54–56] Those studies that used contemporary

interventional techniques (ie, angioplasty and routine stenting) have documented the feasibility of the procedure, with procedural success in more than 98% of patients. The safety of the procedure is reflected by the low rate of periprocedural stroke or TIA (> 2%). In long-term follow-up, the absence of ischemic events and the low rates of restenosis (< 10%) in most series are reassuring.

Estimating the potential risk of not intervening for a symptomatic proximal VA lesion is difficult. Long-term follow-up studies have involved relatively small numbers of patients; have grouped vertebrobasilar artery disease as a single entity, making it impossible to define the risk for proximal VA disease alone; and have not defined the distribution of strokes in follow-up.[60,61] The prognosis for patients with intracranial VA disease is considered worse than in those with proximal VA disease, suggesting that overall estimates tend to exaggerate the risk associated with proximal VA disease. Additionally, in patients with a recent TIA or stroke of the posterior cerebral circulation who are found to have proximal VA disease, associated severe intracranial occlusive disease of the posterior circulation is present in approximately 25% of cases, and further potential causes of stroke are detected in another 25% of cases.[62] In these circumstances, recurrent events may be unrelated to the proximal VA lesion, and the potential benefit of proximal VA intervention on clinical outcome is debatable.

Given these uncertainties, it is best to carefully review all potential VA intervention cases with a cerebrovascular neurologist. Patients with definite symptoms of posterior circulation ischemia may be reasonably offered intervention. In view of the safety of intervention as demonstrated by registry data, it is also reasonable to offer intervention as a primary therapy in asymptomatic patients deemed at high risk based on the appearance of the lesion, the presence of contralateral VA disease, and compromised collateral flow from the carotid circulation. In general however, intervention in asymptomatic patients should be performed with deliberation, because most of these patients have a low risk of future events on medical therapy alone.[63]

【 】 ANATOMY OF VERTEBRAL ARTERY INTERVENTION

The VAs normally arise as the first branch from the proximal third of the subclavian artery (see Figure 53-3). There is usually some asymmetry in the size of the VAs, with the left being larger than the right. Uncommon and rare anomalies of the origin of the VA are recognized and are summarized in Figure 53-11. An awareness of these anomalies is important for all interventionalists participating in diagnostic angiography and intervention of the VAs. The VA is typically divided into four anatomic sections (Figure 53-12):

1. V1: from the origin of the vertebral artery to the point at which it enters the transverse process of the cervical vertebra. This typically occurs at the level of C6 but may occur between C7 and C4.

2. V2: describes the segment of vessel that courses within the transverse processes of the cervical vertebra up to the level of C2.

3. V3: extends between the transverse process of C2 and the foramen magnum. This section of vessel may occasionally give rise to the posterior inferior cerebellar artery (PICA, extracranial). The V1, V2, and V3 segments define the extracranial section of the VA.

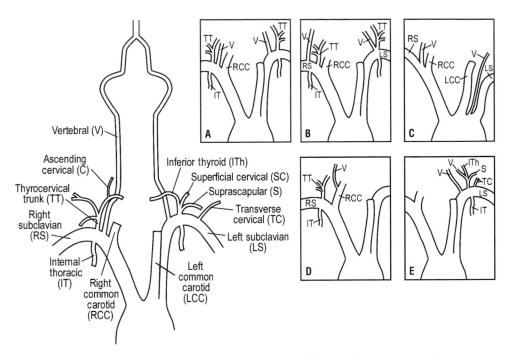

FIGURE 53-11. Normal and variant anatomy of the origin of the vertebral artery. **A.** and **B.** Normal origin of the right and left vertebral artery as the first branch from the proximal subclavian artery. **C.** Origin of the vertebral artery lateral to or as common trunk with the thyrocervical trunk. **D.** Origin of the left vertebral artery from the aortic arch between the origin of the left common carotid and left subclavian arteries. **E.** Origin of the right vertebral artery from right common carotid artery, typically in patients with anomalous origin of the right subclavian artery. **F.** Dual or accessory origin of the vertebral artery from the aortic arch or thyrocervical trunk.

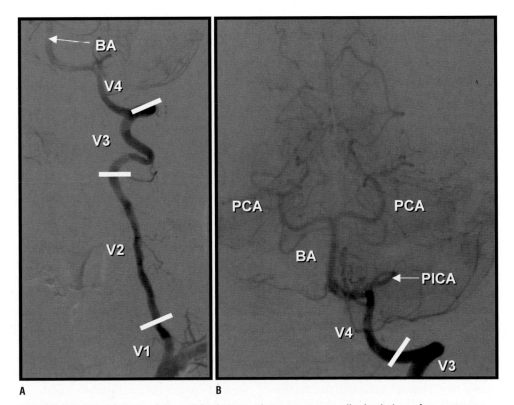

FIGURE 53-12. Anatomy of the vertebral artery. This artery is typically divided into four anatomic sections: V1, V2, V3, and V4 (see text for further details). **A.** Left anterior oblique view of the left vertebral artery. **B.** Posteroanterior cranial view of the distal left vertebral, basilar, and posterior cerebral arteries. BA = basilar artery; PCA = posterior cerebral artery; PICA = posterior inferior cerebellar artery.

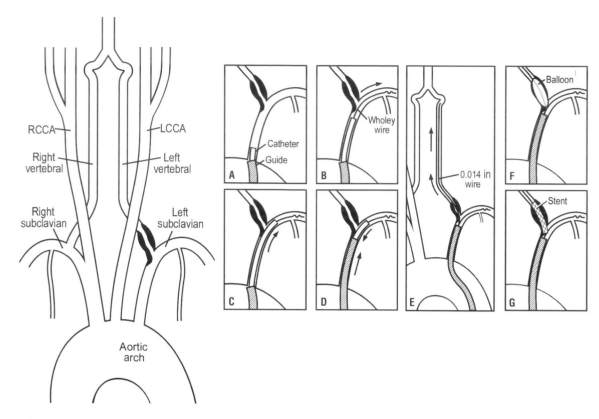

FIGURE 53-13. Schematic of interventional technique to treat proximal vertebral artery disease.

4. V4: defines the intracranial portion of the VA, extending from the foramen magnum to the junction with the contralateral VA to and from the basilar artery. This segment of vessel usually gives rise to the PICA and the anterior spinal artery. The basilar artery supplies branches to the brainstem and cerebellum, giving rise to both posterior cerebral arteries that supply penetrating branches to the diencephalon and midbrain, as well as cortical branches to the occipital, posterior parietal, and medial temporal lobes.

【 】 DIAGNOSTIC ANGIOGRAPHY

An assessment of the aortic arch by conventional or MR angiography is often helpful prior to VA angiography. This helps define the aortic arch type and identifies some of the anomalies in the origin of the VA outlined above. At a minimum, selective engagement of the right or left subclavian artery is required for VA angiography. The origin of the right subclavian artery from the innominate artery makes right-sided VA angiography more challenging. Regardless of arch type, a JR 4 catheter typically engages the left subclavian artery. The aortic arch type heavily influences the catheter choice for right VA angiography. With type I arches, a JR 4 catheter is usually adequate, whereas with type III arches, a Vitek catheter, and rarely a Simmons catheter, is required to engage the innominate artery. Subsequently, the right anterior oblique view typically allows the operator to angiographically separate the origins of the right CCA and right subclavian artery. An 0.035-in wire is then advanced distally into the axillary or brachial artery and the diagnostic catheter advanced over the wire into the proximal subclavian artery. In tortuous anatomy, a stiff-angled glide

wire may be required to accomplish this maneuver. Our practice is to perform nonselective angiography of the respective vertebral artery with a cuff inflated on the arm compressing the brachial artery. This method minimizes the risk of trauma to the ostium of the artery and likely reduces the risk of ischemic events associated with angiography. In general, the contralateral oblique view best defines lesions involving the ostium of the VA. The V2 segment is well visualized in the ipsilateral oblique view. The V3 and V4 segments are typically imaged using the left lateral and steep cranial (~ 40-degree Townes) views.

【 】 INTERVENTIONAL TECHNIQUE (FIGURE 53-13)

VA intervention may be performed using either femoral artery or ipsilateral brachial artery access. Our preference is to use the former. A 6-Fr sheath or 8-Fr guide (typically H-1 or Multipurpose) is positioned in the proximal subclavian artery. The proximal VA lesion is crossed with a soft-tipped coronary 0.014-in wire (eg, Balance Trek, Guidant Corporation; Asahi Soft, Abbott Vascular Devices) that is advanced to the distal portion of the V2 segment of the vessel. Predilation of the lesion is usually performed to facilitate stent delivery. Unless otherwise contraindicated, we stent all proximal VA lesions. In this location, radial strength is important, and hence balloon-expandable stents are used. The type of stent used is heavily influenced by the vessel diameter. For smaller diameter vessels (≤ 3.5-mm), a drug-eluting coronary stent is typically used (Cypher, Cordis Corporation; Taxus, Boston Scientific Ireland Ltd), whereas for larger diameter vessels, a conventional stainless steel peripheral balloon-expandable stent is utilized

(Genesis, Cordis; Herculink, Guidant). Positioning the stent to ensure that the ostium of the VA is covered by stent is of paramount importance and often requires multiple angiographic views of the ostium. Postdilation may be performed to ensure complete stent expansion and minimize any residual stenosis. Final angiographic views of the intracranial VA, basilar artery, and posterior cerebral arteries should be performed to confirm the absence of distal embolization.

CONCLUSION

Interventional cardiologists are well placed to perform carotid and vertebral artery intervention. The foundation for participation in this field is based on a commitment to acquiring a fundamental knowledge of the anatomy, vascular biology, and pathology of these vascular territories, as well as to obtaining appropriate diagnostic and interventional experience in a supervised setting. In the future, the borders between interventional cardiology, interventional radiology, and vascular surgery will become increasingly blurred by the common drive toward endovascular therapies for vascular disease.

REFERENCES

1. Brown MM. Carotid artery stenting–evolution of a technique to rival carotid endarterectomy. *Am J Med.* 2004;116:273.
2. Roubin GS, Yadav S, Iyer SS, et al. Carotid stent-supported angioplasty: a neurovascular intervention to prevent stroke. *Am J Cardiol.* 1996;78:8.
3. Jordan WD, Jr., Voellinger DC, Doblar DD, et al. Microemboli detected by transcranial Doppler monitoring in patients during carotid angioplasty versus carotid endarterectomy. *Cardiovasc Surg.* 1999;7:33.
4. Ohki T, Roubin GS, Veith FJ, et al. Efficacy of a filter device in the prevention of embolic events during carotid angioplasty and stenting: an ex vivo analysis. *J Vasc Surg.* 1999;30:1034.
5. Al-Mubarak N, Roubin GS, Vitek JJ, et al. Microembolization during carotid stenting with the distal-balloon antiemboli system. *Int Angiol.* 2002;21:344.
6. Mas JL, Chatellier G, Beyssen B. Carotid angioplasty and stenting with and without cerebral protection: clinical alert from the Endarterectomy Versus Angioplasty in Patients With Symptomatic Severe Carotid Stenosis (EVA-3S) trial. *Stroke.* 2004;35:e18.
7. Roubin GS, New G, Iyer SS, et al. Immediate and late clinical outcomes of carotid artery stenting in patients with symptomatic and asymptomatic carotid artery stenosis: a 5-year prospective analysis. *Circulation.* 2001;103:532.
8. Mathur A, Dorros G, Iyer SS, et al. Palmaz stent compression in patients following carotid artery stenting. *Cathet Cardiovasc Diagn.* 1997;41:137.
9. Barnett HJ, Taylor DW, Eliasziw M, et al. Benefit of carotid endarterectomy in patients with symptomatic moderate or severe stenosis. North American Symptomatic Carotid Endarterectomy Trial Collaborators. *N Engl J Med.* 1998;339:1415.
10. Randomised trial of endarterectomy for recently symptomatic carotid stenosis: final results of the MRC European Carotid Surgery Trial (ECST). *Lancet.* 1998;351:1379.
11. Mayberg MR, Wilson SE, Yatsu F, et al. Carotid endarterectomy and prevention of cerebral ischemia in symptomatic carotid stenosis. Veterans Affairs Cooperative Studies Program 309 Trialist Group. *JAMA.* 1991;266:3289.
12. Endarterectomy for asymptomatic carotid artery stenosis. Executive Committee for the Asymptomatic Carotid Atherosclerosis Study. *JAMA.* 1995;273:1421.
13. Halliday A, Mansfield A, Marro J, et al. Prevention of disabling and fatal strokes by successful carotid endarterectomy in patients without recent neurological symptoms: randomised controlled trial. *Lancet.* 2004;363:1491.
14. Gray WA. A cardiologist in the carotids. *J Am Coll Cardiol.* 2004;43:1602.
15. Wennberg DE, Lucas FL, Birkmeyer JD, et al. Variation in carotid endarterectomy mortality in the Medicare population: trial hospitals, volume, and patient characteristics. *JAMA.* 1998;279:1278.
16. Ouriel K, Hertzer NR, Beven EG, et al. Preprocedural risk stratification: identifying an appropriate population for carotid stenting. *J Vasc Surg.* 2001;33:728.
17. Ouriel K, Yadav JS. The role of stents in patients with carotid disease. *Rev Cardiovasc Med.* 2003;4:61.
18. Yadav JS. Stenting and angioplasty with protection in patients at high risk for endarterectomy: 30-day results. American Heart Association Scientific Sessions. Chicago, IL; 2002.
19. Yadav JS. Stenting and angioplasty with protection in patients at high risk for endarterectomy: 1-year results. Transcatheter Cardiovascular Therapeutics Meeting. Washington DC; 2003.
20. Featherstone RL, Brown MM, Coward LJ. International carotid stenting study: protocol for a randomised clinical trial comparing carotid stenting with endarterectomy in symptomatic carotid artery stenosis. *Cerebrovasc Dis.* 2004;18:69.
21. Endarterectomy vs. Angioplasty in Patients with Symptomatic Severe Carotid Stenosis (EVA-3S) Trial. *Cerebrovasc Dis.* 2004;18:62.
22. Ringleb PA, Kunze A, Allenberg JR, et al. The Stent-Supported Percutaneous Angioplasty of the Carotid Artery vs. Endarterectomy Trial. *Cerebrovasc Dis.* 2004;18:66.
23. Hobson RW II. Update on the Carotid Revascularization Endarterectomy versus Stent Trial (CREST) protocol. *J Am Coll Surg.* 2002;194:S9.
24. Hobson RW II. Rationale and status of randomized controlled clinical trials in carotid artery stenting. *Semin Vasc Surg.* 2003;16:311.
25. Whitlow PL, Lylyk P, Londero H, et al. Carotid artery stenting protected with an emboli containment system. *Stroke.* 2002;33:1308.
26. Oesterle SN, Hayase M, Baim DS, et al. An embolization containment device. *Cathet Cardiovasc Intervent.* 1999;47:243.
27. Bates MC, Dorros G, Parodi J. Reversal of the direction of internal carotid artery blood flow by occlusion of the common and external carotid arteries in a swine model. *Cathet Cardiovasc Intervent.* 2003;60:270.
28. Adami CA, Scuro A, Spinamano L, et al. Use of the Parodi anti-embolism system in carotid stenting: Italian trial results. *J Endovasc Ther.* 2002;9:147.
29. Bush RL, Lin PH, Bianco CC, et al. Reevaluation of temporary transvenous cardiac pacemaker usage during carotid angioplasty and stenting: a safe and valuable adjunct. *Vasc Endovascular Surg.* 2004;38:229.
30. Mlekusch W, Schillinger M, Sabeti S, et al. Hypotension and bradycardia after elective carotid stenting: frequency and risk factors. *J Endovasc Ther.* 2003;10:851.
31. Mendelsohn FO, Weissman NJ, Lederman RJ, et al. Acute hemodynamic changes during carotid artery stenting. *Am J Cardiol.* 1998;82:1077.
32. Qureshi AI, Luft AR, Sharma M, et al. Frequency and determinants of postprocedural hemodynamic instability after carotid angioplasty and stenting. *Stroke.* 1999;30:2086.
33. Leisch F, Kerschner K, Hofmann R, et al. Carotid sinus reactions during carotid artery stenting: predictors, incidence, and influence on clinical outcome. *Cathet Cardiovasc Intervent.* 2003;58:516.
34. Bove EL, Fry WJ, Gross WS, et al. Hypotension and hypertension as consequences of baroreceptor dysfunction following carotid endarterectomy. *Surgery.* 1979;85:633.
35. Abou-Chebl A, Yadav JS, Reginelli JP, et al. Intracranial hemorrhage and hyperperfusion syndrome following carotid artery stenting: risk factors, prevention, and treatment. *J Am Coll Cardiol.* 2004;43:1596.
36. Sundt TM, Jr., Sharbrough FW, Piepgras DG, et al. Correlation of cerebral blood flow and electroencephalographic changes during carotid endarterectomy: with results of surgery and hemodynamics of cerebral ischemia. *Mayo Clin Proc.* 1981;56:533.
37. Sbarigia E, Speziale F, Giannoni MF, et al. Post-carotid endarterectomy hyperperfusion syndrome: preliminary observations for identifying at risk patients by transcranial Doppler sonography and the acetazolamide test. *Eur J Vasc Surg.* 1993;7:252.
38. Jansen C, Sprengers AM, Moll FL, et al. Prediction of intracerebral haemorrhage after carotid endarterectomy by clinical criteria and intraoperative transcranial Doppler monitoring: results of 233 operations. *Eur J Vasc Surg.* 1994;8:220.
39. McCabe DJ, Brown MM, Clifton A. Fatal cerebral reperfusion hemorrhage after carotid stenting. *Stroke.* 1999;30:2483.
40. Morrish W, Grahovac S, Douen A, et al. Intracranial hemorrhage after stenting and angioplasty of extracranial carotid stenosis. *AJNR Am J Neuroradiol.* 2000;21:1911.
41. Al-Mubarak N, Roubin GS, Vitek JJ, et al. Subarachnoidal hemorrhage following carotid stenting with the distal-balloon protection. *Cathet Cardiovasc Intervent.* 2001;54:521.

42. Caplan LR, Skillman J, Ojemann R. Intracerebral hemorrhage following carotid endarterectomy: a hypertensive complication? *Stroke.* 1978;9:457.

43. Cheung RT, Eliasziw M, Meldrum HE, et al. Risk, types, and severity of intracranial hemorrhage in patients with symptomatic carotid artery stenosis. *Stroke.* 2003;34:1847.

44. Wholey MH, Al-Mubarek N. Updated review of the global carotid artery stent registry. *Cathet Cardiovasc Intervent.* 2003;60:259.

45. Reimers B, Schluter M, Castriota F, et al. Routine use of cerebral protection during carotid artery stenting: results of a multicenter registry of 753 patients. *Am J Med.* 2004;116:217.

46. Schluter M, Tubler T, Steffens JC, et al. Focal ischemia of the brain after neuroprotected carotid artery stenting. *J Am Coll Cardiol.* 2003;42:1007.

47. Wholey MH, Tan WA, Toursarkissian B, et al. Management of neurological complications of carotid artery stenting. *J Endovasc Ther.* 2001;8:341.

48. Endovascular versus surgical treatment in patients with carotid stenosis in the Carotid and Vertebral Artery Transluminal Angioplasty Study (CAVATAS): a randomised trial. *Lancet.* 2001;357:1729.

49. Yadav JS. Stenting and angioplasty with protection in patients at high risk for endarterectomy. American Heart Association Meeting. Chicago, Illinois; 2002.

50. Ansel GM. Treatment of carotid stent restenosis. *Cathet Cardiovasc Intervent.* 2003;58:93.

51. Rocha-Singh K. Vertebral artery stenting: ready for prime time? *Cathet Cardiovasc Intervent.* 2001;54:6.

52. Bhadelia RA, Bengoa F, Gesner L, et al. Efficacy of MR angiography in the detection and characterization of occlusive disease in the vertebrobasilar system. *J Comput Assist Tomogr.* 2001;25:458.

53. Caplan LR. Vertebrobasilar disease. *Adv Neurol.* 2003;92:131.

54. Jenkins JS, White CJ, Ramee SR, et al. Vertebral artery stenting. *Cathet Cardiovasc Intervent.* 2001;54:1.

55. Mukherjee D, Roffi M, Kapadia SR, et al. Percutaneous intervention for symptomatic vertebral artery stenosis using coronary stents. *J Invasive Cardiol.* 2001;13:363.

56. Chastain HD II, Campbell MS, Iyer S, Roubin GS, et al. Extracranial vertebral artery stent placement: in-hospital and follow-up results. *J Neurosurg.* 1999;91:547.

57. Levy EI, Horowitz MB, Koebbe CJ, et al. Transluminal stent-assisted angioplasty of the intracranial vertebrobasilar system for medically refractory, posterior circulation ischemia: early results. *Neurosurgery.* 2001;48:1215.

58. Levy EI, Hanel RA, Bendok BR, et al. Staged stent-assisted angioplasty for symptomatic intracranial vertebrobasilar artery stenosis. *J Neurosurg* 2002;97:1294.

59. Lanzino G, Fessler RD, Miletich RS, et al. Angioplasty and stenting of basilar artery stenosis: technical case report. *Neurosurgery.* 1999;45:404.

60. Whisnant JP, Cartlidge NE, Elveback LR. Carotid and vertebral-basilar transient ischemic attacks: effect of anticoagulants, hypertension, and cardiac disorders on survival and stroke occurrence—a population study. *Ann Neurol.* 1978;3:107.

61. Prognosis of patients with symptomatic vertebral or basilar artery stenosis. The Warfarin-Aspirin Symptomatic Intracranial Disease (WASID) Study Group. *Stroke.* 1998;29:1389.

62. Wityk RJ, Chang HM, Rosengart A, et al. Proximal extracranial vertebral artery disease in the New England Medical Center Posterior Circulation Registry. *Arch Neurol.* 1998;55:470.

63. Moufarrij NA, Little JR, Furlan AJ, et al. Vertebral artery stenosis: long-term follow-up. *Stroke.* 1984;15:260.

PART 6   Complications and Management

CHAPTER (54)

Risk Stratification in Interventional Cardiology

Mandeep Singh, MD

Percutaneous coronary intervention (PCI) has evolved since the introduction of balloon angioplasty by Andreas Gruntzig,[1] with current high procedural success rates and low attendant periprocedural complications.[2] PCI is now the treatment of choice offered to many high-risk subgroups in whom it was previously contraindicated.[3–6]

Evaluation of risk-benefit ratios and risk stratification are important elements in optimizing care for an individual undergoing PCI. Various models for prediction of risks can help physicians, patients, and their families better comprehend attendant risks and provide an objective basis for the most suitable revascularization option. It is paramount for clinicians to become familiar with the available risk scores and apply them in clinical practice. This chapter focuses on the strengths and weaknesses, ease of applicability, and use of risk prediction models in the current environment of PCI.

DEVELOPMENT OF A RISK PREDICTION MODEL: STATISTICAL CONSIDERATIONS

A good predictive model should be accurate and able to discriminate between different levels of risk. An accurate model, on average, is not biased toward over- or underprediction. If the true average risk of an event in a population is 5%, one could achieve accuracy by predicting 5% risk for every patient. Such estimates would lack precision, however, because the same prognosis is given for both low- and high-risk patients. Discriminatory ability is related to precision (distinguishing high- from low-risk patients).

In the context of this chapter, a "prediction" is the probability that an event will occur. A high-risk patient may have a predicted risk of 0.50, but he or she will not suffer a half-event. This may be why assessment of these models tends to focus more on discriminatory ability than accuracy.

Logistic regression is the standard statistical analysis employed for binary outcomes.[7] Harrell and colleagues recommend that the number of explanatory variables considered should not exceed one tenth of the number of events. This set of variables should be determined without knowledge of their relationship to the outcome in the modeling data set. Clinical expertise is essential at this stage of model development. After candidate explanatory variables are chosen, the final model may be determined using automatic selection[8] or bootstrap[9] methods. These methods are intended not only to simplify the model, but also to avoid overfitting. Overfitting occurs when a model reflects anomalous associations specific only to the model-building data, resulting in suboptimal performance in other data sets.

Once a final model is chosen, the Hosmer-Lemeshow goodness-of-fit test may be used to determine if the model adequately reflects the observed data.[10] A significant test result indicates an inadequate fit. Accuracy may be internally validated using data-splitting, cross-validation, or bootstrap methods.[11] However, external validation is more valuable than these methods. Comparison of the observed number of events in the external data set against the events predicted by the model determines the model accuracy.

The discriminatory ability of a model may be quantified by the c-statistic (c stands for concordance).[12] The c-statistic, or area under the receiver operating characteristic (ROC) curve, is the proportion of times that the model correctly ranks the risks for a pair of subjects. That is, if two patients are selected, only one of whom will have an event, it is the rate at which the model assigns a higher level of risk to the patient with the event. Thus, a c-statistic of 0.50 indicates the model performs as well as assigning risk by the toss of a coin. Perfect discrimination results in a c-statistic of 1.00.

The simplification of the statistical model to an additive integer-scoring tool may be useful for patient counseling. The goal is to assign integer coefficients to risk factors significantly associated with an event so that the physician may quickly sum the coefficients for a numerical ranking of the patient's risk. Once the logistic regression model is finalized, the simplified scoring tool may be defined by selecting integer coefficients roughly proportional to the log-odds ratio coefficients (ie, parameter estimates) of the logistic regression model variables.

【 】 RECENT RISK MODELS PREDICTING COMPLICATIONS FOLLOWING PERCUTANEOUS CORONARY INTERVENTIONS

Eight models have been described in the recent literature. They are listed below and compared in Tables 54-1 and 54-2. Another model is described in Ref. 12a.

1. New York (NY) State model.[13,14]
2. American College of Cardiology–National Cardiovascular Data Registry (ACC-NCDR).[15]
3. Northern New England (NNE).[16]
4. Michigan Consortium.[17]
5. William Beaumont Hospital.[18]
6. Cleveland Clinic.[19]
7. Mayo Clinic.[20]
8. Brigham and Women's Hospital.[21]

【 】 VARIABLES INCLUDED IN THE RISK SCORES

All the models incorporated similar demographic features, existing comorbidities, and lesion variables (with the exception of NY State) (see Table 54-2). In general, the risk factors associated with in-hospital complications can be divided into the following broad categories: age, left ventricular function, acuity of presentation, high-risk angiographic features, and additional high-risk demographics (eg, renal failure, peripheral vascular disease, and other variables).

Age

Advancing age is an important risk factor for PCI complication and is universally present in the risk models. Possible explanations include reduced cardiac reserve, presence of multivessel disease, and increased prevalence of comorbidities.[22,23] In all the risk scores, there was a graded increase in the mortality risk with advancing age. Thus, an octogenarian has 2.7 times the risk (Michigan model) as compared with patients between 50 and 59 years of age. The Mayo Clinic risk score extends these observations to composite end points, with an unadjusted odds ratio for these complications of 6.03 in a person older than 80 years or age who undergoes PCI, as compared with a younger patient. Age was considered a binary variable in a recent simplified scoring

system.[18,21] This dichotomous cutoff of age might lead to underestimation of risks from PCI in the very elderly.

Left Ventricular Function

Assessment of left ventricular function is an important variable with prognostic implications during PCI. Various models have measured this risk variable differently. Cardiogenic shock resulting from severe left ventricular systolic dysfunction is the single most important predictor of PCI complications.[3] The mortality in patients presenting with shock in various risk scores ranged from 28% (ACC-NCDR) to 33% (Michigan).[15,17] In the Cleveland and Mayo Clinics models, the odds ratios of in-hospital complications in patients with shock were 12.7 and 4.95, respectively. In the NY State model, reduced ejection fraction and congestive heart failure were independent predictors of death during or after angioplasty. Increased risk of death was associated with patients presenting with New York Heart Classification (NYHA) greater than or equal to 3 in the Mayo model, and in the NNE cardiovascular study group, with an ejection fraction of 40% of less. Similar conclusions were derived from other risk score models. It is, therefore, important to have clinical or objective assessment of left ventricular function at the time PCI is performed.

Acuity of Presentation

Acute myocardial infarction (especially within 24 hours), cardiac arrest, hemodynamic instability during arrhythmia, or cardiogenic shock are important clinical variables that influence the acuity of presentation and adversely affect the outcome of the procedure. Use of intra-aortic balloon pump during an urgent procedure is an important marker for increased mortality risk as seen in the NY State, ACC-NCDR, and NNE models. The odds ratio estimate for complications in urgent or emergent procedures in the Mayo Clinic risk score was 2.13. Similarly, mortality with emergent PCI procedures was high in the other study populations, with rates between 5.8% and 6.35% in the ACC-NCDR and NNE groups, respectively.

High-risk Angiographic Features

Multivessel disease had a higher odds ratio for complications during PCI; 1.54 per extra vessel in the Michigan model, 1.86 in the Mayo Clinic model, and 1.32 per extra vessel in the Cleveland Clinic model. Multivessel angioplasty was a risk factor in the NY State model (OR 1.82) and can influence the prognosis of the patient.[24] Other angiographic risk factors of importance are presence of thrombus (Mayo Clinic and Michigan models), American College of Cardiology/American Heart Association (ACC/AHA) type C lesion classification (ACC-NCDR, NNE, and Cleveland Clinic models), and left main coronary artery disease (ACC-NCDR and Mayo Clinic models) or left main intervention (Brigham and Women's model).

Additional High-Risk Demographics

Renal Failure. Renal failure has been found to be an important predictor of in-hospital complications following PCI.[25,26] The Michigan model had an odds ratio of 5.5 for mortality in patients undergoing PCI who have a creatinine level of more than

TABLE 54-1

Comparison of Available Risk Scores Predicting Complications Following Percutaneous Coronary Interventions in the Current Era

	ACC-NCDR[15]	NY STATE[13,14]	NNE MODEL[16]	MICHIGAN[17]	BEAUMONT HOSPITAL[18]	CLEVELAND CLINIC[19]	MAYO CLINIC[20]	BRIGHAM AND WOMEN'S[21]
Risk(s) studied	Mortality	Mortality	Mortality	Mortality	Mortality	Mortality, Q-MI, emergent CABG	Mortality, Q-MI, emergent CABG, stroke	Mortality, MI, CABG
Study time period	Jan 98–Sep 00	Jan 91–Dec 94	Jan 94–Dec 96	Jul 97–Sep 99	Jan 96–Dec 98	Jul 94–Dec 94	Jan 96–Dec 99	Jan 97–Feb 99
Sample size (model development)	50,123	62,670	15,331	10,729	9954	12,985	5463	1877
Event rate (%)	1.4	0.9	1.1	1.6	1.4	4.5	4.0	6.4
Area under ROC (c) (modeling data set)	0.89	0.892	0.88	0.90	0.87	0.648	0.782	0.767
Internal validation	c = 0.89 Validation set (n = 50130)	NA	c = 0.88 ± 0.02 Bootstrapping	c = 0.92 Validation set (n = 5863)	c = 0.87 Validation set (n = 12005)	c = 0.635 Cross-validation corrected	c = 0.755 Validation set (n = 1781)	0.742 Validation set (n = 1460)
External validation (NHLBI 1997–1999)	n = 4448 Obs = 64, Exp = 603 c = 0.88	n = 4448 Obs = 64, Exp = 69 c = 0.89	n = 4448 Obs = 64, Exp = 60 c = 0.89	n = 4448 Obs = 64, Exp = 47 c = 0.86	NA	NA	n = 3264 Obs = 96, Exp = 93.5 c = 0.76	NA
Simplified scoring tool	No	No	No	Yes	Yes	No	Yes	Yes
Long-term mortality assessment	No	Yes, on external data[7]	No	No	No	No	No	No
Operator volume included in the risk score	No	No	No	No	No	No	No	No

ACC-NCDR = American College of Cardiology-National Cardiovascular Data Registry; CABG = coronary artery bypass grafting; Exp = expected; MI = myocardial infarction; NA = not available; NHLBI = National Heart Lung and Blood Institute; NNE = Northern New England; Obs = observed; ROC = receiver operating characteristics.

TABLE 54-2

Commonly Included Variables in the Currently Available Risk Stratification Models[a]

EVENT	MORTALITY					COMPLICATIONS		
	ACC-NCDR[15]	NY STATE[13,14]	NNE[16]	MICHIGAN[17]	BEAUMONT[18]	CLEVELAND CLINIC[19]	MAYO CLINIC[20]	BRIGHAM AND WOMEN'S[21]
Age								
By decade		1.83					1.37	
Logarithm						24.9		1.35
≥75 y					1.95			
>65 y								
50–59 y	2.61		0.93	1.00				
60–69 y	3.75		1.63	1.00				
70–79 y	6.44		3.32	2.24				
≥80 y	11.3		3.72	2.65				
LV function								
50–59% (EF)	1.00	1.00	2.53	1.00				
40–49%	0.87	1.00	3.32	1.66				
30–39%	0.99	1.49	5.16	1.66				
20–29%	2.04	1.49	5.16	1.66				
10–19%	3.43	3.68	5.16	1.66				
<10%	3.93	3.68	5.16	1.66				
CHF		2.38	3.01				2.11 (NYHA ≥ III)	3.76 (NYHA ≥ III)
Acuity of presentation								
Urgent PCI	1.78		2.19				2.13	
Emergent PCI	5.75		7.71				2.13	
AMI 1–7 d		2.10	1.85		2.14 (<14d)			
AMI 6–23 h	1.31	3.67	(primary therapy)	2.80		4.75		3.15
AMI < 6h	1.31	5.22		2.80		4.75		3.15
Cardiogenic shock	8.49	18.3	6.10	11.5		12.7	4.95	3.15
IABP use	1.68	2.39	3.91					3.47

High-risk angiographic features								
2-VD		1.82 (multivessel intervention)		1.54	2.20	1.32	1.86	
3-VD				2.37	2.20	1.74	1.86	
LM disease	2.04						4.34	2.40 (LM treated)
Thrombus				1.67			1.90	
ACC/AHA B2						1.63		2.58
ACC/AHA C			1.94			2.66		2.58
SCAI II	1.64							
SCAI III	1.87							
SCAI IV	2.11							
Other high-risk clinical features								
Renal failure	3.04	3.51	2.32	5.5	2.06		2.41	1.54
PVD		1.78	2.12	1.57	3.21			
Diabetes mellitus	1.41	1.41			1.54			
Female gender		1.31		1.82	3.57			

^aOdds ratio from logistic regression models.

ACC-NCDR = American College of Cardiology-National Cardiovascular Data Registry; AMI = acute myocardial infarction; CHF = congestive heart failure; IABP = intra-aortic balloon pump; LM = left main; NNE = Northern New England; NYHA = New York Heart Association; PCI = percutaneous coronary intervention; PVD = peripheral vascular disease; SCAI = Society for Cardiac Angiography and Interventions; VD 5 vascular disease.

1.5 mg/dL. Similar findings were noted in all other models except the Cleveland Clinic model. Despite differences in the definition of renal failure, the presence of renal insufficiency clearly increases the risk of complications during PCI. Assessment of renal function before PCI not only helps in prevention and management of contrast-associated renal function deterioration, but also adds this variable to the profile of the patient.

Peripheral Vascular Disease. Peripheral vascular disease is linked to higher mortality with the NNE, Michigan, and Beaumont models. Similar observations were noted in the NY State model (the odds ratio for mortality in patients with femoral popliteal disease was 1.775). This is an important diagnosis and is readily available from history and clinical examination. Peripheral vascular disease is not clearly defined in most of the risk scores; however, any femoral popliteal disease (NY State model), claudication, amputation, peripheral bypass surgery, angioplasty, aortic aneurysm, and history of transient ischemic attacks, stroke, or carotid stenosis (Michigan model), add to the risk of the patient undergoing PCI.

Other Variables. Other predictors (eg, diabetes mellitus [NY State and Beaumont models], and female gender [NY State, Cleveland Clinic, Michigan, and Beaumont models]) are not consistent across all the risk models and have a generally lower, weaker relationship with procedural complications.

[ ] AMERICAN COLLEGE OF CARDIOLOGY/AMERICAN HEART ASSOCIATION LESION CLASSIFICATION

Percutaneous angioplasty techniques have evolved rapidly since the original proposal of this classification in 1986 and its subsequent

modification in 1990.[27,28] It is still the most widely used system used to scorecard the individual operator and the institution. More recently in a new classification system, two variables (nonchronic total occlusion, and degenerated saphenous vein grafts) were significantly correlated with death, non–Q-wave myocardial infarction, and the need for emergency coronary artery bypass grafting (CABG).[29] The Society for Cardiac Angiography and Interventions (SCAI) proposed a simpler classification, collapsing ACC/AHA lesions A, B1, and B2 lesions into non-C category, and then stratifying the lesion by patency (SCAI I = non-C/patent; SCAI II = C/patent; SCAI III = non-C/occluded; SCAI IV = C/occluded) with better, however modest, discrimination (c-statistic 0.665) for prediction of major in-hospital complications as compared with ACC/AHA lesion classification (c-statistic 0.624).[30]

Investigators compared the Mayo Clinic risk score with ACC/AHA lesion classification for prediction of complications following PCI. The ACC/AHA lesion classification was inferior to the Mayo model in predicting the complications from the procedure. In other studies, procedural success is adversely affected by type C lesions.[31,32] Among the type C lesions, chronic total occlusion, and extreme tortuosity are significant lesion variables effecting procedure outcome.[33] Type C lesion was one of the significant variables predictive of the need for emergency CABG following PCI.[2]

PITFALLS IN THE CURRENT RISK SCORE MODELS

Outcome analysis following PCI is an important tool for quality control. However, benchmarking of outcome data is complicated by variations in the case mix, referral patterns, procedural techniques, and operator and hospital volume (Table 54-3). Eight multivariate models that address the prediction of complications following PCI have several limitations.[14–20,34] With the exception of the ACC-NCDR Registry, the other risk scores are derived from either regional (NNE and Michigan Consortium) or single-institution databases (Mayo Clinic, Beaumont, Brigham and Women's), limiting their generalizability. Some data sets antedate current state-of-the-art interventional practice. Important outcome measures such as myocardial infarction, stroke, or need for emergency CABG, can significantly contribute to morbidity, length of hospital stay, and cost, and are not considered in most available models except the Mayo Clinic, Cleveland Clinic, and Brigham and Women's Hospital models. Similarly, operator volume, an important variable predicting outcome following PCI, was not used in most models.[13,35]

[ ] WHICH MODEL TO CHOOSE FOR PREDICTION OF COMPLICATIONS?

The properties of an "ideal" predictive model are highlighted in Table 54-4.[36] All the

⟩ TABLE 54-3

Drawbacks of Available Risk Models for Prediction of Complications Following Percutaneous Coronary Interventions

1. Different definitions of included variables.
2. Risk scores derived from single-center, regional databases have reduced generalizability.
3. Outcome measures other than mortality (myocardial infarction, stroke, and emergency coronary artery bypass surgery) are ignored.
4. Operator and institutional coronary angioplasty volume is not tested.
5. Often-used ACC/AHA lesion classification has only modest discriminatory accuracy for prediction of complications.
6. A lower incidence of events would require an even larger size of the database from which model is derived.
7. Time elapsed between collection of data and analysis compromises applicability of score to contemporary current practice.
8. Newer models, including current definitions of myocardial infarction, are unavailable.
9. Influence of referral bias.

ACC/AHA = American College of Cardiology/American Heart Association.

TABLE 54-4

Characteristics of an Ideal Risk Score Model for Prediction of Complications Following Percutaneous Coronary Interventions[36]

1. It should be derived from simple and easily obtainable variables that are available preprocedure.
2. It should predict not only mortality but also all major procedural complications, including mortality, myocardial infarction, stroke, and need for urgent bypass surgery.
3. It should be validated internally and externally.
4. It should reflect modern practice, which currently includes stent implantation, glycoprotein IIb/IIIa blockers, and post-stent thienopyridine administration.

models described in this chapter have excellent predictive accuracy with c-statistics varying from 0.782 in Mayo Clinic score model to 0.892 in NY State. The c-statistic for combined end points for the Cleveland Clinic model was, however, modest (0.648). The prediction is not a crystal ball; the vast majority of high-risk patients would not have any complication from the procedure. However, the aim of the risk score should be to correctly risk-stratify a patient into low-, moderate-, or high-risk categories. Most of the risk scores with the exception of NY State use both clinical and angiographic variables and, hence, cannot be used

electively for risk stratification at the time of first contact in a patient with unknown angiographic variables.

Most of the mortality models have been externally validated. Holmes and colleagues applied five of these risk models—including NY State, Cleveland Clinic, Michigan, NNE, and ACC-NCDR, developed from different data sets—to patients undergoing PCI in the NHLBI Dynamic Registry.[37] Three models (NY State, Cleveland Clinic, and NNE) predicted mortality rates that were not significantly different than those observed. In both high- and low-risk subgroups, however, the Michigan model slightly underpredicted mortality, and the ACC-NCDR Registry predicted significantly higher mortality than that observed. Potential reasons for this discrepancy were misclassification of renal disease, nonavailability of higher-risk variables (eg, cardiac arrest the strongest prediction in the Michigan model) in the ACC Dynamic Registry. Omission of variables not included in the Dynamic Registry will lead, by default, to underestimation of the mortality risk. Additional limitations are related to clinical definitions, missing data, and how other variables such as renal failure, and ejection fraction are handled.

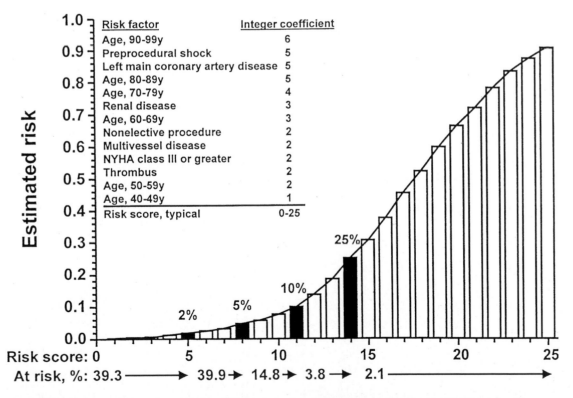

FIGURE 54-1. Mayo Clinic risk score. Complication rates rise with increase in the risk score (*horizontal axis*). Estimated rates of procedural complications for the integer scoring system are depicted. The integers are proportional to the estimated continuous coefficient from the logistic model. Percentages at risk are shown for each of the five risk categories: 2% is very low risk for complications with coronary angioplasty; more than 2% to 5%, low risk; more than 5% to 10%, moderate risk; more than 10% to 25%, high risk; and more than 25%, very high risk. NYHA = New York Heart Association classification. (*Reproduced with permission from Singh M, et al.[20]*)

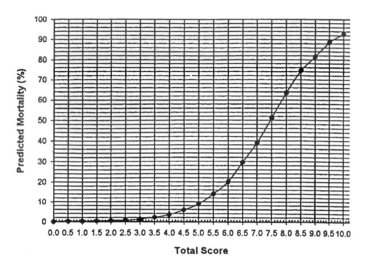

FIGURE 54-2. Michigan risk score. This score is only for in-hospital mortality and is read similar to the Mayo Clinic risk score. To estimate risk, calculate the total score by adding individual scores if comorbidity is present. For number of diseased vessels, add 0.5 for each major epicardial vessel with more than 70% stenosis. Identify the total score on the horizontal axis of the plot and corresponding probability on the vertical axis. Scores of 2.5 or less are associated with risk of death less than 0.8%, whereas scores higher than 7 are associated with risk of death greater than 40%. (*From Ref. 17.*)

The Mayo Clinic, Michigan Consortium, Brigham and Women's, and Beaumont hospital studies[17,18,20,21] have developed risk scores that are easy for an interventionalist to apply at the bedside for rapid risk scoring of the patient. These scores help the physician to triage the patient for the best treatment option, stratify the risk for the PCI procedure, counsel patient and family, and benchmark the outcomes in a more consistent and uniform fashion (Figures 54-1 and 54-2, and Table 54-5).

TABLE 54-5

Michigan Risk Score

VARIABLE	SCORE
Acute MI	1
Shock	2.5
Creatinine > 1.5 mg/dL	1.5
History of cardiac arrest	1.5
No. of diseased vessels	0.5
Age ≥ 70 y	1.0
EF < 50%	0.5
Thrombus	0.5
PVD	0.5
Female sex	0.5
Total Score	—

MI = myocardial infarction; PVD = peripheral *vascular disease*.
Reprinted with permission from Moscucci et al.[17]

SUMMARY

The NNE, Cleveland Clinic, Michigan, NY State, Brigham and Women's, and Mayo Clinic models described in this chapter predict in-hospital complications following PCI in the current era. All the models are robust and represent current PCI practice. The Cleveland Clinic and NY State have also proposed models for both mortality and in-hospital complications. A recent risk score used in the New York State registry showed the power of risk stratification in adjusting hospital mortality following coronary stenting.[12a] Based on the description of strengths and limitations of the currently available models, physicians should be better able to counsel patients and their families about the risks involved in undergoing PCI.

The focus of future studies should be on the uniformity and consensus regarding the definitions of variables used, the outcomes measured, inclusion of post-procedure variables (elevation of cardiac enzymes, stroke, emergency CABG) and operator volume, and a strong national effort to streamline these measures.

REFERENCES

1. Gruntzig AR, Senning A, Siegenthaler WE. Nonoperative dilatation of coronary-artery stenosis: Percutaneous transluminal coronary angioplasty. *N Engl J Med.* 1979;301:61.
2. Seshadri N, Whitlow PL, Acharya N, et al. Emergency coronary artery bypass surgery in the contemporary percutaneous coronary intervention era. *Circulation.* 2002;106:2346.
3. Hochman JS, Sleeper LA, Webb JG, et al. Early revascularization in acute myocardial infarction complicated by cardiogenic shock. SHOCK Investigators. Should We Emergently Revascularize Occluded Coronaries for Cardiogenic Shock? *N Engl J Med.* 1999;341:625.
4. Rihal CS, Sutton-Tyrrell K, Guo P, et al. Increased incidence of periprocedural complications among patients with peripheral vascular disease undergoing myocardial revascularization in the bypass angioplasty revascularization investigation. *Circulation.* 1999;100:171.
5. Singh M, Mathew V, Garratt KN, et al. Effect of age on the outcome of angioplasty for acute myocardial infarction among patients treated at the Mayo Clinic. *Am J Med.* 2000;108:187.
6. Takagi T, Stankovic G, Finci L, et al. Results and long-term predictors of adverse clinical events after elective percutaneous interventions on unprotected left main coronary artery. *Circulation.* 2002;106:698.
7. Walker SH, Duncan DB. Estimation of the probability of an event as a function of several independent variables. *Biometrika.* 1967;54:167.
8. Harrell et al. [R.R. H.] The analysis and selection of variables in linear regression variation of linear analysis. *Biometrics.* 1976;32:1.
9. Sauerbrei W, Schumacher M. A bootstrap resampling procedure for model building: Application to the Cox regression model. *Stat Med.* 1992;11:2093.
10. Hosmer DW LS. A goodness-of-fit test for the multiple logistic regression model. *Communications in Statistics.* 1980;A10:1043.
11. Harrell FE Jr, Lee KL, Mark DB. Multivariable prognostic models: Issues in developing models, evaluating assumptions and adequacy, and measuring and reducing errors. *Stat Med.* 1996;15:361.
12. Hanley JA, McNeil BJ. The meaning and use of the area under a receiver operating characteristic (ROC) curve. *Radiology.* 1982;143:29.
12a. Wu C, Hannan EL, Walford G, et al. A risk score to predict in-hospital mortality for percutaneous coronary interventions. *J Am Coll Cardiol.* 2006; 47:654.
13. Hannan EL, Racz M, Ryan TJ, et al. Coronary angioplasty volume-outcome relationships for hospitals and cardiologists. *JAMA.* 1997;277:892.
14. Holmes DR Jr, Berger PB, Garratt KN, et al. Application of the New York State PTCA mortality model in patients undergoing stent implantation. *Circulation.* 2000;102:517.
15. Shaw RE, Anderson HV, Brindis RG, et al. Development of a risk adjustment mortality model using the American College of Cardiology-National Cardiovascular Data Registry (ACC-NCDR) experience: 1998–2000. *J Am Coll Cardiol.* 2002;39:1104.
16. O'Connor GT, Malenka DJ, Quinton H, et al. Multivariate prediction of in-hospital mortality after percutaneous coronary interventions in 1994–1996.

Northern New England Cardiovascular Disease Study Group. *J Am Coll Cardiol.* 1999;34:681.

17. Moscucci M, Kline-Rogers E, Share D, et al. Simple bedside additive tool for prediction of in-hospital mortality after percutaneous coronary interventions. *Circulation.* 2001;104:263.

18. Qureshi MA, Safian RD, Grines CL, et al. Simplified scoring system for predicting mortality after percutaneous coronary intervention. *J Am Coll Cardiol.* 2003;42:1890.

19. Ellis SG, Weintraub W, Holmes D, et al. Relation of operator volume and experience to procedural outcome of percutaneous coronary revascularization at hospitals with high interventional volumes. *Circulation.* 1997;95:2479.

20. Singh M, Lennon RJ, Holmes DR Jr, et al. Correlates of procedural complications and a simple integer risk score for percutaneous coronary intervention. *J Am Coll Cardiol.* 2002;40:387.

21. Resnic FS, Ohno-Machado L, Selwyn A, et al. Simplified risk score models accurately predict the risk of major in-hospital complications following percutaneous coronary intervention. *Am J Cardiol.* 2001;88:5.

22. Thiemann DR. Primary angioplasty for elderly patients with myocardial infarction: Theory, practice and possibilities. *J Am Coll Cardiol.* 2002;39:1729.

23. Juliard JM, Charlier P, Golmard JL, et al. Age and lack of beta-blocker therapy are associated with increased long-term mortality after primary coronary angioplasty for acute myocardial infarction. *Int J Cardiol.* 2003;88:63.

24. Chaitman BR, Ryan TJ, Kronmal RA, et al. Coronary Artery Surgery Study (CASS): Comparability of 10 year survival in randomized and randomizable patients. *J Am Coll Cardiol.* 1990;16:1071.

25. Best PJ, Lennon R, Ting HH, et al. The impact of renal insufficiency on clinical outcomes in patients undergoing percutaneous coronary interventions. *J Am Coll Cardiol.* 2002;39:1113.

26. Rihal CS, Textor SC, Grill DE, et al. Incidence and prognostic importance of acute renal failure after percutaneous coronary intervention. *Circulation.* 2002;105:2259.

27. Ryan TJ, Faxon DP, Gunnar RM, et al. Guidelines for percutaneous transluminal coronary angioplasty. A report of the American College of Cardiology/American Heart Association Task Force on Assessment of Diagnostic and Therapeutic Cardiovascular Procedures (Subcommittee on Percutaneous Transluminal Coronary Angioplasty). *Circulation.* 1988;78:486.

28. Ellis SG, Vandormael MG, Cowley MJ, et al. Coronary morphologic and clinical determinants of procedural outcome with angioplasty for multivessel coronary disease. Implications for patient selection. Multivessel Angioplasty Prognosis Study Group. *Circulation.* 1990;82:1193.

29. Ellis SG, Guetta V, Miller D, et al. Relation between lesion characteristics and risk with percutaneous intervention in the stent and glycoprotein IIb/IIIa era: An analysis of results from 10,907 lesions and proposal for new classification scheme. *Circulation.* 1999;100:1971.

30. Krone RJ, Shaw RE, Klein LW, et al. Evaluation of the American College of Cardiology/American Heart Association and the Society for Coronary Angiography and Interventions lesion classification system in the current "stent era" of coronary interventions (from the ACC–National Cardiovascular Data Registry). *Am J Cardiol.* 2003;92:389.

31. Block PC, Peterson ED, Krone R, et al. Identification of variables needed to risk adjust outcomes of coronary interventions: Evidence-based guidelines for efficient data collection. *J Am Coll Cardiol.* 1998;32:275.

32. Kastrati A, Schomig A, Elezi S, et al. Prognostic value of the modified American College of Cardiology/American Heart Association stenosis morphology classification for long-term angiographic and clinical outcome after coronary stent placement. *Circulation.* 1999;100:1285.

33. Zaacks SM, Allen JE, Calvin JE, et al. Value of the American College of Cardiology/American Heart Association stenosis morphology classification for coronary interventions in the late 1990s. *Am J Cardiol.* 1998;82:43.

34. Rihal CS, Grill DE, Bell MR, et al. Prediction of death after percutaneous coronary interventional procedures. *Am Heart J.* 2000;139:1032.

35. Malenka DJ, McGrath PD, Wennberg DE, et al. The relationship between operator volume and outcomes after percutaneous coronary interventions in high volume hospitals in 1994–1996: The northern New England experience. Northern New England Cardiovascular Disease Study Group. *J Am Coll Cardiol.* 1999;34:1471.

36. de Feyter PJ, McFadden E. Risk score for percutaneous coronary intervention: Forewarned is forearmed. *J Am Coll Cardiol.* 2003;42:1729.

37. Holmes DR, Selzer F, Johnston JM, et al. Modeling and risk prediction in the current era of interventional cardiology: A report from the National Heart, Lung, and Blood Institute Dynamic Registry. *Circulation.* 2003;107:1871.

CHAPTER (55)

Acute Threatened Coronary Closure

Norman Shaia, MD, and Samuel M. Butman, MD

Abrupt or threatened vessel closure is responsible for many of the critical early complications of percutaneous coronary interventions (PCI). Abrupt closure is recognized as a total or subtotal occlusion of a target vessel during or following PCI. Angiographically, this is associated with Thrombolysis in Myocardial Infarction (TIMI) grade 0 to 1 flow.[1] Clinically, patients often experience ischemic electrocardiographic changes, chest pain, and, if severe, may also develop hemodynamic compromise. Threatened closure is characterized by more than 50% vessel diameter stenosis after an initial successful lesion dilation and is typically associated with reduced flow. Although TIMI grade 2 to 3 flow may be present, the vessel is at increased risk for abrupt closure. However, because of preserved coronary flow, threatened closure may not immediately result in any clinical sequelae.

The incidence of abrupt or threatened closure has previously been reported to be as high as 8.3% of PCI procedures.[2] In an era of improved technologic advances, particularly the coronary stent, the incidence of either threatened or abrupt closure has decreased significantly. However, given the morbidity and mortality associated with this complication, its timely recognition and treatment is vital.

MECHANISM

PCI-induced injury of a coronary artery can trigger a sequence of events that can ultimately lead to abrupt and threatened vessel closure. Balloon dilation results in vessel injury with denudation of the endothelial lining. Disruption of the endothelium with local intima and media fissuring can produce a dissection plane and, depending on the extent of media fissuring, a dissection flap can

lead to significant luminal narrowing. Angiographically, coronary artery dissection can be recognized by curvilinear or spiral-shaped filling defects or extraluminal extravasation of contrast material[3] (Figure 55-1).

In addition, the interruption of the endothelium can result in local activation of the coagulation cascade. Exposure of subendothelial collagen and tissue factor, both highly thrombogenic, stimulates local platelet deposition and subsequent thrombus formation, processes that ultimately may lead to blood stasis and impaired flow (Figure 55-2). In contrast to the angiographic appearance of vessel wall dissection, thrombus may be visualized as one or more progressively enlarging or mobile intraluminal lucencies.[4] A host of vasoactive and proinflammatory substances are often released, frequently resulting in coronary spasm at the site of thrombus formation, as well. These interrelated pathophysiologic processes contribute to abrupt and threatened closure during or after PCI.

ADVERSE CONSEQUENCES

Although recent technologic advances have decreased the incidence of acute vessel closure, it continues to represent the most dangerous hazard of PCI. According to previous National Heart Lung and Blood Institute registries, 48% of coronary bypass procedures, 58% of myocardial infarctions, and 33% of deaths occurred in the 6.8% of patients who experienced abrupt closure during PCI.[5] In addition to the acute complications of vessel closure, long-term vessel patency after PCI has been shown to be diminished, as well. Target lesion revascularization rates are increased secondary to restenosis at 6 months.[6] Although restenosis

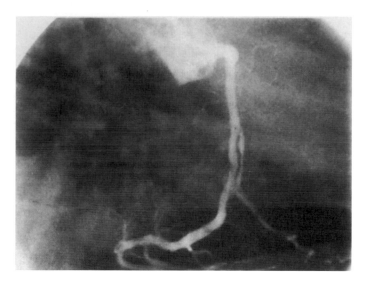

FIGURE 55-1. Typical angiographic appearance of an extensive coronary dissection in the right coronary artery (RAO projection). *(Reproduced with permission from Haase et al.[81])*

does not significantly contribute to increased mortality, the morbidity and increased cost to the health care system can be substantial.

RISK FACTORS

Numerous predictors of abrupt vessel closure have been established. These include various clinical, angiographic, and lesion characteristics. From a clinical standpoint, patients who present with acute coronary syndromes are considered higher risk because of the likely presence of thrombus prior to PCI. Preprocedural presence of thrombus increases the risk for abrupt closure up to ninefold.[7] Balloon inflation can result in further propagation and embolization of preexistent thrombus, resulting in vessel closure. Other clinical predictors include female gender, diabetes mellitus,

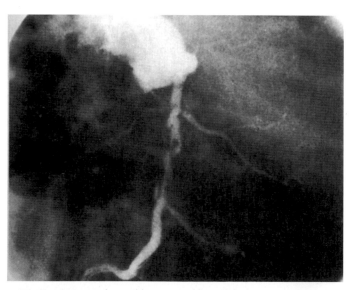

FIGURE 55-2. Intraluminal lucency or filling defect consistent with coronary thrombus as the coronary dissection shown in Figure 55-1 progressed. *(Reproduced with permission from Haase et a.[81])*

TABLE 55-1

Clinical and Angiographic Factors Associated with Abrupt Vessel Closure

Clinical
   Unstable angina
   Female gender
   Acute myocardial infarction
   High surgical risk
Angiographic
   Intraluminal thrombus
   ACC/AHA lesion score
   Multivessel disease
   Multiple stenoses in same vessel
   Lesion length > 10 mm
   Angulated lesion (> 45 degrees)
   Lesion at branch point
   Excessive proximal tortuosity
   Ostial right coronary lesion
   Degenerated saphenous vein graft
   Preprocedure stenosis 90–99%
   Intimal dissection
   Post-procedure stenosis > 35%
   Post-procedure gradient > 20 mm Hg
   Prolonged heparin infusion

ACC/AHA = American College of Cardiology/American Heart Association.
Adapted with permission from Leopold and Jacobs.[8]

and patients at high surgical risk. Unfavorable angiographic lesion characteristics include lesion length greater than 10 mm, angulated lesions greater than 45 degrees, branch-point stenosis, and excessive tortuosity of the vessel[8] (Table 55-1). In addition to pre-PCI lesion morphology, the angiographic appearance after dilation is the most important determinant of a complication. A residual stenosis of more than 35% and the presence of dissection or residual thrombus increases the likelihood of acute closure.[9]

PREVENTATIVE STRATEGIES

Integrating the clinical and angiographic risk factors is vital in predicting the risk of abrupt closure and developing strategies to prevent it from occuring, as well. Because of the significant increase in morbidity and mortality associated with this complication, various preventative strategies have emerged, some now only of historical interest, but others important in the context of the mechanisms involved. These have focused on improved procedural technique as well as adjunctive pharmacologic therapy. The approach to management is discussed later in the chapter.

[ ] MECHANICAL STRATEGIES

The majority of mechanical strategies that have been developed have been aimed at decreasing the frequency of coronary dissection

TABLE 55-2

Reported Mechanical Strategies to Prevent Abrupt Vessel Closure

Appropriate balloon sizing
Long balloons (angulated lesions)
Prolonged balloon inflation
Noncompliant balloon material
Primary stenting

Adapted with permission from Leopold and Jacobs.[8]

(Table 55-2). A thoughtful predilation strategy with appropriate balloon-to-artery sizing has been shown to have a significant impact.[10] Other strategies have included utilizing noncompliant balloons, gradual and prolonged balloon inflations, and longer balloons for angulated lesions.[11,12] In the new device era, primary stenting is frequently employed. Coronary stents result in a greater gain in luminal diameter and eliminate vessel recoil, both important shortcomings of plain old balloon angioplasty.

[ ] PHARMACOLOGIC STRATEGIES

Pharmacologic preventative strategies, on the other hand, have focused on the suppression of thrombus formation before and during PCI (Table 55-3).

Unfractionated Heparin

Unfractionated heparin (UFH) has routinely been used before, during, and after PCI and remains the standard background anticoagulant. Trials of pretreatment have demonstrated a decrease in thrombus formation and consequently a lower incidence of abrupt and threatened closure.[13] Other studies have examined the relationship of the activated clotting time (ACT) during PCI and the risk of closure.[14] Earlier trials, prior to glycoprotein IIb/IIIa (Gp IIb/IIIa) inhibitor use, suggested that maintaining an ACT greater than 300 seconds was associated with a decrease in subacute thrombosis.[15] However, more contemporary trials utilizing additional antiplatelet agents have not shown the same incremental

TABLE 55-3

Pharmacologic Strategies to Prevent Abrupt Vessel Closure

Heparin (unfractionated or low-molecular-weight)
Direct thrombin inhibitors
Aspirin (ASA)
ADP antagonists (eg, clopidogrel)
Glycoprotein IIb/IIIa receptor antagonists
Coronary vasodilators

ADP = adenosine diphosphate; ASA = acetylsalicylic acid.

clinical benefit with higher intraprocedural ACT levels.[16] When used in combination with a Gp IIb/IIIa platelet receptor blocker, the incidence of bleeding is increased with an ACT greater than 300 seconds, and the current recommendation is to maintain an ACT of 200 to 250 during PCI.[17] Post-procedure heparin was routinely used following PCI as a bridge to once necessary combined multiple drug oral anticoagulation. However, the data on the benefit of post-procedure heparin after PCI is less clear and is definitely associated with a higher risk of significant bleeding.[18]

Low-Molecular-Weight Heparin

Two major clinical trials (ESSENCE and TIMI-11B) demonstrated the superiority of low-molecular-weight heparin (LMWH) over UFH in patients with unstable angina and non–ST-segment myocardial infarction.[19,20] However, less than 20% of patients in these two trials underwent PCI. Therefore it is difficult to comment on the effectiveness of LMWH in preventing abrupt or threatened vessel closure in these patient populations.

The more recent National Investigators Collaborating on Enoxaparin (NICE) studies examined the safety and efficacy of planned LMWH in patients undergoing PCI.[21] These nonrandomized trials concluded that enoxaparin could be used alone or with Gp IIb/IIIa inhibitors with similar rates of clinical events and bleeding compared with UFH. In the NICE trials, while not controlled studies, LMWH was as effective in preventing acute and threatened closure when retrospectively compared with standard heparin.

The SYNERGY (Superior Yield of the New Strategy of Enoxaparin, Revascularization and Glycoprotein IIb/IIIa Inhibitors) trial[22] compared the outcomes of patients treated with LMWH versus unfractionated heparin in non–ST-elevation acute coronary syndrome managed with an early invasive approach. Although designed to demonstrate superiority of LMWH, no difference in the primary end point of death or myocardial infarction was observed. In addition, no difference in ischemic events during PCI occurred. The reported incidence of abrupt closure of LMWH and unfractionated heparin was 1.3% and 1.7%, respectively, also not significantly different. Similarly, the rate of threatened closure was 1.1% for LMWH and 1.0% for unfractionated heparin. Although LMWH theoretically offers several advantages when compared with UFH, including a more consistent anticoagulation effect, greater bioavailability, and a greater anti-Xa effect, it appears to be equivalent to unfractionated heparin in contemporary coronary intervention.

Direct Thrombin Inhibitors

Bivalirudin (previously called hirulog), approved by the Food and Drug Administration (FDA) as an antithrombin for use during PCI, is administered as a bolus and infusion during angioplasty procedures.[23] The relationship between abrupt vessel closure and the anticoagulant response to heparin or bivalirudin during PCI was examined in the Hirulog Angioplasty Study.[24] This was a randomized, double-blind comparison of heparin versus bivalirudin in 4312 patients undergoing angioplasty for unstable or postinfarction angina. Abrupt or threatened vessel closure occurred in 9.3% of patients treated with heparin and 9.2% treated with bivalirudin (P = NS). The Randomized Evaluation in Percutaneous Coronary Intervention Linking Angiomax to Reduced Clinical

Events (REPLACE) II trial demonstrated noninferiority of bivalirudin compared with UFH in patients with stable angina undergoing PCI.[23] "Bailout" Gp IIb/IIIa inhibitor use was found to be very low in the bivalirudin arm, suggesting an infrequent occurrence of impending closure during angioplasty.

Aspirin

Aspirin has been shown in several randomized trials to help prevent acute complications associated with PCI.[25] At this time, it is felt to be an important, if not critical, mainstay in periprocedural management.

Clopidogrel

The optimal timing and dosing of clopidogrel, the current oral adenosine diphosphate antagonist of choice, continues to evolve. Clopidogrel is administered as a bolus dose of 300 mg prior to PCI and continued for 1 to 8 months afterward at 75 mg/d.[26] This antiplatelet agent has become an integral part of the pharmacologic armamentarium after PCI because of its ability to decrease post-procedural thrombosis. A transition to double oral antiplatelet therapy in lieu of sodium warfarin and an antiplatelet regimen has been shown to be more effective, as well, in preventing subacute stent thrombosis, a dreaded late complication of a successful intervention.

There is ongoing debate as to the duration of therapy post-PCI, although with the advent of coated stents, 6 to 12 months has become the routine. The CURE (Clopidogrel in USA to Prevent Recurrent Events) and CURE PCI trials of clopidogrel in addition to aspirin demonstrated a decrease in major adverse cardiac events (MACE) up to 8 months after coronary intervention.[27] Its role in helping to prevent intra-procedural thrombosis has not, however, been proven. Furthermore, there are no trials of clopidogrel without a background of aspirin in the prevention of acute or subacute stent thrombosis.

Glycoprotein IIb/IIIa Platelet Receptor Inhibitors

These antiplatelet agents interrupt the final common pathway for platelet aggregation. Several trials have shown their benefit in patients with unstable angina and non–ST-segment myocardial infarction who were managed either medically or with an early interventional approach.[28–31] Among patients with unstable angina who undergo PCI, Gp IIb/IIIa inhibition appears to have a benefit both prior to and during the intervention. The CAPTURE (Chimeric 7E3 AntiPlatelet Therapy in Unstable angina REfractory to standard treatment) trial demonstrated the early benefit with up-front GP IIb/IIIa inhibitor use.[32] Similar low rates of abrupt and threatened closure were also reported with more contemporary trials involving the use of Gp IIb/IIIa inhibitors, such as TACTICS-TIMI 18.[33] For these reasons, these agents have been incorporated as a vital pharmacologic adjunct in patients undergoing PCI. Their role as a bailout agent once abrupt vessel closure occurs is discussed later in the chapter.

Thrombolytic Therapy

Several trials have examined the utilization of thrombolytic therapy in the prevention of abrupt closure. Studies comparing routine administration of systemic urokinase or tissue plasminogen activator before or during PCI versus standard antiplatelet therapy without thrombolytic use were performed in the early 1990s.[34–37] These included both patients presenting for elective angioplasty as well as patients with unstable angina. No significant differences in angioplasty success rates or acute occlusion rates were reported in these trials. In TAUSA (Thrombolysis and Angioplasty in UnStable Angina), the largest of these trials addressing the use of prophylactic urokinase in patients with unstable angina, a paradoxic increase in ischemic complications, as well as abrupt closure, was seen in the patients who received thrombolytic therapy.[38] Prolonged intracoronary urokinase infusions were also studied in patients with chronic total occlusions. Although there has been some variable success in small trials, larger trials have not shown a statistically significant benefit in helping to prevent abrupt and threatened closure during PCI compared with standard therapy.[39–41] Currently, there is no indication for standard use of systemic or intracoronary fibrinolytic agents for the prevention of abrupt vessel closure.

Dipyridamole

This coronary vasodilator, as well as platelet inhibitor, has been studied as a preventative agent in acute vessel closure. In a previous prospective randomized investigation, oral dipyridamole did not prevent acute complications following PCI.[25] However, both oral and intravenous application of dipyridamole is associated with a high level of plasma protein binding. This may counteract a sufficient local concentration at the coronary site, negating any potential therapeutic effect. Heintzen and colleagues examined the effect of intracoronary dipyridamole as a preventative strategy to reduce the incidence of abrupt closure after PCI.[42] Patients were randomized to conventional pretreatment with ASA and heparin versus additional dipyridamole. There was a significant decrease in the incidence of abrupt closure in the dipyridamole arm versus conventional therapy (2.5% and 6.1%, respectively). This reduction was observed in patients with stable angina as well as those who presented with an acute coronary syndrome. These results may be explained by both the vasodilating and possible antithrombotic effects of dipyridamole. Dipyridamole inhibits adenosine reuptake leading to an increased local concentration of adenosine. However, this agent has largely been replaced by the readily available adenosine.

MANAGEMENT

In the event of abrupt and threatened vessel closure, the ultimate goal is to restore normal coronary flow in order to reduce ischemic complications. A comprehensive strategy, including both mechanical and pharmacologic means, is often employed (Table 55-4). Prior to the advent of coronary artery stents, various devices along with numerous pharmacologic agents were utilized. Still important today, these modalities were directed at the treatment of intracoronary thrombus, dissection flaps, and vasospasm in an attempt to maintain vessel patency.

TABLE 55-4

Acute Management of Abrupt and Threatened Vessel Closure

Mechanical
    Autoperfusion balloon
    Directional coronary atherectomy
    Laser angioplasty
    Intra-aortic balloon counterpulsation
    Coronary artery stents
Pharmacologic
    Antithrombotics
    Coronary vasodilators
Coronary artery bypass grafting

【 】 MECHANICAL MEASURES

Autoperfusion Balloon

In the setting of abrupt and threatened vessel closure, prolonged balloon inflation was, and still can be utilized in an attempt to restore vessel patency. Multiple, or more typically prolonged, low pressure dilations with a conventional balloon catheter can be a successful strategy. Although largely supplanted by stents, this strategy is employed in an effort to tack up obstructive intimal flaps and compress intraluminal thrombus. However, this technique is limited by periods of prolonged occlusion and ischemia during balloon inflation. The development of autoperfusion balloon catheters allowed for prolonged dilations while maintaining distal coronary perfusion. Various perfusion balloons were developed, unique in the number of side holes, profile, and flow rates, and were supported by studies confirming a reduction in ischemia during perfusion balloon angioplasty when compared with standard angioplasty.[43,44] A reduction in angina and ST-segment abnormalities, and improved echocardiographic wall motion score, have all been demonstrated.

The clinical utility of autoperfusion balloons has been specifically examined in the setting of abrupt and threatened vessel closure (Table 55-5). Procedural success is achievable in 65% to 80% of patients.[45,46] With regard to long-term efficacy, however, only a few small studies exist on the incidence of angiographic restenosis after utilization of the autoperfusion balloon, best estimated at approximately 40%.[47] This relatively high rate may be explained by a persistence of intimal flaps, and suboptimal results creating a milieu for an accelerated cellular response.

Autoperfusion balloons have several disadvantages in the setting of acute vessel closure. Because they rely on systemic blood pressure to maintain perfusion, they can be ineffective in a hypotensive patient. In addition, these balloons tend to have a higher profile, thus presenting a delivery challenge in complex lesions and anatomy. Finally, extensive dissections that involve one or more large side branches can limit inflation times. For these reasons, autoperfusion balloons continue to have limited use in these bailout situations.

Directional Coronary Atherectomy

Directional coronary atherectomy (DCA) has been used as a treatment modality for failed PCI.[48] DCA has the ability to remove dissection flaps and thrombus, thus helping to restore vessel patency. However, it has numerous limitations that preclude its widespread use for salvage therapy after abrupt closure. Technical considerations such as the lack of prepositioned large sheath and guide placement, as well as difficulty in delivery can be problematic. Coronary perforation remains the dreaded complication with DCA, and the risk is increased with more extensive dissections.[49] Thus, DCA is neither routinely used nor recommended in acute or threatened vessel closure.

Laser Angioplasty

The first applications of laser technology in coronary arteries occurred in the early 1980s.[50,51] Continuous-wave lasers produce visable light or infrared energy to generate local heat. Pulsed-wave lasers soon emerged, which produced high-energy light of a uniform wavelength. The excimer laser is currently available and was

TABLE 55-5

Autoperfusion Balloon for Acute or Threatened Closure

STUDY	PROCEDURAL SUCCESS (%)	RECLOSURE (%)	MI (%)	CABG (%)	DEATH (%)
Saenz et al	22 (100)	1 (4.5)	0	1 (4.5)	0
Landau et al	44 (85)	1 (2)	0	7 (15)	1 (2)
Jackman et al	32 (80)	0	5 (12)	8 (20)	0
Van Lierde et al	16 (67)	0	3 (12)	7 (19)	0
De Muinck et al	26 (65)	0	14 (35)	13 (31)	2 (5)
Seggewiss et al	61 (83)	1 (2)	5 (8)	10 (14)	0
Van der Linden et al	22 (68)	1 (4)	8 (23)	5 (14)	3 (8)

CABG = Coronary artery by pass grafting; MI = myocardial infarction.
Reproduced with permission from De Muinck et al.[59]

first used clinically 1988. The potential niches for the excimer laser were originally thought to be long lesions (> 20 mm), small vessels (< 2.5 mm), and calcified and total coronary occlusions. Although initial trials showed some encouraging results, larger, randomized trials failed to show any superiority over PCI/DCA.[52,53] Its utility in threatened and abrupt closure was investigated in earlier trials. Because the technique of laser balloon angioplasty permitted the heating of vascular tissue, it was thought to seal dissections by thermal welding. However, its unacceptably high rates of coronary perforation and long-term restenosis precluded it as an attractive option for acute vessel closure.

Intra-aortic Balloon Counterpulsation

Patients who develop acute vessel closure after PCI may experience severe hemodynamic compromise. This depends on the patient's baseline cardiac function, the extent of myocardium at risk during PCI, and the number of collateral vessels that supply the treated area. If cardiogenic shock develops, an intra-aortic balloon pump (IABP) is often employed to increase diastolic coronary arterial perfusion and reduce systemic afterload, without increasing myocardial oxygen demand.

The SHOCK (SHould we emergently revascularize Occluded Coronaries for cardiogenic shocK?) trial, which focused on patients with cardiogenic shock in the setting of acute myocardial infarction, reported a significant mortality reduction in patients who received an IABP.[54] Historically, and regardless of the SHOCK trial findings, the IABP is a mainstay in stabilizing patients with abrupt closure until revascularization, be it surgical or percutaneous, is completed.

Coronary Artery Stents

The development of the coronary artery stent in the early 1990s represented a major breakthrough in the field of interventional cardiology. The ability of these stents to scaffold intimal and medial flaps, in addition to limiting elastic recoil, has resulted in a significant decrease in the incidence of abrupt and threatened closure over the past 15 years (Figure 55-3). The Gianturco-Roubin stent was initally studied by Hearn and colleagues in the late 1980s as a mechanical strategy to treat acute vessel closure after unsuccessful PCI.[55] The promising results of this trial, along with other earlier trials, led to FDA approval of this stent for the sole purpose of bailout for abrupt or threatened closure. However, the applicability of stenting has expanded dramatically over the past decade. It has evolved into the gold standard in preventing restenosis as well as in the prevention and treatment of abrupt and threatened closure.

The introduction of coronary artery stents in the early 1990s represented a major breakthrough in the treatment, and more importantly in the prevention of abrupt and threatened vessel closure.[55,56] With the ability to scaffold the arterial wall, secure dissection flaps, and limit elastic recoil, stents produce highly satisfactory angiographic results after abrupt or impending vessel closure.[55–57]

Early Pivotal Trials

Early clinical trials examined the first generation Gianturco-Roubin stent in the treatment of abrupt and threatened closure.

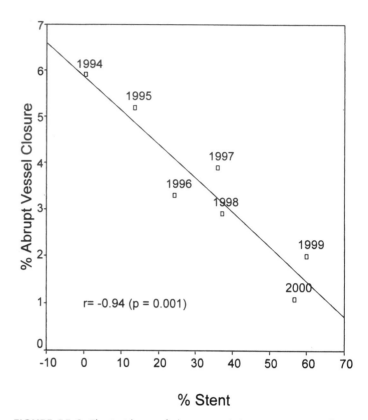

FIGURE 55-3. The incidence of abrupt vessel closure over time with increasing use of coronary stents. *(Reproduced with permission from Almeda et al.[80])*

This was the first FDA-approved stent, and it was specifically approved for the treatment of acute threatened closure. Hearn and colleagues reported single-center experience of this balloon-expandable stent in 116 patients after failed PCI from 1987 through 1990.[55] Stent deployment was successful in approximately 90% of patients and over 70% of patients were spared emergency coronary artery bypass grafting (CABG) after failed PCI. There was an associated decrease in ischemic complications, including death and myocardial infarction. Unfortunately, there was a rather high incidence of subacute thrombosis (8.6%) and angiographic restenosis (53%) at 4 months with this early generation of stent. Similar rates of subacute thrombosis and restenosis with Gianturco-Roubin stents were reported by others, as well.[58]

The early clinical experience with the Palmaz-Schatz stent was very similar to that of the Gianturco-Roubin stent. Although procedural success was very high, this was partly offset by a significant closure rate (2–23%), need for in-hospital CABG (2–18%), and in-hospital myocardial infarction (2–30%)[59,60] (Table 55-6). The frequency of subacute thrombosis, a limitation in earlier stent trials, correlated with incomplete stent coverage of coronary dissections. This was validated in a later pathology study involving detailed postmortem analysis of patients who underwent bailout stenting[61] (Figure 55-4). Stenting after failed PCI restores lumen patency, however, it is the residual dissection in the nonstented segments that results in focal compressions or obstructions.

High angiographic restenosis rates, another concern with earlier stent trials for abrupt vessel closure, were explained by the use of multiple stents to seal coronary dissections. A more recent trial

TABLE 55-6

Palmaz-Schatz Stent for Acute or Threatened Closure

STUDY	PROCEDURAL SUCCESS (%)	RECLOSURE (%)	MI (%)	CABG (%)	DEATH (%)
De Muinck et al	34 (94)	8 (23)	11 (30)	3 (8)	3 (8)
Haude et al	15 (100)	1 (7)	1 (7)	1 (7)	0
Herrmann et al	55 (98)	9 (16)	14 (25)	9 (16)	2 (4)
Kastrati et al	107 (96)	5 (6)	0	20 (18)	0
Maiello et al	30 (94)	1 (3)	2 (6)	2 (6)	1 (3)
Kiemeneij et al	46 (88)	9 (23)	1 (2)	9 (17)	1 (2)
Colombo et al	49 (88)	1 (2)	2 (4)	3 (5)	2 (4)
Alfonso et al	39 (93)	2 (5)	5 (12)	1 (2)	0

CABG = coronary artery by pass grafting; MI = myocardial infarction.
Reproduced with permission from De Muinck et al.[59]

compared the late clinical outcome of patients treated with intracoronary stents in a nonelective, bailout procedure with those undergoing elective stenting.[62] One-hundred and thirty-two patients were prospectively studied and no statistical difference in the primary composite end point of death, myocardial infarction, and the need for repeat revascularization was found between the two groups. Therefore, single and multiple stents could be placed in bailout situations without an increase in either short- or long-term adverse events. These results may also be attributed to improved operator technique and contemporary adjunctive pharmacologic therapy.

As the coronary stent quickly gained widespread acceptance as a treatment of abrupt closure, trials to compare it with older management strategies were conducted. De Muinck and colleagues compared autoperfusion balloon angioplasty with Palmaz-Schatz stent implantation for acute and threatened vessel closure.[47] They reported no difference in clinical success or 3-month event-free survival, but at a higher cost per patient in the stent group. Subsequently, Ray and colleagues demonstrated a much higher procedural success rate with stenting (90%) compared with autoperfusion balloon angioplasty (42%).[63]

Contemporary Trials in PCI

Since the 1990s, coronary artery stenting has been adopted as the main approach for PCI worldwide (Figure 55-5). The benchmark clinical trials, BENESTENT (BElgian NEtherlands STENT) and STRESS (STent REstenosis Study), showed the superiority of stenting over balloon angioplasty alone.[64,65] With that, the incidence

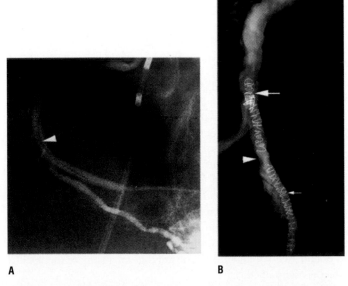

FIGURE 55-4. (A). Spiral dissection (*arrowhead*) after balloon angioplasty of a 90% stenosis in the proximal right coronary artery (RCA). **(B).** Postmortem radiograph demonstrating a 0.5-cm segment (*arrowhead*) of the mid-RCA not covered by stents. *(Reproduced with permission from Farb et al.[61])*

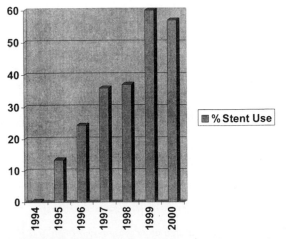

FIGURE 55-5. The past decade has resulted in a steady increase in stent use. *(Reproduced with permission from Almeda et al.[80])*

of abrupt and threatened vessel closure has significantly decreased. In addition, with the advent of novel pharmacologic agents such as Gp IIb/IIIa inhibitors and thienopyridines, periprocedural complications after stenting have decreased as well.[16,26,30,33]

The first few clinical trials incorporating Gp IIb/IIIa use with PCI, EPIC (Evaluation of IIb/IIIa Platelet receptor antagonist 7E3 in Preventing Ischemic Complications) and EPILOG (Evaluation of PTCA to Improve Long-term Outcome by c7E3 GPIIb/IIIa receptor blockade), showed promising results combining these two modalities.[28,29] EPISTENT (Evaluation of Platelet IIb/IIIa Inhibition for Stenting), a larger, randomized trial confirmed the hypothesis that stenting or balloon angioplasty plus Gp IIb/IIIa inhibition was superior to stenting with placebo.[30] The primary end point of death, myocardial infarction, or urgent revascularization occurred least in the group of patients who received stenting plus Gp IIb/IIIa inhibition. Aside from the primary end point, the incidence of abrupt or threatened closure was also the lowest among this group. In fact, 19% of patients who received balloon angioplasty alone had suboptimal results, resulting in a crossover to the stent arm.

ESPRIT (Enhanced Suppression of the Platelet IIb/IIIa Receptor with Integrilin Therapy), another contemporary PCI trial examining the efficacy and safety of eptifibitide, also demonstrated the importance of both stenting and Gp IIb/IIIa inhibition.[16] The trial was terminated early for efficacy because there was such a dramatic benefit in both primary and secondary end points. One of the primary end points was a need for bailout Gp IIb/IIIa inhibitor therapy within 48 hours after randomization. As expected, this occurred more frequently in the placebo arm. Again, periprocedural complications, including abrupt and threatened closure, were reduced with the addition of Gp IIb/IIIa platelet receptor blockade (Figure 55-6). These results were also in accord with the data obtained in the earlier EPISTENT trial.

TARGET (Do Tirofiban And ReoPro Give similar Efficacy Trial) assessed the differences in safety and effiacy between two Gp IIb/IIIa inhibitors, tirofiban and abciximab, in patients undergoing stent implantation.[66] Although the primary end points of death, nonfatal myocardial infarction, and urgent target-vessel revascularization occurred less frequently in the abciximab group, the incidence of abrupt closure (0.8%) was very low in both arms compared with previous trials of balloon angioplasty alone (6.8%). This study confirmed the importance of a combined mechanical and pharmacologic approach to coronary intervention in contemporary practice.

In 2003, the first sirolimus-coated drug-eluting stent was released for clinical use in the United States, and in 2004, a paclitaxel-coated stent was also made available. There have been no unexpected suggestions of increased risk of acute or threatened closure. Despite early concerns, the incidence of procedural of acute stent thrombosis has not increased with the advent of drug-eluting technology, however, the question of a higher risk of late stent thrombosis is dealt with in greater detail in Chapter 10. The approach to recognition and treatment are the same as outlined in this chapter on acute threatened closure. Thus as stent technology and pharmacologic approaches continue to evolve, the incidence of abrupt procedural and late abrupt closure should diminish.

【 】 PHARMACOLOGIC AGENTS

Successful restoration of coronary flow after failed PCI frequently requires both mechanical and pharmacologic interventions. Pharmacologic agents are directed toward treatment of intracoronary thrombus and coronary vasospasm. As with all drug therapy, knowledge of the mechanism of action, dosage, and the best mode of delivery are crucial in optimizing the therapeutic effect.

Antithrombotic Agents

Unfractionated Heparin. Many of the antithrombotic agents mentioned to help prevent clotting are also used to treat acute or threatened closure once it occurs. UFH, the foundation of antithrombotic therapy during these interventions, is still routinely administered during a majority of PCI procedures to prevent intraprocedural thrombosis. As mentioned earlier, an ACT of 200 to 250 seconds appears to be optimal during PCI, when used in combination with Gp IIb/IIIa platelet receptor inhibitors.[16] There have been no data to suggest that achieving a supratherapeutic ACT, once abrupt closure has occurred, is beneficial. However, because heparin may be rapidly consumed due to increased thrombus formation after vessel closure, it is imperative to obtain ACTs frequently to ensure that an adequate therapeutic effect is maintained.

Low-Molecular-Weight Heparin. If LMWH is given prior to or at the time of PCI, one must be able to rapidly confirm and determine the level of anticoagulation if intraprocedural thrombosis occurs. The NICE trials, described earlier, examined dosing

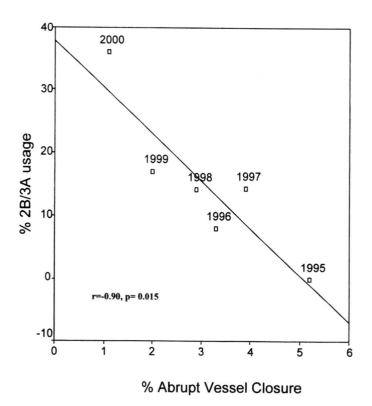

FIGURE 55-6. The relationship of increasing utilization of glycoprotein IIb/IIIa platelet receptor inhibitors and the decreasing incidence of abrupt vessel closure over the past decade. *(Reproduced with permission from Almeda et al.[80])*

regimens based on the degree of anti-Xa/IIa inhibition.[21] Incorporation of the Enox test, a tool used to measure the efficacy of antithrombotic activity of enoxaparin, is invaluable in the catheterization laboratory in managing intraprocedural thrombosis, if enoxaparin is the antithrombotic used.[67] The benefit, if any, of post-PCI administration of LMWH was examined in the ATLAST (Aspirin/Ticlopidine vs. Low molecular weight heparin/Aspirin/ticlopidine high risk Stent Trial) trial.[68] This randomized, double-blind trial investigated whether the addition of LMWH for 14 days post-PCI would reduce MACE compared with placebo. Perhaps due to a surprisingly low rate of MACE (2.3%) at 30 days, no additional benefit of prolonged LMWH was observed in preventing subacute ischemic complications in high-risk patients.

Glycoprotein IIb/IIIa Platelet Receptor Blockers. Haase and colleagues performed an observational trial to assess the efficacy of primary Gp IIb/IIIa antagonist therapy as a bailout procedure after threatened or abrupt closure.[69] PCI was performed in 1332 consecutive patients with stable angina. Abrupt or threatened vessel closure was observed in 63 patients (4.7%). Once recognized, abciximab was administered and early follow-up angiography was performed at 24 hours. Although not a randomized trial, there was a significant increase in TIMI flow grade, accompanied by a decrease in the thrombus score, with low short- and long-term clinical event rates, when compared with previous studies. Muhlestein and colleauges also examined the use of "rescue" abciximab for the dissolution of coronary thrombus when seen as a complication of PCI.[70] Again, abciximab was found to be beneficial as a bailout agent in acute vessel closure. It is difficult to truly assess Gp IIb/IIIa inhibitors as bailout agents in contemporary practice given the infrequent occurrence of abrupt closure with stent implantation. However, based on their mechanism of action and importance in coronary interventions, these agents appear to be valuable pharmacologic adjuncts in these situations.

Thrombolytic Therapy. Trials in the early 1990s examined the use of urokinase for the acute complications of PCI. However, there was significant variability among these trials with regard to procedural success. Although some authors quote success rates of 65% to 90%, others demonstrated more than 50% acute vessel closure 24 to 36 hours after thrombolytic administration.[71] This variability may be explained by the prothrombotic effects of thrombolytic therapy observed in patients with acute coronary syndromes, or the lack of control groups, as well. Thrombolysis activates platelets and exposes clot-bound thrombin, which remains enzymatically active and can lead to thrombosis. Because most patients with acute coronary syndromes have a nonocclusive thrombus in their culprit vessel, the prothrombotic effect of fibrinolytics may result in propagation of thrombus and acute vessel closure.

A meta-analysis of the use of thrombolytic therapy in patients with acute coronary syndromes without ST-segment elevation myocardial infarction has demonstrated increased morbidity and mortality compared with placebo.[72] If extrapolated to patients with threatened closure from formation of a nonocclusive thrombus after PCI, intracoronary fibrinolytic therapy could actually increase the propensity for further deterioration and an adverse outcome.[73,74] At a minimum, when this therapy is used it must be on a background of adequate antiplatelet and antithrombotic therapy. An acceptance or weighing of the increased risk of bleeding is also paramount.

Coronary Vasodilators

Although the etiology of threatened and abrupt vessel closure is frequently coronary thrombosis and dissection, coexisting vasospasm or a reduction in arteriolar flow, or both, may also be present. Intracoronary nitroglycerin or nitroprusside, as well as various calcium channel blockers (verapamil, diltiazem, or nicardipine), are often administered to increase coronary flow once spasm or reduced flow is seen. Adenosine has the capacity to vasodilate at the microvascular level, thus increasing coronary perfusion and facilitating the dispersal of intracoronary thrombi. This mechanism of vasodilation and platelet inhibition may act synergistically in the prevention and possible acute treatment of abrupt vessel closure.

Adenosine. Intracoronary adenosine is often used in clinical practice today and is administered in doses ranging from 10 to 40 µg.

Nitroprusside. This direct donor of nitric oxide is a potent arteriolar vasodilator and is thought to inhibit platelet adhesion as well. Its effect on the microcirculation may help the dispersal of embolized thrombus after PCI in the setting of acute coronary syndrome. Most commonly, an intracoronary dose of 100 to 200 µg is administered for an adequate vasodilatory response.[75] Both adenosine and nitroprusside should be considered as first-line agents once abrupt or threatened closure occurs.

TABLE 55-7

Trends in Incidence of Abrupt Vessel Closure, Urgent CABG Surgery, and the Use of Stents Over Time

YEAR	AVC (N = 103)	URGENT SURGERY (N = 23)	STENTS (N = 1231)	TOTAL PCI (N = 3300)
1994	13 (5.9%)	2 (0.9%)	1 (0.4%)	219
1995	23 (5.2%)	4 (0.6%)	59 (13.5%)	437
1996	15 (3.3%)	4 (0.8%)	110 (24.3%)	452
1997	18 (3.9%)	5 (1.1%)	162 (35.9%)	451
1998	16 (2.9%)	5 (0.9%)	204 (37.1%)	550
1999	11 (2.0%)	2 (0.3%)	329 (60%)	547
2000	7 (1.1%)	1 (0.1%)	366 (56.8%)	644

AVC = abrupt vessel closure; CABG = Coronary artery by pass grafting; PCI = percutaneous coronary intevention.

Reproduced with permission from Almeda et al.[80]

【 】 EMERGENCY CORONARY ARTERY BYPASS SURGERY

If both mechanical and pharmacologic interventions fail in the management of acute vessel closure after PCI, preparations for emergency CABG are vital. CABG should be considered in patients who have refractory myocardial ischemia, high-risk anatomic features such as left main occlusion or compromise, or severely disrupted or unstable angioplasty sites.[76,77] As one would expect, morbidity and mortality rates associated with emergency CABG are significantly higher than those for elective CABG.[78] Predictors of adverse in-hospital outcome after emergency CABG include impaired left ventricular function, multivessel disease, and the presence of hemodynamic instability. In practice, referral for emergency CABG is much less frequent now given the success of stenting as a bailout after an unsuccessful PCI procedure, or the larger reality that coronary stenting is performed in the vast majority of procedures (Table 55-7).

Because of the low frequency of emergent CABG after failed PCI, there has been a growing interest in whether stand-alone angioplasty can be performed safely both in urgent acute myocardial infarction scenarios and in more elective cases in centers without surgical backup on site. A retrospective observational study by Lotfi and colleagues examined this still-evolving issue, using a detailed chart review of all patients who were referred for urgent CABG after failed PCI.[79] From a database of 6582 percutaneous coronary interventions, 45 patients (0.7%) were identified as having urgent CABG after PCI. Using a prespecified set of criteria predicting risk of harm if CABG were to be delayed, 25% of these patients would have potentially been affected. Of concern is that the demographic characteristics of PCI cases requiring emergent CABG were very similar to all PCI cases, highlighting the unpredictability of the need for emergency CABG. Without the presence of on-site surgical backup, patients will likely be affected. However, the absolute risk of potential harm, if CABG were to be delayed remains very low (0.01%). As interventional techniques continue to improve, potential strategies to better identify patients at risk should lead to a growth in stand-alone angioplasty centers. (See Chapter 59.)

SUMMARY

The frequency of abrupt and threatened closure, a dreaded complication during and following PCI, has decreased dramatically over the past 15 years. Significant advances in both the prevention and management of abrupt closure have led to improved outcomes in PCI. The emergence of a combined mechanical and pharmacologic approach has been responsible for minimizing many of the early complications after intervention. As interventional procedural technique improves, the need for emergent CABG after an initial unsuccessful PCI will continue to decline. The favorable impact that drug-eluting stents have had on short- and long-term outcomes continues to be investigated. However, these and other technological and pharmacological improvements in interventional cardiology have forever changed the approach to revascularization in patients with coronary artery disease.

REFERENCES

1. Lincoff AM, Popma JJ, Ellis SG, et al. Abrupt vessel closure complicating coronary angioplasty: Clinical, angiographic and therapeutic profile. *J Am Coll Cardiol.* 1992;19:926.
2. Detre KM, Holmes DR, Holubkov R, et al. Incidence and consequences of periprocedural occlusion: The 1985–1986 National Heart, Lung, and Blood Institute percutaneous transluminal coronary angioplasty registry. *Circulation.* 1990;82:739.
3. Huber MS, Mooney JF, Madison J, Mooney MR. Use of a morphologic classification to predict clinical outcome after dissection from coronary angioplasty. *Am J Cardiol.* 1991;68:467.
4. Goldbaum T, De Sciascio G, Cowley MJ, Vetrovec GW. Early occlusion following successful coronary angioplasty; clinical and angiographic observations. *Cathet Cardiovasc Diagn.* 1989;17:22.
5. Detre KM, Holubkov R, Kelsey S, et al. One-year follow up results of the 1985–1986 National Heart, Lung, and Blood Institute's percutaneous transluminal coronary angioplasty registry. *Circulation.* 1989;80:421.
6. Simptendorfer C, Belardi J, Bellany G, et al. Frequency, management and follow-up of patients with acute coronary occlusions after percutaneous transluminal coronary angioplasty. *Am J Cardiol.* 1987;59:267.
7. Mabin TA, Holmes DR, Smith HC, et al. Intracoronary thrombus: Role in coronary occlusion complicating percutaneous transluminal coronary angioplasty. *J Am Coll Cardiol.* 1985;5:198.
8. Leopold J, Jacobs A. Treatment of closure and threatened closure. In: Ellis SG, Holmes DR, eds. *Strategic Approaches in Coronary Intervention,* 2nd ed. Philadelphia, Pa: Lippincott, Williams and Wilkins; 1999:489.
9. Ellis SG, Roubin GS, King SB III, et al. Angiographic and clinical predictors of acute closure after native vessel coronary angioplasty. *Circulation.* 1988;77:327.
10. Roubin GS, Douglas JS, King SB, et al. Influence of balloon size on initial success, acute complications, and restenosis after percutaneous transluminal coronary angioplasty. *Circulation.* 1988;78:557.
11. Mooney MR, Mooney JF, Longe TF, Brandenburg RO. Effect of balloon material on coronary angioplasty. *Am Heart J.* 1992;69:1481.
12. Tenaglia AN, Quigley PJ, Keriakes DJ, et al. Coronary angioplasty performed with gradual and prolonged inflation using a perfusion balloon catheter: Procedural success and restenosis rate. *Am Heart J.* 1992;124:585.
13. Laskey MAL, Deutsch E, Hirshfeld JW, et al. Influence of heparin therapy on percutaneous transluminal coronary angioplasty outcome in patients with coronary arterial thrombus. *Am J Cardiol.* 1990;65:179.
14. McGarry TF Jr, Gottlieb RS, Morganroth J, et al. The relationship of anticoagulation level and complications after successful percutaneous transluminal coronary angioplasty. *Am Heart J.* 1992;123:1445.
15. Ogilby JD, Kopelman HA, Klein LW, Agarwal JB. Adequate heparinization during PTCA: Assessment using activated clotting times. *Cathet Cardiovas Diagn.* 1989;18:306.
16. ESPRIT Investigators. Novel dosing regimen of eptifibatide in planned coronary stent implantation (ESPRIT): A randomised, placebo-controlled trial. *Lancet.* 2000;356:2037.
17. Tolleson TR, O'Shea JC, Bittl JA, et al. Relationship between heparin anticoagulation and clinical outcomes in coronary stent intervention: Observations from the ESPRIT trial. *J Am Coll Cardiol.* 2003;41:386.
18. Ellis SG, Roubin GS, Wilentz J, et al. Effect of 18–24 hours of heparin administration for prevention of restenosis after uncomplicated coronary angioplasty. *Am Heart J.* 1989;127:777.
19. Cohen M, Demers C, Gurfinkel EP, et al. A comparison of low-molecular weight heparin with unfractionated heparin acutely for unstable coronary artery disease (ESSENCE trial). *N Engl J Med.* 1997;337:447.
20. Antman E, McCabe C, Gurfinkel E, et al. Enoxaparin prevents death and cardiac ischemic events in USA/non-Q-wave MI: Results of the Thrombolysis in Myocardial Infarction (TIMI) 11B trial. *Circulation.* 1999;100:1593.
21. Ferguson JJ, Antman EM, Bates ER, et al; NICE-3 Investigators. Combining enoxaparin and glycoprotein IIb/IIIa antagonists for the treatment of acute coronary syndromes: Final results of the National Investigators Collaborating on Enoxaparin-3 (NICE-3) study. *Am Heart J.* 2003;146:628.
22. The Synergy Trial Investigators. The Superior Yield of the New Strategy of Enoxaparin, Revascularization and GpIIb/IIIa Inhibitors. *JAMA.* 2004;292:45.
23. Lincoff AM, Bittl JA, Harrington RA, et al; REPLACE-2 Investigators. Bivalirudin and provisional glycoprotein IIb/IIIa blockade compared with heparin and planned glycoprotein IIb/IIIa blockade during PCI. *JAMA.* 2003;289:853.

24. Bittl JA, Ahmed WH. Relation between abrupt vessel closure and the anticoagulant response to heparin or bivalirudin during coronary angioplasty. *Am J Cardiol.* 1998;82:50P.

25. Lembo NJ, Black AJR, Roubin GS, et al. Effect of pretreatment with aspirin versus aspirin plus dipyridamole on the frequency and type of acute complications of percutaneous transluminal coronary angioplasty. *Am J Cardiol.* 1990;65:422.

26. Clopidogrel in USA to Prevent Recurrent Events Trial Investigators. Effect of clopidogrel in addition to aspirin in patients with acute coronary syndromes without ST-segment elevation. *N Engl J Med.* 2001;345:494.

27. The PCI Cure Study Investigators. Effect of pretreatment with clopidogrel and aspirin followed by long-term therapy in patients undergoing percutaneous coronary intervention. *Lancet.* 2001;358:1527.

28. The EPIC Investigators. Use of a monoclonal antibody directed against the platelet glycoprotein IIb/IIIa receptor in high-risk coronary angioplasty. The EPIC Investigation. *N Engl J Med.* 1994;330:956.

29. The EPILOG Investigators. Platelet glycoprotein IIb/IIIa receptor blockade and low-dose heparin during percutaneous transluminal intervention. *N Engl J Med.* 1997;336:1689.

30. The EPISTENT Investigators. Randomised placebo-controlled and balloon angioplasty-controlled trial to assess safety of coronary stenting with use of platelet glycoprotein IIb/IIIa blockade. *Lancet.* 1998;352:87.

31. PRISM-PLUS Study Investigators. Inhibition of the platelet glycoprotein IIb/IIIa receptor with tirofiban in unstable angina and non-Q-wave myocardial infarction. *N Engl J Med.* 1998;338:1488.

32. CAPTURE Investigators. Randomized placebo-controlled trial of abciximab before and during coronary intervention in refractory unstable angina: The CAPTURE Study. *Lancet.* 1997;349:1429.

33. TACTICS-TIMI 18B Investigators. Comparison of early invasive versus early conservative strategies in patients with unstable angina and non-ST elevation MI treated with early glycoprotein IIb/IIIa inhibition. *N Engl J Med.* 2001;344:1879.

34. Ambrose JA, Torre SR, Sharma SK, et al. Adjunctive thrombolytic therapy for angioplasty in ischemic rest angina: Results of a double-blind randomized pilot study. *J Am Coll Cardiol.* 1992;20:1197.

35. Topol EJ, Nicklas JM, Kander NH, et al. Coronary revascularization after intravenous tissue plasminogen activator for unstable angina pectoris: Results of a randomized, double-blind, placebo-controlled trial. *Am J Cardiol.* 1988;62:368.

36. Pavlides GS, Schreiber TL, Gangadharan V, et al. Safety and efficacy of urokinase during elective coronary angioplasty. *Am Heart J.* 1991;121:731.

37. The TIMI IIIB Investigators. Effect of tissue plasminogen activator and a comparison of early invasive and conservative strategies in unstable angina and non-Q-wave myocardial infarction: Results of the TIMI IIIB trial. *Circulation.* 1994;89:1545.

38. Ambrose JA, Almedia OD, Sharma SK, et al for the TAUSA Investigators. Adjunctive thrombolytic therapy during angioplasty for ischemic rest angina. Results of the TAUSA trial. *Circulation.* 1994;90:69.

39. Cecena FA. Urokinase infusion after unsuccessful angioplasty in patients with chronic total occlusion of native coronary arteries. *Cathet Cardiovasc Diagn.* 1993;28:214.

40. Grines C, Ajluni S, Savns V, et al. Prolonged urokinase infusion for chronic total native coronary occlusions (abstract). *J Am Coll Cardiol.* 1992; 19: 33A.

41. Zidar F, Schreiber T, Jones D, et al. A prospective trial of prolonged urokinase infusion for chronic total occlusion (CTO) in native coronary arteries [abstract]. *Circulation.* 1993;88(suppl I):I-505.

42. Heintzen MP, Heidland UE, Klimek WJ, et al. Intracoronary dipyridamole reduces the incidence of abrupt vessel closure following PTCA: A prospective randomised trial. *Heart.* 2000;83:551.

43. Quigley PJ, Hinohara T, Phillips HR, et al. Myocardial protection during coronary angioplasty with an autoperfusion balloon catheter in humans. *Circulation.* 1988;78:1128.

44. Turi ZG, Rezkalla S, Campbell CA, Kloner RA. Amelioration of ischemia during angioplasty of the LAD coronary artery with an autoperfusion catheter. *Am J Cardiol.* 1988;62:513.

45. Landau C, Jacobs AK, Currier JW, et al. Long-term clinical follow of patients successfully treated with a perfusion balloon catheter for coronary angioplasty induced dissections or abrupt closure. *Am J Cardiol.* 1994;74:733.

46. Van Lierde JM, Glazier JJ, Stammen FJ, et al. Use of an autoperfusion catheter in the treatment of refractory vessel closure after coronary angioplasty: Immediate and six month follow up results. *Br Heart J.* 1992;68:51.

47. De Muinck ED, van Dijk RB, den Heijer P, et al. Autoperfusion balloon catheter for complicated coronary angioplasty: A prospective study with retrospective controls. *Int J Cardiol.* 1992;37:317.

48. Hirshfeld JW Jr, Ellis SG, Faxon DP. Recommendations for the assessment and maintenance of proficiency in coronary interventional procedures: Statement of the American College of Cardiology. *J Am Coll Cardiol.* 1998;31:722.

49. Bittl JA. Directional coronary atherectomy versus balloon angioplasty. *N Engl J Med.* 1993;329:273.

50. Bittl JA. Clinical results with excimer laser coronary angioplasty. *Semin Interv Cardiol.* 1996;1:129.

51. Holmes DR Jr, Mehta S, George CJ, et al. Excimer laser coronary angioplasty: The new approaches to coronary intervention (NACI) experience. *Am J Cardiol.* 1997;80:99K.

52. Reifart N, Vandormael M, Krajcar M, et al. Randomized comparison of angioplasty of complex coronary lesions at a single center: ERBAC study. *Circulation.* 1997;96:91.

53. Appelman YEA, Piek JJ, Strikwerda S, et al. Randomized trial of excimer laser angioplasty versus balloon angioplasty for treatment of obstructive coronary artery disease. *Lancet.* 1996;347:79.

54. The SHOCK Registry Investigators. Current spectrum of cardiogenic shock and effect of early revascularization on mortality. *Circulation.* 1995;91:873.

55. Hearn JA, King SB 3rd, Douglas JS Jr, et al. Clinical and angiographic outcomes after coronary artery stenting for acute or threatened closure after percutaneous transluminal coronary angioplasty. *Circulation.* 1993;88(pt I):2086.

56. Lincoff AM, Topol EJ, Chapekis AT, et al. Intracoronary stenting compared with conventional therapy for abrupt vessel closure complicating coronary angioplasty: A matched case-control study. *J Am Coll Cardiol.* 1993;21:866.

57. Maiello L, Colombo A, Gianrossi R, et al. Coronary stenting for treatment of acute or threatened closure following dissection after coronary balloon angioplasty. *Am Heart J.* 1993;125:1570.

58. George BS, Voorhoees WD III, Roubin GS, et al. Multi-center investigation of coronary stenting to treat acute or threatened closure after PTCA: Clinical and angiographic outcomes. *J Am Coll Cardiol.* 1993;22:135.

59. de Muinck ED, den Heijer P, van Dijk RB, et al. Distal coronary hemoperfusion during percutaneous transluminal coronary angioplasty. *Cathet Cardiovasc Diagn.* 1996;37:233.

60. Schomig A, Kastrati A, Mudra H, et al. Four-year experience with Palmaz-Schatz stenting in coronary angioplasty complicated by dissection with threatened or present vessel closure. *Circulation.* 1994;90:2716.

61. Farb A, Lindsay J, Virmani R. Pathology of bailout coronary stenting in human beings. *Am Heart J.* 1999;147:621.

62. Amin FR, Yousufuddin M, Stables R, et al. Non-elective intra-coronary stenting: Are the clinical outcomes comparable to elective stenting at 6 months? *Int J Cardiol.* 1999;71:121.

63. Ray SG, Penn IM, Ricci DR, et al. Mechanism of benefit of stenting in failed PTCA. Final results from the Trial of Angioplasty and Stents in Canada (TASC II). *J Am Coll Cardiol.* 1995;25:156A.

64. Serruys PW, de Jaegere P, Kiemeneij F, et al. A comparison of balloon-expandable-stent implantation with balloon angioplasty in patients with coronary artery disease. *N Engl J Med.* 1994;331:489.

65. Fischman DL, Leon MB, Baim DS, et al. A randomized comparison of coronary-stent placement and balloon angioplasty in the treatment of coronary artery disease. *N Engl J Med.* 1994;331:496.

66. TARGET Investigators. Comparison of two platelet glycoprotein IIb/IIIa inhibitors, tirofiban and abciximab, for the prevention of ischemic events with percutaneous coronary revascularization. *N Engl J Med.* 2001;344:1888.

67. Lawrence M, Mixon TA, Cross D, et al. Assessment of anticoagulation using activated clotting times in patients receiving intravenous enoxaparin during percutaneous coronary intervention. *Cathet Cardiovasc Interv.* 2004;61:52.

68. The ATLAST Trial Investigators. A randomized, placebo-controlled trial of enoxaparin after high-risk coronary stenting. *J Am Coll Cardiol.* 2001;38:E1608.

69. Haase KK, Mahrholdt H, Schröder S, et al. Frequency and efficacy of glycoprotein IIb/IIIa therapy for treatment of threatened or acute vessel closure in 1332 patients undergoing percutaneous transluminal coronary angioplasty. *Am Heart J.* 1999;137:234.

70. Muhlestein JB, Karagounis LA, Treehan S, Anderson JL. "Rescue" utilization of abciximab for the dissolution of coronary thrombus developing as a complication of coronary angioplasty. *J Am Coll Cardiol.* 1997;301:1729.

71. Gulba DC, Caniel WG, Rudiger S, et al. Role of thrombolysis and thrombin in patients with acute coronary occlusion during PTCA. *J Am Coll Cardiol.* 1990;16:563.

72. Braunwald E, Mark DB, Jones RH. *Unstable Angina: Diagnosis and Management, Clinical Practice Guideline Number 10.* Rockville, Md: Agency for Health Care Policy and Research and the National Heart, Lung, and Blood Institute, Public Health Service, US Dept of Health and Human Services. 1994.

73. ISIS-2 Collaborative Group. Randomised trial of intravenous streptokinase, oral aspirin, both, or neither among 17, 187 cases of suspected acute myocardial infarction: ISIS-2. *Lancet.* 1988;2:349.

74. Effects of tPA and a comparison of early invasive and conservative strategies in unstable angina and non-Q-wave MI. Results of the TIMI IIIB Trial. Thrombolysis in Myocardial Ischemia. *Circulation.* 1994;89:1545.

75. Hillegas WB, Dean NA, Lino L, Rhinehart RG, Myers PR. Treatment of no-reflow and impaired flow with the nitric oxide donor nitroprusside following percutaneous coronary interventions: Initial human clinical experience. *J Am Coll Cardiol.* 2001;37:1335.

76. Murphy DA, Craver JM, Jones EL, et al. Surgical management of acute myocardial ischemia following PTCA: Role of the IABP. *J Thorac Cardiovasc Surg.* 1984;87:332.

77. Phillips SJ, Kongtahworn C, Zeff RH, et al. Disrupted coronary artery caused by angioplasty: Supportive and surgical considerations. *Ann Thorac Surg.* 1989; 47:880.

78. Buffet P, Danchia N, Villemot JP, et al. Early and long term outcome after emergency CABG after failed coronary angioplasty. *Circulation.* 1991;84(suppl 3):III-254.

79. Lofti M, Mackie K, Dzavik V, Seidelin PH. Impact of delays to cardiac surgery after failed angioplasty and stenting. *J Am Coll Cardiol.* 2004;43:337.

80. Almeda FQ, Nathan S, Calvin JE, et al. Frequency of abrupt vessel closure and side branch occlusion after percutaneous coronary intervention in a 6.5 year period (1994–2000) at a single medical center. *Am J Cardiol.* 2002;89:1151.

81. Haase KH, Mahrholdt H, Schroder S, et al. Frequency and efficacy of glycoprotein IIb/IIIa therapy for treatment of threatened or acute vessel closure in 1332 patients undergoing percutaneous transluminal coronary angioplasty. *Am Heart J.* 1999;137:234.

CHAPTER (56)

Subacute Closure

James L. Orford, MBChB

The major cause of morbidity and mortality associated with balloon angioplasty in the present era was acute closure.[1] Acute closure is commonly defined as angiographically proven occlusion (Thrombolysis in Myocardial Infarction [TIMI] grade 0 flow) at the site of vessel injury, occurring within 24 hours of the index procedure. Acute closure following balloon injury is due primarily to intimal dissection, elastic recoil, and thrombosis. Because most cases of acute closure occurred while the patient was still in the cardiac catheterization laboratory, several interventional techniques were developed in an attempt to treat acute closure and prevent recurrent events.[1,2] The most successful of these interventions was the coronary stent.[3,4] Improved angiographic and clinical outcomes following coronary stenting soon led to the widespread adoption of routine stenting as the preferred treatment strategy for percutaneous revascularization.[5]

Although coronary stenting was certainly an effective treatment for intimal dissection and elastic recoil, thrombosis was not eliminated. It was soon recognized that subacute closure due to stent thrombosis would replace acute closure as the nemesis of the interventional cardiologist.[6] The incidence of stent thrombosis was as high as 20%, depending on clinical, angiographic, and procedural characteristics.[7–9] For example, Serruys and colleagues[8] reported the results of 105 patients who received 117 self-expanding, stainless-steel endovascular stents (Wallstent) in native coronaries (94 stents) or saphenous vein bypass grafts (23 stents). A total of 21 vessel occlusions were documented within the first 14 days, and 25 of 105 patients (24%) had complete occlusion on follow-up angiography 6 months.

DEFINITIONS: SUBACUTE CLOSURE AND STENT THROMBOSIS

Strictly speaking, subacute closure implies angiographically proven vessel occlusion (TIMI grade 0 flow) at the site of vessel injury, occurring between 24 hours and 30 days after the index procedure (in contrast to acute closure, or occlusion that develops within 24 hours). Clinically, stent thrombosis is commonly defined as any of the following occurring within 30 days of the index procedure: angiographically proven vessel occlusion, unexplained sudden death without proof that the stent is patent, myocardial infarction, or urgent target vessel revascularization. However, the terms *subacute closure* and *stent thrombosis* are often used interchangeably, and early stent thrombosis (<24 hours) may be referred to as subacute closure.

EARLY TREATMENT REGIMENS

As mentioned, although it was felt that stent placement adequately prevented elastic recoil and treated flow-limiting dissection, the presence of a foreign body constructed of noncorrosive metallic alloys that are inherently thrombogenic remained problematic. Initial treatment regimens designed to prevent subacute closure included oral antiplatelet agents (aspirin, dipyridamole, and dextran) and oral and intravenous anticoagulants (heparin followed by warfarin).[10] However, despite these complex and intensive periprocedural treatment regimens, large multicenter studies of patients undergoing elective coronary stenting continued to report an incidence of stent thrombosis of 3% to 4%, and the incidence was even higher when coronary stenting was performed as a "bailout" or emergency procedure.[11–13] Furthermore, the incidence of vascular access site and other bleeding complications with these intensive treatment regimens further increased the morbidity of coronary stent procedures.[11,12]

INTRAVASCULAR ULTRASOUND AND HIGH-PRESSURE STENT DEPLOYMENT

At about this time, intravascular ultrasound studies of coronary stenting revealed that, despite an acceptable angiographic result, most stents were not adequately deployed and that stent strut malapposition was common.[14,15] In the light of these findings, and with the understanding that stent thrombosis may in fact, at least in part, be the result of incomplete stent dilation rather than the inherent thrombogenicity of the metallic stent, it was hypothesized that systemic anticoagulation may not be necessary after stent insertion when adequate stent expansion is achieved.

Colombo and colleagues enrolled 359 patients who had undergone successful Palmaz-Schatz coronary stent insertion (<20% stenosis by visual estimation) in a study of intravascular ultrasound optimization of stent deployment.[16] All patients with adequate stent expansion confirmed by ultrasound were treated with antiplatelet therapy alone (either ticlopidine for 1 month with short-term aspirin for 5 days, or only aspirin). With an inflation pressure of 14.9 ± 3.0 atm and a balloon-to-vessel ratio of 1.17 ± 0.19, optimal stent expansion was achieved in 321 of the 334 patients (96%). Despite this limited antiplatelet regimen, only 5 patients suffered stent thrombosis (1.4%) (Figure 56-1). The authors concluded that the use of high-pressure final balloon dilations and confirmation of adequate stent expansion by intravascular ultrasound provides assurance that anticoagulation therapy can

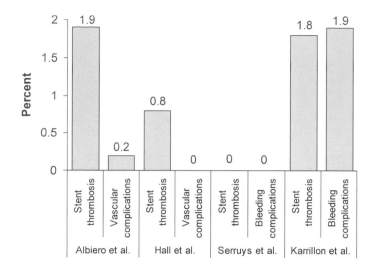

FIGURE 56-2. Stent thrombosis and peripheral vascular or bleeding complication rates in four studies of coronary stenting without intravascular ultrasound guidance and dual oral antiplatelet therapy alone; data from Albiero,[17] Hall,[18] Serruys,[19] and Karrillon et al.[20]

be safely omitted. These results were confirmed in further studies of similar stent deployment technique, with and without intravascular ultrasound guidance[17–20] (Figure 56-2).

DUAL ANTIPLATELET THERAPY

Four randomized, controlled trials compared antiplatelet therapy with conventional anticoagulation regimens[21–24] (Figures 56-3 and 56-4).

Schomig and colleagues randomized 257 patients to dual oral antiplatelet therapy (aspirin plus ticlopidine) and 260 patients to systemic anticoagulation (intravenous heparin, phenprocoumon,

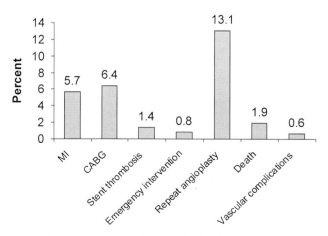

FIGURE 56-1. Six-month event rates following intracoronary stenting without anticoagulation accomplished with intravascular ultrasound guidance; data from Colombo et al.[16] (CABG = coronary artery bypass grafting; MI = myocardial infarction.)

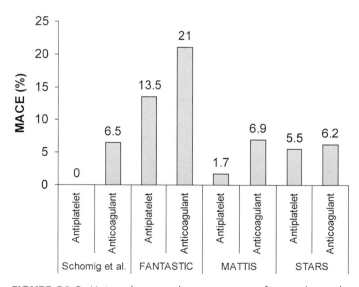

FIGURE 56-3. Major adverse cardiac event rates in four randomized, controlled trials of antiplatelet versus anticoagulant therapy following coronary stenting; data from Schomig,[21] Bertrand,[22] Urban,[23] and Leon et al.[24] (FANTASTIC = Full Anticoagulation Versus Aspirin and Ticlopidine Study; MACE = major adverse cardiac events; MATTIS = Multicenter Aspirin and Ticlopidine Trial after Intracoronary Stenting; STARS = Stent Anticoagulation Restenosis Study Investigators.)

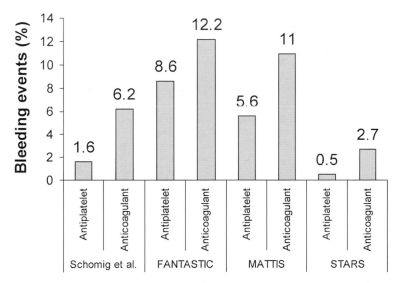

FIGURE 56-4. Bleeding event rates in four randomized, controlled trials of antiplatelet versus anticoagulant therapy following coronary stenting; data from Schomig,[21] Bertrand,[22] Urban,[23] and Leon et al.[24] (FANTASTIC = Full Anticoagulation Versus Aspirin and Ticlopidine Study; MATTIS = Multicenter Aspirin and Ticlopidine Trial after Intracoronary Stenting; STARS = Stent Anticoagulation Restenosis Study Investigators.)

and aspirin).[21] With antiplatelet therapy, there was an 82% lower risk of myocardial infarction, a 78% lower need for repeat target vessel revascularization, and an 87% reduction in the risk of peripheral vascular events. Occlusion of the stented vessel occurred in 0.8% of the dual oral antiplatelet therapy group, as compared with 5.4% of the systemic anticoagulation group (RR = 0.14; 95% CI 0.02, 0.62). Hemorrhagic complications occurred only in the systemic anticoagulation group (6.5%).

The Full Anticoagulation Versus Aspirin and Ticlopidine (FANTASTIC) study randomized 236 patients to anticoagulation (aspirin, heparin and oral anticoagulant) and 249 patients to dual oral antiplatelet therapy (aspirin and ticlopidine).[22] A total of 33 patients (13.5%) in the antiplatelet group and 48 patients (21%) in the anticoagulation group experienced a bleeding or peripheral vascular complication (OR = 0.6; 95% CI 0.36, 0.98). Major adverse cardiac events were less common in the antiplatelet group than in the anticoagulation group (2.4% vs 9.9%; OR = 0.23; 95% CI 0.05, 0.91). Subacute stent occlusion was less common in the antiplatelet group (0.4% vs 3.5%; OR = 0.12; 95% CI 0.01, 0.91).

The Multicenter Aspirin and Ticlopidine Trial after Intracoronary Stenting (MATTIS) study randomized 350 high-risk patients to either antiplatelet therapy (aspirin and ticlopidine) or anticoagulation (aspirin and oral anticoagulation).[24] The primary end point of death, myocardial infarction, or target vessel revascularization at 30 days was reached for 10 patients (5.6%) in the antiplatelet group and 19 patients (11%) in the anticoagulation group (RR = 0.51; 95% CI 0.25, 1.07). Major vascular and bleeding complications were less frequent in the antiplatelet group (1.7%) than in the anticoagulation group (6.9%; RR = 0.24; 95% CI 0.07, 0.85).

The Stent Anticoagulation Restenosis Study (STARS) trial compared three antithrombotic treatment strategies: aspirin alone, aspirin and warfarin, and aspirin and ticlopidine.[23] The primary end point was death, target vessel revascularization, angiographically evident thrombus, or myocardial infarction within 30 days. The primary end point was observed in 20 patients (3.6%) on aspirin alone, 15 patients (2.7%) on aspirin and warfarin, and 0.5% on aspirin and ticlopidine (P = .001 for the comparison of all three groups). Hemorrhagic complications occurred in 10 patients (1.8%) on aspirin alone, 34 patients (6.2%) on aspirin and warfarin, and 30 patients (5.5%) on aspirin and ticlopidine (P < .001 for the comparison of all three groups).

STENT THROMBOSIS IN THE MODERN ERA

A strategy of routine high-pressure coronary stenting and dual oral antiplatelet therapy has since been widely adopted. A pooled analysis of the results of six major randomized clinical trials of coronary stenting and associated nonrandomized registries included 6186 patients who received periprocedural aspirin and ticlopidine.[25] The incidence of stent thrombosis within 30 days was 0.9%. The correlates of stent thrombosis were persistent dissection National Heart, Lung, and Blood Institute grade B or higher, total stent length, and final minimal lumen diameter within the stent.

Similarly, a retrospective analysis of the Mayo Clinic Percutaneous Coronary Intervention database identified 4509 patients who underwent successful coronary stent implantation and were treated with dual antiplatelet therapy (aspirin and a thienopyridine) between July 1, 1994 and April 30, 2000.[26] Stent thrombosis occurred in 23 patients (0.51%; 95% CI 0.32, 0.76) within 30 days of stent placement. Multivariate analysis identified only number of stents placed as an independent correlate of stent thrombosis (OR = 1.80; P < .001).

[ ] STENT THROMBOSIS: CLINICAL OUTCOMES

Stent thrombosis, even in the modern era, is a highly morbid event. The aforementioned pooled analysis[25] reported a 6-month incidence of death of 21% and of death or myocardial infarction of 70% following clinical stent thrombosis. Similarly, the frequency of death and nonfatal myocardial infarction among the 23 patients with stent thrombosis in the Mayo Clinic series was 48% and 39%, respectively.[26]

CLOPIDOGREL

Based on the results of ex vivo studies of platelet inhibition and animal models of platelet deposition and stent thrombosis, and supported by encouraging efficacy data in patients with atherosclerotic vascular disease, many clinicians made the change from the combination of aspirin and ticlopidine to aspirin and clopidogrel.[27,28] This change, without definitive evidence from randomized controlled trials, was prompted by concerns regarding the incidence of neutropenia and thrombotic thrombocytopenic purpura following ticlopidine administration.[27,29]

[ ] OBSERVATIONAL STUDIES

Following this change in clinical practice, several centers analyzed their early experience with this new antiplatelet regimen to determine the relative efficacy of ticlopidine and clopidogrel in patients who received coronary stents. A retrospective analysis of the Mayo Clinic cardiac catheterization database compared the safety and efficacy of ticlopidine (500-mg loading dose, and 250 mg twice daily for 14 days) with clopidogrel (300-mg loading dose immediately prior to stent placement, and 75 mg/d for 14 days) in patients receiving coronary stents.[30] Mortality was 0.4% in clopidogrel patients versus 1.1% in ticlopidine patients, nonfatal myocardial infarction occurred in 0% versus 0.5%, stent thrombosis in 0.2% versus 0.7%, bypass surgery or repeat angioplasty in 0.4% versus 0.5%, and any event occurred in 0.8% versus 1.6% of patients, respectively (*P* = NS). Similar results were reported in patients undergoing PCI with smaller stents (< 3.0 mm).[31]

[ ] RANDOMIZED CONTROLLED TRIALS

The Clopidogrel Aspirin Stent Interventional Cooperative (CLASSIC) study randomized 1020 patients after successful stent placement to a 28-day regimen of either (1) 300-mg clopidogrel loading dose and 325 mg/d aspirin on day 1, followed by 75 mg/d clopidogrel and 325 mg/d aspirin; or (2) 75 mg/d clopidogrel and 325 mg/d aspirin; or (3) 250 mg ticlopidine twice daily and 325 mg/d aspirin.[32] The primary end point of major peripheral or bleeding complications, neutropenia, thrombocytopenia, or early discontinuation of study drug as the result of a noncardiac adverse event during the study-drug treatment period occurred in 9.1% of patients in the ticlopidine group and 4.6% of patients in the combined clopidogrel group (RR = 0.50; 95% CI 0.31, 0.81; *P* = .005). Overall rates of major adverse cardiac events (cardiac death, myocardial infarction, target lesion revascularization) were low and comparable between treatment groups (0.9% with ticlopidine, 1.5% with 75 mg/d clopidogrel, 1.2% with the clopidogrel loading dose; *P* = NS for all comparisons). Similarly, nonsignificant differences in major adverse cardiac events and stent thrombosis were documented in two additional randomized comparisons.[33,34]

[ ] META-ANALYSIS OF TRIAL AND REGISTRY DATA

Bhatt and colleagues performed a formal meta-analysis of published data from trials and registries that compared clopidogrel with ticlopidine in patients receiving coronary stents, identifying 13,955 patients.[35] The pooled rate of major adverse cardiac events was 2.1% in the clopidogrel group and 4.0% in the ticlopidine group (Figure 56-5). After adjustment for heterogeneity in the trials, the odds ratio of having an ischemic event with clopidogrel, as compared with ticlopidine, was 0.72 (95% CI 0.59, 0.89). Mortality was similarly lower in the clopidogrel group (0.48% vs 1.09%; OR = 0.55; 95% CI 0.37, 0.82).

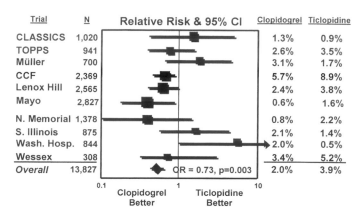

FIGURE 56-5. Meta-analysis of randomized and registry comparisons of ticlopidine with clopidogrel after stenting; data from Bhatt et al.[35] (CCF = Cleveland Clinic Foundation; CLASSICS = Clopidogrel Aspirin Stent International Cooperative Study; TOPPS = Ticlid or Plavix Post-Stents.)

ABCIXIMAB

The glycoprotein IIb/IIIa inhibitor abciximab may also reduce the incidence of stent thrombosis. The randomized, open-label, multicenter Controlled Abciximab and Device Investigation to Lower Late Angioplasty Complications (CADILLAC) trial documented lower rates of stent thrombosis in the study treatment arm that received both abciximab and a coronary stent during primary percutaneous coronary intervention for acute myocardial infarction (0.0%), as compared with balloon angioplasty alone (2.0%), balloon angioplasty with abciximab (0.8%), or coronary stenting alone (1.0%; *P* = .01).[36] These findings are consistent with the previously documented reductions in urgent target vessel revascularization and acute ischemic events following percutaneous coronary intervention with adjunctive intravenous glycoprotein IIb/IIIa inhibition,[37] but the benefit of adjunctive glycoprotein IIb/IIIa inhibitor administration in patients who have been adequately pretreated with dual oral antiplatelet therapy (aspirin and clopidogrel) has recently been questioned. Kastrati and colleagues randomized 2159 low- or intermediate-risk patients due to undergo elective percutaneous coronary intervention to either abciximab or placebo[38]; all patients had been pretreated with a 600-mg dose of clopidogrel at least 2 hours before the procedure. The incidence of the primary end point (the composite of death, myocardial infarction, and urgent target vessel revascularization within 30 days) was 4% (45 patients) in the abciximab group, as compared with 4 percent (43 patients) in the placebo group (RR = 1.05; 95% CI 0.69, 1.59).

HEPARIN-COATED STENTS

A novel approach to prevention of local thrombosis following coronary stenting is the use of a heparin-coated stent. Mehran and colleagues performed a multicenter, nonrandomized pilot study in patients with de novo or restenotic native coronary artery lesions.[39] All patients were treated with aspirin alone; any other antiplatelet or anticoagulation therapy was not permitted. The primary end point of stent thrombosis at 30 days occurred in 2 of 200 patients

(1%): in one after blunt chest trauma and in the other in the setting of essential thrombocytosis. Major adverse cardiac events (death, myocardial infarction, target lesion revascularization, and coronary artery bypass grafting) were observed at 30 days in 5 of 200 patients (2.5%).

INTRACORONARY BRACHYTHERAPY AND LATE STENT THROMBOSIS

Intracoronary brachytherapy for the treatment of in-stent restenosis delays healing following mechanical injury and is associated with late stent thrombosis.[40] This increased rate of stent thrombosis is attenuated with the administration of at least 6 months of dual oral antiplatelet therapy and it is recommended that every effort be made to avoid repeat coronary stenting.[41–43]

DRUG-ELUTING STENTS

The development of drug-eluting stents has revolutionized the practice of interventional cardiology. Angiographic and clinical restenosis rates have been dramatically reduced by the slow release of an antiproliferative agent from the polymer coating on the surface of the stent. But the in vivo effects of the various antiproliferative agents on local platelet activation and aggregation were unclear, and clinicians have been particularly vigilant for increased rates of subacute and even late stent thrombosis. In July 2003, the Cordis Corporation sent a letter to practicing clinicians reporting a number of isolated cases of stent thrombosis following coronary stenting with the Cypher stent.

Several reasons for the possible increased rates of stent thrombosis were proposed. Rapamycin, at serum concentrations similar to that documented following Cypher stent implantation, potentiates agonist-induced platelet aggregation in a time- and dose-dependent manner.[44] Also, antiproliferative agents may promote

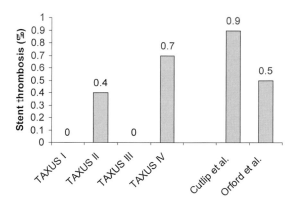

FIGURE 56-7. Stent thrombosis rates in the Taxus trials (I–IV)[54–57] compared with historical controls (bare-metal stents).[26,27]

local thrombosis by inhibiting vascular healing and delaying endothelialization of the injured coronary segment.[45] Loss of the normal antiaggregatory and anticoagulant properties of the healthy endothelium may promote local thrombosis, as is seen following intracoronary brachytherapy.[46] And finally, the rapid adoption of routine use of drug-eluting stents resulted in severe shortages of many stent sizes. Several commentators have suggested that this may have resulted in suboptimal procedural results due to placement of longer stents than necessary, as well as use of smaller-diameter stents that required additional postdilation.[47]

However, an analysis of the randomized, controlled clinical trials that have compared the Cypher stent with traditional bare metal stents has not documented any increased incidence of subacute closure[48–51] (Figure 56-6). Registry data is also reassuring with regards treatment of "real-world" patients[25,26,52,53] (Figure 56-7). Similarly, data evaluating the safety and efficacy of the paclitaxel-eluting Taxus stent has failed to document any increase in the incidence of subacute closure.[54–57] However, these results must be considered within the context of the individual study designs, which required longer periods of dual antiplatelet therapy; the majority of patients received combination oral antiplatelet therapy for at least 2 months, and many for 6 months or longer. In the light of the Clopidogrel in Unstable angina to prevent Recurrent Events (CURE), PCI-CURE and Clopidogrel for the Reduction of Events During Observation (CREDO) trials, it is likely that prolonged (> 6 months) therapy with aspirin and clopidogrel following coronary stenting will become more common, regardless of whether a drug-eluting or bare-metal stent was implanted.[57–59]

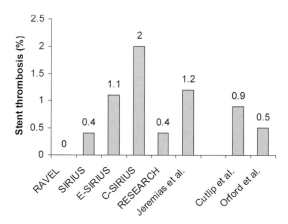

FIGURE 56-6. Stent thrombosis rates in the RAVEL, SIRIUS, C-SIRIUS, and E-SIRIUS randomized controlled trials[48–51] compared with historical controls (bare-metal stents).[25,26] (RAVEL = Randomized Study with the Sirolimus-Coated Velocity Balloon-Expandable Stent in the Treatment of Patients with de Novo Native Coronary Artery Lesions; RESEARCH = Rapamycin-Eluting Stent Evaluated At Rotterdam Cardiology Hospital; SIRIUS = Sirolimus-Eluting Stent in De Novo Native Coronary Lesions.)

TREATMENT OF STENT THROMBOSIS

The diagnosis of stent thrombosis should be considered whenever a patient presents with an acute coronary syndrome following recent coronary stenting. An angiogram should be performed as soon as possible with a view to immediate mechanical reperfusion. Rheolytic thrombectomy may be a particularly useful adjunctive reperfusion modality, facilitating visualization of the treated segment.[60] Intravascular ultrasound may also be useful to confirm adequate stent deployment and strut apposition, as well as exclude edge dissections that may have been overlooked. Gp IIb/IIIa inhibitors may also facilitate reperfusion and should be routinely administered.[60]

FUTURE DIRECTION

【 】 STENT MALAPPOSITION

Although smooth muscle cell proliferation, in excess, is the basis of in-stent restenosis, a certain amount of smooth muscle cell migration and proliferation is necessary for vascular healing. In conjunction with positive remodelling, it was feared that the absence of this physiologic response following drug-eluting stenting might predispose to late stent malapposition and stent thrombosis, as has been documented following intracoronary brachytherapy and placement of radioactive coronary stents.[29,61–64] Fortunately, it does not appear that stent malapposition is a common finding following drug-eluting stenting and is, therefore, unlikely to be a major contributor to subacute closure following treatment with a drug-eluting stent.[61,65] Nevertheless, further refinements of stent technique in the drug-eluting stent era are anticipated following further analysis of the intravascular ultrasound substudies of the aforementioned randomized clinical trials.

【 】 ALTERNATIVE ORAL ANTITHROMBOTIC THERAPIES

Several novel anticoagulant agents are currently under investigation.[65] Two subcutaneously injected synthetic pentasaccharide anticoagulants, fondaparinux and idraparinux, catalyze inactivation of activated factor X (Xa). Melagatran and its orally administered derivative act by directly inhibiting the active site of thrombin and have shown promise as alternatives to heparin. The role of these novel anticoagulants as adjunctive or alternative periprocedural agents following coronary stenting remains to be clarified.

REFERENCES

1. Lincoff AM, et al. Abrupt vessel closure complicating coronary angioplasty: Clinical, angiographic and therapeutic profile. *J Am Coll Cardiol.* 1992;19:926.
2. Scott NA, et al. Recent changes in the management and outcome of acute closure after percutaneous transluminal coronary angioplasty. *Am J Cardiol.* 1993;71:1159.
3. Roubin GS, et al. Intracoronary stenting for acute and threatened closure complicating percutaneous transluminal coronary angioplasty. *Circulation.* 1992;85:916.
4. Sigwart U, et al. Emergency stenting for acute occlusion after coronary balloon angioplasty. *Circulation.* 1988;78(pt 1):1121.
5. Oesterle SN, et al. The stent decade: 1987 to 1997. Stanford Stent Summit faculty. *Am Heart J.* 1998;136(pt 1):578.
6. Herrmann HC, et al. Emergent use of balloon-expandable coronary artery stenting for failed percutaneous transluminal coronary angioplasty. *Circulation.* 1992;86:812.
7. Sigwart U, et al. Intravascular stents to prevent occlusion and restenosis after transluminal angioplasty. *N Engl J Med.* 1987;316:701.
8. Serruys PW, et al. Angiographic follow-up after placement of a self-expanding coronary-artery stent. *N Engl J Med.* 1991;324:13.
9. de Feyter PJ, et al. Emergency stenting for refractory acute coronary artery occlusion during coronary angioplasty. *Am J Cardiol.* 1990;66:1147.
10. Mak KH, et al. Subacute stent thrombosis: evolving issues and current concepts. *J Am Coll Cardiol.* 1996;27:494.
11. Serruys PW, et al. Heparin-coated Palma1z-Schatz stents in human coronary arteries. Early outcome of the Benestent-II Pilot Study. *Circulation.* 1996;93:412.
12. Fischman DL, et al. A randomized comparison of coronary-stent placement and balloon angioplasty in the treatment of coronary artery disease. Stent Restenosis Study Investigators. *N Engl J Med.* 1994;331:496.
13. Schatz RA, et al. Clinical experience with the Palmaz-Schatz coronary stent. Initial results of a multicenter study. *Circulation.* 1991;83:148.
14. Nakamura S, et al. Intracoronary ultrasound observations during stent implantation. *Circulation.* 1994;89:2026.
15. Goldberg SL, et al. Benefit of intracoronary ultrasound in the deployment of Palmaz-Schatz stents. *J Am Coll Cardiol.* 1994;24:996.
16. Colombo A, et al. Intracoronary stenting without anticoagulation accomplished with intravascular ultrasound guidance. *Circulation.* 1995;91:1676.
17. Albiero R, et al. Results of a consecutive series of patients receiving only antiplatelet therapy after optimized stent implantation. Comparison of aspirin alone versus combined ticlopidine and aspirin therapy. *Circulation.* 1997;95:1145.
18. Hall P, et al. A randomized comparison of combined ticlopidine and aspirin therapy versus aspirin therapy alone after successful intravascular ultrasound-guided stent implantation. *Circulation.* 1996;93:215.
19. Serruys PW, et al. A comparison of balloon-expandable-stent implantation with balloon angioplasty in patients with coronary artery disease. Benestent Study Group. *N Engl J Med.* 1994;331:489.
20. Karrillon GJ, et al. Intracoronary stent implantation without ultrasound guidance and with replacement of conventional anticoagulation by antiplatelet therapy. 30-day clinical outcome of the French Multicenter Registry. *Circulation.* 1996;94:1519.
21. Schomig A, et al. A randomized comparison of antiplatelet and anticoagulant therapy after the placement of coronary-artery stents. *N Engl J Med.* 1996;334:1084.
22. Bertrand ME, et al. Randomized multicenter comparison of conventional anticoagulation versus antiplatelet therapy in unplanned and elective coronary stenting. The full anticoagulation versus aspirin and ticlopidine (fantastic) study. *Circulation.* 1998;98:1597.
23. Leon MB, et al. A clinical trial comparing three antithrombotic-drug regimens after coronary-artery stenting. Stent Anticoagulation Restenosis Study Investigators. *N Engl J Med.* 1998;339:1665.
24. Urban P, et al. Randomized evaluation of anticoagulation versus antiplatelet therapy after coronary stent implantation in high-risk patients: The multicenter aspirin and ticlopidine trial after intracoronary stenting (MATTIS). *Circulation.* 1998;98:2126.
25. Cutlip DE, et al. Stent thrombosis in the modern era: A pooled analysis of multicenter coronary stent clinical trials. *Circulation.* 2001;103:1967.
26. Orford JL, et al. Frequency and correlates of coronary stent thrombosis in the modern era: Analysis of a single center registry. *J Am Coll Cardiol.* 2002;40:1567.
27. Berger PB. Clopidogrel instead of ticlopidine after coronary stent placement: Is the switch justified? *Am Heart J.* 2000;140:354.
28. CAPRIE Steering Committee. A randomised, blinded, trial of clopidogrel versus aspirin in patients at risk of ischaemic events (CAPRIE). *Lancet.* 1996;348:1329.
29. Steinhubl SR, et al. Incidence and clinical course of thrombotic thrombocytopenic purpura due to ticlopidine following coronary stenting. EPISTENT Investigators. Evaluation of Platelet IIb/IIIa Inhibitor for Stenting. *JAMA.* 1999;281:806.
30. Berger PB, et al. Clopidogrel versus ticlopidine after intracoronary stent placement. *J Am Coll Cardiol.* 1999;34:1891.
31. Calver AL, et al. Clopidogrel for prevention of major cardiac events after coronary stent implantation: 30-day and 6-month results in patients with smaller stents. *Am Heart J.* 2000;140:483.
32. Bertrand ME, et al. Double-blind study of the safety of clopidogrel with and without a loading dose in combination with aspirin compared with ticlopidine in combination with aspirin after coronary stenting: The clopidogrel aspirin stent international cooperative study (CLASSICS). *Circulation.* 2000;102:624.
33. Muller C, et al. A randomized comparison of clopidogrel and aspirin versus ticlopidine and aspirin after the placement of coronary-artery stents. *Circulation.* 2000;101:590.
34. Taniuchi M, Kurz H, Lasala JM. Randomized comparison of ticlopidine and clopidogrel after intracoronary stent implantation in a broad patient population. *Circulation.* 2001;104:539.
35. Bhatt DL, et al. Meta-analysis of randomized and registry comparisons of ticlopidine with clopidogrel after stenting. *J Am Coll Cardiol.* 2002;39:9.
36. Stone GW, et al. Comparison of angioplasty with stenting, with or without abciximab, in acute myocardial infarction. *N Engl J Med.* 2002;346:957.
37. Bosch X, Marrugat J. Platelet glycoprotein IIb/IIIa blockers for percutaneous coronary revascularization, and unstable angina and non-ST-segment elevation myocardial infarction. *Cochrane Database Syst Rev.* 2001;4:CD002130.

38. Kastrati A, et al. A clinical trial of abciximab in elective percutaneous coronary intervention after pretreatment with clopidogrel. *N Engl J Med.* 2004;350.232.

39. Mehran R, et al. Safety of an aspirin-alone regimen after intracoronary stenting with a heparin-coated stent: Final results of the HOPE (HEPACOAT and an Antithrombotic Regimen of Aspirin Alone) study. *Circulation.* 2003;108:1078.

40. Waksman R, et al. Late total occlusion after intracoronary brachytherapy for patients with in-stent restenosis. *J Am Coll Cardiol.* 2000;36:65.

41. Waksman R, et al. Twelve versus six months of clopidogrel to reduce major cardiac events in patients undergoing gamma-radiation therapy for in-stent restenosis: Washington Radiation for In-Stent restenosis Trial (WRIST) 12 versus WRIST PLUS. *Circulation.* 2002;106:776.

42. Cha DH, et al. Use of restenting should be minimized with intracoronary radiation therapy for in-stent restenosis. *Cathet Cardiovasc Interv.* 2003;59:1.

43. Ajani AE, et al. Have we solved the problem of late thrombosis? *Minerva Cardioangiol.* 2002;50:463.

44. Babinska A, et al. Enhancement of human platelet aggregation and secretion induced by rapamycin. *Nephrol Dial Transplant.* 1998;13:3153.

45. Akselband Y, Harding MW, Nelson PA. Rapamycin inhibits spontaneous and fibroblast growth factor beta-stimulated proliferation of endothelial cells and fibroblasts. *Transplant Proc.* 1991;23:2833.

46. Cheneau E, et al. Time course of stent endothelialization after intravascular radiation therapy in rabbit iliac arteries. *Circulation.* 2003;107:2153.

47. Kereiaks DJ, Choo JK, Young JJ. Thrombosis and drug-eluting stents: A critical appraisal. *Rev Cardiovasc Med.* 2004;5:9.

48. Morice MC, et al. A randomized comparison of a sirolimus-eluting stent with a standard stent for coronary revascularization. *N Engl J Med.* 2002;346:1773.

49. Moses JW, et al. Sirolimus-eluting stents versus standard stents in patients with stenosis in a native coronary artery. *N Engl J Med.* 2003;349:1315.

50. Schampaert E, et al. The Canadian study of the sirolimus-eluting stent in the treatment of patients with long de novo lesions in small native coronary arteries (C-SIRIUS). *J Am Coll Cardiol.* 2004;43:1110.

51. Schofer J, et al. Sirolimus-eluting stents for treatment of patients with long atherosclerotic lesions in small coronary arteries: Double-blind, randomised controlled trial (E-SIRIUS). *Lancet.* 2003;362:1093.

52. Lemos PA, et al. Unrestricted utilization of sirolimus-eluting stents compared with conventional bare stent implantation in the "real world": The Rapamycin-Eluting Stent Evaluated At Rotterdam Cardiology Hospital (RESEARCH) registry. *Circulation.* 2004;109:190.

53. Jeremias A, et al. Stent thrombosis after successful sirolimus-eluting stent implantation. *Circulation.* 2004;109:1930.

54. Grube E, et al. TAXUS I: Six- and twelve-month results from a randomized, double-blind trial on a slow-release paclitaxel-eluting stent for de novo coronary lesions. *Circulation.* 2003;107:38.

55. Colombo A, et al. Randomized study to assess the effectiveness of slow- and moderate-release polymer-based paclitaxel-eluting stents for coronary artery lesions. *Circulation.* 2003;108:788.

56. Tanabe K, et al. TAXUS III Trial: In-stent restenosis treated with stent-based delivery of paclitaxel incorporated in a slow-release polymer formulation. *Circulation.* 2003;107:559.

57. Stone GW, et al. One-year clinical results with the slow-release, polymer-based, paclitaxel-eluting TAXUS stent: The TAXUS-IV trial. *Circulation.* 2004;109:1942.

58. Mehta SR, et al. Effects of pretreatment with clopidogrel and aspirin followed by long-term therapy in patients undergoing percutaneous coronary intervention: The PCI-CURE study. *Lancet.* 2001;358:527.

59. Steinhubl SR, et al. Early and sustained dual oral antiplatelet therapy following percutaneous coronary intervention: A randomized controlled trial. *JAMA.* 2002;288:2411.

60. Rinfret S, et al. Rheolytic thrombectomy and platelet glycoprotein IIb/IIIa blockade for stent thrombosis. *Cathet Cardiovasc Interv.* 2002;57:24.

61. Hong MK, et al. Paclitaxel coating reduces in-stent intimal hyperplasia in human coronary arteries: a serial volumetric intravascular ultrasound analysis from the Asian Paclitaxel-Eluting Stent Clinical Trial (ASPECT). *Circulation.* 2003;107:517.

62. Sousa JE, et al. Sirolimus-eluting stent for the treatment of in-stent restenosis: A quantitative coronary angiography and three-dimensional intravascular ultrasound study. *Circulation.* 2003;107:24.

63. Kalinczuk L, et al. Incidence and mechanism of late stent malapposition after phosphorus-32 radioactive stent implantation. *Am J Cardiol.* 2003;92:970.

64. Dilcher CE, et al. Dose volume histogram assessment of late stent malapposition after intravascular brachytherapy. *Cardiovasc Radiat Med.* 2002;3:190.

65. Degertekin M, et al. Long-term follow-up of incomplete stent apposition in patients who received sirolimus-eluting stent for de novo coronary lesions: An intravascular ultrasound analysis. *Circulation.* 2003;108:2747.

66. Davidson BL. Preparing for the new anticoagulants. *J Thromb Thrombolysis.* 2003;16:49.

CHAPTER (57)

Coronary Artery Perforation

James R. Margolis, MD

In the stent era, coronary artery perforation has become the most serious complication and a leading cause of death in percutaneous coronary intervention (PCI). Although preventable to a great extent, perforations are inevitable in any high-volume center. Prompt recognition and treatment of perforations can make the difference between benign and fatal outcomes. The incidence of coronary artery perforation varies with the complexity of disease under treatment and with the aggressiveness of individual operators. An operator who never experiences a perforation is probably underdilating lesions and underdeploying stents. The reported incidence varies from 0.2% to 0.6%. It is much higher when atheroablative devices are used.[1-3] Although there is no good series reporting the effect of stenting on the incidence of perforation, routine stenting most likely increases the perforation rate.

CLASSIFICATION

The classification of Ellis and colleagues[1] is generally accepted. In this classification, a type I perforation is an extraluminal crater without extravasation (this might also be termed a *pseudoaneurysm*), a type II perforation is a pericardial or myocardial blush without contrast jet extravasation, and a type III perforation is an extravasation through a 1-mm or larger perforation. This classification correlates with prognosis. A fourth category is designated cavity spilling, in which the perforation empties into an anatomic cavity: right ventricle, left ventricle, coronary sinus, and so on. A proposed new classification scheme is listed in Table 57-1. This classification creates categories that relate directly to treatment algorithms.

Small perforations can usually be solved by prolonged balloon inflations combined with reversal of anticoagulation. Large perforations require more sophisticated treatment. Perforations in vein grafts frequently resolve with simple measures. This is because scarring around vein grafts may be enough to limit extravasation.

Perforations in proximal arteries require treatments that will both solve the perforation and preserve antegrade flow. Blocking antegrade flow can sometimes solve more distal perforations. The most practical way to treat perforation in previously occluded arteries is to reocclude the artery. Perforations involving bifurcations are much more difficult to solve, because it may be necessary to stop bleeding in two branches while preserving flow to both branches. Occluding flow is the best way to solve perforations of small branches.

Perforations caused by balloons are relatively easy to solve, whereas those caused by stents are generally more severe and more difficult to treat. Devices are two-edged swords in that debulking prior to stenting may prevent perforations, but the devices themselves can cause very severe and sometimes untreatable perforations.

Guidewire perforations are more frequent, especially when hydrophilic wires are used in complex cases. In the usual scenario, the guidewire migrates distally in a tiny branch and eventually perforates the distal tip of the branch. This complication may not be recognized until after the guidewire has been withdrawn. Although the size of the leaks is generally small, they can lead to cardiac tamponade. In one reported series, 20% of perforations causing cardiac tamponade were the result of guidewire perforations.[4] This is especially a problem in the presence of glycoprotein IIb/IIIa inhibition. Because of relatively small and sometimes unrecognized leaks, guidewire perforation can lead to late cardiac tamponade.

Perforation is a major problem in patients with chronic total occlusions. Guidewire perforations in this setting are seldom a serious problem, unless the perforation is unrecognized and balloon inflation is made over the perforating guidewire. In cases of chronic total occlusion, a guidewire may enter a tiny branch

TABLE 57-1

Classification of Perforations

By size
  Small perforations
  Large perforations
By location
  Native arteries
  Vein grafts
  Proximal arteries
  Distal arteries
  Previously occluded arteries
  Involving bifurcations
  Small branches
By cause
  Balloons
  Stents
  Devices
  Guidewires
Perforations caused during treatment of chronic total
  occlusions

running parallel to the main vessel. If a balloon is inadvertently inflated within this vessel, serious perforation can ensue. Either of the aforementioned circumstances may result in cardiac tamponade and death. This is particularly distressing when the intervention is entirely elective.

HIGH-RISK SITUATIONS

Certain anatomic and morphologic conditions predispose to perforation. Recognition of these circumstances and appropriate adjustments in treatment strategies can prevent problems that would otherwise occur.

[ ] NATIVE ARTERIES

Certain locations in the native coronary arteries represent a higher than standard risk for perforation.

Lesions on Bends

In general, lesions on bends present high risks for dissection with balloons and extreme risks for perforation with atherectomy devices. The curving nature of the right and left circumflex arteries may explain the higher incidence of perforation in these vessels.[3] Excimer laser has the highest perforation risk when used on sharp bends. Excimer laser ablates only in a forward direction. Similar to the headlights on an automobile, laser light points straight when the road turns. Thus, excimer laser invariably causes perforation when used on a sharp bend. Rotablator has some ability to follow bends, but wire bias tends to drive the Rotablator burr toward the outer curvature, thus predisposing to perforation. When using Rotablator on sharp curves, the rule is to undersize

the burr by at least one and preferably two sizes. Directional atherectomy and cutting balloon are less likely to perforate lesions on bends, but the undersize rule is still operative when these devices are used in the curved portions of arteries.

Bifurcation Lesions

Bifurcations are troublesome to treat no matter what the strategy. Because plaque in this location frequently involves both the main artery and the ostium of the branch vessel, debulking strategies are often employed. The problem is that debulking devices may perforate the juncture of the bifurcation, thus producing a very large hole that requires emergent treatment. Treatment of this problem with a covered stent invariably sacrifices the side branch and may not solve the problem. The perforation may involve both branches; therefore, collateral filling of the side branch can lead to continuing leak. Worse, once the stent graft covers the side branch ostium, access to the side branch is longer possible.

The best way to deal with this problem is to avoid it. Theoretically, the bifurcation could be reconstructed with two "kissing" covered stents, but this is technically difficult because of the bulky nature of the stent grafts. In the face of a large perforation at the left anterior descending (LAD)/diagonal bifurcation, it may be best to occlude both branches with kissing balloons and send the patient to surgery.

Lesions in Branches and Distal Vessels

Because of their tapering nature, branches and distal vessels may be prone to rupture during stenting. Stents of appropriate size for proximal branches may be too large distally. This is particularly a problem in the distal LAD, where diffuse negative remodeling may be present. Figure 57-1 is an example of a long, drug-eluting stent in the LAD with a perforation occurring at the distal one third of the stent. With the advent of drug-eluting stents, it is more common to stent more distally and to use longer stents. The best way to approach these tapering vessels is to carefully interrogate them with intravascular ultrasound (IVUS) before and after stenting. Stents should be sized appropriately for the distal vessel, and then postdilated proximally with a short balloon of larger size.

Acute Margin Lesions

Lesions of the right coronary artery (RCA) at the acute margin represent a significant risk for perforation, especially with devices. The problem with this area is that the artery bends more acutely than is generally appreciated in the left anterior oblique projection. Compounding the problem is the bifurcation with the anterior ventricular branch and the propensity for severe stenoses to involve this bifurcation. When devices are used to treat this area, there is a tendency for the device to migrate in the direction of the anterior ventricular branch and thus perforate the artery at the inferior aspect of the bifurcation. This results in extremely large perforations that can become catastrophic if not treated within seconds.

Calcified Vessels

Calcified arteries are noncompliant. When stretched to extreme degrees, they tend to tear, especially at junctures where heavily calcified areas meet relatively normal ones. This is a particular problem

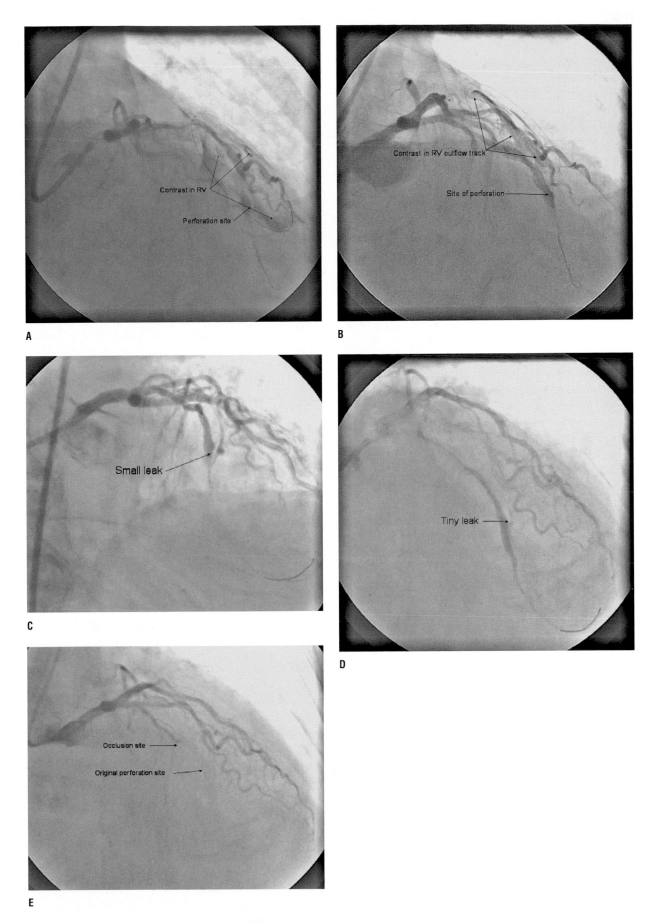

FIGURE 57-1. Type III perforation from the left anterior descending (LAD) coronary artery to the right ventricle (RV) treated with reversal of anticoagulation. (**A**) Type III perforation from mid-LAD to RV. Contrast in RV chamber. (**B**) Contrast seen in RV outflow track. (**C**) Twenty minutes after discontinuing bivalirudin anticoagulation and following 20-minute balloon occlusion, the perforation is almost sealed but a small leak continues. (**D**) Twenty-five minutes after, only a tiny leak remains. (**E**) Thirty minute later, the perforation is completely sealed, but the LAD is occluded.

when stents are placed in these vessels without proper preparation with Rotablator or cutting balloon. When the stents are deployed, they cannot be expanded fully. High-pressure balloons are then used, and the resulting uneven expansion of noncalcified areas leads to perforation or rupture. The mechanisms are similar to those described under vein grafts and eccentric lesions (*vida infra*).

[ ] VEIN GRAFTS

Vein graft perforations generally occur when a resistant lesion suddenly responds to high-pressure balloon inflation. Pathologically, these are tears or ruptures as opposed to discrete holes. These resistant lesions may be the result of old fibrosis, sometimes outside the wall of the vein graft. The vein graft itself is relatively thin walled. Once resistance of the fibrous tissue is overwhelmed, the graft itself ruptures. Clinically, this is seen as an imprint that persists on an inflated balloon despite high pressure. If the imprint suddenly resolves as, for example, a single bar increase in pressure, the operator should be concerned that rupture has occurred. In this instance, it is prudent to inject around the deflated balloon before removing it. If perforation has occurred, the balloon can be reinflated at low pressure while anticoagulation is reversed and preparations are made for stent grafting.

Because vein grafts are normally embedded in scar tissue and there is no pericardium, vein graft perforations usually act differently from those in native vessels. Following perforation of a vein graft, extravasation is generally limited by the dense surrounding cicatrix. This is especially true of vein grafts to the lateral left ventricle and posterior surface of the heart. These perforations can usually be treated with reversal of anticoagulation and observation. There are exceptions to this rule, especially in the proximal and mid-portions of grafts to the LAD and RCA. Vein graft perforations tend to be large. When they do bleed freely, blood loss is extreme and early and effective treatment is mandatory. The first treatment must always be to cover the perforation with an inflated balloon.

[ ] ECCENTRIC LESIONS

Plaque eccentricity is the single most important morphologic feature that portends a propensity to perforation. Thick atheroma on one side and thin, frequently normal, arterial walls on the other characterize eccentric plaques. Balloon inflation and stenting tend to preferentially stretch the thin normal wall while barely affecting the noncompliant plaque. This is especially true when the plaque is diffusely fibrotic or heavily calcified. This is one condition in which preparation of the vessel with cutting balloon or a debulking device prior to stenting may actually reduce the risk of perforation. Routine use of IVUS prior to stenting will identify extreme eccentricity that may not be evident on the angiogram. Sumitsuji and colleagues in the Japanese Intervention and Ultrasound Study group have identified three ultrasound patterns that may predict perforation: (1) severe eccentric calcified plaque with weak segment on the opposite side; (2) severe eccentric fibrous plaque with weak segment on the opposite side; and (3) severe superficial calcium with weak segment in the opposite side.[5]

[ ] GUIDEWIRE PERFORATIONS (FIGURE 57-2)

Guidewire perforations are a product of technologic advance. They occur most frequently with hydrophilic wires. The extreme lubricity

of these wires allows them to migrate distally into and out of the tips of small branches without being noticed. During difficult cases, involving multiple balloon exchanges, it is not unusual to find the tip of a hydrophilic wire several centimeters into the pericardial space. Usually, this does not result in a clinical problem. Occasionally, it can result in a minor or major leak into the pericardium that is difficult or impossible to resolve.

The best way to prevent guidewire perforations is to avoid hydrophilic wires whenever possible, but guidewire perforations can also occur with conventional wires, especially ones with stiffer tips. Unfortunately, hydrophilic wires are most useful in the most difficult cases. In such cases, it is good practice to exchange the hydrophilic wire for a conventional wire at the earliest opportunity. When using hydrophilic wires, it is important to be constantly aware of distal tip position and to guard against distal migration. Problems with guidewire perforation are accentuated in the presence of glycoprotein IIb/IIIa inhibitors. Most guidewire perforations can be easily solved with reversal of anticoagulation. When IIb/IIIa inhibitors are used, anticoagulation reversal is prolonged.

[ ] AORTIC PERFORATIONS

In a single case, my colleagues and I had the experience of a pinhole leak in the aortic root resulting form stenting of the RCA ostium. This occurred in an elderly patient with a calcified aorta. The aortic location of the leak was immediately above the RCA ostium and could not be distinguished angiographically from a proximal RCA perforation. This problem was only identified at surgery after stent grafting of the proximal RCA and its ostium failed to correct the problem. It was possible to suture the small aortic hole without cardiopulmonary bypass and without grafting the coronary artery.

ROLE OF ANTICOAGULATION

Effective management of perforations is greatly dependent on the ability to reverse anticoagulation. Different anticoagulants have different levels of reversibility and differing times required to reverse their effects. All anticoagulants can be reversed with large amounts of fresh frozen plasma and platelets. Unfortunately, the time required to obtain these agents from the blood bank and subsequently administer them is at best 1 hour and usually much longer.

[ ] HEPARIN

Heparin is the anticoagulant most commonly used for PCI. In the case of perforation, it is the anticoagulant that can be most quickly and completely reversed (using protamine). Although protamine reversal should be instantaneous, in reality it takes almost 30 minutes to achieve a normal activated clotting time (ACT) in the setting of perforation. Because protamine titrations are not generally available in the catheterization laboratory, it is necessary to perform a de facto titration by guessing at the initial protamine dose and giving additional protamine after serial ACT measurements. There is a minimum delay of 10 to 15 minutes between doses. If

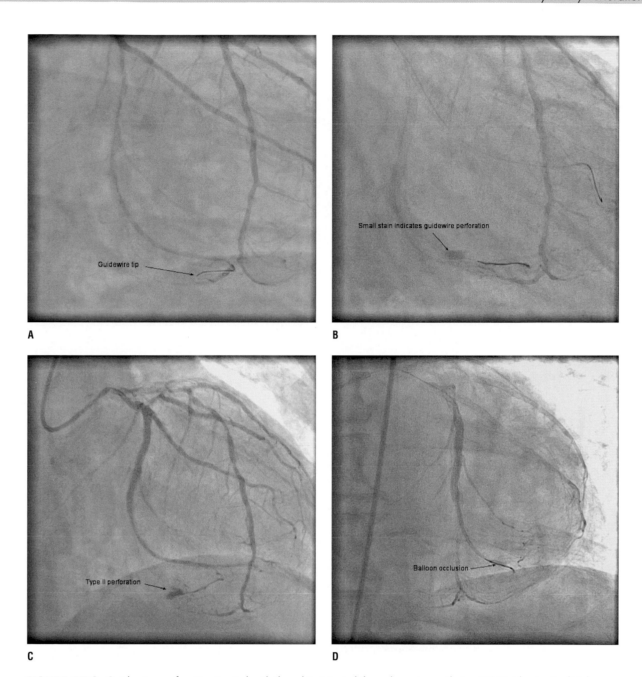

FIGURE 57-2. Guidewire perforation treated with thrombin injected through a microcatheter. (**A**) Guidewire in distal portion of small branch. (**B**) Faint contrast stain during first post-PCI injection. (**C**) Subsequent injection shows type II perforation. (**D**) Balloon inflated at low pressure temporarily stops the leak. (**E**) Post–balloon inflation, the perforation is not fully sealed. (**F**) Type II leak resumes within a few minutes postballoon. (**G**) Post-thrombin, the perforation is sealed without interrupting flow to other branches. (*continued*)

too much protamine is given initially, the protamine itself acts as an anticoagulant, and the operator does not know what to do in the face of a persistently elevated ACT. There is also the problem of reabsorption of heparin from adipose tissue and release of protein-bound heparin. Thus, the theoretically instantaneous reversal of heparin does not take place under real-world conditions. The heparin problem is further complicated by the concomitant use of glycoprotein IIb/IIIa inhibitors. It is extremely difficult to reverse anticoagulation in the presence of these agents.

DIRECT THROMBIN INHIBITION

Direct thrombin inhibition with bivalirudin in lieu of heparin has become increasingly popular in the United States. The advantages of bivalirudin are predictable pharmacokinetics and the ability to avoid concomitant administration of a glycoprotein IIb/IIIa inhibitor. The half-life of bivalirudin is 25 minutes. After two half-lives (50 minutes), anticoagulation is essentially finished. Although there is no readily available antagonist to bivalirudin, its effect is dissipated in less time than it takes to obtain and infuse fresh frozen plasma. Because bivalirudin blocks thrombin-induced

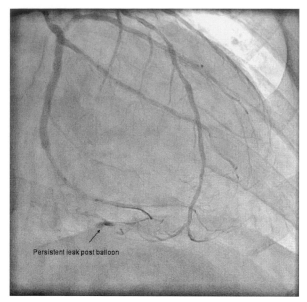

E

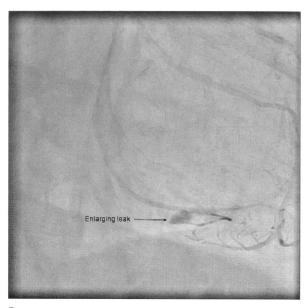

F

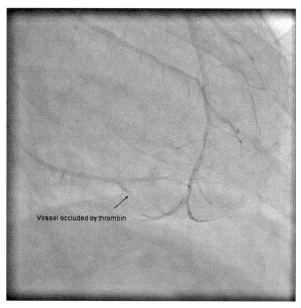

G

FIGURE 57-2. (*continued*)

platelet aggregation, it is unnecessary to give concomitant IIb/IIIa inhibitors, even in the presence of unstable angina.[6] This is a major advantage of bivalirudin, if perforation occurs.

【 】 THIENOPYRIDINES

Theoretically, the presence of thienopyridines should make it difficult to stop bleeding after coronary perforation. There is no specific information on this subject either in the literature or in my personal experience. My colleagues and I give thienopyridines during or immediately after stent procedures; pretreatment is the exception. However, an increasing number of patients undergoing PCI are receiving chronic thienopyridine therapy. In these patients, platelet transfusion would be the only way to completely reverse anticoagulation.

【 】 GLYCOPROTEIN IIB/IIIA INHIBITORS

Glycoprotein IIb/IIIa inhibitors present the greatest problem when attempting to reverse anticoagulation after coronary perforation. Although these agents have relatively short half-lives, their effects generally persist, despite low blood levels.[7] Although there is no series that documents a poorer prognosis in patients with perforation who have been treated with IIb/IIIa inhibitors, it is generally accepted that that these agents complicate the treatment of perforation. There are only three possible solutions: (1) avoid use of IIb/IIIa inhibitors whenever possible; (2) avoid coronary perforation when IIb/IIIa inhibitors must be used; or (3) transfuse platelets when perforation occurs in the presence of IIb/IIIa inhibition. Glycoprotein IIb/IIIa inhibition is truly indicated only in the presence of thrombus (ie, acute coronary syndromes). High-risk situations for perforation occur mostly in chronic settings in which IIb/IIIa inhibition has little rationale. When an operator approaches situations that are high risk for perforation, this risk must be carefully evaluated before administration of these agents.

ROLE OF DEVICES

Devices have been discussed elsewhere in this chapter, especially in relation to lesions on bends, eccentric lesions, and bifurcation lesions. Here, each of the devices is discussed on an individual basis. In general, when used incorrectly, devices can be a source of massive perforation. When used correctly, they can actually prevent perforation by changing the compliance of diseased arteries and allowing ballooning and stenting at lower pressures.

[ ] BALLOONS AND STENTS

Balloons and stents are responsible for more perforations than all other devices combined. The major causes of perforations with balloons and stents are oversizing and stenting of highly eccentric lesions. In the series of Sumitsuji,[5] the stent-artery ratio was 1.25 or more in 67% of perforations, and 72% of perforations occurred when eccentric lesions were treated. IVUS guidance is invaluable in accurately sizing vessels and assessing eccentricity.

[ ] ROTABLATOR

Although Rotablator use has fallen over the past decade, this device is invaluable in the presence of heavy calcification. Perforation secondary to Rotablator occurs mostly with larger burr sizes and when treating lesions on sharp bends. In recent years, I have avoided large burr sizes, because complete debulking is no longer my primary goal. Rather, I am trying to merely change lesion and vessel compliance to permit full stent deployment. This goal can usually be accomplished using burr sizes of 1.5 mm or less—never more than 1.75 mm. With lesions on sharp bends, I invariably start with a 1.25 burr, then check compliance with a balloon before going to larger burr sizes. Compliance is evaluated by the ability to fully inflate a 2.5-mm or 3.0-mm balloon. When a larger stent is contemplated, compliance is verified with a larger balloon. If full balloon inflation is possible, then it should also be possible to fully deploy a stent. If an imprint remains on the balloon, even at high pressure, then further rotational ablation is necessary. I never exceed a burr size of 1.5 mm for lesions on sharp bends.

[ ] EXCIMER LASE

Much of the preceding commentary on Rotablator use is also true for excimer laser. The goal is not massive debulking, but rather compliance changes that will permit full stent deployment. Such compliance changes can frequently be accomplished with very small laser catheters used at higher-than-conventional energies. Excimer laser is absolutely contraindicated for lesions on sharp bends.

[ ] DIRECTIONAL CORONARY ATHERECTOMY

The safety of directional coronary atherectomy (DCA) is highly dependent on operator skill and experience. This method can be

extremely useful in preparing arteries for stenting but extremely dangerous when used overaggressively. Perforations secondary to DCA tend to be massive and possibly untreatable. Again, when the final goal is full stent deployment, aggressive debulking is unnecessary. To avoid perforations from DCA, IVUS guidance is essential.

[ ] CUTTING BALLOON

Cutting balloon is a hybrid between an angioplasty balloon and an atherectomy device. In terms of perforation, it tends to act more like a balloon in that oversizing is the most important cause of perforation. Similar to the debulking devices, the present role of cutting balloon is to change the arterial wall compliance to allow proper stenting. When used properly in this regard, cutting balloon can change lesions from undilatable to easily dilatable and easily stentable. In my practice, cutting balloon has eliminated the necessity for Rotablator in most cases. To avoid perforation from cutting balloon, I tend to slightly undersize the balloon but use relatively high pressures (ie, pressures high enough to fully expand the balloon).

[ ] PROBLEM WITH DEVICES ON BENDS AND AT BIFURCATIONS

As previously noted, cutting and ablating devices must be used with extreme caution when treating lesions on bends and when treating bifurcation lesions. For bifurcation lesions, these devices are especially dangerous when used in the direction of side branches, because side branches generally arise at steep angles.

ROLE OF STENTING

At present, stents are used in nearly 100% of PCI procedures. It is not surprising that they are involved in a high percentage of perforations. Some of these perforations are caused by balloon angioplasty or another device used prior to stenting. When this occurs, deployment of a conventional stent is absolutely contraindicated. Despite reports to the contrary,[8] stent deployment almost invariably worsens the problem and rarely solves it. The stent serves only to enlarge the perforation, thus converting a potentially manageable problem into a disaster. Covered stents, of course, are the exceptions to this rule and are the most useful tools for managing large perforations.

The conundrum of stenting and perforation is that one strives to achieve as large a lumen as possible within the stent, but the larger the stent-artery ratio, the higher the likelihood of perforation. IVUS guidance and proper preparation of arteries prior to stenting are the best ways to prevent perforation. One should aim for stent-artery ratios of 1:1.1.[5] If IVUS suggests poorly compliant plaque (eg, diffuse fibrosis with negative remodeling, heavy calcification, etc) or significant eccentricity, or both, primary stenting should be avoided. In these cases, the arteries need further preparation prior to stenting. This can be done with cutting balloon, undersized balloons at very high pressures, or with cutting or ablating devices. If high stent deployment pressures are anticipated, a slightly undersized stent should be chosen. This stent can be postdilated with a larger balloon once the initial result has been assessed by IVUS.

PREVENTION

Although perforation is a relatively uncommon complication, its sequela is so devastating that all measures must be taken to prevent it. Most perforations are preventable. Operators must be constantly cognizant of high-risk situations and properly prepare arteries prior to stenting. If an artery cannot be properly prepared, stents should not be used. Oversizing must be avoided. In high-risk situations, devices, balloons, and stents should be slightly undersized. Routine IVUS use is integral to each of these disciplines. Guidewire perforations are best prevented by using hydrophilic wires only when necessary, exchanging these wires for conventional wires whenever possible, and being constantly aware of the potential for guidewire perforation in long, complex cases.

MANAGEMENT

Coronary perforation is an emergency. The window of opportunity for effective treatment can be quite short, sometimes less than 1 minute. Treatment delay can mean the difference between life and death. Mortality in type III perforations (large perforations with a jet of contrast) is 19%.[1] When pericardial tamponade occurs, mortality is 42%.[9] When pericardial tamponade occurs in the first 20 minutes, mortality approaches 60%.[9] Appropriate action in the first minute can prevent the occurrence of tamponade. Every catheterization laboratory should have the following basic materials available to treat perforation.

- Angioplasty balloons.
- Pericardiocentesis tray.
- Covered stents.
- ACT machine.

If these materials are not immediately available, the window of opportunity may be lost.

The single most important piece of equipment for the emergency management of perforation is the simple angioplasty balloon. Balloons are the first line of defense, because they are used to temporarily seal the hole while other more definitive measures are prepared. Even in patients who become abruptly hypotensive following perforation, sealing the hole will frequently stabilize blood pressure without concomitant pericardiocentesis or fluid administration. Because the opportunity to stabilize the patient with this approach may last only 30 to 60 seconds, any delay in searching for a balloon outside the catheterization laboratory may result in devastating consequences. Any balloon of any size is satisfactory, and an unprepared balloon is as effective as one that is carefully prepped.

Pericardiocentesis is not infrequently necessary to stabilize blood pressure and preserve cardiac output. Materials for pericardiocentesis must be immediately available.

Covered stents are the definitive treatment for coronary artery perforation. They have revolutionized the treatment of this condition. Covered stents of various sizes and length must be immediately available. Stents that are too short may not cover the hole. Stents that are too long may cover important side branches.

Reversal of anticoagulation is a mainstay of the treatment of perforation. Sometimes this is the only necessary treatment. Satisfactory reversal of anticoagulation is best determined by return of ACT to normal.

Prerequisites for the intermediate treatment of coronary artery perforation include the following:

- A second interventional cardiologist.
- Surgical standby.
- Echocardiography.
- Platelets.
- Coils.

If the patient becomes hemodynamically unstable or pericardiocentesis must be performed, a second experienced physician is invaluable. The second physician also can serve as a sounding board for ideas regarding definitive care. Sometimes it is necessary to invent solutions to individual perforation problems. In such cases, the interchange of ideas between two experienced interventional cardiologists may produce a solution that neither alone could have devised.

Surgical standby has become less and less important during PCI. Some coronary perforations cannot be solved in the catheterization laboratory. Sometimes it is better to stabilize the patient with balloon tamponade of the perforation, with or without pericardiocentesis, and then take the patient to surgery. This is a decision best made by interplay between the interventional cardiologist and surgeon. It is essential that the patient not be taken to surgery while still actively bleeding into the pericardium. The transfer time and time to open the chest and gain control of bleeding exceeds 30 minutes under the best of circumstances. The concomitant blood loss combined with pericardial tamponade during this time may lead to irreversible cardiac end-organ damage. Surgical mortality is high in these very sick patients–18% in one large series.[3] These patients frequently have bleeding into the myocardium, which poses a major surgical problem. All medical efforts to solve the problem should be exhausted before sending a patient to surgery.[3] Specific exceptions to this caveat include certain bifurcation lesions, in which covered stenting will sacrifice one or more large side branches, and perforations that involve the aorta.

The echocardiogram is invaluable in determining the hemodynamic effect of a perforation and whether or not it has been solved. Small or no pericardial effusion suggests that it will be possible to solve the problem in the catheterization laboratory without pericardiocentesis. Large effusions require pericardiocentesis, continuous pericardial drainage, and a possible trip to the operating room.

In the presence of glycoprotein IIb/IIIa inhibitors or thienopyridines, or both, platelet transfusion may be required to reverse anticoagulation. Because there is an inherent delay in obtaining and infusing platelets, the decision to transfuse platelets must be made early in the treatment course. The urgency of the situation must be properly communicated to the blood bank.

Vascular coils may be useful in occluding small branches that have perforated.[10] This is especially true in the case of guidewire perforations. The availability of coils and operator experience with their use can save an otherwise difficult situation. Many interventional cardiologists have no experience with coils. The assistance of an interventional radiologist or neuroradiologist may be required.

It is worthwhile to establish a liaison with such individuals in anticipation of needing their help in an emergency.

TREATMENT ALGORITHM

[ ] STAY COOL AND NEVER LOSE GUIDEWIRE POSITION

There are two absolute caveats in the management of coronary artery perforation: stay cool and never lose guidewire position. These two caveats are grouped together, because if the operator panics when a perforation is first noticed, he or she may by reflex remove the guidewire. Alternatively, if a small perforation is noted, there is a natural tendency to rationalize it away with such thoughts as "it is only a small branch" or "it will stop spontaneously when the anticoagulation goes away." In such cases the guidewire may be removed only to find that the perforation is a much greater problem than originally thought.

A large perforation is a true emergency. However, once bleeding has been controlled (with a balloon), there is usually plenty of time to proceed in an orderly manner. If guidewire position is lost, it may be impossible to control bleeding. Recrossing with a guidewire may not be possible. In this setting, the guidewire tends to exit through the perforation.

[ ] RECOGNIZE PERFORATION IMMEDIATELY

It should be the habit of an interventional cardiologist to be vigilant about looking for perforation after device use, balloon dilation, and stenting. Small perforations recognized early are easy to treat. Even small perforations left untreated can lead to cardiac tamponade and death. When additional balloon dilatation, stenting, or both are performed in the presence of unrecognized small perforations, the perforations invariably enlarge and lead to major bleeding.

First Action: Block the Perforation

As one learns in any elementary first-aid course, it is imperative to control bleeding before undertaking any other treatment. In coronary perforation, inflating a balloon at low pressure across the entrance to the perforation controls bleeding. The essence of this treatment is time. Any balloon—even an unprepped balloon—is suitable. Balloon size is unimportant; the balloon need only be large enough to block the flow of blood. The fastest way to get a balloon in place is to readvance the last balloon used. For this reason it is a good habit to make a post-PCI injection while the balloon is still in the guiding catheter.

With large perforations time is so important that a delay of only 30 seconds may create a downward spiral, leading to death. Following major perforation blood pressure can fall 100 mm Hg in 30 seconds. This is due to a combination of blood loss, pericardial tamponade, and a vagal-mediated reflex from sudden distention of the pericardium. Treatment of this severe hypotension consists of stopping the bleeding and then performing pericardiocentesis. Pericardiocentesis will not be effective if the bleeding is

not controlled. In the 30 seconds necessary to open a pericardiocentesis tray, it should be possible to cross the mouth of the perforation and inflate a balloon at low pressure. On occasion, merely controlling the bleeding will allow the pericardium to accommodate the blood; blood pressure will increase spontaneously, and pericardiocentesis can be avoided.

Once bleeding is controlled, pericardiocentesis, if necessary, can be performed in an orderly manner with proper positioning of the patient and sterile preparation of the chest. Prior to pericardiocentesis, blood pressure should be maintained with intravenous fluids and vasopressors. These two measures are usually effective in maintaining a satisfactory blood pressure for 15 to 30 minutes, as long as bleeding is controlled. During this time, first efforts to reverse anticoagulation must be initiated.

Second Action: Stop and If Possible Reverse Anticoagulation

Although reversal of anticoagulation is fully dependent on the type of anticoagulation in use, the combination of fresh frozen plasma and platelets can be expected to fully reverse virtually any anticoagulant regimen. Procuring and infusing sufficient quantities of these blood products to control bleeding takes more than 1 hour. Therefore, if it appears that blood products will be required, they must be requisitioned at the outset.

Heparin. Protamine is a specific antagonist for heparin. It should be available in all catheterization laboratories where PCI is performed. Immediate administration of protamine is always appropriate when perforation occurs in heparinized patients. The usual initial dose of protamine is 10 to 20 mg, depending on how much heparin has been given and on the ACT level. We tend to err on the low side, because protamine itself is anticoagulant, and too much protamine will be counterproductive. Additional protamine is given, if the ACT is not normalized with the first dose. Titrating protamine administration in this manner usually results in complete reversal of anticoagulation in 30 minutes.

Direct Thrombin Inhibition. Reversal of bivalirudin is less complex. Although fresh frozen plasma is the only way to directly reverse bivalirudin, this is rarely necessary. The short and predictable half-life (25 minutes) of this medication means that merely turning off the infusion will reverse anticoagulation. Normal coagulation should ensue within two half-lives (50 minutes). Figure 57-1 shows a large (type III) perforation from the LAD to the right ventricle. This perforation sealed within 30 minutes after discontinuation of bivalirudin anticoagulation. At 25 minutes, the perforation was essentially sealed and the artery was patent. The operator chose to leave a balloon inflated an additional 5 minutes, during which the mid-LAD occluded within a stent. It is a difficult decision whether to remove the balloon in the presence of a small residual leak and a patent vessel or to proceed with further balloon inflation until the perforation is completely closed. In the former case, there is risk of the perforation's reopening, possibly after the patient has left the catheterization laboratory. In the latter case, there is risk of occluding the stented vessel.

Glycoprotein IIb/IIIa Receptor Inhibitors. These agents are the most problematic when perforation occurs. Reversal of heparin anticoagulation with protamine will normalize the ACT in patients treated with IIb/IIIa inhibitors,[11] but the antiplatelet effect persists. The only effective way to reverse these agents is with platelet transfusion. Theoretically, platelet transfusion is more effective against abciximab than against eptifibatide or tirofiban,[7] but in practice all three agents should be effectively reversed by platelets. Although there is a simple assay to measure platelet function in the catheterization laboratory, it is not available in most labs. From a practical standpoint it takes 1 to 2 hours to obtain and transfuse platelets. Glycoprotein IIb/IIIa receptor inhibitors are most troublesome is small perforations, especially guidewire perforations, which can generally be solved with low-pressure balloon inflations and reversal of anticoagulation. In the presence of IIb/IIIa inhibition, these small perforations can ooze for hours. Occasionally, they will appear to seal while the patient is in the laboratory and then start to bleed again when the patient is returned to the ward. This can lead to slowly developing pericardial tamponade that manifests surreptitiously in the middle of the night.

Despite these reservations, a practical approach to perforation in the presence of glycoprotein IIb/IIIa inhibitors is to reverse concomitant anticoagulation (heparin or bivalirudin), perform prolonged balloon inflation, and observe the results. In some cases, the problem will resolve without further ado.[11] Because of the long lag time in procuring platelets, these should be ordered as soon as the problem is recognized. It the perforation has been solved before platelets become available, so much the better.

Third Action: Solve the Problem

The problem is how to stop bleeding while retaining antegrade flow. In small perforations and guidewire perforations, the problem is frequently solved by reversal of anticoagulation and concomitant prolonged low-pressure balloon inflation.

Covered Stents (Stent Grafts).

When simple measures fail, covered stents are by far the most effective treatment. In the appropriate setting, deployment of a covered stent across the perforation is a simple, quick, and elegant solution. Bleeding stops immediately, even in a fully anticoagulated patient. The problem with stent grafts is that they are much more difficult to use than ordinary stents. Because of their bulk and stiffness, they require 7 French (Fr) guiding catheters, and they may not negotiate tortuous or diffusely diseased vessels. They cannot be used to treat small vessels or branches. In large perforations, there may not be time to do the various maneuvers required to deploy these stents. Side branches represent a major problem for covered stents. If the stent covers the ostium of a side branch, the branch will be sacrificed. If the side branch is small, it can be sacrificed. If the side branch is large, surgery should be considered as an alternative to stent grafting.

Before attempting to deploy a stent graft, it is best to reverse anticoagulation and to minimize bleeding to the greatest extent possible. If it is necessary to switch from a 6-Fr to 7-Fr guiding catheter, this must be done carefully and if possible in an unhurried manner. The exchange is made over a 300-cm guidewire, preferably a stiff wire such as the Ironman or Platinum Plus. Exchange for one of these wires is best accomplished through an over-the-wire or transit-type catheter. Although it may be possible to place the new wire as a "buddy" wire, this is not always easy to do in the presence of perforation. There is a tendency for the wire to migrate through the perforation or into a subintimal space that leads to the perforation. This is especially likely with the stiff wires that must be introduced. An alternative is to leave a partially occlusive balloon to block the perforation while passing the new wire alongside. The most important caveat is never to lose distal guidewire position. There is a strong likelihood that it will not be possible to recross for the previously stated reasons. If this is the case, a fatal outcome may ensue. If an operator is unsure whether he or she has the skills to change the guiding catheter and sheath without losing guidewire position, it may be best to send the patient to surgery with a balloon inflated across the perforation.

With the new guiding catheter and a stiff wire in place, it should be possible to deploy the stent graft without undue difficulty. If significant bleeding has occurred during the guiding catheter exchange, it may be prudent to reintroduce a balloon, tamponade the perforation, and make sure that the patient is hemodynamically stable. If there are signs of cardiac tamponade, it may be possible temporarily to stabilize the hemodynamics with intravenous fluid and pressors. Pericardiocentesis may be necessary at this point. It is better to perform pericardiocentesis during relative calm than to have to do so as an emergency while struggling to deploy a stent graft.

It is imperative to deploy stent grafts at high pressure. These are extremely stiff devices that require a minimum of 14 to 16 atm for proper deployment. To avoid endoleak, the stent graft must be long enough to cover the perforation with 4 mm margins on each side. If a shorter margin is necessary to avoid covering a side branch, the operator needs to weigh the importance of losing the side branch versus the possibility of not sealing the perforation.

Once the stent graft is deployed, bleeding should cease immediately. If bleeding does not stop, the graft is too small or underdeployed, is too short to cover the perforation with adequate margins, or there is a second perforation. Bleeding should again be controlled with a low-pressure balloon while each of these possibilities is considered by careful review of the angiograms. IVUS may be helpful. Even if bleeding is controlled with the covered stent, IVUS should be used to verify full stent deployment. More often than not it will be discovered that the stent graft is underdeployed. Stent grafts available in the United States are "stent sandwiches"–two stainless steel stents with a layer of fabric between. As a result, the outer diameter of these devices is 0.5 mm greater than the inner diameter. Thus, the stent may appear fully deployed on angiogram when it is in fact grossly underdeployed. IVUS will reveal this discrepancy and guide appropriate postdilation. When one has solved a perforation with stent grafting, there is a tendency to finish the case without further ado. This is a mistake. An underdeployed stent graft has a significant probability of subacute thrombosis.

Exotic Solutions.

In some situations, stent grafting will not be possible; these include diffusely diseased arteries, small vessels, and distal branches (including guidewire perforations). In these instances it is necessary to create solutions that fit the actual circumstances. The focus should be on controlling bleeding as opposed to preserving antegrade flow. In most of these situations, the amount of myocardium at risk is relatively small. The general approach to this problem is to permanently block antegrade flow. Although collateral blood flow may allow continuing leakage through the perforation, this is generally small and self-limiting.

When perforations are caused by stents, blocking antegrade flow may be difficult or impossible.

The most effective way to block antegrade flow is through coil embolization. Although this technique is not particularly difficult, it should not be tried for the first time in an emergency situation. If the coils are not deployed precisely, they can occlude the wrong vessel(s). It is worthwhile to learn the technique from an interventional or neuroradiologist, and to know where to obtain coils if they are needed.

An alternative to coils is the intentional underdeployment of a coronary stent. This can be expected to induce thrombosis when anticoagulation has been reversed. Although I have successfully used this approach, coils are a more elegant and more secure approach, when available.

Thrombin Injection. Injection of Gelfoam[12] or thrombin through a microcatheter can be expected to close distal perforations, especially those caused by guidewires. Figure 57-1 shows a distal branch perforation that was closed with thrombin injection. It was possible to close the perforation while preserving flow in all other branches. This would have been difficult to do with coils.

【 】 SURGERY SHOULD BE THE LAST RESORT

Most perforations can be solved with the methods described. If these methods fail, then surgery is the only other option. The cardiac surgeon should be notified as soon as a perforation is recognized and should participate in the decision-making process. Although surgery is best deferred until other measures have been exhausted, one should not wait until a patient is *in extremis* before sending him or her to the operating room. If the previously described approach to treatment is followed, it should be possible to maintain the patient in stable condition. Once the decision is made to go to surgery, preparations must be made to ensure that the patient remains stable during the transfer time and during the time necessary to induce anesthesia and open the chest.

Bleeding must be controlled with an inflated balloon across the perforation. If pericardial tamponade is present, the pericardial cavity must be drained before the patient leaves the catheterization laboratory. Although attention to these matters may create ongoing ischemia, maintenance of hemodynamic stability is of primary importance.

SUMMARY

Perforation as a result of PCI is uncommon but not rare. Any operator who performs several hundred interventions in a year can expect at least one perforation. The best way to prevent perforations is to recognize situations of increased risk and take appropriate precautions. When a perforation does occur, it is mandatory to promptly recognize it, avoid manipulations that make it worse (eg, stenting), and start treatment immediately.

The cornerstones of treatment are maintaining guidewire position and control of bleeding with a low-pressure balloon across the perforation. Prompt control of bleeding can prevent life-threatening complications such as pericardial tamponade. Reversal of anticoagulation is mandatory. Deployment of a covered stent across the perforation is the ultimate solution, but this is seldom easy to do and not always possible.

Surgery in this setting carries a high mortality. Most perforations can be solved without surgery. It is important always to be prepared to treat perforations without delay. This requires appropriate knowledge and skill as well as the immediate availability of the necessary equipment.

REFERENCES

1. Ellis SG, Ajluni SC, Whitlow PL, et al. Increased coronary perforation in the new device era: Incidence, classification, management and outcome. *Circulation.* 1994;90:2725.
2. Dippel EJ, Keriakes DJ, Tramuta DA, et al. Coronary perforations during percutaneous coronary intervention in the era of abciximab platelet glycoprotein IIb/IIIa blockade: An algorithm for percutaneous management. *Catheter Cardiovasc Interv.* 2001;52:279.
3. Gruberg L, Pinnow E, Flood R, et al. Incidence, management and outcome of coronary artery perforation during percutaneous coronary intervention. *Am J Cardiol.* 2000;86:680.
4. von Sohsten R, Kopistansky RN, Cohen M, et al. Cardiac tamponade in the "new device" era: Evaluation of 6999 consecutive percutaneous coronary interventions. *Am Heart J.* 2000;140:279.
5. Sumitsuji S. IVUS predictors of coronary rupture during PCI: Japanese IVUS registry of coronary rupture. Presented at the 19th Annual Interventional Cardiology meeting; March 24, 2004; Snowmass Village, Colo.
6. Lincoff AM, Bittl JA, Harrington RA, et al. Bivalirudin and provisional glycoprotein IIb/IIIa blockade compared with heparin and planned glycoprotein IIb/IIIa blockade during percutaneous coronary intervention: REPLACE-2 randomized trial. *JAMA.* 2003;289:853.
7. Del Campo CD, Zelman R. Successful non-operative management of right coronary artery perforation during percutaneous coronary intervention in a patient receiving abciximab and aspirin. *J Invasive Cardiol.* 2000;12:41.
8. Hammoud T, Tanguay JF, Rios F, et al. Repair of left anterior descending coronary artery perforation by Magic Wallstent implantation. *Catheter Cardiovasc Interv.* 1999;48:304.
9. Fejka M, Dixon SR, Safian RD, et al. Diagnosis, management, and clinical outcome of cardiac tamponade complicating percutaneous coronary intervention. *Am J Cardiol.* 2002;90:1183.
10. Assali AR, Moustapha A, Sdringola S, et al. Successful treatment of coronary artery perforation in an abciximab-treated patient by microcoil embolization. *Catheter Cardiovasc Interv.* 2000;51:487.
11. Keriakes DJ, Broderick TM, Whang DD, et al. Partial reversal of heparin anticoagulation by intravenous protamine in abciximab-treated patients undergoing percutaneous intervention. *Am J Cardiol.* 1997;80:633.
12. Dixon SR, Webster MW, Ormiston JA, et al. Gelfoam embolization of a distal coronary artery guidewire perforation. *Catheter Cardiovasc Interv.* 2000;49:214.

CHAPTER 58

Embolization and No Reflow During Percutaneous Coronary Intervention

Ted Feldman, MD, and Timothy A. Sanborn, MD

EMBOLIZATION IN EXPERIMENTAL STUDIES

The problem of embolization of plaque material during percutaneous catheter angioplasty and stenting has been recognized since the early development of balloon angioplasty. Shortly after the introduction of balloon angioplasty in an experimental model of angioplasty in rabbit aortic and iliac atherosclerosis, effluent debris was collected and analyzed by histologic and polarized light microscopic examinations for gross debris and cholesterol.[1] This study is often widely cited as showing no evidence for significant embolization during balloon angioplasty. A careful review of the results of that paper is prophetic. The authors found microscopically visible atherosclerotic debris in one of eight (about 12%) angioplasty procedures, and thin layer chromatography showed evidence of cholesterol embolization in two of eight (25%) of treated vessels. Although the authors chose to emphasize the proportion of studied vessels in which atheroemboli were not detected, the findings of atherosclerotic debris in between 12% and 25% of treated vessels is completely in line with clinical studies of patients that followed over the next 2 decades.

EMBOLIZATION IN CLINICAL STUDIES

Subsequent clinical work has found remarkably similar levels of evidence for embolization associated with PCI procedures. In the stent era, embolization has been detected in about 20% of simple native vessel stent implantation procedures based on the occurrence of creatine kinase, myocardial bound (CK-MB) enzyme release. For example, in the STARS (Stent Anticoagulation Restenosis Study) trial, patients with type A lesions who had completely uncomplicated, successful stenting with a single stent were included. In this group, the incidence of CK-MB release was 20%.[2] In the STARS registry, which included patients who had dissections, suboptimal stent results, or required additional stents, the incidence of CK-MB release was close to 30%.[3] Similarly, in the STRATAS (Study to Determine Rotablator And Transluminal Angioplasty Strategy) trial, almost 30% of patients had CK-MB release, caused by embolization of plaque debris during the rotational atherectomy procedure.[4] The majority of these enzyme elevations are not associated with clinical events.

Clinically apparent embolization occurs more frequently in saphenous vein graft (SVG) interventions. In-hospital major events occur in almost 15% of these interventions.[5] In contrast to the enzyme elevations seen with PCI in native vessels, these are clinical events. Thus, detectable embolization occurs in 15% to 20% of PCI cases overall.

One of the more severe manifestations of embolization is the no-reflow phenomenon—the failure of restoration of myocardial flow despite removal of the epicardial coronary obstruction. This finding was originally identified in experimental models of myocardial infarction.[6] No reflow occurs infrequently during percutaneous coronary intervention, complicating between 0.5% and 3% of procedures. It is most typically associated with reperfusion after acute myocardial infarction and in SVG interventions. The phenomenon is also relatively more frequent with rotational atherectomy. It occurs rarely in native vessels. The clinical sequelae of the no-reflow phenomenon can be both acutely and chronically severe. Patients have, in the most profound situations, hemodynamic collapse or a severe ischemic syndrome, depending on the size of the affected vessel territory. Both prevention and treatment have been challenging during the development of catheter intervention.

【 】 CLINICAL RELEVANCE

The short-term and long-term consequences of plaque embolization during percutaneous coronary intervention (PCI) have been studied extensively. Acute complications include the no-reflow phenomenon, slow flow in treated vessels, prolonged chest pain, and evidence of myocardial cell necrosis.

In the Primary Angioplasty and Myocardial Infarction (PAMI) trial, no reflow occurred during primary coronary intervention for ST-elevation acute infarction in 1.3% of over 1000 patients. Compared with patients who did not experience the no-reflow phenomenon during PCI, those who did had a significantly higher in-hospital and 6-month mortality rate. The in-hospital mortality rate of 2% for those without versus 13% with no reflow ($P = .04$) and a 6–month rate of 3% without versus 31% with no reflow ($P = .0001$) illustrates the striking clinical importance of this phenomenon.[7]

In another study, data were prospectively collected from more than 4200 consecutive patients undergoing PCI to identify those with no reflow. The phenomenon was identified in 3.2% of patients. Patients with no reflow were more likely to have acute myocardial infarction, unstable angina, and cardiogenic shock, or to have undergone SVG intervention. No reflow in this group was also highly predictive of post-procedural myocardial infarction (17.7% vs 3.5% in patients without no reflow). No reflow was similarly a strong predictor of in-hospital mortality. Administration of calcium-blocking drugs or nitroprusside was not associated with improved in-hospital outcomes in these patients, although antegrade flow rates improved in patients treated with nitroprusside in this group. Mortality was 7.4% in those with no reflow versus 2% in those without ($P < .001$; OR 3.6).[8]

Late consequences of these events have been characterized in numerous studies, suggesting a relationship between in-hospital CK elevations, reflective of embolization, and increased late mortality as long as 3 years after the index interventional procedure.[9]

【 】 PARTICULATE ANALYSIS

Various mechanisms for the clinical effects of embolization during PCI have been elucidated (Table 58-1). Most simply, mechanical disruption of the plaque results in fragmentation of plaque elements.[10] This has been clearly demonstrated in the SAFER (Saphenous Vein Graft Free of Emboli, Randomized) trial, in which particulate could be aspirated from interventional procedures in human saphenous vein graft atherosclerosis. A variety of plaque elements were retrieved, including plaque fragments, cholesterol crystals, foam cells, and amorphous debris.

In a study of the aspirated particles from 23 SVG procedures using the PercuSurge GuardWire system, a mean particle size of

TABLE 58-1

Proposed Mechanisms of No Reflow

Microvascular constriction and vasospasm

Distal embolization of thrombus or atherosclerotic debris, or both

Oxygen free-radical–mediated endothelial injury

Capillary plugging by red blood cells and activated neutrophils

Neutrophil-mediated endothelial cell dysfunction or vasoconstriction

Intracellular and interstitial edema

Intramural hematoma

Loss of capillary integrity due to completed myocardial infarction

Adapted from Klein et al[39] in Catheterization and Cardiovascularization Intervention, *copyright 2003, with permission from J Wiley and Sons, Hoboken, NJ.*

168 μm was noted.[11] The range was large, from a minimal of 6 to a maximum of 815 μm in the minor access, and 7 to 3427 μm in the major access of these particles. Particles were composed of cholesterol clefts, lipid-rich macrophages, fragments of fibrous cap, necrotic lesion core, and fibrin.

Many of the causes of embolization of microscopic debris into the small vessels of the distal microcirculation are well described as well. This is evidenced by studies of rotational ablation.[12,13] Debris of varying sizes of particulate has variable effects on microcirculatory plugging. Rotational atherectomy creates particulate debris with a mean particle size less than 6 μm. These smaller particles pass through the capillary circulation in the same manner as red blood cells. Larger particulate, which comprises about 20% of the rotational atherectomy debris or particle load, is trapped in the microcirculation and contributes to slow flow and CK elevations from this procedure.

Hori and colleagues studied the effective particle size and number in a coronary arterial microsphere embolization perfused canine model.[14] They found that small numbers of 15-μm particle emboli caused patchy myocardial ischemia and a paradoxical regional increase in blood flow from the effect of local adenosine on adjacent areas. Increasing numbers of emboli caused impaired flow reserve and decreased resting flow. For 100- to 300-μm particles, there was a dramatic reduction in the number of emboli needed to cause decreased resting flow.

Studies of embolization in carotid intervention models have been particularly enlightening. Ohki and colleagues used a model in which carotid bifurcation plaques were placed in polytetrafluoroethylene (PTFE) graft material to simulate a carotid plaque.[15] These were connected to a perfusion circuit. Continuous flow was provided through the plaque. A polymeric membrane filter device with multiple micropores was placed beyond the lesion. Angioplasty and stenting was performed using self-expanding stents. The particles released by stenting were captured and analyzed. The filter successfully captured almost 90% of the particulate that was released. The mean and maximum size of the particles that were released during filter passage, missed, and captured by the filter device were 3.1 and 500 μm, 2.8 and 360 μm, and 20.1 and 1100 μm, respectively. This study showed that the filter device in this model markedly decreased the release of embolic material during stenting.

Tubler and colleagues studied the collected aspirate in 54 patients who underwent carotid artery stenting using the PercuSurge GuardWire system for distal protection.[16] The aspirated debris was analyzed for histologic and cytologic findings. The maximum particle size among the three patients who had neurologic events was larger than that seen in patients who did not have events. The total number of particles ranged between 10 and 24 in these three patients. The maximum particle diameter ranged between 1725 and 7301 μm. The total number of particles among patients who did not have neurologic events clustered between 0 and 10 particles, although some of these patients had particle numbers between 10 and 20. Activation of platelets with distal microcirculatory plugging is another important mechanism contributing to distal embolization syndromes.

[ ] ROLE OF THROMBUS

Angiographic thrombus is a powerful predictor of PCI complications. In the clinical setting of acute coronary syndromes, macroembolization of clot is well known among PCI practitioners. Even when not clearly demonstrated, thrombus is usually present. Gross distal embolization is sometimes observed in these procedures. Many practicing interventionalists have had the experience of watching a fragment of clot, or thrombus, visibly embolize downstream during injections in the midst of PCI procedures.

[ ] VASCULAR REACTIVITY

Liberation of vasoactive humoral substances such as serotonin has also been implicated in the genesis of slow flow and no reflow. Serotonin levels have been measured in the distal coronary artery in patients after angioplasty or stenting.[17] Balloon angioplasty caused an increase in coronary sinus serotonin from basal values of 3 ng/mL to almost 30 ng/mL after balloon angioplasty and from 3.5 ng/mL to 114 ng/mL after stenting. This increase in liberation of serotonin was dramatically blunted by the administration of a serotonin antagonist, ketanserin. Coronary cross-sectional area distal to the site of dilation significantly decreased after angioplasty and stenting from 4.33 to 3.3 mm² after balloon angioplasty, and from 4.27 down to 2.86 mm² after stenting, consistent with spasm. Pretreatment with ketanserin diminished this decrease in distal coronary luminal area.

One candidate protein to cause coronary no reflow is tissue factor. This is abundant in atherosclerotic plaque. Scrapings from atherosclerotic carotid arteries have been found to contain tissue factor activity. In one study, coronary blood was drawn from six patients undergoing coronary intervention with a distal protection device PercuSurge, and the particulate material that was recovered from coronary vessels showed tissue factor activity. To examine the role of tissue factor in no reflow, blood was drawn via a catheter from coronary vessels in 13 patients during no reflow and after restoration of flow. Mean tissue factor antigen levels were elevated during no reflow compared with levels after flow restoration (194 pg/mL versus 73 pg/mL; $P = .02$). Tissue factor induced no reflow in a porcine model after selective intracoronary injection of

atherosclerotic material or purified tissue factor. These data suggest that tissue factor is released from dissected coronary plaque and is one of the factors causing the no-reflow phenomenon.[18]

Indirect evidence for the role of vasoactive mediators is seen in the attenuation of rotational ablation flow effects by the use of a vasoactive "cocktail."[19]

PREVENTION OF EMBOLIZATION IN SAPHENOUS VEIN GRAFT INTERVENTIONS

The problem of embolization during PCI became particularly apparent during SVG intervention. Both the volume of SVG atheroma and its nature make it prone to embolization during intervention (Figure 58-1). SVG intervention has become a common procedure due to the large number of patients treated with coronary artery bypass graft surgery. It is well described that beyond 3 years after surgery atherosclerosis of SVG become increasingly frequent.

As many as half of patients with SVGs have angiographic evidence of atherosclerosis at the 5-year mark following surgery. A large proportion of grafts are severely diseased by 7 to 10 years after surgery. In most PCI trials, the mean age at which SVGs undergo percutaneous

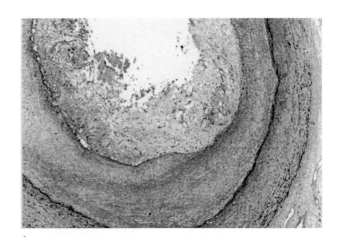

A

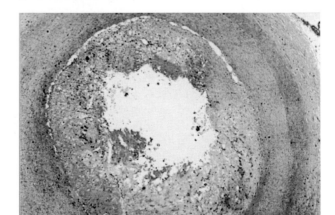

B

FIGURE 58-1. Histologic section from a degenerated saphenous vein graft. The thickened wall of the vessel is easily seen. The volume of plaque material is large, and its friable nature can be seen easily.

intervention is between 8 and 9 years after the original bypass surgery. In addition to the problems presented by the nature of the graft atheroma itself, patients are obviously a decade older than when their initial bypass surgery was done and represent a group with high frequency of congestive heart failure, prior myocardial infarction, depressed left ventricular function, and other comorbid conditions.

During PCI for SVGs, distal embolization is common. Patients who suffer distal embolization during these procedures have significantly poorer outcomes than patients who do not. The proportion of patients with major adverse in-hospital events after embolization approaches 75%, whereas patients without clinical evidence of embolization during their intervention have major adverse event rates in the hospital of less than 20%.[20]

【 】 PLAQUE REMOVAL DEVICES

Early attempts to improve the outcome of intervention in SVGs included the use of plaque removal or debulking using directional coronary atherectomy (DCA). In CAVEAT-2 (Coronary Angioplasty Versus Excision Atherectomy Trial), patients were randomized to receive DCA or plain balloon angioplasty (percutaneous transluminal coronary angioplasty, PTCA).[20] The initial angiographic success rate was improved with DCA (from 79% with PTCA to 89.2% with DCA). Six-month restenosis rates were similar, consisting of 45.6% for DCA and 50.5% for PTCA. Rather than decreasing embolization, distal embolization occurred more frequently with DCA than PTCA (13.4% vs 5.1%; $P =$ .012). Non–Q-wave myocardial infarction was also increased (16.1% vs 11.5%). In this trial, the predictors and sequelae of distal embolization were analyzed carefully. Independent predictors of embolization were the use of DCA and, more importantly, the presence of thrombus. Thirty-nine percent of patients with visible thrombus had embolization compared with 14% of patients without thrombus. Among patients with distal embolization, over 70% had an adverse clinical event during hospitalization, whereas 20% of patients without distal embolization had major adverse events. Two points are notable: embolization occurs frequently during PCI for SVGs, and it is associated with poor outcomes. After 1 year of follow-up in the CAVEAT-2 trial, the composite end point of death, myocardial infarction, repeat intervention, or bypass surgery was worse in the group that suffered distal embolization.

The simplest approach to plaque removal has been guiding catheter aspiration. A simple technique for thrombectomy involves deep seating a guide catheter and aspirating graft or coronary contents. Twenty to 60 mL of blood is typically aspirated, careful study has shown gross macroscopic material in many of the aspirates. Devices constructed specifically for graft aspiration, such as the PercuSurge export catheter, have been employed for this purpose, and recently an aspiration catheter that can be passed monorail over a guidewire has been designed specifically for this purpose[21] (Figure 58-2).

Transluminal extraction, a device that is no longer available, was evaluated in 175 patients.[22,23] No reflow was seen in 19% of patients with thrombus and 5% of patients without thrombus in this experience, and the overall distal embolization rate was 7%. Late complete vessel occlusion was seen in over one third of patients with thrombus. The excimer laser has also been evaluated in vein graft disease. In a series of 495 patients, embolization

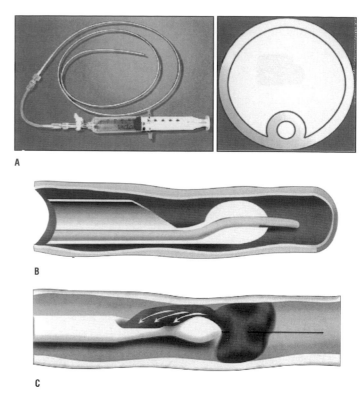

FIGURE 58-2. Simple thrombus aspiration catheter. The catheter passes over a 0.014-in guidewire via the smaller lumen. A syringe is attached to the larger lumen for aspiration. The larger lumen has the capacity to remove a significant volume of thrombus. The two lower panels show the design of the aspiration port of the catheter and, in the lower panel, a schematic illustrates the aspiration of thrombus into the catheter lumen. The system is compatible with a 6-French guide catheter. (*Image of the Pronto catheter used with permission of Vascular Solutions, Inc, Minneapolis, Minn.*)

occurred in only 3.3% of patients and Q-wave infarction in only 2.4% of patients. However, in some laser studies, thrombus-containing lesions were associated with increased rates of embolization and poor clinical outcomes.

Rheolytic thrombectomy, an atherectomy technique that uses high-velocity saline jets directed retrograde into the open mouth of a Bernoulli device, draws thrombus into the catheter tip for maceration and evacuation. In the Vegas II trial, rheolytic thrombectomy in native coronary vessels and SVGs containing thrombus was compared with urokinase bolus of up to 250,000 units, and infusion ranging from 6 to 30 hours. Over half the patients treated had vein graft as opposed to native vessel thrombus-containing lesions. Rheolytic thrombectomy resulted in a significant decrease in major events. Sixteen percent of rheolytic thrombectomy patients had any major adverse event at 30 days, compared with 33% of urokinase patients ($P < .001$). Q-wave infarction occurred in 2% of rheolytic thrombectomy versus 5% or urokinase patients, and non–Q-wave myocardial infarction in 12% versus 25% of patients. Final Thrombolysis in Myocardial Infarction (TIMI) grade 3 flow was present in 89% of the rheolytic thrombectomy patients compared with 83% of urokinase patients. This study demonstrated that thrombus removal lead to significantly better outcomes in thrombotic SVG- or native vessel–containing lesions compared with thrombolytic infusion. Little subsequent study has been made of the efficacy of this form of thrombectomy therapy

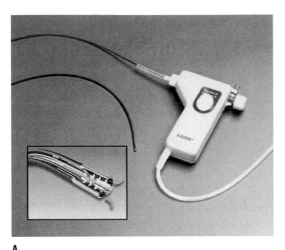
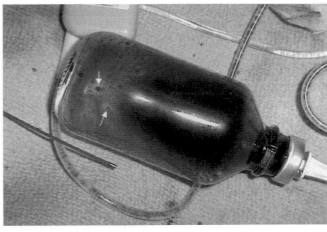

A   **B**

FIGURE 58-3. X-sizer thrombectomy catheter. **(A)** The battery-powered handle with a tube trailing off to the right that attaches to an aspiration bottle. The inset shows the rotating, cutting head that protrudes just slightly from the tip of the catheter; this acts in a corkscrew manner to draw thrombus material into the lumen of the catheter for aspiration. **(B)** A vacuum bottle at the conclusion of an X-sizer procedure. Ground-up thrombus and plaque material (*white arrows*) can be seen adhering to the walls of the vacuum bottle. The device is investigational. *(Image used with permission of EV3, Inc, Plymouth, Minn.)*

for the treatment of degenerated SVG lesions that are predominantly atherosclerotic rather than thrombotic.[24]

A newer form of atherectomy using a cutting device with suction has been evaluated (Figure 58-3). A prospective randomized evaluation of X-Sizer thrombectomy was carried out recently in 60 centers in the United States and Canada. The 797 patients with 839 diseased saphenous grafts with thrombose-containing native coronary arteries were randomized to stent implantation with versus without prior thrombectomy using the X-Sizer device. Periprocedural infarction occurred in 15.8% of X-Sizer patients compared with 16.6% of control patients. The rate of large myocardial infarction, prespecified as the development of new pathologic Q waves or a CK-MB isoenzyme elevation greater than eight times the upper limit of normal, was reduced with the X-Sizer device from 9.6% to 5.5% ($P = .002$). Other major adverse events, including cardiac death, smaller infarction, or repeat target vessel revascularization, occurred in 17% of both groups at 30 days. Thrombectomy with the X-Sizer device, part of stent implantation in high-risk disease SVGs and thrombose-containing native vessels, appeared to reduce the extent, but not the frequency, of myonecrosis.[25,26]

A recent meta-analysis of more than 9000 patients in 16 trials found that ablative devices failed to reduce complications associated with embolization. Periprocedural myocardial infarctions occurred in 4.4% of patients tested with devices versus 2.5% without (OR 1.83, CI 1.43 to 2.34).[27]

PREVENTION OF DISTAL EMBOLIZATION IN SAPHENOUS VEIN GRAFTS

【 】 COVERED STENTS

The use of conventional bare-metal stents improved the results of catheter therapy for obstructive SVGs but did not reduce the restenosis rate. In addition, the potential for liberation of particu-

late degree with embolization seems increased by the use of stenting compared with conventional plain balloon angioplasty.

One of the first concepts tested to diminish the potential for embolization using stenting was evaluation of membrane-covered metal stents compared with bare-metal stents (Figure 58-4). A PTFE membrane–covered balloon expandable stent was compared in a randomized trial with conventional stents.[28] The concept that the PTFE membrane might trap graft atheroma behind the stent and prevents its liberation was assessed. Over 200 patients were randomly assigned to receive either a conventional metal stent or a membrane-covered stent. Neither restenosis nor acute procedural events were diminished by the use of a membrane-covered stent. Restenosis occurred in 20% of the bare stent group compared with 29% of the membrane-covered stent group, which was a nonsignificant difference. This trial experience effectively terminated the development of this device.

【 】 DISTAL OCCLUSIVE DEVICES

Truly effective therapy to prevent the consequences of embolization during PCI for SVG lesions was not available until the introduction of embolic protection devices. Embolic protection devices fall into three categories: distal occlusion,[29–31] filter, and proximal occlusion devices.

The first device to undergo extensive clinical testing was the PercuSurge GuardWire.[29] This device has a distal occlusion balloon mounted on a 0.0.14-in angioplasty wire (Figure 58-5). The system allows recovery of any liberated plaque material by aspiration before balloon deflation and restoration of forward flow in the treated vessel (Figures 58-6 to 58-9).

In the SAFER trial, mentioned earlier, 801 patients were randomized in a multicenter protocol to treatment with balloon occlusion distal embolization protection versus PTCA without embolic protection prior to stent placement. The primary end point of the trial—a composite of death, myocardial infarction, emergency bypass, or target lesion revascularization by 30 days—was

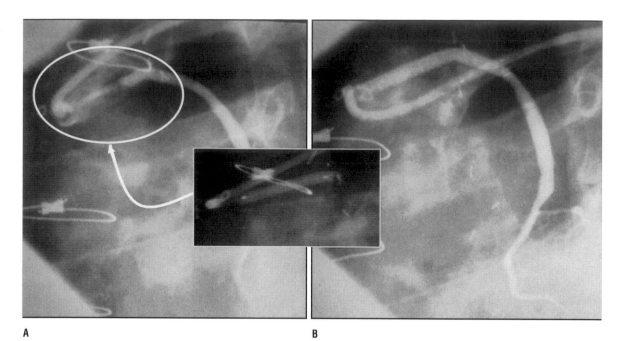

A   **B**

FIGURE 58-4. Angiographic frames from a saphenous vein graft in which a PTFE-covered stent was used. (**A**) A proximal graft lesion, noted by the circle. The inset shows the covered stent being deployed in the lesion. High pressure is required to fully expand the combination of graft membrane and stent material. In this case, 18 atm was necessary for adequate stent expansion. (**B**) The silhouette of the fully expanded stent in the proximal vessel.

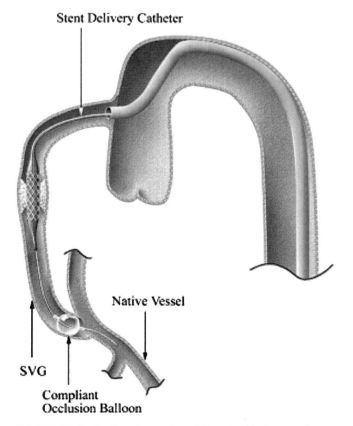

FIGURE 58-5. The PercuSurge GuardWire distal balloon occlusion embolization protection system. A guidewire is passed via the guiding catheter with a compliant distal occlusion balloon. The distal balloon is inflated, creating a static blood column in the saphenous vein graft. A stent can be deployed over this wire, and then an aspiration catheter used to remove the particulate containing blood column. *(Image used with permission from Medtronic, Inc, Minneapolis, Minn.)*

reached by 16.5% of patients assigned to the control group and 9.6% of patients assigned to the embolic protection device arm of the trial ($P = .004$). This represented a 42% relative reduction in major adverse cardiac events and was driven principally by reductions in myocardial infarction (8.6% vs 14.7%; $P = .008$) and no-reflow phenomenon (3% vs 9%; $P = .02$). Clinical benefit was noted even when platelet glycoprotein receptor blockers were administered (61% of patients). The overall composite end points in this subgroup occurred in 10.7% of protection device patients compared with 19.4% of control patients ($P = .008$).

In the SAFER trial, the mean total occlusion time for completion of the procedure was 6.5 minutes. The balloon was inflated in the distal saphenous graft, intervention performed, aspiration of the blood column performed, and then finally the balloon was deflated. This necessitated total cessation of flow to the target perfusion bed of the SVG. Some patients did not tolerate the ischemia.

It was concluded the use of a distal protection total occlusion device during stenting for stenotic SVG disease was associated with a highly significant reduction in major events compared with stenting using a conventional angioplasty guidewire without embolic protection. This represented the first important inroad into preventing the consequences of distal embolization during PCI. This category of graft intervention represents an ideal model for the development of these devices, because there are no proximal side branches into which embolic material can run off during PCI.

【 】 FILTERS

A second class of embolization protection device is filter based. These devices use a wire micropore filter material in the distal target vessel (Figures 58-10 and 58-11). A clear advantage of this category

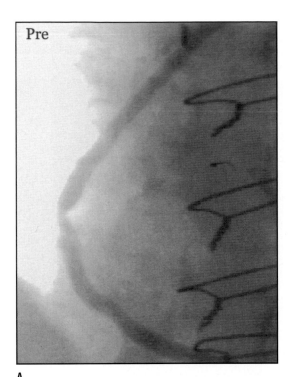

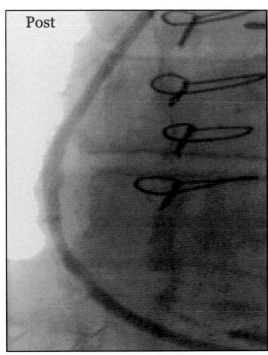

A   **B**

FIGURE 58-6. Focal saphenous vein graft lesion. (**A**) Before intervention, a simple graft lesion is seen midvessel. (**B**) After stenting, an excellent angiographic appearance is noted. This patient was treated with the PercuSurge distal balloon occlusion embolization protection.

of devices is that perfusion is maintained in the distal circulation during the performance of stenting in the vast majority of patients.

The first device in the filter category to complete a large randomized trial is the FilterWire.[32] Six hundred and fifty patients undergoing PCI for SVG lesions were perspectively randomized to treatment with the FilterWire device versus the GuardWire device balloon occlusion and aspiration system in the FIRE (Filterwire Randomized Evaluation) trial. Device success was 95% using the FilterWire compared with 97% using the GuardWire. Measures of

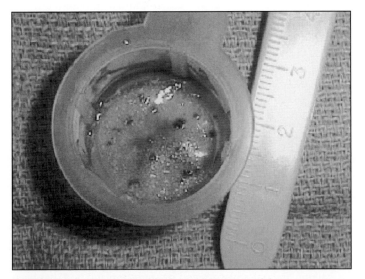

FIGURE 58-7. Aspirated debris from the simple graft lesion seen in Figure 58-6. Even a relatively focal saphenous graft lesion may liberate a great deal of embolic material. The filter here shows multiple particulate elements of highly variable sizes and composition.

epicardial flow and angiographic complications were similar between the two groups. "Bailout" platelet glycoprotein inhibitor use was required less frequently with FilterWire (0% vs 1.5%; $P = .03$). The primary end point, which was a composite of death, myocardial infarction, or target vessel revascularization at 30 days, occurred in 9.9% of FilterWire patients and 11.6% of GuardWire patients. This represents a clear noninferiority result comparing the two devices. It was concluded that distal protection with the FilterWire might be safely used as an adjunctive percutaneous intervention for diseased SVGs and that use of this device, compared with distal protection using the GuardWire occlusion and aspiration system, resulted in similar rates of major adverse cardiac events at 30 days (Figure 58-12).

In the SAFER and FIRE trials, participants were representative of typical SVG intervention patients. They were older and had more comorbidity than patients undergoing native vessel percutaneous coronary intervention.

Despite the great enhancements provided by embolic protection devices, these approaches have some limitations. The major limitation of the balloon occlusion distal embolization protection system is total occlusion of the vessel during stent implantation. In addition, aspiration of the particulate in the fluid column proximal to the inflated balloon is not completely efficient, because events still occur in patients treated with this modality. The balloon and wire system is less steerable than a conventional angioplasty device. Some embolization may occur when the device is passed across the lesion, although the balloon occlusion device has a lower profile than the filter devices. The filter devices require a delivery sleeve to be placed across the filter, increasing their profile. Iterations in device design have made both of these classes of device easier to use with each successive generation.

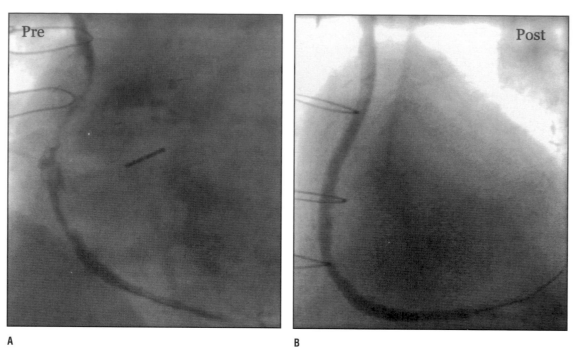

FIGURE 58-8. Thrombotic, complex graft lesion with large thrombus and atherosclerotic burden. **(A)** The patient was treated with the PercuSurge distal balloon occlusion embolization protection. **(B)** The post-stent result is shown.

The filter devices may completely fill with debris, transforming them effectively into occlusion devices. Trying to recapture the filter once it is completely full can be problematic, because particulate embolic material may be suspended in the blood column proximal to the filter. Thus, when a filter device completely occludes, and flow ceases in the target vessel, aspiration of the blood column below the filter with an aspiration catheter similar to that used with the GuardWire system may be important.

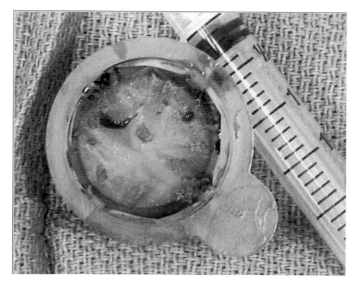

FIGURE 58-9. Debris aspirated from the saphenous vein graft seen in Figure 58-8. In contrast to the aspirate in Figure 58-7 from a simple lesion, the aspirate here shows macroscopic elements of thrombus and plaque, in addition to multiple particles of smaller, variable size.

【 】 PROXIMAL OCCLUSIVE DEVICES

Proximal occlusion devices represent another category of embolization protection devices. An occlusive balloon is inflated in the vessel origin to interrupt flow and create a static blood column distally (Figure 58-13). During intervention any particulate remains in the blood column in the vessel. PCI can be performed through the balloon, and the debris aspirated. These devices have the advantage of causing stasis of blood flow proximal to the origin of side branches. Thus, particulate released during the intervention does not run off into the capillary bed. As a result, this system can be applied in both SVG lesions and also in native vessels.

This device has been tested in a feasibility study in 35 patients with 40 lesions.[33] Both SVG and native vessels (35% of cases) were treated. The overall major adverse cardiac event rate was 5.7% in this nonrandomized group. Embolic material was obtained in the aspirate from all of the patients enrolled.

PREVENTION OF DISTAL EMBOLIZATION IN NATIVE VESSELS: ACUTE MYOCARDIAL INFARCTION

Signs of microvascular hypoperfusion frequently occur after successful PCI for acute myocardial infarction. The large thrombus burden associated with these procedures suggests embolization is a common occurrence. Deterioration of flow after initially successful balloon angioplasty, worsened by stent implantation, has been observed. Stent expansion with mechanical abrasion of the lesion by the stent struts, the so-called *cheese-grater effect,* is probably partially responsible. In a trial evaluating the use of the FilterWire

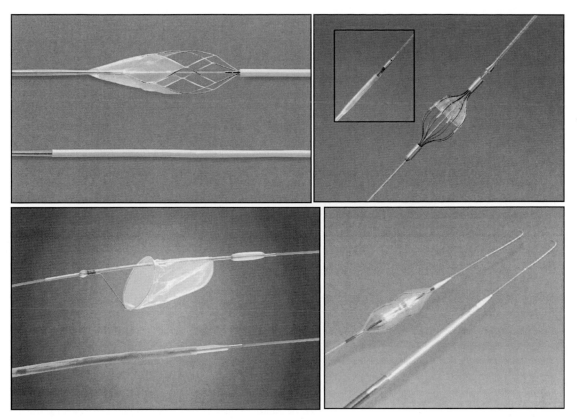

FIGURE 58-10. Currently available embolic filter devices. At the time of writing the Accunet, Angioguard, and Abbott filters are investigational. **Upper left:** Guidant Accunet Filter. The top portion of the panel shows the open filter, and the bottom portion, the filter constrained in a delivery sheath. **Upper right:** Cordis Angioguard filter. **Lower left:** FilterWire EZ, open in the top portion of the panel, and in the retrieval sheath in the bottom portion. **Lower right:** Abbott Emboshield filter in the open and constrained configurations. *(Images used with permission of Guidant, Inc; Cordis, Inc, Warren, NJ; Boston Scientific, Natick, Mass; and Abbott Vascular Devices, Redwood City, Calif.)*

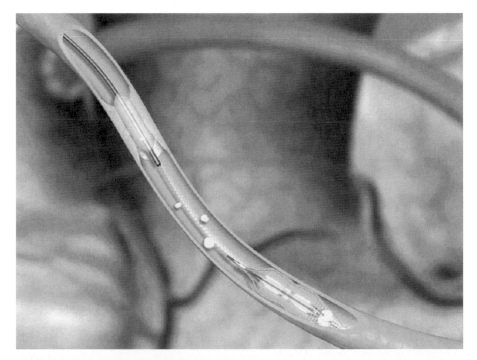

FIGURE 58-11. Schematic showing the Abbott Emboshield in a distal saphenous vein graft during balloon angioplasty with particulate matter traveling downstream toward the filter. The device is investigational. *(Illustration used with permission of Abbott Vascular Devices, Redwood City, Calif.)*

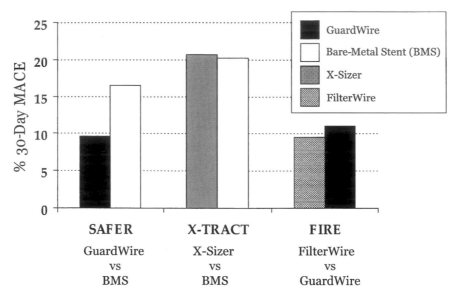

FIGURE 58-12. Comparison of the clinical event rates in three trials of embolization protection devices. (MACE = major adverse cardiac event.)

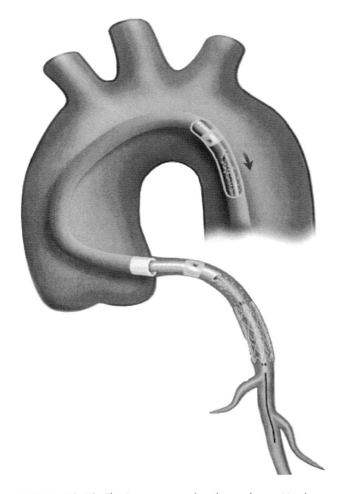

FIGURE 58-13. The Proxis proximal occlusion device. Via the guide catheter, a proximal native coronary soft occlusion balloon is deployed. This creates a static blood column in both the epicardial vessel and the side branches of the distal vessel. Through the occlusion balloon system, conventional stents may be placed. After treatment of the vessel, the blood column can be aspirated through the occlusion catheter. *(Image used with permission of Velocimed, Inc, Minneapolis, Minn.)*

during primary PCI for acute myocardial infarction,[34] 53 patients treated with FilterWire protection were compared with a matched control group. Successful FilterWire positioning was obtained in 89% of cases. Histologic analysis of a selected population of filters showed multiple embolic debris elements in all cases. Use of the FilterWire was associated with a lower postinterventional corrected TIMI frame count (22 vs 31; $P = .005$) and a higher occurrence of grade 3 myocardial blush (66% vs 36%; $P = .006$) and early ST-segment elevation resolution (80% vs 54%; $P = .006$). Using multivariable analysis, FilterWire was the only independent predictor of early ST-segment elevation resolution and of grade 3 myocardial blush. FilterWire patients had lower peak CK-MB release (236 vs 333 ng/mL; $P = .013$). After 1 month, they also had a greater improvement in left ventricular wall motion and ejection fraction (+7% vs +4%; $P = .012$).

A trial of the GuardWire balloon occlusion embolization protection system was recently reported in the setting of acute myocardial infarction. This large, randomized trial failed to show any differences between balloon occlusion embolization protection and conventional PCI and stenting.[35]

As a result of the Enhanced Myocardial Efficacy and Removal by Aspiration of Liberated Debris (EMERALD) trial, 505 patients presenting within 6 hours of onset of acute myocardial infarction were treated with primary or rescue PCI. The end points were ST-segment resolution at 30 minutes and infarct size (assessed by sestamibi imaging) after 1 week. Major events at 30 days were present in 14% of GuardWire patients and 13.1% of controls. Visible debris was removed in 73% of patients in the GuardWire arm. Presence of glycoprotein IIb/IIIa inhibition was about 83% in both groups. TIMI grade 3 flow was present in about 90% of patients in both groups, and TIMI frame counts post-procedure were 22 in the GuardWire group and 23 in the control group. Blush score of 3 was present in 60% of GuardWire and 53% of control patients. This last difference was not statistically significant.

Among patients with ST-elevation myocardial infarction, the use of a distal protection balloon occlusion system was not associated with improvement in the primary end points of ST resolution or infarct size. Despite the capture of visible debris in almost three quarters of patients, no improvements in myocardial perfusion were observed compared with conventional therapy of balloon angioplasty and bare-metal stenting.

Trials evaluating the FilterWire, X-sizer aspiration catheter,[8] and the angiojet have also failed to demonstrate benefits from routine use of embolic protection or thrombectomy in acute MI.

NO-REFLOW PHENOMENON

【 】 SUPPORTIVE MEASURES

Treatment of the no-reflow phenomenon involves basic supportive measures for the patient, including fluid resuscitation, attention to oxygenation, airway management, and blood pressure maintenance with pressors or inotropes (Table 58-2). Maintenance of blood pressure is especially important, because distal perfusion pressure is necessary for recovery from no reflow and also for the delivery of pharmacologic therapy to the distal vascular bed. When no reflow occurs in the right coronary artery or inferior distribution, atropine therapy may be necessary to treat the reflex hypotension and bradycardia that may occur. Intra-aortic balloon pump therapy for blood pressure support is another mainstay of therapy in refractory cases.[36-38]

TABLE 58-2

Initial Evaluation and Treatment of No Reflow

Exclude dissection, thrombus, spasm at lesion site (IVUS, distal contrast injections, or translesion pressure gradient may be useful)

Achieve adequate ACT (250–300 s with unfractionated heparin if a IIb/IIIa inhibitor has been given, >300 s if one has not been given, and 325–375 s with direct thrombin inhibitors)

Ensure sufficient oxygenation and airway management

Treat vagal reactions (IV atropine and fluids)

Maintain adequate perfusion pressure with IV fluids, vasopressors, inotropes, and IABP if necessary

Administer intracoronary nitroglycerin (100–200 μg up to 4 doses) to exclude epicardial spasm

Consider administering a glycoprotein IIb/IIIa receptor inhibitor

Administer pharmacologic agents through an infusion catheter or the central lumen of the balloon catheter to assure drug delivery to the distal bed

ACT = activated clothing times; IABP = intra-aortic balloon pump; IVUS = intravascular ultrasound.

Adapted from Klein et al,[39] in Catheterization and Cardiovascularization Intervention, copyright 2003, with permission from J Wiley and Sons, Hoboken, NJ.

The basis of most therapy for no reflow is intracoronary pharmacotherapy,[39] which often rapidly restores flow and reestablishes a more stable condition. A wide array of pharmacologic agents has been used for this therapy. None are of clear proven therapeutic value in a trial setting. Most of the practice involved with pharmacotherapy for no reflow is based on operator experience and anecdote.

The no-reflow phenomenon is likely to be multifactorial in most cases.[40-48] It is often difficult to distinguish whether large thrombotic occlusion of the distal vessel, dissection, guide catheter damping, or no reflow is the etiology of diminished distal runoff. In many cases, it is necessary to treat all of these possible etiologies. Balloon inflations are frequently necessary in and distal to the lesion to evaluate the potential for dissection and distal large thrombus formation. Occasionally, additional stenting in the inlet or outlet of stented lesions is necessary to eliminate edge dissections as an etiology of diminished blood flow.

【 】 PHARMACOLOGIC THERAPY

Pharmacologic agents are administered into the affected vascular bed through a distal catheter. When drugs are given through a guiding catheter, they will preferentially flow to areas that have preserved runoff. For example, when there is slow flow in the distal circumflex artery, injections into a left system guide catheter will result in the injected agent going to the contralateral vessel and never reaching the target vascular bed. Thus, an infusion catheter or an over-the-wire balloon catheter must be delivered distal to the target lesion into the distal vasculature, and injections given through this catheter. Intracoronary nitroglycerin has been the traditional first-line agent for this therapy. However, the response of the no-reflow phenomenon to nitroglycerin has been poor, and it is not realistic to recommend this as a first-line therapy. Several other agents have shown more promise (Table 58-3).

Agents that have shown positive results in at least small reported series include adenosine, verapamil, and nitroprusside. In addition, the anecdotal experience for these agents has been generally positive. The published evidence for the clinical utility of any of these drugs is remarkably small.

Intracoronary calcium blockers are best described.[49] Piana and colleagues showed that intracoronary verapamil in doses between 50 and 900 μg improved TIMI flow grade in almost 90% of cases.[40] Abbo and associates reported a success rate of two thirds with intracoronary verapamil, especially in cases related to rotational ablation. Kaplan and colleagues compared intragraft verapamil with nitroglycerin and found improvement in all patients who received verapamil, whereas those who received nitroglycerin showed no improvements.[49] Other published reports have shown similar results with calcium blocker therapy. Surprisingly, the total number of reported cases remains relatively small.

Adenosine has similarly been evaluated in a small number of patients with positive results.[50-53] In one series of vein graft intervention, adenosine was successful in the majority of cases.[50] Multiple doses and higher doses of adenosine have been found to be more effective than low doses.

One small experience demonstrating the efficacy of nitroprusside exists.[54] Our own experience with this agent has been extremely positive, even in cases refractory to intracoronary calcium blocker administration.

TABLE 58-3

Intracoronary Drug Therapy for No Reflow

First-Line Management
Adenosine (10–20 μg bolus)
Verapamil (100–200 μg boluses or 100 μg/min up to 1000 μg total dose with temporary pacer on standby)
Nitroprusside (50–200 μg bolus, up to 1000 μg total dose)

Evidence Less Strong
Rapid, moderately forceful injection of saline or blood (to "unplug" microvasculature).
Diltiazem (0.5–2.5 mg over 1 min up to 5 mg)
Papavarine (10–20 μg)
Nicardipine (200 μg)
Nicorandil (2 μg)
Epinephrine (50–200 μg)

Never Shown to Be Effective
Intracoronary nitroglycerin
Coronary artery bypass graftins
Stent placement at site of original stenosis, if widely patent
Thrombolytics (eg, urokinase, tissue plasminogen activator)

Adapted from Klein et al[39] in Catheterization and Cardiovascularization Intervention, *copyright 2003, with permission from J Wiley and Sons, Hoboken, NJ.*

Forceful injection of saline or blood has been described as a method for hydraulically dislodging platelet aggregates or microthrombi from the distal vascular bed. Multiple high-velocity drug doses may be effective as well.

Intravenous and intracoronary platelet glycoprotein IIb/IIIa inhibitors have been described as successful in some cases, but the results seem to be variable.[55–58] A review of the effects of IIb/IIIa agents in more than 4000 patients in the EPIC (Evaluation of IIb/IIIa Platelet receptor antagonist 7E3 in Preventing Ischemic Complications) and EPILOG (Evaluation in PTCA to Improve Long-Term Outcome with Abciximab GP IIb/IIIa Blockade) trials failed to show any benefit from the use of these agents in SVG intervention. Placebo-treated patients had a 16.3% incidence of complications versus 18.6% in those receiving abciximab.[39]

Various other agents have been described, including several other calcium channel blocking drugs.[59–64] Intracoronary epinephrine has been described as effective in this setting, as well, and has an advantage because it will not cause blood pressure decline in patients in whom that is already a problem.[65] Skelding and colleagues identified 29 patients in whom intracoronary epinephrine was administered for refractory no reflow. Administration of a mean dose of 139 ± 189 μg resulted in establishment of TIMI grade 3 flow in 69% of patients. Mean TIMI flow increased from 1 to 2.7 ($P = .0001$). Heart rate increased on average from 72 to 86 beats per minute, but no cases of rhythm disturbance were noted.[49] Nicardipine has been studied in animal models and has

been effective in our experience. Nicorandil has been used with some success intravenously,[64] as has papaverine.[66,67]

Intracoronary thrombolytic agents are ineffective, even when thrombotic embolization is grossly visible.[68] Mechanical disruption of these thromboemboli is probably more effective than use of thrombolytic drugs.

SUMMARY

The no-reflow phenomenon has been a feared complication of PCI since in the inception of balloon angioplasty. No reflow occurs in 0.5% to 3% of cases and is particularly common in interventions for acute myocardial infarction, SVG disease, rotational atherectomy, and, less frequently, in native coronary artery interventions.

Recent advances have made the prevention of no reflow a reality. Embolic protection devices for use in SVG intervention have become routine. Pharmacotherapy for no reflow has similarly improved. Previously, nitroglycerine was the mainstay of intracoronary therapy after no reflow occurred, despite its ineffectuality. More recently, successful therapy with calcium-blocking agents, nitroprusside, adenosine, and possibly epinephrine have proven effective in improving epicardial coronary flow in the no-reflow phenomenon.[69] It remains to be demonstrated whether the acute improvements in epicardial flow correlate with improved late outcomes from no reflow.

It is clear that preventive measures, including embolization protection devices, should be used in high-risk settings for the no-reflow phenomenon. SVG intervention has been proven to be safer with embolization protection, and these devices should be used in conjunction with virtually all SVG interventions. This is akin to wearing seat belts when riding in an automobile. The application of embolization protection devices to other settings, such as acute myocardial infarction, requires further study. Important success has been demonstrated in the carotid circulation, subject of another discussion, and is under study in other peripheral vascular beds.

REFERENCES

1. Sanborn TA, Faxon DP, Waugh D, et al. Transluminal angioplasty in experimental atherosclerosis. Analysis for embolization using an in vivo perfusion system. *Circulation.* 1982;66:917.
2. Leon MB, Baim DS, Popma JJ, et al. A clinical trial comparing three antithrombotic-drug regimens after coronary-artery stenting. Stent Anticoagulation Restenosis Study Investigators. *N Engl J Med.* 1998;339:1665.
3. Cutlip DE, Leon MB, Ho KK, et al. Acute and nine-month clinical outcomes after "suboptimal" coronary stenting: Results from the STent Anti-thrombotic Regimen Study (STARS) registry. *J Am Coll Cardiol.* 1999;34:698.
4. Whitlow PL, Bass TA, Kipperman RM, et al. Results of the study to determine rotablator and transluminal angioplasty strategy (STRATAS). *Am J Cardiol.* 2001;87:699.
5. Keeley EC, Velez CA, O'Neill WW, Safian RD. Long-term clinical outcome and predictors of major adverse cardiac events after percutaneous interventions on saphenous vein grafts. *J Am Coll Cardiol.* 2001;38:659.
6. Kloner RA, Ganote CE, Jennings RB. The "no-reflow" phenomenon after temporary coronary occlusion in the dog. *J Clin Invest.* 1974;54:1496.
7. Mehta RH, Harjai KJ, Boura J, et al, Primary Angioplasty in Myocardial Infarction (PAMI) Investigators. Prognostic significance of transient no-reflow during primary percutaneous coronary intervention for ST-elevation acute myocardial infarction. *Am J Cardiol.* 2003;92):1445.

8. Resnic FS, Wainstein M, Lee MK, et al. No-reflow is an independent predictor of death and myocardial infarction after percutaneous coronary intervention. *Am Heart J.* 2003;145:42.

9. Hong MK, Mehran R, Dangas G, et al. Creatine kinase-MB enzyme elevation following successful saphenous vein graft intervention is associated with late mortality. *Circulation.* 1999;100:2400.

10. Falk E, Thuesen L. Pathology of coronary microembolisation and no-reflow. *Heart (Br Cardiac Soc).* 2003;89:983.

11. Webb JG, Carere RG, Virmani R, et al. Retrieval and analysis of particulate debris after saphenous vein graft intervention. *J Am Coll Cardiol.* 1999;34:468.

12. Safian RD, Niazi KA, Strzelecki M, et al. Detailed angiographic analysis of high-speed mechanical rotational atherectomy in human coronary arteries. *Circulation.* 1993;88:961.

13. Ellis SG, Popma JJ, Buchbinder M, et al. Relation of clinical presentation, stenosis morphology, and operator technique to the procedural results of rotational atherectomy and rotational atherectomy-facilitated angioplasty. *Circulation.* 1994;89:882.

14. Hori M, Inoue M, Kitakaze M, et al. Role of adenosine in hyperemic response of coronary blood flow in microembolization. *Am J Physiol.* 1986;250(pt 2):H509.

15. Ohki T, Roubin GS, Veith FJ, et al. Efficacy of a filter device in the prevention of embolic events during carotid angioplasty and stenting: An ex vivo analysis. *J Vasc Surg.* 1999;30:1034.

16. Tubler T, Schluter M, Dirsch O, et al. Balloon-protected carotid artery stenting: Relationship of periprocedural neurological complications with the size of particulate debris. *Circulation.* 2001;104:2791.

17. Leosco D, Fineschi M, Pierli C, et al. Intracoronary serotonin release after high-pressure coronary stenting. *Am J Cardiol.* 1999;84:1317.

18. Bonderman D, Teml A, Jakowitsch J, et al. Coronary no-reflow is caused by shedding of active tissue factor from dissected atherosclerotic plaque. *Blood.* 2002;99:2794.

19. Cohen BM, Weber VJ, Blum RR, et al. Cocktail attenuation of rotational ablation Flow Effects (CARAFE) pilot study. *Cathet Cardiovasc Diagn.* 1996;(suppl 3):69.

20. Lefkovits J, Holmes DR, Califf RM, et al. Predictors and sequelae of distal embolization during saphenous vein graft intervention from the CAVEAT-II trial. Coronary Angioplasty Versus Excisional Atherectomy Trial. *Circulation.* 1995;92:734.

21. Morales PA, Heuser RR. Guiding catheter aspiration to prevent embolic events during saphenous vein graft intervention. *J Interv Cardiol.* 2002;15:491.

22. Holmes DR Jr, Berger PB. Percutaneous revascularization of occluded vein grafts: Is it still a temptation to be resisted? *Circulation.* 1999;99:8.

23. Braden GA, Xenopolous NP, Young T, et al. Transluminal extraction catheter atherectomy followed by immediate stenting in treatment of saphenous vein grafts. *J Am Coll Cardiol.* 1997;30:657.

24. Kuntz RE, Baim DS, Cohen DJ, et al. A trial comparing rheolytic thrombectomy with intracoronary urokinase for coronary and vein graft thrombus (the Vein Graft AngioJet Study [VeGAS 2]). *Am J Cardiol.* 2002;89:326.

25. Stone GW, Cox DA, Low R, et al, X-TRACT Investigators. Safety and efficacy of a novel device for treatment of thrombotic and atherosclerotic lesions in native coronary arteries and saphenous vein grafts: Results from the multicenter X-Sizer for treatment of thrombus and atherosclerosis in coronary applications trial (X-TRACT) study. *Cathet Cardiovasc Interv.* 2003;58:419.

26. Stone GW, Cox DA, Babb J, et al. Prospective, randomized evaluation of thrombectomy prior to percutaneous intervention in diseased saphenous vein grafts and thrombus-containing coronary arteries. *J Am Coll Cardiol.* 2003;42:2007.

27. Bittl JA, Chew DP, Topol EJ, et al. Meta-analysis of randomized trials of percutaneous transluminal coronary angioplasty versus atherectomy, cutting balloon atherotomy, or laser angioplasty. *J Am Coll Cardiol.* 2004;43:936.

28. Schachinger V, Hamm CW, Munzel T, et al, STENTS (STents IN Grafts) Investigators. A randomized trial of polytetrafluoroethylene-membrane-covered stents compared with conventional stents in aortocoronary saphenous vein grafts. *J Am Coll Cardiol.* 2003;42:1360.

29. Baim DS, Wahr D, George B, et al. Randomized trial of a distal embolic protection device during percutaneous intervention of saphenous vein aorto-coronary bypass grafts. *Circulation.* 2002;105:1285.

30. Shaknovich A, Forman ST, Parikh MA, et al. Novel distal occluder washout method for the prevention of no-reflow during stenting of saphenous vein grafts. *Cathet Cardiovasc Interv.* 1999;47:397.

31. Carlino M, De Gregorio J, Di Mario C, et al. Prevention of distal embolization during saphenous vein graft lesion angioplasty. Experience with a new temporary occlusion and aspiration system. *Circulation.* 1999;99:3221.

32. Stone GW, Rogers C, Hermiller J, et al, FilterWire EX Randomized Evaluation Investigators. Randomized comparison of distal protection with a filter-based catheter and a balloon occlusion and aspiration system during percutaneous intervention of diseased saphenous vein aorto-coronary bypass grafts. *Circulation.* 2003;108:548.

33. Sievert KH, Schuler G, Schofer J, et al. Final results of the FASTER trial using the Proxis embolic protection system; a novel proximal occlusion system for prevention of distal embolization during PCI. *Am J Cardiol.* 2003;92(suppl 6A):32L.

34. Limbruno U, Micheli A, De Carlo M, et al. Mechanical prevention of distal embolization during primary angioplasty: Safety, feasibility, and impact on myocardial reperfusion. *Circulation.* 2003;108:171.

35. Stone GW, Webb J, Cox DA, et al. Enhanced Myocardial Efficacy and Recovery by Aspiration of Liberated Debris (EMERALD) Investigators. Distal microcirculatory protection during percutaneous coronary intervention in acute ST-segment elevation myocardial infarction: a randomized controlled trial. *JAMA.* 2005;293(9):1063.

36. Kern MJ, Aguirre F, Bach R, et al. Augmentation of coronary blood flow by intra-aortic balloon pumping in patients after coronary angioplasty. *Circulation.* 1993;87:500.

37. Port SC, Patel S, Schmidt DH. Effects of intracoronary balloon counterpulsation on myocardial blood flow in patients with severe coronary artery disease. *J Am Coll Cardiol.* 1984;3:1367.

38. O'Murchu B, Foreman RD, Shaw RE, et al. Role of intraaortic balloon pump counterpulsation in high risk coronary rotational atherectomy. *J Am Coll Cardiol.* 1995;26:1270.

39. Klein LW, Kern MJ, Berger P, et al. Society of Cardiac Angiography and Interventions: Suggested management of the no-reflow phenomenon in the cardiac catheterization laboratory. *Cathet Cardiovasc Diagn.* 2003;60:194.

40. Piana RN, Paik GY, Moscucci M, et al. Incidence and treatment of no-reflow after percutaneous coronary intervention. *Circulation.* 1994;89:2514.

41. Abbo KM, Dooris M, Glazier S, et al. No-reflow after percutaneous coronary intervention: Clinical and angiographic characteristics, treatment and outcome. *Am J Cardiol.* 1995;75:778.

42. Feld H, Lichstein E, Schachter J, Shani J. Early and late angiographic findings of the "no-reflow" phenomenon following direct angioplasty as primary treatment for acute myocardial infarction. *Am Heart J.* 1992;123:782.

43. Eeckhout E, Kern MJ. The coronary no-reflow phenomenon: A review of mechanisms and therapies. *Eur Heart J.* 2001;22:729.

44. Gregorini L, Marco J, Kozakova R, et al. Alpha-adrenergic blockade improves recovery of myocardial perfusion and function after coronary stenting in patients with acute myocardial infarction. *Circulation.* 1999;59:482.

45. Asunuma T, Tanabe K, Ochiai K, et al. Relation between progressive microvascular damage and intramyocardial hemorrhage in patients with reperfused anterior myocardial infarction: Myocardial contrast echocardiographic study. *Circulation.* 1997;96:448.

46. Iliceto S, Galiuto L, Marchese A, et al. Functional role of microvascular integrity in patients with infarct-related artery patency after acute myocardial infarction. *Eur Heart J.* 1997;18:618.

47. WU KC, Zerhouni EA, Judd RM, et al. Prognostic significance of microvascular obstruction by magnetic resonance in patients with acute myocardial infarction. *Circulation.* 1998;97:765.

48. Rochitte CE, Lima JAC, Bluemke DA, et al. Magnitude and time course of microvascular obstruction and tissue injury after myocardial infarction. *Circulation.* 1998;98:1006.

49. Kaplan BM, Benzuly KH, Kinn JW, et al. Treatment of no-reflow in degenerated saphenous vein graft intervention: Comparison of intracoronary verapamil and nitroglycerin. *Cathet Cardiovasc Diagn.* 1997;39:113.

50. Fischell TA, Carter AJ, Foster MT, et al. Reversal of 'no-reflow' during vein graft stenting using high velocity boluses of intracoronary adenosine. *Cathet Cardiovasc Diagn.* 1998;45:366.

51. Sdringola S, Assali A, Ghani M, et al. Adenosine use during aortocoronary vein graft interventions reverses but does not prevent the slow-no-reflow phenomenon. *Cathet Cardiovasc Interv.* 2000;51;394.

52. Assali AR, Sdringola S, Ghani M, et al. Intracoronary adenosine administered during percutaneous intervention in acute myocardial infarction and reduction in the incidence of "no-reflow" phenomenon. *Cathet Cardiovasc Interv.* 2000;51:27.

53. Hanna GP, Yhiop P, Fujise K, et al. Intracoronary adenosine administered during rotational atherectomy of complex lesions in native coronary arteries reduces the incidence of no-reflow phenomenon. *Cathet Cardiovasc Interv.* 1999;48:275.

54. Hillegass WB, Dean NA, Liao L, et al. Treatment of no-reflow and impaired flow with the nitric oxide donor nitroprusside following percutaneous coronary interventions. *J Am Coll Cardiol.* 2001;37:1335.

55. Rawitscher D, Levin TN, Cohen I, Feldman T. Rapid reversal of no-reflow using abciximab after coronary device intervention. *Cathet Cardiovasc Diagn.* 1997;42:187.

56. Ellis SG, Lincoff AM, Miller D, et al. Reduction in complications of angioplasty with abciximab occurs largely independently of baseline lesion morphology. EPIC and EPILOG Investigators. Evaluation of 7E3 for the Prevention of Ischemic Complications. Evaluation of PTCA to Improve Long-term Outcome with Abciximab GPIIb/IIIa Receptor Blockade. *J Am Coll Cardiol.* 1998;32:1619.

57. Roffi M, Mukherjee D, Chew DP, et al. Lack of benefit from intravenous platelet glycoprotein IIb/IIIa receptor inhibition as adjunctive treatment for percutaneous interventions of aortocoronary bypass grafts: A pooled analysis of five randomized clinical trials. *Circulation.* 2002;106:3063.

58. Yaryura RA, Zaqqa M, Ferguson JJ. Complications associated with combined use of abciximab and an intracoronary thrombolytic agent (urokinase or tissue-type plasminogen activator). *Am J Cardiol.* 1998;82:518.

59. Pomerantz RM, Kuntz RE, Diver DJ, et al. Intracoronary verapamil for the treatment of distal microvascular coronary artery spasm following percutaneous transluminal coronary angioplasty. *Cathet Cardiovasc Diagn.* 1991;24:283.

60. Taniyama Y, Ito H, Iwakura K, et al. Beneficial effects of intracoronary verapamil on microvascular and myocardial salvage in patients with acute myocardial infarction. *J Am Coll Cardiol.* 1997;30:1193.

61. Weyrens FJ, Mooney J, Lesser J, et al. Intracoronary diltiazem for microvascular spasm after interventional therapy. *Am J Cardiol.* 1995;75:849.

62. Jalinous F, Mooney JA, Mooney MR. Pretreatment with intracoronary diltiazem reduces non-Q wave myocardial infarction following directional atherectomy. *J Invas Cardiol.* 1997;9:270.

63. Fugit MD, Rubal BT, Donovan DJ. Effects of intracoronary nicardipine, diltiazem and verapamil on coronary blood flow. *J Invas Card.* 2000;12:80.

64. Ito H, Taniyama Y, Iwakura K, et al. Intravenous nicorandil can preserve microvascular integrity and myocardial viability in patients with reperfused anterior wall myocardial infarction. *J Am Coll Cardiol.* 1999;33:654.

65. Skelding KA, Goldstein JA, Mehta L, et al. Resolution of refractory no-reflow with intracoronary epinephrine. *Cathet Cardiovasc Interv.* 2002;57:305.

66. Baim DS. Epinephrine: A new pharmacologic treatment for no-reflow? *Cathet Cardiovasc Interv.* 2002;57:310.

67. Ishihara M, Sato H, Tateishi H, et al. Attenuation of the no-reflow phenomenon after coronary angioplasty for acute myocardial infarction with intracoronary papaverine. *Am Heart J.* 1996;132:959.

68. Kloner RA, Alker KJ. The effect of streptokinase on intramyocardial hemorrhage, infarct size, and the "no-reflow" phenomenon during coronary reperfusion. *Circulation.* 1984;70:513.

69. Galiuto L. Optimal therapeutic strategies in the setting of post-infarct no reflow: The need for a pathogenetic classification. *Heart (Br Cardiac Soc).* 2004;90:123.

CHAPTER (59)

Emergency Surgery Following PCI

Michael A. Kutcher, MD

HISTORICAL PERSPECTIVES

As a result of significant technologic improvements over the past 30 years, coronary angioplasty has become an increasingly safe and effective procedure. Along with this maturation, the indications for emergency cardiac surgery for failed angioplasty have been reduced. Nevertheless, some type of surgical backup continues to be a standard of practice for the optimal performance of coronary angioplasty. To understand this evolution, it is appropriate to start this chapter with an historical perspective.

On September 16, 1977, Andreas Gruentzig performed the first percutaneous transluminal coronary angioplasty (PTCA) in Zurich, Switzerland. Elaborate precautions were taken in the event that emergency coronary bypass surgery was necessary to rescue an unstable patient following a failed PTCA. These provisions included a roller pump coronary perfusion device, an open ready operating room, and the presence of a cardiac surgeon and an anesthesiologist in the catheterization laboratory room.[1] Fortunately the procedure was successful and the rest is history. Ironically, the birth of angioplasty would not have been possible without the support and interaction of cardiovascular surgeons. Gruentzig freely credited Ake Senning and Marko Turina, his cardiovascular surgeons in Zurich, with allowing him to develop the technique.

Of Gruentzig's first 50 patients, 7 (14%) needed emergency bypass operations, but surgery was accomplished with no major mortality or morbidity.[2] In June 1979, a PTCA workshop was convened in Bethesda, Maryland, sponsored by the National Institutes of Health, National Heart, Lung and Blood Institute (NIH-NHLBI), at which the initial clinical experience in the technique was discussed. Out of that pivotal meeting, the founding fathers of PTCA took the unprecedented step to commit a fledgling procedure and themselves to a comprehensive multicenter registry that would fairly assess safety and efficacy. As a result, the NIH-NHLBI PTCA Registry[3] was formed, setting the standards for the rigorous analysis of percutaneous coronary interventions (PCI) that continues to this day in various registries and institutional databases. It is with this tradition of information that the evolution of PCI and the role of emergency surgery can be best assessed.

DEFINITIONS

Different degrees and complexity of coronary bypass graft surgery may be necessary following a failed PCI. The most appropriate definitions of urgency are provided by the American College of Cardiology—National Cardiovascular Data Registry (ACC-NCDR) CathPCI Registry.[4]

1. Elective surgery. The patient's cardiac function has been stable in the days prior to the operation. Cardiac surgery could be deferred without risk of compromised cardiac outcome.

2. Urgent surgery. Not elective, not emergency, but the procedure was required during the same hospitalization in order to minimize chance of further clinical deterioration.

3. Emergency surgery. Surgery that must be performed immediately from the catheterization laboratory to the operating room for two major problems:

   a. Ischemic dysfunction, which may involve ongoing ischemia, including rest angina despite maximal medical therapy (medical or intra-aortic balloon pump), acute evolving myocardial infarction (MI) within 24 hours before surgery, or pulmonary edema requiring intubation.

   b. Mechanical dysfunction, which includes shock with or without circulatory support.

4. Emergent salvage surgery. Surgery that is necessary for a patient undergoing actual cardiopulmonary resuscitation en route to the operating room.

This chapter focuses on the above-listed definitions of true emergency and emergent salvage surgery.

The coronary indications for emergency bypass graft surgery include left main dissection, abrupt occlusion, extensive dissection, perforation, cardiac tamponade, retained equipment fragments, and inability to stabilize the affected vessel. Urgent systemic problems to be corrected may include hypoxia, hypotension, acute pulmonary edema, ongoing cardiopulmonary resuscitation, and cardiogenic shock. It should be noted that noncoronary indications may also necessitate emergency cardiac and vascular surgery; these include aortic dissection and severe peripheral vascular access complications.

LOGISTICS

Clarification of the actual logistics and role of the surgeon and the operating room facilities is necessary to avoid confusing terms. Appropriate terminology to differentiate the degree of surgical commitment reflects two levels of support[5]:

- *Surgical standby* indicates a strict arrangement with an open operating room and a surgical team immediately available.

- *Surgical backup* indicates that the cardiac surgery suites are available and emergency surgery cases may be added on to the schedule on a first-case basis.

Logistical arrangements for surgical standby or backup during PCI consist of:

- *On-site.* Surgical facilities are physically present in the medical center facility where PCI is performed.

- *Off-site.* Surgical facilities are present in an institution physically separated by significant distance from the facility where PCI is performed. Timely plans and transportation arrangements are mandatory in the event that a patient requires emergency cardiac surgery for failed PCI.

INCIDENCE, MORTALITY, AND MORBIDITY OF EMERGENCY CARDIAC SURGERY FOR FAILED PERCUTANEOUS CORONARY INTERVENTIONS

From the 14% emergency surgery rate in Gruentzig's first cohort, there has been a significant evolution over the nearly 30 years since, with improvements in success and reductions of both in-hospital mortality and indication for emergency coronary bypass graft surgery. Figure 59-1 summarizes the declining incidence of emergency coronary bypass graft surgery as documented by various major PCI registries over the past two decades.[6–16]

Of note, an analysis from the ACC-NCDR[16] of 100,292 consecutive PCI patients reported an emergency surgery rate of 0.4%. This represents the largest contemporary study to date of this issue. Despite this low incidence, there was an increase in major morbidity for patients who did go on to emergency surgery for failed PCI, as follows: tamponade in 9.4%, Q-wave MI in 6.5%, arrhythmias in 23%, and death in 11%. This appears to confirm a Cleveland Clinic report on 18,593 PCI patients that documented a 0.6% incidence of emergency surgery with a consequence of 12% perioperative MI, 5% cerebrovascular accidents, and 15% mortality.[15] This correlation of lower incidence but higher morbidity was further confirmed in an analysis by the Mayo Clinic of 6,577 patients in the "current stent era" between 2000 to 2003, where the emergency surgery rate was 0.3% but the mortality with emergency surgery was 10% and not significantly different from previous eras.[17]

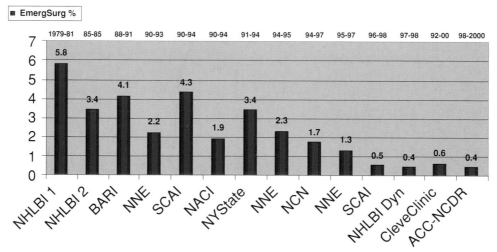

FIGURE 59-1. Incidence of emergency coronary artery bypass surgery in PCI registries. ACC-NCDR = American College of Cardiology-National Cardiovascular Data Registry[16]; BARI = Bypass Angioplasty Revascularization Investigation[7]; CABG = coronary artery bypass grafting; CleveClinic = Cleveland Clinic Registry[15]; NACI = New Approaches to Coronary Intervention Registry[10]; NCN = National Cardiovascular Network Registry[12]; NHLBI 1 and 2 = National Heart Lung Blood Institute Registries 1 and 2[6]; NHLBI Dyn = National Heart Lung Blood Institute Dynamic Registry[14]; NNE = Northern New England Registry[8]; NYState = New York State Database[11]; PCI = percutaneous coronary intervention; SCAI 1990–1994; SCAI 1996–1998 = Society for Cardiac Angiography and Interventions Registry.[9,13]

Multivariant predictors of in-hospital mortality in the ACC-NCDR study were cardiogenic shock, peripheral vascular disease, left main disease, and emergent indications. A disturbing observation was that the ACC and Society for Cardiac Angiography an Interventions Registry (SCAI) lesion identification of low-risk versus high-risk lesions was not a predictor of cases that would go on for emergency surgery. This lack of predictability may be a reflection of the current dominance of stents in coronary interventional procedures. As a result, the traditional lesion risk scores may be less reliable, because they were originally based on data generated from older balloon dilation studies.

An interesting facet of the ACC-NCDR report was that the median procedure volume per hospital was around 600 to 700 cases, which represents high-volume, experienced centers. The question arises whether this degree of safety could be matched in hospitals doing less than 300 procedures a year. Regardless, this recent report and the volume of PCI centers and cases submitting to the ACC-NCDR highlight the Registry as an emerging national standard for the practice of interventional cardiology.

In summary, experience from the various PCI registries indicates that although the incidence of emergency surgery has decreased over the years, when it does occur, the consequences of mortality and morbidity continue to remain high.

FACTORS THAT HAVE REDUCED THE INCIDENCE OF EMERGENCY CARDIAC SURGERY

The best approach to reducing the mortality and morbidity of emergency cardiac surgery for failed PCI would be to avoid the need for emergency surgery altogether. Significant technologic improvements have occurred over the past 30 years to make coronary angioplasty safer and more effective.

There has been a reduction in the French (Fr) size of guiding catheters from 8-, 9-, and 10-Fr to 7-, 6-, and even 5-Fr catheters. The guiding catheters have become much softer, decreasing the likelihood of dissection and complications at the coronary takeoff. Steerable wires have been reduced in diameter size from 0.18-in to the current standard 0.14-in diameter. Various soft steering wire tips are available that reduce the chance of perforation or dissection of the coronary intima. Balloon and dilation shaft profile has been significantly lowered over the years from 1.4-Fr to less than 0.5-Fr diameter in a deflated state.

Along with advances in catheters, there has been a significant improvement in radiologic imaging techniques. Initially biplane fluoroscopy and angiography were thought to be the most effective ways of translating a one-dimensional plane or imaging to at least two dimensions and extrapolating this to three dimensions. The advent of digital fluoroscopic technology has markedly improved our capabilities for visualizing the coronary artery tree and various coronary angioplasty devices.

Adjunctive pharmacotherapies such as direct thrombin inhibitors and platelet glycoprotein IIb/IIIa receptor agents have reduced the thrombotic complications of coronary intervention and the need for emergency surgery. In particular, IIb/IIIa receptor blockers are now a standard of care for acute coronary syndrome patients who undergo PCI.[18]

In the 1990s, the enthusiasm to lower the restenosis rate by using atheroablative devices such as directional coronary atherectomy, rotational atherectomy, transluminal extraction atherectomy, and excimer laser coronary angioplasty was tempered by a higher perforation rate and incidence of emergency surgery.[12] Once experience with the devices became more extensive, the emergency surgery rate was somewhat reduced. However, a recent meta-analysis of multiple trials[19] has confirmed the clinical impression that when atheroablative devices are compared with standard PTCA, there is no reduction in the restenosis rate and an increase in major adverse cardiac events (5.1% vs 3.3%). As a result, the widespread use of atherectomy devices has fallen out of favor, and these devices should be reserved for very select cases.

The introduction of intracoronary stenting in the mid-1990s and eventual refinements in stent technology and pharmacology in the late 1990s resulted in a reduction in the incidence of emergency surgery by providing a more reliable solution to elastic recoil and coronary dissection.[20] In an analysis of the SCAI Registry trends in 16,811 consecutive PCI procedures during this later era, Kimmel and colleagues[21] documented a 0.3% incidence of emergency surgery when stents were used compared with a 0.7% incidence ($P = .002$) with balloon angioplasty.

The development of polytetrafluoroethylene (PTFE)-covered stents (Jomed stent) has provided a better option to seal coronary artery perforations. A European series demonstrated that when perforation occurred as a complication of PCI, use of a PTFE stent reduced the incidence of emergency surgery from 88% to 18%.[22] In addition, even if patients went on to surgery, the PTFE stent served as a valuable supportive device and resulted in a reduction of mortality and morbidity.

The wealth of experience and data in various PCI registries has now permitted risk-adjustment scores, which indicate that hemodynamic instability, disease severity, demographics, and comorbid conditions may predict adverse outcomes, including emergency surgery.[23] Even in the coronary stent era, these assessments may be used to stratify patients according to risk so that more effective strategies and backup may be put in place to reduce adverse events.[11,24]

FACTORS THAT HAVE REDUCED MORTALITY AND MORBIDITY WHEN EMERGENCY CARDIAC SURGERY IS NECESSARY

When all attempts at a percutaneous solution have failed and emergency surgery is necessary, supporting the patient in the catheterization laboratory prior to transfer to the operating suite is crucial to reduce the already evolving higher chance of mortality and morbidity.

Coronary perfusion catheters that allow balloon inflation while still permitting coronary flow via perforated portals in the catheter shaft were a mainstay prior to the development of intracoronary stents.[25] Perfusion catheters still may have role as temporary devices to stabilize dissected coronary flow or to stanch a perforation prior to emergency surgery. As mentioned earlier, PTFE-coated stents also may have a role in stabilizing a coronary perforation prior to going to the operating room.[22]

In addition to mechanical alternatives, attention should be paid to hematologic and hemodynamic instability. There should be a hematologic strategy to stop heparin, consider reversal with protamine, discontinue IIb/IIIa receptor blockers, plan for platelet transfusion, or all of the preceding.[26] When cardiac tamponade is present, percutaneous pericardiocentesis is helpful in reducing this hemodynamic impediment prior to surgery.[27]

The intra-aortic counterpulsation balloon is a mainstay to support patients with cardiovascular hemodynamic compromise who require emergency surgery.[28] Percutaneous cardiopulmonary support has been proposed for catastrophic hemodynamic collapse, but its use has been limited because it requires an experienced standby staff. Nevertheless, it should still be considered as an option in advanced PCI centers, unless immediate transfer to surgery can be assured.[29]

The cardiac surgeon, anesthesiologist, and operating room should be alerted at the first sign that a patient may need emergency surgery. It is better to err on the side of mobilizing the cardiac surgery team even though the event may eventually be controlled and surgery averted. Appropriate anesthesia backup and control of the airway is paramount in providing support of the compromised patient. Advances in surgical technique over the past 20 years have been instrumental in reducing complications following emergency surgery. Having a more stable patient because of the preceding initiatives may also allow arterial conduits, such as the left internal mammary graft vessel, to be used.

Table 59-1 outlines options that should be considered or initiated in the catheterization laboratory to support the patient who requires emergency surgery for failed PCI.

TABLE 59-1

Catheterization Laboratory Support Strategy in Patients Requiring Emergency Surgery

PROBLEM	SUPPORT OPTIONS
Coronary	
Left main dissection	Autoperfusion catheter or stent
Abrupt closure	Autoperfusion catheter or stent
Spiral dissection	Autoperfusion catheter or stent
Perforation	Autoperfusion catheter or covered stent
Systemic	
Hypoxia	Endotracheal intubation
Pulmonary edema	Mechanical ventilation
Hypotension	Intravenous vasopressors
Cardiogenic shock	Intra-aortic balloon pump
Electromechanical dissociation	Percutaneous cardiopulmonary support
Major conduction disorder	Temporary pacemaker
Cardiac tamponade	Pericardiocentesis
Noncoronary	
Aortic dissection	Supportive measures
Vascular accident	Supportive measures
Retained device	Supportive measures
Bleeding	
Heparin therapy	Consider protamine reversal
Glycoprotein IIb/IIIa therapy	Stop infusion
Clopidogrel	Type for platelet transfusion

AMERICAN COLLEGE OF CARDIOLOGY/ AMERICAN HEART ASSOCIATION PERCUTANEOUS CORONARY INTERVENTION GUIDELINES

The American College of Cardiology/American Heart Association/ Society for Cardiovascular Angiography and Interventions (ACC/AHA/SCAI) 2005 Guidelines Update for Percutaneous Coronary Interventions has recommended that a mechanism of quality assurance review be established and ongoing at each institution performing PCI.[30] Operator statistics and institutional data should be reviewed on at least a quarterly basis. Monitoring outcomes by this mechanism assures a mechanism to review cases of mortality, morbidity, or emergency surgery.

Several studies have identified procedural volume as a determining factor for frequency of complications with PCI.[11] An analysis of SCAI registry data confirmed that there was an inverse relationship between the number of angioplasty procedures performed at a hospital and the rate of major complications.[21] Fewer complications occurred in laboratories performing more than 400 angioplasty procedures per year and, conversely, higher rates of emergency coronary bypass graft surgery and death were found in hospitals below this volume. In addition, a volume of 75 Medicare PCIs per physician and 200 per hospital appeared to be a reference mark associated with improved outcomes. Assuming a 35% to 50% ratio of Medicare patients, an appropriate volume to reduce complications would be between 150 and 200 angioplasty procedures per cardiologist and between 400 and 600 per institution per year.[9]

Thus, the most recent ACC/AHA/SCAI revised PCI guidelines[30] recommend that PCI be performed by higher volume operators performing 75 or more cases per year (class I) and that these operators have advanced technical skills and knowledge. Subspecialty certification in interventional cardiology is encouraged. Angioplasties should be performed at institutions with fully equipped interventional laboratories and experienced support staff with the anticipation of performing more than 400 cases per year with an on-site cardiovascular surgical program (class I). The Task Force recommended against angioplasty by low-volume operators (less than 75 cases per year) who work in low-volume institutions (less than 200 cases per year) with or without on-site surgical coverage (class III).

EXPERIENCE IN PERCUTANEOUS CORONARY INTERVENTION WITH OFF-SITE SURGICAL BACKUP

【 】 PRIMARY PCI FOR ACUTE MYOCARDIAL INFARCTION

A recent meta-analysis of 23 randomized trials in acute MI has documented that primary PCI is superior to thrombolytic therapy with significant reductions in death (7% vs 9%), nonfatal reinfarction (3% vs 7%), stroke (1% vs 2%), and combined end point (8% vs 14%).[31] These results are particularly possible if a door-to-balloon time of less than 90 minutes can be achieved. Another meta-analysis of six major MI trials assessing a strategy of transfer for primary PCI versus immediate thrombolysis reaffirmed a significant reduction in morbidity and a trend in reduction of all-cause mortality in the transfer PCI group.[32] These analyses have reaffirmed the favorable risk benefit ratio of primary PCI as the treatment of choice for early acute MI. However, these trials have not tested very early intervention within 1 to 2 hours. Ongoing trials of thrombolysis followed by facilitated coronary angioplasty will contribute additional information to help develop the most comprehensive strategy for acute MI care.

The Primary Angioplasty in Myocardial Infarction Trial-2 (PAMI-2) investigators reported that in 982 patients undergoing primary PCI for acute MI, there was a 0.4% incidence of emergency surgery for failed angioplasty.[33] At the other end of the spectrum, a "real-world" primary PCI registry consisting of a consortium of hospitals in Michigan indicated an emergency surgery rate of 2%, in which there was 20% in-hospital mortality and higher morbidity in the patients who required surgery.[34] The Atlantic Cardiovascular Patient Outcomes Research Team (C-PORT) documented a 0% emergency surgery rate in 225 primary PCI patients at off-site centers.[35] An article by Singh and colleagues[36] from the Mayo Clinic reviewed overall single and multicenter experience with primary PCI at off-site centers and concluded that the risk-benefit ratio for mortality, morbidity, and emergency surgery was favorable. As a result, the 2005 ACC/AHA/SCAI PCI guidelines have agreed that it is appropriate for experienced operators in properly equipped centers without on-site surgical backup to perform direct PCI for acute MI if a moderately large case volume and well-trained staff can be assured.[30]

Wharton and colleagues[37] have proposed criteria for the performance of primary angioplasty at hospitals without on-site cardiac surgery (Table 59-2). In addition, great care should be taken in selecting cases for primary PCI in centers that do not have on-site surgical backup. Table 59-3 is an amalgamation of recommendations from Wharton[37] and the 2005 ACC/AHA/SCAI PCI guidelines[30] regarding patient selection criteria.

At present, the 2005 ACC/AHA/SCAI revised PCI guidelines have designated the strategy of direct PCI in centers with off-site surgical backup as a class IIb indication (conditions for which there is conflicting evidence or a divergence of opinion about the usefulness or efficacy of a procedure or treatment, where the usefulness or efficacy is less well established by evidence or opinion).[30]

【 】 ELECTIVE PCI

Along with the experience of primary PCI for acute MI without on-site surgical backup and with data from Europe regarding elective angioplasty without on-site surgical backup, there is an increasingly spirited debate as to whether low-risk, nonemergency, and elective PCI is appropriate in centers without surgical standby on-site.

A report by Loubeyre and colleagues[38] from a French multicenter registry of 68 centers is a good reflection of the overall European experience with elective PCI in on-site and off-site centers. Only 35% of these centers had on-site surgical backup. Retrospective (1995) and prospective (1996) analysis of more than 50,000 patients undergoing PCI revealed a low 0.38% to 0.32% emergency surgery rate overall but at a consequence of 10% to 17% in-hospital mortality, and 27% to 25% MI. Overall mortality was less in off-site programs (0.41%) versus on-site programs (0.72%). In addition, there was a lower incidence of emergency surgery in off-site centers (0.25%) compared with on-site centers (0.44%), with no difference in subsequent outcome.

The Mayo Clinic has reported on an off-site program in Mankato, Minnesota, linked to a surgical backup center 85 miles away in Rochester, Minnesota.[39] Between 1999 and 2001, 196 patients underwent elective PCI, with success rates of 99.5% and 0.5% in-hospital death. Subsequently, between 2000 and 2001, 89 patients underwent primary PCI for acute MI with success in 93.3% and an in-hospital death rate of 3.4%. There was no emergency

---

◗ **TABLE 59-2**

Criteria for Performing Primary Coronary Angioplasty in Centers with Off-site Surgical Backup[37]

Operator experience: ≥ 75 elective PCI cases per year at on-site center

Institution experience: ≥ 36 primary PCI per year

Catheterization facility service "24/7"

Appropriate supportive equipment

CCU staff experienced in monitoring and IABP

Hospital administration support

Formal written operational protocols

Arrangements for immediate transfer to off-site surgical backup within 1 h

Primary PCI as standard of practice for AMI

Thoughtful case selection

Quality assurance and outcomes analysis program

3–6-month timeline of implementation

AMI = acute myocardial infarction; CCU = critical care unit; IABP = intra-aortic balloon pump; PCI = percutaneous coronary intervention.

TABLE 59-3

Case Selection for Primary Coronary Angioplasty in Centers with Off-site Surgical Backup

Perform in patients with[30]:
　Definite ST-segment elevation on ECG
　Or new left bundle branch block on ECG
　Achievable goal of 90 ± 30 minutes door-to-balloon time

Avoid stable patients with[37]:
　≥ 60% unprotected left main lesions
　Lesions in long or angulated infarct-related vessel with TIMI 3 flow
　Lesions in infarct-related vessel with TIMI 3 flow and triple vessel disease
　Lesions in small or secondary infarct-related vessels
　Lesions in noninfarct vessels

ECG = electrocardiogram; TIMI = Thrombolysis in Myocardial Infarction (trial).

surgery in either the elective or the primary PCI group. This well designed system has been touted as demonstrating the feasibility of elective PCI as the cornerstone of an off-site surgical backup center. However, because there were no emergency surgery cases, the transport system was never really tested.

The ACC-NCDR has recently compared PCI centers with surgery backup on-site to those with surgery off-site in emergency and nonemergency coronary angioplasty cases.[40] This analysis consisted of 278,105 consecutive PCI procedures in 304 centers. Of these, 275,568 patients were from 287 on-site centers compared with 2537 patients in 17 off-site centers. The incidence of emergency surgery in all categories was 0.73% in the on-site group versus 0.39% in the off-site group ($P = .06$). The emergency surgery rate in the subsets of no MI, non-ST- elevation MI or ST-elevation MI was not statistically significant between the two groups. Of those that went on to undergo emergency surgery, there was an 8.7% mortality in on-site centers and no mortality in off-site centers ($P = .68$). Overall in-hospital death regardless of surgery was 1.7% in the off-site centers versus 1.3% in on-site centers ($P = .07$).

However, the off-site emergency group consisted of only 10 patients out of 2537 patients from just 17 centers, which represented only 0.91% of the data and 5.6% of the centers reporting to the ACC-NCDR. The selection of patients at lower risk in off-site centers may have influenced the results. The higher in-hospital mortality in off-site centers may represent a bias against initiating the complex logistics of transport for emergency surgery if PCI was suboptimal or failed.

In general, the initial data from the ACC-NCDR indicates that in selected cases, PCI

centers with off-site surgical backup may perform as well as those centers with on-site surgical backup. However, this is a preliminary report and comprehensive data analysis incorporating more centers is currently underway.

As this chapter has gone to press, a number of publications have reaffirmed the safety of both primary and elective PCI at experienced off-site centers.[41–44] However, an analysis of Medicare data by Wennberg,[45] primarily confined to low volume centers, revealed an increased mortality for elective PCI performed at off-site programs. Since objective peer review is essential to resolve safety issues, off-site PCI centers should be encouraged to participate in registries such as the ACC-NCDR. Additional data elements that should be collected to reflect the unique circumstances of surgical back-up in off-site PCI centers are suggested in Table 59-4.

In summary, it should be emphasized that the current 2005 ACC/AHA/SCAI PCI guidelines[30] still consider elective PCI in facilities with off-site surgical back-up as a class III indication (conditions for which there is evidence or general agreement that

TABLE 59-4

Suggested Additional Database Elements for PCI Programs with Off-site Surgical Backup

Distance: To surgical site (miles)

Transit time: To surgical site (minutes)

Transportation mechanism
　Ground
　Helicopter
　Fixed wing aircraft

Adjunctive support capabilities
　Intra-aortic counterpulsation balloon
　Percutaneous CPS
　Autoperfusion catheter
　Ventilatory support

Training
　Operators
　　Interventional board certified
　　PCI volume per year all centers
　　PCI volume per year at off-site centers
　Catheterization lab staff: rotation at on-site center

Catheterization laboratory facilities
　"24/7" coverage
　Diagnostic volume per year
　PCI volume per year
　　Primary PCI for AMI
　　Elective PCI

If transport for emergency surgery: Time from "decision to transfer" to "open chest/on-pump" (minutes)

AMI = acute myocardial infarction; CPS = cardiopulmonary support; PCI = percutaneous coronary intervention.

the procedure or treatment is not useful or effective, and in some cases may be harmful).

DEBATE OVER ON-SITE VERSUS OFF-SITE SURGICAL BACKUP

The question of whether the development of PCI centers with off-site surgical backup is an appropriate national strategy continues to be a contentious issue, particularly for the performance of elective angioplasty in stable patients. It would seem logical for off-site programs to demonstrate effectiveness on a "24/7" basis in primary PCI for acute MI before expanding to elective PCI. An argument may be made that elective PCI at off-site centers is necessary to assure high institutional and staff skill levels in a less acute setting than acute MI. However, it would seem unacceptable for an off-site PCI center to limit itself to only a "9 to 5" or "boutique" elective program and to not provide "24/7" coverage for primary PCI in acute MI.

Patient selection and prediction of risk are key elements of any PCI program, whether with on-site or off-site surgical backup.[46] Transportation logistics are paramount in any program that does not have on-site surgery. There is a major difference between "off-site" centers across the street or across town versus those that require a helicopter or fixed aircraft transportation system.

Operator qualifications have become a critical issue in the debate about PCI programs without on-site surgical backup. Increased operator volume and institutional volume, as indicated earlier in this chapter, predict higher success and less mortality and morbidity.[11,21,30] Many centers that wish to perform PCI without developing an on-site surgical program tend to be smaller institutions with smaller volume cases. There may be a tendency for less-experienced operators at smaller community hospitals to perform angioplasty procedures. In addition, irrespective of whether a program has on-site or off-site surgical facilities, even an experienced angioplasty operator is no better than the quality of the catheterization laboratory facilities and the experience of the support staff of x-ray technologists and nurses.

The push for PCI centers without on-site surgical backup in elective cases has a disturbing economic incentive that may counteract the best interest of patient care. The medical-legal ramification in the United States of PCI performed in off-site centers is still evolving. Public misperception and the "pseudoscience" of the courtroom serve as sobering reminders of the consequences to operators and the potential liability to institutions that perform elective PCI cases off-site.

Certainly, a very small percentage of PCI cases now require emergency surgical procedures for failed angioplasty. However, when emergency surgery is necessary, the mortality and morbidity are still quite high. Ultimately however, when angioplasty goes awry and appropriate protective options are not in place, the patient suffers. An analogy may be made to the Space Shuttle program, which has had many years of unqualified success punctuated by rare but fatal accidents.

CONCLUSION

The incidence of emergency surgery for failed coronary angioplasty has dropped precipitously over the past 30 years, in parallel with the development of more effective coronary interventional techniques. But the incidence will never be zero, and some form of surgical backup will always be necessary. The interventional cardiologist must ensure that every reasonable, appropriate option is in place to achieve the most effective and safe patient care.

Data are empowering. Interventional cardiologists must continue to actively participate in personal and institutional quality assurance programs and to contribute data to registries such as the ACC-NCDR CathPCI Registry. In that spirit, we may best follow the vision of Andreas Gruentzig, who was courageous in collecting and analyzing the data of a fledgling procedure. This tradition of rigorous self-assessment will continue to result in improved techniques, reassessment of strategies, and reduced mortality and morbidity. In the near future, it is to be hoped, these efforts will result in both an incidence of emergency surgery that is "close to zero" and in significantly reduced consequences to the few patients who require this support mechanism.

REFERENCES

1. Hurst JW. The first coronary angioplasty as described by Andreas Gruentzig. *Am J Cardiol*. 1986;57:185.
2. Gruentzig AR, Senning A, Siegenthaler WE. Nonoperative dilatation of coronary-artery stenosis: Percutaneous transluminal coronary angioplasty. *N Engl J Med*. 1979;301:61.
3. Kent KM, Bentivoglio LG, Block PC, et al. Percutaneous transluminal coronary angioplasty: Report from the Registry of the National Heart, Lung, and Blood Institute. *Am J Cardiol*. 1982;49:2011.
4. American College of Cardiology website. American College of Cardiology-National Cardiovascular Data Registry Module Version 3.04; July 30, 2004. Element 1100, page 31 of 33. Available for download at: http://www.accncdr.com/WebNCDR/NCDRDocuments/datadictdefsonlyv30.pdf.
5. Meier B. Surgical standby for percutaneous transluminal coronary angioplasty. In: Topol EJ, ed. *Textbook of Interventional Cardiology*. Philadelphia, PA: Saunders; 1999:466.
6. Detre K, Holubkov R, Kelsey S, et al. Percutaneous transluminal coronary angioplasty in 1985–1985 and 1977–1981: The National Heart, Lung, and Blood Institute Registry. *N Engl J Med*. 1988;318:265.
7. Feit F, Brooks MM, Sopko G, et al. Long-term clinical outcome in the bypass angioplasty revascularization investigation registry: Comparison with the randomized trial. *Circulation*. 2000;101:2795.
8. McGrath PD, Malenka DJ, Wennberg DE, et al. Changing outcomes in percutaneous coronary interventions: A study of 34,752 procedures in Northern New England, 1990 to 1997. *J Am Coll Cardiol*. 1999;34:674.
9. Grassman ED, Johnson SA, Krone RJ. Predictors of success and major complications for primary percutaneous transluminal coronary angioplasty in acute myocardial infarction: An analysis of the 1990 to 1994 Society for Cardiac Angiography and Interventions registries. *J Am Coll Cardiol*. 1997;30:201.
10. Marks DS, Mensah GA, Kennard ED, et al. Race, baseline characteristics, and clinical outcomes after coronary intervention: The New Approaches in Coronary Interventions (NACI) registry. *Am Heart J*. 2000;140:162.
11. Hannan EL, Racz M, Ryan TJ, et al. Coronary angioplasty volume-outcome relationships for hospitals and cardiologists. *JAMA*. 1997;277:892.
12. Peterson ED, Lansky AJ, Anstrom KJ, et al. Evolving trends in interventional device use and outcomes: Results from the National Cardiovascular Network database. *Am Heart J*. 2000;139:198.
13. Laskey WK, Kimmel S, Krone RJ. Contemporary trends in coronary intervention: A report from the Registry of the Society for Cardiac Angiography and Interventions. *Cathet Cardiovasc Interv*. 2000;49:19.
14. Williams DO, Holubkov R, Yeh W, et al. Percutaneous coronary intervention in the current era compared with 1985–1986: The National Heart, Lung, and Blood Institute Registries. *Circulation*. 2000;102:2945.
15. Seshadri N, Whitlow PL, Acharya N, et al. Emergency coronary artery bypass surgery in the contemporary percutaneous coronary intervention era. *Circulation*. 2002;106:2346.
16. Klein LW, Kutcher MA, Block P, et al. Emergency CABG After failed PCI in contemporary practice: A report from the ACC-NCDR Registry [abstract]. *J Am Coll Cardiol*. 2002;39:8A.

17. Yang EH, Gumina RJ, Lennon RJ, et al. Emergency coronary artery bypass surgery for percutaneous coronary interventions: changes in the incidence, clinical characteristics, and indications from 1979 to 2003. *J Am Coll Cardiol* 2005;46:2004.

18. Boersma E, Harrington RA, Moliterno DJ, et al. Platelet glycoprotein IIb/IIIa inhibitors in acute coronary syndromes: A meta-analysis of all major randomised clinical trials. *Lancet.* 2002;359:189.

19. Bittl JA, Chew DP, Topol EJ, et al. Meta-analysis of randomized trials of percutaneous transluminal coronary angioplasty versus atherectomy, cutting balloon atherotomy, or laser angioplasty. *J Am Coll Cardiol.* 2004;43:936.

20. Haude M, Hopp HW, Rupprecht HJ, et al. Immediate stent implantation versus conventional techniques for the treatment of abrupt vessel closure or symptomatic dissections after coronary balloon angioplasty. *Am Heart J.* 2000;140:e26.

21. Kimmel SE, Localio AR, Krone RJ, et al, for the Registry Committee of the Society for Cardiac Angiography and Interventions. The effects of contemporary use of coronary stents on in-hospital mortality. *J Am Coll Cardiol.* 2001;37:499.

22. Briguori C, Nishida T, Anzuini A, et al. Emergency polytetrafluoroethylene-covered stent implantation to treat coronary ruptures. *Circulation.* 2000;102:3028.

23. Block PC, Peterson EC, Krone, R et al. Identification of variables needed to risk adjust outcomes of coronary interventions: Evidence-based guidelines for efficient data collection. *J Am Coll Cardiol.* 1998;32:275.

24. Holmes DR Jr, Berger PB, Garratt KN, et al. Application of the New York State PTCA mortality model in patients undergoing stent implantation. *Circulation.* 2000;102:517.

25. Ferguson TB Jr, Hinohara T, Simpson J, et al. Catheter reperfusion to allow optimal coronary bypass grafting following failed transluminal coronary angioplasty. *Ann Thorac Surg.* 1986;42:399.

26. Dippel EJ, Kereiakes DJ, Tramuta DA, et al. Coronary perforation during percutaneous coronary intervention in the era of abciximab platelet glycoprotein IIb/IIIa blockade: An algorithm for percutaneous management. *Cathet Cardiovasc Interv.* 2001;52:279.

27. Fejka M, Dixon SR, Safian RD, et al. Diagnosis, management, and clinical outcome of cardiac tamponade complicating percutaneous coronary intervention. *Am J Cardiol.* 2002;90:1183.

28. Craver JM, Weintraub WS, Jones EL, et al. Emergency coronary artery bypass surgery for failed percutaneous coronary angioplasty. A 10-year experience. *Ann Surg.* 1992;215:425.

29. Guarneri EM, Califano JR, Schatz RA, et al. Utility of standby cardiopulmonary support for elective coronary interventions. *Cathet Cardiovasc Interv.* 1999;46:32.

30. Smith SC Jr, Feldman TE, Hirshfeld JW Jr. et al. ACC/AHA/SCAI 2005 guidelines update for percutaneous coronary intervention—summary article: a report of the American College of Cardiology/American Heart Association Task Force on Practice Guidelines (ACC/AHA/SCAI Writing Committee to Update the 2001 Guidelines for Percutaneous Coronary Intervention). *J Am Coll Cardiol.* 2006;47:216.

31. Keeley EC, Boura JA, Grines CL. Primary angioplasty versus intravenous thrombolytic therapy for acute myocardial infarction: A quantitative review of 23 randomised trials. *Lancet.* 2003;361:13.

32. Dalby M, Bouzamondo A, Lechat P, Montalescot G. Transfer for primary angioplasty versus immediate thrombolysis in acute myocardial infarction: A meta-analysis. *Circulation.* 2003;108:1809.

33. Stone GW, Brodie BR, Griffin JJ, et al. Role of cardiac surgery in the hospital phase management of patients treated with primary angioplasty for acute myocardial infarction. *Am J Cardiol.* 2000;85:1292.

34. Moscucci M, O'Donnell M, Share D, et al. Frequency and prognosis of emergency coronary artery bypass grafting after percutaneous coronary intervention for acute myocardial infarction. *Am J Cardiol.* 2003;92:967.

35. Aversano T, Aversano LT, Passamani E, et al. Thrombolytic therapy vs. primary percutaneous coronary intervention for myocardial infarction in patients presenting to hospitals without on-site cardiac surgery: A randomized controlled trial. *JAMA.* 2002;287:1943.

36. Singh M, Ting HH, Berger PB, et al. Rationale for on-site cardiac surgery for primary angioplasty: A time for reappraisal. *J Am Coll Cardiol.* 2002;39:1881.

37. Wharton TP Jr, McNamara NS, Fedele FA, et al. Primary angioplasty for the treatment of acute myocardial infarction: Experience at two community hospitals without cardiac surgery. *J Am Coll Cardiol.* 1999;33:1257.

38. Loubeyre C, Morice MC, Berzin, B et al. Emergency coronary artery bypass surgery following coronary angioplasty and stenting: Results of a French multicenter registry. *Cathet Cardiovasc Interv.* 1999;47:441.

39. Ting HH, Garratt KN, Singh M, et al. Low-risk percutaneous coronary interventions without on-site cardiac surgery: Two years' observational experience and follow-up. *Am Heart J.* 2003;145:278.

40. Kutcher MA, Klein LW, Wharton TP, et al. Clinical outcomes in coronary angioplasty centers with off-site versus on-site cardiac surgery capabilities: A preliminary report from the American College of Cardiology-National Cardiovascular Data Registry [abstract]. *J Am Coll Cardiol.* 2004;43:96A.

41. Wharton TP Jr, Grines LL, Turco MA, et al. Primary angioplasty in acute myocardial infarction at Hospitals with no surgery on-site (the PAMI-No SOS study) versus transfer to surgical centers for primary angioplasty. *J Am Coll Cardiol.* 2004;43:1943.

42. Zavala-Alarcon E, Cecena F, Ashar R, et al. Safety of elective—including "high-risk"—percutaneous coronary interventions without on-site cardiac surgery. *Am Heart J.* 2004;148:676.

43. Paraschos A, Callwood D, Wightman MB, et al. Outcomes following elective percutaneous coronary intervention without on-site surgical backup in a community hospital. *Am J Cardiol.* 2005;95:1091.

44. Ting HH, Raveendran G, Lennon RJ, et al. A total of 1,007 percutaneous coronary interventions without on-site cardiac surgery. Acute and long-term outcomes. *J Am Coll Cardiol.* 2006;47:1713.

45. Wennberg DE, Lucas FL, Siewers AE, et al. Outcomes of percutaneous coronary interventions performed at centers without and with on-site coronary artery bypass graft surgery. *JAMA.* 2004:292:1961.

46. Lotfi M, Mackie K, Dzavik V, Seidelin PH. Impact of delays to cardiac surgery after failed angioplasty and stenting. *J Am Coll Cardiol.* 2004;43:337.

CHAPTER (60)

Complications of Peripheral Procedures

Robert M. Bersin, MD

Percutaneous endovascular intervention has become an established, safe, and effective method to treat a wide variety of vascular diseases. Improvements in devices, techniques, and adjunctive pharmacology have led to marked improvements in not only the clinical effectiveness of these procedures, but also their safety. Nonetheless, complications still occur and vary widely by disease state and vascular bed treated. This chapter highlights the more important complications to be cognizant of, and to carefully avoid, in the performance of endovascular catheter-based interventions.

ACCESS SITE COMPLICATIONS

Access site complications for all endovascular interventions are related to the access site, arteriotomy, and sheath introduction and management. The access site for endovascular interventions is most frequently the common femoral artery, although brachial access is not uncommonly used for lower extremity renal and subclavian intervention. Occasionally, axillary, radial, popliteal, or tibial access sites are employed; these access sites are used less than 5% of the time.

Not only is the femoral access site the most commonly used, it is also associated with the lowest incidence of complications. The most common complication is bleeding and local hematoma formation (3%–6%) followed by pseudoaneurysm formation (1%–2%)[1–7] (Figures 60-1 and 60-2). Surgical repair of the artery is required in approximately 0.5% to 1.0% of procedures. Retroperitoneal hemorrhage is rare with diagnostic procedures (0.2%), but it is greatly increased with high levels of anticoagulation, such as those used in coronary or carotid stent procedures (~3%)[8] (Figure 60-3). The risk of all bleeding complications correlates with the sheath size and level of anticoagulation. Other complications include arterial thrombosis, with or without distal arterial embolization, venous thrombosis, and femoral nerve injury and infection, all of which occur in less than 1% of procedures.[9] Careful attention to detail in achieving access using a single wall technique in the femoral triangle below the inguinal ligament,[10] use of the smallest possible sheath, and frequent monitoring of anticoagulation with measurement of the activated clotting time every 30 minutes during the procedure, along with early sheath removal post-procedure, will minimize the risk of complications. Access site closure devices have been developed for use in the femoral artery, and although they have been demonstrated to shorten the time to ambulation and improve patient comfort, they have not been convincingly demonstrated to reduce major complications.

Access site complications are twice as frequent with use of the brachial artery as with the common femoral artery.[11,12] Because of the smaller size of the brachial artery, arterial thrombosis (Figure 60-4) is the most common complication (~5%), followed by pseudoaneurysm formation (3%–5%). Subclavian artery laceration or rupture has also been reported with brachial access catheter-based intervention, especially in the performance of aortic or thoracic endografting. Major complications such as these, requiring surgical reexploration, have been reported to occur in 5% to 10% of cases involving brachial access. Because thrombosis is the most common complication and is related to the smaller caliber of the brachial artery, it is imperative to minimize the access sheath size during endovascular interventions for this approach, preferably to no larger than 6 French (Fr) but certainly no larger than 8-Fr.

AORTO-ILIAC INTERVENTION

Overall complications of aorto-iliac intervention average 9% to 10%, with little or no difference between percutaneous transluminal

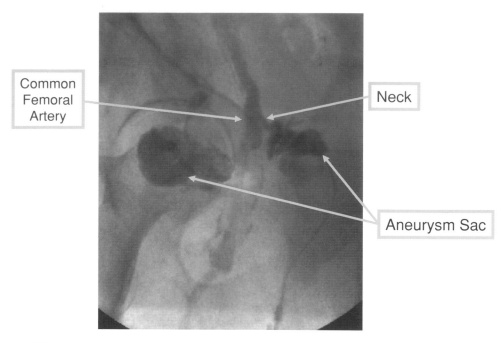

FIGURE 60-1. Common femoral artery pseudoaneurysm. The aneurysm often possesses a neck that leads into an ill-defined sac, which in turn can extend to both sides of the artery.

angioplasty (PTA) and stenting. The majority of complications are related to the access site, as previously discussed.[13] Pseudoaneurysms and acute renal failure related to the administration of large volumes of contrast media are the two most common complications (2%–9% each), followed by acute vessel thrombosis (2.2%), arterial dissection (1.6%), and groin infection (1.3%).[13] Distal embolization is rare (0.3%) and is most commonly seen in the treatment of chronically occluded vessels containing thrombus.[14] Treatment of thromboemboli is problematic in the setting of distal embolization, because most emboli are composed of subacute or chronic thrombus and atheromatous plaque. As a result, the response to thrombolysis has been variable, and the best response observed has been with the performance of rheolytic thrombectomy or surgical embolectomy.

Embolization to the inferior mesenteric artery during aorto-iliac intervention is rare but can be a disastrous complication. Excessive catheter manipulation in a friable aorta has been found to be the strongest correlate of this dreaded complication. Balloon-induced plaque shifting, leading to embolization or occlusion of the inferior mesenteric ostium, has also been observed during balloon angioplasty or stenting of the infrarenal aorta. Although technically challenging, the best technique for avoiding this complication is to minimize catheter manipulation in the diseased infrarenal aorta and to protect the ostium of the inferior mesenteric artery, when it is diseased, with a small 3- to 4-mm, 0.014-in compatible balloon during balloon inflation in the infrarenal aorta.

Iliac artery rupture is also rare (< 0.5%) but can be catastrophic[15] (Figure 60-5). The most common predictors of acute vessel rupture are device oversizing, the heavy presence of calcification at the lesion site, treatment of a chronic total occlusion, or a combination of these. Acute vessel rupture is usually manifested as acute lower abdominal or pelvic pain with attendant hypotension. Contrast extravasation at the site of rupture is usually evident on selective injections; however, it can be obscured, especially if the rupture is angled posteriorly or in the vicinity of a contrast-filled bladder or ureter (see Figure 60-5). The treatment is temporary balloon occlusion with the iliac PTA balloon to temporarily prevent further hemorrhage, followed by

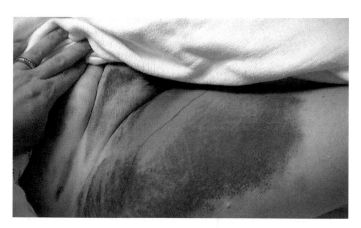

FIGURE 60-2. Large groin hematoma following percutaneous intervention as a result of a common femoral artery pseudoaneurysm.

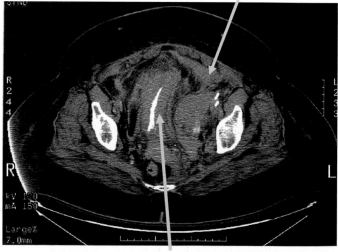

FIGURE 60-3. Extensive retroperitoneal hematoma with resultant extrinsic compression of the bladder.

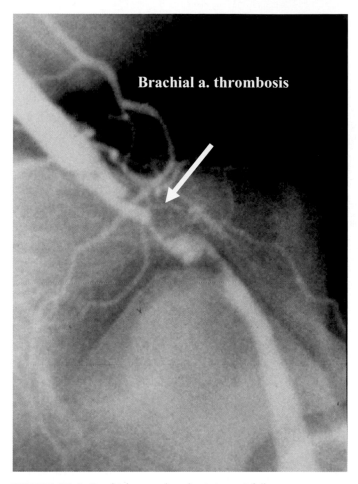

FIGURE 60-4. Brachial artery thrombosis (*arrow*) following percutaneous brachial catheterization.

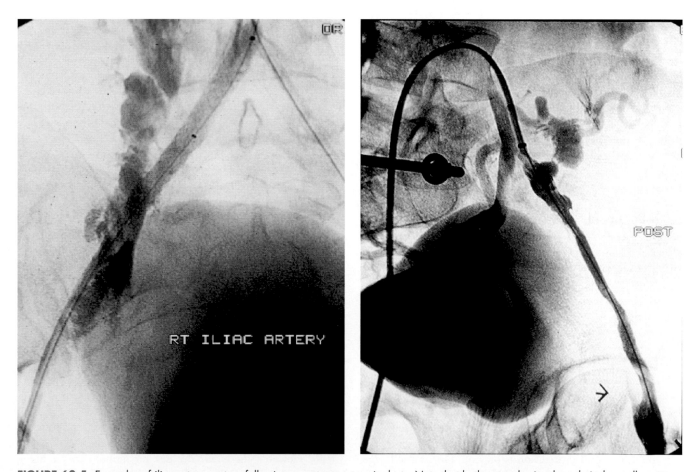

FIGURE 60-5. Examples of iliac artery rupture following percutaneous angioplasty. Note that both examples involve relatively smaller external iliac arteries with diffuse disease.

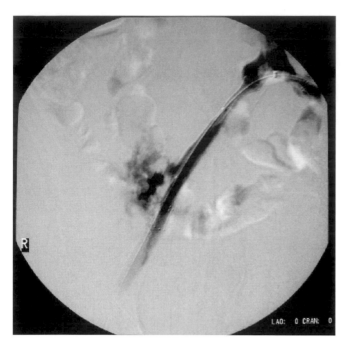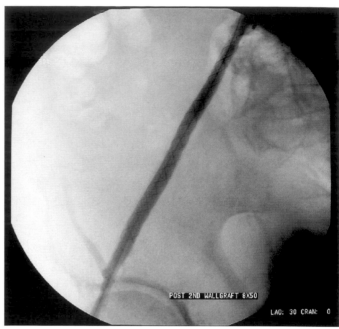

FIGURE 60-6. External iliac artery rupture treated successfully with a WallGraft stent graft device.

placement of a stent graft (Figure 60-6). It is imperative in these situations not to lose wire position from the true lumen when the PTA balloon is exchanged for stent graft placement, and proper care and precautions should be taken to observe that wire compatibilities and lengths are taken into account before the balloons are removed and the stent graft is introduced. Prompt placement of a stent graft has been reported on several occasions to prevent further hemorrhage and obviate the need for urgent surgery.[15]

One additional complication of iliac stenting is inadvertent occlusion of the internal iliac artery. A purposeful covering of the origin of the internal iliac branch is a common occurrence with iliac stent procedures. This rarely has clinical consequences, because the stent itself normally does not occlude the side branch given the large interstices of the iliac stent. However, the internal iliac artery can occlude with some predictability due to plaque shifting during balloon angioplasty or stent deployment, especially if the internal iliac ostium is diseased and the angioplasty procedure is being performed at the transition of the common iliac artery to the external iliac artery. In these situations, patients occasionally become symptomatic with hip or buttock claudication as a result of occlusion of the internal iliac artery.

Rarely, acute myonecrosis and pelvic ischemia can occur if there is sudden occlusion of the internal iliac artery in a vessel without demonstrated collateralization. The clinical impact of this event is greatest if contralateral internal iliac occlusion is also present. In such cases, the sudden development of bilateral internal iliac occlusions can lead to acute pelvic ischemia with disastrous consequences. Therefore, care must be taken in performing iliac angioplasty or stenting at the internal-external iliac bifurcation if a contralateral internal iliac occlusion is present. This is one of the clear indications to protect the internal iliac branch during the

procedure with either wire access, deliberate angioplasty, or stenting of the internal iliac ostium.

INFRA-INGUINAL LOWER EXTREMITY INTERVENTION

Percutaneous transluminal angioplasty of the infra-inguinal vessels has been demonstrated not to be as durable as aorto-iliac interventions, most likely as the result of the smaller vessel sizes, reduced flow rates (often due to poor distal runoff), and lesion length, as well as the presence of diffuse disease.[16,17] Because of these adverse features of the infra-inguinal anatomy, percutaneous interventions in these vessels have expanded broadly to include a rich mixture of new device technologies, including atherectomy devices, laser-assisted angioplasty, cryoplasty, cutting balloon angioplasty, and combinations thereof. The advent of dedicated chronic total occlusion devices and subintimal reentry techniques and devices specifically designed for infra-inguinal use has also spurred the aggressive use of angioplasty techniques for long-segment total occlusions. Any, if not all, of these devices require larger introducer sheaths and longer procedure times.

It is no surprise, therefore, that the potential for access site groin complications is greater in the infra-inguinal procedures (6%), especially if an antegrade common femoral artery or direct superficial femoral artery puncture is employed. Vessel dissection rates with PTA are historically high in the superficial femoral artery and this, coupled with a known high recurrence rate with primary angioplasty, has led to the liberal use of nickel titanium-containing nitinol stents. However, the recurrence rate for nitinol stents is higher in these locations than in any other vascular bed where they are used,

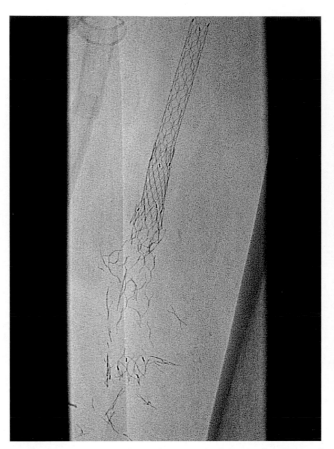
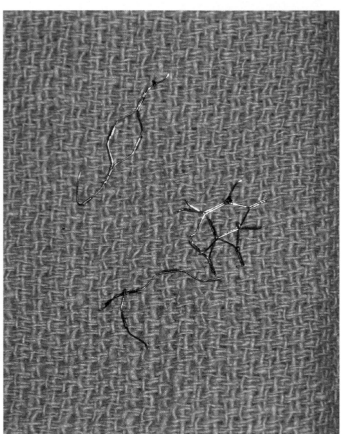

FIGURE 60-7. Fractured nitinol stent in the left superficial femoral artery 2 years after implantation, with surgically removed fragments shown at right. This fracture was associated with a large aneurysm of the vessel at the site of stent implantation.

principally because diffuse disease is often being treated, employing long-segment stenting (16–20 cm of stent length). Stenting of long-segment disease with nitinol stents (≥ 16 cm) has been associated with a high incidence of late stent fracture[18] (Figure 60-8). Stent fractures have been convincingly demonstrated to be associated with restenosis or occlusion in two thirds of the cases.[19,20] Stent fractures

can rarely lead to aneurysmal dilation or rupture of the vessel, necessitating urgent surgery (see Figure 60-7).

Distal embolization has not been systematically studied in lower extremity intervention but is known to occur (Figure 60-9). Clinical consequences can be acute, irreversible limb ischemia often leading to amputation, especially if distal runoff is poor (one vessel or less). Dramatic cases of distal embolization during infra-inguinal intervention have been described in the treatment of long-segment occlusions, particularly with atherectomy and laser devices (2% incidence), but the true incidence of embolization is unknown. Attempts have been made to minimize the risk of distal embolization during complex superficial femoral or popliteal interventions with the use of distal protection devices, principally filters, but this approach has not been systematically studied.

Perforation is uncommon in the treatment of infra-inguinal stenoses (0.5%), even with the liberal use of atherectomy and laser devices, largely because of the lack of vessel tortuosity and lesion angulation (two best correlates of vessel perforation with debulking devices). However, with increasing popularity of the subintimal reentry angioplasty technique for the treatment of chronic total occlusions, the chance for vessel perforation in the subintimal space, especially with the application of atherectomy or laser-assisted angioplasty in these settings, is undoubtedly greater (9% incidence of perforation in the treatment of occlusions with the laser in the PELA [Peripheral Excimer Laser Angioplasty] trial) (Figure 60-8). At times these perforations can be dramatic, requiring stent grafting, embolization, or surgery. This is best avoided by ensuring that the wire passage remains within the true lumen or subintimal space

FIGURE 60-8. Rupture of the superficial femoral artery three days after an otherwise successful percutaneous recanalization and stenting of a chronic total occlusion. Note the rupture is at the point where the stent begins to deviate from the true lumen to the adventitial space.

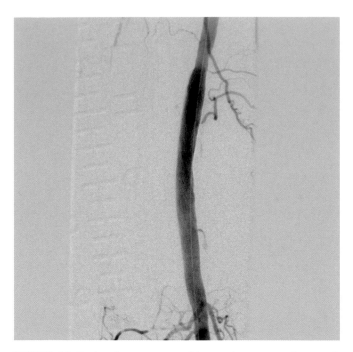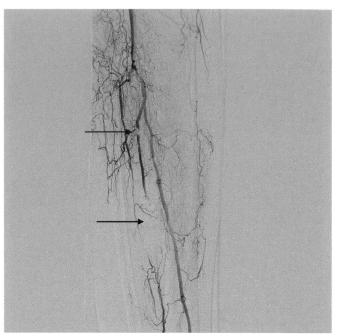

FIGURE 60-9. An otherwise successful stent placement in the superficial femoral artery is complicated by distal embolization to the peroneal artery. Arrows point to embolic occlusions of the peroneal artery.

without traversing adventitia, by avoiding passage of guidewires and devices into bridging collaterals, and by avoiding use of the debulking devices in the subintimal space.

RENAL INTERVENTION

Because of the known effects of renal artery disease on loss of renal mass and renal function, it should not be surprising that the most common complication of renal artery intervention is acute renal failure.[21–24] Acute renal injury is most commonly caused by excessive contrast administration. Because contrast is administered directly into the renal vasculature for these procedures, the volume of contrast needed to produce contrast-induced acute tubular necrosis is generally believed to be less than with other peripheral vascular interventions. The incidence of acute tubular necrosis following renal artery intervention relates to the degree of renal impairment prior to the procedure; the incidence is 10% in patients with creatinine clearances greater than 60 mL/min and 38% for patients with creatinine clearances of 20 mL/min or less.[25]

Techniques to reduce the incidence of contrast-induced acute tubular necrosis include dilution of contrast or saline to minimize the volume administered and measurement of translesion gradients instead of angiograms in borderline lesions to minimize the amount of contrast used. Gadolinium may also be used in lieu of iodinated contrast, but the degree of opacification and image quality will be less because this element is not as radiodense as iodinated contrast. Gadolinium has been demonstrated to be safe, although the absolute volume that can be administered without hepatotoxicity is limited by a per kilogram body weight dosage. Saline or bicarbonate hydration pre- and post-procedure has also been demonstrated to reduce the incidence of contrast-induced

acute tubular necrosis.[26] The use of acetylcysteine is controversial but may be helpful in severe cases where the baseline renal impairment is profound.[27]

Another factor contributing to the development of acute renal failure following renal artery intervention is ischemia related to transient vessel occlusion with the angioplasty balloon catheters. This is not felt to be a major contributor to the development of acute renal failure in most cases, as most renal intervention procedures today are stent placement procedures with short balloon inflation times. However, atheroemboli are felt to be a significant contributor to renal ischemia and do occur with percutaneous renal angioplasty, and especially with renal stent placements (5.3%) (Figure 60-10). In some instances, particularly with long bulky lesions, friable lesions, or vessels with visible thrombus, atheroemboli may contribute significantly to the development of acute renal failure. Distal embolic protection devices have been employed in the renal circulation, and in one prospective study, appeared to reduce the risk of severe and dialysis-dependent acute tubular necrosis following renal angioplasty and stenting.[28] Although dramatic examples of atheroemboli during renal intervention have been observed, the true value of distal protection devices in preventing acute renal failure with renal intervention has not been clearly established and is currently under study.

Other complications of renal intervention include renal artery dissection (6–7%), dissection of the aorta at the renal artery ostium, and renal artery or aortic perforation. These complications are uncommon (≤ 1% each), and are associated with either excessive balloon sizing or severe lesion calcification.[29] Dissections are most common in the distal renal vasculature, particularly the intra-parenchymal branch vessels, which are often prone to spiral dissection. Intervention in these branch vessels is to be avoided unless they have been convincingly demonstrated to be the cause of renal vascular hypertension.

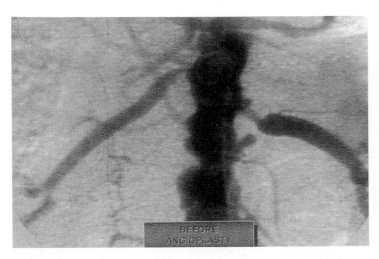
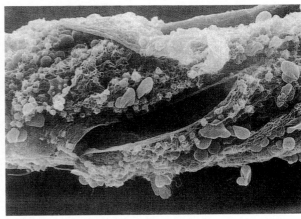

FIGURE 60-10. Atheroemboli recovered with a PercuSurge device following renal artery intervention. *(Courtesy of Henry M, Klonaris C, Henry I, et al. Protected renal stenting with the PercuSurge GuardWire device: A pilot study. J Endovasc Ther. 2001;8:227.)*

CAROTID INTERVENTION

The advent of nitinol stents and distal embolic protection devices (EPDs) has made carotid artery intervention technically feasible and safe. The most important complication of carotid intervention is distal embolization resulting in stroke (Figure 60-11). Although randomized data demonstrating benefit of distal EPDs in the carotid circulation is lacking; single-center studies and multicenter registries suggest that EPDs reduce risk of major and minor stroke and so should be employed wherever feasible. With distal embolic protection, major and minor stroke rates within the first 30 days of the procedure are as low as 1.8%.[30,31]

Techniques to minimize the risk of embolization include minimizing manipulation of the catheter to engage the carotid ostium.

This is accomplished by the performance of a proper aortic arch injection prior to catheter engagement to precisely identify the location of the ostia of the innominate and common carotid vessels and to determine whether disease is present at the ostia. Additionally, proper roadmapping also allows for more direct catheter engagement into the ostium, thus avoiding excessive manipulation of catheters, especially dragging and scraping of the catheters across the aortic arch. Additionally, once the carotid ostium is engaged, care must also be exercised in crossing the carotid lesion with the EPD, preferably without lesion predilation. Once the carotid lesion is crossed, the EPD should then be deployed in a relatively straight segment of the internal carotid artery, avoiding curves or bends, with care taken to assure good apposition of the device against the vessel walls in at least two orthogonal views. Continued monitoring of the EPD for proper apposition is advised at every critical stage of

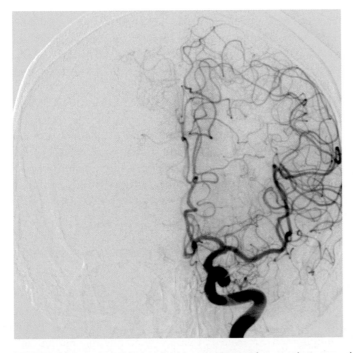
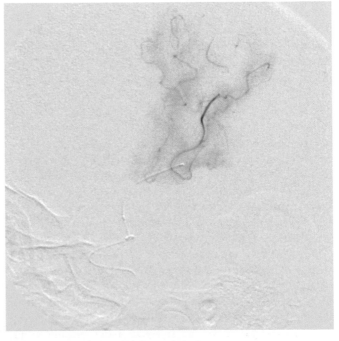

FIGURE 60-11. Distal embolization to the brain after an otherwise technically successful carotid stent procedure.

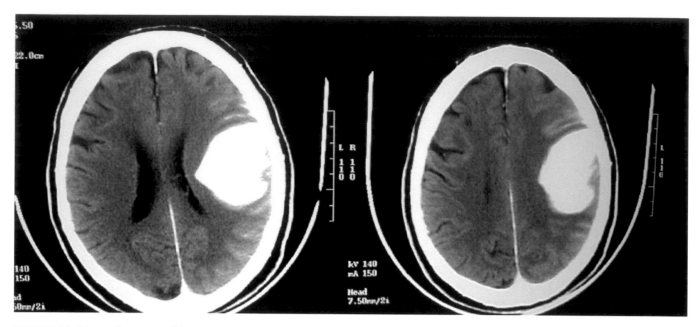

FIGURE 60-12. Fatal intracranial hemorrhage following a carotid stent procedure in a patient with hyperperfusion syndrome.

the procedure, including balloon predilatation, stent deployment, and balloon postdilatation. Finally, equally important is a meticulous recapture and removal of the EPD, taking care not to catch or drag the recapture device against the deployed stent or guiding catheters so as to avoid tearing or snagging the device and potentially liberating the captured embolic debris.

Other significant complications of carotid artery stenting include access site complications (8–10%), systemic hypotension (3.4%), myocardial infarction (2.1–2.6%), and contrast-induced renal failure (1%).[30-34] Contrast-induced acute cerebritis with or without acute renal failure has also been described when contrast volumes are large, particularly in long procedures. For this reason, contrast should be diluted with saline for each injection to minimize the total volume injected directly into the cerebral circulation using digital subtraction angiographic imaging whenever possible.

Acute carotid stent thrombosis or occlusion has also been described, usually in the setting of inadequate anticoagulation, particularly antiplatelet therapy. This risk can be minimized by paying careful attention to preprocedural dosing of aspirin and clopidogrel, and by readministration of loading doses of each agent, even in instances when patients are already on chronic therapy. Careful monitoring of the activated clotting time to ensure therapeutic levels of anticoagulation with heparin or bivalirudin, or both, intraprocedurally is also advised at no more than 30-minute intervals to assure an activated clotting time of at least 275 seconds throughout the procedure. This is important to prevent spontaneous clot formation within the stent or filter during the procedure. The development of acute stent thrombosis may be one of the few indications for the adjunctive administration of a glycoprotein IIb/IIIa antagonist.[35,36]

Intracranial hemorrhage is a rare complication of carotid stenting (< 1%).[30-33] It principally occurs following distal embolization, or in hypertensive patients in whom blood pressure is not adequately controlled prior to the procedure, or in instances where urgent stenting is performed in the setting of an acute neurologic event, especially if a glycoprotein IIb/IIIa antagonist is used.[37]

An extremely rare complication of carotid artery stenting is the hyperperfusion syndrome. This syndrome is characterized by acute cerebral edema, and often hemorrhage, when revascularization is performed in a hemodynamically critical carotid stenosis with an isolated hemisphere.[38] The risk can be minimized by paying careful attention to control of hypertension before and during the procedure, and by careful monitoring of adjunctive anticoagulation to avoid overadministration of either heparin or bivalirudin. Even with proper precautions, spontaneous but rare occurrences of the hyperperfusion syndrome have been described without clear causes. The management includes reversal of anticoagulation and keeping blood pressure in the low normal range. A craniotomy may be necessary to control bleeding. In most instances, the hemorrhage occurring with hyperperfusion syndrome is fatal despite all these measures (Figure 60-12).

Lastly, carotid dissection or rupture is uncommon (< 1% each), because the procedure almost universally involves placement of the self-expanding nitinol stent with minimal predilation and without aggressive postdilation. Vessel dissection can normally be managed with placement of an additional self-expanding stent. However, if vessel rupture occurs, either stent grafting or, more commonly, urgent surgery should be performed if technically feasible.

SUMMARY

As a result of the evolutionary development of vessel-specific techniques and devices, percutaneous vascular interventions are, today, technically successful and safe procedures. The most common complications are related to the access site and the injurious effects of iodinated contrast. The remainder are mechanical in nature and related to the potentially injurious effects of pre-balloon dilation or the ablative effects of mechanical devices, including vessel dissection, perforation, and atheroembolization. Most of these complications can be avoided with meticulous attention to catheterization technique, minimization of catheter manipulation, appropriate device sizing and selection, and careful attention to procedural anticoagulation. However, by far the most important guiding principle is that of appropriate case selection, which, if exercised prudently, can minimize the risk of all potential complications and afford the best outcomes.

REFERENCES

1. Lang EK. A survey of the complications of percutaneous retrograde arteriography. Seldinger technique. *Radiology.* 1963;81:257.
2. Brener BJ, Couch NP. Peripheral arterial complications of left heart catheterization and their management. *Am J Surg.* 1973;125:521.
3. Mortensen JD. Clinical sequelae from arterial needle puncture, cannulation, and incision. *Circulation.* 1967;35:1118.
4. Bourassa MG, Noble J. Complication rate of coronary arteriography. A review of 5250 cases studied by percutaneous femoral technique. *Circulation.* 1976;53:106.
5. Judkins MP, Gander MP. Prevention of complications of coronary arteriography. *Circulation.* 1974;49:599.
6. Adams DF, Frasser DB, Abrams HL. The complications of coronary arteriography. *Circulation.* 1973;48:609.
7. Bogart DB, Bogart MA, Miller JT, et al. Femoral artery catheterization complications: A study of 503 consecutive patients. *Catheter Cardiovasc Diag.* 1995;34:8.
8. Kent KC, Moscucci M, Mansour KA, et al. Retroperitoneal hematoma after cardiac catheterization: Prevalence, risk factors, and optimal management. *J Vasc Surg.* 1994;20:905.
9. Kloster FE, Bristow JD, Griswold HE. Femoral artery occlusion following percutaneous catheterization. *Am Heart J.* 1970;79:175.
10. Schnyder G, Sawhney N, Whisenant B, et al. Common femoral artery anatomy is influenced by demographics and comorbidity: Implications for cardiac and peripheral invasive studies. *Catheter Cardiovasc Interv.* 2001;53:289.
11. Chahine RA, Herman MV, Gorlin R. Complications of coronary arteriography: Comparison of the brachial to the femoral approach. *Ann Int Med.* 1972;76:862.
12. Campion BC, Frye RL, Pluth JR, et al. Arterial complications of retrograde brachial arterial catheterization: A prospective study. *Mayo Clin Proc.* 1971; 46:589.
13. Bosch JL, Hunink MGM. Meta-analysis of the results of percutaneous transluminal angioplasty and stent placement for aortoiliac occlusive disease. *Radiology.* 1997;204:87.
14. Timaran CH, Stevens SL, Freeman MB, et al. Predictors for adverse outcome after iliac angioplasty and stenting for limb-threatening ischemia. *J Vasc Surg.* 2002;36:507.
15. Nyman U, Uher P, Lindh M, et al. Stent-graft treatment of iatrogenic iliac artery perforations: Report of three cases. *Eur J Vasc Endovasc Surg.* 1999;17:259.
16. Sabeti S, Mlekusch W, Amighi J, et al. Primary patency of long-segment self-expanding nitinol stents in the femoropopliteal arteries. *J Endovasc Ther.* 2005;12:6.
17. Gray BH, Sullivan TM, Childs MB, et al. High incidence of restenosis/reocclusion of stents in the percutaneous treatment of long-segment superficial femoral artery disease after suboptimal angioplasty. *J Vasc Surg.* 1997;25:74.
18. Duda SH, Pusich B, Richter G, et al. Sirolimus-eluting stents for the treatment of obstructive superficial femoral artery disease: Six-month results. *Circulation.* 2002;106:1505.
19. Scheinert D, Scheinert S, Sax J, et al. Prevalence and clinical impact of stent fractures after femoropopliteal stenting. *J Am Coll Cardiol.* 2005;45:312.
20. Babalik E, Gulbaran M, Gurmen T, et al. Fracture of popliteal artery stents. *Circ J.* 2003;67:643.
21. Tegtmeyer CJ, Selby JB, et al. Results and complications of angioplasty in fibromuscular disease. *Circulation.* 1991;83(suppl 2):1155.
22. Tegtmeyer CJ, Kellum CD, Ayers C. Percutaneous transluminal angioplasty of the renal artery: Results and long-term followup. *Radiology.* 1984; 153:77.
23. MacLeod M, Taylor AD Baxter G, et al. Renal artery stenosis managed by Palmaz stent insertion: Technical and clinical outcome. *J Hypertens.* 1995; 13:1791.
24. Blum U, Krumme B, Flugel P, et al. Treatment of ostial renal-artery stenoses with vascular endoprostheses after unsuccessful balloon angioplasty. *N Engl J Med.* 1997;336:459.
25. Kennedy DJ, Colyer WR, Brewsster PS, et al. Renal insufficiency as a predictor of adverse events and mortality after renal artery stent placement. *Am J Kidney Dis.* 2003;42:926.
26. Merten GJ, Burgess WP, Gray LV, et al. Prevention of contrast-induced nephropathy with sodium bicarbonate: A randomized controlled trial. *JAMA.* 2004;291:2328.
27. Fishbane S, Durham JH, Marzo K, Rudnick M. N-Acetycysteine in the prevention of radiocontrast-induced nephropathy. *J Am Soc Nephrol.* 2004; 15:251.
28. Holden A, Hill A. Renal angioplasty and stenting with distal protection of the main renal artery in ischemic nephropathy: Early experience. *J Vasc Surg.* 2003; 38:962.
29. Bonelli FS, McKusick MA, Textor SC, et al. Renal artery angioplasty: Technical results and clinical outcome in 320 patients. *Mayo Clin Proc.* 1995; 70:1041.
30. Kastrup A, Groschel K, Krapf H, et al. Early outcome of carotid angioplasty and stenting with and without cerebral protection devices. A systematic review of the literature. *Stroke.* 2003;34:813.
31. Roubin GS, New G, Iyer SS, et al. Immediate and late clinical outcomes of carotid artery stenting in patients with symptomatic and asymptomatic carotid artery stenosis: A prospective 5-year analysis. *Circulation.* 2001; 103:532.
32. Yadav JS, Wholey MH, Kuntz RE, et al for the Stenting and Angioplasty with Protection in Patients at High Risk for Endarterectomy Investigators. Protected carotid-artery stenting versus endarterectomy in high-risk patients. *N Engl J Med.* 2004;351:1493.
33. Wholey MH. The ARCHeR Trial. Prospective clinical trial for carotid stenting in high surgical risk patients. Preliminary 30 day results. Presented at the American College of Cardiology Scientific Sessions; March 30, 2003; Chicago, IL.
34. Tan KT, Cleveland TJ, Berczi V, et al. Timing and frequency of complications after carotid artery stenting: What is the optimal period of observation? *J Vasc Surg.* 2003;38:236.
35. Kittusamy PK, Koenigsberg RA, McCormick DJ. Abciximab for the treatment of acute distal embolization associated with internal carotid artery angioplasty. *Catheter Cardiovasc Interv.* 2001;54:221.
36. Bush RL, Bhama JK, Lin PH, et al. Transient ischemic attack due to early carotid stent thrombosis: Successful rescue with rheolytic thrombectomy and systemic abciximab. *J Endovasc Ther.* 2003;10:870.
37. Moshiri S, Di Marco C, et al. Severe intracranial hemorrhage after emergency carotid stenting and abciximab administration for post-operative thrombosis. *Catheter Cardiovasc Interv.* 2001;53:225.
38. McCabe D, Brown MM, Clifton A. Fatal cerebral reperfusion hemorrhage after carotid stenting. *Stroke.* 1999;30:2483.

PART 7 Medical Management of Risk Factors

CHAPTER (61)

Lipid-Lowering Therapy and the Interventional Cardiologist

R. Scott Wright, MD, and Joseph G. Murphy, MD

Histologically, atherosclerosis is a diffuse inflammatory-proliferative arterial reaction that is initiated by endothelial injury. Although flow-limiting atherosclerotic lesions may appear focal on coronary angiography, their pathologic basis is widespread within the arterial tree. Thus risk factor modification, especially low-density lipoprotein (LDL) cholesterol, high-density lipoprotein (HDL) cholesterol, and triglyceride optimization are mandatory for all patients treated by percutaneous revascularization techniques. Effective lipid-lowering therapy is widely available today for the practicing interventional cardiologist. There are multiple medications from which one can now choose to effectively treat dyslipidemia.[1] Statins, or inhibitors of the 3-hydroxy-3-methyl-glutaryl CoA reductase (HMG) enzyme, are the most widely used agents. Worldwide, consumers spend 15 to 20 billion dollars annually for these agents, with generally good coronary heart disease prevention.[2] Figure 61-1 shows the cardiovascular disease mortality rate in Europe as a function of sales of statins. Many other nonstatin agents are available that compliment the statins or target different pathways altogether, such that it should be rare in today's environment to have a patient whose dyslipidemia cannot be adequately managed. This chapter will focus on the treatment of dyslipidemia in patients with established coronary artery disease (CAD), review the literature in support of the treatment of dyslipidemia, review the available agents which one can use in the treatment of dyslipidemia, review novel and emerging risk factors, and discuss scenarios in the treatment of dyslipidemia.

CLASSIFICATION OF DYSLIPIDEMIA

Dyslipidemia is a heterogeneous disorder with multiple etiologies. The definition of dyslipidemia has undergone revision,[3] and a practical clinical application of the current definitions are depicted in Table 61-1. In western societies, the majority of cases of dyslipidemia are secondary to lifestyle and dietary habits. Physiologic LDL is probably in the range of 50 to 70 mg/mL, as determined by findings in nonwesternized primitive societies where atherosclerosis is unknown. Thus, modern diet and lifestyle (tobacco use, obesity, high fat intake, sedentary activity) are probably the largest contributors to the current epidemic of atherosclerosis. The primary causes of dyslipidemia (Table 61-2) occur rarely and demand the attention of a consulting lipidologist. The many secondary causes of dyslipidemia may exist in the clinical practice of the interventional cardiologist (Table 61-3) and should be addressed concurrently with initiation of pharmacotherapy. The great majority of cases encountered during the daily practice of medicine represent secondary etiologies of dyslipidemia.

It is the rare patient who presents with an isolated pattern of dyslipidemia. Most patients present with a mixed picture of dyslipidemia, such as an elevated LDL cholesterol in combination with a low HDL cholesterol or elevated triglycerides. In addition, many patients with dyslipidemia have multiple confounding medical issues such as diabetes or metabolic syndrome, obesity, hypertension,

Conflict of interest disclosures for Dr. Wright include research grants from Bayer, Merck, Bristol-Myers Squibb, and Centocor; research support from Aventis, Novartis, and Bristol-Myers Squibb; and consultantships with Bristol-Myers Squibb and AstraZeneca.

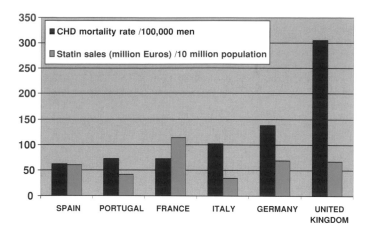

CHD Mortality Compared to Statin Sales 1998-1999

FIGURE 61-1. The coronary heart disease (CHD) mortality rate in Europe as a function of sales of statins. *(From Brady AJB.[2])*

and on occasion obstructive sleep apnea, all of which necessitate treatment. One can also encounter on a rare occasion the patient with an isolated low HDL or isolated hypertriglyceridemia.

The majority of patients can have significant success in managing their dyslipidemia with intensive dietary modification. Reductions in saturated fat and total caloric content typically reduce LDL cholesterol values 10% to 15%, and even better in some situations. Plasma triglycerides can fall 20% to 40% once dietary changes are instituted. Weight loss can result in similar improvements in dyslipidemia. Initiation of a regular, vigorous exercise program can raise HDL cholesterol values by 10% to 15%, comparable to changes induced by pharmacologic therapy yet without any of the potential side effects and economic costs of pharmacologic therapy. Dietary therapy, although undoubtedly effective in the highly motivated individual, fails to achieve goal LDL levels in the majority of patients and often requires the addition of pharmacologic therapies.

TABLE 61-1

Definitions of Dyslipidemia

CATEGORY	VALUE (MG/DL)		
	LDL	HDL	TRIGLYCERIDES
CAD, PVD, CVD	>100	<40	>150
Two NCEP RFs	>130	<40	>150
Less two NCEP RFs	>160	<40	>150
Diabetes mellitus	>100	<40	>150

[a]Risk factors (Rfs) are defined as hypertension, tobacco use, diabetes mellitus, and family history of coronary artery disease. Values listed are for men older than 55 years of age and for women older than 60 years of age.
CAD = coronary artery disease; CVD = cerebrovascular disease; HDL = high-density lipoprotein; LDL = low-density lipoprotein; NCEP = National Cholesterol Education Program; PVD = peripheral vascular disease.

TABLE 61-2

Dyslipidemia: Primary Causes

ELEVATED LDL CHOLESTEROL	LOW HDL CHOLESTEROL
• LDL receptor deficiency • Familial homozygous hyperlipidemia	• Apo A-1 deficiency • Apo A-1 mutations • LCAT deficiency (partial or complete) • Tangier disease • Familial hypoalpaliproteinemia

HDL = high-density lipoprotein; LCAT = lecithin cholesterol acyl transferase LDL low-density lipoprotein.

PHARMACOLOGIC AGENTS FOR THE TREATMENT OF DYSLIPIDEMIA

Drug treatment of dyslipidemia is effective and has been demonstrated to reduce long-term cardiovascular risks.[4–10] The first line of therapy in most patients should be a statin. However, many patients may suffer from mixed dyslipidemias and require combination pharmacotherapy. The approach to the pharmacologic treatment of dyslipidemia should be tailored to correct as much of the total dyslipidemia as possible without inducing drug-related side effects.

TABLE 61-3

Dyslipidemia: Secondary Causes

ELEVATED LDL CHOLESTEROL	LOW HDL CHOLESTEROL
• Obesity • High fat intake • Hypothyroidism • Diabetes mellitus • Nephrotic syndrome • Anabolic steroids • Progestins • Obstructive hepatobiliary disease	• Metabolic syndrome • Diabetes mellitus • Obesity or weight gain • Physical inactivity • Tobacco use • Beta blocker therapy • Low fat or high polyunsaturated fat diets • Anabolic steroids • Progestins • Thiazide diuretics

HDL = high-density lipoprotein; LDL = low-density lipoprotein.

TABLE 61-4

Statins Used to Treat Dyslipidemia

AGENT		CHOLESTEROL EFFECT ↓ LDL (%)	↑ HDL (%)	TRIGLYCERIDE EFFECT ↓ TG (%)
Lovastatin	10 mg	25–30	0–10	0–6
	80 mg	35–40	0–10	19–27
Pravastatin	10 mg	25–30	0–10	11
	40 mg	25–35	0–10	24
Simvastatin	20 mg	25–30	0–10	0–5
	80 mg	40–50	0–10	25–40
Atorvastatin	10 mg	35–40	0–10	19
	40 mg	40–60	0–10	37
Rosuvastatin	5 mg	40–45	0–10	19
	40 mg	50–65	0–10	37

HDL = high-density lipoprotein; LDL = low-density lipoprotein; TG = triglyceride.

[ ] SPECIFIC DRUGS

Statins

Statins function in at least two ways in patients with dyslipidemia. First, statins inhibit the enzyme responsible for the rate-limiting step of cholesterol biosynthesis, HMG coenzyme A reductase, and thus directly inhibit cholesterol biosynthesis. Second, statins promote LDL receptor upregulation of hepatocytes and thus promote the biological clearance of LDL cholesterol. Finally, research has suggested that statins also work by inhibiting the synthesis of prenylated proteins such as geranyl-geranyl pyrophosphate and farnesyl-farnesyl pyrophosphate; this inhibition indirectly mediates intracellular processes that involve cell-signal trafficking and protein synthesis.[11]

TABLE 61-5

Nonstatins Used to Treat Dyslipidemia

AGENT	CHOLESTEROL EFFECT ↓ LDL (%)	↑ HDL (%)	TRIGLYCERIDE EFFECT TG (%)
Resin binding agent	15–20	0–2	5–10 ↑
Ezetamibe	15–20	0–2	0–5 ↑
Sitosterol esters	8–13	0–2	4–8 ↓
Niacin	20–30	20–30	30–40 ↓
Gemfibrozil	10	20	50–60 ↓
Fenofibrate	10–15	5–20	40–50 ↓

HDL = high-density lipoprotein; LDL = low-density lipoprotein; TG = triglyceride.

Statins typically lower LDL cholesterol 25% to 55%, depending on which agent is used (Table 61-4). Statins lower total cholesterol similarly in magnitude to that observed with LDL cholesterol. Statins also raise HDL cholesterol by 5% to 15% and several agents reduce plasma triglycerides 15% to 45%. Table 61-5 shows the efficacy of nonstatin lipid-lowering agents.

Niacin

Niacin is the most potent HDL cholesterol-raising substance currently available. This agent is commonly used and, in most patients, raises HDL cholesterol 20% to 30% and lowers plasma triglycerides 30% to 40%. Niacin also reduces plasma LDL cholesterol an additional 20% to 30%, which is often helpful in the populations in which it is prescribed. Niacin is generally well tolerated if started at lower doses and gradually increased over time. Some clinicians recommend aspirin pretreatment to reduce the risk of flushing and headache that often accompany niacin therapy. Niacin can be used safely in combination with statins, fibrates, and ezetimibe.

Fibrates

Fibrates are potent triglyceride-lowering agents. Currently, two preparations, gemfibrozil and fenofibrate, are available in the United States. Both agents reduce plasma triglycerides 40% to 60% when utilized with appropriate dietary modification. Fibrates also raise HDL cholesterol by an additional 10% to 20% but are generally less effective than niacin for this situation. Fibrates can also lower plasma LDL by only 10% to 15%. Fibrates can be used in combination with statins, but clinicians must exercise caution and judgment when combining pharmacologic agents. Rare but serious cases of rhabdomyolysis have been reported with combination pharmacotherapy. It is generally best to reduce the statin dose prior to addition of a fibrate for combination pharmacotherapy as a safeguard to reduce the risk of rhabdomyolysis.

Ezetimibe

Ezetimibe is a newer agent that works through direct inhibition of cholesterol absorption in the small intestine.[12] It is approved as an agent to add onto an already prescribed statin to further lower plasma LDL cholesterol. Early studies with ezetimibe suggested an additional 15% to 20% lowering of LDL cholesterol. Some patients experiencing further LDL cholesterol reductions of 40% to 50% once ezetimibe is added to statin therapy. A combination pill with simvastatin/ezetimibe for clinical use is available; this should improve patient compliance with combination pharmacotherapy.

Resin-Binding Agents

The resins and bile acid-binding sequestrants cholestyramine and colestipol are well established in the treatment of dyslipidemia. Resin-binding agents reduce total cholesterol and LDL cholesterol by binding bile acids in the intestine to interrupt the enterohepatic circulation of bile acids. This action stimulates a secondary increase in hepatic LDL receptors, which in turn removes LDL cholesterol from the circulation. Resins have no significant effect on HDL but raise plasma triglycerides.

As expected from their mode of action, the major side effects associated with these agents are gastrointestinal intolerance with gas, bloating, constipation, nausea, and esophageal reflux. These agents work well in bringing down LDL cholesterol and, if the dose is slowly incremented, can be reasonably tolerated by patients. A problem with resins is their effect on absorption of vitamin K, especially in patients taking warfarin (Coumadin). Resins also inhibit the absorption of digoxin, warfarin, thyroxine, and diuretics if given simultaneously.

Apo A-1 Milano

The Apo A-1 milano protein, an intravenous agent that is not approved by the Food and Drug Administration (FDA) at the current time, has been demonstrated to mediate regression of atherosclerotic plaque volume when given 3 times a week for several weeks to a small number of patients who were randomized following hospitalization for acute coronary syndrome (ACS).[13] Previous work demonstrated that use of this synthetic protein mediated reductions in arterial thrombosis and clotting time.[14]

【 】 COMPLICATIONS OF PHARMACOLOGIC THERAPY

Most lipid-lowering agents are well tolerated. Nearly every compound can cause myalgias, occasionally with liver transaminase elevation and, rarely, rhabdomyolysis. Patients initiating pharmacotherapy with any of the previously mentioned lipid-lowering agents should be closely and frequently monitored for signs and symptoms of toxicity. They should have periodic assessments of creatine kinase and liver transaminases as well as periodic medical evaluations. It is generally believed that the potential for toxicity increases with the higher doses of any agent and when combination pharmacotherapy is used. However, it is important to realize that toxicity can occur with any dose of these agents, and the treating clinician should maintain a high index of suspicion.

In addition, it is important to watch for significant drug-drug interactions with any of the lipid-lowering agents. Many of the agents are metabolized through the cytochrome P_{450} system and can potentially interact with a number of compounds, including ketoconazole, itraconazole, fluconazole, erythromycin, cyclosporine, digoxin, warfarin, oral contraceptives, amiodarone, and others. It is also important to watch for toxicity and drug interactions whenever combination pharmacotherapy, such as a statin plus fibrate or a

statin plus niacin, is used. As with all prescription medications, it is best to consult the package inserts and manufacturers' labels prior to initiation of therapy.

SECONDARY PREVENTION DATA: WHY TREAT DYSLIPIDEMIA?

A number of clinical trials highlight the secondary prevention benefit of lipid-lowering therapy in patients with CAD (Figure 61-2). Most of these trials have used statin agents for the treatment of dyslipidemia.[6–10] This section highlights results from 5 of these trials, which demonstrate the secondary prevention benefit of lipid-lowering therapy across a variety of clinical situations. Taken together, the data from these studies firmly establish the need for aggressive lipid-lowering in patients with known coronary disease and help us understand the rationale and proper role for treatment of dyslipidemia.

【 】 THE SIMVASTATIN SCANDINAVIAN SURVIVAL STUDY

The Simvastatin Scandinavian Survival Study (4-S) randomized 4444 patients with known CAD whose baseline total cholesterol values were between 200 and 300 mg/dL to simvastatin or placebo daily.[6] Patients randomized to simvastatin (20–40 mg daily) enjoyed significant reductions in risk of overall mortality (~30%), cardiovascular-related mortality (~40%), recurrent myocardial infarction (MI) [~35%], and need for percutaneous and/or surgical coronary revascularization (~40%) (see Figure 61-2). The data from the 4-S trial were the first to report a secondary coronary prevention benefit from statin therapy in patients with CAD and revolutionized the approach to the treatment of dyslipidemia.

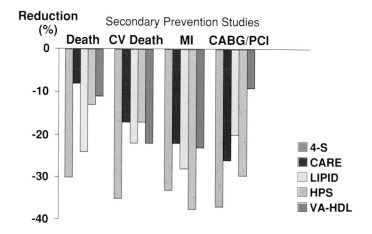

FIGURE 61-2. Pooled efficacy data for five major secondary prevention trials. CV = cardiovascular; MI = myocardial infarction; CABG/PCI = coronary artery bypass graft/percutaneous coronary intervention; 4-S = Simvastatin Scandinavian Survival Study; CARE = Cholesterol and Recurrent Events; LIPID = Long-term Intervention with Pravastatin in Ischemic Disease; HPS = Heart Protection Study; VA-HDL = Veterans' Affairs High-Density Lipoprotein Cholesterol Intervention Trial Study Group.

[ ] LONG-TERM INTERVENTION WITH PRAVASTATIN IN ISCHEMIC DISEASE TRIAL

The Long-term Intervention with Pravastatin in Ischemic Disease (LIPID) trial randomized 9014 patients with coronary disease and hyperlipidemia to pravastatin or placebo and followed them for more than 6 years.[7] Patients in the LIPID trial had lower cholesterol values at entry compared with the 4-S group; total cholesterol values ranged from 155 to 271 mg/dL at the time of randomization. The group randomized to pravastatin had significant reductions in total mortality, cardiovascular mortality, recurrent MI, and the need for surgical or percutaneous coronary revascularization (Figure 61-2).

[ ] CHOLESTEROL AND RECURRENT EVENTS TRIAL

The Cholesterol and Recurrent Events (CARE) trial randomized 4159 patients who were at least 3 months following hospital discharge from an ST-elevation myocardial infarction (STEMI) to pravastatin or placebo and followed them for approximately 5 years.[8] Patients enrolled in the CARE trial needed to have a total cholesterol value of less than or equal to 240 mg/dL to be randomized. The patients randomized to pravastatin in the CARE trial enjoyed reduced risks of cardiovascular mortality, recurrent MI, and need for coronary revascularization (Figure 61-2).

[ ] HEART PROTECTION STUDY

The Heart Protection Study (HPS) randomized 20,536 patients with CAD, vascular disease, or diabetes mellitus to nightly simvastatin (40 mg) or placebo independent of baseline lipid values.[9] Patients were followed an average of 5 years, and those randomized to simvastatin had lower risks of cardiac and noncardiac mortality, MI, stroke, and need for coronary and/or vascular revascularization (see Figure 61-2). The HPS was unique in its design such that it did not prespecify lipid values prior to randomization. The HPS investigators observed a benefit across all LDL subgroups randomized to simvastatin.

[ ] VETERANS' AFFAIRS HIGH-DENSITY LIPOPROTEIN CHOLESTEROL INTERVENTION TRIAL STUDY GROUP

The Veterans Affairs High-Density Lipoprotein Cholesterol Intervention Trial Study Group (VA-HDL) randomized 2531 men with known CAD to gemfibrozil (1200 mg/d) or placebo for slightly more than 5 years and assessed coronary end points.[10] Patients needed an HDL less than or equal to 40 mg/dL and an LDL less than or equal to 140 mg/dL to be eligible for randomization. Randomization to gemfibrozil resulted in a 6% increase in HDL cholesterol values, a 31% decrease in plasma triglycerides, a 4% decrease in total cholesterol values, and no change in LDL cholesterol values. Treatment with gemfibrozil resulted in a significant reduction in the combined end point of cardiac death plus nonfatal MI (21.7% vs 17.3%, P = .006). Of interest, the secondary

prevention benefit observed from treatment with gemfibrozil was essentially independent of change in plasma LDL cholesterol values in this group of patients.

Taken together, data from these 5 studies demonstrate the benefit of aggressive treatment of dyslipidemia in patients with CAD. Appropriate and aggressive treatment results in significant reductions in risk of death, MI, stroke, and need for coronary (surgical or percutaneous) revascularization.

IMPORTANT SUBGROUPS FOR LIPID-LOWERING TREATMENT

[ ] PATIENTS WITH ACUTE CORONARY SYNDROME

A growing body of literature indicates that the use of statin therapy during hospitalization or at discharge from hospitalization for an acute coronary syndrome (unstable angina, non-STEMI or STEMI) is beneficial. Multiple observational studies have demonstrated an association between statin use and improved outcomes.[15–22] Two of the observational studies demonstrated improved outcomes by hospital discharge.[15,16] At least 8 randomized clinical trials have tested the use of statin therapy in ACS, including the Pravastatin Turkish trial (PTT),[23] the FLuvastatin On RIsk Diminishing after Acute myocardial infarction (FLORIDA) trial,[24] The Myocardial Ischemia Reduction by Aggressive Cholesterol Lowering (MIRACL) trial,[25] the Lipid-Coronary Artery Disease (L-CAD) trial,[26] the Prevention of Recurrent Ischemia with Cerivastatin Study (PRINCESS),[27] the Aggrastat to Zocor trial with simvastatin (A to Z),[28] the Pravastatin Acute Coronary Trial (PACT),[27] and the Pravastatin or Atorvastatin Evaluation and Infection Therapy (PROVE-IT) Thrombolysis in Myocardial Infarction-22 (TIMI-22) trial.[29]

The first study, the PTT, randomized 164 patients with STEMI to pravastatin (40 mg) or placebo at the time of intravenous fibrinolytic therapy. The investigators reported on a subset of their original cohort who had undergone percutaneous coronary intervention (PCI) during hospitalization for STEMI.[23] The 80-patient subset revealed that those randomized to pravastatin had fewer recurrent coronary events (32.5%) at 6 months compared with the placebo group (75.6%), P = .0001. The FLORIDA trial randomized 540 patients with STEMI to fluvastatin or placebo within 14 days of the index acute MI, examining a primary end point of reduction in cardiac ischemia on ambulatory Holter monitoring by 6 and 12 weeks following acute MI. No differences in ambulatory ischemia were observed, and there were no differences in death or major adverse cardiac events at 1 year. The MIRACL trial randomized patients with unstable angina, STEMI and non-STEMI to atorvastatin (80 mg) or placebo for 16 weeks and observed a 16% relative reduction in the combined end point of death, recurrent nonfatal acute MI, resuscitated cardiac arrest, or recurrent ischemia requiring repeat hospitalization (atorvastatin group 14.8%, placebo group 17.4%, P = .048, RR = 0.84, 95% CI = 0.70–1.00). The L-CAD trial took patients who had undergone percutaneous coronary revascularization for acute MI or unstable angina and randomized the participants to aggressive lipid-lowering either with pravastatin (20–40 mg) ± cholestyramine and/or nicotinic acid or to usual care. The group randomized to aggressive lipid-lowering had fewer recurrent coronary events at 2 years compared with the usual care group. The PROVE-IT trial took patients with recent hospitalization for acute MI and randomized them to pravastatin (40 mg daily) or atorvastatin (80 mg daily) and followed for cardiovascular outcomes for 2 years. The group randomized to atorvastatin experienced fewer recurrent coronary events (26.3%) compared with the pravastatin group (22.4%, P = .005). Of interest, subgroup analysis demonstrated that patients with STEMI or those on prior statin therapy did not benefit from the aggressive use of atorvastatin. It is also unclear what role suppression of inflammation had in the modulation of cardiovascular outcomes in this study; atorvastatin lowered C-reactive protein (CRP) values more than pravastatin, but no correlation with clinical outcomes was reported.

The PACT trial randomized patients with STEMI and non-STEMI to pravastatin or placebo prior to hospital discharge and examined outcomes as early as 1 month following discharge. The reported results from PACT show an 8% reduction, favoring early statin therapy. It is not known whether the enrollment in PACT was completed or prematurely terminated. The PRINCESS trial randomized approximately 3600 patients with STEMI and non-STEMI to cerivastatin or placebo within 48 hours of admission

and followed them for 4.5 months. The data from PRINCESS are forthcoming. The A to Z trial is testing treatment with simvastatin (80 mg daily) compared to usual care with study randomization occurring at 120 hours after admission with ACS, switching to open-label simvastatin treatment (20 mg daily vs 80 mg daily) at 120 days following randomization. No data from A to Z have yet been reported.

Initiation of lipid-lowering agents during hospitalization for ACS results in achievement of National Cholesterol Education Program (NCEP) lipid treatment targets at a much earlier time. Several reports have suggested that patients who start lipid-lowering therapy during hospitalization are much more likely to achieve target LDL goals at 6 and 12 months following hospital discharge and are more likely to have excellent long-term compliance.[30,31]

In summary, a growing body of evidence suggests that the use of statins at the time of hospitalization for ACS and/or acute MI may offer benefits beyond the role of lipid-lowering. Statins have a variety of pleiotropic actions that may favorably modify the vulnerable plaque, the vulnerable plasma, and the vulnerable patient (Figure 61-3).[32–34] Additionally, patients who are started on these agents before hospital discharge demonstrate better short- and long-term compliance and have more improved LDL values during the first year of hospital follow-up. Figure 61-4 depicts the pooled data regarding efficacy of stains in patients with ACS.

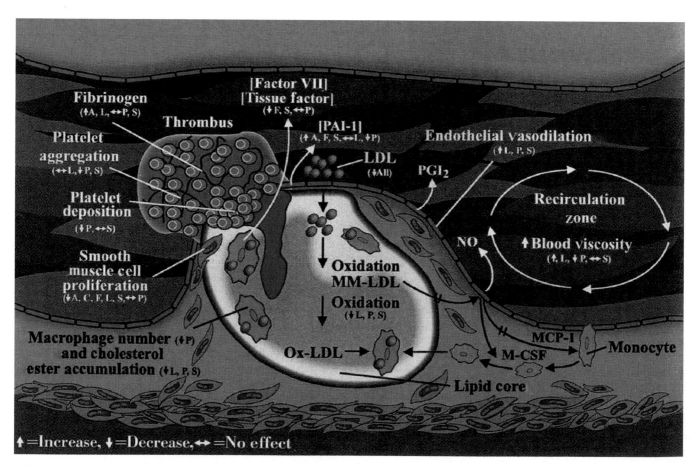

FIGURE 61-3. The potential pleiotropic actions of statins in patients with acute coronary syndromes.

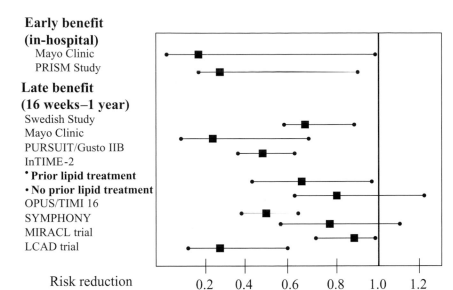

Early benefit (in-hospital)
Mayo Clinic
PRISM Study

Late benefit (16 weeks–1 year)
Swedish Study
Mayo Clinic
PURSUIT/Gusto IIB
InTIME-2
• Prior lipid treatment
• No prior lipid treatment
OPUS/TIMI 16
SYMPHONY
MIRACL trial
LCAD trial

Risk reduction

FIGURE 61-4. Statin therapy and risk reduction in acute coronary syndrome. This figure depicts the pooled data regarding efficacy of statins of affected patients. PRISM = Platelet Receptor inhibition for Ischemic Syndrome Management; PURSUIT = Platelet IIb/IIIa Underpinning the Receptor for Suppression of Unstable Ischemia Trial; GUSTO IIB = Global Use of Strategies To Open Occluded arteries; INTIME-2 = Intravenous nPA for Treatment of Infarcting Myocardium Early-2; OPUS/TIMI 16 = Optimal angioplasty and primary stenting/Thrombolysis in Myocardial Infarction 16; SYMPHONY = Sibrafiban vs aspirin to Yield Maximum Protection from ischemic Heart events postacute coronary syndromes; MIRACL = Myocardial Ischemia Reduction with Aggressive Cholesterol Lowering; L-CAD = Lipid-Coronary Artery Disease.

【 】 PATIENTS UNDERGOING PERCUTANEOUS CORONARY INTERVENTION

There are three studies examining periprocedural statin use that may have direct relevance to the practice of interventional cardiology. The L-CAD study, described above, randomized patients post-PCI for acute MI to statin plus cholestyramine or niacin therapy or to usual care.[26] Those who were randomized to statin therapy experienced far fewer recurrent coronary events compared with the usual care group. The lesson from L-CAD is that patients should be aggressively treated for dyslipidemia before they leave the care of the interventional cardiologist, because those randomized to usual care did not have success with lipid-lowering or with reductions in coronary events. The second study, by Hermann et al,[35] demonstrated that use of a statin agent for 1 week prior to PCI resulted in fewer PCI-related infarcts, as determined on the basis of elevations of cardiac biomarkers. Patients were stratified by whether they had been "pretreated" with a statin prior to elective PCI. Of interest, those who were pretreated had a significantly lower risk of periprocedural rise in creatine kinase, myocardial bound (CK-MB) compared with those who were not pretreated (Figure 61-5). The data from Hermann et al are consistent with recent data revealing that statin therapy at time of hospitalization for acute MI is associated with reduced levels of CK-MB release.[36] The Lescol Intervention Prevention Study (LIPS) randomized 1677 patients from 77 centers to receive fluvastatin 80 mg or placebo following PCI. Adverse coronary events were reduced by 22% at median

follow-up of 3–9 years (26.7% in the placebo group vs 21.4% in the treatment group; $P = .01$).[37] It is therefore indicated to treat patients undergoing PCI with statins unless clinically contraindicated.

【 】 LIPID MANAGEMENT IN PATIENTS WITH HYPERTENSION

Two important studies have demonstrated the importance of lipid lowering therapy in patients with hypertension.[38,39] The Anglo-Scandinavian cardiac outcomes trial (ASCOT) with its accompanying lipid-lowering arm (ASCOT-LLA) along with the Antihypertensive and Lipid-Lowering Treatment to Prevent Heart Attack Trial (ALLHAT) randomized patients with hypertension to statin or placebo to examine if aggressive lipid lowering therapy was associated with improved secondary prevention. Patients in ASCOT-LLA were randomized to atorvastatin (10 mg/day) or placebo, whereas patients in ALLHAT were randomized to pravastatin (40 mg/day) or placebo. The results of the ASCOT-LLA trial was reported before completion of the prespecified amount of time of follow-up because patients randomized to the LLA enjoyed a 36% reduction in nonfatal AMI and CAD-related deaths compared with the placebo group. The ALLHAT trial followed patients for at least 6 years, during which nearly 27% of the placebo group was on open-label statin treatment. This resulted in a mean LDL value of 104.0 mg/dL in the pravastatin group and 121.2 mg/dL in the placebo group. The group randomized to pravastatin had reductions in nonfatal MI and CHD deaths of 95 ($P = .16$). Nonetheless, these data emphasize the importance of aggressive lipid-lowering in patients with hypertension who otherwise are at increased risk of MI, coronary death, and stroke.

Figure 61-6 depicts the beneficial outcomes of patients randomized to statin therapy following PCI in the L-CAD trial.

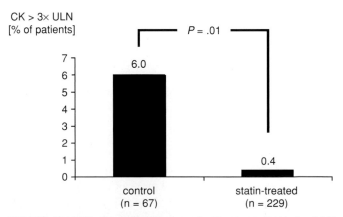

FIGURE 61-5 This figure depicts the reductions in periprocedural CK-MB (creatine kinase, myocardial bound) elevations in patients pretreated with statin agents. ULN = upper limit of normal.

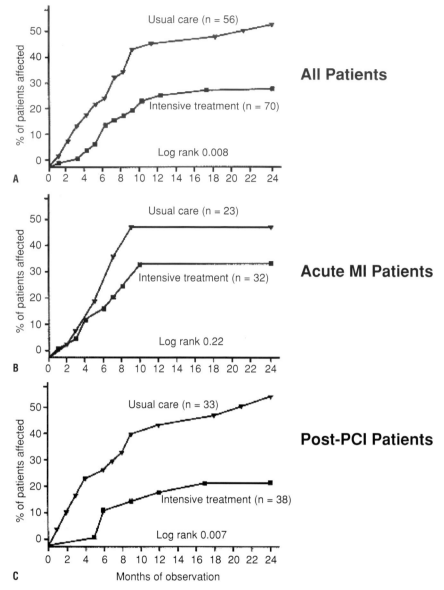

FIGURE 61-6. This figure depicts the beneficial outcomes of patients randomized to statin therapy following percutaneous coronary intervention in the Lipid-Coronary Artery Disease trial. MI = myocardial infarction; PCI = percutaneous coronary intervention.

statins. It is often necessary to treat the elevated Lp(a) pharmacologically before the statin can fully reduce the LDL to less than 100 mg/dL.

Treatment of an elevated Lp(a) is difficult at best.[43] No dietary or lifestyle modification has been demonstrated to effectively lower Lp(a) values. Two agents are somewhat effective at reducing Lp(a). Niacin and fenofibrate have both been demonstrated to reduce Lp(a) and can be safely used in patients in combination with a statin agent. It is important to wait at least 3 months to assess the full treatment effect with these agents. On rare occasion, one could use both niacin and fenofibrate in combination to treat an elevated Lp(a). When using combination pharmacotherapy in the rare patient, it remains important to maintain increased vigilance for side effects and toxicity. Finally, LDL apheresis can also be used to treat elevated Lp(a) values. Statins are useful in this setting to maximally reduce non-Lp(a) LDL.

【 】 HYPERHOMOCYSTEINEMIA

Plasma homocysteine has been epidemiologically linked with increased CAD risk in certain groups of patients.[44-46] Some newer work has suggested that CAD risk may be dependent on which genetic subtype of dihydrofolate reductase is present within the individual.[47] Hyperhomocysteinemia is usually not identified unless specialized testing is ordered. Elevations of plasma homocysteine should be treated equally in patients with CAD and those without CAD given the epidemiologic evidence linking the condition to advanced CAD development. Treatment consists of a daily B-complex vitamin and folic acid (400–1000 μg). The B-complex vitamin is necessary to avoid precipitating pernicious anemia in individuals who have a vitamin B_{12} deficiency and take folic acid as monotherapy. Rare cases of vitamin B_{12} deficiency dementia have been reported when folic acid monotherapy has been administered on a long-term basis in patients with asymptomatic pernicious anemia.

EMERGING RISK FACTORS

【 】 LIPOPROTEIN A

Lipoprotein A [Lp(a)] has emerged as an important risk factor in selected populations.[40,41] It has been associated with accelerated malignant CAD, cerebrovascular disease, and peripheral vascular disease. Lp(a) attaches to the LDL particle via a disulfide bond and promotes atherothrombosis.[42] The Lp(a) moiety facilitates penetration of LDL into the atherosclerotic plaque and alters plasma coagulation and platelet aggregation in ways that promote thrombosis. The presence of an elevated Lp(a) can often be inferred in patients in whom statin therapy does not reduce the LDL cholesterol in the expected manner. It has been our clinical experience to find Lp(a) elevations in patients whose LDL cholesterol values remain greater than 100 mg/dL despite high doses of potent

【 】 C-REACTIVE PROTEIN

Work by Ridker et al first recognized the importance of an elevated CRP with risk of first-time and/or recurrent MI.[48-50] It has become apparent that statin therapy is quite effective in patients with elevations of both LDL cholesterol and CRP. Treatment of the combined dyslipidemia should result in potent reductions in LDL cholesterol and CRP values. Less is known about what the proper treatment decision is with patients who have an elevated CRP but normal LDL cholesterol. Data from the Air Force Coronary/Texas Atherosclerosis Prevention Study (AFCAPS/TexCAPS) trial suggests that an elevated CRP in the setting of an LDL cholesterol less than median represents an atherogenic risk.[50] Patients who were treated with lovastatin in that study had risk reductions of a similar magnitude to that observed in the LDL greater than the median population. There is an ongoing randomized clinical trial testing whether treatment with statins in patients with elevations of CRP but with low LDL cholesterol is beneficial. In the absence of prospective randomized trial data, it is best to individualize treatment decisions in this population.

PHARMACOLOGIC TREATMENT OF HYPERLIPIDEMIA: WHICH AGENT(S) FOR WHICH PATIENTS?

The use of lipid-lowering therapy is based on the underlying type of lipid elevation or abnormality. In the vast majority of patients, treatment should be instituted with one of several FDA-approved statin agents. Figure 61-7 illustrates one approach for treatment.

【 】 ELEVATED LOW-DENSITY LIPOPROTEIN CHOLESTEROL

Statin therapy is the preferred first-line therapy for any patient with an elevated LDL cholesterol. Most patients can achieve the LDL goal with aggressive statin therapy. There may be a need for uptitration of the dose of a particular statin to obtain the target LDL cholesterol.

In the rare patient in whom the LDL goal cannot be achieved with statin monotherapy, it is often necessary to add a second pharmacologic agent. We favor use of ezetimibe in most patients. It is well tolerated, has few side effects, and is potent when added to statin therapy. Other choices include sitostanol esters and/or resin-binding agents. These agents can be used when the patient does not have elevated triglycerides or a low HDL cholesterol. Niacin and fibric acid derivatives are the appropriate choices for addition to statin therapy when the patient has significant elevation of triglycerides (> 150 mg/dL) or a low HDL cholesterol (HDL < 40 mg/dL).

【 】 NORMAL LOW-DENSITY LIPOPROTEIN CHOLESTEROL BUT LOW HIGH-DENSITY LIPOPROTEIN CHOLESTEROL

Patients with known CAD and an LDL cholesterol less than 100 mg/dL may not need pharmacologic treatment unless their HDL cholesterol is less than 40 mg/dL. Niacin and/or a fibrate are appropriate choices to treat isolated low HDL use when wanting to raise HDL cholesterol. A low HDL cholesterol is often associated with elevations in plasma triglycerides, with metabolic states such as diabetes mellitus and obesity, and with patients who have sedentary lifestyles or high-carbohydrate diets. It is crucial to treat the underlying diabetes and obesity aggressively. The patient with diabetes should strive for the best possible glycemic control. Patients who are obese must be encouraged to lose weight and exercise. Vigorous exercise at least 3 times per week has also been demonstrated to raise HDL values, but the increases occur more slowly than with pharmacologic therapy.

【 】 ELEVATED TRIGLYCERIDES AND ELEVATED LOW-DENSITY LIPOPROTEIN CHOLESTEROL

A significant number of patients with CAD have elevations of both LDL cholesterol and plasma triglycerides. A search should be made for metabolic stressors (diabetes, obesity, hypothyroidism), dietary imbalances (excess ethanol ingestion, excessive simple carbohydrate intake), and medication-triggered triglyceride elevations. When medication, dietary, and lifestyle modifications fail to correct the triglyceride elevations, it is necessary to institute pharmacologic therapy. The first line of treatment should be one of the FDA-approved statin agents with potent triglyceride-lowering properties (see Tables 61-1 and Table 61-5). If the triglycerides remain elevated above 150 mg/dL, it is necessary to use niacin or a fibrate. Both niacin and the fibrates are potent triglyceride-lowering agents, often achieving 50% to 60% reductions in patients with hypertriglyceridemia. Resin-binding agents must be avoided in patients with hypertriglyceridemia as these agents will worsen hypertriglyceridemia.

LDL > 100 mg/dL TGs < 150 mg/dL	LDL > 100 mg/dL TGs ≥ 150 mg/dL	LDL > 100 mg/dL HDL < 40 mg/dL	LDL ≤ 100 mg/dL HDL < 40 mg/dL or TG > 150 mg/dL
Statin Goal: LDL < 100 mg/dL	Statin + Fibrate or niacin Goals: • LDL < 100 mg/dL • TGs < 150 mg/dL	Statin Agent +/- Niacin or fibrate Goals: • LDL < 100 mg/dL • HDL > 40 mg/dL	Niacin or fibrate Goals: • HDL > 40 mg/dL • LDL < 100 mg/dL

Assess LFTs every 3 months for first year, then periodically thereafter

• All Patients should be educated on and adhere to the AHA Step 2 diet.
• All Patients should reduce body weight to BMI ≤ 25.
• All Patients should exercise 4–5 times per week for at least thirty minutes per session.
• All Patients should stop using any tobacco products.

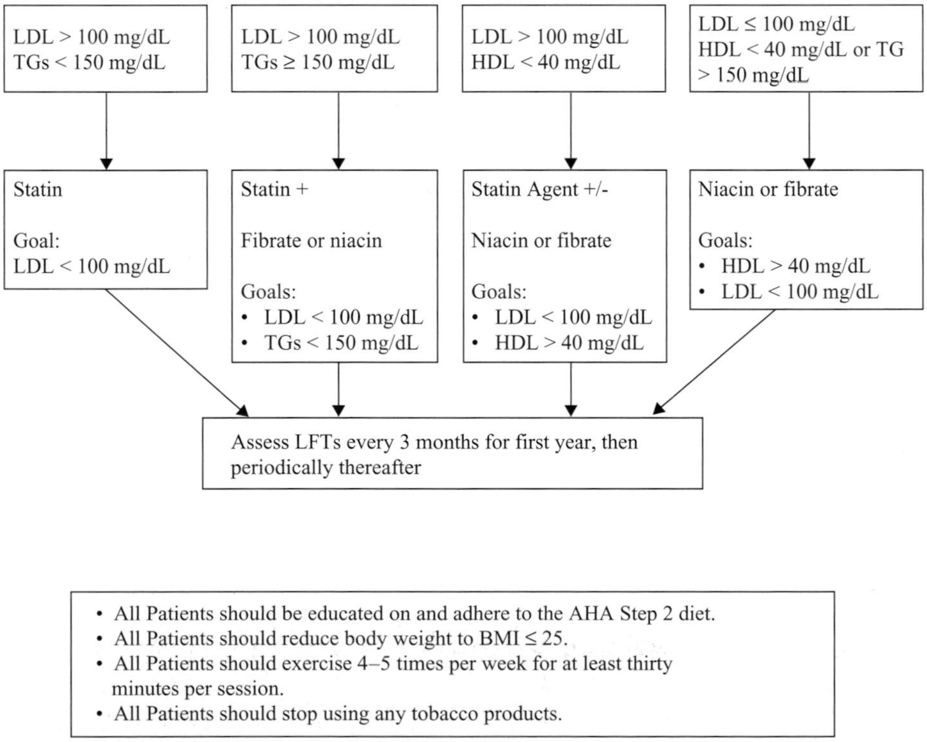

FIGURE 61-7. Treatment algorithm for patients with dyslipidemia. HDL = high-density lipoprotein; LDL = low-density lipoprotein; TG = triglyceride.

SUMMARY

Atherosclerosis is a systemic diffuse disease that may manifest as an angiographically localized coronary, cerebral, mesenteric, renal, and or peripheral arterial stenosis or as diffuse atherosclerosis. Although relief of organ ischemia is frequently possible with percutaneous revascularization, this in itself does not alleviate the long-term risks of disease recurrence or modify the metabolic derangements that promote atherosclerosis. It is critically important for the interventional cardiologist to recognize the need for treatment of dyslipidemia and institute such therapies at the time of percutaneous revascularization.

REFERENCES

1. Wright RS, Kottke TE, Gau GT. Lipid-lowering agents. In: Murphy J, ed. *Mayo Clinic Cardiology Review.* 2nd ed. Philadelphia, Pa: Lippincott Williams & Wilkins; 2000:1301.
2. Brady AJB. Britain: still the sick man of Europe? *Br J Cardiol* 2002;9:7.
3. Executive Summary of the Third Report of the National Cholesterol Education Program (NCEP) Expert Panel on Detection, Evaluation, and Treatment of High Blood Cholesterol in Adults (Adult Treatment Panel III). *JAMA.* 2001;285:2486.
4. Shepherd J, Cobbe SM, Ford I, et al. West of Scotland Coronary Prevention Study Group. Prevention of coronary artery disease with pravastatin in men with hypercholesterolemia. *N Engl J Med.* 1995;333:1301.
5. Downs JR, Clearfield M, Weis S, et al. Primary prevention of acute coronary events with lovastatin in men and women with average cholesterol levels: results of AFCAPS/TexCAPS. *JAMA.* 1998;279:1615.
6. Randomised trial of cholesterol lowering in 4444 patients with coronary artery disease: the Scandinavian Simvastatin Survival Study (4S). *Lancet.* 1994; 344:1383.
7. Long-Term Intervention with Pravastatin in Ischaemic Disease (LIPID) Study Group. Prevention of cardiovascular events and death with pravastatin in patients with coronary heart disease and a broad range of initial cholesterol levels. *N Engl J Med.* 1998;339:1349.
8. Sacks FM, Pfeffer MA, Moye LA, et al. Cholesterol and Recurrent Trial Investigators. The effect of pravastatin on coronary events after myocardial infarction in patients with average cholesterol levels. *N Engl J Med.* 1996; 335: 1001.
9. MRC/BHF Heart Protection Study of cholesterol lowering with simvastatin in 20,536 high-risk individuals: a randomized placebo-controlled trial. *Lancet.* 2002;360:7.
10. Rubins HB, Robins SJ, Collins D, et al, for the Veterans Affairs High-Density Lipoprotein Cholesterol Intervention Trial Study Group. Gemfibrozil for the secondary prevention of coronary heart disease in men with low levels of high-density lipoprotein cholesterol. *N Engl J Med.* 1999;341:410.
11. Khwaja A, Connolly JO, Hendry BM. Prenylation inhibitors in renal disease. *Lancet.* 2000;355:741.
12. Knopp RH, Gitter H, Truitt T, et al, for the Ezetimibe Study Group. Effects of ezetimibe, a new cholesterol absorption inhibitor, on plasma lipids in patients with primary hypercholesterolemia. *Eur Heart J.* 2003;24:729.
13. Nissen SE, Tsunoda T, Tuzcu EM, et al. Effect of recombinant ApoA-1 Milano on coronary atherosclerosis in patients with acute coronary syndromes. *JAMA.* 2003;290:2292.
14. Li D, Weng S, Yang B, et al. Inhibition of arterial thrombus formation by ApoA1 Milano. *Arterioscler Thromb Vasc Biol.* 1999;19:378.
15. Bybee KA, Wright RS, Williams BA, et al. Effect of concomitant or very early statin administration on in-hospital mortality and reinfarction in patients with acute myocardial infarction. *Am J Cardiol.* 2001;87:771.
16. Schiefe R, Gitt AK, Heer T, et al. Early statin use in acute myocardial infarction is associated with a reduced hospital mortality: results of the Mitra-2. *Circulation.* 2000;102:II-435.
17. Stenestrand U, Wallentin L, for the Swedish Registry of Cardiac Intensive Care. Early statin treatment following acute myocardial infarction and 1-year survival. *JAMA.* 2001;285:430.
18. Bybee KA, Wright RS, Powell BD, et al. Differential benefit from treatment with a statin agent at hospital discharge in non-ST elevation MI compared to ST elevation MI [abstract]. *Circulation.* 2000;102(suppl 2):II-614.
19. Aronow HD, Topol EJ, Roe MT, et al. Effect of lipid lowering therapy on early mortality after acute coronary syndromes: an observational study. *Lancet.* 2001;357:1063.
20. Giugliano RP, Antman EM, Thompson SL, et al. Lipid lowering drug therapy initiated during hospitalization for acute MI is associated with lower post-discharge 1-year mortality. *J Am Coll Cardiol.* 2001;37(suppl A):316A.
21. Cannon CP, McCabe CH, Bentley J, et al. Early statin therapy is associated with markedly lower mortality in patients with acute coronary syndromes: observations from OPUS-TIMI 16. *J Am Coll Cardiol.* 2001;37(Suppl A):334A.
22. McGuire DK, Kristinsson A, Bhapkar MV, et al. Early statin use after acute coronary syndromes (ACS) and outcomes at 90-days. *Circulation.* 2001;104: II-343.
23. Kayikcioglu M, Can L, Kultursay H, et al. Early use of pravastatin in patients with acute myocardial infarction undergoing coronary angioplasty. *Acta Cardiol.* 2002;57:295.
24. Van Boven AJ, Liem A. Effects of fluvastatin administration immediately after an acute myocardial infarction on myocardial ischemia (FLORIDA). Presented at: American Heart Association; November 12–15, 2000; New Orleans, La. Available at: http://www.acc.org/education/online/trials/aha00/florida.htm.
25. Schwartz GG, Olsson AG, Ezekowitz MD, et al. Effects of atorvastatin on early recurrent ischemic events in acute coronary syndromes: the MIRACL study. *JAMA.* 2001;285:1711.
26. Arntz HR, Agrawal R, Wunderlich W, et al. Beneficial effects of pravastatin (+/−cholestyramine/niacin) initiated immediately after a coronary event (the randomized Lipid-Coronary Artery Disease [L-CAD] Study). *Am J Cardiol.* 2000;86:1293.
27. Wright RS, Murphy JG, Bybee KA, et al. Statin lipid-lowering therapy for acute myocardial infarction and unstable angina: efficacy and mechanism of benefit. *Mayo Clin Proc.* 2002;77:1085.
28. Blazing MA, de Lemos JA, Dyke CK, et al. The A-to-Z trial: methods and rationale for a single trial investigating combined with use of a low-molecular-weight heparin with the glycoprotein IIb/III inhibitor tirofiban and defining the efficacy of early aggressive simvastatin therapy. *Am Heart J.* 2001;142:211.
29. Cannon CP, Braunwald E, McCabe CH, et al, for the Pravastatin or Atorvastatin Evaluation and Infection Therapy–Thrombolysis in Myocardial Infarction 22 Investigators. *N Engl J Med.* 2004;350:1.
30. Fonarow GC, French WJ, Parsons LS, et al. Use of lipid-lowering medications at discharge in patients with acute myocardial infarction: data from the National Registry of Myocardial Infarction 3. *Circulation.* 2001;103:38.
31. Bybee KA, Powell BD, Williams BA, et al. Superior short-term cholesterol control and achievement of the adult treatment panel III low-density lipoprotein goals with initiation of statin therapy by the time of hospital discharge following acute myocardial infarction. *Am J Cardiol.* 2004;93:776.
32. Rosenson RS, Tangey CC. Antiatherothrombotic properties of statins. Implications for cardiovascular event reduction. *JAMA.* 1998;279:1643.
33. Vaughan CJ, Murphy MB, Buckley BM. Statins do more than lower cholesterol. *Lancet.* 1996;348:1079.
34. Takemoto M, Liao JK. Pleiotropic effects of 3-hydroxy-3-methylglutaryl coenzyme A reductase inhibitors. *Arterioscler Thromb Vasc Biol.* 2001;21:1712.
35. Herrmann J, Lerman A, Baumgarat D, et al. Preprocedural statin medication reduces the extent of periprocedural non-Q wave myocardial infarction. *Circulation.* 2002;106:2180.
36. Bybee KA, Kopecky SL, Williams BA, et al. Reduced creatine kinase release with statin use at the time of myocardial infarction. *Int J Card.* 2004;96:461.
37. Serruys PW, deFeyter P, Macaya C, et al. Fluvastatin for prevention of cardiac events flowing successful first percutaneous coronary intervention: a randomized controlled trial. *JAMA.* 200;287:3215.
38. Sever PS, Dahlof B, Poulter NR, et al, for the ASCOT Investigators. Prevention of coronary and stroke events with atorvastatin in hypertensive patients who have average or lower-than-average cholesterol concentrations, in the Anglo-Scandinavian Cardiac Outcomes Trial-Lipid Lowering Arm (ASCOT-LLA): a multicentre randomized controlled trial. *Lancet.* 2003; 361:1149.
39. The ALLHAT Officers and Coordinators for the ALLHAT Collaborative Research Group. Major outcomes in moderately hypercholesterolemic, hypertensive patients randomized to pravastatin vs usual care. The antihypertensive and lipid-lowering treatment to prevent heart attack trial (ALLHAT-LLT). *JAMA.* 2002;288:2998.
40. Kim C, Gau GT, Allison TG. Relation of high lipoprotein(a) to other traditional atherosclerotic risk factors in patients with coronary heart disease. *Am J Cardiol.* 2003;91:1360.
41. Marcovina SM, Koschinsky ML, Albers JJ, et al. Report of the National Heart, Lung, and Blood Institute Workshop on lipoprotein(a) and cardiovascular disease: Recent advances and future directions. *Clin Chem.* 2003;49:1785.
42. Deb A, Caplice N. Lipoprotein A: new insights into mechanisms of atherogenesis and thrombosis. *Clin Cardiol.* 2004;27:258.
43. van Wissen S, Smilde TJ, Trip MD, et al. Long term statin treatment reduces lipoprotein(a) concentrations in heterozygous familial hypercholesterolaemia. *Heart.* 2003;89:893.
44. Gauthier GM, Keevil JG, McBride PE. The association of homocysteine and coronary artery disease. *Clin Cardiol.* 2003;26:563.
45. Wald DS, Law M, Morris J. Serum homocysteine and the severity of coronary artery disease. *Thromb Res.* 2003;111:55.

46. Matetzky S, Freimark D, Ben-Ami S, et al. Association of elevated homocysteine levels with a higher risk of recurrent coronary events and mortality in patients with acute myocardial infarction. *Arch Intern Med.* 2003;163:1933.

47. Weisberg IS, Park E, Ballman KV, et al. Investigations of a common genetic variant in betaine-homocysteine methyltransferase (BHMT) in coronary artery disease. *Atherosclerosis.* 2003;167:205.

48. Ridker PM, Rifai N, Pfeffer MA, et al, for the Cholesterol and Recurrent Events (CARE) Investigators. Inflammation, pravastatin, and the risk of coronary events after myocardial infarction in patients with average cholesterol levels. *Circulation.* 1998;98:839.

49. Ridker PM, Rifai N, Pfeffer MA, et al. Long-term effects of pravastatin on plasma concentration of C-reactive protein. The Cholesterol and Recurrent Events (CARE) Investigators. *Circulation.* 1999;100:230.

50. Ridker PM, Rifai N, Clearfield M, et al, for the Air Force/Texas Coronary Atherosclerosis Prevention Study Investigators. Measurement of C-reactive protein for the targeting of statin therapy in the primary prevention of acute coronary events. *N Engl J Med.* 2001;344:1959.

CHAPTER (62)

Hypertension

Robert A. Phillips, MD, PhD, and
Joy M. Weinberg, MD

In the first decade of the twenty-first century, evidence-based medicine (EBM) has become the predominant methodology for the education and practice of medicine. In the ascent to this preeminent position, EBM has challenged several methodologies through which medicine was taught and practiced throughout the twentieth century, including: (1) the clinical anecdote, (2) the concept that medicine is an "art," (3) the notion that the physician acts as the filter through which medical knowledge is individualized for the patient, and to some extent (4) the application of principles of pathophysiology to guide individual patient care. Indeed, it appears that in many cases this mechanism-based approach to disease has been replaced by a broad strokes population-based approach based on outcomes research.

However, in medicine, as in law, evidence is open to interpretation, varying opinion, and nuance. Perhaps nowhere is this more evident than in the field of hypertension, which arguably can be credited with developing the field of EBM with randomized clinical trials in the early 1960s[1] and early adaptation and promotion of outcomes based research beginning with the first Joint National Committee Reports on Prevention, Detection, Evaluation and Treatment of High Blood Pressure in the 1970s.[2]

The purpose of this chapter is to review the evidence in the diagnosis and treatment of essential hypertension, focusing on the following areas: (1) use of ambulatory and home blood pressure (BP) monitoring as diagnostic and prognostic tools; (2) recent clinical trials in treatment of essential hypertension that form the basis of evidence-based therapeutics; and (3) presentation of the key features from the Seventh Report of the Joint National Committee on Prevention, Detection, Evaluation and Treatment of High Blood Pressure (JNC 7), which form the current basis of treatment for essential hypertension.

AMBULATORY AND HOME BLOOD PRESSURE MONITORING—TOOLS FOR RISK STRATIFICATION AND EVALUATION OF EFFICACY OF TREATMENT

【 】 TECHNICAL ASPECTS

Ambulatory blood pressure monitoring (ABPM) is a simple but powerful technique. It has many uses across a broad spectrum of patients with hypertension, ranging from determination of whether or not hypertension is even present to guiding intensity of treatment in those with end-organ damage.[3] ABPM began as a research tool in the early 1960s with devices that required the patient to initiate the recording.[4] Over the past 4 decades, extremely lightweight, fully automatic, and quiet devices have been developed for clinical and research applications. A criterion for testing the accuracy of this equipment has been established, and many of the commercially available devices have been validated by independent investigators.[5] BP cuffs are usually designed with either microphones to record Korotkoff sounds or with technology that allows BP measurement with oscillometric methods.

【 】 INDICATIONS FOR AMBULATORY BLOOD PRESSURE MONITORING (TABLE 62-1)

Ambulatory Blood Pressure Monitoring in White Coat Hypertension

The most accepted use for ABPM is to rule in or rule out white coat hypertension. Diagnosis of white coat hypertension is the only reimbursable Medicare code (Health Care Financing

> **TABLE 62-1**
>
> Clinical Indications for Ambulatory Blood Pressure Monitoring
>
> Rule out white coat hypertension[3]
>
> Modification of intensity of antihypertensive therapy[12]
>
> Marked variability of clinic blood pressure (episodic hypertension)
>
> Evaluation of resistant hypertension
>
> Risk assessment (eg, assess potential to develop renal dysfunction in a patient with diabetes)[18]
>
> Determination if neurologic symptoms (eg, episodic dizziness) are related to variability of blood pressure
>
> Detect masked hypertension (ie, normal office blood pressure but elevated ambulatory blood pressure)

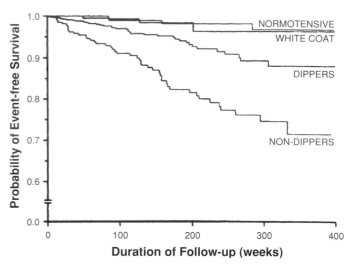

FIGURE 62-1. Probability of event-free survival in 1187 subjects followed for 400 weeks and grouped into 4 categories by pattern of ambulatory blood pressure (BP): normotensive, white coat hypertension, ambulatory hypertension, dipper pattern (ie, sleep BP is 10–20% less than awake BP); nondipper pattern (nocturnal BP < 10% lower than awake BP). Note that there is no difference in survival between the white coat hypertension group and the normotensive group. (*Reprinted with permission from Verdecchia P et al.*[13])

Administration Common Procedure Coding System [HCPCS] code 93788) for ABPM. To be eligible for monitoring under Medicare the patient must fulfill the following 3 criteria: (1) clinic or office BP greater than 140/90 mm Hg on at least 3 separate clinic or office visits, with 2 separate measurements made at each visit; (2) at least 2 documented separate BP measurements taken outside the clinic or office that are less than 140/90 mm Hg; and (3) no evidence of end-organ damage.[6] After monitoring, a patient is defined as having white coat hypertension if his/her clinic BP is persistently greater than 140/90 mm Hg but he/she has a normal ambulatory or home BP, which is defined as less than 135/85 mm Hg during awake hours.[7,8]

White coat hypertension is more common in women and tends to occur in younger patients.[9,10] It can persist over many years.[11] Approximately 20% to 25% of patients who are treated for hypertension have white coat hypertension, and when their medication is withdrawn will have normal ambulatory BP recordings.[12] Because patients with white coat hypertension have the same probability of event-free survival as normotensives[13] (Figure 62-1), the prevailing view is emerging that the patients with white coat hypertension do not require treatment, despite the fact that compared to normotensives left ventricular mass is slightly increased in subjects with white coat hypertension.[14–16]

Risk Stratification With Ambulatory Blood Pressure Monitoring

In addition to white coat hypertension, there are emerging indications to use ABPM to risk stratify patients for future cardiovascular or renal events. For example, at every level of office BP, those with 24-hour ambulatory systolic blood pressure (SBP) less than 135 mm Hg have at least one half the risk of a cardiovascular event as those whose 24-hour systolic BP is 135 mm Hg or greater (Figure 62-2).[17] In patients with diabetes and no prior evidence of renal disease, ambulatory BP monitoring can determine which patients are at risk for deterioration of renal function: blunted dip

in sleep pressure (obtained with ABPM) is highly predictive of development of microalbuminuria.[18] Whether earlier institution of therapy aimed at preventing microalbuminuria will be successful is not yet determined.

Ambulatory Blood Pressure Monitoring in the Elderly

ABPM may also be able to identify patients with stage I and II hypertension who are most likely to benefit from treatment (Figure 62-3). In the Systolic hypertension in elderly in Europe (Syst-Eur)

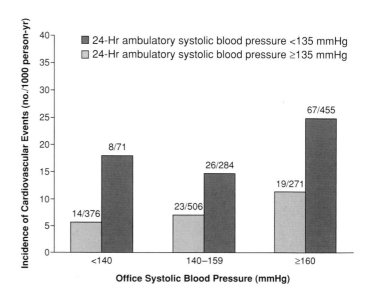

FIGURE 62-2. At each level of office blood pressure (BP), a 24-hour ambulatory systolic BP of 135 mm Hg or more predicted a higher incidence of cardiovascular events than a 24-hour ambulatory systolic BP of less than 135 mm Hg. (*From Clement DL et al.*[17])

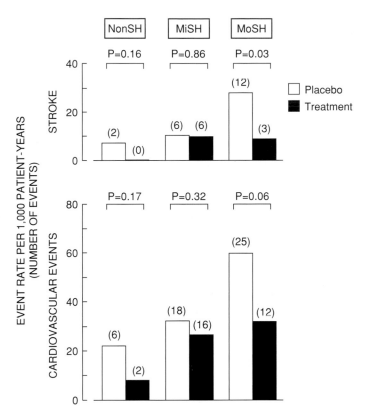

FIGURE 62-3. In the Systolic Hypertension in Elderly in Europe (Syst-Eur) study, elderly participants with white coat hypertension (NonSH group) had few events and treatment did not modify risk. Those with mild systolic hypertension (MiSH group) with elevated office blood pressure (BP) and daytime ambulatory systolic BP of 140 to 159 mm Hg also showed no benefit from treatment. Only those with office hypertension and ambulatory systolic BP greater than 160 mm Hg (MoSH) group showed benefit. (From Fagard et al.[19])

study, a trial of treatment of isolated systolic hypertension in the elderly, the only participants who clearly benefited from treatment were those who not only had office hypertension but whose daytime SBP was 160 mm Hg or greater.[19] It is no surprise that participants in Syst-Eur with white coat hypertension did not benefit from treatment, but it is remarkable that no benefit accrued from treatment in those who had office hypertension and moderately elevated daytime SBP between 140 and 159 mm Hg. Despite this result, until more studies corroborate a lack of benefit associated with treating an ambulatory SBP between 140 and 159 mm Hg in the elderly, it is recommended to continue to treat such patients.

Home Blood Pressure Monitoring and Masked Hypertension

Home BP monitoring can identify patients with normal office BP who are at high risk for cardiovascular events. In a 2004 study of nearly 5000 treated elderly patients, approximately 9% had masked hypertension (ie, treated BP was normal in the office but elevated at home), and the incidence of cardiovascular events was equal to that of those with uncontrolled hypertension.[8] Importantly, in the same study, the incidence of cardiovascular events in patients with white coat effect was similar to patients whose BP was controlled in the office. This confirms the findings of the ambulatory BP studies.

TREATMENT OF HYPERTENSION—CLINICAL TRIAL RESULTS

【 】 KEY LESSONS FROM RECENT CLINICAL TRIALS AND META-ANALYSIS

The publication of the Antihypertensive and Lipid-Lowering Treatment to Prevent Heart Attack Trial (ALLHAT) in late 2002,[20] the JNC 7 in 2003,[21] and the meta-analysis from the Blood Pressure Lowering Treatment Trialists Collaboration[22] led to intensification of the debate that has occupied hypertension specialists over the past decade. First, does it matter how much BP is lowered? Second, does it matter which agent is used as first-line treatment? In 2005, a synthesis of these trials suggests the following answers:

1. The degree of BP-lowering, rather than the class of agent, is the most important factor in reducing cardiovascular events.[22,23]

2. Low-dose diuretic therapy is the platform for treatment of hypertension and is at least as effective as calcium channel blockers and angiotensin-converting enzyme (ACE) inhibitors in preventing cardiovascular death and nonfatal myocardial infarcts.[20] This statement also applies to patients with diabetes.

3. Although overall cardiovascular protection is similar to diuretics, patients treated with calcium channel blockers have greater incidence of congestive heart failure (CHF) than those treated with diuretics or converting enzyme inhibitors.[24,25] On the other hand, calcium channel blockers tend to be associated with better protection against stroke.[22]

4. ACE inhibitors tend to be worse for primary and secondary stroke protection when compared to diuretics and beta-blockers.[22]

5. In Caucasians, angiotensin II receptor blockers (ARBs) are more effective than beta-blockers for reduction of stroke, whereas in African Americans, the opposite may be the case.[6,26] ARBs may be more effective than other regimens in preventing heart failure.

6. In patients with diabetes, coronary artery disease, CHF, and renal disease, blockade of the renin-angiotensin-aldosterone system is often beneficial and has additive value over and above BP reduction. For example, in the Hypertensive Old People in Edinburgh (HOPE) trial, the report of the main results stated that ramipril improved cardiovascular outcomes despite only a 3-mm Hg reduction in office BP.[27] However, the small reduction in office BP may not have reflected the true BP-lowering effect of ramipril. Indeed, in those patients in whom ambulatory BPs were measured, there was a 17-mm Hg reduction in SBP during sleep. Because ramipril was administered prior to sleep in the HOPE trial, its major BP-lowering effect may have occurred during the night, a finding that would not be reflected in the clinic BP. Hence, the ABPM data suggest that the contribution to decreased CV events from ramipril in the HOPE trial was strongly influenced by reduction of nocturnal BP.

Treatment of Uncomplicated Hypertension— Clinical Trial Summary

In studies of uncomplicated hypertension, such as the Swedish Trial in Old Patients with Hypertension-2 (STOP-2),[28] Nordic Diltiazem (NORDIL) study,[25] and International Nifedipine-GITS Study: Intervention as a Goal in Hypertension Treatment (INSIGHT),[24] all drug classes appear to be equally effective in reducing events. In these trials, calcium channel blockers were consistently associated with higher incidence of CHF but appeared to confer protection against stroke and dementia. In this context, the second Australian National Blood Pressure Study (ANBP-2) can be viewed as a trial in uncomplicated hypertension in the elderly, because less than 10% of the population had prior cardiovascular disease.[29] The fact that ACE inhibitor was superior to diuretic in ANBP-2 is not consistent with all of the other trials of uncomplicated hypertension. Rather than view results of ANBP-2 as a reason to use ACE inhibitors in place of diuretics in the elderly, it is probably best to view it as support for using an ACE inhibitor as one of the multiple drugs that is often needed to control BP in the elderly.

【 】 TREATMENT OF PATIENTS WITH HYPERTENSION, RISK FACTORS, AND TARGET ORGAN DAMAGE: THE CASE FOR DIURETICS IN PATIENTS WITH CARDIOVASCULAR DISEASE

In the patient with hypertension as well as cardiovascular disease and diabetes, several lines of evidence suggest that despite the benefits associated with ACE inhibitors and beta-blockers, diuretics should be part of the antihypertensive regimen. In the ALLHAT trial, where more than 50% of the population had atherosclerotic cardiovascular disease, diuretics were equally effective in reducing the primary end point of composite cardiovascular events when compared with ACE inhibitors and calcium channel blockers. In ALLHAT, diuretics demonstrated superiority with regard to prevention of CHF when compared with the calcium channel blocker and were superior to the ACE inhibitor for prevention of heart failure and stroke.[20] Some experts would argue that the inferiority of ACE inhibitors is partially accounted for by less effective lowering of BP. For example, in the ALLHAT trial, there was an increased relative risk of stroke in African Americans treated with the ACE inhibitor compared with those treated with the calcium channel blocker or diuretic.[20] The reason for the increased stroke risk associated with the ACE inhibitor among African Americans could be partially accounted for by a 4-mm Hg less reduction in SBP with lisinopril in comparison to chlorthalidone. The importance of BP reduction with regard to stroke is supported by the Perindopril Protection Against Recurrent Stroke Study (PROGRESS) trial, which was a secondary stroke prevention trial.[30] In that study, an ACE inhibitor prevented recurrent stroke only when it was combined with a diuretic, which led to a further BP reduction of 7/2 mm Hg.

Several other studies support the use of diuretics in patients with cardiovascular disease. In the international verapamil-trandolapril study (INVEST) trial, which enrolled a large number of patients older than 70 years of age with concomitant hyperten-

sion and coronary artery disease, an atenolol-hydrochlorothiazide based strategy was just as effective as the verapamil-trandolapril strategy in preventing death and cardiovascular outcomes in this high-risk population.[31] Similarly, even in the setting of left ventricular hypertrophy (LVH), diabetes, or renal disease, where it appears that treatment of hypertension with blockade of the renin-angiotensin aldosterone system is beneficial with either an ACE inhibitor or an ARB, careful analysis of the studies shows that the overwhelming majority of patients required diuretics for BP control.[32,33] Furthermore, although meta-analysis suggests that ARBs, ACE inhibitors, and calcium channel blockers are superior to diuretics for left ventricular mass regression[34] in the 2 randomized trials of LVH regression in which diuretics were included, the diuretic was superior to other agents for regression of LVH.[5,36]

Clinicians who are cautious about use of diuretics as first-line agents point to the slightly increased risk of developing diabetes associated with diuretic use. However, the emerging debate on the degree to which diuretics cause diabetes should not mean that we take our "eye off the prize"-in randomized controlled clinical trials, diuretic-based therapy consistently lowered cardiovascular risk and therefore should be part of the regimen for treatment unless there are compelling contraindications. Furthermore, it needs to be reemphasized that in ALLHAT, patients with diabetes assigned to the diuretic group had superior protection from combined cardiovascular disease end points than those assigned to the lisinopril group and an equivalent degree of protection as those assigned to the calcium channel blocker group.

Finally, observational studies that suggest adverse outcomes associated with diuretic use in patients with diabetes, such as a recent report from the Progetto Ipertensione Umbria Monitoraggio Ambulatoriale (PIUMA) study (based in Italy) are flawed by selection bias. Using a diuretic in populations where the standard of therapy is a calcium channel blockers or an ACE inhibitor is simply a marker for identifying those patients with more difficult to control hypertension and worse baseline characteristics, such as higher 24-hour BP, more LVH, and more glucose intolerance.[37] The fact that more of such patients go on to develop more diabetes is predictable and not an indictment of diuretics. It is telling that although the PIUMA study showed association between diuretic use and development of diabetes, it failed to make the link between diuretic use and cardiovascular risk. Indeed, although the occurrence of new diabetes was an independent predictor of cardiovascular risk, use of diuretics was not independently associated with cardiovascular risk.

TARGET BLOOD PRESSURE GOALS

【 】 IS A BLOOD PRESSURE OF LESS THAN 140/90 mm Hg A SUFFICIENT GOAL FOR UNCOMPLICATED HYPERTENSION?

The Trial of Mild Hypertension Study (TOMHS) was conducted in patients with State 1 hypertension, and compared 6 antihypertensive regimens–acebutolol, amlodipine, chlorthalidone, doxazosin, enalapril, and placebo in a background of a sustained weight loss intervention program.[35] Over a 4-year follow-up period, there was a sustained 2.6-kg reduction in weight. Participants assigned to drug treatment had greater drop in BP than the placebo (−15.9 vs −9.1 mm Hg for SBP and −12.3 vs −8.6 mm Hg for diastolic BP [DBP], $P < .001$), yielding a difference in treatment BP of 131/81 mm Hg for those assigned to placebo versus 124/74 mm Hg for those assigned to the treatment group. Despite significantly lower BP in the treatment group compared to the placebo (weight loss–only group), there was no difference in the primary end points, which included congestive heart disease (death), myocardial infarction, CHF, aortic aneurysm, coronary artery bypass graft, percutaneous transluminal coronary angioplasty, thrombolysis, or unstable angina. However, after including secondary end points, such as transient ischemic attack and severity of angina or claudication, there were significantly fewer events (11% vs 16%, $P < .05$) in the lower BP group. This trial is the best evidence available that treating to less than 130/80 mm Hg has benefit for uncomplicated hypertension.

The Hypertension Optimal Treatment Trial (HOT) assigned nearly 19,000 participants to 1 of 3 DPB goals: less than 90 mm Hg, less than 85 mm Hg, and less than 80 mm Hg. HOT was designed to determine whether lower DBP goals were associated with improved outcome. Initial treatment consisted of the long-acting calcium channel blocker felodipine. At the end of the 4 years, DBP in the 3 groups was 81 mm Hg, 83 mm Hg, and 85.2 mm Hg, and therefore the less than 80 mm Hg hypothesis was not able to be tested. There were no significant differences between the groups with regard to total cardiovascular events. Those assigned to the less than 80 mm Hg group had fewer myocardial infarctions than those assigned to the less than 90 mm Hg group, but the event rate was low and the P value marginal (2.6 vs 3.6 events per 1000 patient years, $P = .05$). When analyzed from the perspective of the relationship between "achieved" BP and outcome rather than "assigned BP" versus outcome, "optimal" BP was 139/83 mm Hg. If less than 130/80 mm Hg was highly beneficial for patients with hypertension, one would expect to detect the finding in an analysis of "achieved" BP versus events. This is because patients who are able to achieve a lower BP often do not truly have hypertension (ie, have white coat hypertension) and may have intrinsically healthy blood vessels.

TOMHS and HOT study results can be synthesized and a conclusion drawn that in patients with uncomplicated hypertension, there does not appear to be harm in lowering BP to less than 130/80 mm Hg. However, the overwhelming benefit is achieved when BP is lowered to less than 140/90 mm Hg.

【 】 BLOOD PRESSURE GOALS IN PATIENTS WITH DIABETES

According to the guidelines of the National Kidney Foundation, the American Diabetes Association, JNC 7, and others, the target BP should be less than 130/80 mm Hg. Evidence to support the recommendation for a target DBP of less than 80 mm Hg is relatively strong and is derived from observational data and 2 randomized trials, HOT and the Appropriate Blood Pressure Control in Diabetes (ABCD) normotensive study. In HOT, participants with diabetes who were randomized to a goal of less than 80 mm Hg DBP (achieved 82.6 mm Hg) had a 50% reduction in major cardiovascular events compared to those randomized to the less than 90 mm Hg DBP group. The ABCD normotensive study was designed to evaluate the effect of intensive versus moderate DBP control on vascular and renal complications in 480 normotensive patients with type 2 diabetes.[38] Patients were randomized to 1 of 2 BP target groups: either a moderate goal of 80 to 89 mm Hg or a goal of 10 mm Hg below the baseline DBP. After a mean follow-up of 5.3 years, the BP in the groups was 137/81 mm Hg versus 128/75 mm Hg ($P < .0001$). Fewer patients in the intensively

---

● TABLE 62-2

Key Features of JNC 7

Epidemiology

- For persons over age 50, SBP is a more important than DBP as risk factor for CVD.
- Starting at 115/75 mm Hg, CVD risk doubles with each increment of 20/10 mm Hg throughout the BP range.
- Persons who are normotensive at age 55 have a 90% lifetime risk of developing hypertension.
- Those with SBP 120–139 mm Hg or DBP 80–89 mm Hg should be considered prehypertensive and require health-promoting lifestyle modifications to prevent CVD.

Treatment

- Thiazide-type diuretics should be initial drug therapy for most, either alone or combined with drugs from other classes.
- Certain high-risk conditions are compelling indications for use of drugs from other classes.
- Most patients require 2 or more antihypertensive drugs to achieve goal BP.
- If BP is > 20/10 mm Hg above goal, initiate therapy with two agents; one usually should be a thiazide-type diuretic.

Physician-patient relations

- The most effective therapy prescribed by the careful clinician controls hypertension only if patients are motivated.
- Motivation improves when patients have positive experiences with, and trust in, the clinician.
- Empathy builds trust and is a potent motivator.
- The responsible physician's judgment remains paramount.

BP = blood pressure; CVD = cardiovascular disease; DBP = diastolic blood pressure; SBP = systolic blood pressure.

TABLE 62-3

JNC 7 Classification of Blood Pressure and Management in Adults

BLOOD PRESSURE CLASSIFICATION	SBP^a (MM HG)	DBP^a (MM HG)	LIFESTYLE MODIFICATION	INITIAL DRUG THERAPY	
				Without Compelling Indication	With Compelling Indications
Normal	< 120	< 80	Encourage		
Prehypertension	120–139	or 80–89	Yes	No antihypertensive drug indicated.	Drug(s) for compelling indications.^{b}
Stage 1 hypertension	140–159	or 90–99	Yes	Thiazide-type diuretics for most. May consider ACE inhibitor, ARB, beta-blocker, calcium channel blocker, or combination	Drug(s) for the compelling indications.^{b}
Stage 2 hypertension	≥ 160	or ≥ 100	Yes	Two-drug combination for most^c (usually thiazide-type diuretic and ACE inhibitor or ARB or beta-blocker or calcium channel blocker).	Other antihypertensive drugs (diuretic, ACE inhibitor, ARB, beta-blocker, calcium channel blocker) as needed.

^{a}Treatment determined by highest blood pressure category.
^{b}Treat patients with chronic kidney disease or diabetes to blood pressure goal of < 130/80 mm Hg.
^{c}Initial combined therapy should be used cautiously in patients at risk for orthostatic hypotension.
ACE = angiotensin-converting enzyme; ARB = angiotension II receptor blocker.

treated group progressed from normoalbuminuria to microalbuminuria ($P = .012$) and microalbuminuria to overt albuminuria ($P = .028$). There was less progression of diabetic retinopathy ($P = .019$) and a lower incidence of strokes ($P = .03$).

Aside from the ABCD normotensive study, there is no randomized trial clearly demonstrating that lowering SBP to less than 140 mm Hg in patients with diabetes prevents cardiovascular events or progression of renal disease. Because of the uncertainty, there is an ongoing trial of 10,000 patients with diabetes, the Action to Control Cardiovascular Risk in Diabetes (ACCORD), in which participants are randomized to an SBP goal of less than 140 mm Hg versus less than 120 mm Hg.[39] This trial is expected to end in 2010. However, as we await results of this trial, there is data to suggest that lowering blood SBP to less than 130 mm Hg is of benefit in patients with diabetes and hypertension. Much of the enthusiasm for a target SBP of less than 130 mm Hg is derived from the relationship between achieved SBP and cardiovascular outcomes in the UK Prospective Diabetes Study Group study.[40] In that trial, at every level of achieved SBP (including achieved SBP of 110 mm Hg), cardiovascular risk was lower, and no J-curve was observed. However, it is possible that participants who were able to achieve a lower SBP simply had more healthy vasculature, which promoted lower BP and fewer cardiovascular events. Other evidence to support lower

SBP goals and potential benefit of an SBP of less than 130 mm Hg comes from the arm of the ABCD trial that enrolled patients with diabetes with hypertension and randomized them to a target DBP of either 80 to 89 mm Hg or 75 mm Hg. At the end of 5.3 years of follow-up, the mean BP achieved was 138/86 mm Hg in the moderate control group versus 132/78 mm Hg in the intensively treated group. Although there was no difference in cardiovascular or renal outcomes, total mortality was lower in the intensively treated group.[41]

BLOOD PRESSURE GOALS IN PATIENTS WITH HYPERTENSIVE NEPHROSCLEROSIS

Although target BP of less than 125/75 mm Hg for patients with renal disease and proteinuria (> 1 mg/24 h) are relatively well established,[42] the goals for patients with hypertensive renal disease are not as clearcut. The largest trial that specifically addressed this issue is the African American Study of Kidney Disease and Hypertension (AASK), which enrolled patients with hypertension who had mild to moderate renal disease. Patients with overt proteinuria and diabetes were excluded from the study.[43] The study compared the ability of two levels of BP control to blunt progression of renal disease as measured by glomerular filtration rate

TABLE 62-4

Lifestyle Modifications to Prevent and Manage Hypertension[a]

MODIFICATION	RECOMMENDATION	APPROXIMATE SBP REDUCTION (RANGE)[b]
Weight reduction	Maintain normal body weight (body mass index 18.5–24.9 kg/m²).	5–20 mm Hg/10 kg
Adopt DASH eating plan	Consume a diet rich in fruits, vegetables, and low-fat dairy products with a reduced content of saturated and total fat.	8–14 mm Hg
Dietary sodium reduction	Reduce dietary sodium intake to no more than 100 mmol per day (2.4 g sodium or 6 g sodium chloride).	2–8 mm Hg
Physical activity	Engage in regular aerobic physical activity such as brisk walking (at least 30 minutes per day, most days of the week).	4–9 mm Hg
Moderation of alcohol consumption	Limit consumption to no more than 2 drinks (eg, 24 oz beer, 10 oz wine, or 3 oz 80-proof whiskey) per day in most men and to no more than 1 drink per day in women and lighter-weight persons.	2–4 mm Hg

[a]For overall cardiovascular risk reduction, stop smoking.
[b]The effects of implementing these modifications are dose- and time-dependent and could be greater for some individuals.
DASH = Dietary Approaches to Stop Hypertension; SBP = systolic blood pressure.

(GFR) decline or by a composite clinical end points that included any of the following: a GFR event (a confirmed reduction in GFR by 50% or by 25 mL/min per 1.73 m² from baseline), end-stage renal disease (dialysis or transplantation), or death. Participants were randomized to a usual mean arterial BP goal of 102 to 107 mm Hg or to a lower goal of less than 92 mm Hg. Achieved BP averaged 128/78 mm Hg in the lower BP group and 141/85 mm Hg in the usual BP group. A mean separation of approximately 10 mm Hg mean arterial pressure was maintained throughout most of the follow-up period. Despite this marked difference in BP, over a 4-year period, there was no difference in the rate of decline of GFR or in the incidence of clinical composite end points between the low and usual BP control groups. There was a trend favoring the lower BP goal in participants with higher baseline proteinuria and an opposite trend in participants with little or no proteinuria. The study concluded that reduction of BP to levels less than 130/80 mm Hg

was not a strategy to prevent progression of hypertensive nephrosclerosis. Nevertheless, recommendations of the National Kidney Foundation (which were issued prior to the results of the AASK study results)[44] and the JNC 7 both suggest a target BP of less than 130/80 mm Hg in patients with hypertension and decreased renal function.

Whether one accepts a goal of less than 140/90 mm Hg or less than 130/80 for patients with hypertensive renal disease, it is critical that the treating physician use an adequate number of drugs to achieve BP control. Perhaps the greatest legacy of the AASK trial will be the demonstration that excellent BP control is achievable in patients with significant renal dysfunction.[32] It simply requires adequate use of loop diuretics (often 80 mg or greater of furosemide, even in the absence of edema) and at least two other antihypertensive drugs.

【 】 BLOOD PRESSURE GOALS IN OCTOGENARIANS

Several randomized, placebo-controlled trials that included patients older than 80 years of age give us insight into the questions of whether we should even be treating octogenarians, and if so, what BP goal should we seek. The Systolic Hypertension in the Elderly Program (SHEP) found that treatment of hypertension had equivalent reduction in stroke incidence among octogenarians as it did for younger patients.[45] Similarly, STOP-Hypertension demonstrated an effect of antihypertensive treatment on cardiovascular morbidity and mortality as well as total mortality that was discernible up to age 84.[46] In the Surveillance and Control Of Pathogens of Epidemiologic importance (SCOPE) study, in which patients were included up to 89 years of age, the group with the lower BP had fewer nonfatal strokes. In the pilot study of Hypertension in the Very Elderly Trial (HYVET), an ongoing placebo-controlled trial evaluating efficacy of treating hypertension in individuals older than 80 years of age, antihypertensive treatment was associated with a significant reduction in stroke but a nonsignificant trend toward increased mortality.[47]

Another line of evidence to support treating octogenarians is that compared to placebo, antihypertensive treatment leads to an equal relative risk reduction from stroke across age groups and a linear increase in absolute benefit in stroke reduction as a function of the age of the study participant (see Figure 62-1).[48] Therefore, there is no adverse effect observed in treating the elderly (ie, relative risk reduction is equivalent to treating a young person), and more strokes are prevented.

One of the concerns in treating the elderly is that they will have increased falls, fractures, and orthostatic symptoms, or even

TABLE 62-5

Dietary Approaches to Stop Hypertension (DASH) Eating Plan

FOOD GROUP	DAILY SERVINGS	SERVING SIZES	EXAMPLES AND NOTES	SIGNIFICANCE OF EACH FOOD GROUP TO THE DASH DIET PATTERN
Grains and grain products	7–8	• 1 slice bread ½ c dry cereal • ½ c cooked rice, pasta, or cereal	Whole wheat bread. English muffin, pita bread, bagel, cereals, grits, oatmeal	Major sources of energy and fiber
Vegetables	4–5	• 1 c raw leafy vegetable • ½ c cooked vegetable • 6 oz vegetable juice	Tomatoes, potatoes, carrots, peas, squash, broccoli, turnip greens, collards, kale, spinach, artichokes, sweet potatoes, beans	Rich sources of potassium, magnesium, and fiber
Fruits	4–5	• 6 oz fruit juice • 1 medium fruit • ¼ c dried fruit • ½ c fresh, frozen, or canned fruit	Apricots, bananas, dates, oranges, orange juice, grapefruit, grapefruit juice, mangoes, melons, peaches, pineapples, prunes, raisins, strawberries, tangerines	Important sources of potassium, magnesium, and fiber
Low fat or nonfat dairy foods	2–3	• 8 oz milk • 1 c yogurt • 1.5 oz cheese	Skim or 1% milk, skim or low fat buttermilk, nonfat or lowfat yogurt, part skim mozzarella cheese, nonfat cheese	Major sources of calcium and protein
Meats, poultry, and fish	2 or less	• 3 oz cooked meats, poultry, or fish	Select only lean; trim away visible fats; broil, roast, or boil, instead of frying; remove skin from poultry	Rich sources of protein and magnesium
Nuts, seeds, and legumes	4–5 per week	• 1.5 oz or ⅓ c nuts • ½ oz or 2 Tbsp seeds • ½ c cooked legumes	Almonds, filberts, mixed nuts, peanuts, walnuts, sunflower seeds, kidney beans, lentils	Rich sources of energy, magnesium, potassium, protein, and fiber

decreased cerebral blood flow and reduced cognitive function. In SHEP, where the average age of the patients was 72, BP reduction was not associated with more hip fractures, and it did not lead to more orthostatic symptoms.[45] Although treatment in SHEP did not lower the incidence of dementia, in the Syst-Eur study, treatment of isolated systolic hypertension with a long-acting dihydropyridine calcium channel blocker as the initial therapy was associated with a 55% reduction in the risk of dementia.[49]

How low should BP be lowered in the octogenarians? Two lines of evidence suggest than an SBP goal of less than 150 mm Hg is

sufficient. In the SHEP study, reduction in SBP from 170 mm Hg to less than 160 mm Hg lowered stroke rate by 33%, and if BP was lowered to less than 150 mm Hg, stroke rate was reduced an additional 5%.[50] However, in SHEP, those subjects who attained an SBP less than 140 mm Hg showed no further reduction in stroke rate. Furthermore, in SHEP, relative risk of a cardiovascular event appeared to increase in those who achieved a DBP less than 65 mm Hg.[51] The SHEP study may have been underpowered to detect a benefit in subjects who achieved an SBP less than 140 mm Hg, and lower achieved DBP in isolated systolic hypertension

TABLE 62-6

Compelling Indications for Specific Drug Classes

CONDITION	DRUG
Heart failure asymptomatic, demonstrable ventricular function	ACE inhibitors, BBs
Heart failure symptomatic ventricular dysfunction or end-stage heart disease	ACE inhibitors, ARBs, aldosterone blockers, BBs in combination with/loop diuretics
Stable angina	BBs; CCBs are alternatives
Acute coronary syndromes	ACE inhibitors, BBs
Postmyocardial infarction	ACE inhibitors, aldosterone blockers, BBs
High coronary disease risk	ACE inhibitors, BBs, CCBs, thiazide-type diuretics
Diabetes	ACE inhibitors, ARBs, BBs, CCBs, thiazide-type diuretics
Chronic kidney disease	ACE inhibitors, ARBs
Recurrent stroke prevention	ACE inhibitors, thiazide-type diuretics

ACE = angiotension-converting enzyme; ARB = angiotensin II receptor blocker; BB = beta-blocker; CCB = calcium channel blocker.

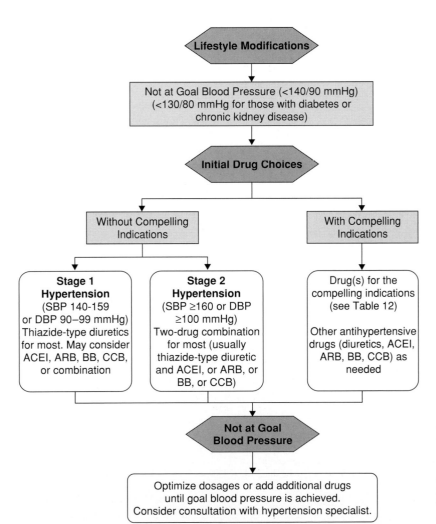

FIGURE 62-4. Algorithm for treatment of hypertension based on Seventh Report of the Joint National Committee on Prevention, Detection, Evaluation and Treatment of High Blood Pressure (JNC 7). ACE = angiotensin-converting enzyme; ARB = angiotensin II receptor blocker; BB = beta-blocker; CCB = calcium channel blocker; DBP = diastolic blood pressure; SBP = systolic blood pressure. (From Chobanian AV et al.[21])

most likely represents "sicker vessels." Nevertheless, we do not have good evidence for lowering BP in the octogenarian with isolated systolic hypertension to less than 150/65 mm Hg.

What about the octogenarian with elevated SPB and DBP? The target BP for the ongoing HYVET trial, which is recruiting patients 80 years of age and older with these parameters, is less than 150/80 mm Hg. Because active treatment to these levels in the pilot trial was associated with stroke reduction, this goal is clearly an appropriate target.

TREATMENT OF HYPERTENSION–AN APPROACH BASED ON JNC 7

The JNC 7, published in 2003, presents a comprehensive approach to diagnosis and treatment of hypertension that is evidence-based. The key messages of JNC 7 are listed in Table 62-2 and are characterized on the basis of new approaches based on epidemiology, randomized clinical trials, and the patient–physician relationship. As compared to previous national guidelines, the major changes in the current approach are the following:

1. Recognition that SBP is a more important risk factor and target for treatment than DBP in persons over age 50.

2. Replacement of the term "borderline hypertensive" with the designation "prehypertensive" in persons with SBP 120-139 mm Hg or DBP 80-89 mm Hg (Table 62-3). This change was effected in order that physicians would advocate health-promoting lifestyle modifications to prevent CVD in these patients.

3. Reemphasis on the importance of lifestyle modification as a means to lower BP (Table 62-4).

4. Endorsement of the Dietary Approaches to Stop Hypertension (DASH) diet as a mechanism to lower BP (Table 62-5).[52]

5. The recommendation that if BP is greater than 20/10 mm Hg above goal, initiate therapy with 2 agents, 1 of which usually should be a thiazide-type diuretic (Figure 62-4).

6. The recognition that most patients require 2 or more antihypertensive drugs to achieve goal BP.

7. Certain patient groups (such as those with CHF) require specific classes of antihypertensive medications, which are considered "compelling indications" (Table 62-6).

REFERENCES

1. Veterans Administration Cooperative Study Group on Antihypertensive Agents. Effects of treatment on morbidity in hypertension: results in patients with diastolic blood pressures averaging 115 through 129 mm Hg. *JAMA.* 1967;202:1028.

2. Report of the Joint National Committee on Detection, Evaluation, and Treatment of High Blood Pressure. A cooperative study. *JAMA.* 1977;237:255.

3. Phillips RA, Diamond JA. Ambulatory blood pressure monitoring and echocardiography–noninvasive techniques for evaluation of the hypertensive patient. *Prog Cardiovasc Dis.* 1999;41:397.

4. Hinman A, Engel BT, Bickford AF. Portable blood pressure recorder. Accuracy and preliminary use in evaluating intradaily variations. *Am Heart J.* 1962;63:663.

5. O'Brien E, Atkins N, Staessen J. Factors influencing validation of ambulatory blood pressure measuring devices. *J Hypertens.* 1995;13:1235.

6. Claims Processing Instructions for Ambulatory Blood Pressure Monitoring. Available at: http://www.cms.hhs.gov/MLNMattersArticles/downloads/MM2726.pdf. Last accessed: July 2006.

7. Pickering TG, for the American Society of Hypertension ad hoc panel. Recommendations for the use of home (self) and ambulatory blood pressure monitoring. *Am J Hypertens.* 1995;9:1.

8. Bobrie G, Chatellier G, Genes N, et al. Cardiovascular prognosis of "masked hypertension" detected by blood pressure self-measurement in elderly treated hypertensive patients. *JAMA.* 2004;291:1342.

9. Pickering TG, James GD, Boddie C, et al. How common is white coat hypertension? *JAMA.* 1988;259:225.

10. Eison H, Phillips RA, Ardeljan M, et al. Differences in ambulatory blood pressure between men and women with mild hypertension. *J Hum Hypertens.* 1990;4:400.

11. Martin KL, Phillips RA, Krakoff LR. Persistent white coat hypertension. *Am J Hypertens.* 1994;7:368.

12. Staessen JA, Byttebier G, Buntinx F, et al. Antihypertensive treatment based on conventional or ambulatory blood pressure measurement. *JAMA.* 1997;278:1065.

13. Verdecchia P, Porcellati C, Schillaci G, et al. Ambulatory blood pressure: an independent predictor of prognosis in essential hypertension. *Hypertension.* 1994;24:793.

14. Kuwajima I, Suzuki Y, Fujisawa A, et al. Is white coat hypertension innocent? Structure and function of the heart in the elderly [see comments]. *Hypertension.* 1993;22:826.

15. Weber MA, Neutel JM, Smith DH, et al. Diagnosis of mild hypertension by ambulatory blood pressure monitoring [see comments]. *Circulation.* 1994;90:2291.

16. Palatini P, Mormino P, Santonastaso M, et al. Target-organ damage in stage I hypertensive subjects with white coat and sustained hypertension: results from the HARVEST study. *Hypertension.* 1998;31:57.

17. Clement DL, De Buyzere ML, De Bacquer DA, et al, for the Office versus Ambulatory Pressure Study Investigators. Prognostic value of ambulatory blood-pressure recordings in patients with treated hypertension. *N Engl J Med.* 2003; 348:2407.

18. Lurbe E. Increase in nocturnal blood pressure and progression to microalbuminuria in type 1 diabetes. *N Engl J Med.* 2002;347:797.

19. Fagard RH, Staessen JA, Thijs L, et al. Response to antihypertensive therapy in older patients with sustained and nonsustained systolic hypertension. *Circulation.* 2000;102:1139.

20. Antihypertensive and Lipid-Lowering Treatment to Prevent Heart Attack Trial (ALLHAT) Officers and Coordinators for the ALLHAT Collaborative Research Group. Major outcomes in high-risk hypertensive patients randomized to angiotensin-converting enzyme inhibitor or calcium channel blocker vs diuretic: ALLHAT. *JAMA.* 2002;288:2981.

21. Chobanian AV, Bakris GL, Black HR, et al. The Seventh Report of the Joint National Committee on Prevention, Detection, Evaluation, and Treatment of High Blood Pressure: The JNC 7 Report. *JAMA.* 2003;289:2560.

22. Turnbull F. Effects of different blood-pressure-lowering regimens on major cardiovascular events: results of prospectively-designed overviews of randomised trials. *Lancet.* 2003;362:1527.

23. Staessen JA, Wang JG, Thijs L. Cardiovascular prevention and blood pressure reduction: a quantitative overview updated until 1 March 2003. *J Hypertens.* 2003;21:1055.

24. Brown MJ, Palmer CR, Castaigne A, et al. Morbidity and mortality in patients randomised to double-blind treatment with a long-acting calcium-channel blocker or diuretic in the International Nifedipine GITS study: intervention as a goal in hypertension treatment (INSIGHT). *Lancet.* 2000;356:366.

25. Hansson L, Hedner T, Lund-Johansen P, et al. Randomised trial of effects of calcium antagonists compared with diuretics and beta-blockers on cardiovascular morbidity and mortality in hypertension: the Nordic Diltiazem (NORDIL) study. *Lancet.* 2000;356:359.

26. Julius S, Alderman MH, Beevers G, et al. Cardiovascular risk reduction in hypertensive black patients with left ventricular hypertrophy: the LIFE study. *J Am Coll Cardiol.* 2004;43:1047.

27. Yusuf S, Sleight P, Pogue J, et al. Effects of an angiotensin-converting-enzyme inhibitor, ramipril, on cardiovascular events in high-risk patients. The Heart Outcomes Prevention Evaluation Study Investigators [see comments]. *N Engl J Med.* 2000;342:145.

28. Hansson L, Lindholm LH, Ekbom T, et al. Randomised trial of old and new antihypertensive drugs in elderly patients: cardiovascular mortality and morbidity the Swedish Trial in Old Patients with Hypertension-2 study [see comments]. *Lancet.* 1999;354:1751.

29. Wing LMH, Reid CM, Ryan P, et al, for the Second Australian National Blood Pressure Study Group. A comparison of outcomes with angiotensin-converting-enzyme inhibitors and diuretics for hypertension in the elderly. *N Engl J Med*. 2003;348:583.

30. PROGRESS Collaborative Group. Randomized trial of a perindopril-based blood-pressure-lowering regimen among 6105 individuals with previous stroke or transient ischemic attack. *Lancet*. 2001;358:1033.

31. Pepine CJ, Handberg EM, Cooper-DeHoff RM, et al. A calcium antagonist vs a non-calcium antagonist hypertension treatment strategy for patients with coronary artery disease: the international verapamil-trandolapril study (INVEST): a randomized controlled trial. *JAMA*. 2003;290:2805.

32. Wright JT Jr, Agodoa L, Contreras G, et al. Successful blood pressure control in the African American Study of Kidney Disease and Hypertension. *Arch Intern Med*. 2002;162:1636.

33. Kjeldsen SE, Dahlof B, Devereux RB, et al. Effects of losartan on cardiovascular morbidity and mortality in patients with isolated systolic hypertension and left ventricular hypertrophy: a Losartan Intervention for Endpoint Reduction (LIFE) substudy. *JAMA*. 2002;288:1491.

34. Klingbeil AU, Schneider M, Martus P, et al. A meta-analysis of the effects of treatment on left ventricular mass in essential hypertension. *Am J Med*. 2003;115:41.

35. Neaton JD, Grimm RH Jr, Prineas RJ, et al. Treatment of mild hypertension study: final results. *JAMA*. 1993;270:713.

36. Gottdiener JS, Reda DJ, Massie BM, et al. Effect of single-drug therapy on reduction of left ventricular mass in mild to moderate hypertension: comparison of six antihypertensive agents. The Department of Veterans Affairs Cooperative Study Group on Antihypertensive Agents [see comments]. *Circulation*. 1997;95:2007.

37. Verdecchia P, Reboldi G, Angeli F, et al. Adverse prognostic significance of new diabetes in treated hypertensive subjects. *Hypertension*. 2004;43:963.

38. Schrier RW, Estacio RO, Esler A, et al. Effects of aggressive blood pressure control in normotensive type 2 diabetic patients on albuminuria, retinopathy and strokes. *Kidney Int*. 2002;61:1086.

39. Action to control cardiovascular risk in diabetes (ACCORD). Available at: http://www.clinicaltrials.gov/ct/show/NCT00000620? order=7. Last accessed: July 2006.

40. UK Prospective Diabetes Study Group. Efficacy of atenolol and captopril in reducing risk of macrovascular and microvascular complications in type 2 diabetes: UKPDS 39. *BMJ*. 1998;317:713.

41. Estacio RO, Jeffers BF, Gifford N, et al. Effect of blood pressure control on diabetic microvascular complications in patients with hypertension and type 2 diabetes. *Diabetes Care*. 2004:B54.

42. Klahr S, Levey AS, Beck GJ, et al, for the Modification of Diet in Renal Disease Study Group. The effects of dietary protein restriction and blood-pressure control on the progression of chronic renal disease. *N Engl J Med*. 1994;330:877.

43. Wright JT Jr, Bakris G, Greene T, et al. Effect of blood pressure lowering and antihypertensive drug class on progression of hypertensive kidney disease: results from the AASK trial. *JAMA*. 2002;288:2421.

44. Bakris GL, Williams M, Dworkin L, et al. Preserving renal function in adults with hypertension and diabetes: a consensus approach. National Kidney Foundation Hypertension and Diabetes Executive Committees Working Group. *Am J Kidney Dis*. 2000;36:646.

45. SHEP Cooperative Research Group. Prevention of stroke by antihypertensive drug treatment in older persons with isolated systolic hypertension: final results of the Systolic Hypertension in the Elderly Program SHEP. *JAMA*. 1991;265:3255.

46. Dahlof B, Lindholm LH, Hansson L, et al. Morbidity and mortality in the Swedish trial in old patients with hypertension (STOP-hypertension). *Lancet*. 1991;338:1281.

47. Bulpitt CJ, Beckett NS, Cooke J, et al. Results of the pilot study for the Hypertension in the Very Elderly Trial. *J Hypertens*. 2003;21:2409.

48. Lever AF, Ramsay LE. Treatment of hypertension in the elderly. *J Hypertens*. 1995;13;571.

49. Forette F, Seux ML, Staessen JA, et al. The prevention of dementia with antihypertensive treatment: new evidence from the Systolic Hypertension in Europe (Syst-Eur) study. *Arch Intern Med*. 2002;162:2046.

50. Perry HMJ, Davis BR, Price TR, et al. Effect of treating isolated systolic hypertension on the risk of developing various types and subtypes of stroke: the Systolic Hypertension in the Elderly Program (SHEP). *JAMA*. 2000;284:465.

51. Somes GW, Pahor M, Shorr RI, et al. The role of diastolic blood pressure when treating isolated systolic hypertension [see comments]. *Arch Intern Med*. 1999; 159:2004.

52. The DASH Eating Plan Available at: http://www.nhlbi.nih.gov/health/public/heart/hbp/dash/new_dash.pdf. Last accessed: July 2006.

CHAPTER (63)

Diabetes and Cardiovascular Disease

Saul M. Genuth, MD

In 1917, in the second edition of his book entitled "Treatment of Diabetes Mellitus," Eliot Joslin recorded the cause of death in 516 patients with diabetes whom he had seen in private practice from 1894 to 1916. Diabetic persons were then defined as people having glycosuria. Sixty percent died of coma, presumably diabetic ketoacidosis, and 11% died of infection. Only 78 patients (14%) died of "cardiorenal causes." Of these, approximately half died of heart disease and approximately one fourth from a cerebral hemorrhage.

Today the picture is completely different. Joslin's patients were obviously mostly type 1, as evidenced by the predominance of coma as the cause of death. Now a large majority, around 90%, of diabetes is type 2, and many cases are diagnosed before their hyperglycemia reaches a level to cause abnormal glycosuria, except after large carbohydrate loads. Estimates vary, but 60% to 75% die of cardiovascular disease (CVD)–mostly coronary artery disease (CAD).[1] People with diabetes have a 2- to 4-fold increased risk of CVD and mortality from CVD,[2-4] and CVD can occur before diabetes is clinically manifest or diagnosed by laboratory means.[5,6] Diabetic patients without a history of prior myocardial infarction (MI) are at the same risk of suffering an MI as nondiabetic persons with a prior history of MI,[7,8] and the same is true for death from CVD.[7,9,10] The extent of CAD is greater in diabetic patients at autopsy[11] or coronary angiography.[12] In the immediate aftermath of an acute MI, diabetic patients have a higher incidence of pulmonary edema and early death[13,14] and late development of congestive heart failure (CHF).[15] Long-term survival is lessened after an MI, especially in those with single vessel disease.[16] After admission for unstable angina and non–Q wave MI, diabetic patients have 1.5 to 2 times the incidence of total mortality, CVD death, new MI, stroke, and CHF.[17] Following coronary artery bypass grafting, diabetic patients, whether or not they have been previously diagnosed, have a poorer prognosis than nondiabetic patients.[18,19,19a] In one series, 27% of diabetic patients suffered stroke, MI, sepsis, and/or death, and these adverse outcomes occurred more often in those with higher perioperative plasma glucose levels.[20] After percutaneous angioplasty, diabetic patients have a higher rate of early restenosis as well as a poorer prognosis,[19a,21-24] although after an acute MI, angioplasty appears to be more effective than thrombolytic therapy.[25] It is therefore vital to the long-term success of coronary revascularization that attention be paid to management of patients' diabetes, which plays a pivotal role in outcome.

Diabetic individuals now comprise 20% to 30% of patients undergoing coronary angiograms,[12] revascularization procedures, and admissions to coronary care units for acute coronary syndromes[26] and MI.[27] Whereas all cause and cancer mortality rates have decreased in the United States over the past 20 years, mortality from diabetes has been increasing (Centers for Disease Control and Prevention and Prevention of Mortality Data Base). During a 10-year period when mortality from CVD or CAD in the general population declined approximately 30%, CVD mortality associated with diabetes declined less in men and actually increased in women.[28] Diabetes accounts for over 50% of CVD deaths.[29]

The major risk factors for CAD in nondiabetic persons, namely hyperlipidemia, hypertension, and smoking, cluster with increased prevalence in diabetic patients.[4,30] Nonetheless, diabetes increases the risk of CVD even after adjustments for these other risk factors have been made.[2,3] Indeed, authorities have recently elevated diabetes to the status of an independent risk factor, equal to that of the others.[31,32] They also emphasize that hyperlipidemia and hypertension need to be treated especially intensively and to stringent targets in diabetic patients.[33,34]

Complicating the problem is the presence of unrecognized MI[35] and of silent myocardial ischemia in diabetic individuals.[36-39]

Abnormal endothelium–mediated coronary circulation responses are also seen in diabetic and prediabetic individuals.[40] Thus screening for coronary artery disease is recommended in patients with even atypical symptoms, abnormal electrocardiograms (EKGs), other occlusive vascular disease, or in patients with at least two of the following risk factors: dyslipidemia, hypertension, smoking, microalbuminuria/proteinuria or family history of premature CAD.[41] Stress perfusion imaging or stress echocardiography are preferred where the presence of CAD is already suspected on clinical or electrocardiographic grounds.[41]

The public health importance of diabetes as a cause or predecessor to CVD has been heightened by the fact that the prevalence and incidence of diabetes are steadily increasing[42–44] following and parallel to serious increases in obesity,[45–48] caloric intake, and sedentary living in the developed world. Obesity is itself a risk factor for death.[49] The prevalence of known diabetes, which was already 5.1%, and of undiagnosed diabetes, 2.7% in the adult US population in 1997,[50] has increased to a total of 21,000,000 in 2005 (one third of cases were still undiagnosed).[44] The prevalence of "prediabetes" in the year 2000 was 12,000,000.[51] For individuals born in the year 2000, there is a 33% individual risk for men and 38% for women of developing diabetes sometime in their lives.[52] Besides the great morbidity this increase will cause, the impact on health care costs will be huge.[26] Most of this cost will be accounted for by CVD hospitalizations, procedures, stents, and drugs.

METABOLIC (INSULIN RESISTANCE) SYNDROME

Clinicians have long noted that obese individuals were more prone to develop diabetes, hypertension, hypercholesterolemia, and CVD than normal-weight individuals. In addition, type 2 diabetes had been called insulin resistance in the 1930s.[53] With the demonstration that obese individuals have higher fasting and postprandial plasma insulin levels than normal weight individuals at comparable plasma glucose levels,[54] the stage was set. In 1988, these observations were pulled together, and a cluster of factors was recognized to constitute an insulin resistance syndrome.[55] This cluster includes resistance to the action of insulin on glucose and fat metabolism with hyperinsulinemia, impaired glucose tolerance or fasting glucose, increased body mass index, abdominal visceral obesity (increased waist circumference), elevated serum triglycerides, low serum high-density lipoprotein (HDL) cholesterol levels, and hypertension. Individuals exhibiting all or parts of this syndrome are at increased risk of developing diabetes and developing CVD.[32] Over time other components (such as microalbuminuria, increased coagulability, and decreased fibrinolysis) have been added by association with the original clinical/biochemical elements. The full syndrome has been most recently named the metabolic syndrome and officially defined by authoritative bodies[33,56] (Table 63-1).

The World Health Organization definition[56] gives primacy to abnormal glucose regulation, whether at the level of impaired fasting glucose (IFG, fasting glucose ≥ 100–125 mg/dL), impaired glucose tolerance (IGT) by oral glucose tolerance testing (OGTT) (2-hour plasma glucose during OGTT ≥ 140–199 mg/dL) or frank diabetes (FPG ≥ 126 mg/dL and/or 2-hour plasma glucose on OGTT ≥ 200 mg/dL). To this is added two or more elements from a group consisting of central adiposity, dyslipidemia, hypertension, and microalbuminuria. The National Cholesterol Educational Program Adult Treatment Panel (NCEP ATP) III definition[33] omits microalbuminuria and defines abnormal glucose regulation only by the fasting plasma glucose level.

Although not as used or essential for the definition, other components of pathophysiological significance to CAD in the metabolic

TABLE 63-1

Definitions of the Metabolic Syndrome

NATIONAL CHOLESTEROL EDUCATION PROGRAM ADULT TREATMENT PANEL III	WORLD HEALTH ORGANIZATION
At least 3 of the following:	Diabetes, IGT or IFG and/or insulin resistance[a] plus at least 2 of the following:
• Fasting plasma glucose ≥ 110 mg/dL	
• Abdominal obesity: waist circumference > 35 inches in women or > 40 inches in men	• Abdominal obesity: waist/hip ratio > 0.85 in women or > 0.9 in men and/or body mass index > 30 kg/m²
• Triglycerides > 150 mg/dL	• Triglycerides > 150 mg/dL and/or HDL < 40 mg/dL in women or < 35 mg/dL in men
• HDL < 50 mg/dL in women or < 40 mg/dL in men	
• Blood pressure ≥ 130/85 mm Hg	• Blood pressure ≥ 140/90 mm Hg
	• Microalbuminuria: urinary albumin excretion ≥ 20 μg/min or albumin/creatinine ratio ≥ 30 mg/g

[a]Insulin resistance assessed as fasting insulin (microunits/mL) × fasting glucose (mmoles/L) ÷ 22.5.
HDL = high-density lipoprotein; IFG = impaired fasting glucose; IGT = impaired glucose tolerance.

syndrome[57] include elevated levels of plasminogen activator inhibitor-1 (PAI-1)[58–60] and of clotting factors[59,61,62] that contribute to an antifibrinolytic and a prothrombogenic state. In diabetic patients, levels of fibrinogen, factor VIII, and von Willebrand factor are associated with coronary heart disease.[63] Hyperinsulinemia is an intrinsic component of the metabolic syndrome that is compensatory to insulin resistance[64] but may only be a marker of that state.[65] On the other hand, hyperinsulinemia is a risk factor for CAD[66] and to some extent can be considered a surrogate for insulin resistance, which in the office or clinic is difficult to measure directly by infusing or injecting insulin and measuring the effect on glucose metabolism. An index of insulin resistance derived from a simultaneous measurement of fasting glucose and fasting insulin called Homeostasis Model Assessment (HOMA) correlates reasonably well with the gold standard insulin clamp method,[67,68] as long as plasma glucose is within normal limits. The plasma level of the beta cell insulin precursor molecule, proinsulin, is also an independent risk factor for CVD.[69]

Insulin resistance and the metabolic syndrome are strong risk factors for both diabetes and cardiovascular disease in many populations,[57,70–72] as are many of their individual components by themselves. For example, in the Framingham Offspring Study, over an 8-year follow-up, the metabolic syndrome by the NCEP criteria increased the relative risk for type 2 diabetes to 6.9 and that of CVD to 2.2, and these risks were noncompeting.[72] Its prevalence in the US population is alarmingly high;[73] however, it is defined.[74,75] Twenty-three percent of adults over age 20 and 40% of those over age 60 have the metabolic syndrome. A rising prevalence in adolescents[76] suggests a further future increase in diabetes and CVD. However defined, the metabolic syndrome doubles the 10-year risk of CVD and mortality from CVD.[77]

In patients with diabetes, insulin resistance correlates directly with total and very-low-density lipoprotein (VLDL) triglycerides, VLDL cholesterol, fibrinogen, PAI-1 and fasting plasma glucose, and correlates inversely with HDL cholesterol and low-density lipoprotein (LDL) particle size.[78] The correlation of insulin resistance, independent of other CVD risk factors, with carotid intimal medial thickness,[79] an indicator of atherosclerosis, suggests that insulin resistance may lead to atheroma formation, but its correlation with thrombogenic and antifibrinolytic factors also suggests that it may cause or contribute to CVD events as well.[80] Markers of inflammation such as C-reactive protein (CRP), interleukin-8 (IL-6), and IL-18 are elevated in the metabolic syndrome.[81] They, along with tumor necrosis factor-α (TNF-α), e-selectin, and soluble intercellular adhesion molecules, are independent risk factors for CAD.[82–84] Some are also risk factors for diabetes[85] and its complications.[86]

The exact cause of the metabolic syndrome remains to be discovered, but it is thought to result from engrafting environmental factors, such as overabundance of available calories and loss of the need to exercise, on genetic factors, such as a postulated "thrifty gene" that is no longer advantageous in today's developed civilizations. A crucial role of visceral adipose tissue in the metabolic syndrome is suggested by the characteristically central nature of the adiposity and by adipocyte secretion of PAI-1 and TNF-α, which promote insulin resistance and adiponectin, which increases insulin sensitivity.[87] Indeed, low plasma levels of adiponectin are present in diabetes[88] and are inversely correlated with insulin resistance.[87]

Should the metabolic syndrome be treated as an entity, and if so, why and how?[89,90] The obvious reasons for treating the metabolic syndrome would be to reduce the risk of progression from IGT or IFG to diabetes and to reduce the incidence of CVD events. Five studies have now shown that progression from a high-risk state to actual diabetes can be prevented or delayed. The Finnish Diabetes Study[91] and the Diabetes Prevention Program (DPP)[92] have both shown that an intensive lifestyle behavioral change resulting in a modest weight loss (7% of body weight) along with increased exercise (150 min/wk of walking at a moderate speed) can reduce the progression to diabetes by 58% over 3 years. Risk factors for CVD were also decreased. A Chinese study has shown similar benefits from diet and exercise.[93] The DPP[92] also simultaneously showed that metformin compared to placebo reduced the risk of progression from IGT to diabetes by 31%. The Swedish Trial in Old Patients-NonInsulin Dependent Diabetes Mellitus (STOP-NIDDM) trial[94] reported a 25% reduction in progression to diabetes with acarbose treatment. Although all these studies began with IGT as the selection criteria for subjects, other elements of the metabolic syndrome, most particularly obesity, were often present. In another group at high risk for diabetes, namely Hispanic American women with a history of gestational diabetes, the thiazolidinedione drug troglitazone reduced progression to diabetes by 55% over 2 1/2 years.[95] In this study, evidence was presented for the persistence of this benefit for eight months after the drug was stopped.

Whether treatment of the metabolic syndrome per se as a global entity with a single drug that reduces insulin resistance (eg, with a thiazolidinedione drug) would decrease CVD risk is completely unknown. For this and other reasons, the American and European Diabetes Associations have issued a joint critical appraisal of the entity, urging caution.[96] They note that the CVD risk predicted by the metabolic syndrome is not necessarily greater than the sum of the individual risks of its components. There is at present no evidence that pharmacologic treatment of the metabolic syndrome would reduce CVD risk more than treatment of its individual high-risk components, such as hypertension and LDL cholesterol. Thus, the most practical present value of defining the syndrome may be to lead physicians to measure the other risk components and treat them aggressively when a single component, such as increased waist circumference, is detected.

Interestingly, therapy directed at nonhyperglycemic components of the metabolic syndrome and its cardiovascular disease risk, such as ramipril[97,98] and pravastatin for dyslipidemia[99] have also decreased the incidence of emerging diabetes during the study. These observations also suggest a strong pathogenic link between diabetes and coronary heart disease. Further follow-up of the large DPP cohort is underway to determine whether intensive lifestyle or metformin treatment will also reduce the future incidence of CVD or its surrogates, such as carotid artery intimal medial thickness, as an index of atherosclerosis. The STOP-NIDDM trial has already reported a sharp decrease in CVD events, especially myocardial infarction, during a three-year interval of taking acarbose.[100] This somewhat surprising early observation in a relatively small number of subjects requires confirmation.

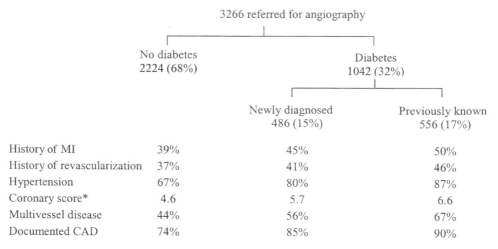

FIGURE 63-1. Clinical data in 3266 patients referred for coronary angiography and screened for diabetes and other risk factors. *(From Hasdai D, Granger CB, Srivatsa SS, et al.[25])*

RELATIONSHIP BETWEEN DIABETES AND CORONARY ARTERY DISEASE

A recent report[12] describes well the relationship between the natural histories of coronary artery disease (CAD) and diabetes and the role of the latter in CAD (Figure 63-1). A total of 3266 consecutive patients referred for coronary angiography were routinely screened for CVD risk factors, including diabetes by OGTT. Thirty-two percent of the total cohort proved to have diabetes, approximately half of whom were previously unknown and newly diagnosed (15% of the total). About half of the newly diagnosed patients were detected by their FPG ($\geq$ 126 mg/dL) and half were identified by a two-hour plasma glucose ($\geq$ 200 mg/dL) on the OGTT. Both groups had an average of 2.1 additional CVD risk factors. Notably, only 1% of the 1024 diabetic patients had type 1 diabetes.

A history of MI and/or prior revascularization, a history of hypertension, and the severity of the CAD on angiography all increased in the sequence: no diabetes, newly diagnosed diabetes, and known diabetes (average duration 11 years in those with and 6 years in those without CAD). After adjusting for other CVD risk factors, newly diagnosed diabetes independently increased the risk for angiographically determined CAD (odds ratio [OR] 1.7, 95% CI 1.3–2.3 and multivessel disease [OR 1.4, 95% CI 1.1–1.8]). Conversely, hypertension (OR 1.8) and CRP greater than 5 mg/L (OR 2.5) were significant predictors of the presence of unrecognized diabetes. In another report, of 181 consecutive admissions to a coronary care unit[27] of people without known diabetes, on OGTT 31% had diabetes at discharge and 25% still had diabetes 3 months later. Another 35% had IGT at discharge and 40% still had IGT at 3 months.

The clinical lesson is that cardiologists need to be on the look-out for undiagnosed diabetes in their CAD patients, at least by screening with an FPG determination, whereas diabetologists should be alert to the presence of CAD in apparently asymptomatic diabetic patients. Cardiologists who find impaired fasting glucose (FPG $\geq$ 100–125 mg/dL) should then perform an OGTT to determine if diabetes itself has developed.

DIABETES AND CARDIOMYOPATHY

The Framingham study[101] first demonstrated an increase in congestive heart failure (CHF) in diabetes. In a recent survey from a health maintenance organization,[102] the prevalence and 2 1/2-year incidence of CHF in type 2 diabetic patients were more than double that of nondiabetic controls (11.8 vs 4.5% and 7.7 vs 3.4%, respectively). On six-year follow-up, the incidence of new CHF was increased (31 cases per 1000 person-years in diabetic patients versus 12.4 in nondiabetic patients; risk ratio 2.5; 95% CI 2.3–2.7).[102a] Moreover, in an analysis of hospital discharges, the odds ratio for idiopathic (nonischemic) cardiomyopathy associated with diabetes was 1.75.[103] CHF is becoming an increasingly common cause of death.[104]

Examination of the mechanisms by which diabetes can lead to cardiac morbidity and mortality, CHF and sudden death reveal multiple factors that can and likely do act in concert (Figure 63-2). A detailed description is beyond the scope of this chapter, but the reader is referred to references 105 to 107a for excellent reviews of this complex and still incompletely understood subject.

Diabetes helps breed atherosclerosis—and thus CAD—by glycation and oxidation of cholesterol-rich lipoproteins, which are more readily taken up by macrophages and deposited in atheromatous plaques. The resultant multivessel CAD, accompanied by both silent and overt MIs, clearly reduces coronary blood flow and oxygen supply and leads to greater loss of myocardium in diabetes. Pulmonary edema and lesser degrees of acute CHF complicate diabetic MIs more than nondiabetic MIs,[10] and both 30-day[10] and long-term[105] mortality are increased. Ischemic heart disease leads to worsening of CHF in diabetes.[109] Hypertensive cardiac disease is often present with diabetic heart disease,[110] and the two share some characteristics, such as early concentric left ventricular hypertrophy and reduced diastolic compliance.[106] Eventually, dilated cardiomyopathy results from accompanying hypertension. In this context, activation of both circulating and local renin angiotensin systems within the heart may stimulate perivascular fibrosis and apoptosis (programmed cell death) of myocytes. Microvascular disease analogous to that of the retina leads to pericyte loss, capillary dropout,

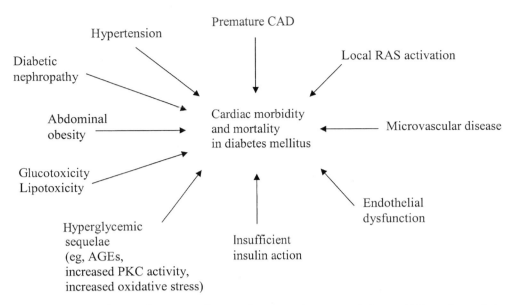

FIGURE 63-2. Mechanistic factors contributing to heart complications in diabetes. AGE = advanced glycation end product; CAD = coronary artery disease; PKC = protein kinase C; RAS = renin–angiotensin system.

and local ischemia. In ways still not well explained, diabetic nephropathy greatly increases CVD, and the latter very frequently is the cause of death in end-stage renal disease.[78] Even incipient nephropathy manifested by microalbuminuria is a major risk factor for CVD events, death, and CHF in diabetes.[111–113]

Endothelial dysfunction has assumed a prominent place in thinking about diabetic cardiopathy.[105,110] There is a decrease in nitric oxide synthesis, which is normally stimulated by insulin, and therefore a decrease in endothelial dependent vasodilation. This decrease in turn is at least partly responsible for a reduction in coronary blood flow reserve, as shown by abnormal responses to the cold pressor test. Endothelial cell dysfunction is also manifest by abnormal activation of some endothelial cell processes, such as increased secretion of von Willebrand Factor, which stimulates adhesion and aggregation of platelets and thereby increases the risk of coronary thrombosis.

Reduced coronary blood flow is also a reflection of loss of or abnormal sympathetic nervous system function.[105] Marked loss of sympathetic innervation due to diabetic neuropathy also causes decreased cardiac output, disordered coronary blood flow with a decrease in coronary blood flow reserve, and orthostatic hypotension, the latter making treatment of hypertension more difficult. Yet there can also be loss of parasympathetic tone in the heart, causing persistent resting tachycardia. Autonomic dysfunction likely plays a role in prolongation of the QTC_c interval on EKG and increased QT dispersion. These predict sudden death and likely contribute to the high mortality rates in patients with severe autonomic neuropathy.[114]

Perhaps the most intriguing causes of cardiomyopathy lie in the diabetic metabolic disturbances themselves, which are attributable to insufficient insulin action on myocardial cells, analogous to that operative in diabetic skeletal muscle. In type 1 diabetes, insulin deficiency and nonphysiologic insulin replacement are to blame. In type 2 diabetes, insulin resistance at a still undetermined locus, accompanied by worsening beta cell insufficiency,[115] is the culprit. The result is inadequate glucose utilization by myocardial cells, despite elevated plasma glucose levels. Free fatty acid levels are also

elevated because insufficient insulin action on adipose cells causes enhanced lipolysis. High free fatty acid levels further inhibit glucose utilization by several biochemical mechanisms that result in decreases in glucose oxidation and glucose transport into cells. Yet elevated glucose levels also impede fatty acid oxidation, so that the overall effect of this complex interrelationship is that the heart starves for energy in the presence of substrate plenty.[106,107]

Chronic elevation of plasma glucose has other noxious effects,[116–118] including increases in glycation of tissue proteins with formation of toxic advance glycation end products (AGEs), increased activity and expression of protein kinase C (PKC), and especially increased production of reactive oxygen species (oxidative stress). The latter has been ascribed to abnormal mitochondrial function.[116] Increased PKC activity leads to excessive formation of extracellular matrix, increased vascular permeability and proliferation, and increased secretion of inflammatory cytokines. Moreover, chronic elevation of free fatty acid levels also leads to formation of intracellular products such as ceramide, which triggers apoptosis (programmed cell death) of myocytes.

Even a superficial consideration of all the ways that the disordered metabolic state of diabetes is bad for the heart, particularly in the presence of ischemia,[109] leads to the conclusion that therapy, whether primary prevention or secondary intervention, must be multifaceted. Not only must hyperglycemia be reversed, but the other cardiac risk factors such as hypertension and dyslipidemia must be aggressively eliminated or minimized.

OVERALL PATHOPHYSIOLOGIC RELATIONSHIP BETWEEN TYPE 2 DIABETES AND CARDIOVASCULAR DISEASE

The exact pathophysiologic relationship between type 2 diabetes and heart disease still remains to be completely elucidated. However, at least two principal overall sequences—with somewhat differing therapeutic implications—can be envisioned (Figure 63-3A).

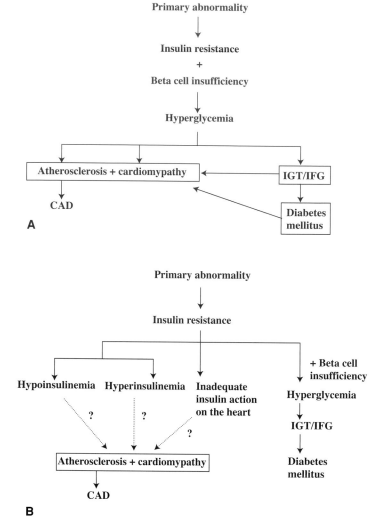

FIGURE 63-3. Alternate pathways leading from insulin resistance to heart disease in diabetes (**A**) through increasing hyperglycemia and (**B**) independent of hyperglycemia. CAD = coronary artery disease; IFG = impaired fasting glucose; IGT = impaired glucose tolerance.

In the first sequence, a primary abnormality, likely genetic, gives rise to insulin resistance with the attendant features of the metabolic syndrome. As beta cells gradually become increasingly less able to compensate for insulin resistance by increasing insulin secretion, hyperglycemia develops (see Figure 63-3A). In at first a subtle way and later as hyperglycemia increases to the level of IGT, IFG, or further to diabetes itself, the high plasma glucose level causes further progressive atherosclerosis and myocardial damage by recruitment of multiple pathogenetic pathways (see Figure 63-3). If this is the actual sequence, therapy aimed at lowering plasma glucose itself should be directly beneficial to the heart.

In the second scenario (Figure 63-3B), insulin resistance is again seen as the primary abnormality accompanied by other components of the metabolic syndrome. However, diabetes and cardiac disease are viewed as parallel consequences not primarily linked in a sequential cause-and-effect manner. Instead, atherosclerosis in the coronary arteries and cardiomyopathy are considered directly consequent to insulin resistance right from the start. Therapy that decreases insulin resistance per se would be beneficial to the heart, even if it did not normalize or even lower plasma glucose.[118a]

Moreover, if insufficient insulin action on the heart muscle were damaging, sufficient exogenous insulin therapy of hyperglycemia would be beneficial, if it were able to overcome the insulin resistance. Exogenous insulin would be even more selectively beneficial if the insulin precursor, proinsulin, were a culprit molecule because exogenous insulin treatment reduces beta cell function.[119]

THE CAUSATIVE ROLE OF HYPERGLYCEMIA

The exact relationship between hyperglycemia and either atherosclerosis or thrombotic CVD events and their outcomes remains incompletely understood. Whether hyperglycemia is a causative risk factor, and if so, by what pathogenetic mechanism, remains unclear and unproven. A large body of cross-sectional and prospective longitudinal epidemiologic data demonstrates associations between plasma glucose or HbA_{1c} levels and current or future risk of CVD and their outcomes.[120–131] The risk of CHF is reported to increase 15% in elderly diabetic patients for every 1% absolute increase in HbA_{1c}.[132] However, there are also reports that weaken the case.[133–137] Of particular importance are associations of hyperglycemia with total mortality,[123] particularly mortality attributed to CVD.[122–126] The Wisconsin Epidemiologic Study of Diabetic Retinopathy[123] showed that in diabetic patients, survival over 10 years decreased with each increasing quartile of Hemoglobin A_{1c} (Figure 63-4). Moreover, ischemic heart disease mortality increased 10% in older onset (type 2) and 18% in younger onset (type 1) with each 1.0% absolute increase in HbA_{1c}. Finnish studies in type 2 diabetes showed an increasing 3.5-year risk of MI[122] and stroke[121] with increasing tertiles of HbA_{1c} at baseline, and a Swedish study[124] showed like results for mortality with increasing fasting plasma glucose. Indeed, even in nondiabetic persons, mortality correlates with blood glucose down into the normal range.[128,129] The Diabetes Epidemiology Collaborative analysis Of Diagnostic criteria in Europe (DECODE) study,[138] however, has shown that the risk of CVD and mortality is more strongly associated with 2-hour plasma glucose after a glucose load than it is with FPG; whereas, in a National Health And Nutrition Examination Survey (NHANES) study, fasting and 2-hour post-challenge glucose levels were equally predictive of mortality.[139] A 1-hour post-breakfast blood glucose predicted death in the Diabetes

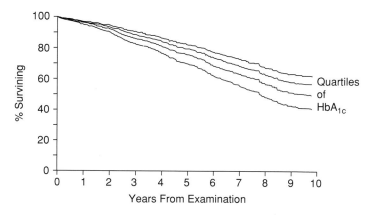

FIGURE 63-4. Survival (total mortality) versus quartiles of HbA_{1c} in older onset (type 2) diabetes. (Reproduced from Moss SE, Klein R, Klein BEK, et al,[23] with permission of the American Medical Association.)

Intervention Study.[140] The debate over whether postprandial hyperglycemia is more harmful to the cardiovascular system than FPG, and independent of chronic glycemia as assessed by hemoglobin A_{1c} (HbA$_{1c}$), has clear therapeutic implications.[141–143]

Hyperglycemia may adversely affect cardiovascular function via many pathways. Both endothelium dependent and independent coronary vasodilation are more than 50% reduced in chronically hyperglycemic type 1 and type 2 diabetic individuals.[144] Infusion of glucose to normal subjects or those with IGT, while preventing the normal insulin response, raised levels of inflammatory cytokines, IL-6, IL-18 and TNF-α, probably by increasing oxidative stress.[145]

Less support for a causative role of hyperglycemia in CVD evidence comes from the Rancho Bernardo Study,[137] the Patient Outcomes Research Team (PORT) Study,[136] and from the Framingham Study.[135] In the latter, HbA$_{1c}$ was only weakly associated with CVD and then only in women. It has also been argued from clinical and pathological evidence that because duration of diabetes does not correlate well with CVD or CAD, prolonged glycemic exposure per se may not be the critical factor leading to an increased prevalence of CVD in diabetes.[146,147] This point of view is reflected in the pathogenetic scheme depicted in Figure 63-3B. If on the other hand, hyperglycemia does cause atherosclerosis and its consequences as depicted in Figure 63-3A, numerous biochemical pathways can be invoked to explain the mechanism(s) that operates.[148,149]

The clearest evidence for the pathogenic importance of hyperglycemia in the increased risk of CVD in type 2 diabetes should come from randomized clinical trials comparing different intensities of glycemic treatment. Thus far, no trials have conclusively proven this point in type 2 diabetes.[150] The first attempt to determine whether more aggressive lowering of blood glucose would reduce the incidence of CVD events and mortality was the University Group Diabetes Program (UGDP);[151] more intensive insulin treatment over 10 years did not lower the cumulative incidence of MI.[152] However, this study was clearly underpowered to detect a meaningful decrease in incidence of MI. The United Kingdom Prospective Diabetes Study (UKPDS) studied an eight-times larger group of newly diagnosed type 2 diabetic patients over a 10-year span and found a suggestive but statistically non-significant ($P = .052$) 16% reduction in MI with intensive diabetes treatment that reduced HbA$_{1c}$ to 7.0% compared to 7.9% with conventional treatment (Figure 63-5).[153] Further follow-up of the UKPDS cohort after the trial has not yet shown a delayed benefit of intensive diabetes treatment on MI. The Veteran's Administration Feasibility Pilot Study found no benefit from intensive compared to conventional glucose lowering (HbA$_{1c}$ 7.1% versus 9.2%), but there were only 2 years of follow-up.[154,155]

In a somewhat puzzling observation, only 3 days of inpatient intravenous insulin infusion during treatment of an acute MI followed by 3 months of outpatient multiple daily injection therapy led to improved survival of type 2 diabetic patients at 1 year[156] and 3.5 years[157] after their MI. The mechanism of such a prolonged benefit resulting from a 3-month course of more aggressive glucose lowering (HbA$_{1c}$ 7.0% vs 7.5% in controls) is obscure. Moreover, an attempt to confirm the results in a larger trial by the same investigator proved negative.[158]

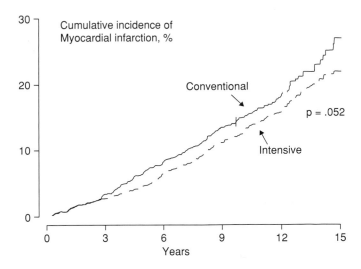

FIGURE 63-5. The effect of intensive versus conventional therapy of hyperglycemia on the cumulative incidence of myocardial infarction in the UKPDS. (Reproduced from UK Prospective Diabetes Study (UKPDS) Group[153] with permission from Lancet.)

It is possible that the benefits of lowering blood glucose on CVD events demonstrated in type 1 diabetes noted below can be extrapolated to type 2 diabetes as well. However, the clear need for an unequivocal resolution of this issue has led the National Heart, Lung and Blood Institute (NHLBI) to sponsor the Action to Control Cardiovascular Risk in Diabetes (ACCORD) trial,[159] which has completed its recruitment of 10,251 type 2 diabetic participants over age 55. They have been randomly assigned to either intensive glycemic treatment aimed at virtual normal glycemia (HbA$_{1c}$ < 6.0%) or conventional glycemic treatment aimed at a HbA$_{1c}$ range of 7.0% to 7.9%. The primary outcome is a composite of CVD death, nonfatal MI, or nonfatal stroke over a planned follow-up of approximately 5.5 years. A vanguard phase has shown that the protocol can be successfully implemented. Results of this hopefully definitive trial should be available in 2010. A Veterans Administration Diabetes Intervention Trial (VADIT) is now also comparing two groups of type 2 diabetic veterans, one maintained around 6.5% and one maintained at 8.0% to 9.0% for 5 to 7 years. A composite CVD event is the primary outcome.[160]

As noted above, insulin resistance may itself be a causative factor for CVD, so that *how* one lowers blood glucose may be as relevant as the *level* of plasma glucose that is reached. The Bypass Angioplasty Revascularization Investigation 2 in Diabetes (BARI 2D) trial,[161] also sponsored by the NHLBI, has randomized 2361 type 2 diabetic patients with angiographically documented CAD into two groups that are treated with two different primary glucose-lowering strategies. One group is primarily receiving the insulin-sensitizing drugs rosiglitazone and metformin, which decrease insulin resistance. The other group is primarily receiving insulin providing drugs (ie, insulin itself, glipizide, and nateglinide). The target HbA$_{1c}$ is less than 7.0% in both groups, so long as that can be achieved with the assigned drug therapy. If HbA$_{1c}$ cannot be kept below 8.0% with the protocol assigned drugs, then a drug from the opposite treatment arm is prescribed. It is hoped that such "cross-overs" can be limited so as to minimize confounding. Planned follow-up is an average of 5 years, and total mortality is the primary outcome.

TYPE 1 DIABETES MELLITUS AND CARDIOVASCULAR DISEASE

Although most of the CVD burden stems from type 2 diabetes, type 1 diabetes also contributes to the incidence of CVD. Type 1 diabetic patients with end-stage renal disease frequently manifest and die of CVD;[162,163] they may suffer from MIs, strokes, and amputations. The risk of CVD is increased some 40-fold overall and 10-fold compared to those without nephropathy.[162] However, even type 1 diabetic patients without demonstrable nephropathy have a 3- to 4-fold increased risk of CVD.[164] In the European Diabetes IDDM Complications (EURODIAB) study, CVD by history or EKG abnormalities was found in 9% of men and 10% of women with type 1 diabetes.[133] The prevalence rose from 6% in the age group 15 to 29 to 25% in the age group 45 to 59.

In a recent large-scale United Kingdom study of type 1 diabetes, standardized mortality ratios (SMRs) were 4.0 for women and 2.7 for men.[165] Thirty-seven percent of all deaths were attributed to CVD and 69% of these to ischemic heart disease (IHD).[166] SMRs due to IHD in women aged 20 to 29 were 45 and in men aged 30 to 39 were 42.[166] Asymptomatic ischemia is reportedly six times more common in type 1 diabetic individuals than in age and gender-matched controls,[167] and coronary artery obstruction on angiography[168] and atherosclerotic plaques on intravenous ultrasound[169] are commonly found. Left ventricular hypertrophy by EKG is three times more prevalent in type 1 diabetes than in the general population.[170] Some studies suggest an association between microvascular complications and death from CVD.[171–175]

The pathogenetic relationship between diabetes and CVD in type 1 diabetes seems at first blush to be more dependent on hyperglycemia and less on insulin resistance than in type 2 diabetes. However, evidence to the contrary is appearing. In the EURODIAB study, high serum triglycerides, low HDL, and body mass index in women were risk factors for CVD, but HbA_{1c} and insulin dose were not.[133] Atherosclerosis measured by carotid intimal medial thickness on ultrasonography in type 1 diabetes was predicted by a positive family history of type 2 diabetes, CVD, or hypertension[176] and was associated with elevated levels of CRP.[177] In the Pittsburgh Epidemiology of Diabetes Complications Study, insulin resistance assessed indirectly—but not HbA_{1c}—was a risk factor for CAD.[134] The metabolic syndrome is present in 20% to 40% of type 1 diabetic patients by age 40[178,179] and in over 20% of the Diabetes Control and Complications Trial/Epidemiology of Diabetes Interventions and Complications (DCCT/EDIC) cohort (personal communication). In the intensively treated DCCT patients, those who gained the most weight and became obese developed hypertension and dyslipidemia.[180] In some studies,[181–183] HbA_{1c} was either not at all or only weakly associated with higher scores or higher prevalence of coronary artery calcification.

These reports not withstanding, glycemic exposure per se does appear to be an independent risk factor for atherosclerosis in type 1 diabetes. In the DCCT/EDIC cohort, prior intensive treatment and a lower HbA_{1c} during the DCCT randomized treatment period were associated with a reduced prevalence of coronary artery calcification eight years later in EDIC[184] as well as a reduced risk of increasing carotid intimal medial thickness from EDIC year 1 to year 6.[185] Patients with HbA_{1c} greater than 7.5% are more likely to show increases in coronary calcification over 3 years than those with HbA_{1c} less than 7.5%.[186] In a Norwegian study assessing coronary artery atheromata by intravenous ultrasound and quantitative coronary angiography, the plaque burden was related to the mean HbA_{1c} over the preceding 18 years.[187] The addition of a pancreas transplant to patients undergoing kidney transplantation restored HbA_{1c} to 6.2%, compared to 8.4% in those patients receiving only a kidney transplant.[188] Subsequently, the much better glycemic controlled pancreatic transplant patients had less carotid intimal medial thickness, a reduced prothrombotic state, and normal endothelial dependent dilation.[188]

Most convincingly, the DCCT/EDIC study has just reported that type 1 diabetic patients treated intensively (mean HbA_{1c} ~ 7%), when compared with patients treated conventionally (mean HbA_{1c} ~ 9%), in the randomized trial from 1983 to 1993, had a 42% reduction in a composite outcome of all CVD events and a 57% reduction in a composite outcome of nonfatal MI, stroke, or CVD death from 1983 to 2005 (Figure 63-6).[189] Most of the

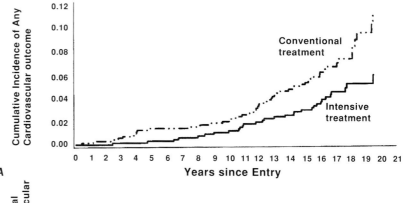

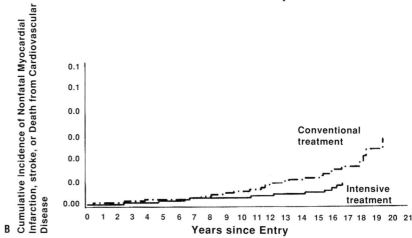

FIGURE 63-6. Cumulative incidence of total CVD events (**A**) and of a composite of stroke, nonfatal MI and CVD death (**B**) in type 1 diabetes participants treated intensively (solid line) or conventionally (dotted line) for 6.5 years during the Diabetes Control and Complications Trial. (*Reproduced from Nathan DM, Cleary PA, Backlund JYC, Genuth SM, et al,[189] with permission of the Massachusetts Medical Society.*)

treatment group effect was attributed to the difference in HbA_{1c} over a mean of 6.5 years of randomized treatment, even after adjustment for differences in nephropathy.

In summary, CVD and in particular CAD are major causes of morbidity and mortality in type 1 diabetes. As early as 8 years after onset, patients may have impaired left ventricular diastolic function.[190] All the usual remediable risk factors warrant aggressive treatment.[191] That diabetic retinopathy is a risk factor for CVD and mortality[192] and augurs badly for the outcome of coronary artery bypass grafting over the long term also suggests a pathogenetic relationship between microvascular complications and CAD.[193] The bulk of the evidence cited suggests that maintaining near-normal glycemia is beneficial for CVD, as it is for microvascular complications,[194] in type 1 diabetes.

MANAGEMENT OF HYPERGLYCEMIA

Until the ACCORD and BARI 2D trials provide us with sorely needed answers, how should glucose-lowering treatment be approached in type 2 diabetes? Given the uncertainties noted above and the wait until ACCORD, VADIT, and BARI 2D hopefully resolve them, how should hyperglycemia be managed in the diabetic age group most likely to have or be at heightened risk for CVD? The DCCT convincingly demonstrated in type 1 diabetes that intensive therapy producing a treatment group mean HbA_{1c} of 7.2% versus a mean HbA_{1c} of 9.0% with conventional therapy greatly reduced the risk of development or progression of retinopathy, nephropathy, and neuropathy by up to 75%.[194] This was confirmed for type 2 diabetes in the UKPDS, where the intensive treatment group with a mean HbA_{1c} of 7.0% versus a conventional treatment group with a mean HbA_{1c} of 7.9%, experienced a 25% reduction in a composite microvascular outcome.[153] The relationship between the mean HbA_{1c} and risk of microvascular complications was similar in the two studies, was exponential in nature, and did not exhibit a glycemic threshold above the nondiabetic range of HbA_{1c}.[132,195,196] Thus, it might seem that normal glycemia should be the goal of glycemic treatment in all diabetic patients.

However, the risk of severe hypoglycemia was increased 2- to 3-fold by intensive treatment (62 vs 19 events per 100 patient-years; 10% vs 5% of patients/year) in the relatively young type 1 diabetic patients in the DCCT.[194] A much lower rate of 2% to 3% of patients per year with intensive insulin treatment was noted in the first 10 years after diagnosis of type 2 diabetes in the UKPDS.[153] However, these data cannot be simply extended to the seventh to ninth decades of life when many CVD events occur, especially because the incidence of severe hypoglycemia is greater over age 75 and it can be associated with serious consequences,[198,199] including silent ischemia.[200] Although type 2 diabetes now accounts for half or more of photocoagulation for retinopathy and chronic dialysis for nephropathy, CVD events and mortality are a greater risk than microvascular complications in the HbA_{1c} range of 6.0% to 8.0%.[132] Physicians should be circumspect about individualizing glycemic targets and treatment in the aged, rather than automatically following authoritative guidelines, particularly those not yet based on clinical trial evidence of CVD benefit.

Lifestyle therapy should emphasize moderate weight loss of 5 to 10% of body weight,[201] which can usually be produced by a daily deficit of 500 to 800 calories. A high soluble fiber intake (50 g/d) is also beneficial.[202] These should be coupled with exercise equivalent to 30 to 45 minutes of walking at a speed and grade that sustains a heart rate 60% to 70% of maximum 5 days per week.[203] This combination reliably improves glycemic control, at least initially, in most patients.[153] Moreover, observational studies suggest that such an exercise program can be expected to reduce CVD events in both women and men with diabetes.[204,205] Patients over age 35 should have a stress test before beginning an exercise program. Patients on treatment with insulin or oral beta cell stimulants should have glucose tablets on their person and should test their blood glucose when exercising long after the last meal.

As adjunctive therapy to a hypocaloric diet and exercise, orlistat (an inhibitor of fat absorption from the gut) and sibutramine (a serotonin and norepinephrine reuptake inhibitor with a satiety effect) can increase the achieved weight loss and plasma glucose reductions somewhat.[206,207] Their long-term efficacy and safety are unproven. Rimonabant, a cannabis receptor antagonist, has demonstrated the ability to augment weight loss on a reduced calorie diet.[207,208] Finally, obese diabetic patients with a body mass index greater than 40 who have failed conservative treatment usually lose large amounts of weight, accompanied by improvement in hyperglycemia and a reduced need for pharmacotherapy, after gastric bypass surgery.[209] Intentional weight loss also is associated with reduced mortality in overweight diabetic individuals.[210]

Over a 10-year period, at least 60% of successfully diet-treated patients escape control of their hyperglycemia due to deterioration of beta cell function.[211] Until recently, when pharmacologic therapy was needed, a single drug was usually prescribed.[212] However, the UKPDS experience showed that with monotherapy using either a sulfonylurea drug or metformin or even insulin, HbA_{1c} rises relentlessly after an initial 1 to 2 years of success.[153] Thus, combinations of oral drugs with or without insulin should be considered earlier in the course of therapy.[213] The commonly employed oral drugs, insulin preparations, and drug combinations have been recently reviewed[214–216] and are shown in Table 63-2.

Metformin[216,217] has probably supplanted sulfonylurea drugs as a starting drug for three reasons: it does not cause hypoglycemia as monotherapy; it does not cause weight gain as sulfonylureas do; and most pertinent to the present context, in the UKPDS, metformin as monotherapy led to decreases in MI and total mortality in obese type 2 diabetic patients.[218] Therefore, it is the preferred starting drug in overweight patients. Metformin acts primarily on the liver, where it lowers hepatic glucose output and FPG, primarily by reducing gluconeogenesis.[216,219,220] It also increases glucose uptake by a modest degree and an unclear mechanism.[219,221] CVD advantages to using metformin include decreases in serum plasminogen activator inhibitor-1 (PAI-1), tissue plasminogen activator, von Willebrand factor, S-vascular cell adhesion molecule (S-VCAM), and e-selectin.[222] Neither CRP nor S-ICAM were affected by metformin in this study.[222] The positive effects of metformin on CVD risk factors were not explained by its lowering of HbA_{1c}.

Metformin can be combined with all other hypoglycemic drug classes and is especially useful with insulin, where it again has the advantage of preventing or limiting weight gain as blood glucose

TABLE 63-2

Drugs for Type 2 Diabetes Mellitus

DRUGS	LOWEST EFFECTIVE SINGLE DOSE (mg)	PRACTICAL MAXIMUM DAILY DOSE (mg)	COMBINATIONS
Sulfonylureas[a]			Sulfonylurea + metformin
Glyburide	1.25	10	Sulfonylurea + thiazolidinedione
Micronized glyburide	1.5	6	Metformin + thiazolidinedione
Glipizide	5	20	Metformin + meglitinide
Glipizide (gastrointestinal therapeutic system)	5	20	Thiazolidinedione + meglitinide
Glimepiride	0.5	8	Sulfonylurea + metformin + thiazolidinedione
Meglitinides			
Repaglinide	0.5	4[b]	Metformin + thiazolidinedione + meglitinide
Nateglinide	60	360	
Biguanides			α-glucosidase inhibitor + any other drug except meglitinide
Metformin	500	2000	
Thiazolidinediones			Insulin + any other drug
Rosiglitazone	2	8	
Pioglitazone	15	45	
α-Glucosidase inhibitors			
Acarbose	25	100[b]	
Miglitol	25	100[b]	
Insulin			
NPH glargine detemir } basal	—	—	
lispro aspart glulisine regular } preprandial	—	—	

[a]Tolbutamide, chlorpropamide, and acetohexamide are also still available.
[b]This maximal dose must be taken each time with meals.

comes down.[221] The main clinical impediment to metformin use is gastrointestinal side effects (nausea, gastric distress, anorexia, diarrhea, and abdominal cramps) in 5% to 15% of patients. Starting with the lowest daily dose of 500 mg and titrating upward every 1 to 2 weeks to a maximum of 2000 mg[223] can prevent these symptoms should they occur, and lowering the dose for a few weeks can remit them.

A more serious concern is renal insufficiency, which causes drug build-up, because excretion in the urine is the main route of elimination. Therefore, serum creatinine levels of 1.5 mg/dL in men and 1.4 mg/dL in women are ordinarily contraindications to metformin use. Lactic acidosis is a very rare complication that occurs mainly when the drug is used inappropriately in the presence of renal insufficiency or ischemic conditions.[224] Among the latter, CHF has until recently been a contraindication. However, two reports now suggest that metformin use is associated with improved outcomes in patients hospitalized with CHF[225] or acute MI.[226] Moreover, subsequent death or acute MI were less frequent after percutaneous revascularization in the Prevention of REStenosis with Tranilast and its Outcomes (PRESTO) trial in patients treated with metformin than in those treated with insulin or sulfonylurea drugs.[227]

Sulfonylurea drugs remain one mainstay of initial monotherapy, especially when insulin deficiency is suspected to be an important contributor to hyperglycemia, as in a normal-weight patient with a history of weight loss and/or slight to moderate ketonuria, but not in ketoacidosis. The earliest widely used sulfonylurea drug was tolbutamide. This agent came under a dark cardiac cloud when the UGDP study reported that its use was associated with an increased cardiovascular mortality rate compared with either placebo or insulin therapy.[228] The UKPDS, however, largely dispelled this cloud by reporting no increase in death rates with either a first-generation (chlorpropamide) or a second-generation (glyburide) sulfonylurea, compared with diet or insulin therapy in a randomized trial.[153] Nonetheless, new retrospective observational studies continue to report that higher doses and exposure to first- or second-generation sulfonylureas are associated with higher mortality than lower doses,[229] and sulfonylurea users have been reported to have higher mortality rates than do metformin users.[230] The addition of metformin to a sulfonylurea in the UKPDS was associated with increased mortality,[218] and this also has been reported in a recent observational study.[231]

TABLE 63-3

Effects of Peroxisome Profilerator Activated Receptors (PPAR) Ligand Drugs

PPAR GAMMA (ADIPOSE TISSUE, MUSCLE, LIVER, BETA CELLS, MACROPHAGES, ENDOTHELIUM)	PPAR ALPHA (LIVER, HEART, MUSCLE)
↑ Insulin sensitivity (↓ Insulin resistance) ↑ Adipose tissue differentiation ↑ Lipogenesis ↑ Glucose uptake & oxidation ↓ Gluconeogenesis ↓ Hepatic glucose output ↓ FFA ↑ Adiponectin ↓ Resistin ↓ TNF alpha ↓ 11-Hydroxysteroid dehydrogenase-1	↑ FFA oxidation ↓ Triglycerides ↑ HDL cholesterol ↑ LDL cholesterol particle size and ↓ density ↓ Inflammation ↓ Atherosclerosis

New theoretical questions have arisen with regard to the safety of sulfonylurea drugs following the discovery that they bind to and inhibit ATP-sensitive potassium channels in the insulin-producing beta cells of the pancreatic islets,[232,233] but moreover in the heart as well.[234,235] One potentially adverse action is impairment of the cardioprotective effect provided by ischemic preconditioning.[236] The clinical consequences of this effect in patients are not completely clear. The latest sulfonylurea, glimepiride, offers the theoretical advantage that it binds less avidly to the cardiac receptor than to the beta cell receptor,[237] and its preferential prescription is prudent. The appropriate use of sulfonylurea drugs remains controversial.[238,239]

Thiazolidinedione drugs (TZDs) are the subject of great interest and intense investigation in treatment of type 2 diabetes, in particular because of their potential to reduce CVD by multiple mechanisms (Table 63-3).[240,241] TZDs work by decreasing insulin resistance in muscle and adipose tissue and to some extent in the liver as well.[242] Thus, they could actually benefit the heart directly in type 2 diabetes (see Figure 63-3B). They are also reported to improve endothelial dysfunction, decrease PAI-1 levels, inhibit progression of carotid atherosclerosis, reduce neointimal hyperplasia after stent placement, decrease vasospastic angina,[243–252] and decrease the levels of such markers of inflammation as CRP, independent of glucose control.[248,253] Effects on serum lipids are mixed, but they are more beneficial than not, as HDL rises and free fatty acids and triglycerides fall.[240,254–256] Blood pressure decreases slightly.[243,254] TZDs do not cause hypoglycemia as monotherapy, but unfortunately they do increase adiposity, although the important abdominal visceral fat depot may decrease.[240,241,257] This is nonetheless a distinct disadvantage in already obese type 2 diabetic patients. Of additional concern are reports of exacerbation of CHF or even precipitation of first episodes of CHF.[256,258] TZDs definitely cause enough fluid retention to produce clinically evident edema in some patients,[214] but whether this is the sole mechanism operating in the infrequent cases of CHF is still debatable. This serious adverse effect of TZDs is mostly seen when they are combined with insulin therapy.[214,255] Although troglitazone, the first TZD to be approved, was later

withdrawn because of serious liver toxicity, the current approved representatives of this drug class, rosiglitazone[259] and pioglitazone,[260] have not evinced serious liver toxicity ascribable to them. However, regular monitoring of serum glutamate pyruvate transaminase (SGPT; alanine aminotransferase) is still called for by the Food and Drug Administration (FDA).

The mechanism of action of TZDs is unique and opens the door to a myriad of metabolic actions and interactions. TZDs are exogenous ligands for a nuclear transcription factor—peroxisome proliferator activated receptor-gamma (PPAR-gamma).[240,241,258] Largely, but not uniquely concentrated in adipose tissue, the natural ligands of PPAR-gamma include fatty acids and their derivatives and prostanoids. The consequences of ligand binding of PPAR-gamma include (see Table 63-3) differentiation of preadipocytes to adipocytes, increases in fat storage and synthesis, enhancement of glucose uptake and oxidation, and sensitization of other pathways of glucose metabolism modulated by insulin. In addition, TZDs regulate adipocyte production and release of adipokines that act like hormones on targets in muscle, liver, and brain. These TZD effects include reduction of resistin—a molecule that causes insulin resistance—and stimulation of adiponectin, a molecule that increases insulin sensitivity. TZDs also decrease cytokines such TNF-α, which can also cause insulin resistance. In animal models, TZDs inhibit the development of atherosclerosis.[261] In humans, they are reported to decrease carotid artery intimal medial thickness[246,252] and to reduce restenosis of coronary artery stents by inhibiting neointimal hyperplasia.[250,251] Most of these effects are exerted through PPAR-gamma receptors.[214,241,243] However, activation of PPAR-alpha receptors (see Table 63-3) by fibrates has also improved insulin sensitivity but decreased adipose tissue.[241,262]

The results of the first direct test of the ability of a TZD to decrease CVD has been inconclusive.[256] The ProActive study, in a randomized trial, compared pioglitazone to placebo in 5238 type 2 diabetic patients who already had evidence of major CVD. Their usual glycemic regimens were maintained. After 3 years of follow-up, the primary outcome—a composite of seven clinical and revascularization end points—was nonsignificantly reduced 10% (95%

CI 80%–102%) by pioglitazone. However, a composite "main secondary endpoint" of all cause mortality or nonfatal and silent MI or stroke, was reduced 16% (95% CI 72%–98%) by the TZD. Strictly interpreted, the latter significant observation can only be considered hypothesis generating, not a conclusion, when the primary outcome test is negative. Moreover, pioglitazone lowered HbA$_{1c}$, systolic blood pressure, and triglycerides, and raised HDL cholesterol more than placebo. Together, these effects could have accounted for any CVD benefit rather than other TZD-specific mechanisms to reduce CVD risk.

As monotherapy, TZDs require 4 weeks to exhibit a modest beneficial effect, and they do not cause hypoglycemia. A midrange dose may be used initially when fasting plasma glucose is above 180 mg/dL if there is no known risk of CHF and insulin is not also being administered. TZDs are especially useful in combination with insulin, sulfonylurea drugs, metformin, and meglitinides.[214] They also hold great potential for preventing the progression of IGT to diabetes[95] not only by decreasing insulin resistance but secondarily by improving the strain imposed on beta cells by insulin resistance.[263] TZDs may possibly also have direct effects through PPAR gamma in the beta cells and thereby improve insulin secretory responses to glucose.[264]

There is no glucose-lowering reason to choose between pioglitazone and rosiglitazone. Pioglitazone has superior antidyslipidemic effects, including lowering triglycerides, raising HDL, and decreasing LDL particle concentration and size.[265] However, the effects in most patients needing amelioration of significant dyslipidemia are not great enough to substitute for statin and fibrate treatment (see below).

Because activation of both PPAR-gamma and PPAR-alpha receptors have hypoglycemic and antiatherosclerotic effects, ligands that activate both receptors offer attractive therapeutic possibilities. Muraglitazar, a dual activator, was tested in drug naïve type 2 diabetic patients for 6 months.[266] In groups with mean baseline HbA$_{1c}$ of 8.0% and 10.6%, muraglitazar lowered HbA$_{1c}$ by 1.2% and 2.6% respectively. Triglycerides were decreased 27% and apolipoprotein B 12%, whereas HDL cholesterol was increased 16% from baseline on a 5-mg dose. Weight increased 2.1 kg, and edema occurred in 11% of cases. Approval by the FDA has been held up by an independent external analysis of all phase 2 and 3 clinical trials,[267] which showed that 1.5% of muraglitazar-treated patients compared to 0.7% of placebo-treated patients had suffered major cardiovascular events, including CHF (risk ratio 2.6, 95% CI 1.4–5.0, P = .004).

The latest oral hypoglycemic drug class, the meglitinides, are acute beta cell stimulants. Repaglinide[269] and nateglinide[270] act at least in part through the sulfonylurea drug receptor to stimulate a release of insulin by the beta cell that peaks 1 hour after drug ingestion and ends after 4 to 5 hours.[269] Thus, these agents mimic the normal mealtime response of beta cells more closely than do most sulfonylurea drugs. Meglitinide drugs must be taken before meals, when they reduce the postprandial hyperglycemia produced by carbohydrate components of the diet. They also have a modest effect on FPG after a period of regular administration. If taken without a meal, repaglinide and nateglinide are apt to cause hypoglycemia. In one head-to-head monotherapy study, both lowered postprandial blood glucose to a similar degree, but repaglinide decreased FPG and HbA$_{1c}$ more than did nateglinide.[271]

The acute beta cell stimulants lower HbA$_{1c}$ modestly as monotherapy.[214] They are best used in combination with metformin or TZD drugs.[270,272] Postprandial hyperglycemia clearly contributes significantly to HbA$_{1c}$ levels.[273] If it finally proves to be a unique causative factor for CVD, independent of overall glycemia as measured by HbA$_{1c}$,[274–280] then these agents may be especially effective in preventing CVD or reducing the risk.

Another means of selectively decreasing postprandial glucose levels is by treatment with α-glucosidase inhibitors. These agents slow the digestion of starches and other complex carbohydrates and thereby slow the rate of absorption of glucose from these dietary sources.[214] Seldom employed thus far as monotherapy, particularly in the United States, they can lower HbA$_{1c}$ levels an additional 0.5% to 0.7% when added to any oral drug or to insulin.[281,282] The common side effect of flatulence and abdominal cramping has limited their acceptability in this country. However, acarbose decreased progression from IGT to diabetes in a recent diabetes prevention trial.[283] Of great interest, a concomitant significant reduction in MI was reported within the first 2 years of acarbose treatment in this trial (1/682 vs 12/686 in a placebo group).[284] However, the data analysis has been severely criticized,[285] and confirmation of this benefit in treatment of diabetes itself awaits a larger trial.

INSULIN

The clearcut proof that intensive insulin therapy reduces the risks of microvascular and neuropathic complications,[194] as well as cardiovascular events[189] in type 1 diabetes, makes it the treatment of choice in those patients.[215] Intensive treatment requires at least three to four blood glucose self-tests a day, a basal insulin such as glargine, detemir, or NPH at bedtime and rapid-acting lispro, glulisine, or aspart insulin before meals.[215] External subcutaneous insulin infusion pumps provide both basal and prandial insulin delivery using only rapid-acting insulin.[215]

About 30% to 40% of type 2 diabetes mellitus patients in the United States are on insulin therapy, alone or in combination with oral drugs. A small proportion of these patients may have delayed-onset type 1 diabetes mellitus and may offer serologic evidence of beta cell autoimmunity. Some of these patients are in the end stage of type 2 diabetes mellitus, when insulin deficiency is almost as profound as in type 1 diabetes. Those exhibiting recent loss of weight and muscle mass (even if still obese), debilitating fatigue and weakness, severe polyuria and polydipsia, severe hypertriglyceridemia, ketonuria, and FPG often exceeding 300 mg/dL should be started on insulin immediately.[286,287] After there has been sufficient clinical and biochemical improvement, these patients can sometimes be tapered off insulin and given a trial of a sulfonylurea drug.

Usually, however, the need for insulin treatment is prompted by failure of oral drug therapy.[288] Normal-weight individuals should generally be switched to insulin. Some patients may be managed on a single dose of basal intermediate- or long-acting insulin (starting dose of NPH or glargine, 0.15–0.20 U/kg) at bedtime to target the FPG and minimize weight gain.[215] Other patients may need intermediate- or long-acting insulin twice a day, in a usual ratio of breakfast dose to bedtime dose of 1:1 to 2:1. Later, glulisine or lispro or aspart insulin must be added before meals, the doses being adjusted by the patient according to the premeal blood glucose level, the carbohydrate content of the meal, or both. These doses may be as low as 1 unit in thin, sensitive patients to as high as 20 units or more in obese, resistant patients.

Stable patients who, because of visual or cognitive impairment, cannot accurately mix different insulins in one syringe may use premixed combinations of NPH with regular or lispro, or aspart, from 50% to 75% NPH and the remainder as short-acting insulin. The disadvantage of such mixtures is that neither the dose of NPH nor the dose of the regular or lispro insulin can be altered individually.

Obese patients with type 2 diabetes mellitus may need extraordinarily large daily doses, which some practitioners are uncomfortable prescribing. Doses of 1 U/kg body weight or more are commonly necessary.[287] As noted above, a concern has arisen that insulin might be atherogenic because plasma insulin is a risk factor for cardiovascular disease in some studies.[66] The results of the UKPDS[153] and the UGDP[151] do not support a reluctance to use exogenous insulin, because patients so treated had no increases in MI or cardiovascular death compared with diet therapy. In two randomized clinical trials,[153,154] the incidence of serious hypoglycemic episodes in patients on insulin treatment was in the range of two to three events per 100 patient-years. However, because one of 20 severe hypoglycemic events in elderly individuals can be accompanied by stroke, transient ischemic attack, MI, injury, or death,[198] patients and families must be educated to recognize and manage hypoglycemia promptly.

In discussing insulin treatment of type 2 diabetes, it is necessary to consider again whether the final effect on CAD and CVD is beneficial or adverse.[289–291] An adverse influence is supported by evidence linking insulin to the degree of angiographically determined CAD,[292] to endothelial dysfunction,[293] and to atherosclerosis in vitro.[294] However, insulin therapy generally improves dyslipidemia.[289] Recently, insulin has also been reported to decrease PAI-1 levels[295] and to have significant anti-inflammatory actions.[296,297] A review[291] shows that studies have demonstrated the acute cardiovascular benefits of aggressive insulin therapy, including a reduction in episodes of ST-segment changes in acute coronary syndromes, a lessening of left ventricular dysfunction, enhanced arterial vasoactivity, a decreased mortality in patients treated with angioplasty during an acute MI, and a decreased mortality after coronary artery bypass graft (CABG). Insulin treatment may also improve myocardial and pulmonary function in CHF. Thus a controversy exists; and only clinical trial data, such as BARI 2D is generating, can settle the longer term clinical issue.

COMBINATION THERAPY

Improved understanding of the pathogenesis of hyperglycemia in type 2 diabetes mellitus, the different modes of action of the hypoglycemic drugs, and the virtual inevitability that monotherapy will fail support earlier use of two or more drug classes simultaneously (eg, reducing insulin resistance in the liver with metformin while increasing insulin secretion with a sulfonylurea or meglitinide; see Table 63-2).[214] Metformin and a TZD also work in triple combination with a sulfonylurea or a meglitinide. Moreover, when monotherapy fails after initial success, substituting another drug from a different drug class has not usually been effective (except for

insulin).[300,301] Pharmaceutical companies have responded to these considerations by marketing a combination pill containing metformin and glyburide and another containing metformin and rosiglitazone for use as initial drug therapy. This single tablet tactic may improve compliance with a two-drug regimen.

The UKPDS found in a randomized substudy that adding metformin to a sulfonylurea led to a significant increase in mortality, compared to continuing the sulfonylurea alone.[218] Two observational studies have confirmed[231,302] and one has refuted[303] this finding. In addition, the UKPDS investigators themselves attributed the increased mortality to chance,[218] and the combination of metformin and a sulfonylurea remains in widespread use.[214]

When combining drugs, particularly with insulin, the lowest dose of the drug should be added and the dose should be increased as though it were being used as monotherapy. Self-blood glucose testing at appropriate times of the day should be used as a guide to efficacy and a safety check. The FBG is most helpful for metformin, TZD drugs, sulfonylureas, and bedtime glargine, detemir, or NPH insulin. Targeting FPG to less than or equal to 100 mg/dL can yield a HbA$_{1c}$ less than or equal to 7.0% in a majority of patients.[304] Postprandial blood glucose levels are important guides to therapy for repaglinide, nateglinide, α-glucosidase inhibitors, premeal regular insulin, lispro, glulisine, or aspart insulin. Patients should be given blood glucose guidelines for when to call the physician (eg, when FBG is consistently > 140 mg/dL or < 100 mg/dL or postprandial blood glucose is consistently > 180 mg/dL). Oral meglitinides for postprandial glucose control may be combined with bedtime insulin for fasting glucose control,[305] and rapid-acting insulin for postprandial glucose control may be combined with oral drugs for fasting glucose control.[306]

The primary aim of combination therapy,[307] which can be quite expensive, should always be to decrease the HbA$_{1c}$. Reduction in insulin dose, number of injections, or both, is sometimes a secondary benefit, when insulin is combined with sulfonylurea drugs,[308,309] metformin,[310,311] or TZDs.[255,311]

NEWLY INTRODUCED ADJUNCTIVE DRUGS[312,317]

Exenatide (Byetta) is a long-acting analog of the incretin, glucagon-like peptide-1 (GLP-1), which has multiple beneficial effects on glucose metabolism. GLP-1 increases insulin synthesis, beta cell replication, and first-phase insulin secretion; concurrently, it inhibits glucagon secretion. Additional actions are to decrease appetite and slow gastric emptying. The net result is to decrease fasting and especially postprandial plasma glucose levels and HbA$_{1c}$ ~ 0.8% when used in type 2 diabetes in combination with metformin, a sulfonylurea, or both. The dose is 5 or 10 (μg injected subcutaneously twice daily within 1 hour before breakfast and dinner. Nausea, vomiting, and diarrhea are the most common side effects. Hypoglycemia may occur when exenatide is added to a sulfonylurea but not to metformin. A small weight loss is an additional benefit.

Pramlintide (Symlin) is a synthetic analog of amylin, a beta cell peptide cosecreted with insulin in response to food. It lowers postprandial plasma glucose by delaying gastric emptying, reducing caloric intake and suppressing glucagon secretion. It is approved for use with (not instead of) insulin in type 1 diabetes and with insulin alone or combined with metformin or a sulfonylurea drug in type 2 diabetes. Pramlintide is injected subcutaneously immediately before meals in a dose of 60 to 120 µg in type 2 diabetes. The starting dose is 15 µg in type 1 diabetes. Premeal rapid-acting lispro, glulisine, or aspart insulin doses should be reduced 50% when starting pramlintide to minimize the risk of hypoglycemia. Nausea is the main side effect, which tends to diminish after 1 week of therapy. There is a mean weight loss of 2 kg, with a HbA_{1c} reduction of 0.6% to 0.9%.

Some patients prefer injecting the above drugs in preference to insulin. Other patients are willing to add one of them in addition to continuing insulin, so as not to increase their doses of insulin. Long-term benefits beyond 2 years of treatment are unknown.

A new form of insulin delivery—pulmonary insulin—has recently been approved by the FDA for use combined with metformin and/or a sulfonylurea drug in type 2 diabetes.[314] It is inhaled from a device and is rapidly absorbed from the lungs. The profile of blood glucose–lowering is similar to that of the rapid-acting insulins lispro and aspart, as is its effect on HbA_{1c}. Its chief advantage seems to be acceptability to patients who would not otherwise inject insulin before meals. A basal insulin, however, still needs to be injected to lower fasting glucose levels. The current formulation has only a slight adverse effect on pulmonary function in 2 years of use, but its long-term safety remains to be determined.

MANAGEMENT OF OTHER CARDIOVASCULAR RISK FACTORS IN DIABETES

Type 2 diabetes, and type 1 diabetes with nephropathy, are notable for the frequent presence of other typical modifiable risk factors for CVD. These include the components of the metabolic (insulin resistance) syndrome. Although hypertension and dyslipidemia are dealt with in detail in Chapters 61 and 62, their management deserves special emphasis in the context of diabetes.

[ ] HYPERTENSION

Hypertension frequently coexists with type 2 diabetes and complicates type 1 diabetes when nephropathy is present. Numerous randomized clinical trials (Table 63-4) either having a significant diabetic subgroup (eg, Systolic Hypertension in the Elderly Program [SHEP]),[315] or being dedicated specifically to diabetic patients (eg, UKPDS),[316] have shown that treating hypertension has as great or greater CVD benefit in patients with diabetes than in the general population. In the SHEP trial, chlorthalidone lowered mean blood pressure from 155/72 mm Hg to 143/68 mm Hg and reduced coronary heart disease events by 56%. The UKPDS reported a 44% reduction in stroke (95% CI, 0.35–0.89) and a 21% reduction in MI (95% CI, 0.59–1.07) when mean blood pressure was lowered from 154/87 mm Hg to 144/82 mm Hg. The benefit was similar whether an angiotensin-converting enzyme (ACE) inhibitor or a beta blocker was used as the primary antihypertensive agent. In the Systolic Hypertension in Elderly in Europe (SYST-EUR) trial,[317] the calcium channel blocker nitrendipine lowered mean blood pressure from 162/82 mm Hg to 153/78 mm Hg and reduced CVD events and stroke by 62%.

The Antihypertensive and Lipid-Lowering treatment to prevent Heart ATtack (ALLHAT) study[318] compared a diuretic (chlorthalidone 12.5–25 mg), an ACE inhibitor (lisinopril 10–40 mg) and a calcium channel blocker (amlodipine 2.5–10 mg) in 33,357 patients, of whom 12,063 (36%) had type 2 diabetes, over 5 years of follow-up. The inexpensive diuretic therapy was as efficacious as the more modern and expensive ACE inhibitor and calcium channel blocker in reducing an aggregate outcome of CVD;

TABLE 63-4

Effects of Antihypertension Therapy on Cardiovascular Disease (CVD) Outcomes in Diabetic Patients in Selected Trials

TRIAL	MEAN BP (mm Hg) LOSE CONTROL	MEAN BP (mm Hg) TIGHT CONTROL	INITIAL DRUG	CVD RISK REDUCTION
SHEP	155/72	143/68	Chlorthalidone	34%
Syst-Eur	162/82	153/78	Nitrendipine	62%
UKPDS	154/87	144/82	Captopril or atenolol	21% (MI) 44% (stroke)
HOT	144/85	140/81	Felodipine	51%
ALLHAT	134/75		Chlorthalidone[a] or lisinopril or amlodipine	1–2% 16–28% (CHF)
LIFE	147/79		Losartan[a] or atenolol	24%
HOPE	143/77	140/77	Ramipril[a] or placebo	25%

[a]drug with lower risk.

ALLHAT = Antihypertensive and Lipid-Lowering treatment to prevent Heart Attack Trial; BP = blood pressure; CHF = congestive heart failure; HOPE = Heart Outcomes Prevention Evaluation; HOT = Hypertension Optimal Treatment; LIFE = Losartan Intervention For Endpoint reduction in hypertension; MI = myocardial infarction; SHEP = Systolic Hypertension in the Elderly Program; Syst-Eur = Systolic Hypertension in Elderly in Europe Trial; UKPDS = United Kingdom Prospective Diabetes Study.

the diuretic decreased the incidence of congestive heart failure more than did the ACE inhibitor (7.1% vs 8.7%) or amlodipine (7.7% vs 10.2%) risk reduction. The results in the diabetic subjects were in all cases similar to the whole cohort. Chlorthalidone increased fasting plasma glucose significantly but only slightly (4 mg/dL). The Hypertension Optimal Treatment (HOT) study[319] directly addressed diastolic blood pressure as a target and demonstrated a 51% reduction in CVD events and a 50% reduction in MI when the target diastolic blood pressure was less than 80 mm Hg (mean achieved 81 mm Hg) compared to a target diastolic blood pressure of less than 90 mm Hg (mean achieved 85 mm Hg). In the Appropriate Blood pressure Control in Diabetes (ABCD) study,[320] a diastolic blood pressure target of 80 to 89 mm Hg was compared to a target of less than 75 mm Hg. With a final achieved mean blood pressure of 132/78 mm Hg versus 138/86 mm Hg, the intensively treated group had a lower all-cause mortality of 5.5% versus 10.7%. However, this benefit could not be accounted for by reductions in MI, CHF, or strokes.

In the Losartan Intervention For Endpoint (LIFE) study,[321] an angiotensin receptor blocker, losartan, was compared to a beta blocker, atenolol, in hypertensive diabetic patients with left ventricular hypertrophy. Over 5 years of follow-up, the relative risk for a composite cardiovascular end point was 0.76 in favor of losartan.

The above record of success has led to repeated lowering of blood pressure targets in diabetes. Thus, the Sixth Report of the Joint National Committee on Prevention, Detection, Evaluation and Treatment of High Blood Pressure (JNC VI) recommended a blood pressure target of less than 130/85 mm Hg, and JNC VII[34] is recommending a blood pressure target of less than 130/80 mm Hg in diabetes. The ACCORD trial is seeking to determine whether a systolic blood pressure target of less than 120 mm Hg is superior to a target of less than 140 mm Hg with regard to CVD and nephropathy.

Diuretics and ACE inhibitors or angiotensin receptor blockers should be the starting drugs, with a preference for ACE inhibitor or angiotensin receptor blocker therapy if microalbuminuria is present; this gains the extra proven benefit of reducing the risk of nephropathy. Beta blockers and calcium channel blockers are next to add when the blood pressure goal is not met. The choice should be made based on other cardiac considerations such as the presence of angina, post-MI status, CHF, and diabetic considerations such as risk of severe hypoglycemia or manifestations of dyslipidemia.

MICROALBUMINURIA

Both ACE inhibitors[322,323] and angiotensin receptor blockers[324,325] decrease microalbuminuria and progression of nephropathy. Because microalbuminuria is an important risk factor for CVD and mortality,[326–329] it is important to take note of the results of the Heart Outcomes and Prevention Evaluation (HOPE) trial,[97] in which the ACE inhibitor, ramipril, was compared to placebo in diabetic patients with one other cardiovascular risk factor. Ramipril decreased the risk of a combined cardiovascular disease end point by 25%, MI by 22%, stroke by 33%, cardiovascular death by 37%, and overt nephropathy by 24%. Adjustment for the lowering of systolic blood pressure by 2.4 mm Hg and diastolic blood pressure by 1.0 mm Hg did not change the results. The effect of reducing the activity of the renin-angiotensin system is

impressive and supports the recommendation for first-line use of an ACE inhibitor in diabetes.

DYSLIPIDEMIA

Dyslipidemia with an atherogenesis-promoting profile frequently accompanies type 2 diabetes, as would be expected because the same dyslipidemia is a component of the metabolic syndrome. A low HDL cholesterol level, elevated triglycerides, elevated apolipoprotein B with increased VLDL and intermediate-density lipoprotein, and increases in the number of small, dense LDL cholesterol-containing particles are typical. LDL cholesterol levels are more often normal than elevated, although women show a tendency toward increased LDL.[30] Diabetic subgroups in primary and secondary intervention trials comparing statin drugs to placebo (Table 63-5) have shown similar relative reductions in CVD events as nondiabetics (17–51%), and the absolute reductions in risk have often been greater in the diabetic participants because of their higher rates on placebo.[330–334] Nonetheless, with statin therapy the absolute event rates in diabetic patients reach only the levels observed in nondiabetic persons on placebo. It is also noteworthy that in diabetic patients, statins used in primary prevention trials reduce absolute risk less than in secondary prevention trials.

The optimum doses and treatment targets for statin therapy are not completely established. In the Treating to New Targets trial, from an LDL baseline of 160 mg/dL, 80 mg of atorvastatin (lowering mean LDL to 77 mg/dL) was more effective than 10 mg (lowering mean LDL to 99 mg/dL); the higher dose lowered CVD events 25%, relative to the lower dose.[335] In the Incremental Decrease in End points through Aggressive Lipid lowering (IDEAL) study of patients with a previous MI, 80 mg of atorvastatin compared to 20 mg of simvastatin produced a nonsignificant 11% reduction in the primary composite outcome of coronary death, nonfatal MI, or cardiac death with resuscitation, but a significant 17% reduction in nonfatal MI.[336] In the Pravastatin or atOrvastatin Evaluation and Infection Therapy (PROVE IT) trial, patients admitted for acute coronary syndromes had 16% fewer major cardiovascular events treated with 80 mg of atorvastatin than 40 mg of pravastatin,[337] with similar results in diabetic as nondiabetic patients. The Collaborative AtoRvastatin Diabetes Study (CARDS) study is of note for having specifically demonstrated a 48% reduction in strokes with only 10 mg of atorvastatin in diabetic patients.[338]

Statin therapy may be effective within 6 months by mechanisms other than lowering LDL cholesterol.[339] In particular, statins have an anti-inflammatory action, demonstrated by lowering C-reactive protein levels.[339,340] This action correlates with the reduction in CVD events, irrespective of whether the LDL level reached is greater or lesser than 70 mg/dL.[340] The third NCEP/ATP panel[33] recommends an LDL target of less than 100 mg/dL in diabetes, even without evidence of CAD. In a later report,[341] the panel stated that "a target of less than 70 mg/dL represents a therapeutic option, ie, a reasonable clinical strategy, for persons at very high risk," including diabetic patients with known CVD. At least a 30% to 40% reduction in LDL cholesterol should be the goal. The long-term safety of very low LDL levels has yet to be rigorously demonstrated;[342] however, in the short term, 34% of PROVE IT subjects with levels of 40 mg/dL to 60 mg/dL and 11% with levels

TABLE 63-5

Effect of Dyslipidemic Therapy on Cardiovascular Disease (CVD) Outcomes in Diabetic Patients in Selected Placebo-controlled Trials

TRIAL	REFERENCE	DRUG	CVD RISK REDUCTION
AFCAPS	330	Lovastatin	43%
4S	331	Simvastatin	51%
HPS	332	Simvastatin	22%
CARE	333	Pravastatin	22%
LIPID	334	Pravastatin	17%
CARDS	338	Atorvastatin	37%
ASCOT-LLA	378	Atorvastatin	23%
VA-HIT	343	Gemfibrozil	22%
DAIS	345	Fenofibrate	23%
FIELD	347	Fenofibrate	11%

AFCAPS/TexCAPS = Air Force Coronary/Texas Atherosclerosis Prevention Study; ASCOT–LLA = Anglo–Scandinavian Cardiac Outcomes Study Trial–Lipid–Lowering Arm; CARDS = Collaborative Atorvastatin Diabetes Study; CARE = Cholesterol and Recurrent Events; DAIS = Diabetes Atherosclerosis Intervention Study; FIELD = Fenofibrate Intervention and Event-Lowering in Diabetes; HPS = Hopkins Precursors Study; LIPID = Long-term Intervention with Pravastatin in Ischemic Disease; 4-S = Scandinavian Simvastatin Survival Study; VA-HIT = Veterans Affairs High-density lipoprotein Intervention Trial study group.

less than 40 mg/dL suffered no more adverse consequences than those with levels of 80 mg/dL to 100 mg/dL.[337]

Whether additional pharmacotherapy specifically aimed at raising HDL cholesterol and lowering triglycerides is mandatory is still somewhat open to question. The results in the diabetic subgroup of the VA-HIT trial offer the best support for adding a fibrate to statin therapy (see Table 63-5). Gemfibrozil decreased triglycerides 25% and increased HDL cholesterol 6%, leading to a decrease of 22% in a composite outcome of CHD death, MI, and stroke.[343] In the Helsinki Heart Study, the number of diabetic participants was too small to conclude benefit from gemfibrozil therapy, although the trend was in that direction.[344] In the Diabetes Atherosclerosis Intervention Study (DIAS), fenofibrate treatment was associated with a 40% to 42% reduction in progression of angiographically measured CAD and decreased events 23%.[345] By contrast, in a secondary intervention trial, bezafibrate failed to decrease CVD event rates.[346]

In the Fenofibrate Intervention and Event Lowering in Diabetes (FIELD) study[347] conducted in nearly 10,000 diabetic subjects, fenofibrate compared to placebo led to a nonsignificant 11% reduction in the primary outcome of CHD death or nonfatal MI. There was a 24% reduction in nonfatal MI alone ($P = 0.01$), and in another secondary outcome, total cardiovascular events (CHD events, total strokes, CVD death, plus coronary or carotid revascularization) were nonsignificantly reduced 11% ($P = 0.35$).

In light of the above, the ACCORD trial is trying to determine definitively the benefit of adding fenofibrate to a fixed dose of simvastatin. The risk of inducing rhabdomyolysis and renal failure is low when fenofibrate is combined with a statin,[348] but this risk still calls for careful monitoring when this combination is employed.

The most potent agent for raising HDL and lowering triglyceride levels is niacin, which acts in part by decreasing free fatty acid levels through interaction with a specific adipose tissue receptor. Niacin is usually avoided in diabetes because of concerns that it will aggravate hyperglycemia by inducing insulin resistance. The possibility of liver toxicity and severe flushing as a side effect also discourages its use. However, in a randomized clinical trial, one extended-release formulation of niacin in a dose of 1500 mg/d increased HDL 10 mg/dL (plus 25% from baseline) while raising HbA$_{1c}$ from only 7.1% to 7.5%, with 30% of the individuals requiring addition or dose increases of hyperglycemic drugs.[349]

In view of the generally positive effects of treating dyslipidemia, it is surprising that until very recently, diabetic patients have been tested[350] and treated[351] no more aggressively and possibly even less aggressively than nondiabetic patients. Some opinion favors treating virtually all adult type 2 nonpregnant diabetic persons with at least statins, irrespective of their LDL levels or CVD status.

[ ] HORMONE REPLACEMENT THERAPY

The virtual cessation of ovarian hormone secretion after the menopause, coupled with a loss of premenopausal cardiovascular protection in women and increasing risk of osteoporosis gave rise to the concept that this "natural sequence" should not be accepted as inevitable when hormone replacement therapy (HRT) became readily available. The use of estrogen ± progesterone routinely after menopause was given a boost by observational studies suggesting that such therapy was associated with a reduction of CHD.[352–354] If that were so, diabetic women already at high risk[355] would be prime candidates for HRT if it were not otherwise contraindicated. However, more recent carefully conducted randomized clinical trials have refuted this hypothesis.[356,357] Compared to placebo, estrogen plus progesterone did not decrease and may even have initially increased the risk of CVD events when given in a primary prevention mode[356] or in a secondary intervention mode.[357] In both studies, the diabetic subgroups, although relatively small, had parallel results to the entire cohorts. Thus according to the best available evidence, diabetic women should not receive HRT explicitly to reduce their risk of CVD. Moreover, prudence suggests that treatment to relieve hot flashes and other difficult-to-tolerate postmenopausal symptoms should be short term. Postmenopausal osteoporosis should be treated by other means whenever possible, such as exercise, calcium, diphosphonates, and parathyroid hormone. If these are ineffective, selective estrogen receptor molecules may be preferable to estrogens.

INPATIENT MANAGEMENT OF HYPERGLYCEMIA

Excessive hyperglycemia is frequently encountered by the cardiologist and other attending physicians during admissions for acute MI, unstable angina, revascularization procedures, and, most strikingly, during and after CABG or complicating infections of the sternum or urinary tract. Elevation of plasma glucose levels occurs in previously known and metabolically stable diabetic patients. However, it can also signal previously unknown type 2 diabetes, which may have been present for months to years but gone undetected because of lack of florid symptoms of hyperglycemia or a failure to perform currently recommended office screening of high-risk individuals for diabetes. Such patients are identified in the hospital by a HbA_{1c} measurement, which usually shows a level greater than 7.0% and may be as high as 15.0%. Even patients who do not have unequivocal diabetes ($HbA_{1c} < 6.0\%$) may acutely exhibit so-called "stress hyperglycemia" caused by increased secretion of all the insulin counterregulatory hormones, namely glucagon, epinephrine, cortisol, and growth hormone. However, those who have positive OGTTs for diabetes 1 week after an MI usually retest positive for diabetes 3 months later[27] or exhibit IGT or IFG.

Diabetic patients whose previous glucose control has been inadequate are already at a disadvantage when admitted for cardiac reasons. For each 1% increase in HbA_{1c} or 18 mg/dL increase in blood glucose, there is a 7% to 8% increase in the relative risk of long-term mortality after an MI.[358] In patients undergoing CABG, of those previously requiring insulin treatment (presumably because of difficulty with glycemic control), 33% suffered a major complication, compared with 20% of those not on prior insulin treatment.[359] Moreover, a high plasma glucose on admission (eg, > 180 mg/dL) for an MI indicates a worsened prognosis for both diabetic and even "nondiabetic" patients.[360–362] Accordingly, lengths of stay in the intensive care unit and for total hospitalization were longer. During a follow-up period of up to 3 years, the insulin-treated group had a 3-fold higher mortality rate.[359] Thus, it behooves cardiologists as well as diabetologists to maintain excellent glucose control in their patients with known CAD, before a need for hospitalization arises.

Typically, patients of all three hyperglycemic categories described above are managed by house officers—countenanced by attending physicians—with the ineffective, but imbedded by tradition, regular insulin sliding scale: 2 units for blood glucose 200 to 250 mg/dL, 4 units for 250 to 300 mg/dL, 6 units for 300 to 350 mg/dL, 8 units for 350 to 400 mg/dL, and call house officer for blood glucose greater than 400 mg/dL.[363] This automatic order does not take into account body size; prior insulin dosage, if any; recent HbA_{1c} level; or history of hypoglycemia and should be condemned. Moreover, this therapeutic approach is reactive rather than proactive and therefore almost guarantees that the blood glucose will exceed 200 mg/dL much of the time. Above this level, infection is fostered by inadequate white blood cell function and immune responses, and wound healing is delayed by negative or insufficiently positive nitrogen balance. The risk of infection after CABG is also increased by perioperative hyperglycemia.[364]

The most effective treatment of hyperglycemia in such acute situations is by intravenous insulin infusion,[365,366] particularly in the patient who is nothing-by-mouth or eats very little. Although various formulas or recipes for infusion rates have been proposed[367,368] based on experience, there is no evidence from randomized clinical trials or good physiologic data from which to predict individual "stress" needs. A starting basal rate of 1 to 2 units of lispro insulin, aspart insulin, or regular insulin with simultaneous infusion of 5 g of glucose per hour (100 mL/h of 5% glucose or 50–100 mL/h of 10% glucose) is conservative and safe. However, the insulin dose in the severely stressed person will usually have to be increased within 1 to 2 hours. It is essential to initially monitor fingerstick blood glucose measurements every hour until a satisfactory blood glucose level is achieved. The target range should be 90 to 130 mg/dL and maintained for 3 to 4 hours. The traditional range of 150 to 250 mg/dL (on surgical services especially) is no longer acceptable. Even in nondiabetic individuals admitted to an acute surgical care unit, a randomized clinical trial has demonstrated a reduction in mortality from 8.0% to 4.2% by maintaining blood glucose between 80 to 110 mg/dL with intensive insulin therapy, compared to maintaining it at 180 to 200 mg/dL.[369] Sepsis was decreased 46% and the need for dialysis or hemofiltration for acute renal failure was decreased by 41%. Researchers have pointed out other beneficial effects of aggressive insulin treatment besides reducing plasma glucose during acute illness.[370]

Insulin infusion rates can be increased by 50% to 100% as needed every 2 hours because the efficacy or lack of efficacy of a given infusion rate is rapidly apparent. During bypass procedures, temporary insulin requirements as high as 100 U/h can be seen. Conversely, if hypoglycemia should occur, an intravenous bolus of 10 to 15 g of glucose (20–30 mL of 50% glucose) to a conscious patient and 25 g (50 mL) to an unresponsive patient, coupled with a prudent decrease in the insulin infusion rate or complete cessation in severe cases (blood glucose < 40 mg/dL, comatose), will correct the situation rapidly. The flexibility and safety of intravenous insulin infusion rates rest on the very short plasma half-life of the hormone (about 5 minutes) and its short biological half-life (30–45 minutes). Cardiac intensive care nurses and house officers should not be apprehensive or reluctant to employ intravenous insulin any more than they are to administer substances such as intravenous nitroglycerine, dopamine, nitroprusside, norepinephrine, and heparin. Monitoring blood glucose frequently in acutely ill or procedurally manipulated diabetic patients deserves the same emphasis as monitoring urine output, blood pressure, and electrolytes.

Another support for controlling blood glucose by insulin infusion comes from the Diabetes and Insulin-Glucose infusion in Acute Myocardial Infarction (DIGAMI) study.[156,157] Diabetic patients admitted for an acute MI were randomly assigned to insulin infusion for 1 to 3 days or "standard coronary care." One third of the patients had been on insulin, one third on oral drugs, and one third had no prior pharmacologic treatment, respectively. Twenty-four hours after admission, the blood glucose was 173 mg/dL in the insulin infusion group and 211 in the standard care group (only 55% of whom received at least one extra insulin injection). During the 3 months following discharge, the insulin infusion group received intensive insulin outpatient treatment with multiple daily injections and the standard care group received conventional diabetes treatment. Although in-hospital morbidity and mortality were similar, the mortality was significantly lower in the insulin infusion group, 18.6% versus 26.1% at 1 year[156] and 33% versus 44% at 3.5 years.[157] Although these results were not confirmed in a larger multicenter trial by the same lead investigator,[158] the reason may lie in the failure to achieve comparable differences in blood glucose between the insulin infusion and control groups.

Despite the bulk of evidence in support of insulin therapy, a recent Canadian survey found that only 2% of diabetic patients admitted to the coronary care unit of a tertiary health facility received intravenous insulin therapy. Moreover, the mean admission HbA$_{1c}$ was 9.1% and the mean glucose was 200 mg/dL. The in-hospital mortality was 21%, double that of nondiabetic individuals.[371]

Finally, any hospitalization offers an opportunity to review the overall diabetic status of each patient and to remediate patient education deficiencies. In newly diagnosed patients, or those whose metabolic control is chronically poor due to self-neglect, it is important to institute a proper outpatient regimen and educate the patient before discharge, if possible. Nothing is more disheartening to a diabetologist or primary care physician than to receive a consultation or phone call on the day of discharge for a patient who up to that moment has received nothing but short-acting insulin on a sliding scale, administered always by nurses, and has never even heard the word "hypoglycemia." In short, the diabetic status of a patient admitted for CAD should be considered from the outset and managed aggressively for optimum results. Subsequent outpatient management should be guided by individual patient characteristics, social circumstances, microvascular complications status, and safety considerations.

CONCLUSION

CVD events and mortality from them can be decreased in diabetes by vigorous attention to reducing blood glucose and blood pressure and by correcting abnormal serum lipids.[372] Yet even in the 1990s, the results of the joint efforts of diabetes care teams (primary care physicians, diabetologists/endocrinologists, cardiologists, nurses and nutritionists) and their patients were far from satisfactory.[373–376] We need to follow the example of Danish investigators, who in a randomized clinical trial treated a group of patients intensively with attention to the major risk factors for 8 years and lowered their incidence of cardiovascular disease by 50% compared to a group of patients treated in the community.[377] The absolute risk reduction was an impressive 20%. Achieving this result required a reduction in systolic and diastolic blood pressure

of 14 mm Hg and 12 mm Hg respectively, a reduction in LDL cholesterol of 47 mg/dL and triglycerides of 41 mg/dL, and a reduction in HbA$_{1c}$ of only 0.5%. The absolute levels of these risk factors that were reached were blood pressure about 130/75 mm Hg, LDL 75 mg/dL and triglycerides 150 mg/dL, and HbA$_{1c}$ 7.5%. These do not seem like unattainable targets in more or even most of our patients, given the necessary will and the essential resources.

REFERENCES

1. Laakso M. Hyperglycemia and cardiovascular disease in type 2 diabetes. *Diabetes.* 1999;48:937.
2. Wilson PW. Diabetes mellitus and coronary heart disease. *Endocrinol Metab Clin North Am.* 2001;30:857.
3. Stamler J, Vaccaro O, Neaton J, et al. Diabetes, other risk factors, and 12-yr cardiovascular mortality for men screened in multiple risk factor intervention trial. *Diabetes Care.* 1993;16:434.
4. Luscher TF, Creager MA. Diabetes and vascular disease: pathophysiology, clinical consequences, and medical therapy: Part II. *Circulation.* 2003;108: 1655.
5. Haffner SM, Stern MP, Hazuda HP, et al. Cardiovascular risk factors in confirmed prediabetic individuals: does the clock for coronary heart disease start ticking before the onset of clinical diabetes? *JAMA.* 1990;263:2893.
6. Stern MP. Do non-insulin-dependent diabetes mellitus and cardiovascular disease share common antecedents? *Ann Intern Med.* 1996;124:110.
7. Haffner SM, Lehto S, Ronnemaa T, et al. Mortality from coronary heart disease in subjects with type 2 diabetes and in non-diabetic subjects with and without prior myocardial infarction. *N Engl J Med.* 1998;339:229.
8. Juutilainen A, Lehto S, Ronnemaa T, et al. Type 2 diabetes as a "coronary heart disease equivalent": an 18-year prospective population-based study in Finnish subjects. *Diabetes Care.* 2005;28:2901.
9. Lotufo PA, Gaziano JM, Chae CU, et al. Diabetes and all-cause and coronary heart disease mortality among US male physicians. *Arch Intern Med.* 2001;161:242.
10. Hu FB, Stampfer MJ, Solomon CG, et al. The impact of diabetes mellitus on mortality from all causes and coronary heart disease in women: 20 years of follow-up. *Arch Intern Med.* 2001;161:1717.
11. Burchfiel CM, Reed DM, Marcus EB, et al. Association of diabetes mellitus with coronary atherosclerosis and myocardial lesions: An autopsy study from the Honolulu Heart Program. *Am J Epidemiol.* 1993;137:1328.
12. Taubert G, Winkelmann BR, Schleiffer T, et al. Prevalence, predictors, and consequences of unrecognized diabetes mellitus in 3266 patients scheduled for coronary angiography. *Am Heart J.* 2003;145:286.
13. Jacoby RM, Nesto RW. Acute myocardial infarction in the diabetic patient: pathophysiology, clinical course and prognosis. *J Am Coll Cardiol.* 1992;20:736.
14. Singer DE, Moulton AW, Nathan DM. Diabetic myocardial infarction: interaction of diabetes with other preinfarction risk factors. *Diabetes.* 1989;38:350.
15. Lewis EF, Moye LA, Rouleau JL, et al. Predictors of late development of heart failure in stable survivors of myocardial infarction. *J Am Coll Cardiol.* 2003;42:1446.
16. Ishihara M, Sato H, Kawagoe T, et al. Impact of diabetes mellitus on long term survival after acute myocardial infarction in patients with single vessel disease. *Heart.* 2001;86:133.
17. Malmberg K, Yusuf S, Gerstein HC, et al. Impact of diabetes on long-term prognosis in patients with unstable angina and non-q-wave myocardial infarction. *Circulation.* 2000;102:1014.
18. Higgins TL, Estafanous FG, Loop FD, et al. Stratification of morbidity and mortality outcome by preoperative risk factors in coronary artery bypass patients. *JAMA.* 1992;267:2344.
19. Lauruschkat AH, Arnrich B, Albert AA, et al. Prevalence and risks of undiagnosed diabetes mellitus in patients undergoing coronary artery bypass grafting. *Circulation.* 2005;112:2397.
19a. Seven-year outcome in the Bypass Angioplasty Revascularization Investigation (BARI) by treatment and diabetic status. *J Am Coll Cardiol.* 2000;35:1122.
20. McAlister FA, Man J, Bistritz L, et al. Diabetes and coronary artery bypass surgery. *Diabetes Care.* 2003;26:1518.

21. Mick MJ, Piedmonte MR, Arnold AM, et al. Risk stratification for long-term outcome after elective coronary angioplasty: a multivariate analysis of 5,000 patients. *J Am Coll Cardiol.* 1994;24:74.

22. Rozenman Y, Sapoznikov D, Mosseri M, et al. Long-term angiographic follow-up of coronary balloon angioplasty in patients with diabetes mellitus: a clue to the explanation of the results of the BARI study. *J Am Coll Cardiol.* 1997;30:1420.

23. Hsu LF, Mak KH, Lau KW, et al. Clinical outcomes of patients with diabetes mellitus and acute myocardial infarction treated with primary angioplasty or fibrinolysis. *Heart.* 2002;88:260.

24. Mathew V, Holmes DR. Outcomes in diabetics undergoing revascularization. *J Am Coll Cardiol.* 2002;40:424.

25. Hasdai D, Granger CB, Srivatsa SS, et al. Diabetes mellitus and outcome after primary coronary angioplasty for acute myocardial infarction: lessons from the GUSTO-IIb Angioplasty Substudy. *J Am Coll Cardiol.* 2000;35:1502.

26. Hurst RT, Lee RW. Increased incidence of coronary atherosclerosis in type 2 diabetes mellitus: mechanisms and management. *Ann Intern Med.* 2003;139:824.

27. Norhammar A, Tenerz A, Nilsson G, et al. Glucose metabolism in patients with acute myocardial infraction and no previous diagnosis of diabetes mellitus: a prospective study. *Lancet.* 2002;359:2140.

28. Gu K, Cowie CC, Harris ML. Diabetes and decline in heart disease mortality in US adults. *JAMA.* 1999;281:1291.

29. Braunwald E, Antman EM, Beasley JW, et al. ACC/AHA guidelines for the management of patients with unstable angina and non-ST-segment elevation myocardial infarction. A report of the American College of Cardiology/American Heart Association Task Force on Practice Guidelines (Committee on the Management of Patients With Unstable Angina). *J Am Coll Cardiol.* 2000;36:970.

30. Resnick HE, Howard BV. Diabetes and cardiovascular disease. *Annu Rev Med.* 2002;53:245.

31. Joint editorial statement by the American Diabetes Association; the National Heart, Lung, and Blood Institute; the Juvenile Diabetes Foundation International; the National Institute of Diabetes and Digestive and Kidney Diseases; and the American Heart Association.Diabetes mellitus: a major risk factor for cardiovascular disease: *Circulation.* 1999;100:1132.

32. Grundy SM, Benjamin IJ, Burke GL, et al. Diabetes and cardiovascular disease: a statement for healthcare professionals from the American Heart Association. *Circulation.* 1999;100:1134.

33. Expert Panel on Detection, Evaluation, and Treatment of High Blood Cholesterol in Adults. Executive summary of the third report of the National Cholesterol Education Program (NCEP) expert panel on detection, evaluation, and treatment of high blood cholesterol in adults (Adult Treatment Panel III). *JAMA.* 2001;285:2486.

34. Chobanian AV, Bakris GL, Black HR, et al. The seventh report of the joint national committee on prevention, detection, evaluation, and treatment of high blood pressure. *JAMA.* 2003;289:2560.

35. Sheifer SE, Manolio TA, Gersh BJ. Unrecognized myocardial infarction. *Ann Intern Med.* 2001;135:801.

36. Koistinen MJ. Prevalence of asymptomatic myocardial ischaemia in diabetic subjects. *BMJ.* 1990;301:92.

37. Naka M, Hiramatsu K, Aizawa T, et al. Silent myocardial ischemia in patients with non-insulin-dependent diabetes mellitus as judged by treadmill exercise testing and coronary angiography. *Am Heart J.* 1992;123:46.

38. Janand-Delenne B, Savin B, Habib G, et al. Silent myocardial ischemia in patients with diabetes. *Diabetes Care.* 1999;22:1396.

39. Wackers FJ, Young LH, Inzucchi SE, et al. Detection of silent myocardial ischemia in asymptomatic diabetic subjects. *Diabetes Care.* 2004;27:1954.

40. Prior JO, Quinones MJ, Hernandez-Pampaloni M, et al. Coronary circulatory dysfunction in insulin resistance, impaired glucose tolerance, and type 2 diabetes mellitus. *Circulation.* 2005;111:2291.

41. American Diabetes Association. Consensus development conference on the diagnosis of coronary heart disease in people with diabetes. *Diabetes Care.* 1998;21:1551.

42. Alexander CM, Landsman PB, Teutsch SM, et al. NCEP-defined metabolic syndrome, diabetes, and prevalence of coronary heart disease among NHANES III patients age 50 years and older. *Diabetes.* 2003;25:1210.

43. King H, Aubert RE, Herman WH. Global burden of diabetes, 1995–2025: prevalence, numerical estimates, and projections. *Diabetes Care.* 1998;21:1414.

44. Steinbrook R. Facing the diabetes epidemic—mandatory reporting of glycosylated hemoglobin values in New York City. *N Engl J Med.* 2006;354:545.

45. Mokdad AH, Serdula MK, Dietz WH, et al. The spread of the obesity epidemic in the United States, 1991–1998. *JAMA.* 1999;282:1519.

46. Mokdad AH, Ford ES, Bowman BA, et al.: Diabetes trends in the U.S.: 1990–1998. *Diabetes Care.* 2000;23:1278.

47. Cho E, Manson JE, Stamper MJ, et al. A prospective study of obesity and risk of coronary heart disease among diabetic women. *Diabetes Care.* 2002;25:1142.

48. Mokdad AH, Ford ES, Bowman BA, et al. Prevalence of obesity, diabetes, and obesity-related health risk factors, 2001. *JAMA.* 2003;289:76.

49. Flegal KM, Graubard BI, Williamson DF, Gail MH. Excess deaths associated with underweight, overweight, and obesity. *JAMA.* 2005;293:1861.

50. Harris MI, Flegal KM, Cowie CC, et al. Prevalence of diabetes, impaired fasting glucose, and impaired glucose tolerance in U.S. adults. *Diabetes Care.* 1998;21:518.

51. Benjamin SM, Valdez R, Geiss LS, et al. Estimated number of adults with prediabetes in the U.S. in 2000. *Diabetes Care.* 2003;26:645.

52. Narayan KM, Boyle JP, Thompson TJ, et al. Lifetime risk for diabetes mellitus in the United States. *JAMA.* 2003;290:1884.

53. Himsworth HP. Diabetes mellitus: its differentiations into insulin-sensitive and insulin-insensitive types. *Lancet.* 1936;1:127.

54. Polonsky KS, Given BD, Van Cauter E. Twenty-four-hour profiles and pulsatile patterns of insulin secretion in normal and obese subjects. *J Clin Invest.* 1988;81:442.

55. Reaven GM. Role of insulin resistance in human disease. *Diabetes.* 1988;37:1495.

56. Alberti KGMM, Zimmet PZ, for the WHO Consultation. Definition, diagnosis and classification of diabetes mellitus and its complications: Part 1—diagnosis and classification of diabetes mellitus provisional report of a WHO consultation. *Diabetic Medicine.* 1998;15:539.

57. Haffner SM, Miettinen H. Insulin resistance implication for type II diabetes mellitus and coronary heart disease. *Am J Med.* 1997;103:152.

58. Juhan-Vague I, Alessi MC, Vague P. Increased plasma plasminogen activator inhibitor 1 levels: a possible link between insulin resistance and atherothrombosis. *Diabetologia.* 1991;34:457.

59. Juhan-Vague I, Thompson SG, Jespersen J. Involvement of the hemostatic system in the insulin resistance syndrome: a study of 1500 patients with angina pectoris. *Arterioscler Thromb.* 193;13:1865.

60. Kohler HP, Grant PJ. Plasminogen-activator inhibitor type 1 and coronary artery disease. *N Engl J Med.* 2000;342:1792.

61. Carroll S, Cooke CB, Butterly RJ. Plasma viscosity, fibrinogen and the metabolic syndrome: effect of obesity and cardiorespiratory fitness. *Blood Coagul Fibrinolysis.* 2000;11:71.

62. Sowers JR. Update on the cardiometabolic syndrome. *Clin Cornerstone.* 2001;14:17.

63. Saito I, Folsom AR, Brancati FL, et al. Nontraditional risk factors for coronary heart disease incidence among persons with diabetes: the Atherosclerosis Risk in Communities (ARIC) Study. *Ann Intern Med.* 2000;133:81.

64. Reaven GM, Laws A. Insulin resistance, compensatory hyperinsulinaemia, and coronary heart disease. *Diabetologia.* 1994;37:948.

65. Jarrett RJ. Why is insulin not a risk factor for coronary heart disease? *Diabetologia.* 1994;37:945.

66. Fontbonne A. Why can high insulin levels indicate a risk for coronary heart disease? *Diabetologia.* 1994;37:953.

67. Matthews DR, Hosker JP, Rudenski AS, et al. Homeostasis Model Assessment (HOMA): insulin resistance and beta cell function from fasting plasma glucose and insulin concentrations in man. *Diabetologia.* 1985;28:412.

68. Wallace TM, Levy JC, Matthews DR. Use and abuse of HOMA modeling. *Diabetes Care.* 2004;27:1487.

69. Alssema M, Dekker JM, Nijpels G, et al. Proinsulin concentration is an independent predictor of all-cause and cardiovascular mortality. *Diabetes Care.* 2005;28:860.

70. Isomaa B, Almgren P, Tuomi T, et al. Cardiovascular morbidity and mortality associated with the metabolic syndrome. *Diabetes Care.* 2001;24:683.

71. Lakka HM, Laaksonen DE, Lakka TA, et al. The metabolic syndrome and total and cardiovascular disease mortality in middle-aged men. *JAMA.* 2002;288:2709.

72. Wilson PWF, D'Agostino RB, Parise H, et al. Metabolic syndrome as a precursor of cardiovascular disease and type 2 diabetes mellitus. *Circulation.* 2005;112:3066.

73. Ford ES, Giles WH, Dietz WH. Prevalence of the metabolic syndrome among US adults: findings from the Third National Health and Nutrition Examination Survey. *JAMA.* 2002;287:356.

74. Ford ES. Prevalence of the metabolic syndrome defined by the international diabetes federation among adults in the U.S. *Diabetes Care.* 2005;28:2745.

75. Hunt KJ, Resendez RG, Williams K, et al. National cholesterol education program versus World Health Organization metabolic syndrome in relation to all-cause and cardiovascular mortality in the San Antonio heart study. *Circulation.* 2004;110:1251.

76. Duncan GE, Li SM, Zhou XH. Prevalence and trends of a metabolic syndrome phenotype among U.S. adolescents, 1999–2000. *Diabetes Care.* 2004; 27:2438.

77. Dekker JM, Girman C, Rhodes T, et al. Metabolic syndrome and 10-year cardiovascular disease risk in the Hoorn study. *Circulation.* 2005;112:666.

78. Haffner SM, D'Agostino R, Mykkänen L, et al. Insulin sensitivity in subjects with type 2 diabetes. *Diabetes Care.* 1999;22:562.

79. Howard G, O'Leary DH, Zaccaro D, et al. Insulin sensitivity and atherosclerosis. *Circulation.* 1996;93:1809.

80. Ginsberg HN. Insulin resistance and cardiovascular disease. *J Clin Invest.* 2000;106:453.

81. Pickup JC, Mattock MB, Chusney GD, et al. NIDDM as a disease of the innate immune system: association of acute-phase reactants and interleukin-6 with metabolic syndrome X. *Diabetologia.* 1997;40:1286.

82. Blake GJ, Ridker PM. Novel clinical markers of vascular wall inflammation. *Circ Res.* 2001;89:763.

83. Esposito K, Ciotola M, Giugliano D. Inflammation warms up the metabolic syndrome. *Arterioscler Thromb Vasc Biol.* 2005;e143.

84. Hansson GK. Inflammation, atherosclerosis, and coronary artery disease. *N Engl J Med.* 2005;352:1685.

85. Pradhan D, Manson JE, Rifai N, et al. C-reactive protein, interleukin 6, and risk of developing type 2 diabetes mellitus. *JAMA.* 2001;286:327.

86. Streja D, Cressey P, Rabkin SW. Associations between inflammatory markers, traditional risk factors, and complications in patients with type 2 diabetes mellitus. *J Diabetes Complications.* 2003;17:120.

87. Kern PA, Di Gregorio GB, Lu T, et al. Adiponectin expression from human adipose tissue: relation to obesity, insulin resistance, and tumor necrosis factor-α expression. *Diabetes.* 2003;52:1779.

88. Hotta K, Funahashi T, Arita Y, et al. Plasma concentrations of a novel, adipose-specific protein, adiponectin, in type 2 diabetic patients. *Arterioscler Thromb Vasc Biol.* 2000;20:1595.

89. Ginsberg HN. Treatment for patients with the metabolic syndrome. *Am J Cardiol.* 2003;91:29e.

90. Davidson MB. Is treatment of insulin resistance beneficial independent of glycemia? *Diabetes Care.* 2003;26:3184.

91. Tuomilehto J, Lindström J, Eriksson JG, et al. Prevention of type 2 diabetes mellitus by changes in lifestyle among subjects with impaired glucose tolerance. *N Eng J Med.* 2001;344:1343.

92. Diabetes Prevention Program Research Group. Reduction in the incidence of type 2 diabetes with lifestyle intervention or metformin. *N Eng J Med.* 2002;346:393.

93. Pan X, Li G, Hu Y, et al. Effects of diet and exercise on preventing NIDDM in people with impaired glucose tolerance. *Diabetes Care.* 1997;20:537.

94. Chiasson J, Josse RG, Gomis R, et al. Acarbose for prevention of type 2 diabetes mellitus: the STOP-NIDDM randomized trial. *Lancet.* 2002;359:2072.

95. Buchanan TA, Xiang AH, Peters RK, et al. Preservation of pancreatic β-cell function and prevention of type 2 diabetes by pharmacological treatment of insulin resistance in high-risk Hispanic women. *Diabetes.* 2002;51:2796.

96. Kahn R, Buse J, Ferrannini E, Stern M. The metabolic syndrome: time for a critical appraisal: joint statement from the American Diabetes Association and the European Associaiton for the Study of Diabetes. *Diabetes Care.* 2005;28:2289.

97. The Heart Outcomes Prevention Evaluation Study Investigators. Effects of an angiotensin-converting-enzyme inhibitor, ramipril, on death from cardiovascular causes, myocardial infarction, and stroke in high-risk patients. *N Eng J Med.* 2000;342:145.

98. Yusuf S, Gerstein H, Hoogwerf B, et al. Ramipril and the development of diabetes. *JAMA.* 2001;286:1882.

99. Freeman DJ, Norrie J, Sattar N, et al. Pravastatin and the development of diabetes mellitus: evidence for a protective treatment effect in the West of Scotland Coronary Prevention Study. *Circulation.* 2001;103:357.

100. Chiasson JL, Josse RG, Gomis R, et al. Acarbose treatment and the risk of cardiovascular disease and hypertension in patients with impaired glucose tolerance. *JAMA.* 2003;290:486.

101. Kannel WB, McGee DL. Diabetes and cardiovascular disease: the Framingham study. *JAMA.* 1979;241:2035.

102. Nichols GA, Hillier TA, Erbey JR, et al. Congestive heart failure in type 2 diabetes: prevalence, incidence, and risk factors. *Diabetes Care.* 2001;24:1614.

102a. Nichols GA, Gullion CM, Koro CE, Ephross SA, Brown JB. The incidence of congestive heart failure in type 2 diabetes: an update. *Diabetes Care.* 2004; 8:1879.

103. Bertoni AG, Tsai A, Kasper EK, et al. Diabetes and idiopathic cardiomyopathy: a nationwide case-control study. *Diabetes Care.* 2003;26:2791.

104. Bell DS. Heart failure: the frequent, forgotten, and often fatal complication of diabetes. *Diabetes Care.* 2003;26:2433.

105. Standl E, Schnell O. A new look at the heart in diabetes mellitus: from ailing to failing. *Diabetologia.* 2000;43:1455.

106. Taegtmeyer H, McNulty P, Young ME. Adaptation and maladaptation of the heart in diabetes: Part 1—general concepts. *Circulation.* 2002;105:1727.

107. Taegtmeyer H, McNulty P, Young ME. Adaptation and maladaptation of the heart in diabetes: part 2—potential mechanism. *Circulation.* 2002;105:1861.

107a. Luscher TF, Creager MA, Beckman JA, Cosentino F. Diabetes and vascular disease: pathophysiology, clinical consequences, and medical therapy: Part I. *Circulation.* 2003;108:1527.

108. Gustafsson P, Hildebrandt M, Seibaeck M, et al. Long-term prognosis of diabetic patients with myocardial infraction: relation to antidiabetic treatment regimen. *Euro Heart J* 2000;21:1937.

109. Dries DL, Sweitzer NK, Drazner MH, et al. Prognostic impact of diabetes mellitus in patients with heart failure according to the etiology of left ventricular systolic dysfunction. *J Am Coll Cardiol.* 2001;38:421.

110. Taylor AA. Pathophysiology of hypertension and endothelial dysfunction in patients with diabetes mellitus. *Endocrinol Metab Clin North Am.* 2001;30:983.

111. Mattock MB, Morrish NJ, Viberti G, et al. Prospective study of microalbuminuria as predictor of mortality in NIDDM. *Diabetes.* 1992;41:736.

112. Dinneen SF, Gerstein HC. The association of microalbuminuria and mortality in non-insulin-dependent diabetes mellitus. *Arch Intern Med.* 1997;157:1413.

113. Gerstein HC, Mann JFE, Yi Q. Albuminuria and risk of cardiovascular events, death, and heart failure in diabetic and non-diabetic individuals. *JAMA.* 2001;286:421.

114. Vinik AI, Maser RE, Mitchell BD, et al. Diabetic autonomic neuropathy. *Diabetes Care.* 2003;26:1553.

115. Kahn SE. The relative contributions of insulin resistance and beta-cell dysfunction to the pathophysiology of type 2 diabetes. *Diabetologia.* 2003;46:3.

116. Nishikawa T, Edelstein D, Du XL, et al. Normalizing mitochondrial superoxide production blocks three pathways of hyperglycaemic damage. *Nature.* 2000;404:787.

117. Brownlee M. Biochemistry and molecular cell biology of diabetic complications. *Nature.* 2001;414:813.

118. Sheetz MJ, King GL. Molecular understanding of hyperglycemia's adverse effects for diabetic complications. *JAMA.* 2002;288:2579.

118a. Davidson MB. Is treatment of insulin resistance beneficial independent of glycemia? *Diabetes Care.* 2003;26:3184.

119. Murayama Y, Kawai K, Nakamura S, et al. The endogenous insulin secretion was suppressed during insulin therapy in NIDDM patients. *Diabetes Res Clin Pract.* 1990;9:129.

120. Usuitupa MIJ, Niskanen LK, Siitonen O, et al. Ten-year cardiovascular mortality in relation to risk factors and abnormalities in lipoprotein composition in type 2 (non-insulin-dependent) diabetic and non-diabetic subjects. *Diabetologia.* 1993;36:1175.

121. Kuusisto J, Mykkänen L, Pyörälä K, et al. Non-insulin-dependent diabetes and its metabolic control are important predictors of stroke in elderly subjects. *Strokes.* 1994;25:1157.

122. Kuusisto J, Mykkänen L, Pyörälä K, et al. NIDDM and its metabolic control predict coronary artery disease in elderly subjects. *Diabetes.* 1994;43:960.

123. Moss SE, Klein R, Klein BEK, et al. The association of glycemia and cause-specific mortality in a diabetic population. *Arch Intern Med.* 1994;154:2473.

124. Andersson DKG, Svärdsudd K. Long-term glycemic control relates to mortality in type II diabetes. *Diabetes Care.* 1995;18:1534.

125. Hanefeld M, Fischer S, Julius U, et al. Risk factors for myocardial infarction and death in newly detected NIDDM: the Diabetes Intervention Study, 11-year follow-up. *Diabetologia.* 1996;39:1577.

126. Wahab NN, Cowden EA, Pearce NJ, et al. Is blood glucose an independent predictor of mortality in acute myocardial infarction in the thrombolytic era? *J Am Coll Cardiol.* 2002;40:1748.

127. de Vegt F, Dekker JM, Ruhé HG, et al. Hyperglycaemia is associated with all-cause and cardiovascular mortality in the Hoorn population: the Hoorn Study. *Diabetologia.* 1999;42:926.

128. Coutinho M, Gerstein HC, Wang Y, et al. The relationship between glucose and incident cardiovascular events: a metaregression analysis of published data from 20 studies of 95,783 individuals followed for 12.4 years. *Diabetes Care.* 1999;22:233.

129. Hoogwerf BJ, Sprecher DL, Pearce GL, et al. Blood glucose concentrations ≤ 125 mg/dL and coronary heart disease risk. *Am J Cardiol.* 2002;89:596.

130. Osende JI, Badimon JJ, Fuster V, et al. Blood thrombogenicity in type 2 diabetes mellitus patients is associated with glycemic control. *J Am Coll Cardiol.* 2001;38:1307.

131. Lehto S, Rönnemaa T, Pyörälä K, et al. Poor glycemic control predicts coronary heart disease events in patients with type 1 diabetes without nephropathy. *Arterioscler Thromb Vasc Biol.* 1999;19:1014.

132. Stratton IM, Adler AI, Neil HAW, et al. Association of glycaemia with macrovascular and microvascular complications of type 2 diabetes (UKPDS 35): prospective observational study. *BMJ.* 2000;321:405.

133. Koivisto VA, Stevens LK, Mattock M, et al. Cardiovascular disease and its risk factors in IDDM in Europe. *Diabetes Care.* 1996;19:689.

134. Orchard TJ, Olson JC, Erbey JR, et al. Insulin resistance-related factors, but not glycemia, predict coronary artery disease in type 1 diabetes. *Diabetes Care.* 2003;26:1374.

135. Singer DE, Nathan DM, Anderson KM, et al. Association of HbA$_{1c}$ with prevalent cardiovascular disease in the original cohort of the Framingham Heart Study. *Diabetes.* 1992;41:202.

136. Meigs JB, Singer DE, Sullivan LM, et al. Metabolic control and prevalent cardiovascular disease in non-insulin-dependent diabetes mellitus (NIDDM): the NIDDM Patient Outcomes Research Team. *Am J Med.* 1997;102:38.

137. Barrett-Connor E. Does hyperglycemia really cause coronary heart disease? *Diabetes Care.* 1997;20:1620.

138. The DECODE Study Group, on behalf of the European Diabetes Epidemiology Group: Glucose Tolerance and cardiovascular mortality: comparison of fasting and 2-hour diagnostic criteria. *Arch Intern Med.* 2001;161:397.

139. Saydah SH, Miret M, Sung J, et al. Postchallenge Hyperglycemia and mortality in a national sample of U.S. adults. *Diabetes Care.* 2001;24:1397.

140. Hanefeld M, Fischer S, Julius U, et al. Risk factors for myocardial infarction and death in newly detected NIDDM: the Diabetes Intervention Study, 11-year follow-up. *Diabetologia.* 1996;39:1577.

141. Ceriello A. The possible role of postprandial hyperglycaemia in the pathogenesis of diabetic complications. *Diabetologia.* 2003;46(suppl 1):M9.

142. Buse JB. Should postprandial glucose be routinely measured and treated to a particular target? No! *Diabetes Care.* 2003;26:1615.

143. Fonseca V. Clinical significance of targeting postprandial and fasting hyperglycemia in managing type 2 diabetes mellitus. *Curr Med Res Opin.* 2003;19:635.

144. Di Carli MF, Janisse J, Grunberger G, et al. Role of chronic hyperglycemia in the pathogenesis of coronary microvascular dysfunction in diabetes. *J Am Coll Cardiol.* 2003;41:1387.

145. Esposito K, Nappo F, Marfella R, et al. Inflammatory cytokine concentrations are acutely increased by hyperglycemia in humans: role of oxidative stress. *Circulation.* 2002;106:2067.

146. Vigorita VJ, Moore GW, Hutchins GM. Absence of correlation between coronary arterial atherosclerosis and severity or duration of diabetes mellitus of adult onset. *Am J Cardiol.* 1980;46:535.

147. Jarrett RJ. Type II (non-insulin-dependent) diabetes mellitus and coronary heart disease—chicken, egg, or neither? *Diabetologia.* 1994;26:99.

148. Libby P, Plutzky J. Diabetic macrovascular disease: the glucose paradox? *Circulation.* 2002;106:2760.

149. King GL, Wakasaki H. Theoretical mechanisms by which hyperglycemia and insulin resistance could cause cardiovascular diseases in diabetes. *Diabetes Care.* 1999;22:C31.

150. Gaster B, IB Hirsch. The effects of improved glycemic control on complications in type 2 diabetes. *Arch Intern Med.* 1998;158:134.

151. The University Group Diabetes Program. Effects of hypoglycemic agents on vascular complications in patients with adult-onset diabetes. VIII. Evaluation of insulin therapy: final report. *Diabetes.* 1982;31:1.

152. Genuth S. Exogenous insulin administration and cardiovascular risk in non-insulin dependent and insulin dependent diabetes mellitus. *Ann Intern Med.* 1996;124:104.

153. UK Prospective Diabetes Study (UKPDS) Group. Intensive blood-glucose control with sulphonylureas or insulin compared with conventional treatment and risk of complication in patients with type 2 diabetes (UKPDS 33). *Lancet.* 1998;352:837.

154. Abraira C, Colwell JA, Nuttall FQ, et al. Veterans affairs cooperative study on glycemic control and complications in type II diabetes (VA CSDM). *Diabetes Care.* 1995;18:1113.

155. Abraira C, Colwell JA, Nuttall FQ, et al. Cardiovascular events and correlates in the Veterans Affairs Diabetes Feasibility Trial. *Arch Intern Med.* 1997;157:181.

156. Malmberg K, Rydén L, Efendic S, et al. Randomized trial of insulin-glucose infusion followed by subcutaneous insulin treatment in diabetic patients with acute myocardial infraction (DIGAMI Study): effects on mortality at 1 year. *J Am Coll Cardiol.* 1995;26:27.

157. Malmberg K. Prospective randomized study of intensive insulin treatment on long term survival after acute myocardial infarction in patients with diabetes mellitus. *BMJ.* 1997;314:1512.

158. Malmberg K, Ryden L, Wedel H, et al. FASTTRACK Intense metabolic control by means of insulin in patients with diabetes mellitus and acute myocardial infarction (DIGAMI 2): effects on mortality and morbidity. *E Heart J.* 2005;26:650.

159. ACCORD Purpose: Protocol Abstract November 14, 2002. Available at http://www.accordtrial.org. Accessed 19 November 2003.

160. Abraira C, Duckworth W, McCarren M, et al. Design of the cooperative study on glycemic control and complications in diabetes mellitus type 2 Veterans Affairs Diabetes Trials. *J Diabetes Complications.* 2003;17:314.

161. Sobel BE, Frye R, Detre KM. Burgeoning dilemmas in the management of diabetes and cardiovascular disease: rationale for the Bypass Angioplasty Revascularization Investigation 2 Diabetes (BARDI 2D) Trial. *Circulation.* 2003;107:636.

162. Jensen T, Borch-Johnsen K, Kofoed-Enevoldsen A, et al. Coronary heart disease in young type 1 (insulin-dependent) diabetic patients with and without diabetic nephropathy: incidence and risk factors. *Diabetologia.* 1987;30:144.

163. Foley RN, Culleton BF, Parfrey PS, et al. Cardiac disease in diabetic-end-stage renal disease. *Diabetologia.* 1997;40:1307.

164. Tuomilehto J, Borch-Johnsen K, Molarius T, et al. Incidence of cardiovascular disease in type 1 (insulin-dependent) diabetic subjects with and without diabetic nephropathy in Finland. *Diabetologia.* 1998;41:784.

165. Laing SP, Swerdlow AJ, Slater SD, et al. The British Diabetic Association cohort study, I: all-cause mortality in patients with insulin-treated diabetes mellitus. *Diabetic Med.* 1999;16:459.

166. Laing SP, Swerdlow AJ, Slater SD, et al. Mortality from heart disease in a cohort of 23,000 patients with insulin-treated diabetes. *Diabetologia.* 2003;46:760.

167. Koistinen MJ. Prevalence of asymptomatic myocardial ischaemia in diabetic subjects. *Br Med J.* 1990;301:92.

168. Senior PA, Welsh RC, et al. Coronary artery disease is common in nonuremic, asymptomatic type 1 diabetic islet transplant candidates. *Diabetes Care.* 2005;28:866.

169. Larsen J, et al. Silent coronary atheromatosis in type 1 diabetic patients and its relation to long-term glycemic control. *Diabetes.* 2002;51:2637.

170. Giunti S, Bruno G, Veglio M, et al. Electrocardiographic left ventricular hypertrophy in type 1 diabetes: prevalence and relation to coronary heart disease and cardiovascular risk factors: the Eurodiab IDDM Complications Study. *Diabetes Care.* 2005;28:2255.

171. Klein R, et al. Association of ocular disease mortality in a diabetic population. *Arch Ophthalmol.* 1999;117:148.

172. Rajala U, et al. High cardiovascular disease mortality in subjects with visual impairment caused by diabetic retinopathy. *Diabetes Care.* 2000;23:957.

173. Ono T, et al. The impact of diabetic retinopathy on long-term outcome following coronary artery bypass graft surgery. *J Am Coll Cardiol.* 2002;40:428.

174. Brown HB, Waugh NR, Jennings PE. Microangiopathy as a prognostic indicator in diabetic patients suffering from acute myocardial infarction. *Scot Med J.* 1992;37:44.

175. Klein BEK, Klein R, McBride PE, et al. Cardiovascular disease, mortality, and retinal microvascular characteristics in type 1 diabetes. *Arch Intern Med.* 2004;164:1917.

176. Mäkimattila S, Ylitalo K, Schlenzka A, et al. Family histories of type II diabetes and hypertension predict intima-media thickness in patients with type I diabetes. *Diabetologia.* 2002;45:711.

177. Hayaishi-Okano R, Yamasaki Y, Katakami N, et al. Elevated C-reactive protein associates with early-stage carotid atherosclerosis in young subjects with type I diabetes. *Diabetes Care.* 2002;25:1432.

178. Reindel J, Zander E, Heinke P, et al. Metabolisches syndrom bei patienten mit diabetes mellitus typ 1. *Herz.* 2004;29:463.

179. Thorn LM, Forsblom C, Fagerudd J, et al. Metabolic syndrome in type 1 diabetes: association with diabetic nephropathy and glycemic control (the FinnDiane study). *Diabetes Care.* 2005;28:2019.

180. Purnell JQ, Hokanson JE, Marcovina SM, et al. Effect of excessive weight gain with intensive therapy of type 1 diabetes on lipid levels and blood pressure. *JAMA.* 1998;280:140.

181. Colhoun HM, Rubens MB, Underwood SR, et al. The effect of type I diabetes mellitus on the gender difference in coronary artery calcification. *J Am Coll Cardiol.* 2000;36:2160.

182. Olson JC, Edmundowicz D, Becker DJ, et al. Coronary calcium in adults with type 1 diabetes. *Diabetes* 2000;49:1571.

183. Starkman HS, Cable G, Hala V, et al. Delineation of prevalence and risk factors for early coronary artery disease by electron beam computed tomography in young adults with type 1 diabetes. *Diabetes Care.* 2003;26:433.

184. Cleary P, Orchard T, Zinman B, et al. Coronary calcification in the Diabetes Control and Complications Trial/Epidemiology of Diabetes Interventions and Complications (DCCT/EDIC) cohort for the DCCT/EDIC study group. *Diabetes.* 2003;52:A152.

185. The Diabetes Control and Complications Trial/Epidemiology of Diabetes Interventions and Complications Research Group. Intensive diabetes therapy and carotid intima-media thickness in type 1 diabetes mellitus. *N Eng J Med.* 2003;348:2294.

186. Snell-Bergeon JK, Hokanson JE, Jensen L, et al. Progression of coronary artery calcification in type 1 diabetes: the importance of glycemic control. *Diabetes Care.* 2003;26:2923.

187. Larsen J, Brekke M, Sandvik L, et al. Silent coronary atheromatosis in type 1 diabetic patients and its relation to long-term glycemic control. *Diabetes.* 2002;51:2637.

188. Fiorina P, La Rocca E, Venturini M, et al. Effects of kidney-pancreas transplantation on atherosclerotic risk factors and endothelial function in patients with uremia and type 1 diabetes. *Diabetes.* 2001;50:496.

189. Nathan DM, Cleary PA, Backlund JYC, Genuth SM, et al. Intensive diabetes treatment and cardiovascular disease in patients with type 1 diabetes: the Diabetes Control and Complications Trial/Epidemiology of Diabetes interventions and complications study research group. *N Engl J Med.* 2005;353:2643.

190. Raev DC. Which left ventricular function is impaired earlier in the evolution of diabetic cardiomyopathy? An echocardiographic study of young type I diabetic patients. *Diabetes Care.* 1994;17:633.

191. Orchard TJ, Forrest K, Kuller LH, et al. Lipid and blood pressure treatment goals for type 1 diabetes. *Diabetes Care.* 2001;24:1053.

192. van Hecke MV, Dekker JM, Stehouwer CDA, et al. Diabetic retinopathy is associated with mortality and cardiovascular disease incidence: the EURO-DIAB prospective complications study. *Diabetes Care.* 2005;28:1383.

193. Ono T, Kobayashi J, Sasako Y, et al. The impact of diabetic retinopathy on long-term outcome following coronary artery bypass graft surgery. *J Am Coll Cardiol.* 2002;40:428.

194. The Diabetes Control and Complications Trial Research Group. The effect of intensive treatment of diabetes on the development and progression of long-term complications in insulin-dependent diabetes mellitus. *N Eng J Med.* 1993;329:977.

195. The Diabetes Control and Complications Trial Research Group. The relationship of glycemic exposure (HbA$_{1c}$) to the risk of development and progression of retinopathy in the Diabetes Control and Complications Trial. *Diabetes.* 1995;44:968.

196. The Diabetes Control and Complications Trial Research Group. The absence of a glycemic threshold for the development of long-term complications: the perspective of the Diabetes Control and Complications Trial. *Diabetes.* 1996;45:1289.

197. Leese GP, Wang J, Broomhall J, et al. Frequency of severe hypoglycemia requiring emergency treatment in type 1 and type 2 diabetes: a population-based study of health service resource use. *Diabetes Care.* 2003;26:1176-1180.

198. Shorr RI, Ray WA, Daugherty JR, et al. Incidence and risk factors for serious hypoglycemia in older persons using insulin or sulfonylureas. *Arch Intern Med.* 1997;157:1681.

199. Holstein A, Plaschke A, Egberts EH. Clinical characterisation of severe hypoglycaemia: a prospective population-based study. *Exp Clin Endocrinol Diabetes.* 2003;111:364.

200. Desouza C, Salazar H, Cheong B, et al. Association of hypoglycemia and cardiac ischemia: a study based on continuous monitoring. *Diabetes Care.* 2003;26:1485.

201. Wing RR, Koeske R, Epstein LH, et al. Long-term effects of modest weight loss in type II diabetic patients. *Arch Intern Med.* 1987;147:1749.

202. Chandalia M, Garg A, Lutjohann D, et al. Beneficial effects of high dietary fiber intake in patients with type 2 diabetes mellitus. *N Engl J Med.* 2000;342:1392.

203. Hamdy O, Goodyear LJ, Horton ES. Diet and exercise in type 2 diabetes mellitus. *Endocrinol Metab Clin North Am.* 2001;30:883.

204. Tanasescu M, Leitzmann MF, Rimm EB, et al. Physical activity in relation to cardiovascular disease and total mortality among men with type 2 diabetes. *Circulation.* 2003;107:2435.

205. Hu FB, Stampfer MJ, Solomon C, et al. Physical activity and risk for cardiovascular events in diabetic women. *Ann Intern Med.* 2001;134:96.

206. Scheen AJ, Ernest PH. New antiobesity agents in type 2 diabetes: overview of clinical trials with sibutramine and orlistat. *Diabetes Metab (Paris.)* 2002;28:437.

207. Padwal R, Majumdar S. Metabolic risk factors, drugs, and obesity. *N Engl J Med.* 2006;354:975.

208. Pi-Sunyer FX, Aronne LJ, Heshmati HM, et al. Effect of rimonabant, a cannabinoid-1 receptor blocker, on weight and cardiometabolic risk factors in overweight or obese patients: RIO-North America: a randomized controlled trial. *JAMA.* 2006;295:761.

209. Pinkney JH, Sjöström CD, Gale EAM. Should surgeons treat diabetes in severely obese people? *Lancet.* 2001;357:1357.

210. Williamson DF, Thompson TJ, Thun M, et al. Intentional weight loss and mortality among overweight individuals with diabetes. *Diabetes Care.* 2000;23:1499.

211. Levy J, Atkinson AB, Bell PM, et al. Beta-cell deterioration determines the onset and rate of progression of secondary dietary failure in type 2 diabetes mellitus: the 10-year follow-up of the Belfast Diet Study. *Diabetic Med.* 1998;15:290.

212. Genuth S. Diabetes mellitus in adults (type 2 diabetes). In: Rakel RE, Bope ET (editors). *Conn's Current Therapy 2001.* Philadelphia, Pa: WB Saunders: 2001;573.

213. Turner RC, Cull CA, Frighi V, et al. Glycemic control with diet, sulfonylurea, metformin, or insulin in patients with type 2 diabetes mellitus. *JAMA.* 1999;281:2005.

214. Inzucchi SE. Oral antihyperglycemic therapy for type 2 diabetes: scientific review. *JAMA.* 2002;287:360.

215. DeWitt DE, Hirsch IB. Outpatient insulin in therapy in type 1 and type 2 diabetes mellitus. *JAMA.* 2003;289:2254.

216. DeFronzo RA. Pharmacologic therapy for type 2 diabetes mellitus. *Ann Intern Med.* 1999;131:281.

217. Setter SM, Iltz JL, Thams J, Campbell RK. Metformin hydrochloride in the treatment of type 2 diabetes mellitus: a clinical review with a focus on dual therapy. *Clin Therap.* 2003;25:2991.

218. UK Prospective Diabetes Study (UKPDS) Group. Effect of intensive blood-glucose control with metformin on complications in overweight patients with type 2 diabetes (UKPDS 34). *Lancet.* 1998;352:854.

219. Bailey CJ: Biguanides and NIDDM. *Diabetes Care.* 1992;15:755.

220. Wiernsperger NF, Bailey CJ. The antihyperglycaemic effect of metformin. *Drugs.* 1999;58:31.

221. Cusi K, DeFronzo RA. Metformin: a review of its metabolic effects. *Diabetes Rev* 1998;6:89.

222. de Jager J, Kooy A, Lehert PH, et al. Effects of short-term treatment with metormin on markers of endothelial function and inflammatory activity in type 2 diabetes mellitus: a randomized, placebo-controlled trial. *J Int Med.* 2005;257:100.

223. Garber AJ, Duncan TG, Goodman AM, et al. Efficacy of metformin in type II diabetes: results of a double-blind, placebo-controlled, dose-response trial. *Am J Med.* 1997;102:491.

224. Misbin RI. The phantom of lactic acidosis due to metformin in patients with diabetes. *Diabetes Care* 27:1791-1793, 2004.

225. Masoudi FA, Inzucchi SE, Wang Y, et al. Thiazolidinediones, metformin, and outcomes in older patients with diabetes and heart failure: an observational study. *Circulation.* 2005;111:583.

226. Inzucchi SE, Masoudi FA, Wang Y, et al. Insulin-sensitizing antihyperglycemic drugs and mortality after acute myocardial infarction: insights from the National Heart Care Project. *Diabetes Care.* 2005;28:1680.

227. Kao J, Tobis J, McClelland RL, et al. Relation of metformin treatment to clinical events in diabetic patients undergoing percutaneous intervention. *Am J Cardiol.* 2004;93:1347.

228. Klimt C, Knatterud GL, Meinert CL, et al. A study of the effects of hypoglycemic agents in vascular complications in patients with adult-onset diabetes. *Diabetes.* 1970;19:747.

229. Simpson SH, Majumdar SR, Tsuyuki RT, et al. Dose-response relation between sulfonylurea drugs and mortality in type 2 diabetes mellitus: a population-based cohort study. *CMAJ* 2006;174:169.

230. Johnson JA, Majumdar SR, Simpson SH, Toth EL. Decreased mortality associated with the use of metformin compared with sulfonylurea monotherapy in type 2 diabetes. *Diabetes Care.* 2002;25:2244.

231. Mannucci E, Monami M, Masotti G, Marchionni N. All-cause mortality in diabetic patients treated with combinations of sulfonylureas and biguanides. *Diabetes Metab Res Rev.* 2004;20:44.

232. Ashcroft S, Ashcroft FM. The sulfonylurea receptor. *Biochim Biophys Acta.* 1992;1175:45.

233. Ashcroft FM. Mechanisms of the glycaemic effects of sulfonylureas. *Horm Metab Res.* 1996;28:456.

234. Leibowitz G, Cerasi E. Sulphonylurea treatment of NIDDM patients with cardiovascular disease: a mixed blessing? *Diabetologia.* 1996;39:503.

235. Brady P, Terzic A. The sulfonylurea controversy: more questions from the heart. *J Am Coll Cardiol.* 1998;31:950.

236. Scognamiglio R, Avogaro A, Vigili de Kreutzenberg S, et al. Effects of treatment with sulfonylurea drugs or insulin on ischemia-induced myocardial dysfunction in type 2 diabetes. *Diabetes.* 2002;51:808.

237. Klepzig H, Kober G, Matter C, et al. Sulfonylureas and ischaemic preconditioning: a double-blind, placebo-controlled evaluation of glimepiride and glibenclamide. *Eur Heart J.* 1999;20:403.

238. Brady PA, Jovanovic A. The sulfonylurea controversy: much ado about nothing or cause for concern?. *J Am Coll Cardiol.* 2003;42:1022.

239. Bell DSH. Do sulfonylurea drugs increase the risk of cardiac events? *CMAJ.* Jan 17;174(2):185-6, 2006.

240. Vasudevan AR, Balasubramanyam A. A review of their mechanisms of insulin sensitization, therapeutic potential, clinical efficacy, and tolerability. *Diabetes Technol Ther.* 2004;6:850.

241. Yki-Järvinen HY. Thiazolidinediones. *N Engl J Med.* 2004;351:1106.

242. Inzucchi SE, Maggs DG, Spollett GR, et al. Efficacy and metabolic effects of metformin and triglitazone in type II diabetes mellitus. *N Engl J Med.* 1998;338:867.

243. Parulkar AA, Pendergrass ML, Granda-Ayala R, et al. Nonhypoglycemic effects of thiazolidinediones. *Ann Intern Med.* 2001;134:61

244. Kotchen TA, Zhang HY, Reddy S, et al. Effect of pioglitazone on vascular reactivity in vivo and in vitro. *Am J Physiol.* 1996;270:R660.

245. Kruszynska YT, Yu JG, Olefsky JM, et al. Effects of troglitazone on blood concentrations of plasminogen activator inhibitor 1 in patients with type 2 diabetes and in lean and obese normal subjects. *Diabetes.* 2000;49:633.

246. Minamikawa J, Satsuki T, Yamauchi M, et al. Potent inhibitory effects of troglitazone on carotid arterial wall thickness in type 2 diabetes. *J Clin Endocrinol Metab.* 1998;83:1818.

247. Takagi T, Akasaka T, Yamamuro A, et al. Troglitazone reduces neointimal tissue proliferation after coronary stent implantation in patients with non-insulin dependent diabetes mellitus: a serial intravascular ultrasound study. *J Am Coll Cardiol.* 2000;36:1529.

248. Haffner SM, Greenberg AS, Weston WM, et al. Effect of rosiglitazone treatment on nontraditional markers of cardiovascular disease in patients with type 2 diabetes mellitus. *Circulation.* 2002;106:679.

249. Murakami T, Mizuno S, Ohsato K, et al. Effects of troglitazone on frequency of coronary vasospastic-induced angina pectoris in patients with diabetes mellitus. *Am J Cardiol.* 1999;84:92.

250. Choi D, Kim SK, Choi SH, et al. Preventative effects of rosiglitazone on restenosis after coronary stent implantation in patients with type 2 diabetes. *Diabetes Care.* 2004;27:2654.

251. Marx N, Wöhrle J, Nusser T, et al. Pioglitazone reduces neointima volume after coronary stent implantation: a randomized, placebo-controlled, double-blind trial in nondiabetic patients. *Circulation.* 2005;112:2792.

252. Langenfeld MR, Forst T, Hohbert C, et al. Pioglitazone decreases carotid intima-media thickness independently of glycemic control in patients with type 2 diabetes mellitus: results from a controlled randomized study. *Circulation.* 2005;111:2525.

253. Pfützner A, Marx N, Lubben G, et al. Improvement of cardiovascular risk markers by pioglitazone is independent from glycemic control: results from the Pioneer Study. *J Am Coll Cardiol.* 2005;45:1925.

254. Granberry MC, Fonseca VA. Cardiovascular risk factors associated with insulin resistance: effects of oral intidiabetic agents. *Am J Cardiovasc Drugs.* 2005;5:201.

255. Schwartz S, Raskin P, Fonseca V, et al. Effect of troglitazone in insulin-treated patients with type II diabetes mellitus. *N Eng J Med.* 1998;338:861.

256. Dormandy JA, Charbonnel B, Eckland DJ, et al. Secondary prevention of macrovascular events in patients with type 2 diabetes in the PROACTIVE Study (PROspective pioglitAzone Clinical Trial In macroVascular Events: a randomised controlled trial. *Lancet.* 2005;366:1279.

257. Kelly IE, Han TS, Walsh K, et al. Effects of a thiazolidinedione compound on body fat and fat distribution of patients with type 2 diabetes. *Diabetes Care.* 1999;22:288.

258. Tang WHW, Francis GS, Hoogwerf BJ, et al. Fluid retention after initiation of thiazolidinedione therapy in diabetic patients with established chronic heart failure. *J Am Coll Cardiol.* 2003;41:1394.

259. Lebovitz HE, Kreider M, Freed MI. Evaluation of liver function in type 2 diabetic patients during clinical trials: evidence that rosiglitazone does not cause hepatic dysfunction. *Diabetes Care.* 2002;25:815.

260. Mudaliar S, Henry RR. New oral therapies for type 2 diabetes mellitus: the glitazones or insulin sensitizers. *Annu Rev Med.* 2001;52:239.

261. Li AC, Brown KK, Silverstre MJ, et al. Peroxisome proliferator-activated receptor γ ligands inhibit development of atherosclerosis in LDL receptor-deficient mice. *J CLin Invest.* 2000;106:523.

262. Guerre-Millo M, Gervois P, Raspé E, et al.: Peroxisome proliferator-activated receptor γ activators improve insulin sensitivity and reduce adiposity. *J Biol Chem.* 2000;275:16638.

263. Wallace TM, Levy JC, Matthews DR. An increase in insulin sensitivity and basal beta-cell function in diabetic subjects treated with pioglitazone in a placebo-controlled randomized study. *Diab Med.* 2004;21:568.

264. Shimabukuro M, Zhou Y-T, Levi M, et al. Fatty acid-induced β cell apoptosis: a link between obesity and diabetes. *Proc Natl Acad Sci USA.* 1998;95:2498.

265. Goldberg RB, Kendall DM, Deeg MA, et al. A comparison of lipid and glycemic effects of pioglitazone and rosiglitazone in patients with type 2 diabetes and dyslipidemia. *Diabetes Care.* 2005;28:1547.

266. Buse JB, Rubin CJ, Frederich R, et al. Muraglitazar, a dual (alpha/gamma) PPAR activator: a randomized double-blind, placebo-controlled, 24-week monotherapy trial in adult patients with type 2 diabetes. *Clin Ther.* 2005;27:1181.

267. Nissen SE, Wolski K, Topol EJ. Effect of muraglitazar on death and major adverse cardiovascular events in patients with type 2 diabetes mellitus. *JAMA.* 2005;294:2581.

268. Wolffenbuttel BHR, Landgraf R, on behalf of the Dutch and German Repaglinide Study Group. A 1-year multicenter randomized double-blind comparison of repaglinide and glyburide for the treatment of type 2 diabetes. *Diabetes Care.* 1999;22:463.

269. Schmitz O, Lund S, Anderson PH, et al. Optimizing insulin secretagogue therapy in patients with type 2 diabetes: a randomized double-blind study with repaglinide. *Diabetes Care.* 2002;25:342.

270. Horton ES, Clinkingbeard C, Gatlin M, et al. Nateglinide alone and in combination with metformin improves glycemic control by reducing mealtime glucose levels in type 2 diabetes. *Diabetes Care.* 2000;23:1660.

271. Rosenstock J, Hassman DR, Madder RD. Repaglinide versus nateglinide monotherapy: a randomized, multicenter study. *Diabetes Care.* 2004;27:1265.

272. Moses R, Slobodniuk R, Boyages S, et al. Effect of repaglinide addition to metformin monotherapy on glycemic control in patients with type 2 diabetes. *Diabetes Care.* 1999;22:119.

273. Monnier L, Lapinski H, Colette C. Contributions of fasting and postprandial plasma glucose increments to the overall diurnal hyperglycemia of type 2 diabetic patients: variations with increasing levels of HbA1c. *Diabetes Care.* 2003;26:881.

274. American Diabetes Association. Postprandial blood glucose. *Diabetes Care.* 2001;24:775.

275. Gerich JE. Clinical significance, pathogenesis, and management of postprandial hyperglycemia. *Arch Intern Med.* 2003;163:1306.

276. Barrett-Connor E, Ferrara A. Isolated postchallenge hyperglycemia and the risk of fatal cardiovascular disease in older women and men: the Rancho Bernardo Study. *Diabetes Care.* 1998;21:1236.

277. Smith NL, Barzilay JI, Shaffer D, et al. Fasting and 2-hour postchallenge serum glucose measures and risk of incident cardiovascular events in the elderly: the Cardiovascular Health Study. *Arch Intern Med.* 2002;162:209.

278. Meigs JB, Nathan DM, D'Agostino RB, et al. Fasting and postchallenge glycemia and cardiovascular disease risk. *Diabetes Care.* 2002;25:1845.

279. Saydah SH, Miret M, Sung J, et al. Postchallenge hyperglycemia and mortality in a national sample of U.S. adults. *Diabetes Care.* 2001;24:1397.

280. Balkau B, Forhan A, Eschwège E. Two hour plasma glucose is not unequivocally predictive for early death in men with impaired fasting glucose: more results from the Paris Prospective Study. *Diabetologia.* 2002;45:1224.

281. Coniff RF, Shapiro JA, Robbins D, et al. Reduction of glycosylated hemoglobin and postprandial hyperglycemia by acarbose in patients with NIDDM. *Diabetes Care* 18:817, 1995.

282. Chiasson JL, Josse RG, Hunt JA, et al. The efficacy of acarbose in the treatment of patients with non-insulin-dependent diabetes mellitus: a multicenter controlled clinical trial. *Ann Intern Med.* 1994;121:935.

283. Chiasson JL, Josse RG, Gomis R et al. Acarbose for prevention of type 2 diabetes mellitus: the STOP-NIDDM randomized trial. *Lancet.* 359:2072.

284. Chiasson JL, Josse RG, Gomis R, et al. Acarbose treatment and the risk of cardiovascular disease and hypertension in patients with impaired glucose tolerance. *JAMA.* 2003;290:486.

285. Kaiser T, Sawicki PT. Acarbose for prevention of diabetes, hypertension and cardiovascular events? A critical analysis of the STOP-NIDDM data. *Diabetologia.* 2004;47:575.

286. Hayward RA, Manning WG, Kaplan SH, et al. Starting insulin therapy in patients with type 2 diabetes. *JAMA.* 1997;278:1663.

287. Genuth S. Insulin use in NIDDM. *Diabetes Care.* 1990;13:1240.

288. Genuth S. Management of the adult onset diabetic with sulfonylurea drug failure. *Endocrinol Metab Clin North Am.* 1992;21:351.

289. Boyne MS, Saudek CD. Effect of insulin therapy on macrovascular risk factors in type 2 diabetes. *Diabetes Care.* 1999;22(suppl 3):C45.

290. Fonseca VA. Management of diabetes mellitus and insulin resistance in patients with cardiovascular disease. *Am J Cardiol.* 2003;92(S):50J.

291. Panunti B, Kunhiraman B, Fonseca V. The impact of antidiabetic therapies on cardiovascular disease. *Curr Atheroscler Rep.* 2005;7:50.

292. Spallarossa P, Cordera R, Andraghetti G, et al. Association between plasma insulin and angiographically documented significant coronary artery disease. *Am J Cardiol.* 1994;74:177.

293. Arcaro G, Cretti A, Balazano S, et al. Insulin causes endothelial dysfunction in humans: sites and mechanisms. *Circulation.* 2002;105:576.

294. Stout RW. Insulin and atheroma: an update. *Lancet.* 1987;1:1077.

295. Jain SK, Nagi DK, Slavin BM, et al. Insulin therapy in type 2 diabetic subjects suppresses plasminogen activator inhibitor (PAI-1) activity and proinsulin-like molecules independently of glycaemic control. *Diabetic Med.* 1993;10:27.

296. Dandona P, Alijada A, Mohanty P. The anti-inflammatory and potential anti-atherogenic effect of insulin: a new paradigm. *Diabetologia.* 2002;45:924.

297. Dandona P, Aljada A, Chaudhuri A, et al. The potential influence of inflammation and insulin resistance on the pathogenesis and treatment of atherosclerosis-related complications in type 2 diabetes. *J Clin Endocrinol Metab.* 2003;88:2422.

298. Guazzi M, Tumminello G, Matturri M, et al. Insulin ameliorates exercise ventilatory efficiency and oxygen uptake in patients with heart failure–type 2 diabetes comorbidity. *J Am Coll Cardiol.* 2003;42:1044.

299. Levy WC, Hirsch IB. Diabetes and heart failure: is insulin therapy the answer? *J Am Coll Cardiol.* 2003;42:1051.

300. Multicenter Metformin Study Group. Efficacy of metformin in patients with non-insulin-dependent diabetes mellitus. *N Eng J Med.* 1995;333:541.

301. Horton ES, Whitehouse F, Ghazzi MN, et al. Troglitazone in combination with sulfonylurea restores glycemic control in patients with type 2 diabetes. *Diabetes Care.* 1998;21:1462.

302. Fisman EZ, Tenenbaum A, Boyko V, et al. Oral antidiabetic treatment in patients with coronary disease: time-related increased mortality on combined glyburide/metformin therapy over a 7.7-year follow-up. *Clin Cardiol.* 2001;24:151.

303. Johnson JA, Majumdar SR, Simpson SH, et al. Decreased mortality associated with the use of metformin compared with sulfonylurea monotherapy in type 2 diabetes. *Diabetes Care.* 2002;25:2244.

304. Riddle MC, Rosenstock J, Gerich J, on behalf of the Insulin Glargine 4002 Study Investigators. The treat-to-target trial: randomized addition of glargine or human NPH insulin to oral therapy of type 2 diabetic patients. *Diabetes Care.* 2003;26:3080.

305. Furlong NJ, Hulme SA, O'Brien SV, et al. Comparison of repaglinide vs. gliclazide in combination with bedtime NPH insulin in patients with type 2 diabetes inadequately controlled with oral hypoglycaemic agents. *Diabet Med.* 2003;20:935.

306. Poulsen MK, Henriksen JE, Hother-Nielsen O, et al. The combined effect of triple therapy with rosiglitazone, metformin, and insulin aspart in type 2 diabetic patients. *Diabetes Care.* 2003;26:3273.

307. Yki-Jarvinen H. Combination therapy with insulin and oral agents: optimizing glycemic control in patients with type 2 diabetes mellitus. *Diabetes Metab Res Rev.* 2002;18:S77.

308. Genuth S. Treating diabetes with both insulin and sulfonylurea drugs: what is the value? *Clin Diabetes.* 1987;5:73.

309. Riddle MC, Schneider J. Beginning insulin treatment of obese patients with evening 70/30 insulin plus glimepiride versus insulin alone. The Glimepiride Combination Group. *Diabetes Care.* 1998;21:1052.

310. Tong PC, Chow CC, Jorgensen LN, et al. The contribution of metformin to glycaemic control in patients with type 2 diabetes mellitus receiving combination therapy with insulin. *Diabetes Res Clin Pract.* 2002.57:93.

311. Strowig SM, Aviles-Santa M, Raskin P. Comparison of insulin monotherapy and combination therapy with insulin and metformin or insulin and troglitazone in type 2 diabetes. *Diabetes Care.* 2002;25:1691.

312. Hussar DA. New drugs: exenatide, pramlintide acetate, and micafungin sodium. *J Am Pharm Assoc* 2005;45:636.

313. Uwaifo GI, Ratner RE. Novel pharmacologic agents for type 2 diabetes. *Endocrinol Metab Clin North Am.* 2005;34:155.

314. Rosenstock J, Ninman B, Murphy LJ, et al. Inhaled insulin improves glycemic control when substituted for or added to oral combination therapy in type 2 diabetes: a randomized, controlled trial. *Ann Intern Med.* 2005;143:549.

315. Curb JD, Pressel SL, Cutler Jam et al. Effect of diuretic-based antihypertensive treatment on cardiovascular disease risk in older diabetic patients with isolated systolic hypertension. *JAMA.* 1996;276:1886.

316. UK Prospective Diabetes Study Group. Tight blood pressure control and risk of macrovascular and microvascular complications in type 2 diabetes: UKPDS 38. *BMJ.* 1998;317:703.

317. Tuomilehto J, Rastenyte D, Birkenhager WH, et al. Effects of calcium-channel blockade in older patients with diabetes and systolic hypertension: systolic hypertension in Europe trial. *N Eng J Med.* 1999;340:677.

318. The ALLHAT Officers and Coordinators for the ALLHAT Collaborative Research Group. Major outcomes in high-risk hypertensive patients randomized to angiotensin-converting enzyme inhibitor or calcium channel blocker vs diuretic. *JAMA.* 2002;288:2981.

319. Hansson L, Zanchetti A, Carruthers SG, et al. Effects of intensive blood-pressure lowering and low-dose aspirin in patients with hypertension: principal results of the Hypertension Optimal Treatment (HOT) randomized trial. HOT Study Group. *Lancet.* 1998;351:1755.

320. Schrier RW, Estacio RO, Jeffers B. Appropriate blood pressure control in NIDDM (ABCD) Trial. *Diabetologia.* 1996;39:1646.

321. Lindholm LH, Ibsen H, Dahlöf B, et al. Cardiovascular morbidity and mortality in patients with diabetes in the Losartan Intervention For Endpoint reduction in hypertension study (LIFE): a randomized trial against atenolol. *Lancet.* 2002;359:1004.

322. Ravid M, Brosh D, Levi Z, et al. Use of enalapril to attenuate decline in renal function in normotensive, normoalbuminuric patients with type 2 diabetes mellitus. *Ann Intern Med.* 1998;128:982.

323. The Euclid Study Group. Randomised placebo-controlled trial of lisinopril in normotensive patients with insulin-dependent diabetes and normoalbuminuria or microalbuminuria. *Lancet.* 1997;349:1787.

324. Zandbergen AA, Baggen MG, Lamberts SW, et al. Effect of losartan on microalbuminuria in normotensive patients with type 2 diabetes mellitus: a randomized clinical trial. *Ann Intern Med.* 2003;139:90.

325. Tütüncü NB, Gürlek A, Gedik O. Efficacy of ACE inhibitors and ATII receptor blockers in patients with microalbuminuria: a prospective study. *Acta Diabetol.* 2001;38:157.

326. Mogensen CE. Microalbuminuria predicts clinical proteinuria and early mortality in maturity onset diabetes. *N Engl J Med.* 1984;310:356.

327. Messent JW, Elliott TG, Hill RD, et al. Prognostic significance of microalbuminuria in insulin-dependent diabetes mellitus: a twenty-three year follow-up study. *Kidney Int.* 1992;41:836.

328. Deckert T, Yokoyama H, Mathiesen E, et al. Cohort study of predictive value of urinary albumin excretion for atherosclerotic vascular disease in patients with insulin dependent diabetes. *BMJ.* 1996;312:871.

329. Dinneen SF, Gerstein HC. The association of microalbuminuria and mortality in non-insulin-dependent diabetes mellitus: a systematic overview of the literature. *Arch Intern Med.* 1997;157:1413.

330. Downs JR, Clearfield M, Weis S, et al. Primary prevention of acute coronary events with Lovastatin in men and women with average cholesterol levels: results of AFCAPS/TexCAPS. *JAMA.* 1998;279:1615.

331. Haffner SM, Alexander CM, Cook TJ, et al. Reduced coronary events in simvastatin-treated patients with coronary heart disease and diabetes or impaired fasting glucose levels: subgroup analyses in the Scandinavian Simvastatin Survival Study. *Arch Intern Med.* 1999;159:2661.

332. Heart Protection Study Collaborative Group. MRC/BHF Heart Protection Study of cholesterol lowering with simvastatin in 20,536 high-risk individuals: a randomised placebo-controlled trial. *Lancet.* 2002;360:7.

333. Goldberg RB, Mellies MJ, Sacks FM, et al. Cardiovascular events and their reduction with pravastatin in diabetic and glucose-intolerant myocardial infarction survivors with average cholesterol levels: subgroup analyses in the cholesterol and recurrent events (CARE) trial. The Care Investigators. *Circulation.* 1998;98:2513.

334. LIPID (Long-Term Intervention with Pravastatin in Ischemic Disease) Study Group: Prevention of cardiovascular events and death with pravastatin in patients with coronary heart disease and a broad range of initial cholesterol levels. *N Engl J Med.* 1998;339:1349.

335. Shepherd J, Barter P, Carmena R, et al. Effect of lowering LDL cholesterol substantially below currently recommended levels in patients with coronary heart disease and diabetes: the Treating to New Targets (TNT) study. *Diabetes Care.* 2006;29:1220.

336. Pederson TR, Faergeman O, Kastelein JJ, et al. High-dose atorvastatin vs usual-dose simvastatin for secondary prevention after myocardial infarction: the IDEAL study: a randomized controlled trial. *JAMA.* 2005;294:2437.

337. Wiviott SD, Cannon CP, Morrow DA, et al. Can low-density lipoprotein be too low? The safety and efficacy of achieving very low low-density lipoprotein with intensive statin therapy: a PROVE IT-TIMI 22 substudy. *J Am Coll Cardiol.* 2005;46:1411.

338. Colhoun HM, Betteridge DJ, Durrington PN, et al. Primary prevention of cardiovascular disease with atorvastatin in type 2 diabetes in the Collaborative Atorvastatin Diabetes Study (CARDS): multicentre randomized placebo-controlled trial. *Lancet* 2004;364:685.

339. Nissen SE. High-dose statins in acute coronary syndromes: not just lipid levels. *JAMA*. 2004;292:1365.

340. Ridker PM, Cannon CP, Morrow D, et al. C-reactive protein levels and outcomes after statin therapy. *N Engl J Med*. 2005;352:20.

341. Grundy SM, Cleeman JI, Merz NB, et al. Implications of recent clinical trials for the national cholesterol education program adult treatment panel III guidelines. *Circulation*. 2004;110:227.

342. Efficacy and safety of cholesterol-lowering treatment: prospective meta-analysis of data from 90,056 participants in 14 randomised trials of statins. *Lancet*. 2005;366:1267.

343. Rubins HB, Robins SJ, Collins D, et al. Gemfibrozil for the secondary prevention of coronary heart disease in men with low levels of high-density lipoprotein cholesterol. Veterans Affairs High-Density Lipoprotein Cholesterol Intervention Trial Study Group. *N Engl J Med*. 1999;341:410.

344. Frick MH, Elo O, Haapa K, et al. Helsinki Heart Study: primary-prevention trial with gemfibrozil in middle-aged men with dyslipidemia: safety of treatment, changes in risk factors, and incidence of coronary heart disease. *N Engl J Med*. 1987;317:1237.

345. Diabetes Atherosclerosis Intervention Study Investigators. Effect of fenofibrate on progression of coronary-artery disease in type 2 diabetes: the Diabetes Atherosclerosis Intervention Study, a randomised study. *Lancet*. 2001;357:905.

346. Anonymous. Secondary prevention by raising HDL cholesterol and reducing triglycerides in patients with coronary artery disease: the Bezafibrate Infarction Prevention (BIP) study. *Circulation*. 2000;102:21.

347. Effects of long-term fenofibrate therapy on cardiovascular events in 9795 people with type 2 diabetes mellitus (the FIELD study): randomised controlled trial. *Lancet*. 2005;366:1849.

348. Taher TH, Dzavik V, Reteff EM, et al. Tolerability of statin-fibrate and statin-niacin combination therapy in dyslipidemic patients at high risk for cardiovascular events. *Am J Cardiol*. 2002;89:390.

349. Grundy SM, Vega GL, McGovern ME, et al. Efficacy, safety, and tolerability of once-daily niacin for the treatment of dyslipidemia associated with type 2 diabetes: results of the Assessment of Diabetes Control and Evaluation of the Efficacy of Niaspan Trial. *Arch Intern Med*. 2002;162:1568.

350. Massing MW, Henley NS, Carter-Edwards, L, et al. Lipid testing among patients with diabetes who receive diabetes care from primary care physicians. *Diabetes Care*. 2003;26:1369.

351. Massing MW, Foley KA, Sueta CA, et al. Trends in lipid management among patients with coronary artery disease: has diabetes received the attention it deserves? *Diabetes Care*. 2003;26:991.

352. Grodstein F, Manson JE, Colditz GA, et al. A prospective, observational study of postmenopausal hormone therapy and primary prevention of cardiovascular disease. *Ann Intern Med*. 2000;133:933.

353. Psaty BM, Heckbert SR, Atkins D, et al. The risk of myocardial infarction associated with the combined use of estrogens and progestins in postmenopausal women. *Arch Intern Med*. 1994;154:1333.

354. Newton KM, LaCroix AZ, Heckbert SR, et al. Estrogen therapy and risk of cardiovascular events among women with type 2 diabetes. *Diabetes Care*. 2003;26:2810.

355. Lee WL, Cheung AM, Cape D, et al. Impact of diabetes on coronary artery disease in women and men: a meta-analysis of prospective studies. *Diabetes Care*. 2000;23:962.

356. Manson JE, Hsia J, Johnson KC, et al. Estrogen plus progestin and the risk of coronary heart disease. *N Engl J Med*. 2003;349:523.

357. Hodis HN, Mack WJ, Azen SP, et al. Hormone therapy and the progression of coronary-artery atherosclerosis in postmenopausal women. *N Engl J Med*. 2003;349:535.

358. Malmberg K, Norhammar A, Wedel H, et al. Glycometabolic state at admission: important risk marker of mortality in conventionally treated patients with diabetes mellitus and acute myocardial infarction—long term results from the Diabetes and Insulin-Glucose Infusion in Acute Myocardial Infarction (DIGAMI) Study. *Circulation*. 1999;99:2626.

359. Luciani N, Nasso G, Gaudino M, et al. Coronary artery bypass grafting in type II diabetic patients: a comparison between insulin-dependent and non-insulin-dependent patients at short- and mid-term follow-up. *Ann Thorac Surg*. 2003;76:1149.

360. Capes SE, Hunt D, Malmberg K, Gerstein HC. Stress hyperglycaemia and increased risk of death after myocardial infarction in patients with and without diabetes: a systematic overview. *Lancet*. 2000;355:773.

361. Kosiborod M, Rathore SS, Inzucchi SE, Masoudi FA, et al. Admission glucose and mortality in elderly patients hospitalized with acute myocardial infarction: implications for patients with and without recognized diabetes. *Circulation*. 2005;111:3078.

362. Stranders I, Diamant M, van Gelder RE, et al. Admission blood glucose level as risk indicator of death after myocardial infarction in patients with and without diabetes mellitus. *Arch Intern Med*. 2004;164:982.

363. Genuth S. The automatic (regular insulin) sliding scale or 2,4,6,8 call HO. *Clin Diabetes*. 1994;12:40.

364. Guvener M, Pasaoglu I, Demircin M, et al. Perioperative hyperglycemia is a strong correlate of postoperative infection in type II diabetic patients after coronary artery bypass grafting. *Endocr J*. 2002;49:531.

365. Trence DL, Kelly JL, Hirsch IB. The rationale and management of hyperglycemia for in-patients with cardiovascular disease: time for change. *J Clin Endocrinol Metab*. 2003;88:2430,.

366. Furnary AP, Guangqiang G, Grunkemeier GL, et al. Continuous insulin infusion reduces mortality in patients with diabetes undergoing coronary artery bypass grafting. *J Thorac Cardiovasc Surg*. 2003;125:1007.

367. Goldberg PA, Sakharova OV, Barrett PW, et al. Improving glycemic control in the cardiothoracic intensive care unit: clinical experience in two hospital settings. *J Cardiothorac Vasc Anesth*. 2004;18:690.

368. Ku SY, Sayre CA, Hirsch IB, Kelly JL. New insulin infusion protocol improves blood glucose control in hospitalized patients without increasing hypoglycemia. *Jt Comm J Qual Patient Saf*. 2005;3:141.

369. Van den Berghe G, Wouters P, Weekers F, et al. Intensive insulin therapy in critically ill patients. *N Engl J Med*. 2001;345:1359.

370. Pantaleo A, Zonszein J: Using insulin as a drug rather than as a replacement hormone during acute illness: a new paradigm. *Heart Dis*. 2003;5:323.

371. Imran SA, Cox JL, Ur E. Diabetes control among patients presenting with acute myocardial infarction in a Canadian tertiary health care setting. *Can J Cardiol*. 2003;19:1407.

372. Huang ES, Meigs JB, Singer DE. The effect of interventions to prevent cardiovascular disease in patients with type 2 diabetes mellitus. *Am J Med*. 2001;111:633.

373. Saaddine JB, Engelgau MM, Beckles GL, et al. A diabetes report card for the United States: quality of care in the 1990s. *Ann Intern Med*. 2002;136:565.

374. McFarlane SI, Jacober SJ, Winer N, et al. Control of cardiovascular risk factors in patients with diabetes and hypertension at urban academic medical centers. *Diabetes Care*. 2002;25:718.

375. George PB, Tobin KJ, Corpus RA, et al. Treatment of cardiac risk factors in diabetic patients: how well do we follow the guidelines? *Am Heart J*. 2001;142:857.

376. Saydah SH, Fradkin J, Cowie CC. Poor control of risk factors for vascular disease among adults with previously diagnosed diabetes. *JAMA*. 2004;291:335.

377. Gæde P, Vedel P, Larsen N, et al. Multifactorial intervention in cardiovascular disease in patients with type 2 diabetes. *N Engl J Med*. 2003;348:383.

378. Sever PS, Poulter NR, Dahlof B, et al. Reduction in cardiovascular events with atorvastatin in 2,532 patients with type 2 diabetes: Anglo-Scandinavian Cardiac Outcomes Trial-Lipid-Lowering Arm (ASCOT-LLA). *Diabetes Care*. 2005;28:1151.

CHAPTER (64)

Nontraditional Risk Factors for Atherosclerosis

Iftikhar J. Kullo, MD

Assessment of the risk of coronary heart disease (CHD) in an individual is an important first step in primary prevention and helps determine the intensity of therapy needed to reduce CHD risk. Currently 2 algorithms for assessing CHD risk are recommended in the National Cholesterol Education Program guidelines.[1] The first algorithm estimates the 10-year probability of CHD using the Framingham risk score. The second algorithm identifies the presence of the metabolic syndrome. The currently available predictive models have less-than-desired accuracy in predicting CHD risk, thereby stimulating the search for new tools to refine risk stratification (Figure 64-1). In particular, there is an intense interest in evaluating circulating biomarkers related to the atherosclerotic process that might improve CHD risk stratification.

The concept of cardiovascular risk factors arose from the Framingham Heart Study, a landmark study in cardiovascular disease epidemiology that established age, male sex, diabetes, hypertension, dyslipidemia, and smoking as the major risk factors for CHD. Subsequent advances in our understanding of the pathogenesis of atherosclerotic vascular disease have led to considerable interest in the so-called nontraditional risk factors for CHD.[2] The study of these risk factors is important for at least 3 reasons.

1. Not all cardiovascular events can be explained on the basis of conventional risk factors. Indeed, cardiovascular events can occur in the absence of or with relative paucity of conventional risk factors, and these risk factors may have limited sensitivity and specificity for predicting events, particularly among younger subjects.[3]

2. Conventional risk factors explain less than 50% of the variability in measures of atherosclerotic vascular disease (assessed by coronary angiography or electron-beam computed tomography).[4] Other biochemical and genetic factors are likely to be associated

with the residual variability in measures of atherosclerotic vascular disease.

3. Nontraditional risk factors may partly explain the variation in CHD risk among different ethnic groups. The Seven Countries Study, another landmark study in cardiovascular epidemiology, confirmed the results of the Framingham study, but whole populations as well as individuals differed in the burden of CHD at any given level of risk factors.[5] An example is the elevated CHD risk of individuals of people of south Asian descent living in western countries at any given level of conventional risk factors. In this ethnic group, nontraditional risk factors such as insulin resistance, lipoprotein(a) [Lp(a)], and homocysteine may be important in causation of atherosclerosis.[6]

An American Heart Association statement[7] has suggested a new classification of risk factors (Table 64-1) with 3 main categories. A fourth category that can be added is that of emerging risk factors. The conventional risk factors appear to have a direct causal role in atherogenesis. Predisposing factors, including obesity, family history of premature atherosclerotic vascular disease, and sedentary lifestyle, mediate some of their risk through the causal factors but may have independent effects as well. The conditional risk factors are associated with an increased risk of CHD although whether these have a causal and independent contribution to CHD is not well established. The 6 conditional risk factors are homocysteine, fibrinogen, Lp(a), triglycerides, small low-density lipoprotein (LDL) particle size, and C-reactive protein (CRP). Some of the emerging risk factors include lipoprotein-associated phospholipase A_2,[8] asymmetric dimethyl arginine,[9] pregnancy-associated plasma phosphatase,[10] markers of oxidative stress,[11] and myeloperoxidase.[12]

At present, other than for CRP, there are no specific guidelines for the use of nontraditional risk factors in clinical practice.

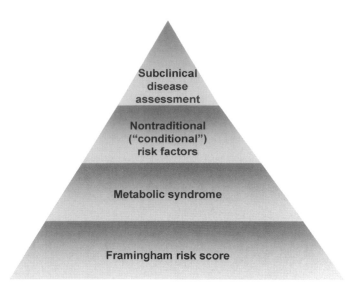

FIGURE 64-1. The coronary heart disease (CHD) risk assessment pyramid. *(From Kullo IJ, Ballantyne CM. Conditional risk factors for atherosclerosis. Mayo Clin Proc. 2005, 80:219. Used with permission of Mayo Foundation for Medical Education and Research.)*

Identifying nontraditional or conditional risk factors may increase the accuracy of risk stratification of individual subjects and thereby facilitate targeted strategies for primary or secondary prevention.[13] Such knowledge may also further our understanding of the pathogenesis of atherosclerotic vascular disease and help uncover new targets for therapeutic intervention. This review provides an update on the current state of knowledge about the clinical relevance of the conditional risk factors (except triglycerides, the subject of multiple previous reviews). For each risk factor, the mechanisms of atherogenicity, available assays, evidence for association with cardiovascular events, and clinical and therapeutic implications will be considered. The review will focus mainly on the potential utility of these risk factors in the prediction of risk of cardiovascular events in asymptomatic subjects.

HOMOCYSTEINE

Homocysteine is a thiol-containing amino acid intermediate formed during the metabolism of methionine, an essential amino acid. Plasma homocysteine levels are normally between 5 and 15 μmol/L in the fasting state. Markedly elevated plasma homocysteine levels, in excess of 100 to 200 μmol/L, are found in inborn errors of homocysteine metabolism, such as cystathionine β-synthase deficiency.[14] McCully[15] demonstrated the presence of atherosclerosis in children and young adults with these enzyme deficiencies, and his work raised the possibility that mild to moderate elevations in homocysteine could contribute to atherosclerotic vascular disease. Such increases in plasma homocysteine levels can occur with aging, menopause, chronic renal insufficiency, low plasma levels of vitamin cofactors (B_6, B_{12}, and folic acid), and cardiac transplantation. Genetic variation in enzymes involved in homocysteine metabolism may also lead to increased levels. One such polymorphism (677C →T) in methylene tetrahydrofolate reductase (MTHFR), an enzyme that metabolizes homocysteine, is associated with mild to moderate elevations in plasma homocysteine levels, particularly in the setting of low dietary folate intake.[16] Because nearly 15% of the white population may be homozygous for this polymorphism, it is an important determinant of plasma homocysteine levels in the population.

[ ] MECHANISMS OF INCREASED RISK

Although considerable evidence links elevated plasma homocysteine levels to an increased risk of atherosclerotic vascular disease, the role of homocysteine in atherogenesis is yet to be established. Whether homocysteine is a causal risk factor for atherogenesis or simply a marker of existing vascular disease continues to be a matter of debate.[17,18] Experimental data suggest several potential mechanisms of vascular damage mediated by elevated plasma homocysteine. These include endothelial cell damage, stimulation

TABLE 64-1

Categories of Risk Factors

CONVENTIONAL	PREDISPOSING	CONDITIONAL	EMERGING
Cigarette smoking	Overweight and obesity	Homocysteine	Lipoprotein-associated phospholipase A₂[8]
Elevated blood pressure	Physical inactivity	Fibrinogen	
Elevated serum cholesterol	Male sex	Lipoprotein (a)	Asymmetric dimethyl arginine[9]
Low HDL-C	Family history of early-onset CHD	Small LDL particle size	Pregnancy-associated plasma Phophatase[10]
Diabetes mellitus		Triglycerides	
	Socioeconomic factors	C-reactive protein	Plasminogen activator inhibitor-1
	Behavioral factors		Measures of oxidative stress[11]
	Insulin resistance		Myeloperoxidase[12]
			Candidate gene polymorphisms

CHD = coronary heart disease; HDL-C = high-density lipoprotein cholesterol; LDL = low-density lipoprotein.
Modified from Smith et al.[7] By permission of American Heart Association, Inc.

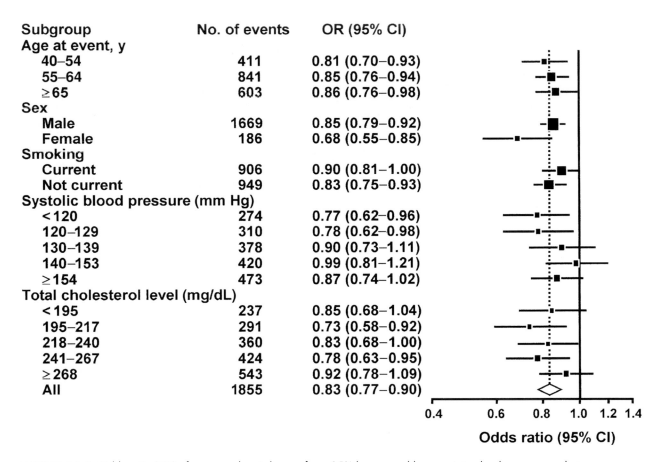

Subgroup	No. of events	OR (95% CI)
Age at event, y		
40–54	411	0.81 (0.70–0.93)
55–64	841	0.85 (0.76–0.94)
≥65	603	0.86 (0.76–0.98)
Sex		
Male	1669	0.85 (0.79–0.92)
Female	186	0.68 (0.55–0.85)
Smoking		
Current	906	0.90 (0.81–1.00)
Not current	949	0.83 (0.75–0.93)
Systolic blood pressure (mm Hg)		
<120	274	0.77 (0.62–0.96)
120–129	310	0.78 (0.62–0.98)
130–139	378	0.90 (0.73–1.11)
140–153	420	0.99 (0.81–1.21)
≥154	473	0.87 (0.74–1.02)
Total cholesterol level (mg/dL)		
<195	237	0.85 (0.68–1.04)
195–217	291	0.73 (0.58–0.92)
218–240	360	0.83 (0.68–1.00)
241–267	424	0.78 (0.63–0.95)
≥268	543	0.92 (0.78–1.09)
All	1855	0.83 (0.77–0.90)

Odds ratio (95% CI)

FIGURE 64-2. Odds ratio (OR) of coronary heart disease for a 25% lower usual homocysteine level among people in prospective studies. Data were adjusted for study, sex, and age at enrollment. Studies are grouped by age at event, sex, smoking history, and quintiles of systolic blood pressure and total cholesterol level. A global test for heterogeneity between all these subgroups was not significant ($\chi^2_{16} = 14$; $P = .60$). The size of the square is inversely proportional to the variance of the log of the OR. The horizontal lines indicate the 95% confidence intervals (CIs). The diamond indicates the total and its 95% CI. To convert cholesterol to mmol/L, multiply by 0.02586. *(From Homocysteine Studies Collaboration.[24] Used with permission of American Medical Association.)*

of vascular smooth muscle proliferation, activation of factor V, inhibition of protein C, enhanced platelet aggregation, and endothelial dysfunction.[19,20] See Figure 64–2.

[ ] ASSAYS

Methods of measurement of plasma homocysteine levels include high-pressure liquid chromatography, enzyme-linked immunosorbent assay (ELISA), and mass spectrometry. Levels are measured in the fasting state, but even nonfasting plasma homocysteine levels have been shown to be related to future cardiovascular events.[21] Postmethionine load homocysteine levels may classify an additional 27% to 40% of patients with CHD as having abnormal methionine metabolism.[22] However, at present, the clinical utility of the methionine load test is unclear.

[ ] EVIDENCE OF ASSOCIATION

Most (but not all) prospective studies of homocysteine and cardiovascular risk show homocysteine to be predictive of cardiovascular events. A 1995 meta-analysis of 27 studies indicated that an

elevation of homocysteine levels (> 15 μmol/L) is associated with increased risk of CHD, peripheral arterial disease, stroke, and venous thromboembolism;[23] a 5-μmol/L increment increased CHD risk as much as a 20-mg/dL elevation in total cholesterol. A 2002 meta-analysis suggests a modest increase in the risk of cardiovascular events attributable to elevated homocysteine (Figure 64-2).[24] After adjustment for traditional cardiovascular risk factors and regression dilution bias in the prospective studies, a 25% lower homocysteine level was associated with an 11% lower CHD risk and 19% lower stroke risk.

Genetic variation in enzymes participating in homocysteine metabolism seems to influence CHD risk, suggesting a causal role for homocysteine in vascular disease. Two large 2002 meta-analyses of the studies of association of MTHFR 677 T→C polymorphism with CHD suggest that the TT genotype is associated with a modest but statistically significant increase in the risk of cardiovascular events.[25,26] The genotype relative risk (TT vs CC) in the 2 meta-analyses was 1.21 (95% CI, 1.06–1.39)[25] and 1.16 (95% CI, 1.05–1.28).[26] The risk appeared to be higher in patients with low folic acid levels.

Another 2002 study implicates plasma homocysteine as a risk factor for restenosis after percutaneous coronary intervention.[27]

Homocysteine-lowering treatment significantly reduced the rate of restenosis[28] and the incidence of major adverse events 1 year after percutaneous coronary intervention.[29] Subsequent data from a randomized controlled study of 626 patients treated with folic acid and vitamin B supplements after percutaneous coronary intervention found increased rates of restenosis and major adverse cardiac events in the vitamin treatment group after 6 months of follow-up.[30] Further work is needed to clarify the role of homocysteine in restenosis after percutaneous coronary intervention.

[ ] CLINICAL IMPLICATIONS

Doses of 1 mg of folic acid in conjunction with vitamin B_{12} and vitamin B_6 supplements are likely to be effective in lowering plasma homocysteine in most individuals. In patients with renal failure, much higher doses (up to 20 mg) of folic acid are often needed to lower homocysteine levels.[31] In refractory cases, betaine, a cofactor in homocysteine metabolism pathway, may be efficacious.[32] Since January 1998, cereal grain or flour is being fortified with 140 mg of folic acid per 100 g of flour to reduce the incidence of neural tube defects. Malinow and colleagues[33] suggest that such supplementation may not be adequate to reduce coronary risk.

Although folic acid supplementation is postulated to have a beneficial effect on atherosclerotic vascular disease, prospective randomized trials are needed to prove this. The results of three large randomized controlled trials indicate that lowering of plasma homocysteine with folic acid and B vitamins does not reduce cardiovascular events. The possibility that folic acid supplementation of flour may reduce the power of some of these trials has been raised.[34]

FIBRINOGEN

Fibrinogen is essential to the coagulation cascade and a major determinant of plasma viscosity. Plasma levels of fibrinogen are in part genetically determined.[35] Increasing age and adiposity, smoking, diabetes mellitus, and menopause are associated with increased plasma levels.[36] African Americans tend to have higher levels than whites.[37]

[ ] MECHANISMS OF INCREASED RISK

Fibrinogen may be proatherogenic by increasing plasma viscosity, promoting platelet aggregability, and stimulating smooth muscle proliferation.[38] Fibrinogen is also a marker of inflammation and it is now established that atherosclerosis is an inflammatory process. During an acute-phase response, hepatic synthesis of fibrinogen can increase severalfold.

[ ] ASSAYS

The main assay types are immunoassays and a functional clotting-time–based assay, also known as the Clauss assay.[39] In the Framingham Offspring Population study, fibrinogen levels measured by immunoprecipitation showed a stronger association with cardiovascular events than levels measured by the Clauss method.[40] The use of fibrinogen in cardiovascular risks' stratification is hampered by the variability in assays and by lack of established cutoffs to discriminate between gradations of risk.

[ ] EVIDENCE OF ASSOCIATION

Fibrinogen has been consistently associated with risk of cardiovascular events in multiple studies.[39,41] Fibrinogen levels are associated with several conventional CHD risk factors, but even after statistical adjustment for these risk factors, the association between fibrinogen and cardiovascular disease remains significant.[36] A meta-analysis of 6 prospective epidemiologic studies found that increased fibrinogen levels were associated with subsequent myocardial infarction or stroke (Figure 64-3).[36] Individuals with levels in the upper tertile had a relative risk of future cardiovascular events 2.3 times higher than that of individuals with levels in the lowest tertile. Results from 2 meta-analyses confirm a near doubling of risk for individuals in the upper tertile of baseline fibrinogen concentration compared with those in the lower tertile.[39,42]

Fibrinogen is a risk factor for peripheral arterial disease as well and is included in the Framingham equation to estimate the risk of intermittent claudication.[43] In addition to being a predictor of cardiovascular events, fibrinogen is associated with subclinical atherosclerotic burden.[44,45] Elevated fibrinogen levels may interact with other risk factors in increasing the risk of cardiovascular events. Thus, elevated fibrinogen levels appear to increase the risk in subjects with elevated LDL cholesterol[46] and elevated Lp(a).[47]

[ ] CLINICAL IMPLICATIONS

Measuring fibrinogen levels may be helpful in risk stratifying patients, but lack of a standardized assay has diminished its potential clinical value in this context. There is no evidence yet to suggest that reduction of fibrinogen levels alters clinical outcome. Fibrinogen levels are reduced by smoking cessation, exercise, alcohol, and estrogens. Drugs that specifically lower fibrinogen levels are not yet available. The fibrates have potent fibrinogen-lowering effects,[48] but because they concomitantly modify plasma lipids, these drugs are not suitable for examining the specific effect of fibrinogen lowering.

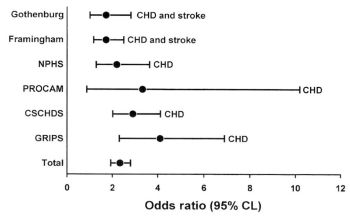

FIGURE 64-3. Odds ratio (and 95% confidence interval [CI]) for cardiovascular events in persons with fibrinogen levels in the upper tertile compared with the lower tertile in 6 prospective epidemiologic studies. CSCHDS = Caerphilly and Speedwell Collaborative Heart Disease Studies; GRIPS = Gottingen Risk, Incidence, and Prevalence Study; CHD = coronary heart disease; NPHS = Northwick Park Heart Study; PROCAM = Prospective Cardiovascular Munster Study. *(From Ernst and Resch.[36] Used with permission of American College of Physicians.)*

LIPOPROTEIN A

Lp(a) is a circulating lipoprotein that resembles LDL cholesterol in core lipid composition and in having apolipoprotein B-100 (apo B-100) as a surface apolipoprotein. In addition, it has a unique glycoprotein, apo(a), which is bound to apo B-100 by a disulfide bond. Its physiologic function remains obscure, although a role in wound healing has been proposed. Plasma levels vary widely between individuals on the order of a 1000-fold but are stable within individuals, suggesting a strong heritable component.[49] Levels are generally unrelated to those of other lipoproteins and apolipoproteins.[49] Nongenetic mechanisms that regulate serum Lp(a) levels are unknown. Lp(a) levels are increased in renal insufficiency, nephrotic syndrome, diabetes mellitus, and menopause. Ethnicity influences Lp(a) levels, and African Americans on average have 2- to 3-fold higher levels of Lp(a).[50]

【 】 MECHANISMS OF INCREASED RISK

Multiple mechanisms have been implicated to explain the potential atherogenicity of Lp(a). Its LDL cholesterol-like properties may allow delivery of cholesterol at sites of vessel injury. The apo(a) moiety is structurally similar to plasminogen but lacks fibrinolytic activity. By competing with plasminogen in binding to fibrin, Lp(a) may hinder endogenous fibrinolysis.[51] Lp(a) has been shown to stimulate the growth of human vascular smooth muscle cells in vitro and enhance expression of adhesion molecules in endothelial cells.

【 】 ASSAYS

Lp(a) levels may range up to 300 mg/dL in the population, with a frequency distribution that is skewed toward higher concentrations. Risk of cardiovascular events appears to be increased when levels exceed 20 to 30 mg/dL. Most of the assays for Lp(a) are immunoassays, including ELISA and immunoturbidimetric methods. An alternative to immunoassays is the measurement of the amount of cholesterol associated with Lp(a) by lipoprotein electrophoresis. Information about apo(a) size isoforms may be relevant; in some studies, elevated plasma Lp(a) levels were associated with CHD only among carriers of small apo(a) isoform sizes.[52]

【 】 EVIDENCE OF ASSOCIATION

A series of cross-sectional and retrospective case-control studies implicate Lp(a) as a risk factor for CHD. In most retrospective studies, higher levels of plasma Lp(a) have been found in patients with CHD than in controls. Several prospective studies have found Lp(a) to be related to future cardiovascular events.[53–55] However, in the Physicians' Health Study, Lp(a) levels failed to predict cardiovascular events.[56] The conflicting data from the prospective studies may be attributable to variability in the methods used to determine Lp(a) levels and the fact that different isoforms of the apo(a) component of Lp(a) might have different atherogenic potential. In 2000, a meta-analysis of 27 prospective studies of 5000 subjects with a mean follow-up of 10 years concluded that Lp(a) was an independent risk factor for future cardiovascular events (Figure 64-4).[57] Among individuals participating in the population-based studies, patients with

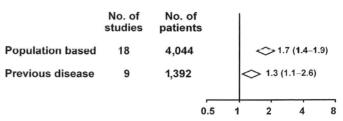

	No. of studies	No. of patients	Risk ratio (95% CI) (top third vs bottom third)
Population based	18	4,044	1.7 (1.4–1.9)
Previous disease	9	1,392	1.3 (1.1–2.6)

FIGURE 64-4. Prospective studies of lipoprotein(a) and coronary heart disease. Risk ratios compare top and bottom thirds of baseline measurements. Diamonds indicate the combined risk ratio and its 95% confidence interval (CI) for each grouping. *(Modified from Danesh et al.[57] Used with permission of American Heart Association, Inc.)*

baseline Lp(a) values in the top tertile had a 70% greater risk than those in the bottom tertile.

Although African Americans have a higher median plasma Lp(a) concentration than white individuals, this difference does not seem to translate into an increased risk of CHD.[50] CHD risk may be increased synergistically in patients with elevated Lp(a) levels and low levels of high-density lipoprotein (HDL) cholesterol.[58,59] However, no such interaction was observed in the Framingham Offspring Study.[60] In a large cohort of subjects who underwent percutaneous coronary intervention and stent placement, Lp(a) levels did not influence the 1-year clinical and angiographic outcome.[61]

【 】 CLINICAL IMPLICATIONS

Pharmacologic therapy of elevated Lp(a) levels is challenging, and plasma apheresis appears to be the most effective therapeutic modality. Although statins do not lower Lp(a) levels, lowering LDL cholesterol levels may decrease the atherogenicity of Lp(a). Maher and colleagues[62] found that, in patients with combined elevations of LDL cholesterol and Lp(a), a reduction in angiographic progression of CHD as well as in clinical event rates occurred with use of a statin, without any change in Lp(a) levels. Estrogens decrease plasma Lp(a) concentration, and a posthoc analysis from the Women's Health Study found that estrogens had a favorable impact on cardiovascular events in women who had elevated Lp(a) levels.[63] Niacin has been shown to have Lp(a)–lowering effects.[64] The effect of fibrates and omega-3 fatty acids on Lp(a) levels is yet to be established.

Lack of a standardized assay and limited therapeutic options in the treatment of elevated levels have impeded more widespread use of serum Lp(a) measurement in risk assessment. Measurement of Lp(a) levels may be useful in subjects with early-onset CHD or a family history of early-onset CHD or those who develop CHD in the absence of the conventional risk factors. Levels may need to be measured only once because of little variability within an individual. If elevated levels are detected, testing and counseling of family members may be warranted. The detection of high Lp(a) levels in a patient with CHD or at risk of developing CHD may be an indication for more aggressive therapy and may motivate patients to make lifestyle changes. The most common approaches to treatment are the use of statins to aggressively lower LDL cholesterol or initiation of niacin.

LOW-DENSITY LIPOPROTEIN PARTICLE SIZE

LDL particles differ in size and density. Two distinct phenotypes have been described: pattern B with a predominance of small LDL particles and pattern A with a higher proportion of large, more buoyant LDL particles.[65] Small LDL particles tend to coexist with elevated triglycerides and low HDL cholesterol. This trait has been called "atherogenic dyslipidemia" and appears to be highly heritable.[65] A predominance of small LDL particles is associated with a number of other cardiovascular risk factors, including metabolic syndrome, type 2 diabetes, and postprandial hypertriglyceridemia.[66]

【 】 MECHANISMS OF INCREASED RISK

Animal and in vitro studies suggest that small LDL particles are more atherogenic than larger LDL particles. This may be attributable to greater susceptibility to oxidation, increased binding to intimal proteoglycans, increased ability to cross into the subintimal space, and reduced affinity for the LDL receptor.[67]

【 】 ASSAYS

The standard for measurement of LDL particle size is analytical ultracentrifugation.[68] However, this is a difficult and time-consuming method. Density ultracentrifugation,[69] nondenaturing gradient gel electrophoresis,[70] and nuclear magnetic resonance[71] are used more commonly.

【 】 EVIDENCE OF ASSOCIATION

Several retrospective studies suggest that the small LDL particle size is associated with an increased risk for CHD.[70,72–74] These studies, however, do not clearly establish whether this risk is mediated independent of the coexisting lipoprotein abnormalities. Prospective studies are also not consistent for LDL particle size as an independent risk factor. A nested case-control study from the Stanford Five City Project showed that LDL particle size is associated inversely with CHD but not after the findings were adjusted for the ratio of total cholesterol to HDL cholesterol.[75] In the Physicians' Health Study, LDL particle size was associated with increased risk of myocardial infarction but not after adjustment for the triglyceride level.[76] In the Quebec Cardiovascular Study,[77] men in the first tertile of LDL particle size had a 3.6-fold increase in the risk of CHD compared with those in the third tertile. The relationship remained significant after adjustment for variations in LDL cholesterol, triglycerides, HDL cholesterol, and apo B concentrations.

【 】 CLINICAL IMPLICATIONS

Whether measurement of LDL particle size will improve the ability to predict risk of CHD in an individual patient needs to be clarified by further clinical and epidemiologic studies. Modification of LDL particle size may involve different approaches than those typically taken to lower LDL cholesterol.[78] An increase in LDL particle diameter has been seen after an intensive exercise training program.[79] Statins do not appear to alter LDL particle size,[80]

whereas ciprofibrate[81] and niacin[78] have been shown to increase LDL particle size. Because these interventions are also likely to alter other lipoprotein levels, prospective trials to determine outcomes after altering LDL particle size are not yet feasible. Interventions that reduce insulin resistance may also favorably impact LDL particle size. Thiazolidinediones have been shown to increase LDL particle size and increase resistance of LDL particles to oxidation in obese subjects.[82]

C-REACTIVE PROTEIN

Interest is increasing in the potential use of plasma levels of markers of inflammation in assessing risk of cardiovascular events. Because specific markers of atherosclerotic plaque inflammation are not available at present, circulating markers of systemic inflammation have been studied as surrogates. An acute-phase reactant that reflects systemic inflammation, CRP is the most widely studied of the inflammatory markers. It is a trace protein in healthy subjects, with a median concentration of around 1 mg/L.

【 】 MECHANISMS OF RISK

Inflammation in the arterial wall, inflammation elsewhere in the body, or both have been postulated to result in elevated CRP. CRP is associated with traditional risk factors such as diabetes mellitus, smoking, low HDL cholesterol, and obesity.[83] Other as yet unknown or unmeasured risk factors acting on the vessel wall may also influence CRP levels. The possibility has been raised that pathogens may be responsible for the elevation in CRP. However, CRP levels do not correlate with serologic markers of *Helicobacter pylori* or *Chlamydia pneumoniae* infection in the general population.[84]

It remains to be established whether CRP itself is atherogenic. CRP may be prothrombotic by increasing expression of tissue factor.[85] Transgenic mice that overexpress CRP are more prone to develop thrombosis after arterial injury.[86] CRP has been shown to activate complement,[87] decrease nitric oxide production,[88] and be associated with endothelial dysfunction.[89]

【 】 ASSAYS

CRP exhibits minimal diurnal or seasonal variation and is stable in blood samples even after prolonged storage. Relatively sensitive and inexpensive assays are commercially available. When interpreting levels, one needs to consider the presence of other risk factors as possibly influencing the CRP level. These include obesity, tobacco use, type 2 diabetes, hormone replacement therapy, and female sex. Recent cutoffs for CRP levels suggested by the Centers for Disease Control and Prevention-American Heart Association (CDC-AHA) guidelines, however, do not require consideration of these factors.[83]

【 】 EVIDENCE OF ASSOCIATION

In recent years, several prospective studies have related baseline CRP levels to the future risk of cardiovascular events. In the Multiple Risk

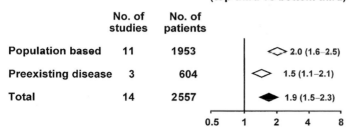

	No. of studies	No. of patients	Risk ratio (95% CI) (top third vs bottom third)
Population based	11	1953	2.0 (1.6–2.5)
Preexisting disease	3	604	1.5 (1.1–2.1)
Total	14	2557	1.9 (1.5–2.3)

0.5   1   2   4   8

FIGURE 64-5. Prospective studies of C-reactive protein and coronary heart disease. Risk ratios compare top and bottom thirds of baseline measurements. The combined risk ratio and its 95% confidence interval (CI) are indicated by unshaded diamonds for subtotals and a shaded diamond for total. All studies included in the meta-analysis were adjusted for age, sex, smoking history, and other conventional vascular risk factors. (Modified from Danesh at al.[84] Used with permission of BMJ Publishing Group.)

Factor Interventional Trial, increased CRP levels were associated with increased risk of CHD.[90] However, this relationship was detected only in smokers. In the Physicians' Health Study, baseline levels of CRP were predictive of future risk of myocardial infarction, thromboembolic stroke, and peripheral artery disease.[91,92] The risk of future events associated with CRP was independent of conventional risk factors as well as Lp(a), fibrinogen, and homocysteine. A meta-analysis by Danesh et al[42] reported a pooled relative risk of 1.9 (95% CI, 1.5–2.3) for the highest versus lowest thirds of the distribution of CRP (Figure 64-5). More recently, in a study of nearly 28,000 women followed up for an average of 8 years, CRP in the highest quintile was associated with a doubling of the risk of a cardiovascular event after adjustment for traditional risk factors.[93]

【 】 CLINICAL IMPLICATIONS

Recent CDC-AHA guidelines suggest optional use of CRP determination in patients at intermediate risk of CHD (based on the Framingham risk equation).[83] Widespread CRP screening is not recommended. People who are at very low risk or high risk are unlikely to benefit from further testing. Levels higher than 15 mg/L may indicate a "subclinical" infection or inflammation or other chronic disease and need to be evaluated appropriately.

If CRP is in the elevated range, then lifestyle changes should be the initial approach, including attempted weight reduction, low-fat diet, smoking cessation, and regular exercise. Recently, a diet containing several components that are known to lower serum cholesterol was shown to lower CRP.[94] Moderate alcohol consumption has been associated with a lower plasma CRP.[95] Statins have been shown to reduce CRP. Other medications that may lower CRP include fibrates and fish oil. Aspirin does not appear to affect CRP levels.

A reduction in CRP has not shown to be associated with a decrease in cardiovascular events. There is currently no drug that selectively lowers CRP. Whether statin therapy based on CRP levels will result in a reduction of cardiovascular events is not yet known. To answer this question, a trial is under way that will randomize 15,000 patients with elevated CRP values and LDL cholesterol levels less than 100 mg/dL to treatment with a statin or to placebo;[96] these patients would not therefore qualify for lipid-lowering therapy.

CONCLUSION

The importance of conventional risk factors in increasing the burden of atherosclerosis in the general population is well known. Efforts need to be intensified to treat these risk factors or prevent their onset. Although most patients who have cardiovascular events have 1 or more of the conventional risk factors,[97] the number and severity of the risk factors may not explain entirely the development of cardiovascular events in an individual. Atherosclerosis is a complex multifactorial disease process involving many pathways and both genetic and environmental factors. Estimation of the CHD risk in an individual on the basis of information derived from large epidemiologic studies, although helpful, is likely to be imprecise to varying degrees.

Clearly further work is needed to refine assessment of CHD risk in an individual. This includes continued research into the role of newer risk factors and the genetic epidemiology of atherosclerotic vascular disease. Advances in genomics and proteomics will likely lead to newer markers of atherosclerotic vascular disease. Such research will help unravel the web of causation of atherosclerotic vascular disease. For the newer markers to be clinically relevant, however, several criteria will need to be met, as outlined by Mosca[98] and Manolio.[99]

In the meantime, measurement of the nontraditional risk factors discussed herein may be useful in several clinical settings (Figure 64-6). The information derived may help motivate patients to make lifestyle changes and help physicians adjust the threshold for treatment of conventional risk factors. Pharmacologic as well as nonpharmacologic therapy may also be used, although evidence that such an approach would lead to reduction in cardiovascular events has not yet been produced.

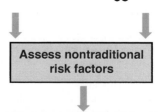

PRIMARY PREVENTION
- Family history of early-onset CHD
- Intermediate 10-y CHD risk

SECONDARY PREVENTION
- Early-onset CHD
- CHD in absence of conventional risk factors
- "Aggressive" disease

Assess nontraditional risk factors

- Motivate patient to make lifestyle changes
- Aggressive treatment of conventional risk factors
- Pharmacologic/nonpharmacologic treatment

FIGURE 64-6. A potential algorithm for the use of nontraditional risk factors. CHD = coronary heart disease.

REFERENCES

1. Expert Panel on Detection Evaluation, Treatment of High Blood Cholesterol in Adults. Executive Summary of The Third Report of The National Cholesterol Education Program (NCEP) Expert Panel on Detection, Evaluation, and Treatment of High Blood Cholesterol in Adults (Adult Treatment Panel III). *JAMA.* 2001;285:2486.

2. Ross R. Atherosclerosis: an inflammatory disease. *N Engl J Med.* 1999;340:115.

3. Akosah KO, Schaper A, Cogbill C, et al. Preventing myocardial infarction in the young adult in the first place: how do the National Cholesterol Education Panel III guidelines perform? *J Am Coll Cardiol.* 2003;41:1475.

4. Kullo IJ, McConnell JP, Bailey KR, et al. Relation of C-reactive protein and fibrinogen to coronary artery calcium in subjects with systemic hypertension. *Am J Cardiol.* 2003;92:56.

5. Kimura N, Keys A. Coronary heart disease in seven countries: X. Rural southern Japan. *Circulation.* 1970;41(suppl 4):I101.

6. Reddy KS, Yusuf S. Emerging epidemic of cardiovascular disease in developing countries. *Circulation.* 1998;97:596.

7. Smith SC Jr, Greenland P, Grundy SM. AHA Conference Proceedings. Prevention conference V: beyond secondary prevention: identifying the high-risk patient for primary prevention: executive summary. *Circulation.* 2000; 101:111.

8. Packard CJ, O'Reilly DS, Caslake MJ, et al, for the West of ScotlandCoronary Prevention Study Group. Lipoprotein-associated phospholipase A2 as an independent predictor of coronary heart disease. *N Engl J Med.* 2000;343:1148.

9. Miyazaki H, Matsuoka H, Cooke JP, et al. Endogenous nitric oxide synthase inhibitor: a novel marker of atherosclerosis. *Circulation.* 1999;99:1141.

10. Bayes-Genis A, Conover CA, Overgaard MT, et al. Pregnancy-associated plasma protein A as a marker of acute coronary syndromes. *N Engl J Med.* 2001; 345:1022.

11. Patrono C, FitzGerald GA. Isoprostanes: potential markers of oxidant stress in atherothrombotic disease. *Arterioscler Thromb Vasc Biol.* 1997;17:2309.

12. Brennan M-L, Penn MS, Van Lente F, et al. Prognostic value of myeloperoxidase in patients with chest pain. *N Engl J Med.* 2003;349:1595.

13. Grundy SM, Pasternak R, Greenland P, et al. Assessment of cardiovascular risk by use of multiple-risk-factor assessment equations: a statement for healthcare professionals from the American Heart Association and the American College of Cardiology. *Circulation.* 1999;100:1481.

14. Mudd SH, Skovby F, Levy HL, et al. The natural history of homocystinuria due to cystathionine beta-synthase deficiency. *Am J Hum Genet* 1985;37:1.

15. McCully KS. Homocystinuria, arteriosclerosis, methylmalonic aciduria, and methyltransferase deficiency: a key case revisited. *Nutr Rev* 1992;50:7.

16. Jacques PF, Bostom AG, Williams RR, et al. Relation between folate status, a common mutation in methylenetetrahydrofolate reductase, and plasma homocysteine concentrations. *Circulation.* 1996;93:7.

17. Ueland PM, Refsum H, Beresford SA, et al. The controversy over homocysteine and cardiovascular risk. *Am J Clin Nutr.* 2000;72:324.

18. Brattstrom L, Wilcken DE. Homocysteine and cardiovascular disease: cause or effect? *Am J Clin Nutr.* 2000;72:315.

19. Welch GN, Loscalzo J. Homocysteine and atherothrombosis. *N Engl J Med.* 1998;338:10428.

20. Woo KS, Chook P, Lolin YI, et al. Hyperhomocyst(e)inemia is a risk factor for arterial endothelial dysfunction in humans. *Circulation.* 1997;96:2542.

21. Bostom AG, Silbershatz H, Rosenberg IH, et al. Nonfasting plasma total homocysteine levels and all-cause and cardiovascular disease mortality in elderly Framingham men and women. *Arch Intern Med.* 1999;159:1077.

22. Bostom AG, Jacques PF, Nadeau MR, et al. Post-methionine load hyperhomocysteinemia in persons with normal fasting total plasma homocysteine: initial results from the NHLBI Family Heart Study. *Atherosclerosis.* 1995;116:147.

23. Boushey CJ, Beresford SA, Omenn GS, et al. A quantitative assessment of plasma homocysteine as a risk factor for vascular disease: probable benefits of increasing folic acid intakes. *JAMA.* 1995;274:1049.

24. Homocysteine Studies Collaboration. Homocysteine and risk of ischemic heart disease and stroke: a meta-analysis. *JAMA.* 2002;88:2015.

25. Klerk M, Verhoef P, Clarke R, et al, and the MTHFR Studies Collaboration Group. MTHFR 677C→T polymorphism and risk of coronary heart disease: a meta-analysis. *JAMA.* 2002;288:2023.

26. Wald DS, Law M, Morris JK. Homocysteine and cardiovascular disease: evidence on causality from a meta-analysis. *BMJ.* 2002;325:1202.

27. Schnyder G, Roffi M, Flammer Y, et al. Association of plasma homocysteine with restenosis after percutaneous coronary angioplasty. *Eur Heart J.* 2002;23:726.

28. Schnyder G, Roffi M, Pin R, et al. Decreased rate of coronary restenosis after lowering of plasma homocysteine levels. *N Engl J Med.* 2001;345:1593.

29. Schnyder G, Roffi M, Flammer Y, et al. Effect of homocysteine-lowering therapy with folic acid, vitamin B_{12}, and vitamin B_6 on clinical outcome after percutaneous coronary intervention: the Swiss Heart study: a randomized controlled trial. *JAMA.* 2002;88:973.

30. Lange HW, Dambrink JH, Pasalary M. Folate therapy increases in stent restenosis: results from the Folate After Coronary Intervention Trial (FACIT). Presented at: American College of Cardiology 52nd Annual Scientific Session; March 30–April 2, 2003; Chicago, Ill.

31. Bostom AG, Shemin D, Lapane KL, et al. High dose-B-vitamin treatment of hyperhomocysteinemia in dialysis patients. *Kidney Int.* 1996;9:147.

32. Wilcken DE, Wilcken B, Dudman NP, et al. Homocystinuria: the effects of betaine in the treatment of patients not responsive to pyridoxine. *N Engl J Med.* 1983;309:448.

33. Malinow MR, Duell PB, Hess DL, et al. Reduction of plasma homocyst(e)ine levels by breakfast cereal fortified with folic acid in patients with coronary heart disease. *N Engl J Med.* 1998;338:1009.

34. Bostom AG, Selhub J, Jacques PF, et al. Power shortage: clinical trials testing the "homocysteine hypothesis" against a background of folic acid-fortified cereal grain flour. *Ann Intern Med.* 2001;135:133.

35. Hamsten A, Iselius L, de Faire U, et al. Genetic and cultural inheritance of plasma fibrinogen concentration. *Lancet.* 1987;2:988.

36. Ernst E, Resch KL. Fibrinogen as a cardiovascular risk factor: a meta-analysis and review of the literature. *Ann Intern Med.* 1993;118:956.

37. Folsom A. Fibrinogen and cardiovascular risk in the Atherosclerosis and Risk in Communities (ARIC) study. In: Ernst E, ed. *Fibrinogen, A 'New Cardiovascular Risk Factor.'* Wein, Blackwell; 1992.

38. Ernst E. The role of fibrinogen as a cardiovascular risk factor. *Atherosclerosis.* 1993;100:1.

39. Maresca G, Di Blasio A, Marchioli R, et al. Measuring plasma fibrinogen to predict stroke and myocardial infarction: an update. *Arterioscler Thromb Vasc Biol.* 1999;19:1368.

40. Stec JJ, Silbershatz H, Tofler GH, et al. Association of fibrinogen with cardiovascular risk factors and cardiovascular disease in the Framingham Offspring Population. *Circulation.* 2000;102:1634.

41. Ma J, Hennekens CH, Ridker PM, et al. A prospective study of fibrinogen and risk of myocardial infarction in the Physicians' Health Study. *J Am Coll Cardiol.* 1999;33:1347.

42. Danesh J, Collins R, Appleby P, et al. Association of fibrinogen, C-reactive protein, albumin, or leukocyte count with coronary heart disease: meta-analyses of prospective studies. *JAMA.* 1998;279:1477.

43. Murabito JM, D'Agostino RB, Silbershatz H, et al. Intermittent claudication: a risk profile from the Framingham Heart Study. *Circulation.* 1997;96:44.

44. Tracy RP, Bovill EG, Yanez D, et al. Fibrinogen and factor VIII, but not factor VII, are associated with measures of subclinical cardiovascular disease in the elderly: results from the Cardiovascular Health Study. *Arterioscler Thromb Vasc Biol.* 1995;15:1269.

45. Levenson J, Giral P, Megnien JL, et al. Fibrinogen and its relations to subclinical extracoronary and coronary atherosclerosis in hypercholesterolemic men. *Arterioscler Thromb Vasc Biol.* 1997;17:45.

46. Heinrich J, Balleisen L, Schulte H, et al. Fibrinogen and factor VII in the prediction of coronary risk: results from the PROCAM study in healthy men. *Arterioscler Thromb.* 1994;14:54.

47. Cantin B, Despres JP, Lamarche B, et al. Association of fibrinogen and lipoprotein(a) as a coronary heart disease risk factor in men (The Quebec Cardiovascular Study). *Am J Cardiol.* 2002;89:662.

48. Ernst E. Lowering the plasma fibrinogen concentration with drugs. *Clin Pharmacol.* 1992;11:968.

49. Scanu AM. Lipoprotein(a): a genetic risk factor for premature coronary heart disease. *JAMA.* 1992;267:3326.

50. Moliterno DJ, Jokinen EV, Miserez AR, et al. No association between plasma lipoprotein(a) concentrations and the presence or absence of coronary atherosclerosis in African-Americans. *Arterioscler Thromb Vasc Biol.* 1995;15:850.

51. Hajjar KA, Gavish D, Breslow JL, et al. Lipoprotein(a) modulation of endothelial cell surface fibrinolysis and its potential role in atherosclerosis. *Nature.* 1989;339:303.

52. Sandholzer C, Saha N, Kark JD, et al. Apo(a) isoforms predict risk for coronary heart disease: a study in six populations. *Arterioscler Thromb.* 1992;12:1214.

53. Assmann G, Schulte H, von Eckardstein A. Hypertriglyceridemia and elevated lipoprotein(a) are risk factors for major coronary events in middle-aged men. *Am J Cardiol.* 1996;77:1179.

54. Cremer P, Nagel D, Labrot B, et al. Lipoprotein Lp(a) as predictor of myocardial infarction in comparison to fibrinogen, LDL cholesterol and other risk factors: results from the prospective Gottingen Risk Incidence and Prevalence Study (GRIPS). *Eur J Clin Invest.* 1994;24:444.

55. Schaefer EJ, Lamon-Fava S, Jenner JL, et al. Lipoprotein(a) levels and risk of coronary heart disease in men: the Lipid Research Clinics Coronary Primary Prevention Trial. *JAMA*. 1994;271:999.

56. Ridker PM, Hennekens CH, Stampfer MJ. A prospective study of lipoprotein(a) and the risk of myocardial infarction. *JAMA*. 1993;270:2195.

57. Danesh J, Collins R, Peto R. Lipoprotein(a) and coronary heart disease: meta-analysis of prospective studies. *Circulation*. 2000;102:1082.

58. Solymoss BC, Marcil M, Wesolowska E, et al. Relation of coronary artery disease in women <60 years of age to the combined elevation of serum lipoprotein (a) and total cholesterol to high-density cholesterol ratio. *Am J Cardiol*. 1993;72:1215.

59. von Eckardstein A, Schulte H, Cullen P, et al. Lipoprotein(a) further increases the risk of coronary events in men with high global cardiovascular risk. *J Am Coll Cardiol*. 2001;37:434.

60. Bostom AG, Cupples LA, Jenner JL, et al. Elevated plasma lipoprotein(a) and coronary heart disease in men aged 55 years and younger: a prospective study. *JAMA*. 1996;276:544.

61. Wehinger A, Kastrati A, Elezi S, et al. Lipoprotein(a) and coronary thrombosis and restenosis after stent placement. *J Am Coll Cardiol*. 1999;33:1005.

62. Maher VM, Brown BG, Marcovina SM, et al. Effects of lowering elevated LDL cholesterol on the cardiovascular risk of lipoprotein(a). *JAMA*. 1995;274:1771.

63. Shlipak MG, Simon JA, Vittinghoff E, et al. Estrogen and progestin, lipoprotein(a), and the risk of recurrent coronary heart disease events after menopause. *JAMA*. 2000;283:1845.

64. Kashyap ML, McGovern ME, Berra K, et al. Long-term safety and efficacy of a once-daily niacin/lovastatin formulation for patients with dyslipidemia. *Am J Cardiol*. 2002;89:672.

65. Austin MA, Brunzell JD, Fitch WL, et al. Inheritance of low density lipoprotein subclass patterns in familial combined hyperlipidemia. *Arteriosclerosis*. 1990;10:520.

66. Roheim PS, Asztalos BF. Clinical significance of lipoprotein size and risk for coronary atherosclerosis. *Clin Chem*. 1995;41:147.

67. Griffin BA. Lipoprotein atherogenicity: an overview of current mechanisms. *Proc Nutr Soc*. 1999;58:163.

68. Lindgren FT, Jensen LC, Wills RD, et al. Flotation rates, molecular weights and hydrated densities of the low-density lipoproteins. *Lipids* 1969;4:337.

69. Krauss RM, Burke DJ. Identification of multiple subclasses of plasma low density lipoproteins in normal humans. *J Lipid Res*. 1982;23:97.

70. Austin MA, Breslow JL, Hennekens CH, et al. Low-density lipoprotein subclass patterns and risk of myocardial infarction. *JAMA*. 1988;260:1917.

71. Otvos JD, Jeyarajah EJ, Bennett DW, et al. Development of a proton nuclear magnetic resonance spectroscopic method for determining plasma lipoprotein concentrations and subspecies distributions from a single, rapid measurement. *Clin Chem*. 1992;38:1632.

72. Campos H, Blijlevens E, McNamara JR, et al. LDL particle size distribution: results from the Framingham Offspring Study. *Arterioscler Thromb*. 1992;12:1410.

73. Coresh J, Kwiterovich PO Jr, Smith HH, et al. Association of plasma triglyceride concentration and LDL particle diameter, density, and chemical composition with premature coronary artery disease in men and women. *J Lipid Res*. 1993;34:1687.

74. Griffin BA, Freeman DJ, Tait GW, et al. Role of plasma triglyceride in the regulation of plasma low density lipoprotein (LDL) subfractions: relative contribution of small, dense LDL to coronary heart disease risk. *Atherosclerosis*. 1994;106:241.

75. Gardner CD, Fortmann SP, Krauss RM. Association of small low-density lipoprotein particles with the incidence of coronary artery disease in men and women. *JAMA*. 1996;276:875.

76. Stampfer MJ, Krauss RM, Ma J, et al. A prospective study of triglyceride level, low-density lipoprotein particle diameter, and risk of myocardial infarction. *JAMA*. 1996;276:882.

77. Lamarche B, Tchernof A, Moorjani S, et al. Small, dense low-density lipoprotein particles as a predictor of the risk of ischemic heart disease in men: prospective results from the Quebec Cardiovascular Study. *Circulation*. 1997;95:69.

78. Superko HR, Krauss RM. Differential effects of nicotinic acid in subjects with different LDL subclass patterns. *Atherosclerosis*. 1992;95:69.

79. Dreon DM, Fernstrom HA, Miller B, et al. Low-density lipoprotein subclass patterns and lipoprotein response to a reduced-fat diet in men. *FASEB J*. 1994;8:121.

80. Gaw A. Can the clinical efficacy of the HMG CoA reductase inhibitors be explained solely by their effects on LDL-cholesterol? *Atherosclerosis*. 1996;125:267.

81. Gaw A, Packard CJ, Caslake MJ, et al. Effects of ciprofibrate on LDL metabolism in man. *Atherosclerosis*. 1994;108:137.

82. Tack CJ, Smits P, Demacker PN, et al. Troglitazone decreases the proportion of small, dense LDL and increases the resistance of LDL to oxidation in obese subjects. *Diabetes Care*. 1998;21:796.

83. Pearson TA, Mensah GA, Alexander RW, et al. Markers of inflammation and cardiovascular disease: application to clinical and public health practice: a statement for healthcare professionals from the Centers for Disease Control and Prevention and the American Heart Association. *Circulation*. 2003;107:499.

84. Danesh J, Whincup P, Walker M, et al. Low grade inflammation and coronary heart disease: prospective study and updated meta-analyses. *BMJ*. 2000;321:199.

85. Cermak J, Key NS, Bach RR, et al. C-reactive protein induces human peripheral blood monocytes to synthesize tissue factor. *Blood*. 1993;82:513.

86. Danenberg HD, Szalai AJ, Swaminathan RV, et al. Increased thrombosis after arterial injury in human C-reactive protein-transgenic mice. *Circulation*. 2003;108:512.

87. Wolbink GJ, Brouwer MC, Buysmann S, et al. CRP-mediated activation of complement in vivo: assessment by measuring circulating complement-C-reactive protein complexes. *J Immunol*. 1996;157:473.

88. Verma S, Wang CH, Li SH, et al. A self-fulfilling prophecy: C-reactive protein attenuates nitric oxide production and inhibits angiogenesis. *Circulation*. 2002;106:913.

89. Fichtlscherer S, Rosenberger G, Walter DH, et al. Elevated C-reactive protein levels and impaired endothelial vasoreactivity in patients with coronary artery disease. *Circulation* 2000;102:1000.

90. Kuller LH, Tracy RP, Shaten J, et al. Relation of C-reactive protein and coronary heart disease in the MRFIT nested case-control study: Multiple Risk Factor Intervention Trial. *Am J Epidemiol*. 1996;144:537.

91. Ridker PM, Cushman M, Stampfer MJ, et al. Inflammation, aspirin, and the risk of cardiovascular disease in apparently healthy men. *N Engl J Med*. 1997;336:973.

92. Ridker PM, Cushman M, Stampfer MJ, et al. Plasma concentration of C-reactive protein and risk of developing peripheral vascular disease. *Circulation*. 1998;97:425.

93. Ridker PM, Rifai N, Rose L, et al. Comparison of C-reactive protein and low-density lipoprotein cholesterol levels in the prediction of first cardiovascular events. *N Engl J Med* 2002;347:1557.

94. Jenkins DJ, Kendall CW, Marchie A, et al. Effects of a dietary portfolio of cholesterol-lowering foods vs lovastatin on serum lipids and C-reactive protein. *JAMA*. 2003;290:502.

95. Sierksma A, van der Gaag MS, Kluft C, et al. Moderate alcohol consumption reduces plasma C-reactive protein and fibrinogen levels: a randomized, diet-controlled intervention study. *Eur J Clin Nutr*. 2002;56:1130.

96. Ridker PM. Should statin therapy be considered for patients with elevated C-reactive protein? The need for a definitive clinical trial. *Eur Heart J*. 2001;22:2135.

97. Greenland P, Knoll MD, Stamler J, et al. Major risk factors as antecedents of fatal and nonfatal coronary heart disease events. *JAMA*. 2003;290:891.

98. Mosca L. C-reactive protein: to screen or not to screen? *N Engl J Med*. 2002;347:1615.

99. Manolio T. Novel risk markers and clinical practice. *N Engl J Med*. 2003;349:1587.

PART 8 Preclinical and Clinical Trials

CHAPTER (65)

Preclinical Laboratory Functions

Keith A. Robinson, PhD, Nicolas A. F. Chronos, MD, and Robert S. Schwartz, MD

Although ideas for novel interventional cardiology devices and therapies may initially be conceived in the mind of the physician, scientist, or engineer from experiences and observations in the clinical setting, it is within the boundaries of the preclinical laboratory where those ideas are realized. This venue is the site of device or treatment testing, development, and retooling; it also represents the means for final entry into clinical evaluation. For fulfilling both of these vital roles, the preclinical laboratory is a crucial link in the process of translating basic discoveries and engineering concepts into clinical practice for the improvement of cardiovascular patient care.

Although the reality of the assertions mentioned here is understood intuitively, the subtleties of preclinical laboratory functions and the details and requirements of laboratory daily operations are not so readily appreciated. The intent of this chapter is to introduce the scope of those functions and operations, as well as to convey insights into some of the processes of translational research. It is hoped that both fledgling investigators as well as seasoned veterans find informative content herein.

HISTORICAL FOUNDATIONS OF THE INTERVENTIONAL PRECLINICAL LABORATORY

One may reasonably trace the roots of the interventional preclinical laboratory back through the millennia, past William Harvey, whose experiments on both human and lower-animal subjects in the 17th century established modern concepts of the physiology of blood circulation and the function of the heart[1]; before the work of the great anatomist Andreas Vesalius, who defined human anatomy based in part on dissections of animals[2]; back even to

Galen and before the founding of civilization to the curiosity of our species for the workings of the body and the means to treat disease. However, our heritage is most directly linked to the first interventional cardiologist, Andreas Gruentzig, the inventor of coronary angioplasty and the founder of the field of catheter-based coronary intervention. It was Gruentzig who reported in 1976 on an animal experiment conducted in Zurich, Switzerland, that demonstrated the utility and feasibility of his prototype balloon catheter system for the percutaneous transluminal dilatation of a coronary stenosis (Figure 65-1).[3]

In that study, Gruentzig used a canine preparation of coronary artery catheterization. His surgical collaborator, Marko Turina, performed a thoracotomy and tied a partial ligature around the left circumflex artery. Gruentzig performed angiography measuring proximal and distal diameters and the coronary stenosis, as well as transstenotic pressure gradient, then maneuvered his balloon catheter into position and inflated it to break the ligature, relieving the stenosis and normalizing the distal coronary pressure. Through this straightforward experiment, the new technique of coronary angioplasty was invented and the field of coronary intervention was born. Without a preclinical evaluation of some type and involving the support and participation of his surgical collaborator, it is doubtful that translation of Gruentzig's ideas into clinical reality would ever have occurred.

From that time forward, numerous interventional cardiology preclinical laboratories emerged and flourished worldwide. Many have contributed significantly to the field of coronary and peripheral vascular intervention, and the world literature, as well as the revolutionary advances of the medical device, pharmaceutics, and biotechnology industries echoes the contributions these labs and their investigators and technologists have made.[4–9] With the progress of history into the present, some laboratories recently

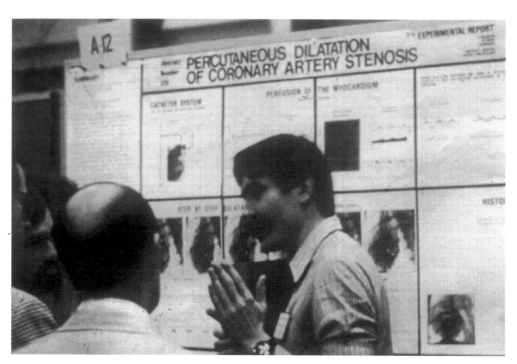

FIGURE 65-1. Andreas Gruentzig explaining his novel balloon catheter angioplasty system to a captivated audience at the 1976 American College of Cardiology Scientific Sessions. *(Photo courtesy of Spencer B. King, III, MD.)*

(1) small exploratory "proof-of-concept" studies to evaluate the feasibility of a prototype cardiovascular device; (2) larger studies to determine efficacy of a potential new therapy in an animal model of disease; and (3) safety studies intended for submission to the US Food and Drug Administration (FDA) as part of investigational new device (IND) or drug filings.

None of these three types of studies fit easily into the research bureaucracies of large academic medical institutions, which are fashioned primarily to accommodate the aforementioned government- or agency-sponsored programs. Signing of confidentiality and research contract agreements, concern for intellectual property and confidentiality, institutional animal care and use committee review and approval, indirect cost assessments, and other aspects of the university administrative processes can be agonizingly slow and financially onerous to the device and drug industry sponsors who often are in fast-paced competition to produce marketable products within a limited research and development (R & D) budget. Furthermore, the tight control of the research process and personnel necessary for studies compliant with Good Laboratory Practice (GLP) mandated by the FDA for preclinical studies intended for filing submissions is not typically possible in the university setting.

Although some academic centers understand the importance and benefits of such research and are devising new means to accommodate research needed by corporate entities, many are either unable or unwilling to make the necessary adjustments. Contract research laboratories, however, which are GLP compliant and operate in businesslike fashion for budgeting and contracting, are often tailored primarily for toxicology/pathology studies in rodents and other species. The specialized types of animal preparations and equipment, as well as personnel with scientific acumen and technical expertise for catheter-based procedures that are needed in interventional research, may be either unavailable or suboptimal in for-profit contract labs. Consequently, independent nonprofit research institutions are an attractive alternative to academic medical centers and contract laboratories for performance of interventional preclinical studies. Such environments can be designed and developed with the needs of the biomedical device, pharmaceutics, and biotechnology industries considered, and maintain high academic standards as well.

evolved into quite different organizations than they were even several short years ago, as technology and science continually push the edges of the clinical envelope even further.

ENVIRONMENT FOR THE INTERVENTIONAL PRECLINICAL LABORATORY

Many, if not most, interventional cardiology animal laboratories either currently operate or had their origin in the setting of medical academia. This environment is in most instances highly conducive to the pursuit of both basic and clinical research. Knowledge transfer from mentors and interaction with colleagues is readily available and there is access to various support services particularly in the form of libraries, presentation formats, laboratory animal care resources, and, often, laboratory space and equipment. In addition, the administrative components usually provide services for regulatory compliance, as well as contractual arrangements with entities sponsoring research projects.

There are, however, impediments to the research conducted in interventional animal labs as experienced in the academic institutions. Large academic medical centers have traditionally been oriented toward support of basic research sponsored by government agencies such as the National Institutes of Health, National Science Foundation, and private nonprofit agencies such as the American Heart Association, the Howard Hughes Foundation, and others. Yet, more often than not, the majority of research carried out in the interventional lab has focus that is quite different from large, agency-sponsored basic research. Frequently, research projects for interventional labs are sponsored by medical device, biotechnology, or pharmaceutics companies and fall into one of three categories:

FACILITIES AND EQUIPMENT

The physical facilities of the interventional preclinical lab depend on the scope of research to be conducted. At a minimum, a large-animal cardiac catheterization suite is needed, because the core of

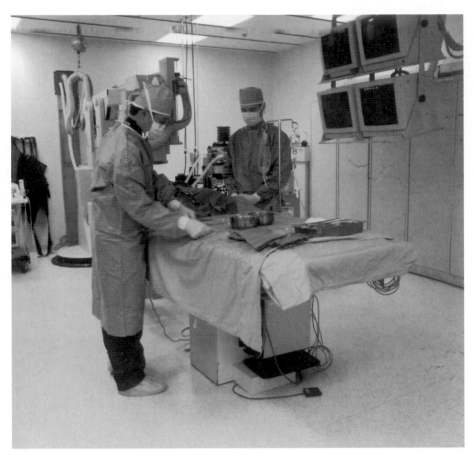

FIGURE 65-2. Research fellow Dr. Takafumi Ueno and technologist Pat Mulkey performing pig cardiac catheterization. The animal cath lab houses a Phillips OM200 cinefluoroscope with online quantitative angiography system, a Marquette MacLab electrocardiography and hemodynamic monitor, Acuson echocardiography machine, ancillary equipment and supplies.

measurements. Many minor equipment items such as tabletop centrifuges, activated clotting time (ACT) machines, infusion pumps, and similar apparatus complete the laboratory's capabilities. Overall, the appearance of the preclinical interventional laboratory resembles that of a clinical cardiac catheterization laboratory.

A variety of ancillary laboratories may be developed to extend the research capacities of the preclinical operation. The types of equipment needed may vary widely, and for investigators in an academic environment, these resources might be available through collaboration rather than within the scope of the interventional cardiology division. Histology processing and light microscopy are the most commonly needed components (Figure 65-5), because histologic evaluations of blood vessels, myocardium, and other tissues implanted with devices such as stents or otherwise affected by experimental treatments frequently provide the critical dependent variables of preclinical research studies. Facilities for necropsy and tissue harvest with apparatus and supplies for initial sample preparation by chemical fixation or other means are clearly necessary. Automated tissue processors are a practical means to efficiently dehydrate and infiltrate large numbers of samples, saving labor and supplies. Embedding stations and standard rotary microtomes enable preparation of paraffin sections useful for a variety of

translational research in our field is the testing of interventional vascular devices and associated drug or biotechnology therapies in clinically relevant, large-animal preparations. Fluoroscopy remains the fundamental means for performance of catheterization, angiography and ventriculography, and experimental intervention (Figure 65-2). Quantitative angiography is essential for accurate vessel measurement in the sizing of stent implants and angioplasty balloon catheters, which should be maintained within narrow limits to reduce variability of vascular responses (Figure 65-3). Echocardiography is an increasingly useful adjunct both for the analytical assessment of cardiac function and dimensions as well as guidance for catheter-based procedures such as endoventricular intramyocardial injections (Figure 65-4). Intravascular ultrasound is also useful for certain applications. Physiologic monitoring equipment for basic electrocardiography and comprehensive hemodynamic assessment, including left and right side cardiac and vascular pressures, the first derivative pressure measurements of ventricular systolic contractility and diastolic relaxation ($+d\,P/dt$ and $-d\,P/dt$, respectively), and cardiac output is a core requirement and can be used not only for diagnostics in performance of catheterization procedures but for basic safety determinations as well. More complex systems for evaluation of global and regional ventricular performance, such as sonomicrometry, have become increasingly more useful as the current era of cardiac cell therapy and tissue engineering virtually mandates these more precise

purposes; however, for sectioning of stented arteries or tissue with other metal implants, methacrylate plastic embedding will be needed requiring sections to be prepared with precision saw-and-grinding or heavy-duty microtome (see Figure 65-5). Preparation of quality sections using these techniques is no trivial task; the equipment, supplies, technologic expertise, and labor involved represent a substantial investment of finances, time, and effort.

Light microscopy is best performed using modern systems with digital imaging and analysis. An upright brightfield or combined brightfield and epifluorescence microscope with a range of objective lenses and filters, digital camera, and computer with capture board and software for image processing and measurement fulfill the most basic requirements (Figure 65-6).

Other laboratory environments and equipment may be sought to support a range of investigational outcomes. These may include capabilities to evaluate device or vessel thrombogenicity and vasomotor reactivity; assess biochemical components; perform cell and tissue culture; determine gene expression patterns; and potentially fulfill other research needs. Each of these requires facilities and equipment unique to the particular analytic approach; and the extent of environment and facilities varies depending on the sophistication applied into the study design.

For example, thrombogenicity of a novel stent or stent coating could be assessed in a variety of ways. One of the easiest would require little in terms of facilities, equipment, or labor. Stents could

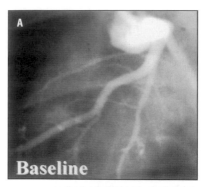
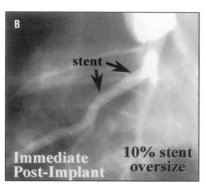
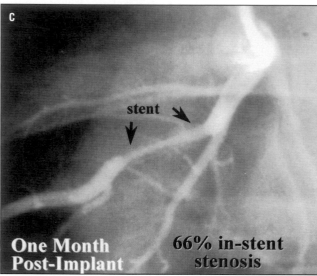

FIGURE 65-3. Angiography of polymer membrane—covered stent placement in pig left anterior descending coronary artery. Oversizing of the covered stent by 10% resulted in a tubular 66% stenosis at 1-month follow-up.

simply be weighed and placed in a tube of human or animal blood for a given time, removed, and then weighed and photographed; thrombus weight and scoring of thrombus severity would be the dependent variables for this analysis and only test tubes, an analytic balance, and a camera are needed. However, this design is inferior since it does not approach replicating the in vivo conditions of stented arteries. In this experiment, blood is static rather than flowing, is not under the influence of systemic conditions (eg, temperature, gas exchange, neurohumoral factors), and is affected in unpredictable ways by exposure to anticoagulants and other variables. All these characteristics of the test system not only render a set of circumstances far removed from the physiologic milieu, but also introduce artifacts that confound interpretation of results.

Improvements could and should be made in both the experimental setup as well as the analytic techniques, but necessarily implicate increased expense in equipment and supplies as well as greater investment of personnel. The next level of improvement in this example might involve deployment of the stents within silicone rubber tubing with perfusion of blood through the tubing using an apparatus consisting of a roller pump and fluid reservoir. Enhancement of this basic setup might be achieved by use of a water bath to maintain physiologic temperature in the system, and maintenance of physiologic gas pressures and pH using aeration with 95%-air/5%-CO_2 and frequent sampling to adjust acid–base balance as needed. Improvement in the measurement tools might

consist of obtaining both wet and dry thrombus weights to help control for variability in water content that could develop from differences in hydrophilicity of thrombus components, or embedding and sectioning the thrombus-containing stents to measure thrombus cross-sectional area using histomorphometry.

The final evolution of design for this type of experiment would be the use of an exteriorized arteriovenous shunt with on-line quantitative imaging of thrombus using cumulative serial gamma camera scans in the conscious non-human primate.[15] Isolation, radioisotopic labeling, and reinfusion of autologous platelets in this test system allows precise determination of platelet accumulation on a stent or other device interposed in tubing with blood flowing from the femoral artery to femoral vein; this measures the primary element of arterial thrombus formation. Fibrinogen can also be labeled to determine fibrin deposition providing a method for measurement of this important thrombus component that can reveal subtle differences in the pathways to thrombosis. Correlative morphologic observations such as macroscopy and scanning electron microscopy of the subsequently perfusion-fixed samples enable a thorough interpretation of results from a highly reproducible experimental system, regarding the performance of biomimetic stent coatings or other technological developments.[16] Variability within groups is reduced when different devices can be run on sequential days in the same animal under similar conditions. Although this approach is clearly the most precise means available for assessing vascular device thrombogenicity, the facilities, equipment, and personnel necessary represent a substantial commitment beyond the capacities of most interventional laboratories and thus requiring collaboration or subcontracting with a fully developed and staffed laboratory.

To summarize, the facilities and equipment in and around the interventional preclinical laboratory reflect a synthesis of the interests and specializations of the investigators coupled with and balanced by the resources at their disposal.

PERSONNEL

An integral component of the preclinical lab is the personnel who staff it. Dedication, commitment, experience, intelligence, team spirit, problem-solving skills, adaptability, an appetite for hard work, and a thirst for knowledge are some of the personal characteristics that enable individual workers to contribute to a successful laboratory operation. It is essential that senior personnel establish a positive, organized work environment and lead the team by example.

REGULATORY COMPLIANCE

Preclinical research is bound and governed by guidelines established and maintained by a number of regulatory agencies and accreditation organizations. In the United States, the use of

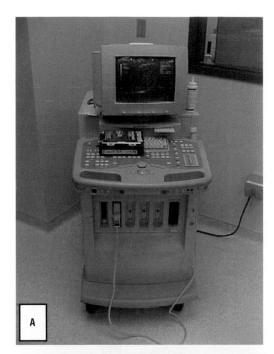

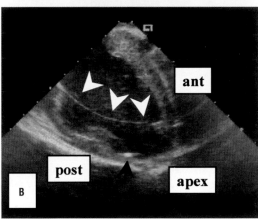

FIGURE 65-4. Echocardiography in the preclinical interventional laboratory. (**A**) Acuson echocardiography machine. (**B**) Intracardiac echocardiography (ICE) long-axis image showing intramyocardial injection catheter (*white arrowheads*) in left ventricle, during injection in anteroapical region; bright spot (*black arrow*) is the site of previous injection.

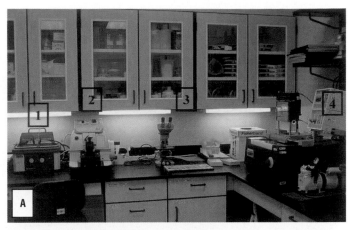

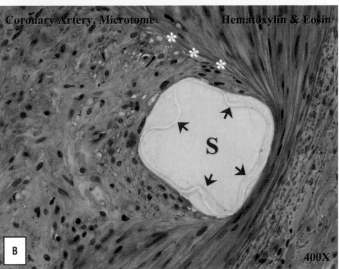

FIGURE 65-5. Histology of stented arteries. (**A**) Portion of plastic-slide histotechnology laboratory: (1) water bath; (2) Leica heavy-duty microtome; (3) slide review station; (4) Exakt precision grinder. (**B**) light microscopy of H & E-stained methacrylate section of pig coronary artery fixed 1 month after implant of polymer-coated metal stent; remnant of polymer coating (*arrows*) is seen in stent-strut void (S). * = internal elastic lamina.

experimental animals is ruled by federal laws (Animal Welfare Act)[17] and overseen by the US Department of Agriculture (USDA). The National Research Council publishes a guidance document that has been a fundamental basis for animal research in this country since the 1960s.[18] Any organization, whether academic or commercial, that performs experimentation involving the use of live animals is required to comply with these guidelines and must register with the USDA. Any entity performing research on live animals that is supported by the Public Health Service (ie, National Institutes of Health) must comply with the PHS Policy on Humane Care and Use of Laboratory Animals, mandated by the Health Research Extension Act of 1985 (Public Law 99–158, section 495). This document, published by the Office of Laboratory Animal Welfare (OLAW), provides resources for infrastructure development related to preclinical research, including documents pertaining to the staffing and operation of the

institutional animal care and use committee (IACUC). An annual compliance report resulting from oversight of animal care and use by the IACUC is required by OLAW.

The highest standard of laboratory animal use is upheld by the Association for the Assessment and Accreditation of Laboratory Animal Care International (AAALAC International).[19] This organization is not a government body, but an independent agency that provides a system of guidelines and inspections targeted to develop and maintain animal research facilities at an advanced level of operation. Certain funding agencies such as the American Heart Association require proof of certification by AAALAC before providing grant support for studies involving use of experimental animals.

Research intended for submission by a sponsoring for-profit corporate entity toward an investigational new device or drug filing to the FDA must adhere to the guidelines governing nonclinical research (laboratory animal or in vitro studies). The FDA is a branch of the federal government that, among other functions, is responsible for the oversight of research supporting these submissions. A document describing the requirements for such research to be

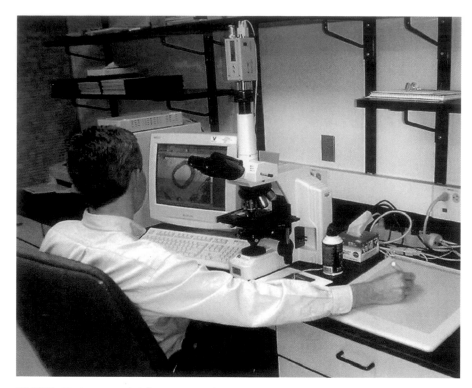

FIGURE 65-6. Research fellow Dr. Patrick Coussement traces section of balloon-injured irradiated pig coronary artery. Microscopic morphometry system displays image on high-resolution monitor enabling measurements from 12-in. tracing tablet.

conducted according to these guidelines (Good Laboratory Practice, GLP) is available.[20] A part of the regulatory requirement for adherence to GLP is the monitoring of research activities by an independent quality assurance unit, reporting to a management distinct from the study directorship.

ACADEMIC MISSION

In the face of many challenges, including financial burdens, personnel management, operations complexities and compliance with federal regulations, it is of central importance to the preclinical laboratory that its primary mission remains intact and at the forefront. For most interventional cardiology labs, this means that research is targeted toward improving the care of patients suffering from cardiovascular disease. In a word, the research is "translational," which is that its focus is on translating new discoveries in science, engineering, and related technologies into novel devices, drugs, and other therapies that have a direct and positive impact on the quality and diversity of treatments available to patients. In the end, it is hoped that our efforts will contribute to the well-being of global society, a lofty but attainable goal, as proved by the historical and ongoing contributions of preclinical interventional laboratories worldwide.[3,6-14,16]

REFERENCES

1. Harvey W. *An Anatomical Essay Concerning the Movement of the Heart and the Blood in Animals.* 1628.

2. Vesalius A. *De Humani Corporis Fabrica.* 1543.
3. Gruentzig AR, Turina M, Schneider JA. Experimental percutaneous dilatation of coronary artery stenosis (abstract). *Circulation.* 1976;53(suppl II):II–81.
4. Karas SP, Gravanis MB, Santoian EC, et al. Coronary intimal proliferation after balloon injury and stenting in swine: an animal model of restenosis. *J Am Coll Cardiol.* 1992;20:467–74.
5. Schwartz RS, Huber KC, Murphy JG, et al. Restenosis and the proportional neointimal response to coronary artery injury: results in a porcine model. *J Am Coll Cardiol.* 1992;19:267–74.
6. Waksman R, Robinson KA, Crocker IR, et al. Endovascular low dose irradiation inhibits neointima formation after coronary artery balloon injury in swine: a possible role for radiation therapy in restenosis prevention. *Circulation.* 1995;91:1533–1539.
7. Ishiwata S, Verheye S, Robinson KA, et al. Inhibition of neointima formation by tranilast in the pig coronary artery after balloon angioplasty and stent implantation. *J Am Coll Cardiol.* 2000;35:1331–1337.
8. Oberhoff M, Kunert W, Herdeg C, et al. Inhibition of smooth muscle cell proliferation after local drug delivery of the antimitotic drug paclitaxel using a porous balloon catheter. *Bas Res Cardiol.* 2001;96:275–282.
9. Kuiper KK, Robinson KA, Chronos NA, et al. Phosphorylcholine-coated metallic stents in rabbit iliac and porcine coronary arteries. *Scand Cardiovasc J* 1998;32:261–268.
10. Carter AJ, Laird JR, Bailey LR, et al. Effects of endovascular radiation from a beta-particle-emitting stent in a porcine coronary restenosis model: a dose-response study. *Circulation.* 1996;94:2364–2368.
11. Rogers C, Tseng DY, Squire JC, et al. Balloon-artery interactions during stent placement: a finite element analysis approach to pressure, compliance, and stent design as contributors to vascular injury. *Circ Res.* 1999;84:378–383.
12. Wilensky RL, March KL, Gradus-Pizlo I, et al. Vascular injury, repair, and restenosis after percutaneous transluminal angioplasty in the atherosclerotic rabbit. *Circulation.* 1995;92:2995–3005.
13. Christen T, Verin V, Bochaton-Piallat M, et al. Mechanisms of neointima formation and remodeling in the porcine coronary artery. *Circulation.* 2001;103:882–888.
14. Schwartz RS, Edelman ER, Carter A, et al. Consensus Committee. Drug-eluting stents in preclinical studies: recommended evaluation from a consensus group. *Circulation.* 2002;106:1867–1873.

15. Hanson SR, Harker LA. Ex vivo and in vivo evaluation of drugs that inhibit platelet function. *Ann NY Acad Sci.* 1983;416:642–650.

16. Verheye S, Markou CP, Salame MY, et al. Reduced thrombus formation by hyaluronic acid coating of endovascular devices. *Arterioscler Thromb Vasc Biol.* 2000;20:1168–1172.

17. Animal Welfare Act of 1966 (PL 89-544); Animal Welfare Act of 1970 (PL 91–579).

18. Institute of Laboratory Animal Resources, Commission on Life Sciences, National Research Council. *Guide for Care and Use of Laboratory Animals.* National Academy Press, Washington, DC, 1996.

19. http://www.aaalac.org/index.cfm

20. The Code of Federal Regulations Title 21. *Food and Drugs, Part 58: Good Laboratory Practice for Non Clinical Laboratory Studies.* (Revised as of April 1, 2003). GMP Publications, Inc.

CHAPTER 66

The Core Laboratory: Quantitative Coronary Angiography

Alexandra J. Lansky, MD, Ricardo A. Costa, MD, Johan H. Reiber, PhD

BASIC PRINCIPLES OF CORONARY ANGIOGRAPHY AND IMAGING

Coronary angiography remains the gold standard for imaging the coronary anatomy and defining the extent and precise location of coronary artery disease. Optimal coronary angiography is dependent on a thorough knowledge of coronary anatomy and its variations, and a systematic imaging sequence protocol that enables visualization of all coronary segments, particularly areas of vessel overlap, bifurcations, or tortuous anatomy. A basic map of the coronary anatomy is delineated in Figure 66-1 and the optimal views for imaging each coronary segment are summarized in Table 66-1 (Figures 66-2 through 66-5). Although standard views are generally consistent from one patient to the next, the precise angulations tend to vary based on the variations in anatomic orientations. A number of coronary segment numbering systems have been established; the most commonly used is the Coronary Artery Surgery Study (CASS) numbering system derived from the BARI study,[1] which assigns a unique number to each coronary vessel segment and its branch vessels, and has gained wide acceptance in interventional clinical trials (Table 66-2).

[ ] DEFINING SIGNIFICANT AND NONSIGNIFICANT CORONARY ARTERY DISEASE

Coronary atherosclerosis, with progression and regression of coronary atherosclerotic lesions, the healing of lesions, and the development of new ones, is a dynamic process.[2,3] A complicating factor in the angiographic evaluation of the severity and extent of the degree of coronary atherosclerosis is the occurrence of compensatory mechanisms, known as *coronary artery remodeling*, characterized by a compensatory enlargement of the atherosclerotic coronary artery that occurs in the early stages of plaque formation.[4,5] This compensatory enlargement results in the preservation of a nearly normal lumen cross-sectional area (and angiographic appearance), so that the early atherosclerotic plaque has less hemodynamic effects. As the maximal stretching capacities of the vessel are reached, the expansion of the vessel stops, and further plaque deposition begins to impinge on the lumen. Once the lumen of the vessel becomes compromised, it becomes visible on x-ray arteriography, which visualizes only the two-dimensional contrast-filled lumen.

Typically, atherosclerosis is characterized angiographically as a series of focal narrowings on a background of diffuse atherosclerosis within

TABLE 66-1

Views for Optimal Visualization of the Coronary Anatomy

	AP	LAO	RAO	LEFT LATERAL
Left Main	Optimal view for LM	LAO/caudal: bifurcation of LAD, LCx, and Ramus		
LAD	AP/cranial	LAO/cranial: proximal LAD, diagonals, septals Straight LAO: Mid and distal LAD	RAO/cranial or caudal: mid, distal LAD; diagonals	Mid and distal LAD
LCx		Steep LAO/cranial: proximal LCx	RAO/caudal: proximal, mid LCx;OMs	
RCA		Steep LAO: ostial, proximal RCA LAO/Cranial: Distal RCA, PDA, crux, and PLSA	Straight RAO: mid RCA RAO/Cranial for PDA and PLSA	Mid and distal RCA, PDA

LAO = left anterior oblique; LAD = left anterior descending (artery); RAO = right anterior oblique; RCA = right coronary artery; PDA = peripheral distal artery; PLSA = posterolateral spinal artery.

the entire coronary artery system. Because x-ray arteriography depicts only the coronary lumen, it tends to underestimate the presence of diffuse atherosclerosis and is essentially unable to detect the early stages of coronary atherosclerosis. Cross-sectional imaging of the coronary arteries is better assessed in these early stages by intravascular ultrasound (IVUS), which can provide real-time high-resolution cross sections of the arterial wall and demonstrate the presence or absence of plaque deposition and compensatory arterial enlargement.

[ ] QUALITATIVE ANGIOGRAPHY

Qualitative Assessment of Lesion Morphology

Several angiographic morphologic characteristics have been identified that have short- and long-term prognostic implications on outcome after coronary intervention with balloon angioplasty and new-device angioplasty.[6] Recent studies evaluating the prognostic implication of morphologic characteristics on patients undergoing intracoronary stenting demonstrate that these remain predictors of angiographic success, but not clinical outcome. Specific lesion morphologic criteria that contribute to the complexity of a lesion include: (1) the lesion location (proximal, mid, distal, ostial, or anastomotic), where ostial lesions begin within 3 mm of the origin of a major epicardial artery and anastomotic lesions begin within 3 mm of the insertion of a saphenous vein graft (SVG) or arterial conduits into the native vessel; (2) the lesion length, which is classified as discrete (< 10 mm in length), tubular, (10–20 mm in

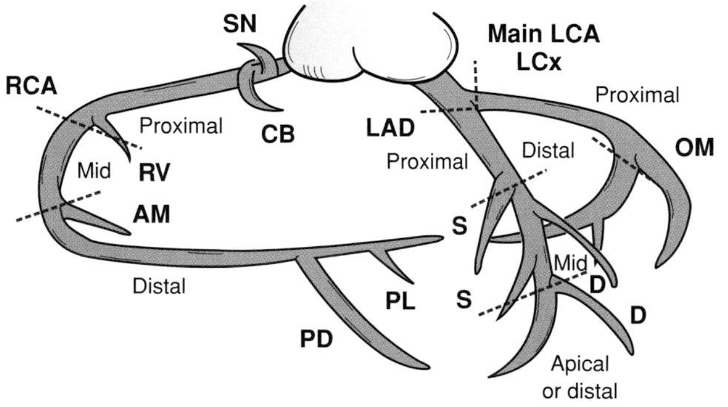

FIGURE 66-1. Schematic diagram of the coronary anatomy. RCA = right coronary artery; SN = sinus nodal artery; CB = conus branch; RV = right ventricular artery; AM = acute marginal artery; PD = posterior descending artery; PL = posterior lateral artery; LCA = left coronary artery; LAD = left anterior descending artery; S = septal branch; D = diagonal branch; LCx = left circumflex; OM = obtuse marginal artery.

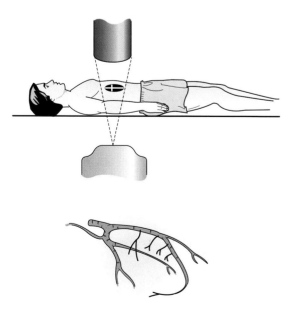

FIGURE 66-2. Anteroposterior (AP) view of the LCA. Ideal view to visualize the left main coronary segment.

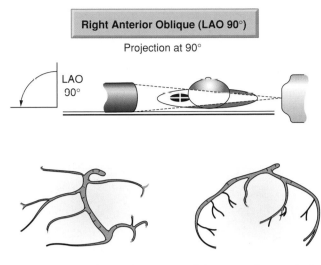

Right Anterior Oblique (LAO 90°)

Projection at 90°

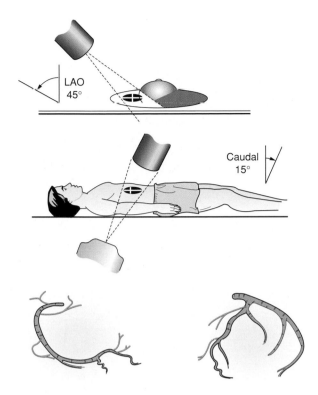

FIGURE 66-5. Left lateral (LLat) view of the LCA and RCA. Ideal view to visualize the mid- and distal segments of the LAD and RCA.

FIGURE 66-3. Left anterior oblique (LAO) view of the left and right coronary arteries. Ideal view to visualize the mid- and distal LAD and RCA.

length), or diffuse (≥ 20 mm in length); (3) the eccentricity of the lesion; (4) the angulation of the lesion (Figure-66-6), classified as mild (< 45°), moderate (45°–89°), or severe (≥ 90°); (5) the presence of thrombus (Figure-66-7); (6) vessel tortuosity (Figure 66-8) classified by the number of bends present before reaching the target lesion, none/mild (< two bends), moderate (two bends > 75° or one bend > 90°), or severe (two bends > 90°); (7) calcification; (8) ulceration defined by the presence of a crater or lumen flap in

the area of the stenosis; (9) aneurysm defined by a lumen expansion of at least 50% in the region of maximum stenosis (Figure 66-9); and (10) the presence of a bifurcation of the parent vessel with a branch vessel. These criteria have been used to define the complexity of a lesion and are the basis of the modified AHA/ACC complexity score.[7] Type A lesions are characterized by focal (< 10 mm length) concentric lesions with smooth contours, little or no calcification, less than totally occlusive, nonangulated (< 45° bend), not ostial, without major side branch involvement, and without thrombus. Type B lesions are categorized as type B1 or B2 lesions depending on whether a single or more than one B characteristic is present. These include tubular lesions (10–20 mm length), with moderate to severe calcification, eccentric plaque, moderate proximal tortuosity, irregular contour, angulation 45° or more and less than 90°, ostial location, involving a bifurcation, or containing thrombus. Type C lesions have one or more of the following complex characteristics: diffuse (≥ 2 cm length), degenerated SVG, total occlusion, excessive proximal tortuosity, extreme angulation (≥ 90°).

Assessment of Collaterals

Many factors contribute to the growth of collaterals, including hypoxemia and the release of angiogenic factors. Collateral identification and quantification is important in the context of clinical trials assessing growth factors. Collaterals are defined by their site of origin as ipsilateral (collateral between the left anterior descending [LAD] artery and LCx or vice versa), as bridging (collateral originates from the same coronary artery) (Figure 66-10), or contralateral (collateral from the left to right coronary artery or vice versa). The Rentrop Collateral Classification grades the collateral according to the extent of filling of the major epicardial vessel the collateral is supplying.[8] Other less well-validated parameters that have been used for assessing collaterals include the collateral size; the collateral frame count, measured by the number of frames from opacification of the guiding catheter to the filling of the collaterals; and collateral density, measured as the number of collaterals (> 1 mm) per square centimeter in a region of interest.[9]

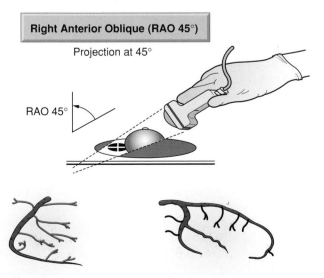

Right Anterior Oblique (RAO 45°)

Projection at 45°

RAO 45°

FIGURE 66-4. Right anterior oblique (RAO) view of the LCA and RCA. Ideal view to visualize the LCx and mid-right coronary artery.

TABLE 66-2

Coronary Artery Surgery Study Numbering System

SEQMENT	CASS NUMBER
RCA, proximal	1
RCA, mid	2
RCA, distal	3
PDA	4
PLSA	5
RPL1	6
RPL2	7
RPL3	8
RPL4	9
RV	10
Left main	11
LAD, proximal	12
LAD, mid	13
LAD, distal	14
Diagonal 1	15
Diagonal 2	16
Septal	17
Left circumflex, proximal	18
Left circumflex, distal	19
Obtuse marginal 1	20
Obtuse marginal 2	21
Obtuse marginal 3	22
LPL1	23
LPL2	24
LPL3	25
Left PDA	27
Ramus (optional)	28

RCA = right coronary artery; PDA = peripheral distal artery; RV = right ventricle.

A prefix of "1" is added to the CASS segment to designate saphenous vein grafts and numbered according to the location of the distal anastomotic insertion site of the conduit; a prefix of "2" is affixed to designate an arterial grafts.

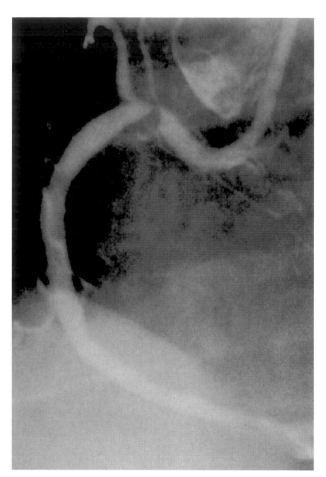

FIGURE 66-6. LAO view of the RCA. Demonstrates a moderately angulated stenosis on a 90° bend.

Assessment of Flow

The traditional method for assessing and grading epicardial flow was defined by the Thrombolysis in Myocardial Infarction study (TIMI) group,[10] and was graded according to the following criteria: *Grade O* refers to no anterograde flow beyond the point of arterial occlusion; *Grade 1* is defined by the appearance of contrast beyond the point of arterial obstruction but fails to opacify the entire distal coronary bed; *Grade 2* is defined by contrast opacification of the entire coronary bed distal to the stenosis but at a rate of entry and/or clearance that is slower than in the other epicardial vessels unaffected by the stenosis. In TIMI grade 2, complete filling of the artery and its major and minor branches occurs after more than three full cardiac cycles, or alternatively, delayed contrast washout in the target lesion territory may occur, compared with comparable areas of myocardium not perfused by the target lesion. TIMI *Grade 3* refers to complete or normal perfusion, with anterograde flow of contrast and complete filling of the artery with its major and minor branches within three full cardiac cycles.[10] Other measures of epicardial perfusion include continuous variables. The TIMI frame count is defined by the number of frames necessary for the contrast column to completely fill the coronary artery at a constant acquisition frame rate. The corrected TIMI frame count is a similar measure that corrects for variability in coronary lengths by using specific anatomic landmarks and specifically corrects for the longer length of the left anterior descending coronary artery.[11]

Finally, a more recent assessment of myocardial perfusion has been defined: the myocardial blush score. Myocardial blush has important prognostic implications in patients with acute myocardial infarction undergoing reperfusion treatment. The myocardial blush scoring system is based on the extent of ground glass appearance within the myocardial territory subtended by the coronary artery of interest (Figure 66-12). A blush grade of 0 suggests no ground-glass appearance, blush grade of 1 is minimal ground-glass appearance, blush grade of 2 incomplete opacification of

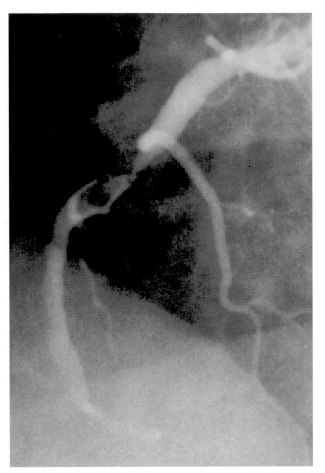

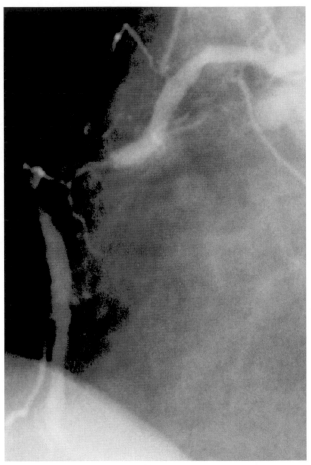

FIGURE 66-7. LAO view of the RCA. This view demonstrates a classic large globular thrombus at the lesion site.

FIGURE 66-8. LAO view of the RCA. This view demonstrates a moderate to severely tortuous vessel with two bends more than 90° prior to reaching the stenosis.

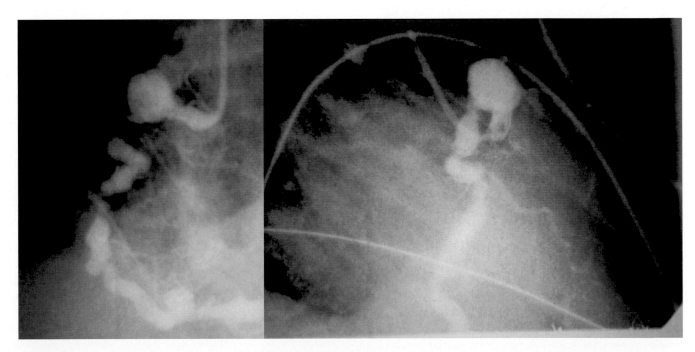

FIGURE 66-9. LAO and RAO views of the RCA. This view demonstrates a large coronary aneurysm in the proximal segment of the RCA.

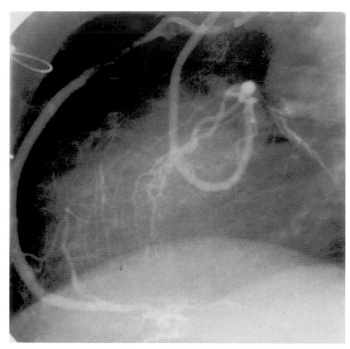

FIGURE 66-10. Simultaneous injection of the saphenous vein graft (SVG) to the distal RCA and LAD. This view demonstrates an occluded native RCA and an occluded proximal LAD with an extensive collateral network between the left and the right system.

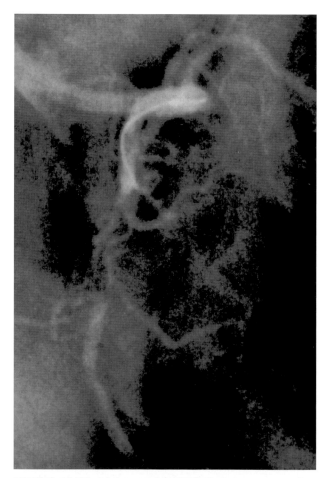

FIGURE 66-11. RAO view of the RCA. Demonstrates a total occlusion in the mid-RCA, with bridging right to right collaterals filling the distal vessel.

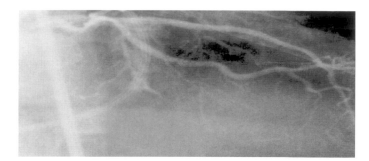

A

B

FIGURE 66-12. RAO view of the LCA after primary intervention for acute myocardial infarction of the LAD. (**A**) Region of interest demonstrates minimal myocardial blush in the myocardial territory of the LAD (blush score = 0/1). (**B**) Region of interest demonstrates normal myocardial blush (ground-glass appearance) in the myocardial territory of the LAD (blush score = 3).

myocardium, and blush grade of 3 is normal myocardial opacification. This scoring system has been shown to have independent prognostic value in both thrombolytic and primary angioplasty reperfusion trials in predicting mortality.[12–14]

The prognostic importance of establishing TIMI-3 flow in patients with acute myocardial infarction has been demonstrated to be the predominant determinant of survival[15] after thrombolytic and primary intervention reperfusion strategies.[16,17] Patients reperfused with primary angioplasty within 2 hours of symptom onset have lower mortality and greater myocardial salvage after primary percutaneous transluminal coronary angioplasty (PTCA) than patients with delayed reperfusion.[18] The importance of early reperfusion is also emphasized in patients spontaneously achieving TIMI-3 flow prior to primary PTCA, as demonstrated in between 10% and 20% of patients at the time of initial angiography. Factors influencing early spontaneous reperfusion may include endogenous fibrinolysis and/or pre-treatment with aspirin, ADP antagonists, and heparin.[19–27] In an analysis of the 2507 patients from the four major Primary Angioplasty in Myocardial Infarction (PAMI) trials, TIMI-3 flow was present at initial angiography (spontaneous reperfusion) in 16% of patients. No baseline demographic characteristics clearly predicted spontaneous reperfusion, however, early reperfusion with initial TIMI-3 flow prior to PTCA was a powerful and independent predictor of in-hospital and late survival in patients undergoing a mechanical reperfusion strategy. The independent impact of initial TIMI-3 flow on survival persisted even when corrected for postprocedural TIMI-3 flow.[28] This observation

TABLE 66-3

Risks of Cardiac Catheterization and Angiography

Mortality	0.11%
Myocardial infarction	0.05%
Cerebrovascular accidents	0.07%
Vascular complications	0.38%
Contrast reaction	0.43%
Hemodynamic complications	0.37%
Perforation of heart chamber	0.03%
Overall complications	1.70%

suggests that early pre-PTCA reperfusion has benefits independent of promoting the ultimate restoration of TIMI-3 flow. Studies evaluating pharmacologically mediated reperfusion prior to intervention, the so-called facilitated primary PTCA strategy, have begun. In the Plasminogen-activator Angioplasty Compatibility Trial (PACT), 606 patients with AMI were randomized to low dose t-PA versus placebo prior to catheterization and angioplasty, when appropriate.[29] This study demonstrated that patients achieving early TIMI-3 flow (whether spontaneously or pharmacologically mediated) had improved myocardial salvage compared to patients in whom TIMI-3 flow was restored by PTCA alone.[29] Rather than using higher doses of thrombolytic agents to achieve greater rates of TIMI-3 flow prior to PTCA, current interest has shifted to the combination of glycoprotein IIb/IIIa receptor inhibitors plus reduced dose thrombolytic therapy, which in dose ranging studies has been found to promote earlier and more complete reperfusion than full-dose thrombolytics alone.[30,31] The safety of these combination regimens has not yet been established, and a careful risk–benefit analysis requires larger randomized trials to determine whether the benefits of early reperfusion outweigh the potential risks of intracranial hemorrhage, access site bleeding, and additional costs. (See Table 66-3.)

PRINCIPLES OF VENTRICULOGRAPHY AND ANALYSIS CONSIDERATIONS

Left venticulography is most accurately performed using a 30° right anterior oblique (RAO) and a 60° straight left anterior oblique (LAO) (to minimize overlap of the apex and the diaphragm) projection. To evaluate function and wall motion abnormalities quantitatively, the end-diastolic and end-systolic frames with the minimum and maximum volumes are selected from a well opacified normal (non-premature ventricular contraction) sinus beat. The frames are digitized for analysis and the endocardial contours can be traced using commercially available software. Wall motion is most commonly measured by the centerline method along 100 chords constructed perpendicular to a centerline midway between the end-systolic and end-diastolic contours, and normalized by the end-diastolic perimeter to standardize chord lengths.[32] This results in a dimensionless shortening fraction, a linear equivalent of the volume ejection fraction. Abnormality in chord motion is reported in units of standard deviation from the mean of normal biplane left ventriculograms, with negative values indicating hypokinesis and positive values indicating hyperkinesis. The centerline method has been extensively validated.[32,33] To minimize measurement variability and increase sensitivity and specificity using this method, wall motion in each territory is computed from the average motion of the chords confined to the most abnormally contracting 50% of the territory. The region of the left ventricle in the RAO and LAO projections considered the territory of each coronary artery has been defined from patients with isolated stenoses and infarcts of the LAD, the right coronary artery (RCA), and the LCx (Table 66-4). LCx disease results in widely variable hypokinesis over the entire contour of the left ventricle that spans both anterior and inferior distributions. This is a consequence of the variable anatomy of the LCx, with left dominant systems exhibiting inferior distribution hypokinesis, and right or balanced systems exhibiting anterior hypokinesis. Extended search chord regions have been identified based on patients with known LCx infarcts to increase the sensitivity of detecting LCx regional hypokinesis.[34] In the 30° RAO view, chords 48–80 are specific to the LCx (chords 0–21 and 81–100 are

TABLE 66-4

Left Ventriculography Centerline Method: Defining Arterial Territories Based on Chords Numbers

CORONARY ARTERY	CHORD NUMBER DELIMITING THE TERRITORY		
	30° RAO biplane	30° RAO single	30° LAO plane
LAD	12–68	10–67	50–100
RCA	52–84	51–80	38–74
LCx Rt dominant	12–68	(LAD like)	10-100[a]
LCx Lft dominant	52–84	(RCA 48–80 Like)	10-100[b]

[a]LAO best for evaluation LCx of Rt dominant system behaves more like LAD).

[b]Extended search chords for LCx territory (original limited to chords 19–67).

LAO = left anterior oblique; LAD = left anterior descending (artery); RAO = right anterior oblique; RCA = right coronary artery.

excluded because of variability associated with overlap from RCA and LAD territories, making these regions nonspecific to the LCx). The RAO view is less specific than the LAO view for assessing LCx disease. In the 60° LAO view, LCx infarcts result in longer regions of hypokinesis compared to the RAO view, with extended LCx specific chords spanning from chords 10 through 100 being more sensitive than the previously defined limited chord region 19–67.[34] The LAO view is more specific and sensitive in evaluating the LCx in a right dominant coronary system.

PRINCIPLES OF QUANTITATIVE CORONARY ANGIOGRAPHY

The field of quantitative coronary angiography (QCA) has evolved tremendously since the mid-1980s.[35,36] First-generation QCA systems, developed in the 1980s, were based on 35-mm cine-film analysis. Second-generation systems (1990–1994) had further improvements in the quality of the edge detection, more frequently applied to digital images (which is not a mere application of the algorithm for cine-based analysis to digital analyses), and included corrections for the overestimation of small vessel sizes (< ~1.2 mm).[37] Third-generation (1995–1998) QCA systems provided solutions for the quantitative analysis of complex lesion morphology using, for example, the Gradient Field Transform (GFT)[38] and improved diameter function calculations.[39] Fourth-generation QCA systems, available since 1999, are characterized by simplified portability to digital DICOM (Digital Imaging and Communication in Medicine) viewers, network connectivity, improved reporting and database facilities, and options for specialized QCA functions, such as brachytherapy and drug-eluting stent analyses.[40] Although most modern QCA packages are based on the linear programming approach (ie, minimal cost algorithm) for contour detection, there are still differences in the qualities of these packages that must be documented by extensive validation reports.[41]

【 】 BASIC PRINCIPLES OF QUANTITATIVE CORONARY ARTERIOGRAPHY

For a QCA package to be applicable in a routine clinical or research environment, a number of requirements must be met, which include the following: (1) minimal user interaction in the selection and processing of the coronary segment to be analyzed; (2) minimal editing of the automatically determined results; (3) short analysis time (10 sec or less); (4) provide highly accurate and precise results, with small systematic and random errors. These criteria should be demonstrated by extensive validation studies using phantom and routinely acquired clinical studies.

Basic Principles of Automated Contour Detection

The general principles and characteristics of a modern QCA software package that satisfies these requirements are best illustrated by the QCA-CMS (Clinical Measurement Solutions, MEDIS) algorithms.[42–44] The QCA operator selects (Figure 66-13A) the coronary segment to be analyzed by defining the start and end points of the arterial segment. An arterial pathline through the arterial segment is computed automatically (Figure 66-13B).[43] The contour-

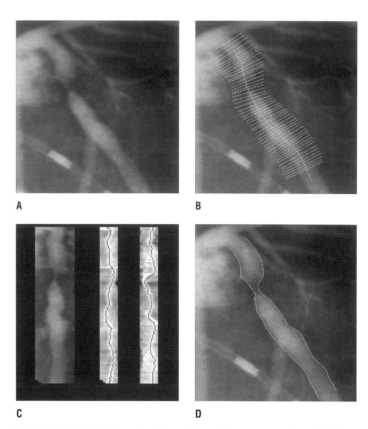

FIGURE 66-13. Basic principles of the minimum cost analysis (MCA) contour-detection algorithm. (**A**) Initial segment. (**B**) Scanlines defined. (**C**) Straightened for analysis; contours calculated. (**D**) Contours returned to initial image; diameter measurements performed.

detection procedure is carried out in two iterations relative to a model. In the first iteration, the detected pathline is the model. To detect the contours, scanlines are defined perpendicular to the model (Figure 66-13B). For each point or pixel along such a scanline, the corresponding *edge-strength value* (local change in brightness level) is computed as the weighted sum of the corresponding values of the first- and second-derivative functions applied to the brightness values along these scanlines (Figure 66-14). The resulting edge-strength values are input to the minimal cost analysis (MCA) contour-detection algorithm, which searches for an optimal contour path along the entire segment (Figure 66-13C). The individual left and right vessel contours detected in the first iteration now serve as models in the second iteration, in which the MCA contour-detection procedure is repeated relative to the new models.

To correct for the limited resolution of the entire x-ray system, the MCA algorithm is modified in the second iteration based on an analysis of the quality of the imaging chain in terms of its resolution, which is of particular importance for the accurate measurement of small diameters, as in coronary obstructions. If such a correction were not applied, significant overestimation of vessel sizes smaller than approximately 1.2 mm would occur. If the QCA operator does not agree with one or more parts of the detected contours, they can be edited in various ways. However, each manual editing is followed by a local MCA iteration, so that the newly detected contours are truly based on the local brightness information. In other words, the operator indicates roughly where the contour should be detected, and the MCA algorithm searches for the final contour based on the available image information (Figure 66-13D).

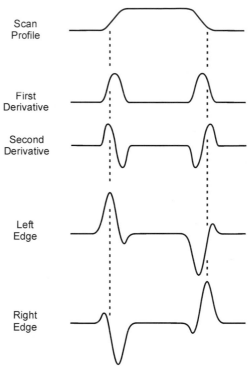

FIGURE 66-14. Schematic presentation of the brightness profile of an arterial vessel assessed along a scanline perpendicular to the local pathline direction and the computed first derivative, second derivative, and the combinations of these first and second derivative functions; the maximal values of the last functions determine the edge positions.

Calibration Procedure

Image calibration is performed on a non-tapered portion of the contrast-filled catheter using an MCA edge-detection procedure similar to that applied to the arterial segment. In this case, however, additional information is used in the edge-detection process because this part of the catheter is characterized by parallel boundaries. Catheter calibration is frequently the weakest link in the analysis chain because of the variable image quality of the displayed catheters, and the potential problem of out-of-plane magnification, which can occur when the catheter and the coronary segment are positioned at different distances from the image intensifier. Biplane calibration can overcome this limitation,[44–46] but is rarely applied in routine QCA.

Coronary Segment Analysis

A diameter function is determined from the contours of the arterial segment (Figure 66-15). Calculation of the width of a vessel segment along its trajectory is not a trivial task, especially not in a situation of complex anatomy.[39] Pincushion distortion caused by the convex input screen of the image intensifier may influence diameter calculations. Correction for this distortion should not be applied routinely in single-plane QCA, as this may introduce more artifacts rather than resolve problems.[47] Pincushion distortion is minimal in modern image intensifiers, and absent in the latest solid-state flat-panel image intensifiers.

The most widely used parameter to describe the severity of a coronary obstruction is the percentage of diameter narrowing. Calculation of this parameter requires computation of a reference diameter, which can be derived in one of two ways: (1) a "user-defined" reference diameter is identified by the user at a so-called normal portion of the vessel, or (2) the interpolated reference diameter value, requiring no user interaction and accounts for vessel

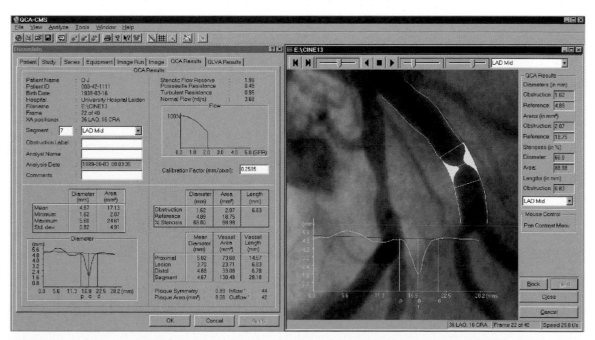

FIGURE 66-15. The results of the minimal cost analysis, including the reconstructed original vessel contours, plaque area (shaded), and the diameter function, are presented for QCA-CMS V4.0. All the derived absolute and relative QCA parameters are presented in the QCA DICOM-box (*left*).

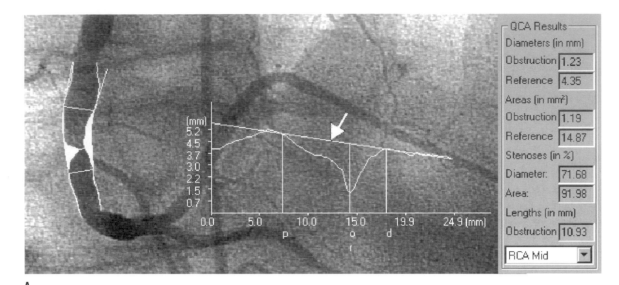

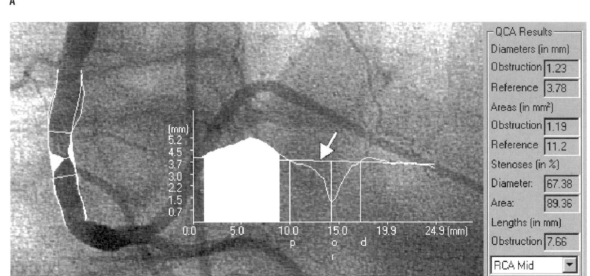

FIGURE 66-16. Example of a vessel with an ectatic area. (**A**) Straightforward application of the reference diameter function would lead to arbitrary, erroneous results; in this case, in significant tapering of the reference diameter function (*arrow*). (**B**) By "flagging" the proximal ectatic area, a nontapering reference diameter function (*arrow*) results and appropriately reconstructed vessel reference contours.

taper. The interpolated reference diameter function is calculated by an iterative regression technique that excludes the influence of obstructions or ectatic segments. In cases of extensive ectatic segments, the user can "flag" the portion of the vessel segment (Figure 66-16B), and the corresponding diameter values are excluded in the subsequent calculation of the reference diameter function. The interpolated reference is therefore displayed as a straight line, and represents the best approximation of the vessel size before the occurrence of any focal narrowing or dilation. However, correction cannot be made in the presence of diffuse atherosclerosis along the vessel segment, because angiography is a two-dimensional lumenogram. The difference in area between the detected lumen contours and the interpolated reference contours is a measure for the atherosclerotic plaque Figure 66-15.

The interpolated reference diameter value corresponding to an obstruction is taken as the value of the reference diameter function

at the site of the obstruction, thereby neither overestimating nor underestimating the reference. From the reference diameter value and the obstruction diameter, the percentage diameter narrowing is calculated. This automated approach has been found to be very reproducible.

From the calculated diameter function, many parameters including obstruction symmetry, inflow and outflow angles, the area of the atherosclerotic plaque, and functional information, such as the stenotic flow reserve (SFR) can be derived. The SFR describes, on the basis of a mathematical/physiologic model, how much the flow can possibly increase under maximal hyperemic conditions in that particular coronary segment as a result of that single obstruction; it can also be described as a wind-tunnel test of the stenosis under standardized conditions (Figure 66-15).[48] In a disease-free segment, the SFR equals 4–5, a value that decreases as the severity of the obstruction increases.

Complex Vessel Morphology

Modern contour detection approaches are based on the MCA algorithm, which has been demonstrated to be fast and robust for images that may vary significantly in image quality. This approach has been shown to work very well as long as the vessel and lesion outlines are relatively smooth. However, complex vessel morphology may occur before (ulcerated lesions) and after coronary intervention (dissections).

In its design, the MCA technique is limited when tracing very irregular and complex boundaries as the MCA algorithm can select only one point per scanline, and the edge strength or derivative values can be calculated only along the direction of the scanlines, despite the fact that the highest edge-strength values may occur in other directions in complex lesions with irregular boundaries. The Gradient Field Transform (GFT) was developed to circumvent these limitations Figure 66-17.[38] Scanlines are defined perpendicular to the pathline as in standard MCA. Whereas MCA would consider only three potential points, the GFT considers eight neighboring points. Each branch from a particular scan point to a neighboring scan point is assigned a different cost value (a mathematical technique), which is a function of its edge strength and the angle between the direction of the edge and the direction of the branch. The goal of the algorithm now is to find an optimal path between one node on the first scanline of the vessel segment and one node on the last scanline of this segment.

In practice, the entire contour detection procedure is applied twice to a coronary segment: the first time the detected pathline is used as a model and the GFT is carried out. In the second iteration, the initially detected contours are again used as models for the subsequent detection of the arterial boundaries, this time using the standard MCA algorithm. This approach enables the GFT to follow more irregular arterial boundaries and even reverse direction of the contour, for example, to follow flaps or dissections. An illustrative example of the GFT is given in Figure 66-18.

The obstruction diameters of complex lesions assessed by GFT analysis are, on the average, 0.25 mm smaller than those detected by the MCA algorithm.[38] The detected contours tend to be more irregular because the algorithm is more sensitive to noise in all possible spatial directions. However, these data tend to represent a

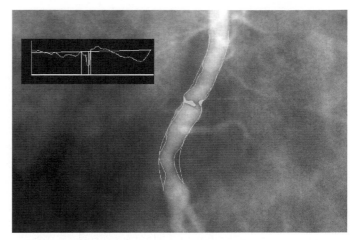

FIGURE 66-18. Example of outcome of GFT analysis on a vessel segment with very severe complex stenosis. Conventional approaches with the MCA algorithm are not able to follow automatically the abrupt changes in morphology.

more accurate reflection of the vessel's morphology, and may also provide prognostic information.[49]

Densitometry

Because the x-ray arteriogram is a two-dimensional projection image of a three-dimensional structure, measured vessel sizes may be of limited value in vessels with very irregular cross-sections. Many efforts have been devoted to deriving information from densitometric measures based on the brightness within the coronary arteries. If a valid relation between density and arterial dimensions could be established, other parameters such as the arterial cross-sectional area could be derived from a single angiographic view.

Unfortunately, densitometry has not provided reliable results, particularly from cine film,[50] and as a result, the interest in it has largely diminished. It may be of interest to revisit the densitometric approaches for the digital systems in which the entire transfer function of the x-ray system is better controlled and more stable than with the use of cine film.

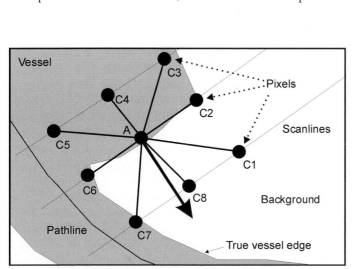

FIGURE 66-17. Schematic representation of a vessel with its pathline, the scanlines, and the search directions for the GFT algorithm.

DIGITAL VERSUS DIRECT ANGIOGRAPHY

Cinefilm based x-ray systems are rapidly being replaced by complete digital systems. The DICOM-3 standard, initially developed to allow compatibility and networking of digital x-ray images, was accepted by the American College of Cardiology in 1995 as the digital standard for cardiac angiography, ensuring that all manufacturers conform to a single interchangeable standard.[51] The recordable compact disk (CD-R) was the chosen medium of exchange, with sufficient storage capacity for 99% of interventional procedures (assuming at most 1200 MB of digital data). Current digital cardiac angiography systems use a matrix of at least 512 × 512 pixel with 8 bits/pixel providing 2^8 (256) gray levels. The matrix size, bit depth, and underlying noise are the major determinants of the digital image quality. The wide acceptance of the cineless cardiac catheterization laboratory has been spurred by several advantages, including a reduction in radiation exposure necessary for equivalent image processing, reduction in storage space with on-line image archiving and retrieval, and universal networking.[52] With now more than 60% cineless cardiac catheterization laboratories in the United States, the impact of digitally acquired images on results of randomized clinical trials using quantitative angiography as surrogates of clinical endpoints has required specific definition, in terms of the comparability of quantitative angiographic (QA) results obtained from cineangiograms and DICOM-3 compatible digital CD-R media. Based on the analysis of simultaneously acquired cine and digital angiograms, repeated measures obtained from digital images are better correlated and have a higher precision than repeated measures obtained from the analysis of cineangiograms, without apparent systematic overestimation or underestimation of measurements.

【　】 DIFFERENCES BETWEEN CINE AND DIGITAL QUANTITATIVE ANGIOGRAPHY

Figure 66-19 outlines the differences between the cine film and digital techniques in the image acquisition and analysis portions of the x-ray imaging chains. For QCA purposes, the cine film is mounted on a cine-video converter, which features optical magnification and an analog or digital video camera for conversion of the images into video format. The converters must satisfy specific requirements for QCA applications, such as zooming capabilities (minimally 1- to 3-fold continuous), high spatial resolution of the optical chain, even brightness distribution over the field-of-view, high quality of the video camera, and so forth. To analyze a selected coronary segment, a region of interest (ROI) encompassing the coronary segment or catheter is magnified optically approximately 2.3-fold, such that pixel sizes in the range of 0.08–0.10 mm are obtained after digitization; this range of pixel sizes has been found to be optimal for contour detection approaches. The video signal from the camera in the cine-film projector is digitized (A/D conversion; eg, at a resolution of 512 × 512 pixels × 8 bits) and stored in the workstation for subsequent analysis.

In the digital approach, the output image of the image intensifier is projected onto the input target of a video camera. The analog video output signal is modified electronically in the so-called white compression unit, resulting in greater contrast differences in the parts with high x-ray absorption (eg, vertebrae and contrast-filled arteries or the ventricle) and lower contrast differences in the areas with low x-ray absorption (eg, lung area). This markedly improves the image quality of the images. Next, the resulting video signal is digitized at a resolution of 512 × 512 pixels × 8 bits on most x-ray systems or up to 1024 × 1024 pixels × 12 bits on some other x-ray systems and stored on the high-speed disks (RAID system) of the digital imaging system for subsequent review and quantitative analysis. Because optical magnification is not possible in this approach, the pixel size in the standard 512 × 512 × 8 bits mode is markedly larger than achievable with the cine film.

New developments in the image intensifier technology will lead to a replacement of the conventional vacuum tube to a completely digital flat panel image intensifier or digital detector. Typical matrix size of the flat panel for the GE system is 1000 × 1000 pixels, but the actual image matrix size varies between 600 × 600 for a 12-cm field-of-view (FOV) to 836 × 836 for a 17-cm FOV with 12 bits depth for cardiac acquisitions. These flat panels are characterized by linear system responses and absence of geometric distortions.

From the user's point of view, the analysis of digital images on the QCA workstation is similar to the analysis of cine-film frames. However, there are a number of important differences between cine-film and digital media: (1) Cine film has a nonlinear density function (H & D curve), which differs between hospitals and may differ slightly from day to day or week to week. Digital systems are characterized by well-defined and constant nonlinear functions (the white compression); (2) cine-film is hampered by film grain noise, which is absent on the digital systems; (3) on cine-film, the vessels are visible as bright structures on a dark background, whereas in the digital images, they are dark structures on a bright background; and (4) edge enhancement is not possible on cine-film. It is frequently used on digital images.

【　】 IMPACT OF IMAGE PROCESSING ON QUANTITATIVE ANGIOGRAPHIC ANALYSIS

One limitation of the cineless catheterization laboratory is the vast volume of digital data required for storage and real-time retrieval. On average, a single interventional case requires a 7.5 MB/sec transfer rate.[52] Data compression and subsequent decompression may minimize archiving space and data transfer time. Compression can be achieved using the Joint Photographic Experts Group (JPEG) standard, where lossless compression of up to 3-fold can be completely recovered on retrieval of the image, and where lossy compression results in irretrievable loss of data. In clinical practice, JPEG lossy compression up to 15:1 has been shown not to affect identification of dissections, thrombus, or the presence of intracoronary stents, and is therefore deemed acceptable for clinical decision making during coronary interventions.[53,54] Before the wide acceptance of data compression for archiving and storage purposes, the impact of irreversible compression on quantitative angiographic measurements and the results of randomized clinical trials that use angiographic surrogate endpoints

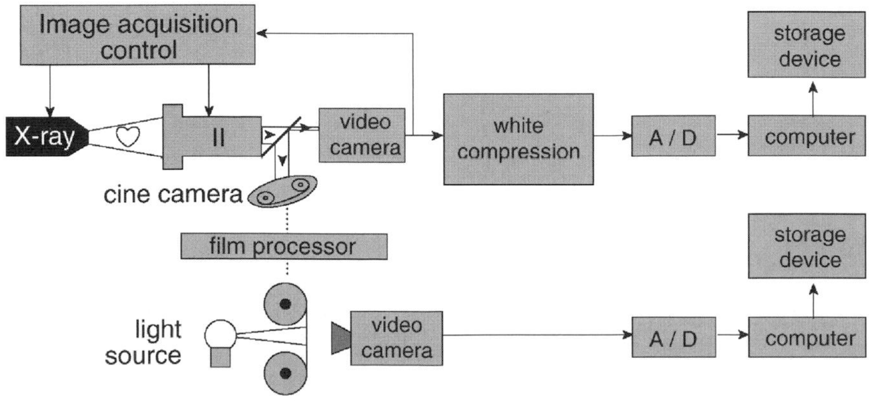

FIGURE 66-19. Block diagram of combined film-based and digital angiographic system.

requires further definition. Quantitative angiographic analysis of 5:1, 8:1, and 12:1 lossy JPEG compression was shown in one study[55] to result in higher intraobserver variability (0.23–0.31 mm) compared to original images (< 0.13 mm), and is therefore not recommended for QCA in clinical trials. However, a recent study comparing QCA measurements of 96 digital angiograms with 15:1 lossy JPEG compression to the original images resulted in excellent correlation ($r = 0.99$) for vessel measurements ranging from 0.69 to 5.08 mm (56).

FUTURE DIRECTIONS

Further development and refinements of networking capability from the catheterization laboratory to the cardiologist's office and referring hospitals will have major implications on the rapidity and cost of transfer of vital patient information in the form of electronic patient records (EPR), for improved patient care, clinical research, and patient and physician education. Integration of other quantitative modalities such as QCA, quantitative intravascular ultrasound (QCU),[44] and in the future, novel diagnostic modalities such as intravascular thermography and infrared imaging will facilitate and guide the optimal interventional therapy for patients with established obstructive coronary disease and vulnerable plaque. Other angiographic measurement options including objective myocardial perfusion parameters based on densitometry and the area of the myocardial muscle at risk,[50] three-dimensional reconstruction,[44,57] and other derived data such as wall shear stress based on computational fluid dynamics, stress and strain on the vessels in relation to the sites of the development of local atherosclerosis[59] will further complement derived patient-specific data parameters to optimize therapeutic decision making and outcomes.

REFERENCES

1. Ringqvist I, Fisher LD, Mock M, et al. Prognostic value of angiographic indices of coronary artery disease from the Coronary Artery Surgery Study (CASS). *J Clin Invest.* 1983;71:1854.
2. Bruschke AVG, Wijers TS, Kolsters W, Landmann J. The anatomic evolution of coronary artery disease demonstrated by coronary arteriography in 256 non-operated patients. *Circulation.* 1981;63(3):527.
3. Jukema JW, Bruschke AVG, Reiber JHC. Lessons learned from angiographic coronary atherosclerosis trials. In: Reiber JHC, van der Wall EE, eds. *Cardiovascular Imaging.* Kluwer Academic Publishers, 1996:119.
4. Glagov S, Weisenberg E, Zarins CK, Stankunavicius R, Kolettis GJ. Compensatory enlargement of human atherosclerotic coronary arteries. *N Engl J Med.* 1987;316(22):1371.
5. Stiel GM, Stiel LS, Schofer J, Donath K, Mathey DG. Impact of compensatory enlargement of atherosclerotic coronary arteries on angiographic assessment of coronary artery disease. *Circulation.* 1989;80(6):1603.
6. Ellis SG, Vanddormeal M, Cowley M, et al. Coronary morphologic and clinical determinants of procedural outcome with angioplasty with for multivessel coronary disease. Implications for patient selection. *Circulation.* 1990;82:1193.
7. Ryan T, Faxon D, Gunnar R, et al. Guidelines for percutaneous transluminal coronary angioplasty. *J Am Coll Cardiol.* 1998;12:529.
8. Rentrop KP, Feit F, Sherman W, et al. Serial angiographic assessment of coronary artery obstruction and collateral flow in acute myocardial infarction. *Circulation.* 1989;80:1166.
9. Gibson CM, Ryan K, Sparano A, et al. Angiographic methods to assess human coronary angiogenesis. *Am Heart J.* 1999;137:169.
10. Sheehan FH, Braunwald E, Canner P, et al. The effect of intravenous thrombolytic therapy on left ventricular function: A report on tissue type plasminogen activator and streptokinase from the Thrombolysis in Myocardial Infarction (TIMI) Phase I trial. *Circulation.* 1987;72:817.
11. Gibson CM, Sandor T, Stone PH, et al. Quantitative angiographic and statistical methods to assess serial changes in coronary luminal diameter and implications for atherosclerosis regression trials. *Am J Cardiol.* 1992;69:1286.
12. van't Hof AWJ, Liem A, Suryapranata H, et al. Angiographic assessment of myocardial reperfusion in patients treated with primary angioplasty for acute myocardial infarction–myocardial blush grade. *Circulation.* 1998;97:2302.
13. Stone GW, Peterson MA, Lansky AJ, et al. Impact of normalized myocardial perfusion after successful angioplasty in acute myocardial infarction. *J Am Coll Cardiol.* 2002;39:591.
14. Gibson CM, Cannon CP, Murphy SA, et al. Relationship of TIMI myocardial perfusion grade to mortality after administration of thrombolytic drugs. *Circulation.* 2000;101:125.
15. Stone GW, Brodie B, Griffin J, et al. Should the risk of delaying reperfusion prohibit inter-hospital transfer to perform primary PTCA in acute myocardial infarction? *Circulation.* 1996;94(suppl I):I-331. Abstract.
16. Braunwald E. Myocardial reperfusion, limitation of infarct size, reduction of left ventricular dysfunction, and improved survival: should the paradigm be expanded? *Circulation.* 1989;79:441.
17. Califf RM, Topol EJ, Gersh BJ. From myocardial salvage to patient salvage in acute myocardial infarction: the role of reperfusion therapy. *J Am Coll Cardiol.* 1989;14:1382.
18. Brodie BR, Stuckey TD, Wall TC, et al. Importance of time to reperfusion for 30-day and late survival and recovery of left ventricular function after primary angioplasty for acute myocardial infarction. *J Am Coll Cardiol.* 1998;32:1312.
19. Stone GW, Grines CL, Topol EJ. Update on percutaneous transluminal coronary angioplasty for acute myocardial infarction. In: Topol E, Serruys P, eds. *Current Review of Interventional Cardiology,* 2nd ed. Current Medicine. 1995:1–56.
20. Cannon CP, Gibson CM, Lambrew CT, et al. Relationship of symptom onset-to-balloon time and door-to-balloon time with mortality in patients undergoing angioplasty for acute myocardial infarction. *JAMA.* 2000;283:2941.
21. Grines CL, Browne KF, Marco J, et al. A comparison of immediate angioplasty with thrombolytic therapy for acute myocardial infarction. *N Engl J Med.* 1993;328:673.
22. Stone GW, Grines CL, Browne KF, et al. Predictors of in-hospital and 6 month outcome after acute myocardial infarction in the reperfusion era: the Primary Angioplasty in Myocardial Infarction (PAMI) Trial. *J Am Coll Cardiol.* 1995;25:370.
23. Stone GW, Marsalese D, Brodie BR, et al. A prospective, randomized evaluation of prophylactic intraaortic balloon counterpulsation in high risk patients with acute myocardial infarction treated with primary angioplasty. *J Am Coll Cardiol.* 1997;29:1459.
24. Grines CL, Marsalese D, Brodie B, et al. Safety and cost effectiveness of early discharge after primary angioplasty in low risk patients with acute myocardial infarction. *J Am Coll Cardiol.* 1998;31:967.
25. Stone GW, Brodie BR, Griffin JJ, et al. A prospective, multicenter study of the safety and feasibility of primary stenting in acute myocardial infarction: in-hospital and 30 day results of the PAMI Stent Pilot Trial. *J Am Coll Cardiol.* 1998;31:23.
26. Stone GW, Brodie BR, Griffin JJ, et al. Clinical and angiographic follow-up after primary stenting in acute myocardial infarction: the Primary Angioplasty in Myocardial Infarction (PAMI) Stent Pilot Trial. *Circulation.* 1999;99:1548.
27. Grines CL, Cox D, Stone GW, et al. A randomized trial of primary angioplasty compared to heparin-coated stent implantation for acute myocardial infarction: coronary angioplasty with or without stent implantation for acute myocardial infarction. *N Engl J Med.* 1999;341:1949.
28. Stone GW, Cox D, Garcia E, et al. Normal flow (TIMI 3) before mechanical reperfusion therapy is an independent determinant of survival in acute myocardial infarction. Analysis from the Primary Angioplasty in Myocardial Infarction Trials. *Circulation.* 2001;104:636.
29. Ross AM, Coyne KS, Reiner JS, et al. A randomized trial comparing primary angioplasty with a strategy of short-acting thrombolysis and immediate planned rescue angioplasty in acute myocardial infarction: the PACT trial. *J Am Coll Cardiol.* 1999;34:1954.
30. Strategies for Patency Enhancement in the Emergency Department (SPEED) Investigators. Trial of abciximab with and without low-dose reteplase for acute myocardial infarction. *Circulation.* 2000;101:2788.
31. Antman EM, Giugliano RP, Gibson CM, et al. Abciximab facilitates the rate and extent of thrombolysis: results of the thrombolysis in myocardial infarction (TIMI) 14 trial. *Circulation.* 1999;99:2729.
32. Sheehan FH, Bolson EL, Dodge HT, Mathey DG, Schofer J, Woo HW. Advantages and applications of the centerline method for characterizing regional ventricular function. *Circulation.* 1986;74:293.

33. Sheehan FH, Schofer J, Mathey DG, Kellett MA, Smith H, Bolson EL, Dodge HT. Measurement of regional wall motion from biplane contrast ventriculograms: a comparison of the 30 degree right anterior oblique and the 60 degree left anterior oblique projections in patients with acute myocardial infarction. *Circulation.* 1986;74:796.

34. Sheehan FH. Left ventricular dysfunction in acute myocardial infraction due to isolated left circumflex coronary artery stenosis. *Am J Cardiol.* 1998;64:440.

35. Brown BG, Bolson E, Frimer M, Dodge HT. Quantitative coronary arteriography: estimation of dimensions, hemodynamic resistance, and atheroma mass of coronary artery lesions using the arteriogram and digital computation. *Circulation.* 1977;55(2):329.

36. Reiber JHC, Booman F, Tan H, et al. A cardiac image analysis system. Objective quantitative processing of angiocardiograms. *IEEE Comp Cardiol.* 1978;XX:239.

37. Reiber JHC, von Land CD, Koning G, et al. Comparison of accuracy and precision of quantitative coronary arterial analysis between cine film and digital systems. In: Reiber JHC, Serruys PW, editors. *Progress in Quantitative Coronary Arteriography.* Kluwer Academic Publishers, 1994:67.

38. van der Zwet PM, Reiber JHC. A new approach for the quantification of complex lesion morphology: The gradient field transform; basic principles and validation results. *J Am Coll Cardiol.* 1994;24(1):216.

39. Reiber JHC, Schiemanck L, van der Zwet PM, et al. State of the art in quantitative coronary arteriography as of 1996. In: Reiber JHC, van der Wall EE, eds. *Cardiovascular Imaging.* Kluwer Academic Publishers, 1996:39.

40. Lansky AJ, Desai KJ, Koning G, Reiber JHC. Quantitative coronary angiography in vascular brachytherapy trials. In: Ron Waksman, ed. *Vascular Brachytherapy,* 3rd ed. Futura Publishers, 2001.

41. Reiber JHC, Koning G, von Land CD, van der Zwet PM. Why and how should QCA systems be validated? In: Reiber JHC, Serruys PW, eds. *Progress in Quantitative Coronary Arteriography.* Kluwer Academic Publishers, 1994:33.

42. Reiber JHC, Serruys PW, Kooijman CJ, Wijns W, Slager CJ, Gerbrands JJ et al. Assessment of short-, medium-, and long-term variations in arterial dimensions from computer-assisted quantitation of coronary cineangiograms. *Circulation.* 1985;71(2):280.

43. Reiber JHC, van der Zwet PM, Koning G, et al. Accuracy and precision of quantitative digital coronary arteriography: observer-, short-, and medium-term variabilities. *Cathet Cardiovasc Diagn.* 1993;28(3):187.

44. Reiber JHC, Koning G, Dijkstra J, et al. Angiography and intravascular ultrasound. In: Sonka M, Fitzpatrick JM, editors. *Handbook of medical imaging–Volume 2: Medical image processing and analysis.* SPIE Press, 2001:711.

45. Büchi M, Hess OM, Kirkeeide RL, et al. Validation of a new automatic system for biplane quantitative coronary arteriography. *Int J Card Imag.* 1990;5(2–3):93.

46. Wahle A, Wellnhofer E, Mugaragu I, Sauer HU, Oswald H, Fleck E. Assessment of diffuse coronary artery disease by quantitative analysis of coronary morphology based upon 3D reconstruction from biplane angiograms. *IEEE Trans Med Imag.* 1995;14:230.

47. van der Zwet PM, Meyer DJ, Reiber JHC. Automated and accurate assessment of the distribution, magnitude, and direction of pincushion distortion in angiographic images. *Invest Radiol.* 1995;30(4):204.

48. Kirkeeide RL. Coronary obstructions, morphology and physiologic significance. In: Reiber JHC, Serruys PW, eds. *Quantitative Coronary Arteriography.* Kluwer Academic Publishers, 1991:229.

49. Kalbfleisch SJ, McGillem MJ, Simon SB, DeBoe SF, Pinto IM, Mancini GB. Automated quantitation of indexes of coronary lesion complexity. Comparison between patients with stable and unstable angina. *Circulation.* 1990;82(2):439.

50. Reiber JHC. An overview of coronary quantitation techniques as of 1989. In: Reiber JHC, Serruys PW, eds. *Quantitative Coronary Arteriography.* Kluwer Academic Publishers, 1991:55.

51. Group, ACC/ACR/NEMA Ad Hoc, American College of Cardiology, American College of Radiology, and industry develop satndard for digital transfer of angiographic images. *J Am Coll Cardiol.* 1995;25:800.

52. Holmes DR, Wondrow MA, Bell MR, Nissen SE, Cusma JT. Cine film replacement: digital archival requirements and remaining obstacles. *Cathet Cardiovasc Diagn.* 1998;44(3):346.

53. Baker WA, Hearne SE, Spero LA, et al. Lossy (15:1) JPEG compression of digital coronary angiograms does not limit detection of subtle morphological features. *Circulation.* 1997;96:1157.

54. Silber S, Dorr R, Zindler G, Muhling H, Diebel T. Impact of various compression rates on interpretation of digital coronary angiograms. *Int J Cardiol.* 199760(2):195.

55. Koning G, Beretta P, Zwart P, Hekking E, Reiber JH. Effect of lossy compression on quantitative coronary measurements. *Int J Card Imag.* 199713(4):261.

56. Rigolin VH, Robiolio PA, Spero LA, et al. Compression of digital coronary angiograms does not affect visual or quantitative assessment of coronary artery stenosis severity. *Am J Cardiol.* 199678(2):131.

57. Dumay ACM, Reiber JHC, Gerbrands JJ. Determination of optimal angiographic viewing angles: Basic principles and evaluation study. *IEEE Trans Med Imag.* 1994;13:13.

58. Seiler C, Kirkeeide RL, Gould KL. Basic structure-function relations of the epicardial coronary vascular tree. Basis of quantitative coronary arteriography for diffuse coronary artery disease. *Circulation.* 1992;85(6):1987.

59. Chen SJ, Carroll JD. 3-D reconstruction of coronary arterial tree to optimize angiographic visualization. *IEEE Trans Med Imag.* 2000;19(4):318.

CHAPTER (67)

Reading Clinical Trials

Manesh R. Patel, MD, David E. Kandzari, MD, and Robert A. Harrington, MD

INTERVENTIONAL CARDIOLOGY AND CLINICAL TRIALS

On September 16, 1977, Andreas Gruntzig performed the first coronary angioplasty on a 38-year-old businessman with unstable angina and a discrete proximal left anterior descending (LAD) artery lesion. The procedure was a success, and on subsequent angiograms at 10 years and 23 years the patient continues to have a patent artery.[1,2] Gruntzig reported his first series of favorable results and immediately called for a prospective randomized trial comparing it to bypass surgery.[3,4] The field of interventional cardiology was born, and percutaneous transluminal coronary angioplasty (PTCA) quickly spread, with multiple operators in many countries gaining experience.

Today, percutaneous coronary intervention (PCI) is the dominant form of coronary revascularization. The practice of interventional cardiology has changed dramatically to include numerous diagnostic, pharmacologic, and technologic advances. The challenge for the practicing interventionalist is deciding when to adopt new therapies or technologies, in which patients and clinical situations, and at what cost. Fortunately, in keeping with Gruntzig's initial emphasis, the field now requires rigorous scientific studies to evaluate these new therapies and technologies. As a consequence, the interventional cardiologist is faced with a large body of medical literature of varying quality.

Therefore, a framework for reading and evaluating the medical literature is necessary to make the best decisions for patient care. This practice, termed *evidence-based medicine,* is defined by Sackett et al[5] as "the conscientious, explicit, and judicious use of current best evidence in making decisions about the care of individual patients." Much of the general framework used in this chapter and in most of the current practice of evidence-based medicine has been adapted from the in-depth guide on evaluating and teaching the medical literature provided by Sackett et al[6] The goal of this chapter is to provide some tools and specific examples that help the reader become facile at reading and evaluating the medical literature, specifically clinical trials with a focus on interventional cardiology.

Three steps have been identified by Sackett et al as integral to the practice of evidence based medicine. They are as follows: (1) asking a clinical question and finding an answer, (2) reading the answer article, and (3) applying the results to individual patient care. The first step, asking a clinical question and finding an answer, is not addressed directly in this chapter. With the increase in electronic resources, including PubMed, MEDLINE, and Cardiosource, most clinicians have access to the medical literature. The majority of the discussion focuses on reading the clinical trial answer article. Finally, there is a section on applying the results to the care of the individual patient. Many of the principles used in this chapter for evaluating the medical literature can be found in detail in the *JAMA User's Guide to the Medical Literature* series.[7-10]

【 】 CASE SCENARIO

You are in the cardiac catheterization lab with a cardiology fellow seeing a 62-year-old businessman with hypertension. The patient recently presented with increasing angina, for which he was admitted to the hospital and ruled out for a myocardial infarction. He was treated with 300 mg of clopidogrel on the night of admission, and is now referred for cardiac catheterization. After discussing the diagnostic and potential interventional procedure with the patient, the fellow asks you if it would be all right to treat the patient with bivalrudin and provisional glycoprotein 2b/3a inhibitor, because she recently read a trial on its benefits. You tell the fellow that is a good question, and she should bring the REPLACE-2 article to the next cath lab meeting for discussion.

【 】 DOES THIS ARTICLE ADDRESS THE QUESTION?

In order to determine if an article answers a clinical question, a clearly defined clinical question is required. The clinical question is made up of four parts: the population or clinical problem, the intervention, the control, and the outcome of interest.[11]

The population or clinical problem should be defined as clearly as possible. For instance, in the case presented earlier, this could be a patient with unstable angina and obstructive coronary artery disease. The intervention should be easy to define in many of the clinical situations in interventional cardiology. These can range from pharmacologic to device therapies. Again, in this case the intervention is percutaneous intervention with bivalirudin and provisional glycoprotein (GP) 2b/3a inhibitor use. The comparison group may either be a placebo or the current standard of care. This also may be a pharmacologic therapy, interventional device, or usual standard care practices. In this case, the comparison group is heparin and GP 2b/3a inhibitor use. Finally, the outcome of interest can be many things. Often, the reader can determine if the outcome measure used in the clinical trial is of interest and clinical importance. Death, myocardial infarction (MI), need for urgent target vessel revascularization, or bleeding might all be considered important outcomes for this clinical situation.

In this example, the clinical question could be phrased as, "In patients with coronary artery disease, does percutaneous intervention with bivalirudin and provisional GP 2b/3a inhibitor use compared to heparin and GP 2b/3a inhibitor use decrease death, myocardial infarction, urgent target vessel revascularization, or bleeding?" Using these simple criteria, many clinicians will be able to glance quickly through article titles to determine if the question is addressed. Once this first step in reading a clinical trial is accomplished, the reader can move to step two, determining if the results are valid.

【 】 ARE THE RESULTS VALID?

Determining if the results reported in a clinical trial are valid is the most important and time-consuming step in reading an article. The goal of determining the validity of a study design is to ensure the results reported are accurate. If the experiment or the clinical trial was set up in an appropriate manner, then the results are believable. However, if there is a major flaw in the experimental design, then the reader may interpret the results cautiously and potentially disregard the results. Unfortunately, for many clinical questions about therapeutics, there is no perfect clinical trial design. Therefore, many trials have some aspects that are well done and others that are not. The practice of applying the rigorous criteria for validity and determining each trial's strengths and weaknesses helps lend weight to findings and ultimately helps makes clinical decisions. This ability to weigh different study results helps the reader practice the "judicious use of the best available evidence."

In addition, understanding clinical trial design helps put future clinical trial results into the context of prior findings with an understanding of previous limitations in the medical literature. The criteria for evaluating the validity of a study depend on the type of study question: therapy, prevention, diagnosis, etiology, or

harm. In this section, we review the validity methodology for therapy questions, as these are the most common questions addressed in the medical literature. However, the criteria for the other types of studies are also easily available for review in the *JAMA* series on the using the medical literature.[10,12,13]

Step 1

The first step in determining the validity of a clinical trial evaluating a therapy is to determine if the study was randomized and follow-up was complete. Randomization is a crucial step in evaluating a therapy and should be considered one of the cornerstones of good trial design. Randomization assures the equal distribution of both measured and unmeasured characteristics that may have an affect on the measured outcome. Not all methods of randomization are the same. Patients can be randomized to a therapy by simple, block, and stratified randomization methods.

Simple randomization is random allocation of either the experimental therapy or the control therapy to the patients. This is usually accomplished with computer-generated random numbers. However, in trials with smaller numbers of patients, there can sometimes be imbalances in the number of patients in each arm of the trial depending on where in the random number sequence enrollment is completed. For this reason, block randomization is used. Block randomization creates blocks (eg, of 4 or 6) in which there are equal numbers of patients receiving the experimental or control therapy. In this fashion, even if enrollment stops in the middle of a block, the imbalance between the numbers of patients in each group is limited.

Stratified randomization is used to achieve balance between important characteristics that may affect the outcome without losing the benefits of randomization. For example, the number of diabetic patients receiving an interventional therapy such as a type of stent may play an important role on the rate of restenosis, the outcome of interest. In this case, a separate randomization sequence would be developed for diabetic and non-diabetic patients. In this manner, the trial would continue to be randomized and have equal numbers of diabetic patients in each group.

The value of randomization cannot be emphasized enough, particularly in interventional cardiology trials. Numerous unmeasured variables that may effect the pharmacologic and device therapies used in addition to the experimental therapy are best controlled for with randomization. Without randomization, observational cohorts must attempt to control for these factors by first identifying all of the variables and then applying statistical methods. For this reason, studies evaluating therapies without randomization must be seen as describing associations and not reflecting true effect. Several examples exist in which the findings from observational data were not confirmed in randomized controlled trials, the most notable of which is the effect of estrogen replacement therapy on cardiovascular outcomes.

After randomization is determined, the reader must focus on accounting for the patients in the trial. In accordance with the CONSORT guidelines for reporting randomized controlled trials, many trials now provide a diagram showing the flow of all patients in a clinical trial. This helps the reader quickly determine the dropout rate and follow-up of the study. If 500 patients are randomized to a particular interventional device and only 400 are seen in follow-up, then a potential for an unmeasured effect of the therapy exists. Even if the patients are not able to undergo all follow-up exams and procedures, the investigators must be able to report the outcome of these patients. In trials where a considerable number of patients (~20%) are lost to follow-up, significant caution must be used in interpreting the results.

Step 2

The second step in evaluating the validity of clinical trial design in testing a therapy is in determining blinding. The goal of blinding is to ensure that once randomized, patients get care that is similar outside of the studied or control therapy. Blinding should be applied to as many potential parties as possible. In the case of pharmacologic therapies, the medial staff providing care, the patients, and the outcomes assessors can and should all be blinded. This becomes more difficult in trials evaluating devices in interventional cardiology. It may not be feasible to blind the operator to the type of stent or the use of an atherectomy device. However, the patients, the other medical staff, the clinicians that see the patients in follow up, the interventionalists that perform repeat angiograms, and the outcomes assessors can all be blinded to the therapy.

In the example case, the investigators in the REPLACE-2 trial went to great lengths to retain blinding. Prior to randomization, the interventionalist specified a preference for abciximab or eptifibatide as the GP 2b/3a inhibitor of choice for the intervention. Each patient then received three infusions. In one arm they received bivalirudin, heparin placebo, and GP 2b/3a inhibitor placebo, and in the other arm they received bivalirudin placebo, active heparin, and GP 2b/3a inhibitor. A blinded activated clotting time (ACT) was then performed and active drug was given if the ACT was less than 225 sec. Finally, if the interventionalist determined that provisional GP 2b/3a inhibitor was required, the active bivalirudin arm received active GP 2b/3a inhibitor while the heparin and GP 2b/3a inhibitor arm received placebo GP 2b/3a inhibitor. In this fashion, blinding of the patients and medial staff was retained and helped ensure patients in both arms of the trial received similar care during the procedure and afterward.

The next step is to determine if the patients were similar at the start of the trial. Most clinical trials present the baseline characteristics of the patients in the first table. If randomization was successful, the patients should be similar with regard to most characteristics. As mentioned earlier, some important characteristics that affect the outcome may have been stratified, thus ensuring equal numbers of patients in each group. In smaller trials, there are often small differences in the groups. However, we would caution against making any significant conclusions from these differences and would continue to lend weight to the process of randomization. At best, differences in the groups and direction of potential effect on the results should be noted prior to reading the results.

The last part of the second step should be to determine how the patients were evaluated at the end of the trial. Specifically, was the analysis of the patients done based on the groups they were randomized at the start of the trial, regardless of any crossover or dropout? This is defined as the *intention to treat principle,* and is crucial in interventional clinical trials. This must be differentiated from an analysis of patients who received successful treatment. For example, if a group of patients were randomized to stent implantation or angioplasty, but the analysis for the outcome of urgent target vessel revascularization was carried out only in the group of patients who successfully underwent stent implantation, then the results would be biased toward the stent group. The stent may be difficult to deliver, and those patients who were unable to undergo stent implantation may have higher rates of the desired outcome. Therefore, in both pharmacologic and device trials in interventional cardiology, the intention to treat principle is critical because it provides a conservative view of the benefit of a therapy, one that may be closer to actual practice.

Step 3

The third step in determining the validity of a clinical trial is assessing the analysis plan. The analysis plan starts with the intended comparison. When the clinical trial is set up and reported, the investigators should specify the intended comparison groups clearly. In addition, when more than one therapy is being tested, the comparison groups must be pre-specified and appropriate.

For example, the Controlled Abciximab and Device Investigation to Lower Late Angioplasty Complications (CADILLAC) trial compared angioplasty with stenting, with or without abciximab, in patients with acute myocardial infarction (MI).[14] Patients were randomized in a two-by-two factorial design, meaning that patients were randomized to angioplasty or stenting and then each group was randomized again to abciximab use or not. The results are that some patients received angioplasty alone, angioplasty with abciximab, stenting alone, and stenting with abciximab. This design conserves resources and addresses two questions: the value of angioplasty or stenting and the value of abciximab or not.

However, to answer these questions appropriately, the correct groups must be compared. To answer the utility of PTCA versus stenting in acute MI, the comparison in the trial should be all patients who received PTCA (50% of the patients) versus stenting (50% of the patients). Likewise, when answering the question of the utility of abciximab, the comparison groups must be all patients who received abciximab, irrespective of PTCA or stent status (50% of the patients), versus all patients who did not receive abciximab (50% of the patients). When this latter comparison was carried out, the value of abciximab was found to be significant.[15]

Aside from not performing the correct comparisons, another pitfall is making multiple comparisons at the conclusion of a clinical trial. The power, or ability to detect a difference between therapies, is calculated for the primary analysis. Multiple comparisons that are performed after the completion of the trial may not have the power to detect a difference, or they may find a difference by chance. A classic example of the multiple comparisons yielding a chance finding is the published report from the ISIS-2 investigators that patients with the astrologic sign Libra did not gain a benefit from the use of aspirin at the time of acute MI.[16] This example clearly does not have physiologic basis, but demonstrates the ability of multiple comparisons (12 astrologic signs) to uncover a false finding. Therefore, findings from subgroup analysis should be considered similar to observational analysis. They are hypothesis generating, but do not indicate a true effect and should be viewed with caution in trials that demonstrate a consistent benefit of a therapy.

After determining the comparison groups, the analysis plan must be reviewed. A contemporary trial design in interventional cardiology to account for the rapidly changing pharmacologic and device therapies is the *non-inferiority analysis plan*. In order to understand non-inferiority, we must first review the classic superiority trial design. Traditionally, when therapy A was compared against placebo or usual care, the trial was set up to test whether the therapy improved outcome. In order to do this, the investigators generally postulate that therapy A will lead to a prespecified percentage improvement in the outcome; for example, 30% improvement in the rate of restenosis. Then the power calculation is used to determine the number of patients required to demonstrate that percentage improvement. If the findings are statistically significant, then the therapy has lead to at least the prespecified degree of improvement, if not more. If the results are not statistically significant, then the therapy has been found to not improve outcomes by the prespecified amount, less than 30% improvement in restenosis in the previous example. Although this design allows the evaluation of potential superiority of one therapy, this trial design does not answer if the two therapies being tested are similar with regard to the therapeutic effects.

In contrast to the classic superiority clinical trial design, the non-inferiority trial design attempts to test if a new experimental therapy is not inferior to a control therapy by retaining a prespecified percentage of the effect of the control therapy. In the case of the REPLACE-2 trial comparing bivalirudin to heparin and GP 2b/3a inhibitor, *non-inferiority* was defined as the ability of bivalirudin to retain 50% of the benefit of GP 2b/3a inhibitor therapy. Hence, based on the previous studies, the upper confidence interval for 50% of the benefit of GP 2b/3a inhibitor plus heparin versus heparin therapy was set at an OR of 0.92 (Figure 67-1). If the effect of bivalirudin crosses this upper boundary, then the conclusion would be that bivalirudin does not meet the prespecified non-inferiority criteria, and bivalirudin may indeed be inferior to GP 2b/3a inhibitor therapy. The findings of the REPLACE-2 trial did find bivalirudin to not be inferior to GP 2b/3a inhibitor plus heparin therapy. However, there are examples of trials that have demonstrated the superiority of a therapy, even when the initial trial design is non-inferiority.

A notable example in interventional cardiology includes the randomized trial of tirofiban versus abciximab in patients undergoing percutaneous revascularization.[17] Using a two-tailed analysis of the 95% confidence interval found tirofiban to have a hazard ratio of 1.01–1.57 compared to abciximab, demonstrating the superiority of abciximab.

As point of clarification, it should be noted that equivalence does not carry the same meaning as non-inferiority with regard to clinical trial design. In order to establish the equivalence between two therapies, both non-inferiority and non-superiority must be established. This means that the effect of a new therapy and its confidence intervals on both sides must be similar to the control therapy. In fact, the effect of the new therapy could be less than or greater than the control therapy. In order to demonstrate this, significantly more patients are required to prove true equivalence. It is for this reason that many clinical trials comparing two therapies are designed as non-inferiority trials, especially when one therapy is the standard of care.

Non-inferiority trials will continue to occur in interventional cardiology as newer therapies and devices are discovered. As each new therapy is found with some specific advantage, such as cost, ease of use, and safety, trials are required to demonstrate that the therapy is as least as effective as the prior standard of care. This was the driving force for the design for the TARGET trial that was designed specifically to demonstrate the tirofiban was non-inferior to abciximab because of its considerable cost benefit. Finally, it should be noted that there is no current consensus on the exact boundaries that are pre-specified for non-inferiority trials.

Design Issues Specific to Interventional Cardiology. Many of the validity criteria described for evaluating the methodology of therapy clinical trials thus far should be applied to all interventional cardiology trials. However, there are trial issues specific to the field of interventional cardiology that require discussion.

In addition to the non-inferiority design already discussed, interventional trials require specific consideration when dealing with devices. In order to understand the total effect of a new device, the safety and the therapeutic effect must be understood. Also, the learning curve required to be able to successfully use the experimental device must also be investigated.

Currently, a new device goes through significant study in the steps prior to the phase 3 efficacy trial. Along the way, the device is tested in pre-clinical, phase 1, and phase 2 optimal use or "dose-ranging" studies. The safety of the device can be evaluated by combining all the data. In addition, a sense of the clinical learning curve is also demonstrated.

Finally, the large phase 3 therapeutic efficacy trials address many of these same issues. However, as stated earlier, these trials can often not be blinded. Therefore, particular attention must be paid to postapproval surveillance. Often, rate adverse events can be detected only by this method. Unfortunately, complication rates for postapproval device therapy may be vastly underreported, making evaluation of new devices difficult. Both the United States Food and Drug Administration (FDA) and industry are working hard to standardize the process for both this special type of therapy trial and postapproval monitoring.

Step 4

The fourth and final step in evaluating the validity of a clinical trial design is to determine a validity score. No clinical trial design is absolutely ideal, and no clinical trial design is absolutely without merit. However, there may be some clinical trials that have fatal flaws in their design that may preclude reviewing the results. In fact, the entire exercise of the determining the validity of a clinical

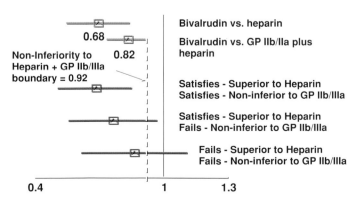

FIGURE 67-1. Non-inferiority design for REPLACE-2

trial design and methodology is to assess the strength with which the reader may feel the results mirror actual truth. Therefore, we have found it helpful to stop after reviewing the validity of a clinical trial design and answer two simple questions. The first is, "Should the results be viewed?" If the trial is set up with such a fatal flaw, the therapies were not randomized or blinded, for example, then the reader should consider not reviewing the results at all. The second question is on a scale of 1–10, with 10 being the ideal clinical trial design for the specific question, "How well was the trial set up?" We have found that putting a numeric value on the validity of the trial design helps indeed in the future when weighing the results and applying them to patient care.

WHAT ARE THE RESULTS?

Once the reader determines that the trial was set up with suitable methodology, then the results should be interpreted. In general, the results of the treatment effect are presented with regard to pre-specified primary outcome measure.

For example, the SIRIUS trial evaluated the sirolimus-eluting stent versus a standard, bare-metal BX velocity stent in 1058 patients with a newly diagnosed coronary lesion in a native coronary artery.[18] The primary outcome was *failure of the target vessel,* defined as a composite of death from cardiac causes, myocardial infarction, and repeated percutaneous or surgical revascularization of the target vessel. The rate of target vessel failure occurred in 21.0% of the patients in the standard stent group and 8.6% of the sirolimus-eluting stent group ($p < .001$). The investigators report that this difference was driven largely by a decrease in the need for target vessel revascularization (16.6% in the standard stent group vs 4.1% in the sirolimus-eluting stent group [$p < .001$]).[18] These results are significant and may be better understood in terms of absolute risk reduction.

〖 〗 ABSOLUTE RISK REDUCTION

The absolute risk reduction (ARR) is a simple calculation that can be performed for any outcome, and it can provide a sense of the overall magnitude of effect. The absolute risk reduction is defined as the difference in the rates of outcomes for the tested therapy versus the control therapy. In the example of the SIRIUS trial described earlier, the absolute risk reduction associated with a sirolimus-eluting stent compared to a standard stent for the outcome of target vessel failure is 21.0% − 8.6% = 12.4%. This means 12.4% fewer patients treated with sirolimus-eluting stents will have target vessel failure compared to standard stent therapy.

The ARR can used to calculate the *number needed to treat (NNT)*. The NNT is calculated as 1/ARR, or, in the earlier example, 1/0.124 = 8. The NNT can be used to express the results of a trial and its magnitude in terms of patients required to demonstrate the desired outcome. In our example, this would be stated as 8 patients must be treated with sirolimus-eluting stent to prevent 1 episode of target vessel failure at 9 months, the duration of follow-up in the clinical trial.

Once multiple trial results are converted to NNTs for each outcome, then it becomes easier to determine the weight of findings from each clinical trial finding. Similar to the SIRIUS trial, the results of the landmark ISIS-2 trial evaluating aspirin, streptokinase, both, or neither in patients with acute MI can also be summarized using NNT.[16] The number of patients with acute MI who must be treated with 162 mg of aspirin or streptokinase compared to placebo to prevent one vascular death at 5 weeks is 36. In addition, 19 patients must be treated with the combination of aspirin and streptokinase to prevent one death within 30 days. These numbers underscore both the strength of the clinical trial findings and the synergy of the therapies when used in combination.

〖 〗 RELATIVE RISK REDUCTION

A cautionary note should be made with regard to relative risk reduction. In contrast to absolute risk reduction, the relative risk reduction takes into account the actual rate of an outcome. Specifically, the relative risk reduction is calculated by dividing the difference between the therapies by the control event rate (Table 67-1). For example, the CAPRIE trial evaluated 75 mg of clopidogrel a day versus 325 mg of aspirin to reduce the risk of a composite outcome comprised of ischemic stroke, myocardial infarction, or vascular death.[19] In total, 19,185 patients were randomized, and the event

〖 〗 TABLE 67-1

Calculating Absolute and Relative Risk Reductions

EXAMPLE RATES		OUTCOME (ie, RESTENOSIS)
Therapy A (for Patients Undergoing Cardiac Catheterization)		3%
Control Therapy (Standard Therapy for Patients Undergoing Catheterization)		5%
MEASUREMENT	**FORMULA**	**RESULT**
ARR	Control event rate − experimental event rate	5% − 3% = 2%
RRR	Control event rate − experimental event rate/ control event rate	5 − 3/5 × 100 = 40%
Number needed to treat	1/ARR	1/0.02 = 50

ARR = absolute risk reduction; RRR = relative risk reduction.

rate of 5.32% in the clopidogrel-treated patients versus 5.83% in the aspirin-treated patients. This difference was found to be statistically significant ($p = .043$). The investigators correctly report an 8.7% relative risk reduction in favor of the clopidogrel-treated patients. However, the absolute risk reduction (5.83% − 5.32%) is 0.51%. This translates to an NNT of 196. This means the clinician would have to treat 196 patients with clopidogrel instead of aspirin for at least 1 year to prevent 1 ischemic stroke, myocardial infarction, or death. Hence, this example demonstrates how the NNT and ARR may provide a better view of the overall strength of trial results compared to relative risk reduction calculations. The use of these terms may help the clinician determine whether the clinical trial findings are clinically important.

【 】 STATISTICAL SIGNIFICANCE VERSUS CLINICAL SIGNIFICANCE

Statistical significance is a mathematical evaluation. Clinical trials set out to answer a question by determining the magnitude of effect that would be meaningful to practicing clinicians. They then determine the number of patients needed to adequately address the question with a specific degree of certainty, also known as the *power of the trial*. Finally, the results are said to meet statistical significance if the findings have less than 5% chance of representing a chance finding. It should be noted that the p value of .05 is an arbitrary standard, and certainly the level of significance for secondary analyses may require more rigorous statistical standards.[20]

In contrast, clinical significance may vary tremendously. The trial assumptions, including the magnitude of the effect, the cost of the therapy, and the outcome tested, may all affect the individual clinician's determination of clinical significance. The CAPRIE trial, mentioned earlier, did not lead to a change from aspirin to clopidogrel for patients with atherosclerotic disease. However, the CURE trial, which evaluated clopidogrel plus aspirin versus aspirin alone and found a 2.1% ARR in a composite of death from cardiovascular causes, non-fatal myocardial infarction, and stroke in patients with acute coronary syndromes, did lead to a change in practice.[21] Finally, clinical significance may vary depending on the location of practice. The GUSTO trial demonstrated an ARR of 1% in death at 30 days for tPA with intravenous heparin, compared to streptokinase and intravenous heparin in patients with acute MI.[22] This changed clinical practice in the United States, but was not immediately adopted in other parts of the world.

【 】 WHAT ARE THE ADVERSE EFFECTS?

The last part of evaluating the results of a clinical trial includes determining any adverse events. Most trials report the rate of adverse events with indication of whether the results are significant. For instance, in the GUSTO trial, tPA resulted in a 0.23% increase in hemorrhagic stroke compared to streptokinase. This percentage can be termed a *0.23% absolute risk increase* in hemorrhagic stroke in patients treated with tPA, correlating to a number needed to harm (NNH) of 434. Restated, 434 patients with acute MI must be treated with tPA versus streptokinase to lead to one additional hemorrhagic stroke. In this manner, adverse effects of therapies can be put into context with the therapeutic benefits so that clinicians can weigh all the risks and benefits prior to determining clinical significance.

CONCLUSIONS

We reviewed a method for reading clinical trials involving therapies with an emphasis on interventional cardiology. The process of determining if the trial answers your clinical question, evaluating the trials for valid methodologic design, and reviewing the results should help provide a framework for a lifelong review of the medical literature. The process of reading the medical literature ends with applying the results to the patient care.

In applying the results to patient care, special emphasis should be placed on whether relevant outcomes, both beneficial and adverse, were considered. Restenosis rates in trials with drug-eluting stents seem like reasonable outcomes. However, practicing clinicians may not routinely perform cardiac catheterizations on asymptomatic patients at 6 months, and this may indeed inflate the rate of the outcome of interest. Also, clinicians must weigh the risks and benefits of each individual therapy with patient characteristics and preferences. This is the art of medicine, and improving one's ability to appraise the literature critically should only help with this process.

It is hoped that we provided some helpful tips and warnings about pitfalls that should help with the critical appraisal of the literature. With the ever-changing face of interventional cardiology; our review of clinical trial design, including non-inferiority trial design; valid trial methodology, including randomization and blinding; and assessment of trial results using absolute risk reduction and number needed to treat should provide the tools to continue to stay abreast of an ever-changing scientific field.

REFERENCES

1. Meier B, Bachmann D., Luscher T. 25 years of coronary angioplasty: almost a fairy tale. *Lancet.* 2003;361(9356):527.
2. King SB, 3rd, Meier B. Interventional treatment of coronary heart disease and peripheral vascular disease. *Circulation.* 2000;102(20 Suppl 4):IV81.
3. Gruntzig A., Transluminal dilatation of coronary-artery stenosis. *Lancet.* 1978;1(8058):263.
4. Gruntzig AR, Senning A, Siegenthaler WE. Nonoperative dilatation of coronary-artery stenosis: percutaneous transluminal coronary angioplasty. *N Engl J Med.* 1979;301(2):61.
5. Sackett DL, Rosenberg WM, Gray JA, et al. Evidence based medicine: what it is and what it isn't [Editorial]. *BMJ.*1996;312(7023):71–2.
6. Sackett DL, Richardson WS, Rosenberg WMC, Haynes RB. *Evidence-Based Medicine: How to Practice and Teach EBM* 2nd ed. 2000; Churchill Livingston.
7. Oxman AD, Sackett DL, Guyatt GH. Users' guides to the medical literature. I. How to get started. The Evidence-Based Medicine Working Group. *JAMA.* 1993;270(17):2093.
8. Guyatt GH, Rennie D. Users' guides to the medical literature. *JAMA.* 1993;270(17):2096.
9. Guyatt GH, Sackett DL, Cook DJ. Users' guides to the medical literature. II. How to use an article about therapy or prevention. A. Are the results of the study valid? Evidence-Based Medicine Working Group. *JAMA.* 1993;270(21):2598-601.
10. Guyatt GH, Sackett DL, Cook DJ. Users' guides to the medical literature. II. How to use an article about therapy or prevention. B. What were the results and will they help me in caring for my patients? Evidence-Based Medicine Working Group. *JAMA.* 1994;271(1):59.
11. Richardson WS, Wilson MC, Nishikawa J, Hayward RS. The well-built clinical question: a key to evidence-based decisions [Editorial]. *ACP J Club.* 1995;123(3):A12.
12. Jaeschke R, Guyatt GH, Sackett DL. Users' guides to the medical literature. III. How to use an article about a diagnostic test. B. What are the results and will they help me in caring for my patients? The Evidence-Based Medicine Working Group. *JAMA.* 1994271(9):703.

13. Oxman AD, Cook DJ,, Guyatt GH. Users' guides to the medical literature. VI. How to use an overview. Evidence-Based Medicine Working Group]. *JAMA.* 1994;272(17):1367.

14. Stone GW, Grines CL, Cox DA, et al. Comparison of angioplasty with stenting, with or without abciximab, in acute myocardial infarction. *N Engl J Med.* 2002;346(13): 957.

15. Tcheng JE, Kandzari DE, Grines CL, et al. Benefits and risks of abciximab use in primary angioplasty for acute myocardial infarction: the Controlled Abciximab and Device Investigation to Lower Late Angioplasty Complications (CADILLAC) trial. *Circulation.* 2003;108:1316.

16. Anonymous. Randomised trial of intravenous streptokinase, oral aspirin, both, or neither among 17,187 cases of suspected acute myocardial infarction: ISIS-2. ISIS-2 (Second International Study of Infarct Survival) Collaborative Group. *Lancet.* 1988;2(8607):349-60.

17. Topol EJ, Moliterno DJ, Hermann HC, et al. Comparison of two platelet glycoprotein IIb/IIIa inhibitors, tirofiban and abciximab, for the prevention of ischemic events with percutaneous coronary revascularization.[see comment]. *N Engl J Med.* 2001;344(25):1888.

18. Moses JW, Leon MB, Popma JJ, et al. Sirolimus-eluting stents versus standard stents in patients with stenosis in a native coronary artery. *N Engl J Med.* 2003;349(14):1315.

19. Anonymous. A randomised, blinded, trial of clopidogrel versus aspirin in patients at risk of ischaemic events (CAPRIE). CAPRIE Steering Committee. [see comment]. *Lancet.* 1996;348(9038):1329.

20. Moye LA. *P*-value interpretation and alpha allocation in clinical trials. *Ann Epidemiol.* 19988(6):351.

21. Yusuf S, Zhao F, Mehta SR, et al. Effects of clopidogrel in addition to aspirin in patients with acute coronary syndromes without ST-segment elevation. [erratum appears in *N Engl J Med.* 2001;345(23):1716]. *N Engl J Med.* 2001; 345(7):494.

22. Anonymous. An international randomized trial comparing four thrombolytic strategies for acute myocardial infarction. The GUSTO investigators. *N Engl J Med.* 329(10):673.

PART 9　Reimbursement

CHAPTER (68)

Cost-Effectiveness

Uwe Siebert, MD

For decades, health-care costs have been rising in the United States. Among many factors, the rapid advance in expensive medical technologies is a major cause for this rise. Meanwhile, issues surrounding health-care costs have captured the attention of the public, policymakers, health-care providers, industry, and policymakers. More than most other areas in medicine, cardiology has been affected by the continued technologic progress leading to the development of new and effective technologies such as percutaneous coronary intervention (PCI), implantable defibrillators, heart transplantation, and various sophisticated diagnostic procedures, with an even larger class of medical treatments. The American Heart Association estimated an overall cost of $368.4 billion for cardiovascular disease in the US.[1] In 1999, $26.3 billion in payments were made by the Medicare program to acute care hospitals, for a principal diagnosis of cardiovascular disease.[1] Therefore, it is not surprising that the field of cardiology has become one of the areas where economic issues are now raised continuously.

In an environment of economic limitations, rising health care expenditures have led decision makers to question whether these technologies are worth the cost. Cost effectiveness analyses represent an attempt to compare the overall costs of an intervention with a measure of clinical benefit, which is meaningful to the patient, clinician or health-care payer.

The first part of this chapter reviews the key concepts and methods in economic evaluation. The second part presents four examples of cost-effectiveness studies to illustrate how these approaches can be applied to evaluate the cost-effectiveness of prevention, diagnosis, and treatment of cardiovascular disease. Finally, the chapter briefly discusses the limitations and challenges we confront in the field of cost-effectiveness analysis.

CONCEPTS AND METHODS IN HEALTH ECONOMICS

【 】 DEFINITION OF ECONOMIC EVALUATION

We usually express costs in monetary terms (eg, dollars). A health economist, however, has a different concept of costs. A fundamental premise in economics is that any utilization of resources in the production of goods or services is accompanied by foregone opportunities to produce some other goods or services with those resources.[2] This concept is referred to as *opportunity costs,* which are "the value of resources when put to their next best alternative use."[3] This principle is linked directly to another premise in economic reasoning: Society's resources are finite and can never satisfy all societal needs. Resources that are used for health care cannot be used for other purposes such as public education, transportation, defense, and other priorities. Similarly, given a fixed health-care budget, resources applied to the treatment of one disease (eg, hospital space, material, personnel time, the human effort to develop and produce drugs and devices) are lost for the treatment of another disease. For example, the resources devoted to PCI within a health-care system might be used for alternative interventions such as cancer screening programs or vaccination. Therefore, it is critical to use resources for preventive, diagnostic, and therapeutic health-care interventions in a way that balances the costs and health benefits of any of these strategies when compared to alternative strategies. Thus, one of the goals of health economics is to determine the most efficient use of the resources available to provide health care to a population. Economic evaluation aims at providing structured information in order to guide decision makers to make choices.

Economic evaluation is defined as the comparative analysis of alternative courses of action in terms of both their costs and consequences.[2] Applied to health care, in most cases, this concerns the comparison between a new intervention and the current clinical standard of care.

[ ] TYPES OF ECONOMIC EVALUATIONS

Economic evaluations that focus only on costs and not on health benefits or evaluate the costs and health outcomes (eg, mortality) of one intervention without comparing it to the other available options are designated "partial evaluations." In contrast, a "full economic evaluation" considers both costs and health outcomes of two or more alternative interventions.[2] There are four basic types of full economic evaluations (Table 68-1):

1. Cost-minimization analyses.

2. Cost-benefit analyses.

3. Cost-effectiveness analyses.

4. Cost-utility analyses.

A cost minimization analysis can be used when the health consequences of alternative interventions are equivalent. In this case, the economic analysis is essentially a search for the least expensive alternative, and therefore, confined to comparing the costs of the alternative interventions.

In a cost–benefit analysis, both costs and health gains are valued in monetary terms. The results are usually reported as net economic cost or net economic benefit. If the net benefit of an intervention is positive, this intervention "pays" for itself (in economic terms). Although this study type has the advantage of combining an intervention's effects on all outcomes, the analyst must assign a monetary value to health gains such as reduction of pain or increase of life expectancy. However, the concept of placing a monetary value on a human life is highly controversial, especially among physicians.

A cost-effectiveness analysis can be applied to comparisons of interventions that have a common outcome of interest, such as reduction of restenosis risk or life-years gained. If the more effective therapy is also the more expensive one, an incremental cost-effectiveness ratio (ICER) is calculated, that is, the additional cost per additional health gain. The policymaker must then decide whether the incremental health gain achieved with the more effective therapy is worth the additional cost.

Finally, a cost-utility analysis compares the difference in cost between strategies with the net clinical benefit as measured in terms of generic health outcome measures such as quality-adjusted life years (QALYs), which can be compared across different interventions and diseases (see later for a more detailed description of this concept). In cases where the more effective therapy is more expensive, the incremental cost-utility ratio expresses the additional cost per QALY gained. Again, the question is then whether the extra cost of the more effective intervention is justified by the QALY gain.

In most of the cardiology literature and in this chapter, economic evaluations are used to compare a proposed new strategy with the appropriate reference strategy. Usually, new strategies in cardiology differ from previous strategies in costs and health outcomes, and therefore, cost-minimization analyses are rare in the field of cardiology. After Weinstein and Stason introduced the concept of cost-effectiveness in economic health-care evaluation,[4] most economic evaluations have been either cost-effectiveness studies or cost-utility studies. Therefore, this chapter focuses on these types of economic evaluations, and refers to both study types as *cost-effectiveness analyses*.

Table 68-2 describes the possible results of comparing a new intervention with the current standard of care. The new technology could be better, equal, or worse than the standard treatment, when comparing clinical effectiveness, and the costs of the new technology could be higher than, equal to, or lower than those of the standard treatment. This leads to nine possible results of the comparison. If a treatment strategy A is less costly and leads to equal or better clinical outcomes than the alternative strategy B, A is the obvious choice, and A is said to "dominate" B and is cost-saving. If two strategies yield the same costs, the method that offers the better clinical outcomes is preferred and dominates the other without being cost saving. The most interesting and challenging situation is when the clinically superior strategy is also more expensive. In this case, the question is whether the improved health outcome is worth the additional costs, and the incremental cost-effectiveness (or cost-utility) ratio is a useful measure to guide the decision maker in choosing the preferred strategy.[5]

TABLE 68-1

Study Types and Outcome Measures of Economic Evaluations

TYPE OF ECONOMIC ANALYSIS	OUTCOME MEASURE	FORMULA
Cost-minimization analysis	Net costs $=$	$Cost_1 - Cost_2$
Cost-benefit analysis	Net economic cost $=$	$(Cost_1 - Cost_2) - (Benefit_1 - Benefit_2)$
Cost-effectiveness analysis	Incremental cost-effectiveness ratio $=$	$\dfrac{Cost_1 - Cost_2}{Effectiveness_1 - Effectiveness_2}$
Cost-utility analysis	Incremental cost-utility ratio $=$	$\dfrac{Cost_1 - Cost_2}{U_1 - U_2}$

U: quality-adjusted life-years (QALY) or other generic health outcome measures used as utility.

TABLE 68-2

Possible Results of Comparing a New Intervention with Current Standard of Care

	$EFF_1 < EFF_2$	$EFF_1 = EFF_2$	$EFF_1 > EFF_2$
$Cost_1 > Cost_2$	(1) Int_1 dominant and cost-saving	(2) Int_2 dominant and cost-saving	(3) CEA
$Cost_1 = Cost_2$	(4) Int_2 dominant, but not cost-saving	(5) Indifference	(6) Int_1 dominant, but not cost-saving
$Cost_1 < Cost_2$	(7) CEA	(8) Int_1 dominant and cost-saving	(9) Int_1 dominant and cost-saving

Indices 1 and 2 indicate intervention 1 (new technology) and intervention 2 (current standard of care).
Eff: effectiveness; Int: intervention; CEA: cost-effectiveness analysis.

[ ] MEASURING COSTS

A fair economic evaluation should completely account for all relevant costs.[2] Besides the costs of the treatment itself, costs for adjunctive therapy, treatment of complications, hospitalization, and the costs for follow-up and treatment of late adverse events have to be considered. Therefore, the time horizon of the economic evaluation should be long enough to capture all relevant events and related costs of the health-care intervention.

The identification and determination of costs is usually a highly complex task. Critical to any economic analysis is how the costs are defined. Costs are usually divided into "direct" and "indirect" costs. Whereas "direct" generally refers to costs attributable to the intervention, "indirect" is often used to refer to productivity gains or losses caused by morbidity or death. Another distinction is made between medical and nonmedical costs. *Direct medical costs* include the costs of tests, drugs, supplies, health-care personnel, and medical facilities. Costs arising from the initial intervention and subsequent hospitalizations have to be included as well as follow-up visits and procedures during a predefined period when complications from the index procedure are expected.[6,7] For example, an economic evaluation of treating acute myocardial infarction (MI) should include the cost of the initial intervention (eg, streptokinase), treatment of complications induced (eg, bleeding, stroke) and averted (eg, congestive heart failure) by the intervention, as well as concomitant treatments (eg, coronary stent implantation).[8]

Direct non-medical costs are those associated with the intervention but not related to health care. Examples are child-care costs for a parent undergoing a coronary angiography, the increase in total costs required by a dietary prescription, the transportation to and from the hospital, chronic nursing care, or an equivalent reflecting services by unpaid family members.[6]

Indirect costs refer to the societal costs associated with gains or loss of productivity related to illness or death. As the term *indirect* has many other interpretations (eg, in accounting, it is used to describe overhead or fixed costs), it has been suggested to use the term productivity costs instead.[6] *Productivity costs* are costs associated with lost or impaired ability to work or to engage in leisure activities as a result of morbidity and lost economic productivity because of death.[9] Because it is a major cause of disability and death, cardiovascular disease has a substantial economic impact on productivity. For example, when comparing stent implantation versus coronary artery bypass surgery, one must consider the fact that bypass surgery is, on average, associated with a longer hospital stay and recovery period, and thus, a longer absence from work than after stenting. This component of productivity costs has also been referred to as *morbidity costs*.[9] Changes in life expectancy as a result of an intervention can lead to changes in economic productivity as well. For example, when a patient dies from the complications of a PCI, the goods this person would have produced during his or her lifetime are lost to society. This component of productivity costs has been referred to as *mortality costs*.[9] The Panel on Cost-Effectiveness in Health and Medicine, which was convened by the US Public Health Service in 1993,[6] recommends that productivity costs associated with morbidity be included in the denominator of an incremental cost–utility ratio; that is, they should be incorporated in the quality-of-life measure (and excluded from the numerator to avoid double counting). Mortality effects are by convention included in the denominator (QALY) of an incremental cost–utility ratio, and therefore should not be included in the numerator (costs). The same applies to incremental cost-effectiveness ratios if the measure of effectiveness is life expectancy. However, reporting the gains or losses in productivity costs may be of particular interest in some analyses, and could be reported separately. If the analyst wishes to incorporate the monetary value of productivity costs into the calculation, this could be done by cost–benefit analysis.[9] Other time costs have previously been included under the heading of indirect costs, such as the value of the time individuals devote to the care of sick friends and relatives. The US Panel on Cost-Effectiveness in Health and Medicine suggests that these latter components of time cost be included as direct costs in the numerator of the cost-effectiveness ratio.[10]

For the collection of cost data, it is useful to think about the cost of a health-care product or service as a function of both the resources used to produce it and the price of each of those resources.[11] For example, the cost of stent implantation should include the stent and other supplies used in the procedure; the amount of time spent by physicians, nurses, and technicians; and the cost of using the catheterization laboratory facility with its equipment.

There are two major methods to measure costs in clinical studies, "bottom-up" and "top-down."[12] The bottom-up approach is based on the assessment of the utilization of key resources (eg, tests, drugs, procedures, hospital days, office visits) and calculates costs by multiplying resources by prices or item costs. This approach may be preferred in large studies and in settings in which patients are not billed for services.[13]

The second approach to collecting economic data in clinical studies is the top-down approach, which establishes costs based on billing and financial records. This approach has the practical limitation that obtaining copies of bills for every service is labor intensive and records can be incomplete. Moreover, charges for a health-care service are often a poor reflection of its actual cost.[14] In particular, cardiac interventions are profitable under most insurance systems, whereas many other types of interventions are not. Using charge data may serve to make cardiac interventions look less cost-effective, because charges may overestimate the real resources being used to produce the medical care.[15] This limitation has been addressed by using standardized methods to convert charges to costs, based on "cost-to-charge ratios" published in each hospital's annual Medicare Cost Report, which is available to the public.[13,16] An alternative cost estimation method, which does not depend on the conversion of hospital charge data, is the use of diagnosis-related group (DRG) reimbursement rates. This system assigns the hospital costs based on the DRG of the individual patient.[12] For physician's fees, no cost-to-charge ratios are available. Some countries (eg, United States, Canada) have developed Physician Fee Schedules reflecting the long-term cost of services provided by physicians.[17] The Medicare fees of the United States are linked to the physician's Current Procedural Terminology (CPT), a classification system developed by the American Medical Association that codes for different physician services.[12]

Finally, in some studies, it is feasible to collect economic data by accessing computerized databases used by hospitals, insurers or health-care systems, such as the Centers for Medicare and Medicaid Services (CMS) in the United States, or private insurance databases. However, this approach requires permission to access these databases, which can be difficult given the concerns about the privacy of medical records. Furthermore, the fact that the United States has no national health insurance limits the generalizability of the conclusions of such studies.

A recent study compared four different methods for measuring costs from multicenter clinical trials to determine the extent to which the methodology affects results.[18] Using patient-level data ($n = 1849$) from three multicenter clinical trials of percutaneous coronary revascularization, the investigators compared the following approaches: (1) hospital charges; (2) hospital charges converted to costs by use of hospital-level cost-to-charge ratios; (3) hospital charges converted to costs by use of department-level cost-to-charge ratios; and (4) itemized catheterization laboratory costs with nonprocedural hospital costs generated from department-level cost-to-charge ratios. In this study, charges were approximately twice as high as hospital cost estimates, and thus, the magnitude of absolute and incremental cost estimates varied considerably by method. However, the method used to approximate costs did not affect the main results of the economic comparisons for any of the trials. The authors emphasized the importance of a detailed description of cost derivation, particularly when the absolute magnitude of the cost estimates is important to decision makers.[18]

MEASURING EFFECTIVENESS

All economic evaluations involve the selection of relevant endpoints for measuring the clinical benefits of the health-care interventions under comparison. One way of measuring the health effect of the compared interventions is to use a common endpoint of interest that can be expressed in "natural units," such as cholesterol levels for lipid-lowering therapies, blood pressure for antihypertensive treatments, or prevented revascularizations for PCIs. Furthermore, outcomes such as major cardiac events, rehospitalizations, deaths, disease-free survival, or life expectancy have been used to compare different cardiologic interventions.

In many cases, however, none of these endpoints captures all relevant dimensions that the decision maker wants to incorporate in the decision. For example, patients do not directly perceive surrogate endpoints such as cholesterol levels and blood pressure. Furthermore, few new therapies in interventional cardiology have been shown to substantially extend life, but they may improve health-related quality of life, and therefore, survival and health-related quality of life should be combined in a single metric. The most commonly used approach in cost–utility analyses is the metric of QALYs. QALYs are calculated by combining duration and quality of life by weighting (ie, multiplying) the length of time a person survives in a specific health state with a quality-of-life index (ie, utility) assigned to this health state. The utility weight reflects the individual's preference for a specific health state relative to perfect health (utility = 1) and death (utility = 0).

Utilities can be measured indirectly with instruments such as the Health Utility Index[19] or the EuroQol,[20] or with direct preference-based assessment methods such as the Standard Gamble[21] or the Time Trade-off.[22] Indirect utility assessments are based on interviews or questionnaires, which assign ordinal levels of different quality-of-life dimensions (eg, mobility, emotion, cognition, pain) to the health state of interest and weight these levels with empirical values derived from large surveys. Preference-based methods ask the individuals how many years of life they would give up or what level of instantaneous mortality risk they would accept to achieve perfect health.

PERSPECTIVE

Most common perspectives are societal, third-party payer (eg, Medicare, managed care organization), government, provider (hospital, clinic, physician), and patient. If a cost-effectiveness analysis is intended to inform resource allocation decisions, it should be conducted from the societal perspective, because it accounts for benefits, harms, and costs to all parties, and therefore allows for comparisons across interventions and patient groups.[23] For reasons of comparability, the standard approach is to adopt the societal perspective, and also use other perspectives when those are of particular interest to the analyst.[24,25]

TIME HORIZON

The time horizon adopted in a cost-effectiveness analysis should be long enough to capture all relevant future effects of a health-care intervention. For example, using a drug-eluting stent imposes higher initial costs than a bare metal stent, but the drug-eluting stent reduces the number of patients with subsequent clinical restenosis, and repeat revascularization procedures. A fair economic evaluation must thus include these downstream costs.

Costs and effectiveness may also vary over time. In surgical or invasive interventions such as coronary bypass or PCIs, initial costs are higher than costs of treatment maintenance. In contrast, costs for medical treatments (eg, for hypercholesterolemia or hypertension) differ less over time. Effectiveness may also differ over time. All invasive interventions have initial (periprocedural) mortality risks, whereas the mortality risk during initiation of pharmaceutic treatment is virtually zero. Therefore, in all comparisons of invasive versus noninvasive treatments, the comparison is biased against the invasive procedure if the analytic time horizon is too short. Finally, costs and benefits can occur at different points in time. In the economic evaluations of preventive interventions or diagnostic procedures, the costs occur immediately, whereas the benefit may be observed years or even decades later. Consequently, in a cost-effectiveness study comparing different strategies for diagnosis of coronary artery disease (CAD) in patients presenting with chest pain, the analysts used a lifetime horizon so as to capture even very late effects.[26]

[ ] DISCOUNTING

A key economic notion is that future benefits and costs are not valued the same as those in the present. Therefore, economists express future costs and health outcomes as "present value." This technique, called *discounting*, gives less weight to future costs compared to present costs, and allows the analyst to calculate the present value from a stream of costs (and health outcomes) that occur over a period of time. The rationale for discounting costs is illustrated easily by determining the present value of having $100 in 10 years from now translates to the following question: How much must be invested today in order to receive $100 in 10 years? Assuming a positive interest rate, the present value of $100 in 10 years would be significantly less than $100. Discounting is less intuitive when it is applied to health effects. However, health gains in the present are generally preferred over those in the future. Furthermore, it has been shown that welfare theory supports discounting of health outcomes,[27] and not discounting health outcomes would lead to logical inconsistencies regarding the choice of interventions.[28]

It should be noted that discounting is distinct from inflation. Whereas discounting reflects real-time preferences (even in the absence of inflation), inflation does not affect the present value. However, if cost data are obtained from historical cost studies, these figures must be corrected for inflation. Usually, the medical care component of the Consumer Price Index (CPI) published by the Bureau of Labor Statistics is used for this adjustment.

[ ] WHEN IS A HEALTH-CARE INTERVENTION CONSIDERED TO BE COST-EFFECTIVE?

A recurring theme in medicine is that medical advances occur at an increase in cost. What cost-effectiveness analyses attempt to do is estimate the additional cost required to achieve the additional health gain of interest when introducing a new technology. The interested parties (ie, health-care provider, insurance company,

government agency, or society) must then determine whether the health gain achieved through a new technology is worth the additional cost compared to the current standard of care.

Different societies have different thresholds regarding what is considered to be cost-effective. Wealthier countries are usually willing to spend more money to improve health than are poorer countries. In the United States, a cost-effectiveness ratio of less than $50,000 per QALY gained has generally been considered to be economically attractive. This threshold value has been cited in numerous cost-effectiveness studies and textbook chapters, and methodologic journal articles on cost-effectiveness analysis also make reference to the threshold.[29] However, it is important to recognize that this value is somewhat arbitrary, because formal attempts to measure the maximum acceptable ICER are still lacking.[21,30,31] It is therefore important that, in practice, the ICER of a health technology should be compared to the ICERs of other well-accepted health technologies.[6]

Common examples of therapies with ICERs less than $50,000 per life year or QALY gained include coronary bypass surgery for left main disease,[4] beta-blocker therapy after myocardial infarction,[32] thrombolytic therapy for acute myocardial infarction,[33] and drug-eluting stent implantation in de novo native coronary artery lesions.[34,35] These procedures are considered economically attractive because the health gains associated with these interventions have been deemed by society to be "worth the additional cost."[36]

In interventional cardiology, few interventions have been shown to truly save lives and the formal evaluation of quality of life is often problematic. For therapies that reduce coronary restenosis, Cohen et al.[37] hence recently proposed that a disease-specific cost-effectiveness ratio of $10,000 per repeat revascularization avoided may be a reasonable threshold for the societal willingness-to-pay within the US health-care system. Avoidance of repeat revascularization as a measure of clinical benefit is justified based on previous studies showing a close association between clinical restenosis and impaired quality of life during the first year after PCI.[38–40] The disease-specific cost-effectiveness threshold of $10,000 per repeat revascularization avoided is based on the observation that cardiovascular interventions with an ICER below this value have generally been widely adopted and reimbursed within the US health-care system and other industrialized countries within recent years. For example, economic evaluation of coronary stenting versus balloon angioplasty in the Benestent II trial yielded an ICER of about $11,000 per repeat revascularization procedure avoided.[41] Similarly, the Stent-PAMI trial estimated the cost-effectiveness of stenting versus PTCA in acute MI as about $10,000 per repeat revascularization procedure avoided.[42] Because both of these forms of therapy are currently well accepted in the US health-care system, a reasonable cost-effectiveness threshold of $10,000 per repeat revascularization avoided may be inferred.

This reasoning is supported by two health technology assessments (HTA) performed by National Health Technology Assessment Agencies that estimate that incremental cost-effectiveness ratios below $10,000–15,000 per clinical restenosis avoided can be considered cost-effective, under the assumption that an incremental cost–utility ratio of about $50,000 per QALY gained is used as societal willingness-to-pay threshold.[43,44]

[ ] ECONOMIC EVALUATION ALONGSIDE CLINICAL TRIALS

Two approaches are commonly used in economic evaluations of health care[2]: first, economic evaluation alongside clinical trials, and second, decision–analytic modeling (covered in the next section).

In economic evaluation alongside clinical trials, both clinical endpoints and resource utilization are directly assessed in a trial population. For example, Cohen and colleagues[35] performed a cost-effectiveness analysis along the SIRIUS trial[45] comparing PCI with drug-eluting stent (DES) versus bare metal stent (BMS) implantation. Clinical outcomes, resource use, and costs were assessed prospectively for all patients over a 1-year follow-up period. Because the major benefit of the drug-eluting stent was a reduction in the need for repeat revascularization, the authors chose the incremental cost per repeat revascularization avoided as primary endpoint of the cost-effectiveness analysis. Initial hospital costs were increased by $2881 per patient with DES. Over the 1-year follow-up period, the use of DES led to substantial reductions in repeat revascularization rates. Although follow-up costs were reduced by $2571 per patient with DES, total 1-year costs remained $309 higher per patient. The ICER for DES was $1650 per repeat revascularization avoided. In a secondary analysis, the authors assumed that there would be no differences in long-term survival or quality of life beyond the first year of follow-up and used QALYs at 1-year of follow-up as the effectiveness measure. This analysis resulted in an ICER for DES versus BMS of $27,540 per QALY gained.[35]

This approach of economic evaluation alongside clinical trials offers certain advantages by completely relying on empirical data, and therefore minimizing assumptions and the need for modeling. Disadvantages of the empirical approach include differences between protocol driven care and routine care, and limited generalizability of the highly selected clinical trial population. In addition, the time horizon of the study may not be long enough to fully assess the health benefits or risks of a procedure.[13,46]

[ ] DECISION-ANALYTIC MODELING

The other approach to economic evaluation uses mathematical models to project and compare clinical and economic outcomes of different interventions over the time horizon of interest. These decision-analytic models allow the analyst to combine data from different credible sources including patient level data from clinical trials as well as aggregated data from the published literature (eg, meta-analyses of trials, epidemiologic studies, quality-of-life studies, resource utilization assessments).

Several definitions have been offered for the term *model* as it applies to the context of health care. The International Society for Pharmacoeconomics and Outcomes Research (ISPOR) Task Force on Good Research Practices–-Modeling Studies defines a health-care evaluation model as "an analytic methodology that accounts for events over time and across populations, that is based on data drawn from primary and/or secondary sources, and whose purpose is to estimate the effects of an intervention on valued health consequences and costs."[47] Buxton and colleagues[48] defined models in scientific disciplines as "a way of representing the complexity of the real world in a more simple and comprehensible form." Other definitions have been given and summarized previously.[49]

Decision analysis is defined as the application of explicit and quantitative methods to analyze decisions under conditions of uncertainty.[50,51] Decision analysis is naturally suited for decisions in the prevention, diagnosis, and treatment in cardiovascular disease because usually multiple alternative options are available with complex and uncertain outcomes. Decision analysis allows the analyst to compare the expected consequences of different strategies after considering all relevant events and complications with their probabilities and weighing all relevant clinical outcomes and costs. The results of such analyses can inform a decision both for an individual patient and a health-care policy.[52,53] Depending on the purpose of the analysis, different perspectives can be chosen, such as the patient's perspective or the perspective of society or a national health authority.[2]

Whereas clinical decision analysis focuses solely on clinical outcomes such as success rates, complication rates, survival, life-expectancy, and health-related quality of life associated with the compared strategies, economic decision modeling is often used to estimate the long-term consequences (beyond the time horizon of a clinical trial) and cost-effectiveness of health-care technologies.[49]

There are two basic forms of decision-analytic models: decision trees and Markov models. A *decision tree* is a visual representation of all the possible options and the consequences that may follow each health-care strategy.[54] Each alternative strategy is followed by branches representing the possible events with their respective probabilities. Probabilities may depend not only on the different strategies, but also on patient characteristics (eg, subgroups with different risk-factor profiles). At the end of the tree, each path leads to an outcome, such as symptoms, classification of disease severity (eg, NYHA stage, left ventricular ejection fraction), survival, death, and so on. For each alternative strategy, the expected value of the clinical outcome can be calculated as a weighted average of all possible outcomes, applying the path probabilities as weights. Decision trees work well when analyzing events with limited recursion and a fixed time horizon.

In chronic diseases such as cardiovascular disease, model parameters such as progression rates, quality-of-life measures (utilities), or costs may change over time, the time-to-event or time-to-progression plays an important role, and events may also recur. Under these circumstances, Markov models are usually the preferred method to evaluate interventions.[55,56] Markov models offer a straightforward methodology for considering extended (variable) time horizons, timing of events, and recurring events.[54] In a Markov model, a hypothetic cohort of patients moves through defined health states, and time is represented in cycles during which patients can (1) remain in their current health states, (2) move to another health state, or (3) die, according to certain transition probabilities. During this process, cumulative life years, QALYs, and costs can be accumulated in each of the interventions and then compared among the interventions.[55,56]

Situations that call for the use of decision-analytic modeling have been described earlier.[49] Table 68-3 lists some of the most important purposes. In most of these situations, decision models are used for either combining/linking data from different research areas and sources or for transferring/extrapolating results from one time, place, population or setting to another.

TABLE 68-3

When Should Decision-Analytic Modeling be Used in Economic Evaluation of Health Care?[49]

- Combining evidence from short-term clinical trials and long-term epidemiologic studies
- Assessment of screening programs and diagnostic procedures
- Extrapolating efficacy beyond the time horizon of a clinical trial
- Informing decisions in the absence of clinical trial data
- Considering patient preferences
- Generalizing from efficacy to routine effectiveness
- Transferring the evidence from one health care system or country to another
- Resource allocation decisions
- Fine-tune single features of health care technologies, tailor technologies for subgroups, and inform clinical guidelines
- Value-of-information analysis
- Health policy models and national projections
- National Health Technology Assessments (HTA)

【 】 SELECTED STATISTICAL ISSUES AND TECHNIQUES

This section covers selected statistical topics that may be helpful to understand and handle the issues emerging with analyzing cost data as well as dealing with the uncertainty surrounding empirical data used in cost-effectiveness analysis.

Cost Distributions

One of the technical difficulties in statistical analysis of economic data originates from the shape of the distribution of costs. As most patients use few resources and only few patients use many resources, cost distributions are usually skewed to the right. Therefore, statistical tests comparing across groups that assume normal distributions should not be used and (nonparametric) ranking tests must be used instead. For example, a cost-effectiveness analysis alongside a randomized clinical trial (RCT) comparing total cost for two different interventions should be analyzed using the nonparametric Mann-Whitney-Wilcoxon U-Test rather than the Student's t Test, because the latter is based on the assumption of normality. Similarly, in comparisons across more than two groups the nonparametric Kruskal-Wallis test should be used rather than analysis of variance. Although ranking tests are a valid approach for obtaining statistic p values in hypothesis testing, they do not provide our estimate of interest, the difference in expected (ie, mean) cost.

An alternative approach is, therefore, to transform the cost data to a less-skewed distribution. For this purpose, often the log-transformation is used, because it allows us to describe the effect as a cost ratio with confidence intervals and can also be used in multivariate regression models to identify multiple predictors of healthcare costs (eg, age, gender, disease stage, type of intervention). If the dataset contains some cost values of zero, a small constant (eg,

$1) can be added to all costs before the log-transformation, to enable the mathematical operation, that is, transformed cost = log(cost + $1).

Survival Curves and Cumulative Cost Curves

If a clinical trial has a relatively short and fixed follow-up period, calculation of effectiveness and costs are straightforward. Survival and complication-free survival can be expressed as proportions and resource utilization as mean cumulative costs at end of follow-up. However, it is often useful to describe events and costs as a function of time over the follow-up period. For example, Figure 68-1 shows the mean cumulative cost curves over the 1-year follow-up period of a cost-effectiveness analysis along the SIRIUS trial.

However, the estimation of survival and cumulative costs becomes more difficult when the trial has a long period of patient accrual and different patients contribute different durations of observation to the analysis. Similarly, a long follow-up period with a non-negligible number of losses to follow-up or deaths leads to variable lengths of observation time. In these situations, observations of mortality or other events may be censored, which led to the development of actuarial methods such as the Kaplan-Meier sample-average estimator and the Logrank Test. These methods take into account the censored nature of the data and the variable lengths of follow-up. Similarly, in cost-effectiveness analyses, cost curves can be adjusted for censored data by dividing

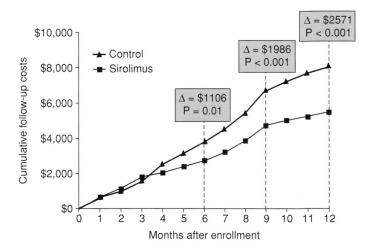

FIGURE 68-1. Mean cumulative cost curves of the SIRIUS trial according to treatment group (drug-eluting stent vs. bare metal stent) over 1-year follow-up period excluding initial hospital costs. Cost differences at 6, 9, and 12 months are indicated in shaded boxes. *(Used by permission from: Cohen DJ, Bakhai A, Shi C, et al. Cost-effectiveness of sirolimus-eluting stents for treatment of complex coronary stenoses: results from the sirolimus-eluting balloon expandable stent in the treatment of patients with de novo native coronary artery lesions (SIRIUS) trial. Circulation. 2004;110(5):508–514.)*

the follow-up period into intervals and weighting the mean cost in each interval with the proportion of survivors in that interval.[57]

Handling Uncertainty

Most data used for determining the ICER of a health technology are surrounded by uncertainty, either caused by systematic bias or random error. One way to address this problem is to perform one-way or multiway sensitivity analyses, presenting the ICER (eg, graphically) as a function of variables that are varied across plausible ranges to assess the robustness of the results or potential threshold at which decisions would change.

Another way to address random error is to consider sampling uncertainty in a formal statistical fashion and to summarize this uncertainty as a confidence interval (CI). For example, in an economic evaluation along a clinical trial, the standard error of the differences in effects and costs between two interventions as well as the correlation between effect and cost differences can be derived from the observed trial data. However, as the ICER is a ratio statistic, the estimation of its variance is problematic. Various approaches based on different assumptions have been suggested in the health economics literature. These include the confidence box,[58] the Delta method,[58] the confidence ellipse,[59] Fieller's theorem,[60] and nonparametric bootstrapping.[61] An excellent overview on these approaches and their underlying assumptions and limitations has been presented by Briggs.[62] Different methods for estimating confidence intervals may give different answers, and the results of simulations show which methods have the best coverage properties.[62] Figure 68-2 shows the cost-effectiveness plane and confidence ellipses for the incremental cost-effectiveness of heparin-coated Palmaz-Schatz stent implantation compared with

balloon angioplasty in the Benestent II trial. The diagonal line indicates a threshold ICER of Dfl 19,358 per event-free survival (ie, < $10,000).

Another statistical approach to represent the uncertainty concerning the cost-effectiveness of health-care interventions is the method of cost-effectiveness acceptability curves (CEAC). This approach was originally introduced as an alternative to confidence intervals around ICERs in the context of decisions involving two interventions.[59] The CEAC plots the probability that one treatment strategy is more cost-effective than another, as a function of the threshold willingness to pay for one additional unit of effectiveness.[63]

Figure 68-3 shows the CEAC for the cost-effectiveness analysis along the SIRIUS trial as described earlier. The probability for the use of drug-eluting stents being cost-effective is represented as a function of the dollars the decision maker is willing to spend to avoid one additional repeat revascularization. Based on other well-accepted interventions, the authors assumed a willingness to pay of $10,000 per repeat revascularization avoided, which led to a probability of 98.2% of DES being cost-effective. With a willingness to pay of only $5,000 per repeat revascularization avoided, this probability would be only about 82%. The point estimate of the ICER was $1,150 per repeat revascularization avoided.[35] If effectiveness is measured in terms of QALYs gained, the threshold willingness to pay should be expressed in this unit, for example, $50,000 per QALY gained (see the section entitled "When Is a Health-care Intervention Considered to Be Cost-Effective?" for the threshold discussion).

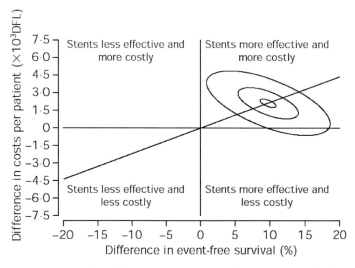

FIGURE 68-2. Cost-effectiveness plane and confidence ellipses for the incremental cost-effectiveness comparing heparin-coated Palmaz-Schatz stent implantation with balloon angioplasty in selected patients with stable or stabilized unstable angina; based on the BENESTENT II trial data. Outer/middle/inner ellipse = 95%/50%/5% confidence ellipse, respectively. Center of ellipses = point estimate of both incremental costs and incremental effects. *(Used by permission from: Serruys PW, van Hout B, Bonnier H, et al. Randomised comparison of implantation of heparin-coated stents with balloon angioplasty in selected patients with coronary artery disease (Benestent II). The Lancet. 1998;352(9129):673–681.)*

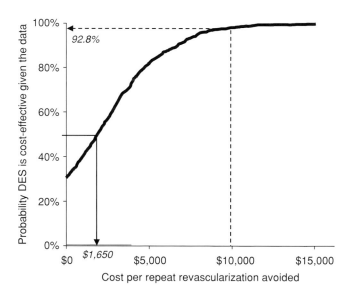

FIGURE 68–3. Cost-effectiveness acceptability curve for the incremental cost-effectiveness of drug-eluting stenting versus bare metal stenting based on bootstrap analysis of primary SIRIUS results. As indicated by the dotted arrow, 98.2% of bootstrapped incremental cost-effectiveness ratios were less than $10,000 per repeat revascularization avoided. The solid arrow (50% point) indicates the point estimate of the incremental cost-effectiveness ratio of $1,650 per repeat revascularization avoided. *(Modified with permission from: Cohen DJ, Bakhai A, Shi C, et al. Cost-effectiveness of sirolimus-eluting stents for treatment of complex coronary stenoses: results from the Sirolimus-Eluting Balloon Expandable Stent in the Treatment of Patients with De Novo Native Coronary Artery Lesions (SIRIUS) trial. Circulation. 2004;110(5):508–514.)*

The CEAC is derived from the joint density of incremental costs and incremental effects for the intervention of interest. There are parametric and nonparametric ways to generate the joint density. For example, integrating a given joint normal distribution of incremental costs and incremental effects can generate it. In the context of a cost-effectiveness analysis alongside a clinical trial, nonparametric bootstrapping can be used to resample patient level data. In the context of decision-analytic modeling, there are generally certain model parameters whose values are not known precisely. It may then be important to assess the sensitivity of model results to variation in those parameters. Probabilistic sensitivity analysis is a method that allows the analyst to simultaneously vary multiple model parameters by assigning distributions around model parameters (eg, based on standard errors or confidence intervals), and then performing a Monte Carlo simulation, that is, repeatedly drawing from these distributions, in order to generate the joint density of incremental costs and incremental effectiveness.[64] The cost-effectiveness plane and the CEAC can then be plotted based on the joint distribution of incremental costs and incremental effects generated in the Monte Carlo simulation.

Value-of-Information Analysis

Usually there are two conceptually separate research questions that must be answered in health-care decision making: (1) Given the available information, should the new technology be adopted?; and (2) Should more information be obtained to inform (ie, confirm or change) this decision in the future?[65,66] Value-of-information (VOI) analysis is concerned with the second question, and usually is done in the context of decision-analytic modeling. Howard Raiffa[50] described the concept of VOI as the difference between the expected consequences (utility) of a decision guided by a particular piece of information and the respective expected consequences without the information. This concept is directly applicable to the assessment of whether more empirical information is justified including such information that can reduce uncertainty about decision parameters. Deferring approval of a drug until more empirical information about the magnitude or duration of its effect is available may include the possibilities of either gaining or losing health benefits and resources in the interim. After estimating the expected value of perfect information for each parameter of a decision model, the analyst can identify those parameters for which more precise estimates would be most valuable and determine the optimal sample size for an empirical study from a societal perspective based on the incremental cost and incremental benefit of the sample information.[67]

Although VOI analyses have not been used frequently in the past, they may play an important role in future sample-size calculations and decision making on research priorities, for example, in national Health Technology Assessment Programs.

CASE STUDIES IN CORONARY ARTERY DISEASE AND PERCUTANEOUS CORONARY INTERVENTION

In this section, four cases of cost-effectiveness studies are discussed. They represent health technologies in the prevention, diagnosis, and treatment of cardiovascular disease, and cover devices as well as pharmaceutics. The focus of the discussion is on the different purposes of these studies and the different methodologic approaches.

The first case represents an example of an economic evaluation alongside a clinical trial investigating the cost-effectiveness of routine intravascular ultrasound (IVUS) guidance for provisional stenting. The second case is an example of a diagnostic Markov model used for the economic evaluation of coronary pressure–based fractional flow reserve in patients without documented ischemia. In the third case, a decision-analytic treatment model is presented that consists of three submodels, two short-term decision trees, and one long-term Markov model. It was used for the clinical and economic evaluation of coronary stent implantation versus conventional angioplasty. The fourth case demonstrates the use of a different model type, a health policy model. The example shows how the population-based Coronary Heart Disease (CHD) Policy Model was used to evaluate the effectiveness and cost-effectiveness of cholesterol-lowering therapies depending on risk-factor profiles in the entire US population between ages 35 and 84.

【 】 CASE 1: ECONOMIC EVALUATION ALONGSIDE CLINICAL TRIALS— INTRAVASCULAR ULTRASOUND GUIDANCE FOR PERCUTANEOUS CORONARY INTERVENTIONS

Intravascular ultrasound (IVUS) allows the interventional cardiologist to assess vascular dimensions, the extent of vessel remodeling, and plaque morphology, and thereby has advanced knowledge in many areas of interventional cardiology. Although some studies have shown the potential of IVUS guidance to improve procedural results and reduce the need for subsequent target vessel revascularization after PCI, a multicenter study failed to show a statistically significant benefit of IVUS guidance for primary stenting.[68] In the short term, IVUS guidance is costly because of the additional expense for the IVUS catheter, the IVUS console, extra balloons and/or stents that are used to fulfill IVUS criteria, and the extra personnel time in the catheterization laboratory needed to optimize results with multiple catheter exchanges.

In the following example, Mueller and colleagues[69] performed an economic evaluation alongside a randomized clinical trial to investigate the cost-effectiveness of routine IVUS guidance of provisional stenting.

【 】 METHODOLOGIC APPROACH

This study was a classic prospective cost-effectiveness study alongside a randomized clinical trial. In this study, 296 consecutive patients with 356 lesions were randomly assigned to receive provisional stenting with IVUS guidance or with angiographic guidance only. The time horizon was 2 years. The primary clinical endpoint was survival free of major adverse cardiac events (MACE, ie, death, nonfatal myocardial infarction, or clinically driven target vessel revascularization) at 2 years. Costs were based on direct costs for IVUS-related supplies and devices, personnel time, cardiac medication, initial hospitalization and cardiac-related hospitalizations during 2 years of follow-up, and indirect costs for the 2-year follow-up period. A 3% annual discount rate was used.

Incremental cost-effectiveness was expressed as additional costs per MACE avoided. The investigators used bootstrapping techniques to assess the uncertainty surrounding costs, effectiveness, and incremental cost-effectiveness.

In this trial, the 2-year major adverse cardiac event-free survival was significantly higher in the IVUS-guided group (80% vs. 69%, $p < .04$). In-hospital costs for equipment and personnel were higher in the IVUS group, but were offset by lower costs for inpatient care and urgent target vessel revascularization in the IVUS group. Total costs over the 2-year period were nearly identical ($15,947 and $16,103 per patient for IVUS-guided and angiography-guided strategy, respectively, $p = .89$). Therefore, based-on the empirical data, the IVUS-guided strategy dominated the intervention with angiographic guidance only. Figure 68-3 shows the results from 5000 bootstrap replications with 95% and 50% confidence ellipses, respectively, for the incremental cost-effectiveness of IVUS guidance compared with angiographic guidance only. In 55.3% of bootstrapping replications, IVUS was less expensive and more effective (ie, dominated the angiography-guided procedure). Please note that in Figure 68-4, the dots on the left side (ie, negative effectiveness values) represent bootstrap samples in which IVUS guidance was more effective than angiographic guidance only.

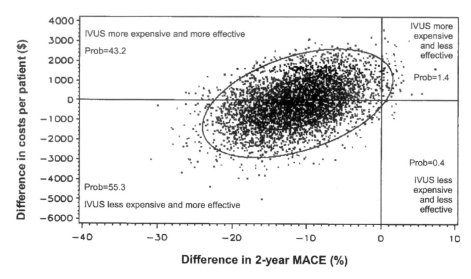

FIGURE 68-4. Incremental cost-effectiveness of intravascular ultrasound (IVUS) guidance for percutaneous coronary interventions. Results from 5000 bootstrap replications with 95% confidence region (outer ellipse) and 50% confidence region (inner ellipse) for incremental cost-effectiveness of IVUS guidance compared with angiographic guidance only. The center of the ellipse represents the point estimate of incremental costs and effects. Prob = estimated probability that the incremental cost-effectiveness of IVUS guidance obtained from a bootstrap sample lies in the respective quadrant (in percentages); MACE = major adverse cardiac events. *(Used by permission from: Mueller C, Hodgson JM, Schindler C, Perruchoud AP, Roskamm H, Buettner HJ. Cost-effectiveness of intracoronary ultrasound for percutaneous coronary interventions. Am J Cardiol. 2003;91(2):143–147.)*

CONCLUSIONS

This study demonstrates how an economic evaluation can be performed alongside a single clinical trial and uncertainty can be addressed by bootstrapping methods. The advantage of this approach is that the results are based entirely on the empirical data observed in the study, and no further modeling assumptions need to be made. The downside, however, is that the time horizon of the economic evaluation was relatively short (compared to lifetime as in many decision models) and the outcome was intermediate (ie, MACE), and quality of life was not considered. Moreover, the analysis does not take into account data from other trials that have less positive results.

In this regard, it is worth noting that two National Health Technology Assessments, one commissioned by the German Federal Ministry of Health[44,70] and another commissioned by the National Institute for Clinical Excellence (NICE) in the United Kingdom,[43] evaluated this topic systematically and stated that a major part of IVUS-related costs may be offset by savings from reductions in early and late complications. However both groups concluded that because of insufficient data, no final conclusion could be achieved.

CASE 2: DIAGNOSTIC ASSESSMENT TO GUIDE THE DECISION TO PERFORM PERCUTANEOUS CORONARY INTERVENTION—CORONARY PRESSURE–BASED FRACTIONAL FLOW RESERVE

It is generally accepted that decisions regarding coronary revascularization in patients with chest pain should be based not only on the presence of coronary stenosis at angiography, but also on the results of noninvasive tests for reversible ischemia.[71] Even so, many patients are referred and accepted for PCI solely on the basis of an angiogram, whereas noninvasive tests were negative, equivocal, or not performed at all.[72] In such patients, it remains unproved if the chest pain is the result of coronary stenosis or whether PCI would improve survival or quality of life.[73] Coronary pressure–based fractional flow reserve (FFR) is an accurate invasive test for myocardial ischemia.[74] A decision-analytic model has been used to evaluate the long-term effectiveness, costs, and cost-effectiveness of FFR testing to guide the decision for PCI versus universal performance of PCI in all patients with moderate coronary stenosis.[75,76] The impact of using drug-eluting stents rather than bare metal stents in such patients has also been investigated.

METHODOLOGIC APPROACH

A short-term decision tree was linked to a lifetime Markov model to project clinical and economic outcomes for patients with one-vessel coronary stenosis and mild angina, but without proven myocardial ischemia (Figure 68-5). The strategies considered were (1) Universal PCI (UNIV) without FFR testing, and (2) FFR testing

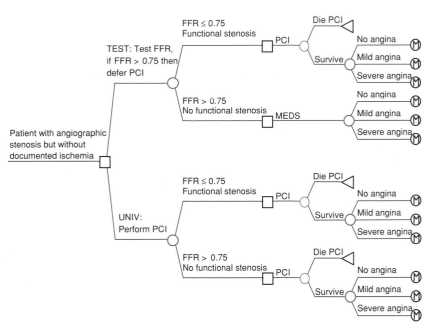

FIGURE 68-5. Decision tree for measuring FFR to guide the decision to perform PCI (TEST) versus universal performance of PCI (UNIV). Patients in the universal PCI strategy are stratified by underlying FFR, which will not be revealed. Patients in the FFR-guided strategy undergo PCI only if the FFR is equal or less than 0.75. Patients surviving PCI are assigned to the corresponding angina status immediately after treatment. At the end of each branch, survivors enter a Markov cycle tree (M) that models their lifetime cost and prognosis. FFR = fractional flow reserve; PCI = percutaneous coronary intervention; MEDS = medical treatment. Decision nodes are indicated by squares, chance nodes by circles, terminal nodes by triangles, and Markov model by circles with the letter M.

followed by PCI only for those with FFR of 0.75 or less (TEST). A cost-effectiveness analysis was performed in age (30–70 years) and gender subgroups. Prevalence of functional stenosis (FFR ≤ 0.75) and risk ratios for major adverse cardiac events were based on the original data of a randomized clinical trial.[77] Long-term clinical outcomes of PCI and medical management including recurrence rates, disease progression, and quality of life (utilities) were derived from the published literature. The relative efficacy of drug-eluting stents versus bare metal stents was determined using a fixed effects meta-analysis.

Overall, men and women showed similar patterns, with the FFR-guided strategy as the less costly but slightly less effective strategy. Regardless of the type of stent (bare metal or drug-eluting), measuring FFR to guide the decision to perform PCI led to significant cost savings. Even under very optimistic assumptions regarding the mortality benefits and restenosis rates for drug-eluting stents, the incremental cost–utility ratio of universal PCI without FFR testing was greater than $50,000 per QALY gained, when compared with the FFR-guided strategy.

[ ] CONCLUSIONS

Outcomes of randomized clinical trials in interventional cardiology are often intermediate (short-term) outcomes, such as restenosis or other nonfatal adverse cardiac events. This example shows how decision-analytic models can be

used to extrapolate results from a randomized clinical trial to long-term outcomes such as life expectancy, quality-adjusted life expectancy, and lifetime costs, and furthermore, consider emerging technologies in a decision-analytic framework.

[ ] CASE 3: LONG-TERM EFFECTS OF INVASIVE TREATMENT— CORONARY STENT IMPLANTATION

When stent implantation was introduced into interventional cardiology in the early 1990s, there was intense interest in assessing the relation between clinical gains from stenting and the related costs of this procedure.[78] Although intracoronary stenting was a promising procedure with the potential of reducing restenosis rates[79] at the time of this analysis, several investigators cautioned that widespread application of coronary stenting may have a deleterious impact on national health-care expenditures.[80,81] Although several randomized clinical trials had assessed the short-term effectiveness of stenting on angiographic and clinical restenosis rates, long-term effectiveness and costs remained unclear.

To address this question, in 1994 Cohen et al.[82] developed a detailed decision-analytic model predicting quality-adjusted life expectancy and lifetime treatment costs for patients with symptomatic, single-vessel coronary disease treated by either Palmaz-Schatz stenting or conventional balloon angioplasty. The model combined results from clinical trials and long-term follow-up studies as well as utilities and cost data. Although this model was developed in the mid-1990s and many of its parameters may differ today, the basic structure of the model is still valid. This model has been chosen to illustrate how evidence on initial, short-term, and long-term events and costs can be linked in a modular decision model.

[ ] METHODOLOGIC APPROACH

The decision model developed by Cohen and colleagues[82] is one of the most comprehensive models for the clinical and economic pathways of patients undergoing PCI. The model consists of two decision trees for the initial and short-term periods linked with a Markov model for the long-term prognosis (Figure 68-6). The first

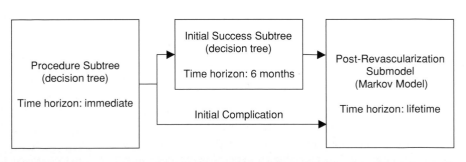

FIGURE 68-6. Components of the decision-analytic stenting model developed by Cohen and colleagues.[82] The model consists of two decision trees and one Markov model.

decision tree (*procedure subtree*) reflects the initial therapeutic decision and the immediate outcomes of the chosen procedure, such as success, abrupt closure, procedural failure, emergency procedures, or death. The second decision tree (*initial success subtree*) tracks the first 6 months and reflects short-term events, including subacute thrombosis or restenosis, leading to subsequent procedures, stable post-procedure state, complications, or death. The third submodel (*post-revascularization Markov model*) covers the remaining life after successful single-vessel PCI or coronary artery bypass graft. During repeated cycles of 6 months, patients could remain asymptomatic, develop symptoms, experience an event (ie, myocardial infarction, repeat PCI, or bypass surgery), develop chronic angina pectoris, or die. Transition probabilities for each event were a function of the particular health state and the time interval after procedures.

Cohen et al.[82] demonstrated that despite the higher cost, elective coronary stenting was a cost-effective treatment for selected patients with single-vessel coronary disease. In sensitivity analyses, the investigators showed that low risk of restenosis and expected stenting costs had a substantial impact on cost-effectiveness.

[ ] CONCLUSIONS

This example demonstrates how a decision-analytic model with a modular design allows the investigator to link short-term evidence from randomized clinical trials and results from long-term cohort studies. Moreover, it allows for the combination of these data with quality-of-life measures and cost data to determine the long-term effectiveness and cost-effectiveness of a medical technology. This is crucial information for those who make health-care policy decisions as well as for patients and their physicians.

[ ] CASE 4: HEALTH POLICY MODELS— EVALUATION OF ASPIRIN AND CLOPIDOGREL USING THE CORONARY HEART DISEASE POLICY MODEL

So-called Health Policy Models in cardiovascular disease are used to simulate the epidemiologic and economic effects of health technologies on a heterogeneous population (eg, the entire patient cohort of a specific country, over a specified period of time).[83–85] Therefore, these types of models often simulate "open" cohorts, in which members are allowed to enter and exit from the simulated population according to demographic projections and disease-specific events. One of the best known examples of a detailed health-policy model is the Coronary Heart Disease Policy Model, which was developed to project the future mortality, morbidity, and cost of CHD in the United States.[83] Since this model was created, it has been used extensively in the evaluation of CHD-related interventions.[86–102]

Gaspoz and colleagues[102] used the Coronary Heart Disease Policy Model to perform an incremental cost-effectiveness analysis of the long-term use of aspirin, clopidogrel, or both for secondary prevention in patients with known coronary disease. This analysis was motivated by the results of studies that demonstrated that both aspirin[103] and clopidogrel[104,105] were effective in reducing cardiovascular events and/or mortality in patients with prior cardiovascular disease.

[ ] METHODOLOGIC APPROACH

The Coronary Heart Disease Policy Model is a computer simulation Markov model of CHD in US residents aged 35 through 84 years who are initially without coronary heart disease.[83] It includes variables for CHD event rates, case fatality rates, and costs. The model consists of three submodels: (1) demographic–epidemiologic submodel, (2) bridge submodel, and (3) disease history submodel.

In the demographic–epidemiologic submodel, an individual develops CHD depending on his or her individual risk factor profile, ie, age, gender, smoking status, diastolic blood pressure, serum cholesterol level, and high-density lipoprotein level (240 risk subgroups). When coronary disease develops in an individual, the model classifies the presentation as cardiac arrest, acute myocardial infarction, or angina, and the individual moves into the bridge submodel, which represents the clinical outcomes, deaths, and health-care costs during the first 30 days after the initial CHD event. Individuals who survive the first 30 days with CHD move to the disease history submodel, which simulates the subsequent events after the initial CHD event, including revascularization procedures and CHD-specific and non-CHD-related mortality. Incidence of CHD and mortality of non-CHD have been determined by multivariate risk functions. Each individual is assigned an annual cost on the basis of his or her history and on additional costs related to any new events.[83]

Gaspoz and colleagues[102] used the Coronary Heart Disease Policy Model to compare four strategies regarding clinical and economic outcomes in patients with CHD from 2003 to 2027: (1) aspirin for all eligible patients (ie, those who were not allergic to or intolerant of aspirin), (2) aspirin for all eligible patients plus clopidogrel for patients who were ineligible for aspirin, (3) clopidogrel for all patients, and (4) the combination of aspirin for all eligible patients plus clopidogrel for all patients. The investigators showed that the extension of aspirin therapy from the current levels of use to all eligible patients during the 25-year time horizon would have an ICER of about $11,000 per QALY gained. The stream of costs because of aspirin use, CHD, and non-CHD is shown in Figure 68-7. Adding

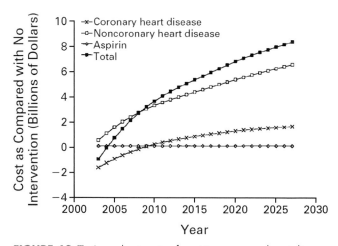

FIGURE 68-7. Annual net costs of aspirin, coronary heart disease, and noncoronary heart disease with routine aspirin use for secondary prevention in patients 35 to 84 years of age during 2003 to 2027 in the United States. *(Used by permission from: Gaspoz JM, Coxson PG, Goldman PA, et al. Cost effectiveness of aspirin, clopidogrel, or both for secondary prevention of coronary heart disease. N Engl J Med. 2002;346(23):1800–1806.)*

clopidogrel for the 5% of patients who are ineligible for aspirin would cost about \$31,000/QALY. The remaining strategies (ie, clopidogrel alone in all patients or in combination with aspirin) had ICERs of more than \$130,000/QALY in the base-case analysis. The authors concluded that increased prescription of aspirin for the secondary prevention of CHD is cost-effective, and clopidogrel, as currently priced, is not attractive from a cost-effectiveness perspective, unless its use is restricted to patients who are ineligible for aspirin.[102]

【 】 CONCLUSIONS

One of the specific strengths of a health policy model is its ability to simulate costs and health outcomes for an entire population over a long time horizon while considering demographic changes. As such, the CHD Health Policy model demonstrates the important role of such models in targeting medical interventions to those who benefit most when compared to the resources used. Thus, decision modeling can be an important aide to clinical guideline development and efficient resource allocation, when different subgroups and variants/combinations of interventions are considered in the decision analysis.

LIMITATIONS, CHALLENGES, AND CLOSING REMARKS

In the current health-care environment, decisions about new technologies and treatment paradigms cannot be made on clinical grounds alone. In 2004, the estimated direct and indirect cost of cardiovascular disease was \$368.4 billion. Currently, 64.4 million Americans (22.6%) suffer from one or more types of cardiovascular disease.[1] The aging of the population will undoubtedly result in an increased incidence of cardiovascular disease. In addition, the alarming increase in unattended risk factors in younger generations will continue to fuel the cardiovascular epidemic for years to come. An estimated 6.2 million inpatient cardiovascular operations and procedures were performed in the United States in 2001.[1] Therefore, even modest additional expenditures for diagnostic or therapeutic technologies have the potential to increase overall health-care expenditures substantially. Nevertheless, effective treatment of cardiovascular disease is of paramount importance for patients as well as for society. Nearly 50% of deaths are related to major cardiovascular disease or stroke, and eliminating all forms of these diseases would increase the average life expectancy by almost 7 years. As demonstrated in this chapter, cost-effectiveness analysis represents an important tool for evaluating choices among competing alternatives in the armamentarium of the interventional cardiologist.

Although the field of economic technology assessment in health care is still relatively young, many high-quality economic studies have been performed to evaluate new techniques or treatment strategies in cardiology. As several reviews of economic evaluations in cardiology have shown, most new technologies in cardiology that improve clinical outcomes also tend to increase costs compared with the established alternatives. Nonetheless, cost-effectiveness analyses incorporating the results of such studies suggest that the majority of treatments shown to improve health outcomes have been found to be reasonably cost-effective as well. For example, drug-eluting stent implantation increases overall costs for most patients, but is associated with such improved outcomes as reduced restenosis rate and increased quality of life compared with bare metal stent implantation. Formal cost-effectiveness analysis suggests that these benefits are "worth the cost" when compared with other well-accepted interventions in cardiology or other areas of medicine and health care. However, invasive diagnostic tests such as coronary pressure–based FFR measurement may be an efficient tool to guide physicians in selecting patients who are expected to benefit from stent implantation. In this case, the economic analysis suggests that the additional costs of the test will be more than offset by the savings because of the reduced number of stent implantations.

In the future, economic evaluations are likely to play an integral role in the development of optimal treatment strategies, guidelines, and health-care management for incorporation of new technologies and treatment paradigms in the treatment of patients with cardiovascular disease. In particular, as the field of decision-analytic modeling (methods and applications) continues to advance, decision-analytic models will play an even more important role in cost-effectiveness analysis. Most economic studies already involve the use of decision-analytic modeling techniques to synthesize data from various sources to estimate the cost-effectiveness ratio. For example, only 6% of cost-effectiveness studies published in 1996 were conducted alongside a clinical trial, whereas 85% were primarily modeling studies.[106] Given the limited time horizon and scope of most clinical trials, some form of modeling is usually required to progress from the within-trial results to incremental cost-effectiveness ratio of interest.[49,62] In this chapter, several additional situations are described in which decision modeling is needed to produce the economic results of interest, and case examples have been used to demonstrate the value of modeling techniques as a tool for health-care evaluation. Decision-analytic models have a long history in cardiology outcomes research. They may aid clinical decisions affecting individual patients as well as inform clinical policy decisions and decisions regarding national health policy. Decision models can be applied to preventive strategies as well those aimed at diagnosis and treatment. Several of the Agency for Health Care Policy and Research's patient outcomes research teams[107] used such models to combine clinical outcome data and cost information from various sources, to summarize existing cost-effectiveness relationships for important patient populations and subgroups, to guide research agendas, and to inform clinical practice guidelines.[108]

With increasing computing power and speed, it is now possible to use increasingly sophisticated methods for model simulation (eg, extensive Monte Carlo simulations are necessary for probabilistic sensitivity analysis). As outlined by a panel of experts during the Methods Symposium, "Probabilistic Sensitivity Analysis: Is It Useful and Should It Be Mandatory?" at the 26th Annual Meeting of the Society of Medical Decision Making in Atlanta, Georgia, probabilistic sensitivity analysis has many advantages. For example, it can be used for integrating high levels of subgroup heterogeneity, performing multi-way sensitivity analyses, evaluating statistical inference, and prioritizing future research through value-of-information analysis. However, this advance comes with new challenges. For example, a thorough and valid probabilistic sensitivity analysis requires information on the joint distribution of multiple model parameters reflecting their interdependence, but this information is usually lacking in economic modeling studies. This example shows that it is questionable whether each statistical advance in modeling techniques can be applied in routine technology assessment and lead to practical advances.

Moreover, as we increasingly rely on such quantitative and formal studies, we must not forget that cost-effectiveness is constructed to identify interventions that produce the most health with the resources available, which is only one dimension in the overall evaluation of new medical technologies. For example, issues of equity and distributive justice, which include the distribution of health across different subpopulations, are not yet consistently integrated in the traditional concept of cost-effectiveness analysis.[109]

Therefore, despite its utility, cost-effectiveness analysis is not a complete procedure for determining resource allocation decisions in health care, because it cannot incorporate all the values and criteria relevant to such decisions. Rather, it should be used as an aid in the complex decision-making process.[23] In addition to the criterion of maximizing the overall health of a population, health policymakers must often consider other ethical criteria to comply with societal preferences. Finally, we must recognize that as physicians our primary goal remains to deliver high quality of health care, extend patients' life expectancy, and improve their quality of life. Cost-effectiveness analysis should thus be used to support the development of rational guidelines for application of existing and emerging health technologies but should not be used to constrain physician practice within the limits of those guidelines.

REFERENCES

1. American Heart Association. *Heart Disease and Stroke Statistics—2004 Update.* Dallas, Texas: American Heart Association; 2004.
2. Drummond MF, O'Brien B, Stoddart GL, Torrance GW. *Methods for the Economic Evaluation of Health Care Programmes,* 2nd ed. New York: Oxford University Press; 1997.
3. Mills A, Drummond MF, Economic evaluation of health programmes: Glossary of terms. *World Health Stat.* 1985;Q 38:432–434.
4. Weinstein MC, Stason WB. Cost-effectiveness of coronary artery bypass surgery. *Circulation.* 1982;66(5 Pt 2):III56–66.
5. Mark DB, Simons TA. Economics and cost-effectiveness in evaluating the value of cardiovascular therapies. Fundamentals of economic analysis. *Am Heart J.* May 1999;137(5):S38–40.
6. Gold MR, Siegel JE, Russell LB, Weinstein MC. *Cost-Effectiveness in Health and Medicine.* New York: Oxford University Press; 1996.
7. Shroff AR, Cohen DJ. Cost-effectiveness of coronary stenting. In: Stone GW, Leon MB, eds. *The Textbook of Coronary Stenting.* Philadelphia: WB Saunders; 2007 [in press].
8. Hlatky MA, Mark DB. Economics and cardiovascular disease. In: Braunwald E, Zipes D, Libby P, eds. *Heart disease: a textbook of cardiovascular medicine,* 6th ed. Philadelphia: WB Saunders Company; 2001:19–26.
9. Luce BR, Manning WG, Siegel JE, Lipscomb J. Estimating costs in cost-effectiveness analysis. In: Gold MR, Siegel JE, Russell LB, Weinstein MC, eds. *Cost-effectiveness in Health and Medicine.* New York: Oxford University Press; 1996:176–213.
10. Sculpher M. The role and estimation of productivity costs in economic evaluation. In: Drummond MF, McGuire A, eds. *Economic Evaluation in Health Care. Merging Theory with Practice.* New York: Oxford University Press; 2001:94–112.
11. Hlatky MA. Economic endpoint in clinical trials. *Epidemiol Rev.* 2002; 24(1):80–84.
12. Mark DB. Medical economics in cardiovascular medicine. In: Topol EJ, ed. *Textbook of Cardiovascular Medicine,* 2nd ed. Philadelphia: Lippincott Williams & Wilkins; 2002:957–979.
13. Mark DB, Hlatky MA. Medical economics and the assessment of value in cardiovascular medicine: Part I. *Circulation.* 2002;106(4):516–520.
14. Finkler SA. The distinction between cost and charges. *Ann Intern Med.* 1982; 96(1):102–109.
15. Kupersmith J, Holmes-Rovner M, Hogan A, Rovner D, Gardiner J. Cost-effectiveness analysis in heart disease, Part I: General principles. *Prog Cardiovasc Dis.* 1994;37(3):161–184.
16. Shwartz M, Young DW, Siegrist RB. The ratio of costs to charges: how good a basis for estimating costs? *Inquiry.* 1995;32:476–481.
17. Hsiao W, Braun P, Yntema D, Becker E. Estimating physicians' work for a resource-based relative-value scale. *N Engl J Med.* 1988;319(13):835–841.
18. Taira DA, Seto TB, Siegrist R, Cosgrove R, Berezin R, Cohen DJ. Comparison of analytic approaches for the economic evaluation of new technologies alongside multicenter clinical trials. *Am Heart J.* 2003; 145(3): 452–458.
19. Furlong W, Feeny D, Torrance GW, et al. *Multiplicative Multi-Attribute Utility Function for the Health Utilities Index Mark 3 (HUI3) System: A Technical Report.* McMaster University Centre for Health Economics and Policy Analysis. 1999;98–11.
20. Anonymous. EuroQol—a new facility for the measurement of health-related quality of life. The EuroQol Group. [see comment]. *Health Pol.* 1990;16(3):199–208.
21. Torrance GW. Measurement of health state utilities for economic appraisal. *J Health Econ.* 1986;5(1):1–30.
22. Torrance GW, Thomas WH, Sackett DL. A utility maximization model for evaluation of health care programs. *Health Serv Res.* 1972;7(2):118–133.
23. Russell LB, Gold MR, Siegel JE, Daniels N, Weinstein MC. The role of cost-effectiveness analysis in health and medicine. Panel on Cost-Effectiveness in Health and Medicine.[see comment]. *JAMA.* 1996;276(14): 1172–1177.
24. Torrance GW, Siegel JE, Luce BR. Framing and designing the cost-effectiveness analysis. In: Gold MR, Siegel JE, Russell LB, Weinstein MC, eds. *Cost-Effectiveness in Health and Medicine.* New York: Oxford University Press. 1996;54–81.
25. Gold M. Panel on cost-effectiveness in health and medicine. *Med Care.* 1996;34(12 Suppl):DS197–199.
26. Kuntz KM, Fleischmann KE, Hunink MG, Douglas PS. Cost-effectiveness of diagnostic strategies for patients with chest pain. *Ann Intern Med.* 1999;130(9):709–718.
27. Weinstein MC, Stason WB. Foundations of cost-effectiveness analysis for health and medical practices. *N Engl J Med.* 1977;296(13):716–721.
28. Keeler EB, Cretin S. Discounting of live-saving and other nonmonetary effects. *Manag Sci.* 1983;29:300–306.
29. Laufer FN. On the cutting edge. *Soc Med Dec Mak News.* 2004;16(4):4.
30. Garber AM, Phelps CE. Economic foundations of cost-effectiveness analysis. *J Health Econ.* 1997;16(1):1–31.
31. Siegel JE, Clancy CM. Using economic evaluations in decision making. In: Haddix AC, Teutsch SM, Corso PS, eds. *Prevention Effectiveness: A Guide to Decision Analysis and Economic Evaluation,* 2nd ed. New York: Oxford University Press; 2003.
32. Goldman L, Sia ST, Cook EF, Rutherford JD, Weinstein MC. Costs and effectiveness of routine therapy with long-term beta-adrenergic antagonists after acute myocardial infarction. *N Engl J Med.* 1988;319(3):152–157.
33. Krumholz HM, Pasternak RC, Weinstein MC, et al. Cost effectiveness of thrombolytic therapy with streptokinase in elderly patients with suspected acute myocardial infarction. *N Engl J Med.* 1992;327(1):7–13.
34. Cohen DJ, Cosgrove RS, Berezin RH, et al. Cost-effectiveness of gamma radiation for treatment of in-stent restenosis: results from the Gamma-1 trial. *Circulation.* 2002;106(6):691–697.
35. Cohen DJ, Bakhai A, Shi C, et al. Cost-effectiveness of sirolimus-eluting stents for treatment of complex coronary stenoses: results from the Sirolimus-Eluting Balloon Expandable Stent in the Treatment of Patients with De Novo Native Coronary Artery Lesions (SIRIUS) trial. *Circulation.* 2004;110(5):508–514.
36. Cohen DJ, Krumholz HM, Sukin CA, et al. In-hospital and one-year economic outcomes after coronary stenting or balloon angioplasty. Results from a randomized clinical trial. Stent Restenosis Study Investigators. *Circulation.* 1995;92(9):2480–2487.
37. Seto T, Cohen DJ. Cost-effectiveness of adjunctive intracoronary brachytherapy for the treatment of in-stent restenosis. *Vasc Radiother Mon.* 2001;4:9–15.
38. Rinfret S, Grines CL, Cosgrove RS, et al. Quality of life after balloon angioplasty or stenting for acute myocardial infarction: One-year results from the Stent-PAMI trial. *J Am Coll Cardiol.* 2001;38(6):1614–1621.

39. Weaver WD, Reisman MA, Griffin JJ, et al. Optimum percutaneous transluminal coronary angioplasty compared with routine stent strategy trial (OPUS-1): a randomised trial. *The Lancet*. 2000;355(9222):2199–2203.

40. van Hout BA, Goes ES, Grijseels EW, van Ufford MA. Economic evaluation in the field of cardiology: theory and practice. *Prog Cardiovasc Dis*. 1999;42(2):167–173.

41. Serruys PW, van Hout B, Bonnier H, et al. Randomised comparison of implantation of heparin-coated stents with balloon angioplasty in selected patients with coronary artery disease (Benestent II). *The Lancet*. 1998; 352(9129):673–681.

42. Cohen DJ, Taira DA, Berezin R, et al. Cost-effectiveness of coronary stenting in acute myocardial infarction: results from the stent primary angioplasty in myocardial infarction (stent-PAMI) trial. *Circulation*. 2001;104(25): 3039–3045.

43. Berry E, Kelly S, Hutton J, et al. Intravascular ultrasound-guided interventions in coronary artery disease: a systematic literature review, with decision-analytic modelling, of outcomes and cost-effectiveness. *Health Tech Assess*. 2000;4(35).

44. Siebert U, Aidelsburger P, Peeters J, et al. *Intravascular Ultrasound in Diagnostic and Therapeutic Heart Catheterization. A Health-Economic HTA Report. Health Technology Assessment (Series of the German Institute for Medical Documentation and Information commissioned by the Federal Ministry of Health and Social Security)*. Vol 27. St. Augustin: Asgard; 2003.

45. Moses JW, Leon MB, Popma JJ, et al. Sirolimus-eluting stents versus standard stents in patients with stenosis in a native coronary artery.[see comment]. *N Engl J Med*. 2003;349(14):1315–1323.

46. Meltzer MI. Introduction to health economics for physicians. [see comment]. *Lancet*. 2001;358(9286):993–998.

47. Weinstein MC, O'Brien B, Hornberger J, et al. Principles of good practice for decision analytic modeling in health-care evaluation: report of the ISPOR Task Force on Good Research Practices–Modeling Studies. [comment]. *Val Health*. 2003;6(1):9–17.

48. Buxton MJ, Drummond MF, Van Hout BA, et al. Modelling in economic evaluation: an unavoidable fact of life. *Health Econ*. 1997;6(3):217–227.

49. Siebert U. When should decision-analytic modeling be used in the economic evaluation of health care? [Editorial]. *Euro J Health Econ*. 2003;4(3): 143–150.

50. Raiffa H. *Decision Analysis: Introductory Lectures on Choices under Uncertainty*. Reading, MA: Addison Wesley; 1968.

51. Weinstein MC, Fineberg HV, Elstein AS, et al. *Clinical Decision Analysis*. Philadelphia: WB Saunders Company; 1980.

52. Eddy DM. Clinical decision making: from theory to practice. Designing a practice policy. Standards, guidelines and options. *JAMA*. 1990;263(22):3077,3081,3084.

53. Richardson WS, Detsky AS. Users' Guides to the Medical Literature: VII. How to Use a Clinical Decision Analysis. A: Are the Results of the Study Valid? Evidence Based Medicine Working Group. *JAMA*. 1995;273(16): 1292–1295.

54. Hunink MG, Glasziou PP, Siegel JE, et al. *Decision Making in Health and Medicine. Integrating Evidence and Values*. Cambridge, Mass: 4 Cambridge University Press; 2001.

55. Beck JR, Pauker SG. The Markov process in medical prognosis. *Med Decis Making*. 1983;3(4):419–458.

56. Sonnenberg FA, Beck JR. Markov models in medical decision making: a practical guide. *Med Decis Making*. 1993;13(4):322–338.

57. Etzioni R, Urban N, Baker M. Estimating the costs attributable to a disease with application to ovarian cancer. *J Clin Epidemiol*. 1996;49(1):95–103.

58. O'Brien BJ, Drummond MF, Labelle RJ, Willan A. In search of power and significance: issues in the design and analysis of stochastic cost-effectiveness studies in health care. *Med Care*. 1994;32(2):150–163.

59. van Hout BA, Al MJ, Gordon GS, Rutten FF. Costs, effects and C/E-ratios alongside a clinical trial. *Health Econ*. 1994;3(5):309–319.

60. Fieller EC. The distribution of an index in a normal bivariate population. *Biometrika*. 1932;24:428–440.

61. Efron B, Tibshirani R. *An Introduction to the Bootstrap*. New York: Chapman & Hill; 1993.

62. Briggs AH. Handling uncertainty in economic evaluation and presenting the results. In: Drummond M, McGuire A, eds. *Economic Evaluation in Health Care. Merging Theory with Practice*. New York: Oxford University Press; 2001:172–214.

63. Berger ML, Bingefors K, Hedblom EC, Pashos CL, Torrance GW, eds. *Health Care Cost, Quality, and Outcomes. ISPOR Book of Terms*. Lawrenceville, NJ: International Society for Pharmacoeconomics and Outcomes Research; 2003.

64. Doubilet P, Begg CB, Weinstein MC, Braun P, McNeil BJ. Probabilistic sensitivity analysis using Monte Carlo simulation. A practical approach. *Med Decis Making*. 1985;5(2):157–177.

65. Claxton K, Neumann PJ, Araki S, Weinstein MC. Bayesian value-of-information analysis. An application to a policy model of Alzheimer's disease. *Int J Tech Assess Health Care*. 2001;17(1):38–55.

66. Weinstein MC, Toy EL, Sandberg EA, et al. Modeling for health care and other policy decisions: uses, roles, and validity. *Val Health*. 2001;4(5): 348–361.

67. Ades AE, Lu G, Claxton K. Expected value of sample information calculations in medical decision modeling. *Med Dec Mak*. 2004;24(2):207–227.

68. Mudra H, di Mario C, de Jaegere P, et al. Randomized comparison of coronary stent implantation under ultrasound or angiographic guidance to reduce stent restenosis (OPTICUS Study). *Circulation*. 2001;104(12):1343–1349.

69. Mueller C, Hodgson JM, Schindler C, Perruchoud AP, Roskamm H, Buettner HJ. Cost-effectiveness of intracoronary ultrasound for percutaneous coronary interventions. *Am J Cardiol*. 2003;91(2):143–147.

70. Peeters J, Siebert U, Aidelsburger P, et al. *Intravascular Ultrasound in Diagnostic and Therapeutic Heart Catheterization: A Clinical HTA Report. Health Technology Assessment (Series of the German Institute for Medical Documentation and Information commissioned by the Federal Ministry of Health and Social Security)*. Vol 26. St. Augustin: Asgard; 2003.

71. Wilson RF. Assessing the severity of coronary-artery stenoses. *N Engl J Med.*. 1996;334(26):1735–1737.

72. Topol EJ, Ellis SG, Cosgrove DM, et al. Analysis of coronary angioplasty practice in the United States with an insurance-claims data base. *Circulation*. 1993;87(5):1489–1497.

73. Scanlon PJ, Faxon DP, Audet AM, et al. ACC/AHA guidelines for coronary angiography: executive summary and recommendations. A report of the American College of Cardiology/American Heart Association Task Force on Practice Guidelines (Committee on Coronary Angiography) developed in collaboration with the Society for Cardiac Angiography and Interventions. *Circulation*. 1999;99(17):2345–2357.

74. Pijls NH, De Bruyne B, Peels K, et al. Measurement of fractional flow reserve to assess the functional severity of coronary-artery stenoses. *N Engl J Med*. 1996;334(26):1703–1708.

75. Siebert U, Cohen D, Kuntz KM. Clinical and economic evaluation of coronary pressure measurement in patients with unclear coronary stenosis. The role of Markov Models in the development of clinical guidelines. *Drug Res*. 2002;52(4):38.

76. Siebert U, Greenberg D, Kuntz KM, Cohen DJ. Cost-effectiveness of measuring pressure-derived fractional flow reserve to guide coronary interventions in the drug-eluting stent era: Insights from a decision-analytic model. *Circulation*. 2003;108(17):356.

77. Bech GJ, De Bruyne B, Pijls NH, et al. Fractional flow reserve to determine the appropriateness of angioplasty in moderate coronary stenosis: a randomized trial. *Circulation*. 2001;103(24):2928–2934.

78. Dick RJ, Popma JJ, Muller DW, Burek KA, Topol EJ. In-hospital costs associated with new percutaneous coronary devices. *Am J Cardiol*. 1991;68(9):879–885.

79. Serruys PW, Strauss BH, Beatt KJ, et al. Angiographic follow-up after placement of a self-expanding coronary-artery stent. *N Engl J Med*. 1991;324(1):13–17.

80. Serruys PW, Strauss BH, van Beusekom HM, van der Giessen WJ. Stenting of coronary arteries: has a modern Pandora's box been opened? *J Am Coll Cardiol*. 1991;17(6 Suppl B):143B–154B.

81. Block PC. Coronary-artery stents and other endoluminal devices. *N Engl J Med*. 1991;324(1):52–53.

82. Cohen DJ, Breall JA, Ho KK, et al. Evaluating the potential cost-effectiveness of stenting as a treatment for symptomatic single-vessel coronary disease. Use of a decision-analytic model. *Circulation*. 1994;89(4):1859–1874.

83. Weinstein MC, Coxson PG, Williams LW, Pass TM, Stason WB, Goldman L. Forecasting coronary heart disease incidence, mortality, and cost: the Coronary Heart Disease Policy Model. *Am J Public Health*. 1987;77(11): 1417–1426.

84. Matchar DB, Samsa GP, Matthews JR, et al. The Stroke Prevention Policy Model: linking evidence and clinical decisions. *Ann Intern Med*. 1997;127(8 Pt 2):704–711.

85. Mui SL. Projecting coronary heart disease incidence and cost in Australia: results from the incidence module of the Cardiovascular Disease Policy Model. *Aust N Z J Pub Health*. 1999;23(1):11–19.

86. Goldman L, Weinstein MC, Williams LW. Relative impact of targeted versus populationwide cholesterol interventions on the incidence of coronary heart disease. Projections of the Coronary Heart Disease Policy Model. *Circulation*. 1989;80(2):254–260.

87. Edelson JT, Weinstein MC, Tosteson ANA, Williams L, Lee TH, Goldman L. Long-term cost-effectiveness of various initial monotherapies for mild to moderate hypertension. *JAMA*. 1990;263:408–413.

88. Tosteson AN, Weinstein MC, Williams LW, Goldman L. Long-term impact of smoking cessation on the incidence of coronary heart disease. *Am J Pub Health*. 1990;80(12):1481–1486.

89. Goldman L, Weinstein MC, Goldman PA, Williams LW. Cost-effectiveness of HMG-CoA reductase inhibition for primary and secondary prevention of coronary heart disease. *JAMA*. 1991;265(9):1145–1151.

90. Tsevat J, Weinstein MC, Williams LW, Tosteson AN, Goldman L. Expected gains in life expectancy from various coronary heart disease risk factor modifications. *Circulation*. 1991;83(4):1194–1201.

91. Tsevat J. Impact and cost-effectiveness of smoking interventions. *Am J Med*. 1992;93(1A):43S–47S.

92. Goldman L, Gordon DJ, Rifkind BM, et al. Cost and health implications of cholesterol lowering. *Circulation*. 1992;85(5):1960–1968.

93. Goldman L, Goldman PA, Williams LW, Weinstein MC. Cost-effectiveness considerations in the treatment of heterozygous familial hypercholesterolemia with medications. *Am J Cardiol*. 1993;72(10):75D–79D.

94. Stinnett A, Mittleman A, Weinstein M, et al. The cost-effectiveness of dietary and pharmacologic therapy for cholesterol reduction in adults. In: Gold MR, Siegel JE, Russell LB, Weinstein MC, eds. *Cost-Effectiveness in Health and Medicine: Report on the Panel of Cost-Effectiveness in Health and Medicine*. New York: Oxford University Press; 1996:349–391.

95. Hunink MGM, Goldman L, Tosteson AN, et al. The recent decline in mortality from coronary heart disease, 1980–1990. The effect of secular trends in risk factors and treatment. *JAMA*. 1997;277(7):535–542.

96. Tosteson AN, Weinstein MC, Hunink MG, et al. Cost-effectiveness of populationwide educational approaches to reduce serum cholesterol levels. *Circulation*. 1997;95(1):24–30.

97. Goldman L, Coxson P, Hunink MGM, et al. The relative influence of secondary versus primary prevention using the National Cholesterol Education Program Adult Treatment Panel II guidelines. *J Am Coll Cardiol*. 1999;34(3):768–776.

98. Prosser LA, Stinnett AA, Goldman PA, et al. Cost-effectiveness of cholesterol-lowering therapies according to selected patient characteristics. *Ann Intern Med*. 2000;132(10):769–779.

99. Phillips KA, Shlipak MG, Coxson P, et al. Health and economic benefits of increased beta-blocker use following myocardial infarction. *JAMA*. 2000;284(21):2748–2754.

100. Goldman L, Phillips KA, Coxson P, et al. The effect of risk factor reductions between 1981 and 1990 on coronary heart disease incidence, prevalence, mortality and cost. *J Am Coll Cardiol*. 2001;38(4):1012–1017.

101. Tice JA, Ross E, Coxson PG, et al. Cost-effectiveness of vitamin therapy to lower plasma homocysteine levels for the prevention of coronary heart disease: effect of grain fortification and beyond. *JAMA*. 2001;286(8):936–943.

102. Gaspoz JM, Coxson PG, Goldman PA, et al. Cost effectiveness of aspirin, clopidogrel, or both for secondary prevention of coronary heart disease. *N Engl J Med*. 2002;346(23):1800–1806.

103. Anonymous. Collaborative overview of randomised trials of antiplatelet therapy–I: Prevention of death, myocardial infarction, and stroke by prolonged antiplatelet therapy in various categories of patients. Antiplatelet Trialists' Collaboration [see comment] [erratum appears in *Br Med J*. 1994;308(6943):1540]. *Br Med J*. 1998;106:81–106.

104. Anonymous. A randomised, blinded, trial of clopidogrel versus aspirin in patients at risk of ischaemic events (CAPRIE). CAPRIE Steering Committee.[see comment]. *Lancet*. 1996;348(9038):1329–1339.

105. Yusuf S, Zhao F, Mehta SR, et al. Effects of clopidogrel in addition to aspirin in patients with acute coronary syndromes without ST-segment elevation.[see comment][erratum appears in *N Engl J Med*. 2001;345(23):1716]. *N Engl J Med.*. 2001;345(7):494–502.

106. Posnett J, Jan S. Indirect cost in economic evaluation: the opportunity cost of unpaid inputs. *Health Econ*. 1996;5(1):13–23.

107. Sonnenberg FA, Roberts MS, Tsevat J, Wong JB, Barry M, Kent DL. Toward a peer review process for medical decision analysis models. *Med Care*. 1994;32(7 Suppl):JS52–64.

108. Eisenstein EL, Mark DB, Califf RM. Importance of cost and quality of life in decisions about routine angiography after acute myocardial infarction. The role of cost-effectiveness models.[comment]. *Circulation*. 1996;94(5):869–871.

109. Marckmann G, Siebert U. [Cost-Effectiveness as criterion for resource allocation in health care]. *Zeitsch Med Ethik*. 2002;48(2):171–190.

CHAPTER 69

Quality Assurance and Quality Improvement in Interventional Cardiology

Mauro Moscucci, MD

Historians would agree that Wednesday, December 18, 1991, was a landmark day in world history. As shown in the cover of that day's issue of the New York City newspaper *Newsday* (Figure 69-1), this was the day that Yeltsin and Gorbachev agreed to dissolve the Soviet Union and proclaim the New Commonwealth. In addition, it also marked the first time ranking of physicians was published in a newspaper. In that issue of *Newsday,* names of cardiac surgeons performing coronary artery bypass surgery in New York State were published, together with the hospital where they were practicing and their mortality statistics.

The background of that publication can be traced back to 1987, another landmark year in the history of scorecard cardiovascular medicine and of public reporting. In that year, Medicare released for the first time mortality statistics for coronary artery bypass surgery. In 1988, mortality statistics for percutaneous transluminal coronary angioplasty (PTCA) were released. Following those reports, New York State began collecting mortality data for cardiac surgeons performing coronary artery bypass surgery. *Newsday* asked New York State to release those mortality data, but the State refused. *Newsday* sued the State, and, under the Freedom of Information Act, New York State was ordered by the Supreme Court to release those mortality statistics, which were then published in on December 18, 1991. In the same year, two studies had been published side-by-side in the *Journal of the American Medical Association.* The first report, from the Northern New England Cardiovascular Study group, showed that differences in mortality rates among institutions could not be explained solely on the basis of disease severity.[1] The second report, from Pennsylvania, confirmed the results of the first report.[2] Both reports were noticed by the public and generated a vivid debate.

As a result of the increased scrutiny of surgical and percutaneous coronary procedures following those initial reports, the years since 1991 have been characterized by a major effort toward a better understanding of factors related to adverse outcomes, and by a movement toward measurement and improvement of quality of care. A push toward public reporting of physicians' and hospitals' scorecards has been an important component of this movement.[3–6] Therefore, establishment of a process for quality assessment and quality improvement should be a key element of contemporary invasive and interventional cardiology practice.

FACTORS RELATED TO ADVERSE OUTCOMES OF PROCEDURES

There are several factors that might relate to adverse outcomes of diagnostic cardiac catheterization and of percutaneous coronary interventions (PCI). These factors can be grouped in three categories: (1) equipment limitations, (2) human error, and (3) patients' comorbidities.

〖 〗 EQUIPMENT LIMITATIONS

Since the mid-1980s, improvement in catheter technology and the introduction of breakthrough mechanical and pharmacologic interventions have resulted in a progressive increase in the safety of PCI and in improved outcomes. For example, although the incidence of emergency coronary bypass surgery following contemporary PCI is estimated to be approximately 0.5% today,[7,8] prior to

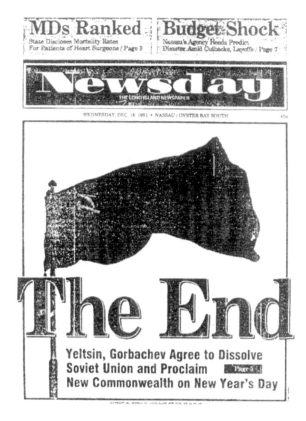

The table within the figure image reads:

mortality rate Physician	Hospital		Cases	Deaths	
Smith C	Presbyterian	159	1	1.05
Major W	Millard Fillmore	153	3	2.52
Nelson R	North Shore	151	14	5.42
Guarino R	Millard Fillmore	148	4	4.16
Griepp R	Beth Israel/Mt. Sinai	145	1	0.68
Williams L	Winthrop-University	144	5	4.10
Stewart S	Strong Memorial	143	12	9.12
Sabado M	Maimonides Medical Center	138	6	1.86

FIGURE 69-1. Cover of the December 18, 1991, issue of *Newsday*. The title on the top left announces ranking of cardiac surgeons and hospitals according to mortality rates for coronary artery bypass surgery.

the introduction of coronary stenting, the incidence of emergency bypass surgery was as high as 6%. In addition, the introduction of new pharmacologic agents such as GPIIb/IIIa receptor blockers and ADP receptor blockers resulted in further improvement in acute and long-term outcomes of PCI.

Yet the adoption of new technology is often characterized by the introduction of new complications, such as coronary perforation with rotational atherectomy, subacute stent thrombosis with coronary stenting, or late stent thrombosis in patients undergoing brachytherapy and not treated with dual antiplatelet therapy. The prevention of these complications requires appropriate modification of the process of care through the application of standing orders, critical pathways, and guidelines, as well as careful monitoring of clinical outcomes. In addition, the laboratory should be equipped with devices that have been shown to reduce complication rates in selected patient groups, or that can be used for bailout situations, such as snares, distal embolic protection devices, or thrombectomy devices.

[ ] HUMAN ERROR AND OPERATOR EXPERIENCE

After the first report by Luft et al.[9] on the empirical relationship between surgical volume and mortality, numerous studies have shown a direct relationship between operator or institutional volume and outcomes of surgical or percutaneous procedures. Whereas for coronary artery bypass surgery the continued importance of this relationship was confirmed using contemporary clinical[10] and claims data,[11] for PCI the majority of the studies available either predate the widespread use in interventional practice

of coronary stenting and glycoprotein receptor blockers, or were obtained through analysis of Medicare claims. Recognized limitations related to the use of Medicare data include the need to extrapolate total number of procedures from the number of Medicare procedures, the often incomplete reporting in Medicare claims of comorbidities that have been shown to be important risk factors for adverse outcomes,[4,12] and the possible miscoding of complications as comorbidities.[13]

Ellis el al.[14] analyzed clinical data from a quality-controlled, multi-institutional clinical database of percutaneous coronary interventions. The patient population included patients treated in 1993 and 1994, a time period preceding the widespread use of coronary stents and of glycoprotein IIb/IIIa receptor blockers. Operators performing less than 70 procedures per year had significantly worse outcomes than the reminder of the group, whereas the best outcomes were observed in a high-volume group of operators performing more than 270 procedure year. Similar results were reported by Hannan et al.[15] in an analysis of 1991–1994 data from the New York State Department of Health Coronary Angioplasty Reporting System, and by Jollis et al.[16,17] in two separate analyses of claims data from the Medicare database. These analyses also predated the widespread use of coronary stents and of glycoprotein IIb/IIIa receptor blockers in interventional practice. Both analyses showed better outcomes with high volume operators. In the analysis by Hannan et al.,[15] an important interaction between operator volume and institution volume was also identified, with worse outcomes observed for low-volume operators performing procedures in low-volume institutions. More recently, McGrath et al.[18] analyzed relatively contemporary data (calendar year 1997) from the Medicare database. As in previous reports, better outcomes were observed in patients treated by high-volume operators when compared to patients treated by low-volume operators.

Similar results were obtained in an analysis of data collected from 107, 713 procedures performed in 34 hospitals in New York State from 1998–2000,[18a] and in a second analysis including 18,504 procedures performed in Michigan in the calendar year of 2002.[18b] Using contemporary clinical data collected in the era of coronary stenting, both studies showed once again worse outcomes in patients treated by low-volume.

Against this extensive evidence supporting a relationship between volume and outcome, there have been two studies that found no such relationship. The first study was an analysis from a single high-volume center. In that analysis, no direct relationship was observed between volume and outcome.[19] The second analysis was from the Northern New England Cardiovascular Consortium.[20] Although that analysis did not demonstrate a relationship between operator annual volume of PCI and outcomes, it should be noted that all institutions in the study were high volume institutions (> 600 procedures/year), and that the "low volume operators" group from this collaborative registry had a relatively high procedure volume (average of 68 procedures/year and median of 75 procedures/year).

Although most studies have documented a volume–outcome relationship, there is little question that procedure volume is only a poor surrogate of quality and outcomes. It does not take into account prior operator experience or number of years in practice; it does not differentiate between low-volume operators who still have good outcomes and low-volume operators who provide poor care; and, more important, it does not take into account severity of illness. In other words, quantity does not necessarily equate to quality.

Since the mid-1990s, there has been substantial progress in refining the scientific rigor of clinical risk adjustment. Factors related to in-hospital mortality following PCI are now well defined,[21–24] and progress has been made in developing statistical models for other outcomes. As the methodology for risk adjustment continues to evolve, procedure volume will likely no longer be used as a replacement or a surrogate for appropriately risk-adjusted outcomes. However, procedure volume is easy to measure, and its potential implications are easily understood by patients undergoing PCI. Thus, all considered, implementation of minimal volume standards seems prudent.

[ ] PATIENTS' COMORBIDITIES

For decades it has been known that patients' comorbidities might relate to adverse outcomes. More recently, we have learned that the relationship between an explanatory variable, such as advanced age or diabetes, and an outcome such as in-hospital mortality can be estimated using statistical techniques. These statistical techniques have allowed the development of mathematical models (ie, risk adjustment models) that, by adjusting for patients' comorbidities and other confounding factors, can be used to compare the results of different operators, for the assessment of the results of quality improvement efforts, and as an aid in the prediction of individual patient prognosis.

As of today, the methodology of risk adjustment for the prediction of in-hospital mortality following contemporary PCI appears secure. Models for in-hospital PCI mortality have been developed from regional and national databases, and they have been internally or externally validated.[14,15,22–26] These models have been used for

public reporting of institutions and operators outcomes, for quality improvement efforts, and for the prediction of individual patient prognosis.[24] Clinical variables included in the leading risk adjustment mortality models are listed in Table 69-1. As shown in the table, the models have several similarities. Thus, the requirement for appropriately risk-adjusted mortality data can be fulfilled through the collection of a relatively modest number of variables.

Although risk factors for other outcomes such as vascular complications,[27–32] contrast nephropathy,[33–36] stroke,[37–40] and major adverse events have been identified,[41] less progress has been made in the development of validated risk adjustment models that can be used for quality-assurance and quality-improvement programs. Nonetheless, it is expected that the same progress that has been made in the development of the mortality models will soon be made in the development of models for nonfatal complications.

QUALITY ASSURANCE

Major domains pertaining to quality assurance in the cardiac catheterization laboratory are listed in Table 69-2.

[ ] CREDENTIALING

Criteria for training and credentialing of physicians performing diagnostic and therapeutic catheterization have been recommended by the American College of Cardiology Task Force on Clinical Expert Consensus Documents, and have been endorsed by the Society of Coronary Angiography and Intervention.[42] Training should include a detailed curriculum on topics ranging from vascular biology to clinical management strategies (Table 69-3). This curriculum should be part of a dedicated fourth year of training in interventional cardiology. According to the American Council on Graduate Medical Education (ACGME), during this fourth year the trainee should perform a minimum of 250 coronary interventional cases.

The relationship between operator volume and outcomes has been previously discussed. Recent analyses suggest that this relationship still exists with contemporary PCI. In particular, worse outcomes have been observed with low-volume operators performing procedures in low-volume institutions. Therefore, a minimum of 75 procedures per year per operator is currently recommended.[43] It has been recommended that operators performing fewer than 75 procedures per year should work under the supervision of high-volume operators, and in an environment that supports close monitoring of clinical outcomes.[44] Board certification in cardiovascular disease and interventional cardiology is also advisable, and it is currently part of the credentialing process in our laboratory. Recommended criteria for credentialing of a catheterization laboratory ("cath lab") director in a lab performing interventional procedures include a minimum of 5 years in practice and board certification in cardiovascular disease and interventional cardiology.

The prior guidelines for cardiac catheterization recommended a minimum of 150 diagnostic cardiac catheterizations per year as part of the recredentialing process. However, this threshold was derived arbitrarily and, currently there has been no study that has shown a relationship between procedure volume and outcomes of diagnostic catheterization. Therefore, minimum volume standards for diagnostic cardiac catheterization have been removed from the most recent guidelines for cardiac catheterization standards.[42]

TABLE 69-1

Clinical Variables Included in Leading Risk Adjustment Models for In-Hospital Mortality and Corresponding Coefficients

VARIABLE	RISK ADJUSTMENT MODEL				
	MICHIGAN (24)	NORTHERN NEW ENGLAND (22)	CLEVELAND CLINIC (14)	ACC/NCDR (74)	NEW YORK (15)
Age (Continuous)			3.21 (log)		0.06
50–59		−0.07		0.97	
60–69		0.49		1.32	
70–79	0.81	1.19		1.86	
>80	0.97	1.31		2.43	
Female gender	0.59				0.26
Male Gender			−0.6		
PVD	0.46	0.74			0.57
Chronic lung disease				0.28	
Use of thrombolytic				0.34	
CHF		1.10			0.86
Creatinine >1.5 mg/dL	1.7				
Creatinine >2.0 mg/dL		0.84		1.11	1.25
Diabetes				0.34	0.34
Prior PCI					−0.53
Prior open heart					0.35
2 or 3 vessels					0.59
MI	1.03	0.6	1.56	0.27	
<6h					1.65
6–23h					1.30
1–7 d					0.74
Hemodynamic Instability					1.42
Shock	2.44	1.80	2.54	2.13	2.90
Salvage				2.59	
Cardiac Arrest	1.29				
Emergency		2.04		1.67	
Urgency		0.78		0.54	
IABP		1.36		0.47	0.87
Thrombus	0.52				
Type C lesion		0.66			
Type BC lesion			0.49		
SCAI II-IV				0.49–0.74	
Left Main Disease				0.68	
				0.26	
Prox LAD lesion					

TABLE 69-1

Clinical Variables Included in Leading Risk Adjustment Models for In-Hospital Mortality and Corresponding Coefficients (*continued*)

| | RISK ADJUSTMENT MODEL | | | | |
VARIABLE	MICHIGAN (24)	NORTHERN NEW ENGLAND (22)	CLEVELAND CLINIC (14)	ACC/NCDR (74)	NEW YORK (15)
EF					
<50%	0.51				
50–59%		0.92			
40–49%		1.20			
<40%		1.64			
20–39%					0.39
<20%					1.30
40–50%				−0.17	
30–39%				−0.01	
20–29%				0.70	
10–19%				1.18	
<10%				1.41	
# of Diseased vessels	0.44		0.28		

TABLE 69-2

Major Domains for Quality Assurance in the Cardiac Catheterization Laboratory

Credentialing
Catheterization laboratory personnel
Radiation safety
Equipment maintenance
Costs
Clinical appropriateness
Outcome assessment
Post-procedure and long-term follow-up care

[ ] CATHETERIZATION LABORATORY PERSONNEL

Performance of diagnostic and therapeutic cardiac catheterization requires familiarity with complex radiologic equipment and monitoring systems, as well as familiarity with ancillary equipment, advanced techniques, and therapeutic interventions. There are currently no set standards for training of catheterization laboratory personnel. Cardiac cath lab staff includes cardiovascular technicians (CVT), who undergo specific training and pass the CVT examination; nurses; radiology technicians; and technicians who have been trained "on the job." Thus, the background experience and knowledge among personnel might vary significantly, and strict internal protocols must be developed both for training and for assessment of proficiency on a continuous basis. The develop-

ment of a "clinical ladder" that provides recognition of clinical expertise and corresponding compensation can be used as an incentive toward professional growth. In addition, the designation of a technical leader in charge of training, assurance of proficiency, and who is designated as "go-to" person plays an important role in the development of the appropriate environment for training and for quality assurance of laboratory procedures. As part of proficiency assessment and maintenance, in our institution we require Advanced Cardiac Life Support certification for all cath lab personnel involved with direct patient care.

[ ] RADIATION SAFETY

Radiation exposure guidelines for medical workers have been provided by the National Council on Radiation Protection and Measurement (NCRPM). As recommended by the American College of Cardiology Task Force for Cardiac Catheterization Standards,[42,45] quality assurance in the cardiac cath lab should include: (1) ongoing educational programs concerning radiation safety and appropriate use of x-ray equipment; (2) accurate monitoring and timely reporting of personnel exposure; and (3) modification of procedural conduct in cases where exposure levels are concern.

The maximum permissible dose (MPD) for radiation has been set to ensure that the risk of working with radiation is similar to the risk of other occupations.[46–49] Currently, the MPD is an average of 10 millisieverts (mSv) per year for radiation workers and 1 mSv/year for nonradiation workers.[47,49] Educational programs on radiation safety should focus on the "as low as reasonably achievable" (ALARA) principle to reduce the total dose to a fraction of the MPD, and to minimize the risk of stochastic effects (cancer and genetic defects) to levels that are similar to other risks of general workers.[49] Training on the use of optimal angiographic and fluoro-

TABLE 69-3

Training Requirement for Operators Performing Adult Diagnostic Cardiac Catheterization and Coronary Intervention

LEVEL	PROFICIENCY LEVEL	MONTHS OF TRAINING	N OF DIAGNOSTIC CARDIAC CATHETERIZATION	N OF CORONARY INTERVENTIONS
Level 1	Basic training required of all trainees to be competent, consulting cardiologist	4 Months	100	
Level 2	Additional training required to perform diagnostic procedure	12 months	300, with 200 as primary operator	
Level 3	Advanced training in interventional cardiac catheterization	12 months		250 as primary operator

scopic techniques and on the optimal use of shielding, including the use of mobile shielding,[47] is a key component of such program.

It is the policy at the University of Michigan to distribute dosimeters once monthly to cath lab personnel, trainees, and attending physicians. In the past we observed a poor compliance in returning the dosimeters to the radiation safety office. This compliance issue was resolved in our institution by posting a board in the cardiac cath lab that includes names of all personnel involved with the use of x-ray equipment, including trainees. New dosimeters are attached to the names at each cycle and can be easily picked up by the cath lab personnel. The used dosimeters are returned in a bin located near the board. Operators who have not returned their used dosimeters are reminded repeatedly by a staff member in charge of ensuring compliance until they have returned their dosimeters. A policy of suspending cardiac cath lab privileges of noncompliant personnel is often used in other institutions.

[ ] EQUIPMENT MAINTENANCE

The modern cardiac catheterization laboratory is a complex technical environment that requires a rigorous equipment maintenance program to prevent unscheduled down times and equipment failures resulting in adverse outcomes. It is recommended that the x-ray equipment and hemodynamic monitoring system be checked at the beginning of each day to ensure appropriate operation.

Scheduled assessment of the image quality and of the image chain should not be overlooked. In a recent study,[50] two measures of fluoroscopic image quality were assessed in 64 interventional cardiology cath labs. Both measures revealed significant variation and relevant limitations in performance. In addition, under simulated conditions, 50% of systems failed to detect a wire of 0.017-in. diameter. These data support the need for scheduled assessment of the image chain and quality of images, and for scheduled assessment of natural wear and tear, which require recalibration or preventive replacement of components of the image chain.[51,52]

Other areas pertaining to equipment maintenance include the routine calibration of coagulation monitoring devices and the routine assessment of appropriate operation of diagnostic and therapeutic devices (eg, IVUS, Rheolytic thrombectomy devices, rotational atherectomy devices).

[ ] COST CONTAINMENT

Since the mid-1990s, the financial pressure from variations in reimbursement and payer mix combined with escalating costs of a rapidly evolving technology has forced health-care institutions in the United States to seek options for cost savings. As a major cost (and profit) center for many US hospitals, the cardiac cath lab has been a prime candidate for these efforts. Methods to reduce costs of PCI include implementation of critical pathways for reduction of complications and of postprocedure length of stay,[53,54] reuse of balloon catheters[55,56] percutaneous revascularization performed at the same time of diagnostic catheterization,[57,58] reduced anticoagulation and early sheath removal (leading to shorter length of hospital stay),[59,60] and the use of new pharmacologic interventions such as IIb/IIIa antagonists to reduce acute complications.

In addition, the implementation of competitive bidding for cath lab supplies represents a key opportunity for costs savings in interventional cardiology.[53,54,61] It is important to underscore that an essential aspect of a successful competitive bidding process is a unified approach by both the physicians and the purchasing department. Lack of communication between purchasers and users has been identified as a problem affecting cost-effectiveness in both health care and other industries. This lack of communication may result in decreased efficiency, and may lead to increased costs as a result of a decrease in quality. This aspect is particularly important in a technology-dependent field such as interventional cardiology, where the difference between a successful or unsuccessful procedure may sometimes depend predominantly on equipment selection. Providing feedback to physicians on resource utilization and procedure costs and a close partnership between hospital adminis-

Blue Cross Blue Shield of Michigan
Cardiovascular Consortium

09/1/2001

Patient Demographics Report (*sample*)

Hospital Code: **99**

Physician's ID: **9999**

Patient Variable	Collaborative		Hospital		Physician	
Patients Enrolled		n= 492		n= 45		n= 10
Average Age	63.5	+/- 12.2	64.1	+/- 12.8	63.8	+/- 13.1
Gender: (# + % Males)	330	67.1%	30	66.7%	9	90.0%
Hypertension	345	70.1%	32	71.1%	7	70.0%
Diabetes	122	24.8%	9	20.0%	1	10.0%
Hx CHF	61	12.4%	8	17.8%	1	10.0%
COPD	51	10.4%	2	4.4%	0	0.0%
CVD	44	8.9%	4	8.9%	1	10.0%
Hx Cardiac Arrest	8	1.6%	2	4.4%	1	10.0%
Prev MI:	148	30.1%	11	24.4%	4	40.0%
Prev PTCA	176	35.8%	12	26.7%	4	40.0%
Prev CABG (>0)	90	18.3%	8	17.8%	5	50.0%

FIGURE 69-2. Sample of quarterly patient demographic report currently distributed to all operators participating in the Blue Cross/Blue Shield of Michigan Cardiovascular Consortium.

trators and physicians are additional important aspects of the overall approach toward financial issues in the cardiac cath lab.

[ ] OUTCOMES ASSESSMENT

Prospective evaluation of clinical outcomes through an internal data collection process and benchmarking through participation to a national or regional PCI registry are a must for any interventional cardiology program that seeks to maintain and improve quality. The data collection process should include collection of comorbidities, procedure variables, and outcomes variables. Figure 69-2 shows a sample report of clinical outcomes that are currently collected by the Blue Cross/Blue Shield of Michigan Cardiovascular consortium.[62,63] The quality-assurance program should also include an assessment of the quality of the data collected through random audits and ascertainment of inclusion of consecutive cases.[63] Our outcome assessment program at the University of Michigan currently includes biannual morbidity and mortality conferences during which summary statistics for all cases are reviewed. During the conference, any in-hospital deaths and any cases associated with an unforeseen or rare complication are also reviewed.

[ ] APPROPRIATE UTILIZATION OF PROCEDURES AND ETHICAL ISSUES

Appropriateness of surgical and percutaneous coronary interventions recently received the attention of health policymakers and health services researchers. Although advances in catheter technology and the introduction of new pharmacologic interventions

resulted in increased safety of PCI, the procedure is still associated with a small but real risk of fatal and nonfatal complications, including vascular complications (~3.0%), emergency coronary artery bypass graft surgery (CABG) (~0.5%),[7] and in-hospital death (0.8%–1.6%). In addition, subacute stent thrombosis can occur in up to 0.9%–1% of cases, and it is associated with a 15% rate of Q-wave myocardial infarction (MI) and a 20% 6-month mortality rate.[64] It is estimated that nearly 900,000 stenting procedures are performed each year in the United States alone. A conservative 5% inappropriate procedure rate would result in a total of 225 cases of emergency CABG, 450 subacute stent thrombosis, 67 Q-wave MIs, and 90 deaths. Thus, inappropriate procedures expose a large number of patients who are unlikely to benefit from the procedure to a risk of fatal and nonfatal complications

Appropriateness criteria for diagnostic cardiac catheterization and for PCI were first proposed by the American College of Cardiology/AHA task force in 1993.[65] Revised guidelines were published in 2001,[66] and a further update with incorporation of the results of the latest clinical trials was released in 2005.[65a] The guidelines provide a detailed classification of appropriateness criteria. Although prospective application of the guidelines might be challenging, a quality-assurance program for interventional cardiology should nonetheless incorporate some assessment of clinical appropriateness. Such assessment can include prospective discussion of cases where the clinical decision-making process might be considered controversial. Combined cardiac surgery/interventional cardiology conferences where cases can be discussed prospectively appear an ideal setting for such evaluation. At the University of Michigan, a combined interventional cardiology/cardiac surgery clinical conference is

Blue Cross Blue Shield of Michigan
Cardiovascular Consortium

09/1/2001

Outcomes Prior to Discharge / Length of Stay *(sample)*

Hospital ID: **99**

Physician ID   **999**

Outcome Variable:	Collaborative		Hospital		Physician	
Patients Enrolled:	n= 492		n= 45		n= 10	
Reocclusion (Ver 5) (Used in v5)	1	0.2%	0	0.0%	0	0.0%
Acute Closure (Ver 4.0 and before) (Used in v4 and before)	0	0.0%	0	0.0%	0	0.0%
Emergent CABG	0	0.0%	0	0.0%	0	0.0%
Non Emergent CABG	7	1.4%	1	2.2%	0	0.0%
Q MI	1	0.2%	0	0.0%	0	0.0%
Stroke	2	0.4%	0	0.0%	0	0.0%
TIA	1	0.2%	0	0.0%	0	0.0%
Nephropathy req. Dialysis	4	0.8%	0	0.0%	0	0.0%
Vasc. Complication	8	1.6%	0	0.0%	0	0.0%
Transfusion	17	3.5%	1	2.2%	0	0.0%
Death	7	1.4%	1	2.2%	0	0.0%
Length of stay (Avg)	3.0	+/- 3.0	3.7	+/- 3.9	1.9	+/- 1.3
Post procedure length of stay	2.4	+/- 3.1	2.3	+/- 3.3	1.2	+/- 0.4

FIGURE 69-3. Sample of quarterly outcome report currently distributed to all operators participating in the Blue Cross/Blue Shield of Michigan Cardiovascular Consortium.

held every other week. The focus of the conference is to discuss clinical cases in an open forum in order to reach a consensus pertaining medical, surgical, or percutaneous management.

[ ] POSTPROCEDURE AND LONG-TERM FOLLOW-UP CARE

The importance of postprocedure and long-term follow-up care as an integral part of quality of any interventional cardiology program cannot be overemphasized. For example, the beneficial effect of lipid lowering therapy and in particular of statins has been well documented in numerous studies and patient populations, including patients undergoing PCI for de novo coronary artery stenosis.[67] More recent data also suggest that initiating statin therapy at the time of hospitalization might have an important impact on long-term compliance.[68–70] In one study,[71] 91% of patients who were started on statins in the hospital were on a statin at 1-year follow-up, compared to only 10% of patients who were not started on statins during initial hospitalization. Of the patients started on a statin during the initial hospitalization, 58% had LDL cholesterol less than 100 mg/dL at 1 year compared

with only 6% of patients who were not started on statins. These data suggest that if secondary prevention is not started at the time of initial hospitalization, the likelihood that it will ever be started after hospital discharge is relatively low.[72] Therefore, as interventional cardiologists, we should not miss the opportunity to have an important impact on long-term outcomes beyond the effect of the PCI itself. Establishing the foundation of appropriate long-term care during the initial encounter with the patient might be just what is needed.

QUALITY IMPROVEMENT

In the manufacturing industry, assessment of the quality of a product requires measurement of failure rates and of prespecified characteristics of the product, whereas improving the quality of the product requires modification of the process that leads to the product. The same concepts can be applied to the health-care industry and interventional cardiology. Thus, starting points for quality improvement programs in interventional cardiology include baseline measurement of the outcome of interest and a detailed analysis of the process of care.

Benchmarking is one of the most important first steps toward improving patients' outcomes. Many complications are relatively rare, and therefore there is insufficient data for any single hospital to perform a meaningful statistical analysis. Merging data across institutions allows the development of robust datasets that can be used to understand the link between process and outcomes through solid statistic analysis. Comparing performance across institutions then allows the identification of opportunities for improvement.

There are currently several national and regional registries that provide benchmarking in interventional cardiology and that have been developed with different goals. Data collection in the ACC National Cardiovascular Data Registry (ACC-NCDR) began in 1998.[73–75] Participation in the registry is voluntary. Although the registry currently does not audit data submitted, it provides an overview of contemporary PCI practice in the United States. In addition, the national registry has the important benefit of providing standardized definitions of comorbidities and of procedure and outcome variables that can then be used for standardization of data collection across different registries. The New York State Data Registry is a regional registry with mandatory participation in New York State.[25] The Northern New England Cardiovascular Consortium[76] and the Blue Cross/Blue Shield of Michigan Cardiovascular Consortium[62] are two regional registries developed with the primary goal of improving outcomes of PCI. Participation in the national registry and in regional registries are not mutually exclusive. The regional registries traditionally include direct quality improvement programs, a data monitoring process, and promote exchange of information across institutions in a rapid cycle that involves benchmarking, data feedback, working group meetings and site visits. Figures 69-2 and 69-3 show sample reports from the Blue Cross/Blue Shield of Michigan Cardiovascular Consortium. As shown in the figures, the reports have three columns. The first column includes data from a collaborative group, the second column includes data from a hospital, and the third column includes physician data. The purpose of these reports is to provide feedback to participating physicians and to allow the physicians to compare their practices with the practice in their own institution and in the larger consortium.

【 】 QUALITY IMPROVEMENT PHASES

Quality improvement efforts can be divided into three major phases. The first phase includes baseline data collection for measurement of the outcome of interest, benchmarking for the comparison of clinical outcomes and process of care, and identification of targets for improvement.

The second phase includes the intervention aimed toward modification of the process of care. The process of care should be broken down into detailed components so that areas for changes can be identified. Changes can then be implemented through application of critical pathways and standing orders, modification of procedural protocols, training of physicians and cardiac cath lab personnel, and by providing continuous feedback on data. The quality improvement process should then be followed by a third phase with collection of follow-up data and analysis of risk-adjusted data to assess the effect of the intervention.

BMC² POCKET GUIDE
Risk prediction tool for nephropathy requiring dialysis and guidelines for prevention

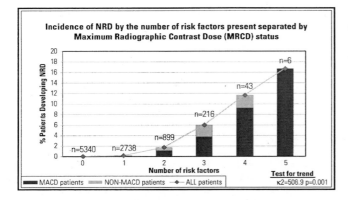

Incidence of nephropathy requiring dialysis (NRD) by number of risk factors present and the effect of exceeding a weight and creatinine adjusted Maximum Radiographic Contrast Dose (MRCD).
The risk factors for NRD include 1) Diabetes mellitus 2) Creatinine > 2 mg/dl 3) Peripheral Vascular Disease 4) Cardiogenic shock 5) History of congestive heart failure. Within each risk factor number group, the relative proportion of patients exceeding a weight and creatinine adjusted Maximum Radiographic Contrast Dose (MRCD) is represented by the darker bar.

High Risk Patient Characteristics For Contrast Nephropathy

Diabetes
Creatinine ≥2 mg/dl
Peripheral vascular disease
Cardiogenic shock
Congestive heart failure

Proposed Guidelines For High Risk Patients

A) Aggressive hydration **before** contrast administration. Measuring the LVEDP or PCWP before contrast administration might help in further determining volume status. It is not uncommon to find low PCWP/LVEDP in patients who have been admitted for pre-procedure "I.V. Hydration".

B) Determine "maximum allowed contrast dose" according to the following formula:

5cc x kg body weight/creatinine

C) Avoid exceeding this amount. Use of biplane coronary angiography and avoidance of unnecessary images (i.e. left ventriculogram or other images) might help in minimizing total amount of contast used.

D) Consider staged procedures. When planning a staged procedure, current recommendations are to perform the second procedure several days after the first.

E) Use of smaller catheters might help in decreasing amount of contrast.

F) Use of low osmolar or non-ionic contrast might decrease the risk in high risk patients.

G) In view of a recent study showing a significant benefit from acetylcysteine, and given its safety, consider acetylcysteine 600 mg bid on the day before and on the day of contrast administration (NEJM, 2000; 343: 180-184).

Email: evakline@umich.edu
moscucci@umich.edu

REV: 07/01; NRD

FIGURE 69-4. Risk prediction tool for nephropathy requiring dialysis. Courtesy of reference 81.

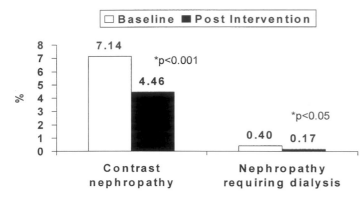

FIGURE 69-5. Frequency of contrast nephropathy and nephropathy requiring dialysis at baseline (1998) and at follow-up (2002) in a consortium of five hospitals in Michigan. *Contrast nephropathy* is defined as an increase of serum creatinine of more than 0.5 mg/dL over baseline following PCI.

Contrast nephropathy can be used as an example of outcome variable that might be modified through the application of the process previously described. Contrast nephropathy and nephropathy requiring dialysis are rare complications of PCI, but are associated with a high risk of morbidity and mortality.[33,36] Prior studies[33,36,77] have shown that among other risk factors, the total amount of contrast media used during the procedure and, in particular, exceeding a weight- and creatinine-based contrast volume threshold are important determinants for the development of contrast nephropathy.[33,78] In addition, appropriate hydration prior to contrast administration continues to be a key intervention in the prevention of contrast nephropathy.[79,80]

In view of these data, a risk prediction tool for nephropathy requiring dialysis and guidelines for its prevention was developed in our regional consortium and distributed to all participating physicians (Figure 69-4). On one side, the tool lists risk factors for nephropathy requiring dialysis and frequency of nephropathy requiring dialysis depending on number of risk factors present. The other side of the tool has recommendations for its prevention. Since about 2000, we have observed in our consortium a progressive decrease in the incidence of contrast nephropathy and nephropathy requiring dialysis in association with modification of procedure strategies adopted in participating institutions (Figure 69-5). This example, although derived from observational, nonrandomized data, suggests that application of an aggressive quality improvement process with inclusion of feedback on risk adjusted outcomes and modification of the processes of care can result in improved outcomes.

CONCLUSION

The years since the mid-1990s have been characterized by major advancements of diagnostic and therapeutic interventions for patients with cardiac disease, and by a progressive shift of focus toward outcomes assessment, quality indicators, and performance assessment. As a result of these developments, a quality assurance program in interventional cardiology requires a multidisciplinary team approach that includes physicians, nursing staff, and cath lab personnel, and integration of technical, administrative, and clinical data in a continuous rapid cycle that should go well beyond the environment of the cardiac catheterization laboratory.

REFERENCES

1. O'Connor GT, Plume SK, Olmstead EM, et al. A regional prospective study of in-hospital mortality associated with coronary artery bypass grafting. The Northern New England Cardiovascular Disease Study Group. *JAMA.* 1991;266:803-9.
2. Williams SV, Nash DB, Goldfarb N. Differences in mortality from coronary artery bypass graft surgery at five teaching hospitals. *JAMA.* 1991;266:810–815.
3. Hannan EL, Kumar D, Racz M, Siu AL, Chassin MR. New York State's Cardiac Surgery Reporting System: four years later. *Ann Thorac Surg.* 1994;58:1852–1857.
4. Hannan EL, Kilburn H, Jr., Lindsey ML, Lewis R. Clinical versus administrative data bases for CABG surgery. Does it matter? *Med Care.* 1992;30:892–907.
5. Hibbard JH, Stockard J, Tusler M. Does publicizing hospital performance stimulate quality improvement efforts? *Health Aff (Millwood).* 2003;22:84–94.
6. Lee TH, Meyer GS, Brennan TA. A middle ground on public accountability. *N Engl J Med.* 2004;350:2409–2412.
7. Seshadri N, Whitlow PL, Acharya N, Houghtaling P, Blackstone EH, Ellis SG. Emergency coronary artery bypass surgery in the contemporary percutaneous coronary intervention era. *Circulation.* 2002;106:2346–2350.
8. Moscucci M, O'Donnell M, Share D, et al. Frequency and prognosis of emergency coronary artery bypass grafting after percutaneous coronary intervention for acute myocardial infarction. *Am J Cardiol.* 2003;92:967–969.
9. Luft HS, Bunker JP, Enthoven AC. Should operations be regionalized? The empirical relation between surgical volume and mortality. *N Engl J Med.* 1979;301:1364–1369.
10. Hannan EL, Wu C, Ryan TJ, et al. Do hospitals and surgeons with higher coronary artery bypass graft surgery volumes still have lower risk-adjusted mortality rates? *Circulation.* 2003;108:795–801.
11. Birkmeyer JD, Stukel TA, Siewers AE, Goodney PP, Wennberg DE, Lucas FL. Surgeon Volume and Operative Mortality in the United States. *N Engl J Med.* 2003;349:2117–2127.
12. Birkmeyer JD, Siewers AE, Finlayson EV, et al. Hospital volume and surgical mortality in the United States. *N Engl J Med.* 2002;346:1128–1137.
13. Hannan EL, Racz MJ, Jollis JG, Peterson ED. Using Medicare claims data to assess provider quality for CABG surgery: does it work well enough? *Health Serv Res.* 1997;31:659–678.
14. Ellis SG, Weintraub W, Holmes D, Shaw R, Block PC, King SB, 3rd. Relation of operator volume and experience to procedural outcome of percutaneous coronary revascularization at hospitals with high interventional volumes. *Circulation.* 1997;95:2479–2484.
15. Hannan EL, Racz M, Ryan TJ, et al. Coronary angioplasty volume-outcome relationships for hospitals and cardiologists. *JAMA.* 1997;277:892–898.
16. Jollis JG, Peterson ED, DeLong ER, et al. The relation between the volume of coronary angioplasty procedures at hospitals treating Medicare beneficiaries and short-term mortality. *N Engl J Med.* 1994;331:1625–1629.
17. Jollis JG, Peterson ED, Nelson CL, et al. Relationship between physician and hospital coronary angioplasty volume and outcome in elderly patients. *Circulation.* 1997;95:2485–2491.
18. McGrath PD, Wennberg DE, Dickens JD, Jr., et al. Relation between operator and hospital volume and outcomes following percutaneous coronary interventions in the era of the coronary stent. *JAMA.* 2000;284:3139–3144.
18a. Hannan EL, Wu C, Walford G, et al. Volume—outcome relationships for percutaneous coronary interventions in the stent era. *Circulation.* 2005;112:1171–1179.
18b. Moscucci M, Share D, Smith D, et al. Relationship between operator volume and adverse outcome in contemporary percutaneous coronary intervention practice: an analysis of a quality-controlled multicenter percutaneous coronary intervention clinical database. *J Am Coll Cardiol.* 2005;46:625–632.
19. Klein LW, Schaer GL, Calvin JE, et al. Does low individual operator coronary interventional procedural volume correlate with worse institutional procedural outcome? *J Am Coll Cardiol.* 1997;30:870–877.
20. Malenka DJ, McGrath PD, Wennberg DE, et al. The relationship between operator volume and outcomes after percutaneous coronary interventions in

high volume hospitals in 1994–1996: the northern New England experience. Northern New England Cardiovascular Disease Study Group. *J Am Coll Cardiol.* 1999;34:1471–1480.

21. Holmes DR, Selzer F, Johnston JM, et al. Modeling and risk prediction in the current era of interventional cardiology: a report from the National Heart, Lung, and Blood Institute Dynamic Registry. *Circulation.* 2003;107:1871–1876.

22. O'Connor GT, Malenka DJ, Quinton H, et al. Multivariate prediction of in-hospital mortality after percutaneous coronary interventions in 1994-1996. Northern New England Cardiovascular Disease Study Group. *J Am Coll Cardiol.* 1999;34:681–691.

23. Moscucci M, O'Connor GT, Ellis SG, et al. Validation of risk adjustment models for in-hospital percutaneous transluminal coronary angioplasty mortality on an independent data set. *J Am Coll Cardiol.* 1999;34:692–697.

24. Moscucci M, Kline-Rogers E, Share D, et al. Simple bedside additive tool for prediction of in-hospital mortality after percutaneous coronary interventions. *Circulation.* 2001;104:263–268.

25. Hannan EL, Arani DT, Johnson LW, Kemp HG, Jr., Lukacik G. Percutaneous transluminal coronary angioplasty in New York State. Risk factors and outcomes. *JAMA.* 1992;268:3092–3097.

26. Holmes DR, Jr., Berger PB, Garratt KN. Application of the New York State PTCA mortality model in patients undergoing stent implantation. *Circulation.* 2000;102:517–522.

27. Randomized trial of ridogrel, a combined thromboxane A2 synthase inhibitor and thromboxane A2/prostaglandin endoperoxide receptor antagonist, versus aspirin as adjunct to thrombolysis in patients with acute myocardial infarction. The Ridogrel versus Aspirin Patency Trial (RAPT). *Circulation.* 1994;89: 588–595.

28. Blankenship JC, Balog C, Sapp SK, et al. Reduction in vascular access site bleeding in sequential abciximab coronary intervention trials. *Cath Cardiovasc Interv.* 2002;57:476–483.

29. Blankenship JC, Hellkamp AS, Aguirre FV, Demko SL, Topol EJ, Califf RM. Vascular access site complications after percutaneous coronary intervention with abciximab in the Evaluation of c7E3 for the Prevention of Ischemic Complications (EPIC) trial. *Am J Cardiol.* 1998;81:36–40.

30. Piper WD, Malenka DJ, Ryan TJ, Jr., et al. Predicting vascular complications in percutaneous coronary interventions. *Am Heart J.* 2003;145:1022–1029.

31. Moscucci M, Mansour KA, Kent KC, et al. Peripheral vascular complications of directional coronary atherectomy and stenting: predictors, management, and outcome. *Am J Cardiol.* 1994;74:448–453.

32. Popma JJ, Satler LF, Pichard AD, et al. Vascular complications after balloon and new device angioplasty. *Circulation.* 1993;88:1569–1578.

33. Freeman RV, O'Donnell M, Share D, et al. Nephropathy requiring dialysis after percutaneous coronary intervention and the critical role of an adjusted contrast dose. *Am J Cardiol.* 2002;90:1068–1073.

34. Mehran R, Aymong ED, Nikolsky E, et al. A simple risk score for prediction of contrast-induced nephropathy after percutaneous coronary intervention: development and initial validation. *J Am Coll Cardiol.* 2004;44:1393–1399.

35. McCullough PA, Sandberg KR. Epidemiology of contrast-induced nephropathy. *Rev Cardiovasc Med.* 2003;4 Suppl 5:S3–S9.

36. Rihal CS, Textor SC, Grill DE, et al. Incidence and prognostic importance of acute renal failure after percutaneous coronary intervention. *Circulation.* 2002;105:2259–2264.

37. Fuchs S, Stabile E, Kinnaird TD, et al. Stroke complicating percutaneous coronary interventions: incidence, predictors, and prognostic implications. *Circulation.* 2002;106:86–91.

38. Brown DL, Topol EJ. Stroke complicating percutaneous coronary revascularization. *Am J Cardiol.* 1993;72:1207–1209.

39. Cubo E, Estefania CM, Monaco M, et al. Risk factors of stroke after percutaneous transluminal coronary angioplasty. *Eur J Neurol.* 1998;5:459–462.

40. Bittl JA, Caplan LR. Stroke after percutaneous coronary interventions. *J Am Coll Cardiol.* 2004;43:1168–1169.

41. Singh M, Lennon RJ, Holmes DR, Jr., Bell MR, Rihal CS. Correlates of procedural complications and a simple integer risk score for percutaneous coronary intervention. *J Am Coll Cardiol.* 2002;40:387–393.

42. Bashore TM, Bates ER, Berger PB, et al. American College of Cardiology/Society for Cardiac Angiography and Interventions Clinical Expert Consensus Document on cardiac catheterization laboratory standards. A report of the American College of Cardiology Task Force on Clinical Expert Consensus Documents. *J Am Coll Cardiol.* 2001;37:2170–2214.

43. Smith SC, Jr., Dove JT, Jacobs AK, et al. ACC/AHA guidelines of percutaneous coronary interventions (revision of the 1993 PTCA guidelines)–executive summary. A report of the American College of Cardiology/American Heart Association Task Force on Practice Guidelines (committee to revise the

1993 guidelines for percutaneous transluminal coronary angioplasty). *J Am Coll Cardiol.* 2001;37:2215–2239.

44. Hirshfeld JW, Jr., Ellis SG, Faxon DP. Recommendations for the assessment and maintenance of proficiency in coronary interventional procedures: Statement of the American College of Cardiology. *J Am Coll Cardiol.* 1998;31:722–743.

45. Hirshfeld JW, Jr., Balter S, Brinker JA, et al. ACCF/AHA/HRS/SCAI clinical competence statement on physician knowledge to optimize patient safety and image quality in fluoroscopically guided invasive cardiovascular procedures. A report of the American College of Cardiology Foundation/American Heart Association/American College of Physicians Task Force on Clinical Competence and Training. *J Am Coll Cardiol.* 2004;44:2259–2282.

46. Balter S. An overview of radiation safety regulatory recommendations and requirements. *Cath Cardiovasc Interv.* 1999;47:469–474.

47. Balter S. Radiation safety in the cardiac catheterization laboratory: operational radiation safety. *Cath Cardiovasc Interv.* 1999;47:347–353.

48. Balter S. Radiation safety in the cardiac catheterization laboratory: basic principles. *Cath Cardiovasc Interv.* 1999;47:229–236.

49. Sinclair WK. Radiation protection recommendations on dose limits: the role of the NCRP and the ICRP and future developments. *Int J Radiat Oncol Biol Phys.* 1995;31:387–392.

50. Laskey WK, Stueve R, Wondrow M, Grill D, Holmes D. Image quality assessment in contemporary interventional cardiology laboratories: spatial and low-contrast video resolution. *Cath Cardiovasc Interv.* 2000;50:257–263.

51. Laskey WK, Holmes DR, Kern MJ. Image quality assessment: a timely look. *Cath Cardiovasc Interv.* 1999;46:125–126.

52. Wondrow MA, Laskey WK, Hildner FJ, Cusma J, Holmes DR, Jr. Cardiac catheterization laboratory imaging quality assurance program. *Cath Cardiovasc Interv.* 2001;52:59–66.

53. Eagle KA, Moscucci M, Kline-Rogers E, et al. Evaluating and improving the delivery of heart care: the University of Michigan experience. *Am J Manag Care.* 1998;4:1300–1309.

54. Moscucci M, Muller DW, Watts CM, et al. Reducing costs and improving outcomes of percutaneous coronary interventions. *Am J Manag Care.* 2003;9: 365–372.

55. Plante S, Strauss BH, Goulet G, Watson RK, Chisholm RJ. Reuse of balloon catheters for coronary angioplasty: a potential cost-saving strategy? *J Am Coll Cardiol.* 1994;24:1475–1481.

56. Rozenman Y, Gotsman MS. Reuse of balloon catheters for coronary angioplasty. *J Am Coll Cardiol.* 1995;26:840–841.

57. Rozenman Y, Gotsman MS, Penchas S. Single-stage coronary angiography and angioplasty: a new standard. *Am J Cardiol.* 1995;76:1321.

58. O'Keefe JH, Jr., Gernon C, McCallister BD, Ligon RW, Hartzler GO. Safety and cost effectiveness of combined coronary angiography and angioplasty. *Am Heart J.* 1991;122:50–54.

59. Friedman HZ, Cragg DR, Glazier SM, et al. Randomized prospective evaluation of prolonged versus abbreviated intravenous heparin therapy after coronary angioplasty. *J Am Coll Cardiol.* 1994;24:1214–1219.

60. Rabah M, Mason D, Muller DW, et al. Heparin after percutaneous intervention (HAPI): a prospective multicenter randomized trial of three heparin regimens after successful coronary intervention. *J Am Coll Cardiol.* 1999;34: 461–467.

61. Eagle KA, Knight BP, Moscucci M, et al. Competitive bidding for interventional cardiology supplies: lessons learned during round 2. *Am J Manag Care.* 2002;8:384–388.

62. Moscucci M, Share D, Kline-Rogers E, et al. The Blue Cross Blue Shield of Michigan Cardiovascular Consortium (BMC2) collaborative quality improvement initiative in percutaneous coronary interventions. *J Interv Cardiol.* 2002;15:381–386.

63. Kline-Rogers E, Share D, Bondie D, et al. Development of a multicenter interventional cardiology database: the Blue Cross Blue Shield of Michigan Cardiovascular Consortium (BMC2) experience. *J Interv Cardiol.* 2002;15:387–392.

64. Cutlip DE, Baim DS, Ho KK, et al. Stent thrombosis in the modern era: a pooled analysis of multicenter coronary stent clinical trials. *Circulation.* 2001;103:1967–1971.

65. Guidelines for percutaneous transluminal coronary angioplasty. A report of the American College of Cardiology/American Heart Association Task Force on Assessment of Diagnostic and Therapeutic Cardiovascular Procedures (Committee on Percutaneous Transluminal Coronary Angioplasty). *J Am Coll Cardiol.* 1993;22:2033–2054.

65a. Smith SC Jr, Feldman TE, Hirshfeld JW Jr, Jacobs AK, Kern MJ, King SB III, Morrison DA, O'Neill WW, Schaff HV, Whitlow PL, Williams DO. ACC/AHA/SCAI 2005 guideline update for percutaneous coronary intervention:

a report of the American College of Cardiology/American Heart Association Task Force on Practice Guidelines (ACC/AHA/SCAI Writing Committee to Update the 2001 Guidelines for Percutaneous Coronary Intervention). © 2005 by the American College of Cardiology Foundation and the American Heart Association, Inc. Available at: http://www.acc.org/clinical/guidelines/percutaneous/update/index.pdf.

66. Smith SC, Jr., Dove JT, Jacobs AK, et al. ACC/AHA Guidelines for Percutaneous Coronary Intervention (Revision of the 1993 PTCA Guidelines). A report of the American College of Cardiology/American Heart Association Task Force on Practice Guidelines (committee to revise the 1993 guidelines for percutaneous transluminal coronary angioplasty). *J Am Coll Cardiol.* 2001;37:2239i–224lxvi.

67. Serruys PW, De Feyter PJ, Benghozi R, Hugenholtz PG, Lesaffre E. The Lescol(R) Intervention Prevention Study (LIPS): a double-blind, placebo-controlled, randomized trial of the long-term effects of fluvastatin after successful transcatheter therapy in patients with coronary heart disease. *Int J Cardiovasc Intervent.* 2001;4:165–172.

68. Mukherjee D, Fang J, Chetcuti S, Moscucci M, Kline-Rogers E, Eagle KA. Impact of combination evidence-based medical therapy on mortality in patients with acute coronary syndromes. *Circulation.* 2004;109:745–749.

69. Aronow HD, Topol EJ, Roe MT, et al. Effect of lipid-lowering therapy on early mortality after acute coronary syndromes: an observational study. *Lancet.* 2001;357:1063–1068.

70. Chan AW, Bhatt DL, Chew DP, et al. Early and sustained survival benefit associated with statin therapy at the time of percutaneous coronary intervention. *Circulation.* 2002;105:691–696.

71. Fonarow GC, Gawlinski A, Moughrabi S, Tillisch JH. Improved treatment of coronary heart disease by implementation of a Cardiac Hospitalization Atherosclerosis Management Program (CHAMP). *Am J Cardiol.* 2001;87: 819–822.

72. Aronow HD, Novaro GM, Lauer MS, et al. In-hospital initiation of lipid-lowering therapy after coronary intervention as a predictor of long-term utilization: a propensity analysis. *Arch Intern Med.* 2003;163:2576–2582.

73. Brindis RG, Fitzgerald S, Anderson HV, Shaw RE, Weintraub WS, Williams JF. The American College of Cardiology-National Cardiovascular Data Registry (ACC-NCDR): building a national clinical data repository. *J Am Coll Cardiol.* 2001;37:2240–2245.

74. Shaw RE, Anderson HV, Brindis RG, et al. Development of a risk adjustment mortality model using the American College of Cardiology–National Cardiovascular Data Registry (ACC-NCDR) experience: 1998–2000. *J Am Coll Cardiol.* 2002;39:1104–1112.

75. Shaw RE, Anderson HV, Brindis RG, et al. Updated risk adjustment mortality model using the complete 1.1 dataset from the American College of Cardiology National Cardiovascular Data Registry (ACC-NCDR). *J Invasive Cardiol.* 2003;15:578–580.

76. Malenka DJ. Indications, practice, and procedural outcomes of percutaneous transluminal coronary angioplasty in northern New England in the early 1990s. The Northern New England Cardiovascular Disease Study Group. *Am J Cardiol.* 1996;78:260–265.

77. McCullough PA, Manley HJ. Prediction and prevention of contrast nephropathy. *J Interv Cardiol.* 2001;14:547–558.

78. Cigarroa RG, Lange RA, Williams RH, Hillis LD. Dosing of contrast material to prevent contrast nephropathy in patients with renal disease. *Am J Med.* 1989;86:649–652.

79. Goldenberg I, Shechter M, Matetzky S, et al. Oral acetylcysteine as an adjunct to saline hydration for the prevention of contrast-induced nephropathy following coronary angiography. A randomized controlled trial and review of the current literature. *Eur Heart J.* 2004;25:212–218.

80. Mueller C, Buerkle G, Buettner HJ, et al. Prevention of contrast media-associated nephropathy: randomized comparison of 2 hydration regimens in 1620 patients undergoing coronary angioplasty. *Arch Intern Med.* 2002;162: 329–336.

81. Moscucci M, Rogers EK, Montoye C, et al. Association of a continuous quality improvement initiative with practice and outcome variations of contemporary percutaneous coronary interventions. *Circulation* 2006;113: 814–822.

PART 10   Principles of Innovation

CHAPTER 70

Innovation and Interventional Cardiology: Looking Back, Thinking Ahead

William R. Overall, PhD

Paul G. Yock, MD

Interventional cardiology has been shaped by innovative physicians. Pioneers such as Andreas Gruentzig, Tom Fogarty, John Simpson, and Julio Palmaz conceived of and developed technologies that have revolutionized cardiovascular care. Technology continues to evolve faster in cardiology than in any other specialty, stimulated by a culture of innovation among cardiologists and sustained by the large size of the cardiovascular health market and the highly developed industry in this sector. As one measure of the rate of technology innovation in our field, cardiovascular devices account for more than half of all devices receiving premarket approval from the FDA (Figure 70-1).[1] In this and the next chapter, we explore the landscape of innovation in our field, first by examining the common characteristics of successful innovators and then by providing some of the essential tools required for developing and assessing new cardiovascular technologies.

BACKGROUND OF INNOVATION

【 】 THE PIONEERS

The culture of innovation in interventional cardiology owes much to Andreas Gruentzig himself—the dynamic, free-spirited physician who launched the field of interventional cardiology with his invention of coronary balloon angioplasty in 1975. Gruentzig provided a role model for much of what was to occur at the interface of innovation, entrepreneurship, and practice in interventional cardiology. He was a principal figure in the company that produced his

balloon catheter; for a while, he personally approved which physicians could purchase the devices. Gruentzig was also known for his charismatic and enthusiastic style as a clinician and teacher. He pioneered the live-demonstration course, which has become the defining educational and cultural event in the field and serves as a showcase for new technologies.

Many of the other early practitioners of angioplasty were also inventive and entrepreneurial. As a young field, interventional cardiology was particularly well suited to mechanical innovations that could be conceptualized by inventive clinicians. The pioneers seized this opportunity, designing and helping test catheters that carried their names. These individuals also helped found and grow start-up companies that competed to develop the best new technologies. The industry expanded rapidly, and the unusually close interaction between physicians and companies was reinforced by clinical and financial success on all sides. Young interventionalists learned from their mentors how to interface with companies, providing the basis for a next generation of innovators. A growing number of interventionalists became involved in device testing in preclinical and clinical trials.

These individuals and the culture they created have brought interventional cardiology to a unique position at the epicenter of technical innovation and entrepreneurship in modern medicine. With the tragic exception of Gruentzig, who died in a plane crash in 1984, the pioneers of our field remain actively engaged in the invention and development of new technologies. They have also helped mentor a new generation of innovators and entrepreneurs who are actively identifying unmet clinical needs, testing and refining their concepts, and bringing new technologies forward into clinical practice.

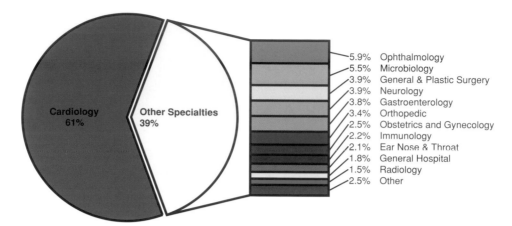

FIGURE 70-1. Breakdown of FDA premarket approvals for medical devices according to specialty from 1/1/2005 through 7/5/2005. *(Reproduced from the US Food and Drug Administration. PMA Database Search. Available at:* http://www.accessdata.fda.gov/scripts/cdrh/cfdocs/cfPMA/pma.cfm. *Accessed July 5, 2003.)*

【 】 COMMON QUALITIES OF SUCCESSFUL INNOVATORS

Careful examination of the lives and careers of these early innovators reveals a number of shared characteristics and character traits that contributed to their success. In many cases, these qualities contradict commonly held ideas about the characteristics required in the typical innovator. In this section, we outline some of the key factors that lead to important innovations–and in the process, highlight some potential misconceptions and myths about the development of new technologies.

Focus on the Patient

Myth: Medical technology innovators are born tinkerers; success requires an engineering background.

Fact: Successful medical innovators identify important clinical problems and seek to solve them; success requires focus on the patient.

The familiar image of a great inventor is someone with extraordinary technical expertise—the type of person who spent his or her childhood taking apart clocks and calculators to see how they work. Indeed, many of the world's inventors are innate tinkerers. In order to apply their analytic minds to the solution of everyday problems, these individuals often choose engineering or another technical profession. However, the inventor of medical devices and medical products may be cut from a different mold. The critical characteristic of the medical innovator is a keen understanding of the shortcomings of current medical practice.

John Simpson is a good example (see inset). Simpson is responsible for the original over-the-wire angioplasty system, directional atherectomy, and several other key innovations, but he would characterize himself as an inherently nontechnical person. He spent much of his childhood on a farm and never developed an interest in taking things apart or any of the other childhood activities normally associated with inventors. During his education, Simpson pursued a PhD in immunology as well as his medical training, but stayed away from engineering and technological fields. Other

physician–innovators, including Thomas Fogarty (see inset) and Julio Palmaz (see inset), come closer to the tinkerer mold, but they also acknowledge that it is the identification of important clinical needs that makes a great inventor of medical technologies. As Simpson himself says succinctly, "You fix the patient and you win."[2]

Another common misconception about physician–innovators is that in order to be successful, they must also be shrewd businessmen. Julio Palmaz cites his own experience as a counterexample: he was unable to convince his university that his invention of the stent was worth patenting and he was not successful in attracting financial backing until he partnered with Richard Schatz.

In fact, the critical aspect of medical technology innovations is that they solve a true problem in clinical practice. Clearly, other concerns must be addressed before a product can ultimately be successful, but the clinical need forms the foundation on which a successful business opportunity lies. The fundamental intellectual discipline is needs finding (see Chapter 71).

Relationships

Myth: Successful physician–innovators are lone geniuses who single-handedly bring a concept to life.

Fact: Successful physician–innovators know their own limitations and build a team of talented individuals to surround them.

As with any other professional undertaking, relationships are essential to the success of the physician–innovator. For the young innovator, the most important early relationship is with a mentor. Successful medical inventors can all point to a number of mentors whose support and enthusiasm was instrumental to their success. Andreas Gruentzig was training at the Ratchow Clinic in Darnstadt, Germany, when he first heard a talk on an early method of peripheral recanalization. Gruentzig was extremely interested in this subject, but his chief at the time was upset by the very concept, and vowed that such treatments would not take place in his hospital. As a result, Gruentzig moved on to University Hospital in Zurich, where he was able to find several mentors who were much more supportive. Among these were the chief of medicine,

Tom Fogarty, MD

While an OR scrub technician in the late 1950s, a young Tom Fogarty removed the finger from a surgical glove and tied it to the end of a ureteral catheter. With this crude bit of engineering, Fogarty invented the first balloon catheter for the vascular system. The resulting device, the Fogarty embolectomy catheter (Figure 70–2), eventually became the standard of care for surgical embolectomy. Since then, Dr. Fogarty has received more than 70 patents for a range of surgical and interventional products, including balloons used for laparoscopic hernia repair, a device for minimally invasive breast cancer diagnosis and therapy, and a self-expanding stent graft for percutaneous abdominal aortic aneurysm repair. In his distinguished career, Dr. Fogarty has founded or cofounded more than 30 medical–technology companies, and serves as a scientific advisor to numerous others.

Notable inventions:

- Embolectomy catheter
- Atraumatic clamps
- Minimally invasive device for breast cancer diagnosis
- Self-expanding AAA stent graft

Dr. Fogarty is also the Founder/Director of

- General Surgical Innovations, Inc.
- AneuRx
- CTS
- Biopsys
- Bentley Labs
- Hancock Labs
- Three Arch Partners
- Fogarty Engineering
- Thomas Fogarty Winery and Vineyards

Quotes by Dr. Fogarty[4]:

. . . on the patient:	If you start off with an overwhelming desire to start a company to make money, you'll probably not be in the business of medical devices because . . . you've got to really know what works for the patient.
. . . on relationships:	If you think just because you had the idea you brought all the value, you're not going to get there because . . . one individual can't do it.
. . . on the landscape:	I think it's become extremely difficult by comparison; . . . there are just a lot more things that you have to deal with now, versus what you could do then.

Dr. Walter Siegenthaler, and the head of cardiology, Dr. Wilhelm Rutishauser. Dr. Rutishauser assisted Gruentzig in his critical move from the department of radiology into cardiology, which was a political and practical necessity for him to initiate his research program in angioplasty.[3] There is, of course, no formal educational process that teaches the skills of innovation. Mentors fill this gap. In the words of Tom Fogarty, "Being in the environment promotes [innovation]; it's more of a mentoring issue than it is reading a book on how to innovate."[4]

As a project begins to take shape, a different relationship—partnering with experts in other areas—becomes a critical component of success. Even the most iconic medical innovators are quick to acknowledge scores of colleagues who brought key abilities to their fledgling companies. Success comes from identifying and acknowledging areas of personal limitation and enlisting the aid of those who can be most helpful. There is a broad range of skills and experience required. According to Fogarty, "If you think just because you had the idea you brought all the value, you're not going to get there because . . . one individual can't do it."[4] For a medical tech-

nology venture, success requires people with expertise in engineering, medicine, regulatory affairs, reimbursement, fundraising, finance, managing, marketing, sales, as well as other areas.

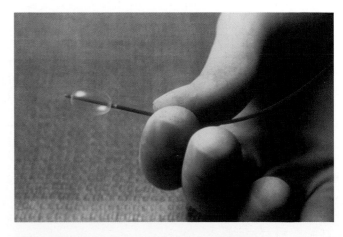

FIGURE 70-2. The Fogarty embolectomy catheter.

John Simpson, MD, PhD

John Simpson began his career as a physician innovator by inventing the over-the-wire angioplasty catheter, a device that formed the basis for Advanced Cardiovascular Systems (ACS, now Guidant). Later, Dr. Simpson invented the Simpson AtheroCath, the first catheter for directional atherectomy (see Figure 70–3). Since then, Dr. Simpson has helped found numerous other companies in interventional cardiology, including Perclose, LuMend Inc., and Fox Hollow Technologies. Dr. Simpson is also a founding partner at De Novo Ventures, a medical–technology venture capital fund in Menlo Park, California.

Notable inventions:

- Over-the-wire angioplasty catheter
- Suture-based interventional closure device
- Simpson AtheroCath
- Directional atherectomy

Dr. Simpson is also the Founder/Director of

- Advanced Cardiovascular Systems (ACS)
- Devices for Vascular Intervention (DVI)
- Perclose
- LuMend
- Fox Hollow Technologies
- De Novo Ventures

Quotes by Dr. Simpson[3];

. . . on relationships:	I'm sure there are some special visionaries and I might even put Fogarty and Julio Palmaz in that domain, but for me, I'm not that smart and it's got to be a team effort.
. . . on perseverance:	If you've got people that bring some commitment and some special willingness to persevere in adversity, then you can make really special things happen, if you stay focused on doing something really clinically relevant.
. . . on the future:	I remain committed to the concept that material that's in the coronary artery, it doesn't belong there.

Julio Palmaz, MD

After attending a lecture by Andreas Gruentzig on the advantages and limitations of balloon angioplasty in 1978, Julio Palmaz invented the idea of the balloon-expandable stent (see Figure 70–4). Although his path was not easy, Dr. Palmaz eventually convinced Johnson & Johnson to acquire his technology, which formed the basis for the Johnson & Johnson Interventional Systems division. Dr. Palmaz was also a key inventor of the endovascular stent graft for treatment of abdominal aortic aneurysms. More recently, Dr. Palmaz has worked to improve the materials used for stenting and has been an active proponent of implantable nanodevices for in vivo diagnostics.

Notable inventions:

- Balloon-expandable vascular stent
- Endovascular AAA stent graft

Quotes by Dr. Palmaz[6]:

. . . on independent thinking:	[In the early eighties, physicians] thought that metals did not have a future as a vascular implant. There were so many other techniques that were being evaluated at the time that stents had to wait their turn.
. . . on the landscape:	The Europeans are not embracing drug-eluting stents widely, based on cost considerations, and in the States, I think it'll be less of an impact.
. . . on the future:	My opinion is that drug-eluting stents may be actually useful in certain patient subsets in the future, but not for widespread application.

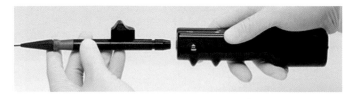

FIGURE 70-3. The Fox Hollow Technologies atherectomy device.

The story of Gruentzig's development of the first coronary balloon provides a good example of the need to partner for key expertise. During the early development of angioplasty balloons, Gruentzig experimented with a number of materials, all of which proved to be too compliant to be effective in dilating arterial stenoses. The breakthrough came when he approached a professor emeritus of chemistry, Dr. Andreas Hopf, who introduced Gruentzig to polyvinylchloride.

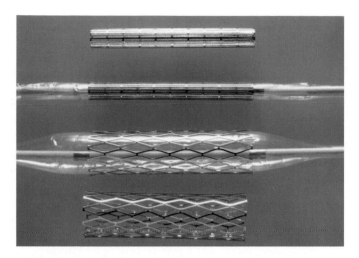

FIGURE 70-4. An early Palmaz-Schatz stent before and after balloon deployment.

Using this material, Gruentzig was able to make the thin-walled non-compliant balloons necessary for angioplasty.

As innovator–entrepreneurs progress in their careers, they typically develop significant networks of individuals with diverse areas of expertise. These networks can be enormously helpful to the aspiring inventor in the process of building a good team.

Independent thinking

Myth: Successful physician–innovators pursue a concept only after receiving consensus approval from colleagues in their field.

Fact: Successful physician–innovators often encounter significant disbelief and discouragement from their colleagues and the medical establishment.

The typical physician is not especially adept at identifying which promising medical technologies will ultimately be successful. This phenomenon is not unique to medicine—many design and consulting firms exist on the principle that innovation is best done using the unique perspective of an outsider. Experience teaches people to view their profession only as it exists today without questioning its foundations in any meaningful way. Telegraph operators, for example, notoriously failed to appreciate the changes in behavior that would result from voice transmissions.

Physicians are particularly susceptible to this professional conservatism because the format of medical school tends to discourage the inquisitiveness required of an innovator. Fogarty says, "You do no harm by doing what you've always done before, and . . . in the field of medicine, I think the way we're taught certainly deters innovation."[4] Much of medical training is devoted to learning the current standard of care in terms of symptoms and treatment guidelines. Because of the volume of information to be learned, little time remains to question the status quo.

The medical culture also affects the would-be innovator in the early stages of testing and promoting an idea. Most successful innovators have numerous stories of the initial disbelief and discouragement that they faced from their peers. Thomas Fogarty invented his thrombectomy balloon during a time when it was widely believed that any manipulation of the intima would result in additional thrombosis. Fogarty's balloon, designed to rub across the intima in order to remove clot, was therefore considered to be unsafe. Even after collecting clinical data to support his claims, Fogarty was unable to even publish his work; three journals rejected his manuscript for publication because his results defied conventional wisdom. Eventually, the volume of data that Fogarty and others generated in support of the thrombectomy balloon forced a change in thinking, and the technique became accepted.

The physician–innovator must avoid professional conservatism in order to be successful. Innovation occurs when an individual champions a new technique, despite initial unpopularity, until sufficient data exists to convince the medical community of its merit. For this reason, the typical inventor needs independent-thinking skills sufficient to identify promising new technologies and the perseverance to pursue them despite an initial lack of acceptance.

Perseverance

Myth: The best innovators succeed because they do not allow failures to occur.

Fact: Successful innovators accept that setbacks occur, and are driven to persevere because of a strong belief in their concept.

Disbelief from the medical community is only the beginning of the hardships that the typical medical technology venture may face. Fundraising, design development, clinical trials, and business development each may result in setbacks. The successful entrepreneur accepts this uncertainty and is driven to persevere, motivated by the clinical need and a belief in a particular solution.

Julio Palmaz's experience with the coronary stent provides an excellent example of this quality of the innovator. At the time of his invention, implantation of metallic structures into arteries was so novel that most physicians were unable to imagine its success. They understood the potential structural benefits of a stent, but they believed that any foreign structure placed within the artery would thrombose. When early human trials showed a high risk of thrombosis,[5] many physicians believed that their fears had been affirmed. Undeterred, Palmaz revised the implantation technique to include anticoagulation, and other investigators (notably Antonio Colombo) modified the implantation technique so that thrombosis became a manageable issue.

Due in part to these clinical issues, Palmaz also encountered difficulties in obtaining funding. In Palmaz's words, "There were so many other techniques that were being evaluated at the time that stents had to wait their turn."[6] Alternatives to angioplasty from atherectomy to brachytherapy had the attention of funding agencies, leaving Palmaz unable to obtain grant support or private funding.

In the course of pursuing an innovation, setbacks naturally occur. One approach for managing this is, simply, persistence. When Palmaz and his associates approached established vascular device companies with his initial stent results, the response was uniformly negative. None of these companies were willing to shoulder the significant risk that remained in getting the stent to market. After months of trying, the stent team finally found a backer in Johnson & Johnson, which was just trying to enter the catheterization market at the time. The support of this company was sufficient to bring the product to market, and all of the rejections leading up to that point became an interesting footnote.

Every major development program experiences one or more significant changes in direction, some of which can be drastic.

Entrepreneurs should avoid becoming so enamored of their invention in its original form that they are unable to adapt to new developments.

PREPARING FOR A FUTURE IN INNOVATION

With these qualities of successful physician–innovators in mind, how can a physician entering the specialty of interventional cardiology prepare to become a part of the culture of innovation? To answer this question, we interviewed a number of interventional cardiologists who have made names for themselves in various areas of innovation. Their insights and recommendations were often unique to their own experience, but even so, a number of suggestions emerged consistently from one physician to the next. Often, these insights reinforce the importance of the character traits mentioned previously. In this section, we explore their insights and provide concrete advice for those wishing to join this innovative culture. (See Table 70-1.)

【　】 TRAINING FOR INNOVATION

As discussed in the previous section, the most important characteristic of the successful physician innovator is a strong focus on the needs of the patient. Our interviewees echoed this sentiment, recommending that would-be physician–innovators take an active interest in their patients. In the words of Jay Yadav (September 12, 2003), "If you just try to stay in an ivory tower and are not hands-on, chances are you're not going to find the right problems and what are acceptable solutions. There are a lot of solutions that sound great on paper, but are not really implementable in a clinical setting."

In order to be innovative, an individual must often synthesize knowledge over more than one discipline in order to solve a clinical problem in a new way. Early innovations in interventional cardiology were technologically straightforward, so physicians with little additional training were able to make those leaps single-handedly. As the field matures, the physicians we interviewed envision that the technical and scientific knowledge required for successful innovations will steadily increase. Several interviewees felt particularly strongly that basic science will play a significant role in future innovations, and should be emphasized in training whenever possible:

> I think over time we're going to see some problems with the current approach. I would encourage future inventors to understand the biology as much as they can and certainly sit down with people with expertise in, say, inflammation, if that was an important area. I don't think that people like ourselves are ever going to become experts in inflammation, but at least [we can understand] the implications for other biological processes.
>
> Nick Chronos
> September 11, 2003

> Training at physiology and at all of the basic sciences should be in-depth. . . . There should be a sound interest and desire to know what is the basis of things, why is some part of the body made, what is the task of every part of the body, why is a particular process in physiology going on. By sound physiologic thinking, . . . the need for new inventions will be created.
>
> Nico Pijls
> October 20, 2003

Although a solid foundation in basic science was perceived as critical to the future of innovation in the field, the interviewees were less eager to recommend conventional engineering training for physicians. There was a perception that the physician's time is better spent outside an engineering classroom:

> The technologies in the next decade are going to change and they're going to be complicated. I'm not sure that picking up an engineering course is going to be enough. . . . I would probably suggest that they start reading things like *New Scientist* or *In Vivo*, because it gives you a much better idea of what's out there in the way of technology that can be applied.
>
> Steve Oesterle
> September 22, 2003

> It's not so much if you're an engineer or not; you can always hire engineers. Really the key thing is to look at the thing that everybody else is looking at, but do it with a questioning mind.
>
> Jay Yadav
> September 12, 2003

In additional to scientific skills, several of the successful entrepreneurs recommended business training for the aspiring physician–innovator. None recommended a formal business degree, instead believing that the necessary skills could be learned through a short course or on the job:

> I think most interventional cardiologists can learn business if they have an interest and an aptitude for it. I think that's much more learnable, in some ways, than some of the engineering and physics parts of it.
>
> Tim Fischell
> October 14, 2003

> It's a useful background, particularly as people try to start businesses, to understand what it really costs, what is the opportunity cost, utility cost, and I don't think you need to go two years to do that. Some fundamental accounting background and understanding accounting rules would be pretty helpful; you could do that in a 2- to 3-week course, frankly.
>
> Steve Oesterle
> September 22, 2003

Thus, innovative physicians should focus on being physicians first, emphasizing good patient care and thorough knowledge of the underlying science. If possible, reading medical-device journals and acquiring basic business knowledge could also be valuable.

【　】 THE CHANGING LANDSCAPE

The experts also commented on changes that they perceive are occurring in the field of medical-technology entrepreneurship. In order to navigate the ever-more complicated landscape of innovation, the panel echoed the importance of a team approach. Early formation of a strong team provides the entrepreneurial effort with proficiency across a range of disciplines.

Broadly, there is a perception that true innovation is becoming more difficult because of changes in the nature of technologies themselves as well as the increasing need to integrate device development with clinical trials and regulatory and reimbursement approvals. Tim Fischell (October 14, 2003) describes a well-known example:

TABLE 70-1

Anticipating the Future[a]

Atherosclerosis	People are going to go to areas that traditionally have not been ideal for revascularization, but subtends an area of the myocardium that is clearly hibernating or potentially viable. With the pandemic of heart failure that we're going to see, we're going to actually have to start thinking about how to improve pump function. *Nick Chronos*	I see a further less-invasive treatment, maybe a combination of interventional cardiology to treat the symptoms, and medical treatment to improve the prognosis. Ultimately, I am optimistic that we will defeat atherosclerosis within ten years or so. *Nico Pijls*
Vulnerable Plaque	I think that targeting vulnerable plaque is a very formidable challenge, because of the very dynamic, episodic nature of the disease, and the likelihood that you'll have to be intravascular to do it. What I favor is treating plaque burden, and conceding that we don't know what part of the plaque is vulnerable and what's not, but we definitely know where plaque is. *Steve Oesterle*	What's the life cycle of [a vulnerable plaque]? There's definitely a process that will be discovered in the next one or two decades. And ensuing from that will be chemical testing; BNP-like markers; diagnostic testing. . . . Then there will be a form of therapy depending upon what the pathophysiology is. So this whole thing that we have laid the foundation over the last three years in the literature, with very little evidence; a lot of talk and very little science, will, I believe, mature. *Maurice Buchbinder*
Congestive Heart Failure	Witness the advents of bi-ventricular pacemakers and defibrillators in that population as evidence of what fairly simple device development in that area can do to affect a huge cohort of patients. Futuristic therapies-cell therapy and other pro-systolic therapies of one kind or another-have incredible potential markets, therefore are incredible potential areas for device development. *Campbell Rogers*	Earlier diagnosis is important, better monitoring is very important. It's a chronic disease, so I think like the diabetes model, we'll have ways of monitoring the disease state of the patient at home, suggest medications and so forth to prevent decompensation. This will segue into other types of monitoring technologies, communication systems, using the internet, etc. *Jay Yadav*
Valvular Disease	I see little reason to doubt that within ten to fifteen years, most valves will be treated percutaneously, either through ways to decalcify them, or ways to repair them, or ways to replace them. All of these technologies are existent today that make sense and have shown reasonable feasibility; I think that will only get better. *Steve Oesterle*	The calcified aortic valve is a real challenge, and I don't know how you deal with that. If I were a heart surgeon, I certainly would be happy to continue to do aortic valve surgery. I think mitral valve surgery, on the other hand, is going to dramatically change. . . . I think that technologies that move toward repair rather than replacement are going to be very important. *Nick Chronos*

TABLE 70-1

Anticipating the Future (*continued*)

Atrial Fibrillation	As we understand atrial arrhythmias better, we're going to see our EP colleagues doing better and better having less scarring. They'll figure out ways to make a better catheter-based maze burning of the pulmonary veins to prevent re-entry. I think we're going to have catheter-based cures that will be safe and effective in maybe 80% of people with atrial fibrillation.	What I'm most excited about is a field that is being ignored, which is the left-atrial appendage. . . . I think atrial fibrillation anticoagulation, mechanical suppression or elimination of coagulation, if we have a left-atrial appendage closure approach that is sound and effective, is a major frontier to be conquered.
	Tim Fischell	*Maurice Buchbinder*

*September–October, 2003.

In the last three years, Johnson & Johnson spent millions of dollars working on aligning with [Medicare] on reimbursement for drug-eluting stents in parallel with clinical trials, in parallel with economic data-collection, to prove that this technology would be cost-neutral or cost-beneficial to the health-care system. If you want to bring a new technology to the market, especially if it's an expensive technology, you better have some data that the new bell or whistle reduces health-care costs or does something good and is cost-neutral.

The US Food and Drug Administration (FDA) in particular has been lauded for their efforts in the rapid approval of the drug-eluting stent. Hope is strong that the speed and cooperation with Medicare that the FDA demonstrated with the initial drug-eluting stent approval will continue:

I think the drug-eluting stents have really changed the landscape of how the FDA views and is viewed in this field. They're held now and they hold themselves to a much higher standard than was the case two or three years ago in terms of the rapidity of turnaround and the timeliness of review. I think that now that the dam has broken, they're going to continue to be held to those really speedy responses.

Campbell Rogers
September 11, 2003

At the same time, experts warned not to be too optimistic about any further changes in regulatory policy:

No matter what the FDA commissioners come up and say, "We have to be kindler and gentler and we have to be more compliant," the FDA is the FDA and it remains for the foreseeable future a gating mechanism.

Maurice Buchbinder
September 8, 2003

The consensus is that the US FDA has become more responsive to speedy device approvals, and concurrent Medicare reimbursement for those devices may also be possible. Further changes in policy, however, are not envisioned in the near future.

In addition to these policy changes, the interviewees each had a number of comments to make about the future of clinical practice in areas ranging from atherosclerosis to rhythm management. The experts agreed in very broad terms about the current challenges facing cardiology, but each had a unique view of what the future holds for clinical care (see inset). Innovation by its very nature is unexpected, so it should come as no surprise that even respected authorities in the field would disagree on the devices that will be adopted into clinical practice in the future!

SUMMARY

In this chapter, we have described a number of traits held in common among the most successful physician–innovators and provided advice directly solicited from a number of contemporary inventors and entrepreneurs. The key messages are simple:

• Focus on the patient and the clinical need.

• Build a good team.

• Be persistent in the face of disbelief and discouragement.

As interventional cardiologists we are in a privileged position of being in an environment of major clinical needs every day. The skills required to identify these needs and create significant new technological solutions are in fact very similar to those we have already developed in our training and practice.

Tom Fogarty, MD

REFERENCES

1. US. Food and Drug Administration. PMA Database Search. Available at: http://www.accessdata.fda.gov/scripts/cdrh/cfdocs/cfPMA/pma.cfm Accessed July 5, 2006.
2. Simpson J. *From the Innovator's Workbench.* Interview by David Cassack, March 3, 2003.
3. Klaidman S. *Saving the Heart: The Battle to Conquer Coronary Disease.* New York; Oxford University Press, 2000.
4. Fogarty T. *From the Innovator's Workbench.* Interview by David Cassack, January 27, 2003.
5. Serruys PW, Strauss BH, Beatt KJ et al. Angiographic follow-up after placement of a self-expanding coronary-artery stent. *N Engl J Med.* 1991;324(1):13–17.
6. Palmaz J. *From the Innovator's Workbench.* Interview by David Cassack, February 10, 2003.

CHAPTER (71)

Principles of Innovation: Transforming Clinical Needs into Viable Inventions

Joshua Makower, MD, and
Asha Nayak, MD, PhD

Nowhere is the opportunity to innovate as inviting as in the field of medicine, and no specialty has been as productive in the development of new technologies as cardiology. Because heart disease remains the most common cause of death in the United States, new developments in cardiology can affect an especially large population and have a tremendous impact. Advances in our understanding of human physiology, genetics, and molecular biology continue to define the fundamental mechanisms responsible for disease. Through these insights, we gain new perspectives and tools with which to create novel solutions. Regardless of the specific clinical problem to be solved, a common approach to innovation can be applied. It is this basic knowledge base of tools and techniques required to create new medical technologies that we hope to convey within this chapter.

To the many important disciplines discussed in this book, a dedicated section on innovation has been added this year. This is because, although these skills are not taught in medical school, they have been critical to the advancement of medicine, especially in interventional cardiology. It is generally difficult for people in medicine to learn these principles especially of innovation, as they are usually taught only in engineering programs at leading universities. This trend has just begun to change, and several programs have begun offering curricula targeted at this very issue.[1-3] As history has demonstrated many times, clinicians and scientists make very good innovators. Although it is important for engineers to be skilled in these principles, it is even more important for clinicians and scientists to understand and implement them during the first steps of concept creation.

Developing a new medical technology is a rewarding but often arduous process. The greatest success comes to those who understand the many necessary steps and can develop a strategy to approach each efficiently.

INNOVATION: THE BASIC STEPS

Innovation is defined as the process of creating something new. As developers of a medical technology, we seek to address a real clinical need with the goal of not only creating something new, but creating something better as well. The basic process of focused innovation is very simple, and is summarized in Figure 71-1.

Although this process is one that may be used by someone new to a field (top orange arrow), you may enter this process at any stage (orange arrows). In general, it is best to run this process rigorously from beginning to end without skipping steps to avoid the biases that come with arriving at a solution too soon. Regardless of where you enter, awareness of all steps and sensitivity to the need for iteration (blue arrows) can further improve on a good initial idea. As such, each step is briefly described.

【 】 STEP 1: OBJECTIVE DEFINITION

Starting with a clearly defined objective is critically important to keep you on the path to focused innovation. Being focused can prevent wasting time and energy on creative but tangential ideas that do not meet the intended objective. A well-defined need (eg, to create a significant improvement in minimally invasive mitral valve repair) limits one's focus to a reasonably sized clinical area where the application of time, research, and creative energy is likely to yield a real outcome. It is a good idea to write this goal down and refer back to it occasionally as a project takes shape, so that the statement of objective becomes a mission statement for the project. In some cases, it may become clear during the development of the project that the overall goal must change.

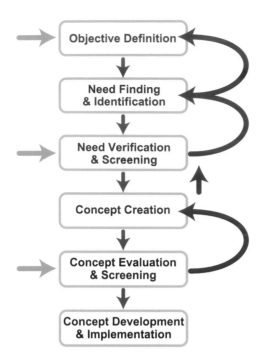

FIGURE 71-1. A process for innovation. Orange arrows indicate entry points; blue arrows indicate iterative loops.

Although focus, at any one time, on a single need is ideal, it is also important to engage others with different backgrounds in your investigation. Medicine itself is a broad field in which an in-depth understanding of different disciplines (eg, anatomy, physiology, pathophysiology) is required to understand a problem and arrive at meaningful solutions. However, a mastery of other fields (eg, physics, electronics, engineering, mechanics) and how they may be applied to solve medical problems can yield some of the most novel inventions with greater impact. For these reasons, the ideal team is a multidisciplinary one that is diverse but remains focused on the defined objective.

Another advantage of defining an objective at the start of the innovation sequence is a practical one—in general, innovators work best within a defined area of expertise. Although there are examples of wildly creative individuals[1,2] whose inventions span many disciplines and technologies, it is difficult with this type of approach to develop the depth necessary to reliably generate significant advances in medicine. More commonly, this broad style of inventorship results in patents that lie in wait for science to catch up to what has been proposed ("submarine patents"). This approach can be financially rewarding in some situations, but generally does not provide an effective pathway to technology innovation.

【 】 STEP 2: IDENTIFICATION OF AN UNMET CLINICAL NEED

Most successful medical technology inventors would say that identifying an important clinical need is the single most essential step in innovation. Clinical needs can be identified in many different ways. Often they are recognized by a clinician involved in patient care when a frustrated physician wishes for a better solution to a clinical problem (eg, "If only we could have repaired this mitral

valve with a catheter-based approach, sparing the patient major surgery"). Needs can also be recognized by those not within the field of medicine, or by those who are actively seeking unmet clinical needs (eg, an entrepreneur). Such an intentional innovator must do exhaustive research and observation to evaluate a clinical problem and all existing solutions to it, carefully understanding the strengths and limitations of each. Here again, it is often helpful to involve people of different backgrounds who may not have the biases of an expert deeply entrenched in the conventions of a particular specialty. An outsider to the field is likely to question even the most basic of assumptions and may uncover a true need that is not apparent, even to the specialist (*latent needs*).[3] Finding clinical needs is a fundamental skill that improves with experience. Some of the most notable innovators in cardiology have demonstrated their abilities as serial need finders (Dotter, Simpson, Fogarty, Imran; see Chapter 70).

The characteristics of a "good" need depend on personal and professional objectives. If one were to have the opportunity to choose from an array of needs, the magnitude of the potential patient outcome benefit and the size of the available market/population would certainly top the list of considerations. Although one could list many other factors, such as accessibility of the market, reimbursement, or regulatory environment, having a burning passion for the need is probably the single most important factor for success.

Once a need area has been identified, it is critically important to precisely define the need by producing a *need statement*. A need statement can be deceptively simple: It is a one-line description of the clinical problem, stated as clearly as possible. Although at first it seems like an unnecessarily formal exercise to write down a need statement, it is an absolutely essential step to really understanding the need and communicating it effectively to others. Following are some examples of need statements from interventional cardiology:

- A less invasive approach to reduce mitral regurgitation in patients with congestive heart failure.

- A better technique for directing a guidewire safely and efficiently across a chronic total occlusion.

- A minimally invasive method for restoring myocardial contractile function after myocardial infarction.

It is important to differentiate carefully between needs and solutions, and focus on understanding the clinical needs first. This includes paying close attention to the way in which the need and its attributes are described, as this can substantially narrow or bias subsequent efforts. For example, the statement "The need for a more torqueable Teflon catheter to perform balloon angioplasty" is heavily biased. Solutions to this need would clearly be restricted to catheter-based solutions and those using Teflon materials. More importantly, these solutions would exclude even superior concepts that employ something besides a catheter. It is also a useful technique to both focus in and zoom back from the central problem. The result should be a set of need statements that clearly outline the clinical problems and suggest several pathways for creative improvement. An example of a focused need statement might be: "A way to prevent smooth muscle cell migration in response to stenting"; whereas a more global need statement may read more like: "A better way to prevent restenosis after stenting." Finding the appropriate level of specificity of a need may take some time, and brainstorming at every level can be a very useful exercise. The most productive level of focus usually becomes clear only later, once solutions have been proposed and fertile ground for invention has been exposed.

STEP 3: NEED VERIFICATION AND SCREENING

Once you have identified one or more unmet clinical needs, the verification process begins. In this stage, you must validate that the needs you found are indeed experienced by others and characterize the features of the ideal solution. By the end of your verification process you should have an array of information about each need. Such information could include the size and features of the population affected, problems with current solutions, and the impact of the unmet clinical need (ie, morbidity, mortality, and cost) on society and the patient. The ideal solution should include parameters defined by the patient (eg, risk–benefit, comfort, efficacy, fit), physician (eg, ease of use, complications), hospital (eg, cost tolerance), payer (eg, cost vs. future cost savings), and other stakeholders. This detailed examination of a need is called its *need specification*. With this constellation of information, the process of needs screening may now begin. The goal of this process is to identify objectively the most optimal need to be addressed, given the criteria developed during need finding and validation. One method is to define categories such as those listed earlier and create some sort of ranking system. A spreadsheet can simplify your assessment and enable you to make rapid updates as new information becomes available.

STEP 4: CONCEPT CREATION

With the need specification process completed, it is time to create potential solutions. This stage of the process is widely misunderstood. The popular model for the concept creation process is some mystical "aha" by the lone, brilliant inventor (see Chapter 70). In fact, brainstorming is best done with a team. Selecting the right people to brainstorm with is one of the key determinants of success. Generally, such people should be highly creative, cooperative, and experienced in the technical and/or clinical area of interest. The team members should understand that they may be helping create some new intellectual property that may ultimately be of financial value, but that the brainstorming stage is only a small part of the process of invention, which includes the substantial work of need finding, verification, and specification that has gone on before.

There are several rules for successful brainstorming.[4] Perhaps most important is that the participants should create a positive session that encourages open thinking and wild ideas. Critical comments and judgment should be held back until later in the process. Participants should build on the ideas of others; the collective strength of the team carries it much further than any individual can alone. Another important tip is to have the group focus on generating as many ideas as possible, regardless of how unrealistic they may seem; the goal at this stage is quantity over quality. A typical 60- or 90-minute brainstorming session should generate as many as a hundred or more different ideas, which may be grouped in clusters of concepts. Some groups like to use *concept mapping* techniques to record the branching pattern of new idea creation visually. It is certainly helpful to have a large whiteboard or other writing surface and encourage participants to draw their concepts. It may even be useful to have some materials on hand—cardboard, clay, foam board—to create very quick and rough conceptual prototypes.

It may often be necessary to have several brainstorming sessions on a given need. It may also be useful to have different people involved in these sessions. Remember throughout the process of inventing that it is critical to document the evolution of new ideas and their anticipated applications. Any significant writing on a whiteboard should be copied or photographed; any rough models should be saved. This helps organize and build mature ideas and enables the inventors to substantiate their rights to intellectual property.

STEP 5: CONCEPT EVALUATION AND SCREENING

Successful brainstorming produces a large array of potential solutions to a need. The next step is to distinguish the ideas worth pursuing from those that are not. Although the brainstorming process is unconstrained and strives for quantity of ideas, concept evaluation and screening introduces reality into the equation. The goal is to have the winning solution emerge from the list and to understand the features of that solution that need improvement in order to become successful.

The most important metrics for the first screening should already be at hand, and they are the same characteristics of the ideal solution developed for the need specification (see Step 3). A simple rating of how well each of the concepts fits these characteristics results in an initial ranking. Often, this process permits the inventor to reevaluate the merits of each solution, suggesting modifications or improvements. From the highest-ranking ideas, one can further screen out the best solution by imposing additional metrics. Some examples of these might include: an assessment of the technical feasibility of the idea, the likelihood of adoption, potential ease-of-use, or the expected timeline of clinical trials and regulatory approval. Developing a reproducible scoring system helps keep this process objective. Some research may be necessary to support the scoring process, and often iteration of the process and idea is required. This type of process is an adaptation of "The House of Quality."[5]

STEP 6: CONCEPT DEVELOPMENT AND IMPLEMENTATION

Once you have selected your target concept, you can now begin the exciting journey toward making it a reality. Some important questions to pose at this stage are as follows: Is this an idea that is so significant that it could be the foundation of a company, or is it simply an incremental improvement that is better licensed off to an existing manufacturer? Are the clinical and technical foundations established enough to justify bringing in investors, or is this still a research project that requires further development in an academic setting? To answer these questions, it is helpful to look at comparable companies or projects at similar stages. If you are working in a university setting, much of the work at this stage may be performed by the technology licensing office, but if you truly want to establish this invention as a reality, it is often necessary for the inventor to take a pivotal driving role. To move your idea from this point, it is now necessary to dig into your med-tech inventor's toolkit (described next) and pull all the pieces into place.

Whatever approach the technology takes, the inventor has the opportunity to play a central role in the early development and implementation of the technology. The next section describes the essential tools to make this a productive experience.

THE MED-TECH INVENTOR'S TOOLKIT

【 】 THE TEAM

Regardless of the fact that many famous and successful inventors like to work alone, the benefits of working with multidisciplinary teams have been extolled in many texts.[6] Even those who choose to invent alone realize that a team is almost always necessary to take their invention to the next level. The most important thing you can do as an innovator is understand your personal strengths and weaknesses. Assemble your team based on how the additional members complement your abilities. It is also important that your team fit the task at hand. Initially, you may not need much help, but as the project moves forward, you must bring in other people to accomplish the next set of goals. Once you lay out a plan for your business (Figure 71–2), the evolving set of requirements logically translates into a sequence of skills necessary to move the project forward, and you then can build your team on that basis.

【 】 INTELLECTUAL PROPERTY

The Basics

At the core of any great company or new product is its intellectual property. *Intellectual property (IP)* is defined as any creation of the human mind or intellect that has some value in the marketplace, and that ultimately can be reduced to a tangible form. IP can be an idea, invention, expression, unique name, business method, industrial process, or even a chemical formula. IP can take on many forms. One, called the *utility patent,* is most commonly used in the medical industry. A utility patent describes a novel invention that can be used to perform a task. Typically it details a device (eg, surgical instrument) or method (eg, procedure or manufacturing process).

A patent gives its assignee the right to exclude others from practicing an invention. In receiving that right, the assignee must permit disclosure of the invention openly to the public (hence the name *patent,* which means "to open"). In the United States and internationally, a patent term is 20 years from the *filing date* (date the patent application was filed with the US Patent and Trademark Office [USPTO]).

The Laboratory Notebook

Legally, a properly maintained notebook is the gold standard used by the courts to determine when and how an individual developed an invention. The more detailed and well maintained your notebook is, the more valuable it is in supporting your claim of invention. Following are a few key points to remember:

1. Get a bound notebook with numbered pages. Although it is allowable to paste in material on existing, bound pages, never tear out or try to add pages.

2. Date and sign each page. Never ever backdate! Even if an idea occurred on a previous day, always date your notebook with the actual date matching the signature. It may be important to add an explanation for the delay in writing an entry into your notebook, but do not falsify. Dishonesty here is fraud.

3. Have a noninventor witness and date each page. Do this every few weeks; it doesn't need to be each day. Ideally, this person would be skilled enough in the art to understand the invention.

4. Sign over the edge of material that you paste or tape into the notebook, so that your signature or initials span both the bound page and the pasted-in material.

5. Cross out blank spaces to ensure that no retroactive entries could be made.

6. Never whiteout anything! Use a single line to strike through any errors and initial the correction.

Inventorship and Ownership

Legally, the definition of *inventor* is a very specific one. To be an inventor, one must have contributed (partially or totally) to the

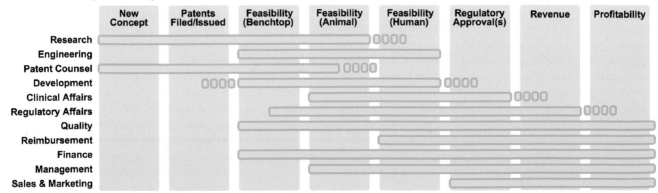

FIGURE 71-2. Milestones and expertise sequence.

invention and participated in its reduction to practice. If you invent something on your own, then you are considered the sole inventor, as long as this work was not performed as a "work for hire" or bound by some other contractual obligation. If someone adds to any part of a claim, then they are a joint inventor, regardless of whether their contribution was large or small. Unless bound by other contractual arrangements, rights to the patent are shared equally by all inventors. This means that each inventor can use the invention, but neither can exclude the other inventor(s). It is very important to include each inventor when filing a new patent. If inventors are not properly acknowledged, a patent may be declared invalid, rendering it of no value to any party involved.

It is very important to document and date your ideas as soon as you have them. If you compete with someone else who filed a patent at the same time, the courts turn first to your notebooks to determine who had the idea first. In the United States, which will be a substantial portion of your market, it is the inventor who shows documented proof of earliest invention that receives patent rights. Thus, in the United States, a notebook that substantiates your patent application is critical in the patenting process. In contrast, internationally, the notebook carries less weight. Outside the United States, it is the first to file an application for a patent that is awarded the rights of first inventorship, regardless of when the idea was first conceived or documented. Thus, as a general rule, documenting and filing your ideas with the patent office as soon as possible is highly advisable.

Many physicians are asked to speak publicly about their research. *Public disclosure* is defined as disclosure done outside the terms of a confidentiality agreement (see next section). Be aware that public disclosure has important patent consequences. If you disclose your invention prior to filing a patent application, you have 1 year to file a patent application in order to obtain rights over this invention. However, if someone else files a patent application on this idea before you do, you lose international (not United States) rights. In this way, public disclosure opens up the possibility for you to lose international rights. Because of this issue, it is always a good idea to file a provisional or full patent application before disclosure to the public.

Confidentiality

Inventors often must define the difficult balance between secrecy and disclosure while trying to advance their ideas. It is necessary to disclose your ideas to others to build your team and teach others in your field, but such disclosures put your ideas at risk. Confidentiality agreements can be used to discourage others from sharing or using your ideas, but often these agreements are very difficult to enforce. In general, it is always a good practice to limit your disclosure to nonconfidential matters until you have placed the receiving party under a confidentiality agreement.

How to Get Started

Start the process by going online and searching for evidence of your idea in the literature or patent archive. Medline, MEdical Subject Help (MESH), and other online medical resources are available through several providers, and the US Patent and Trademark Office (USPTO) has a very easy-to-use website for searching US patents as well. Several commercial providers offer the ability to download full patents and articles at the touch of a button, making this process fast and easy. After searching the literature and relevant patent databases,[7] if the idea still appears to be novel, the next step is to file either a provisional or a full patent application. All patents ultimately require a full application for consideration, but provisional patents offer a low-cost way to protect your idea. A full patent application includes the following:

- An abstract: a brief description of the invention.
- The specification: text in which the background of the idea, the idea itself, and its various uses are described in detail. This includes drawings that are included in the application.
- The claims: a numbered list of the exact characteristics of the invention that the applicant believes are novel and for which the applicant is seeking legal rights.

Because the legal phrasing in the application is so important, it is recommended that you work with a patent lawyer to assemble the application. The cost of creating and filing a full patent application in the United States is usually $5,000–$15,000, most of which is the cost of legal counsel. After filing, the USPTO responds to the claims in the application, making arguments for or against rights to each of the claims individually. This process is called *patent prosecution* and can often be a substantial process that can last for months or years. Finally, if the patent is granted (usually in a revised form), it is called an *issued patent,* and you or the organization that owns the patent are designated as the *assignee.*

A provisional patent application (PPA) is a type of fast-track submission for inventors who want to get the earliest possible file date without having to commit the investment necessary for a full patent application. The PPA can be a much more informal application than the full patent. Legal wording is not as essential, and many inventors generate their own PPAs without hiring legal counsel. The cost of the application is $100, and it does not undergo any formal review or approval process by the USPTO. It merely serves to hold the filing date. As long as the inventors submit a full patent application within 1 year of filing the PPA, they are granted the earlier PPA filing date for both.

One concept concerning patent rights is often misunderstood: the difference between patentability and the ability to practice. An invention is patentable if it has at least one claimed element that is novel. Although a patent grants permission to exclude others from practicing an invention as described in the claims, it does not necessarily provide its inventor the *freedom to practice* (ie, manufacture or sell the technology or perform the procedure) the invention without infringement. To *infringe* a patent means that one has literally followed every step claimed by an existing patent. So, for example, if your invention incorporates another invention (in its entirety), but builds on it with a novel addition, it may be necessary for you to license rights to the other patent before practicing your invention.

For more information on the mechanics of filing patents and the legal aspects of creating new companies and technologies, there are several excellent references specifically for new inventors.[8,9]

MARKET ASSESSMENT

It is best to make an early assessment of the market to determine the potential size of the opportunity in order to ensure that it warrants investing significant time and resources. The essential steps are to characterize and quantify the potential customers and understand how the demand for the new technology may evolve over time. A well-developed market analysis is an essential part of a business plan.

To properly assess the value of an idea, it is necessary to define its application in some detail. If the concept is a "disposable" or "implantable," its use is defined by the number of procedures or patients in which it is used. Alternatively, if it is a reusable product, the market depends on the number of hospitals or operating rooms that use it. A good starting point is to estimate from the literature the number of treatable patients within a typical year. This number multiplied by the estimated price per use serves as the total

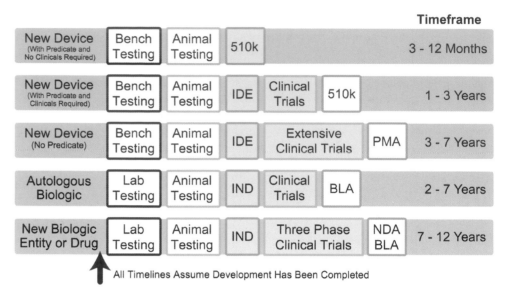

FIGURE 71-3. Sample processes toward approval of medical products in the United States. IDE = Investigational Device Exemption; IND = Investigational New Drug; PMA = Pre-Market Approval; BLA = Biologic License Application; NDA = New Drug Application.

potential market per year. Demographic changes, preventive measures, access to the appropriate healthcare providers, and other factors that affect the size of the future patient population should be considered when rendering these types of estimates. Physician adoption rates vary widely between specialties, and the best estimates of these rates can be determined by examining comparable technologies. If, however, no such comparable technologies are available, a model can be derived by considering several factors: the severity of the clinical need, risk tolerance of the patient and physician population, appropriate patient inclusions/exclusions, other available competitive treatment options, and the risk–benefit profile of your technology.

When conducting market research, physician feedback can be very valuable. However, one must recognize that customers (physicians) often do not recognize their own needs, particularly considering breakthrough technologies. More often than not, they adapt to available technologies and are relatively comfortable with what is at hand. Also, one must consider physician culture; some specialties embrace new ideas (interventional cardiology is a prime example), whereas others reproach them. Although customer input is very helpful in this assessment, it is important to weigh and filter these factors carefully to differentiate between negative feedback that is fundamental and that which simply reveals resistance to change.

CLINICAL, REGULATORY, AND REIMBURSEMENT CONSIDERATIONS

Health-care technologies are highly regulated, and thus, it is very important to understand the various paths to approval and reimbursement before spending significant resources to develop an idea. Although the fundamental aspects are not likely to change soon, specific regulations and reimbursement parameters can change dramatically over time and can be heavily linked to current sociopolitical issues. It is therefore essential that one consult with

experienced professionals in the field before casting one's plan into action.

In the United States, the Food and Drug Administration (FDA) oversees all commercial medical devices, biotechnology, and pharmaceutical products. In other countries there are similar regulatory bodies, although their roles vary widely. Although the focus of US regulators is often to prove efficacy equal to or beyond that of existing technologies, the CE mark process (the approval pathway for the European Union) is more focused on safety and quality. Figure 71-3 is a chart showing a few typical paths a new medical device, biologic, or drug might take through the US FDA or European Competent Authority process. These are just a few examples; the actual process must be customized as appropriate for every individual technology.

The litigious nature of the US market demands a higher level of scrutiny on behalf of the FDA in comparison to the situation in Europe. Thus, quite often devices and drugs can be tested on humans and commercialized much sooner outside the US than within. There are important philosophic and ethical issues that this disparity creates. Overseas patients have access to the latest and potentially greatest medical advances much earlier; however, Americans benefit from the knowledge resulting from repeated human experience and follow-up before these new approaches are released to the US population. Until there is normalization in the way different cultures approach risk, these regulatory differences are likely to remain.

Product labeling is a significant element of the regulatory process, and is fundamentally important when formulating a clinical development strategy. The claim a manufacturer makes regarding the performance of a technology is the key factor that determines how regulatory bodies determine the product must be tested. Whatever is claimed must be proven; therefore, if this proof is derivable only through extensive and expensive clinical testing, then that is dictated by the nature of the claims. Often, manufacturers choose initial labeling that results in the most straightforward pathway to approval; they may seek subsequent amendments or expansions of the labeling based on trials conducted after the initial indication has been approved. In other cases, manufacturers may instead choose to never seek these expanded approvals, allowing physicians to use the product "off-label"; that is, outside of the recommendations specified in the Instructions for Use insert that is included with the product. Although off-label use is not illegal when performed by physicians, it is illegal for companies to promote that use in any way. Many books and websites detail these regulations and policies.[10,11]

Having a reimbursement strategy for a new technology is equally as important as the regulatory issues in designing an approach to clinical trials. A clinical trial must be designed and powered to demonstrate that the new technology is worth reimbursing. If the reimbursement process has not been carefully considered early on, the costs required to commercialize the product can be grossly underestimated, and expensive clinical trials may need to be repeated.

Regulatory and reimbursement pathways that appear to be particularly difficult discourage investors or potential corporate partners. Those who understand how to navigate the process successfully can wield a significant competitive advantage. For those who do not have this experience readily at hand, there are many high-quality consulting firms that specialize in these fields, as well as recruiters available to help you add this expertise to your team.

ETHICAL CONSIDERATIONS

It is critically important to be aware of the potential conflicts of interest involved in bringing a new, for-profit technology forward into a health-care setting. At every stage in the development process you should evaluate choices against your own values. For example, when one identifies a clinical need to address, it is appropriate to ask several questions, such as:

- Should I work on this problem?
- Am I trying to increase the quality or duration of life?
- What impact would that have on the patient, caregiver, family, society, and the health care system?

For example, reducing mortality after major stroke seems like a noble goal, but one should consider the impact on the size and debility of the affected patient group. Environmental issues also come into play: What are the implications of disposable versus reusable products? In manufacturing, consider the ramifications of manufacturing risk on employees (safety), the product being sold (integrity), and so on. In forming a business strategy, to what extent should consideration be given to access by people of different geographic and socioeconomic groups? Clearly, these and related questions can be difficult to answer, but it is essential to raise these issues early and reflect on the core values behind the technology that is being created.

A common ethical dilemma facing clinician inventors is the balance between financial gain from the application of a new technology and the responsibilities of ethical patient care. Many academic, hospital, and corporate organizations are wrestling with this delicate balance. Without the clinical leadership provided by physician inventors, many of our most significant technologies would not be available today. At the same time, there are clearly

examples of perceived financial conflict of interest and, arguably, situations in which patients have been put at risk inappropriately. With proper oversight by independent ethical review boards and rigorous scientific peer review, it is possible to proceed wisely on a case-by-case basis. Establishing a credo is a good way to acknowledge these issues and generate the open discussion necessary to establish balance. Corporations such as Johnson & Johnson and Medtronic have integrated their credo deeply into their culture and the way they do business.[12] Although this credo can functions effectively for corporations, such a document can also provide value for organizations operating in university or not-for-profit settings.[13]

COMMUNICATION TOOLS

There are three main communication tools that are important in the successful communication of a new technology: prototypes, business plans, and presentations. Prototypes serve a multitude of early-stage functions. However crude they may be, prototypes communicate an invention to others, help determine its feasibility, and identify challenges that may arise as it is developed further (eg, scaling it up or down, fitting it to different anatomies, manufacturing it). A tangible model is far more useful than a description or drawing of an invention. Those reviewing a technology (eg, investors, physicians) will be able to provide much better feedback with a real, three-dimensional prototype. Placing a prototype into the hands of an end-user can also be very informative. By observing how they handle the device and what features give them the greatest satisfaction or difficulty, it is possible to learn important lessons unachievable through other means.

Business plans are another powerful communication tool. Developing and writing a plan enhances the likelihood of success of any technology development program. Although the business plan is useful to potential investors, the process of creating a plan is even more important to the innovator because it forces one to think strategically about the project that is about to be launched. A plan must tell a story. It should explain the primary motivation, the unmet clinical need, market opportunity, and the proposed business solution. Once the solution is established and clearly described, the plan should outline the development path and basics of how the company or group will bring the technology to market. Important issues should be identified and addressed, but the explanations and text should be succinct. A clear, well-organized, and concise plan communicates as much about the innovator as it does the project, and can be an important step to successful financing. An outline of a typical med-tech business plan is presented in Table 71-1. The plan must communicate clearly why someone should be interested in the technology and describe succinctly a compelling strategy for sustainable competitive advantage and profitability. Most audiences prefer a shorter plan (10–15 pages) than a longer one. For more detailed suggestions on how to write a winning plan, there are many sources available.[14,15]

The third main communication tool is the presentation, or the "pitch." The innovator must always be prepared to present his/her idea. Chance provides encounters with people whose feedback or support may be important. For these occasions, it is important to

TABLE 71-1

Business Plan Outline

Executive Summary

Background and Clinical Need Being Addressed

The Market

The Proposed Idea and Business Model

Research and Development

Regulatory, Reimbursement, and Clinical
  Pathway/Strategy

Intellectual Property

Competition

Proposed Use of Funds

Financials

have a prepared, up-to-date, "30-second elevator pitch"—a rehearsed summary of the idea that communicates all its salient aspects succinctly. There should be different pitches for different anticipated audiences. Eventually, when it is time to present the concept more formally (eg, to potential investors), a polished presentation is required. Typically, these presentations are given to a wide audience including non-clinicians/non-scientists. It is important to determine in advance exactly who will be in your audience, their backgrounds, interests, and concerns, and tailor the presentation specifically to each unique audience. Detail the clinical need, the strategy for developing a sustainable competitive advantage toward profitability, and explain clearly what is being asked from the audience, as well as any returns they might gain from participating. Fundamentally, if your business plan tells a compelling story, it will be of great interest to investors.

FINANCIAL CONSIDERATIONS

Once the basic business plan is formulated, the innovator must develop a financing plan to get it off the ground. By examining the most significant value-building milestones at each stage, it is possible to determine approximately how much funding is necessary initially and how many infusions of capital may be required over the life of the business. It is rare that one is able to obtain enough capital to finance an entire venture in a single round of financing. Usually, new ventures are funded in stages, providing an opportunity to reassess the progress and value of the venture at each stage, essentially lowering the risks for investors. The chart in Figure 71-4 illustrates a few typical examples of how value roughly tracks with milestones and cash requirements.

ASSESSING CASH REQUIREMENTS

The skill required to estimate accurately the cash required to launch a new venture can be gained only by experience. Overestimating these costs can discourage potential investors; on the other hand,

underestimating costs may cause the business to fail simply because of lack of funds. Med-tech venture start-up costs can vary significantly, depending on the size and scope of the project. For example, a simple class I surgical instrument provider may be able to start-up with less than $1 million, whereas a typical medical device or biotech company often requires tens to hundreds of millions of dollars to reach profitability. Over the life of a new company, the expenses and sources of risk shift from development costs to more standard execution costs such as sales, marketing, and manufacturing. It is often the earlier, more risky expenses that are the hardest to assess, and thus, usually after all the expected expenses are tabulated, most entrepreneurs expand the amount of funding that they seek to offset the impact of the unknown.

FUNDING SOURCES AND FINANCING STRATEGY

Finding resources can be the most challenging and daunting task for the innovator. Following is a list of the most common funding strategies as well as their pros and cons.

【 】 GOVERNMENT OR OTHER GRANTS

Government funding through small business innovation research grants (SBIRs), the advanced technology program (ATV), the National Institutes of Health (NIH), or other such grants are an excellent way to fund highly research-oriented projects. Although some grant processes can be highly political and burdened with bureaucracy, innovators rarely sacrifice any ownership or loss of control in the process.[16]

【 】 ANGEL INVESTORS AND SELF-FUNDING

At the earliest stage, it is very common to draw funding from friends and family, self-funding, or "angel" investors. These resources are best applied to the initial patent and feasibility work, and can often help an entrepreneur frame the opportunity better for more professional investors. If access to such resources or contacts is not immediately available, there are some well-known angel investor groups that can be approached.[17] Although some of these groups have been moving into larger and later-stage financing, financing your company exclusively with angel money through several rounds can make later-stage financing more difficult when cash requirements exceed those of your angel network. Angels typically demand less of the company early on, and tend to be more flexible than other investors; however, companies without professional investors risk a significant value reset later if early valuations were set outside of prevailing market conditions.

【 】 VENTURE CAPITAL

Venture capital is the source that is usually tapped for cash-intensive opportunities that require substantial cash and time investment before returning profits. A complete list of venture groups and their interest areas can be obtained from the National Venture Capital Association (NVCA) or one of the many available handbooks on venture capital.[18] Access to venture capital is rarely obtained through a "cold call" or an uninvited business plan. The

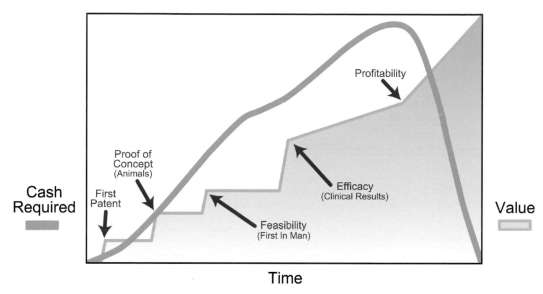

FIGURE 71-4. Value creation, milestone, and cash requirement chart.

vast majority of venture groups rely on their extensive network of contacts to establish the credibility of incoming ideas and entrepreneurs. These contacts cut across academic, industry, and investment domains, and your reputation and demonstrated ability to advance such ventures can have enormous impact. It is therefore very important for the innovator to develop these relationships or find ways of accessing this network of people. Once those links are established, it is much easier to gain access to the venture capital community. Venture capitalists (VCs) add discipline and focus to a business as well as financial resources, but in return they often require substantial percentages of the company as well as other conditions that further limit their risk and increase their control. Unlike angels, who may be happy to invest in a long-standing business that throws off dividends, VCs make their returns through "exits" or liquidity events (such as acquisitions or initial public offerings [IPOs]). It is very important that the goals of the innovator align with the goals of the investors, particularly with venture capitalist investors, because most of them play an active and pivotal role in the decision making for the company.

【 】 BANKS

Although banks are good places to get equity loans on your house, they are traditionally not good places to obtain financing for new businesses that are far from profitability. Banks have a much lower risk tolerance, and do not usually place very much value on intangibles such as IP or technology.

【 】 VENDORS

Vendors, customers, or other business partners can be very creative and strategic sources of capital. In general, these relationships are best structured once you have something to offer in return (eg, purchased services or other rights), but it is still possible to arrange preferred pricing or other cash-relief arrangements. These relationships vary widely, and offer an alternative to traditional financing approaches by minimizing cash requirements.

【 】 CORPORATE PARTNERSHIPS

Corporate or strategic investors can be an excellent source of capital and other resources for a new or developing business. In general, strategic investors tend to be less price-sensitive and more interested in the strategic value to their own businesses. It is usually better to bring such investors into the picture later, because the involvement of such players in a business can have a direct impact on the liquidity options later. Although each deal is different, traditionally, these partnerships can involve the corporation gaining access to equity, intellectual property, distribution, or development rights in exchange for cash or other resources. Many of the larger corporations (eg, Johnson & Johnson, Pfizer, Medtronic) have groups dedicated to partnerships that can be approached easily.

【 】 PUBLIC EQUITY

Under current market conditions, public equity accessed via an initial public offering (IPO) in the stock market or acquisition of a corporation is an option generally reserved either for biotech companies that have passed into phase III testing, or medical device companies with revenue growth and profits. This threshold can change dramatically with market conditions. Several investment banks (eg, Piper Jaffray, JP Morgan, UBS Securities) have developed specialized practices focused on the med-tech space and are essential for any company contemplating this pathway. Online resources such as the Electronic Data Gathering, Analysis, and Retrieval System (EDGAR) can be used to study recent IPO activity and easily allows users to compare the fundamentals of these businesses.[19]

【 】 INCUBATORS

Since the mid-1990s, several incubator companies have been formed to help early innovators bring their new concepts forward. These entities, such as ExploraMed, the Foundry, In-Cube, the Innovation Factory, and SyneCor, focus on identifying new ideas themselves or working with clinicians/scientists with ideas who do not wish to commercialize them alone. In general, incubators combine these ideas with funding, appropriate staff, and expertise in return for a significant portion of the equity of resulting companies.

KEY RESOURCES

There are many other sources to turn to for more specific information and advice. Undoubtedly, the most useful resource is a mentor who has succeeded in developing new technologies in a given area. There are plenty of resources even if a mentor is not available, especially with the availability of the Internet. Following are a few suggestions:

- Offices of Technology Licensing: For those affiliated with an academic or government medical center, the technology licensing office can provide support in filing patents. They often finance the patent application process and explain how to license technology in order to start up a new business.

- The National Center for Biologic Information (NCBI) (www.ncbi.nlm.nih.gov): The NCBI has an extensive publicly available database that permits users to search articles, books, and other media covering almost all areas that relate to the field of medicine.

- The Food and Drug Administration (FDA) (www.fda.gov): The FDA's website can help with regulatory and clinical trial strategy. It provides guidelines (required performance, safety, efficacy, and preclinical and clinical data) for different types of devices. The website also provides a more detailed description of the regulatory process and up-to-date information on the approval status of existing and emerging devices.

- The US Patent and Trademark Office (USPTO) (www.uspto.gov): The USPTO's website allows users to search issued and filed patents on-line for free.

FINAL THOUGHTS

In this chapter, we have provided a basic primer on how to take a new technology idea to the next level. There are several excellent references cited here that are useful for those who wish to develop a deeper understanding of the issues. Just as in clinical medicine, however, the best source of expertise is experience.

Clinicians and biomedical scientists have the enormous advantage of being on the front lines of need finding, where technology opportunities present themselves. The technology innovation process does not require mystical insight—just the willingness to work hard and pay attention to some of the fundamentals we have outlined here. The biggest mistake is not taking the first step.

REFERENCES

1. Peter Wilk—More than 365 US patents issued as of January 1, 2004.
2. Jerome Lemelson—326 US patents issued.
3. Leonard D, Rayport JF. Spark innovation through empathic design. *Harv Bus Rev.* Reprint 97606, November–December 1997;102–113.
4. Kelley T, Littman J. *The Art of Innovation.* New York:Doubleday; 2001.
5. Hausner J, Clausing D. The House of Quality. *Harv Bus Rev.* May–June, 1988;3–13.
6. Schrage M. *Shared Minds.* New York: Random House; 1990.
7. http://www.uspto.gov
8. Pressman D. *Patent It Yourself,* 7th ed. Berkeley, Calif: Nolo Press; 1999.
9. Bagley CE, Dauchy C. *The Entrepreneur's Guide to Business Law,* South Western College Publishing, July 22, 2002.
10. http://www.fda.gov
11. Harnack G. *Mastering and Managing the FDA Maze: Medical Device Overview: A Training and Management Desk Reference for Manufacturers Regulated by the Food and Drug Administration.* American Society for Quality, March 1999.
12. http://www.jnj.com/our_company/our_credo, http://www.medtronic.com/corporate/mission.html
13. http://innovation.stanford.edu/jsp/program/credo.jsp
14. Pinson L. *Anatomy of a Business Plan,* 5th ed. Chicago, III:Dearborn Trade Publishing, August 30, 2001.
15. Rich SR. *Business Plans That Win $$$: Lessons from the MIT Enterprise Forum,* Perennial; Reprint edition. February 18, 1987.
16. Government grant information: http://www.evelexa.com/resources/gov_grants.cfm
17. Nationwide Directory of Angel Funds: http://www.inc.com/articles/2001/09/23461.html
18. National listing of venture groups: National Venture Capital Association (NVCA), http://www.nvca.org
19. http://www.edgar-online.com

Note: Page numbers followed by f indicate figures; those followed by t indicate tables.